THE AMERICAN PSYCHIATRIC PUBLISHING

TEXTBOOK OF GERIATRIC NEUROPSYCHIATRY

THIRD EDITION

THE AMERICAN PSYCHIATRIC PUBLISHING

TEXTBOOK OF GERIATRIC NEUROPSYCHIATRY

THIRD EDITION

Editors

C. Edward Coffey, M.D.

Jeffrey L. Cummings, M.D.

Associate Editors

Mark S. George, M.D.

Daniel Weintraub, M.D.

American Psychiatric Publishing, Inc.

Washington, DC
London, England

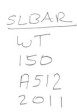

Manufactured in the United States of America on acid-free paper
15 14 13 12 11 5 4 3 2 1
Third Edition

Typeset in Adobe's Delta and Minion.

American Psychiatric Publishing, Inc.
1000 Wilson Boulevard
Arlington, VA 22209–3901
www.appi.org

Library of Congress Cataloging-in-Publication Data
The American psychiatric publishing textbook of geriatric neuropsychiatry / edited by C. Edward Coffey, Jeffrey L. Cummings ; associate editors, Mark S. George, Daniel Weintraub. — 3rd ed.
p. ; cm.
Textbook of geriatric neuropsychiatry
Rev. ed. of: The American Psychiatric Press textbook of geriatric neuropsychiatry. 2nd ed. 2000.
Includes bibliographical references and index.
ISBN 978-1-58562-371-6 (hardcover : alk. paper)
1. Geriatric neuropsychiatry. 2. Clinical neuropsychology. I. Coffey, C. Edward, 1952– II. Cummings, Jeffrey L., 1948– III. American Psychiatric Publishing. IV. American Psychiatric Press textbook of geriatric neuropsychiatry. V. Title: Textbook of geriatric neuropsychiatry.
[DNLM: 1. Aged. 2. Mental Disorders. 3. Aging—physiology. 4. Geriatric Psychiatry—methods. 5. Neuropsychiatry—methods. WT 150]
RC451.4.A5A516 2011
618.97'689—dc22

2011006284

British Library Cataloguing in Publication Data
A CIP record is available from the British Library.

Contents

Contributors

Olusola Ajilore, M.D., Ph.D.
Assistant Professor, Department of Psychiatry, University of Illinois at Chicago, Chicago, Illinois

Karen E. Anderson, M.D.
Clinical Assistant Professor of Psychiatry and Neurology, University of Maryland School of Medicine, Baltimore, Maryland

Carmen Andreescu, M.D.
Assistant Professor, Department of Psychiatry, University of Pittsburgh, Pittsburgh, Pennsylvania

David B. Arciniegas, M.D., F.A.N.P.A., C.B.I.S.T.
Michael K. Cooper Professor of Neurocognitive Disease; Director, Neurobehavioral Disorders Program; and Associate Professor of Psychiatry and Neurology, University of Colorado School of Medicine, Aurora, Colorado

Alon Y. Avidan M.D., M.P.H.
Associate Professor of Neurology; Neurology Residency Program Director; Director, UCLA Neurology Clinic; Associate Director, Sleep Disorders Center, University of California, Los Angeles, California

John J. Campbell III, M.D.
Associate Clinical Professor of Psychiatry, Tufts University School of Medicine, Boston, Massachusetts

Michael R. Clark, M.D., M.P.H.
Associate Professor and Director, Adolf Meyer Chronic Pain Treatment Services, Department of Psychiatry and Behavioral Sciences, The Johns Hopkins Medical Institutions, Baltimore, Maryland

C. Edward Coffey, M.D.
Vice President, Henry Ford Health System; Chief Executive Officer, Behavioral Health Services; Kathleen and Earl Ward Chair of Psychiatry, Henry Ford Hospital; Director, Center for Brain Stimulation Therapies, Henry Ford Hospital; Professor of Psychiatry and of Neurology, Wayne State University (Henry Ford Campus), Detroit, Michigan

M. Justin Coffey, M.D.
Chief, Electroconvulsive Therapy Service and Associate Director, Center for Brain Stimulation Therapies, Behavioral Health Services, Henry Ford Health System, Detroit, Michigan

Paul T. Costa Jr., Ph.D.
Scientist Emeritus, National Institute on Aging, National Institutes of Health, U.S. Department of Health and Human Services, Baltimore, Maryland

Jeffrey L. Cummings, M.D.
Director, Cleveland Clinic Lou Ruvo Center for Brain Health; Andrea and Joseph Hahn Chair of Neurotherapeutics, Cleveland Clinic Neurological Institute, Las Vegas, Nevada; Cleveland, Ohio; Westin, Florida

D.P. Devanand, M.D.
Professor of Clinical Psychiatry and Neurology and Director, Division of Geriatric Psychiatry, New York State Psychiatric Institute and College of Physicians and Surgeons, Columbia University, New York, New York

Marie A. DeWitt, M.D.
Staff Psychiatrist, Atlanta VA Medical Center; Assistant Professor, Department of Psychiatry and Behavioral Sciences, Emory University School of Medicine; Adjunct Clinical Assistant Professor, Department of Psychiatry and Behavioral Sciences, Morehouse School of Medicine, Atlanta, Georgia

Amelia N. Dubovsky, M.D.
Resident, Department of Psychiatry, Harvard University and Massachusetts General Hospital, Boston, Massachusetts

Steven L. Dubovsky, M.D.
Professor and Chair, Department of Psychiatry, University at Buffalo, Buffalo, New York; Adjoint Professor of Psychiatry and Medicine, Departments of Psychiatry and Medicine, University of Colorado, Denver, Colorado

Richard B. Ferrell, M.D.
Associate Professor of Psychiatry, Dartmouth Medical School, Lebanon, New Hampshire

Norman L. Foster, M.D.
Director, Center for Alzheimer's Care, Imaging and Research; Professor, Department of Neurology; Senior Investigator, The Brain Institute, University of Utah, Salt Lake City, Utah

Mark S. George, M.D.
Distinguished Professor of Psychiatry, Radiology, and Neuroscience; Founding Director, MUSC Center for Advanced Imaging Research; Co-Director, SC Brain Imaging Center of Economic Excellence; Director, Brain Stimulation Laboratory, Medical University of South Carolina and Ralph H. Johnson VA Medical Center, Charleston, South Carolina

Stacey Gramann, D.O., M.P.H.
Psychosomatic Medicine Fellow, Oregon Health and Science University, Portland, Oregon

Edmund S. Higgins, M.D.
Clinical Associate Professor of Family Medicine and of Psychiatry, Medical University of South Carolina, Charleston, South Carolina

Ricardo E. Jorge, M.D.
Associate Professor, Department of Psychiatry, Carver College of Medicine, The University of Iowa and VA Medical Center, Iowa City, Iowa

Jennifer M. Keller, Psy.D.
Clinical Neuropsychologist, VA Pittsburgh Healthcare System, Pittsburgh, Pennsylvania

Charles H. Kellner, M.D.
Professor of Psychiatry and Director, Division of Geriatric Psychiatry, Mount Sinai School of Medicine; Director, ECT Service, Mount Sinai Hospital, New York, New York

Anand Kumar, M.D.
Professor and Chair, Department of Psychiatry, University of Illinois at Chicago, Chicago, Illinois

Eric J. Lenze, M.D.
Associate Professor, Department of Psychiatry, Washington University School of Medicine, St. Louis, Missouri

Daniel C. Marson, J.D., Ph.D.
Professor, Department of Neurology, and Director, Alzheimer's Disease Center, University of Alabama at Birmingham, Birmingham, Alabama

Thomas W. McAllister, M.D.
Millennium Professor of Psychiatry, Dartmouth Medical School, Lebanon, New Hampshire

Robert R. McCrae, Ph.D.
Senior Investigator, Personality, Stress and Coping Section, Laboratory of Personality and Cognition, National Institute on Aging, National Institutes of Health, U.S. Department of Health and Human Services, Baltimore, Maryland

Glenise McKenzie, R.N., Ph.D.
Assistant Professor, School of Nursing, Oregon Health and Science University, Ashland, Oregon

Mario F. Mendez, M.D., Ph.D.
Professor of Neurology and Psychiatry and Biobehavioral Sciences, David Geffen School of Medicine at UCLA; Director, Neurobehavior, VA Greater Los Angeles (VAGLA) Healthcare System, Los Angeles, California

Ziad H. Nahas, M.D.
Associate Professor of Psychiatry and Neuroscience, Medical University of South Carolina, Charleston, South Carolina

David W. Oslin, M.D.
VA Associate Chief of Staff for Behavioral Health and Director, VISN 4 Mental Illness, Research, Education and Clinical Center (MIRECC), Philadelphia Veterans Administration Medical Center; Associate Professor of Psychiatry, University of Pennsylvania School of Medicine, Philadelphia, Pennsylvania

Kenneth Podell, Ph.D.
Director, Division of Neuropsychology, Henry Ford Health System; Clinical Associate Professor, Department of Psychiatry, Wayne State Unviversity, Detroit, Michigan

Richard E. Powers, M.D.
Professor, Department of Neurology, School of Medicine, University of Alabama at Birmingham, Birmingham, Alabama; Medical Director, Alabama Department of Mental Health, Montgomery, Alabama

John M. Ringman, M.D., M.S.
Interim Director, Mary S. Easton Center for Alzheimer's Disease Research; Associate Clinical Professor, UCLA Department of Neurology, Los Angeles, California

Robert G. Robinson, M.D.
Paul W. Penningroth Chair and Professor and Head, Department of Psychiatry, Carver College of Medicine, The University of Iowa, Iowa City, Iowa

Adam Rosenblatt, M.D.
Associate Professor of Psychiatry; Director of Neuropsychiatry; Clinical Director, Baltimore Huntington's Disease Center; Johns Hopkins School of Medicine, Baltimore, Maryland

Quincy M. Samus, Ph.D.
Assistant Professor, Department of Psychiatry, Johns Hopkins School of Medicine, Baltimore, Maryland

Douglas W. Scharre, M.D.
Director, Division of Cognitive Neurology, and Assistant Professor of Cognitive Neurology, Department of Neurology, The Ohio State University, Columbus, Ohio

Andrew D. Siderowf, M.D., M.S.C.E.
Associate Professor of Neurology at the Hospital of the University of Pennsylvania, Philadelphia, Pennsylvania

Andrea C. Solomon, Ph.D.
Neuropsychology Postdoctoral Fellow, Department of Neurology, Alzheimer's Disease Center, University of Alabama at Birmingham, Birmingham, Alabama

Linda Teri, Ph.D.
Professor and Interim Chair, Department of Psychosocial and Community Health; Director, Northwest Research Group on Aging, University of Washington School of Nursing, Seattle, Washington

Alexander I. Tröster, Ph.D., A.B.P.P.(CN)
Professor of Neurology and Codirector, National Parkinson Foundation Center of Excellence, The University of North Carolina at Chapel Hill School of Medicine, Chapel Hill, North Carolina

Larry E. Tune, M.D., M.A.S.
Professor, Departments of Psychiatry and Behavioral Sciences and Neurology; Vice Chair, Investigational Review Board, Emory University School of Medicine, Atlanta, Georgia

Harry V. Vinters, M.D.
Professor of Pathology and Laboratory Medicine and of Neurology, and Daljit S. and Elaine Sarkaria Chair in Diagnostic Medicine, David Geffen School of Medicine at UCLA, Los Angeles, California

Elena Volfson, M.D., M.P.H.
Addiction Psychiatrist, Philadelphia VA Medical Center; Assistant Professor of Psychiatry, University of Pennsylvania School of Medicine, Philadelphia, Pennsylvania

Julie Loebach Wetherell, Ph.D.
Associate Professor, Department of Psychiatry, University of California, San Diego; Staff Psychologist, VA San Diego Healthcare System, San Diego, California

Daniel Weintraub, M.D.
Associate Professor of Psychiatry at the Hospital of the University of Pennsylvania, Philadelphia, Pennsylvania

Hal S. Wortzel, M.D.
Director, Neuropsychiatric Consultation Services and MIRECC Psychiatric Fellowship, Denver Veterans Hospital; Assistant Professor of Psychiatry, University of Colorado–Denver School of Medicine, Denver, Colorado

Disclosure of Interests

The following contributors to this book have indicated a financial interest in or other affiliation with a commercial supporter, a manufacturer of a commercial product, a provider of a commercial service, a nongovernmental organization, and/or a government agency, as listed below:

Alon Y. Avidan M.D., M.P.H.—*Speaker's bureau:* Cephalon, Sanovian, Takeda Pharmaceuticals; *Consultant:* Best Doctors, Merck

Michael R. Clark, M.D., M.P.H.—*Consultant:* Eli Lilly and Company

Paul T. Costa Jr., Ph.D.—*Royalties:* Revised NEO Personality Inventory (NEO-PI-R)

Jeffrey L. Cummings, M.D.—*Consultant (pharmaceutical companies):* Abbott, Acadia, Acerra, ADAMAS, Astellas, Avanir, Bristol-Myers Squibb, CoMentis, Eisai, Elan, Eli Lilly and Company, EnVivo, Forest Laboratories, Genentech, GlaxoSmithKline, Janssen, Lundbeck, Medivation, Medtronics, Merck, Merz, Myriad, Neuren, Neurokos, Novartis, Noven, Orion, Pfizer, Prana, reMYND, Schering Plough, Signum Bioscience, Sonexa, Takeda, Toyama, Wyeth; *Consultant (assessment companies):* Avid, Bayer, GE, MedAvante, Neurotrax, UBC; *Stock:* ADAMAS, MedAvante, Neurokos, Neurotrax, Prana, Sonexa; *Speaker/lecturer:* Eisai, Forest Laboratories, Janssen, Lundbeck, Merz, Novartis, Pfizer; *Copyright:* Neuropsychiatric Inventory; *Expert witness/legal consultation* provided regarding olanzapine and ropinirole

D.P. Devanand, M.D.—*Consultant:* Bristol-Myers Squibb (Advisory Board), Sanofi-Aventis (Data and Safety Monitoring Board member); *Research support:* Eli Lilly and Company, National Institute on Aging, Novartis

Steven L. Dubovsky, M.D.—*Research support:* Cardiokine, Eli Lilly and Company, Otsuka, Pfizer

Norman L. Foster, M.D.—*Consultant:* GE Healthcare, Janssen Alzheimer Immunotherapy; *Investigator:* clinical trials sponsored by Baxter Bioscience, Eli Lilly and Company, Janssen Alzheimer Immunotherapy, Pfizer

Mark S. George, M.D.—Dr. George reports no equity or other direct financial investment in any device or pharmaceutical firm. Within the past 3 years he has served as a paid consultant to Cyberonics, GlaxoSmithKline, Jazz Pharmaceuticals, Neuropace; received research grants from Brainsway, GlaxoSmithKline, Jazz Pharmaceuticals; served as an unpaid consultant to Brainsonix, Brainsway, Neuronetics, NeoStim; and served as the editor-in-chief of the journal *Brain Stimulation* published by Elsevier. MUSC holds patents in the area of combining TMS with functional brain imaging. The total compensation from any company in a single year has been less than $10,000. The total combined compensation from all consulting activities is less than 10% of his university salary.

Eric J. Lenze, M.D.—*Research support:* Bristol-Myers Squibb (medication for federal study only), Forest Laboratories, National Institute of Mental Health, Veterans Medical Research Foundation, Wyeth (medication for federal study only); *Consultant:* Fox Learning Systems, National Institutes of Health

Daniel C. Marson, J.D., Ph.D.—*Royalties:* Capacity to Consent to Treatment Instrument (CCTI)

Robert R. McCrae, Ph.D.—*Royalties:* Revised NEO Personality Inventory (NEO-PI-R)

Richard E. Powers, M.D.—*Board* (unpaid position): Alzheimer's Foundation of America [501(c)(3) organization]

Robert G. Robinson, M.D.—*Consultant:* Avanir Pharmaceuticals

Andrew D. Siderowf, M.D., M.S.C.E., is supported by a Morris K. Udall Parkinson's Disease Research Center of Excellence grant from NINDS (NS-053488) and has been supported by SAP4100027296, a health research grant awarded by the Department of Health of the Commonwealth of Pennsylvania from the Tobacco Master Settlement Agreement under Act 2001-77. He has received consulting fees from Teva Neurosceince, Supernus Pharmaceuticals, Schering-Plough, and Merck Serono. He has receved speaking honorarium from Teva Neuroscience and research support from Avid Radiopharmaceuticals.

Alexander I. Tröster, Ph.D., A.B.P.P.(CN)—*Consultant:* Boston Scientific, Medtronic, St. Jude Neuromodulation; *Grants:* Medtronic; *Speaker fees:* Medtronic

Julie Loebach Wetherell, Ph.D.—*Research support:* Forest Laboratories

The following contributors to this book have indicated no competing interests to disclose during the year preceding manuscript submission:

Olusola Ajilore, M.D., Ph.D.
Carmen Andreescu, M.D.
David B. Arciniegas, M.D., F.A.N.P.A., C.B.I.S.T.
John J. Campbell III, M.D.
C. Edward Coffey, M.D.
M. Justin Coffey, M.D.
Amelia N. Dubovsky, M.D.
Richard B. Ferrell, M.D.
Stacey Gramann, D.O., M.P.H.
Edmund S. Higgins, M.D.
Ricardo E. Jorge, M.D.
Jennifer M. Keller, Psy.D.
Glenise McKenzie, R.N., Ph.D.
David W. Oslin, M.D.
Kenneth Podell, Ph.D.
Douglas W. Scharre, M.D.
Andrea C. Solomon, Ph.D.
Linda Teri, Ph.D.
Larry E. Tune, M.D., M.A.S.
Elena Volfson, M.D., M.P.H.
Daniel Weintraub, M.D.
Hal S. Wortzel, M.D.

Preface

Geriatric neuropsychiatry is a clinical subspecialty devoted to the diagnosis and treatment of psychiatric or behavior disorders in aging patients with disturbances of brain function. Such disturbances are common in older individuals, and the continued expansion of the elderly segment of our population gives special importance to the study of neuropsychiatric illness associated with brain aging. Optimal care of older persons with brain disease is a medical-social-political imperative.

The first edition of the *The American Psychiatric Press Textbook of Geriatric Neuropsychiatry* was published in 1994, and the second edition in 2000. Since then, we have witnessed a continued explosion in neuroscience research and in our understanding of human behavior. In addition, the proportion of seniors in the population is growing, and just as importantly, the definition of "senior" continues to be pushed to higher limits—age 65 is the new 55.

The third edition of the *The American Psychiatric Publishing Textbook of Geriatric Neuropsychiatry* takes to heart the advice of our previous readers and advisors, embraces the "graying" of our population, and incorporates the very latest in neuroscience research in an updated text designed for clinicians interested in brain-behavior relations. The third edition of the *The American Psychiatric Publishing Textbook of Geriatric Neuropsychiatry* bridges the fields of geriatric neurology and geriatric psychiatry, and it emphasizes the relationships that exist between neuropsychiatric illness and aging of the nervous system. The book is intended for health care professionals—psychiatrists, neurologists, psychologists, geriatricians, and other clinicians—who desire to understand and manage disturbed behavior in the elderly through a comprehensive approach based on a thorough knowledge of contemporary neuroscience. This volume endeavors to establish a link between the neurobiology of idiopathic psychiatric illness and the neurobiology of neurological disorders that cause disturbed behavior in the elderly, and in so doing, to stimulate consideration of fundamental brain-behavior relationships.

A number of changes have been incorporated in the third edition of the *The American Psychiatric Publishing Textbook of Geriatric Neuropsychiatry.* The text has been reduced by almost a third, from 41 chapters to 29, and the reference sections have been revised to make them representative but not comprehensive—all in an effort to keep the book within the price range of our entire audience. In response to feedback requesting more clinical application, the chapters now have a sharper focus on the *health care* of patients with neuropsychiatric illness. Still, the authors have gone to great lengths to ensure that such care is informed by scientific evidence, and as such, all chapters have been extensively revised and updated with the latest in published research.

The book is organized into four parts, each of which is edited by one or more of the *Textbook's* editors or associate editors. The section editors have assembled an outstanding collection of world-renowned neuropsychiatrists and neuroscientists, who in turn have produced chapters that impart clinically relevant information within the context of the very latest in neuroscience research.

Part I, "Introduction to Geriatric Neuropsychiatry," begins with an overview of the clinical subspecialty of geriatric neuropsychiatry and the epidemiology of age-related neuropsychiatric illness, followed by a chapter on the neurobiology of brain aging to update the reader on the latest research into normal, usual, and pathological aging. The final chapter in this section provides an integrative model linking neurobiology with behavior and thus sets the stage for the subsequent parts in the book.

Part II, "Neuropsychiatric Assessment," comprises two practical chapters on the clinical and neuropsychological examination of the elderly and two chapters on the role of advanced brain imaging technologies in the evaluation of the aging patient. This section accomplishes the essential and fundamental task of defining the acceptable limits of "normal aging" as assessed at the bedside and in the clinical neuroscience laboratory.

Part III, "Principles of Neuropsychiatric Treatment," emphasizes the principles and special considerations that are essential for safe and effective treatment of neuropsychiatric disorders in the elderly. This section features up-to-date chapters on interactions between aging and psychosocial, family, neuropharmacological, and brain stimulation therapies (electroconvulsive therapy, vagus nerve stimulation, transcranial magnetic stimulation, and deep brain stimulation). Three additional chapters provide important updates on genetic interventions; behavioral and cognitive rehabilitation; neuropsychiatry in the extended care setting; and ethical, medicolegal, and forensic issues related to the care of the elderly with neuropsychiatric illness. The discussions and recommendations for treatment are anchored as much as possible in a firm foundation of clinical science research. The chapters in this section acknowledge the increasingly complex ethical, social, and forensic issues arising in the health care of the elderly.

Part IV, "Neuropsychiatric Syndromes and Disorders," provides the clinical core of the book and focuses on the essential neuropsychiatric syndromes and disorders commonly seen in the elderly. The comprehensive chapters in this section highlight the influence of the aging nervous system on the pathophysiology, neuropsychiatric manifestations, clinical course, and prognosis of neurological and psychiatric illness in the elderly.

We wish to acknowledge the associate editors, Mark S. George, M.D., and Daniel Weintraub, M.D., for the amazing effort they devoted to the *Textbook*. They join us in thanking all of the chapter authors for their contributions—such quality work requires thought, time, and energy, all of which must be redirected from other pressing demands. We also are very appreciative of the staff at American Psychiatric Publishing (APPI), including Ann Eng, Senior Editor; Greg Kuny, Managing Editor; John McDuffie, Editorial Director; and Robert E. Hales, M.D., Editor-in-Chief, for their heroic efforts in bringing this book to publication. They provided much guidance and were always available to assist with the many issues that invariably arise with a project of this scale. We are grateful for all of these collaborators—the associate editors, chapter authors, and APPI staff—who shared our vision and made this textbook a priority.

We also acknowledge with special appreciation Mark Kelley, M.D., and the Henry Ford Medical Group, as well as the Board of Trustees of Henry Ford Behavioral Health, all of whom understand and value the importance of science in the enterprise of clinical medicine. We acknowledge Mike Modic and colleagues in the Cleveland Clinic Lou Ruvo Center for Brain Health for their support and for their leadership in providing optimal care for patients with neurodegenerative disorders.

Finally, this project was ultimately made possible by the understanding, patience, and support of our families.

C. Edward Coffey, M.D.
Jeffrey L. Cummings, M.D.
September 2010

PART I

Introduction to Geriatric Neuropsychiatry

1

Geriatric Neuropsychiatry

Jeffrey L. Cummings, M.D.
C. Edward Coffey, M.D.

Our challenge is to insure that an extended life span is accompanied by an extended brain span.

Meryl Comer

Neuropsychiatry is the discipline devoted to understanding the neurobiological basis of human behavior. Neuropsychiatry has patient care, research, and educational dimensions, which emphasize, respectively, the application, generation, and dissemination of neuropsychiatric knowledge. The growth of neuropsychiatry has been stimulated by advances in basic neurobiology, neurogenetics, neuroimaging, neuropsychopharmacology, geriatrics, and psychiatry. *Geriatric neuropsychiatry* represents the application of neuropsychiatry to older individuals. Geriatric neuropsychiatry is an integrative discipline bridging the fields of psychiatry, neurology, neuroscience, and geriatrics. The emergence of geriatric neuropsychiatry is a response to the increasing size of the elderly population and the high prevalence of brain diseases and behavioral disorders among those older individuals. The practice of geriatric neuropsychiatry reflects commitment to the principle that improved understanding of brain-behavior relationships can lead to a higher quality of life for older individuals through minimization of excess disability, early recognition of diseases, and improved therapeutic interventions in brain diseases and behavioral disturbances.

The American Psychiatric Publishing Textbook of Geriatric Neuropsychiatry and its authors are devoted to the discipline of geriatric neuropsychiatry. This text is intended to serve as a guide to the practice and further development of this area of health care and research. In this introductory chapter, we review the major issues in geriatric neuropsychiatry. Our purpose is to provide a neurobiological perspective on behavioral disturbances in elderly individuals, to create a context for the remaining chapters of this book, and to define and describe geriatric neuropsychiatry. In this chapter, we also review important aspects of training and research in geriatric neuropsychiatry.

Geriatric Neuropsychiatry as a Discipline

Most subspecialization or growth of an area of specific knowledge results from concentration on a small part of a parent discipline. With the explosion of information relevant to behavioral alterations in elderly individuals, however, the emergence

Dr. Cummings is supported by National Institute on Aging Alzheimer's Disease Center Grant P50 AG16570, an Alzheimer's Disease Research Center of California grant, the Sidell-Kagan Foundation, and the Jim Easton Gift. Dr. Coffey is supported by the Mental Illness Research Association, Detroit, MI.
The source for the epigraph is a private conversation in 2009 between Dr. Cummings and Meryl Comer.

of geriatric neuropsychiatry arises from a different imperative. Geriatric neuropsychiatry is an integrative specialty that draws from a diversity of fields (psychiatry, neuropsychiatry, neurology, neuroscience, neuroimaging, neuropsychopharmacology, neuropsychology, gerontology, geriatrics, and geriatric psychology) with the intent of improving the health care of elderly individuals with behavioral disorders and to stimulate research in this critical area (Figure 1–1).

The clinical practice of geriatric neuropsychiatry depends on distinguishing normal age-related changes from those of disease and disordered brain function. Slowing of cognition, diminished access to specific bits of memory (e.g., names), and reduced cognitive flexibility may occur in the course of normal aging (Van Gorp and Mahler 1990) (see Chapter 5, "Neuropsychological Assessment"). These changes must be differentiated from the effects of dementia, depression, and systemic illness. Geriatric neuropsychiatry provides expertise in this area.

Neuropsychiatry and Geriatric Neuropsychiatry

Neuropsychiatry is actually an old discipline that has been resurrected to assume a prominent place in contemporary psychiatry and neurology. There is no consensus definition of *neuropsychiatry*. Lishman (1992) suggested that it is the aspect of psychiatry that seeks to advance understanding of behavioral problems through increased knowledge of brain structure and function. Yudofsky and Hales (1989a, 1989b) defined *neuropsychiatry* as the discipline concerned with the assessment and treatment of patients with psychiatric illnesses or symptoms associated with brain abnormalities. Trimble (1993) emphasized that neuropsychiatry attempts to understand the effects of central nervous system structural or functional change on behavior, recognizing the essentially dynamic and individualistic nature of behavioral dispositions. More recently, Lee et al. (2008) described neuropsychiatry as the interface between neurology and psychiatry—the intersecting field of inquiry embracing both brain and mind. The underlying premise of neuropsychiatry is that neurological and psychiatric disorders share a common anatomical and neuronal substrate. Lee et al. observed that the field is growing in the wake of the unprecedented progress in the neurosciences, including molecular biology, genetics, and neuroimaging. Northoff (2008) suggested that neuropsychiatry represents a bridge between neuroanatomy and psychopathology; it is poised between strictly localizable neurological functions and strictly holistic psychological processes. Indeed, functional neuroanatomy is a key conceptual underpinning of contemporary neuropsychiatry and has been informed by advances in systems neuroanatomy and functional imaging.

We view neuropsychiatry as an umbrella discipline under which geriatric neuropsychiatry is subsumed. Geriatric neuropsychiatry, however, integrates information from geriatrics, gerontology, and aging research not specifically relevant to all areas of the broader discipline of neuropsychiatry. The knowledge framework of geriatric neuropsychiatry applies to older individuals.

Geriatric Neuropsychiatry and Geriatric Psychiatry

Geriatric neuropsychiatry has a wide interface with geriatric psychiatry and can be regarded as a synthesis of geriatric psychiatry and neuropsychiatry. Both geriatric psychiatry and geriatric neuropsychiatry are concerned with care, education, and research related to behavioral disturbances in elderly individuals. The principal difference between the two is one of emphasis. The emphasis in geriatric neuropsychiatry is on the relationship among the neurosciences, the application of pharmacological treatments, and the assessment and management of psychiatric aspects of neurological diseases in older patients. Geriatric neuropsychiatry is committed to the proposition that the cure of neuropsychiatric disorders of elderly persons, improved management of behavioral disturbances, and amelioration of adverse age-related changes in brain function are all linked to advances in neuroscience, as well as to progress in psychology, sociology, and related disciplines. While accepting the incontestable importance of social, cultural, and psychological aspects of aging and diseases of the elderly population, geriatric neuropsychiatry emphasizes integrating and developing neuroscience information with the goal of better understanding and treatment of brain disorders of elderly patients.

Geriatric Neuropsychiatry and Behavioral Neurology

No definitional boundaries exist between neuropsychiatry and behavioral neurology or between geriatric neuropsychiatry and behavioral neurology. Traditionally, behavioral neurology has been devoted to the study of "deficit disorders" (negative symptoms) such as aphasia, amnesia, agnosia, and apraxia, whereas neuropsychiatry has been concerned with the diagnosis and management of syndromes with "productive symptoms" (positive symptoms) such as hallucinations, delusions, and mood changes. In addition, behavioral neurologists usually have been trained in neurology, whereas neuropsychiatrists usually have had a background in psychiatry. Neither neurology nor psychiatry, however, completely prepares a clinician for the broad range of behavioral disorders associated with acquired and idiopathic brain dysfunction. Both disciplines produce behavioral neuroscientists who use

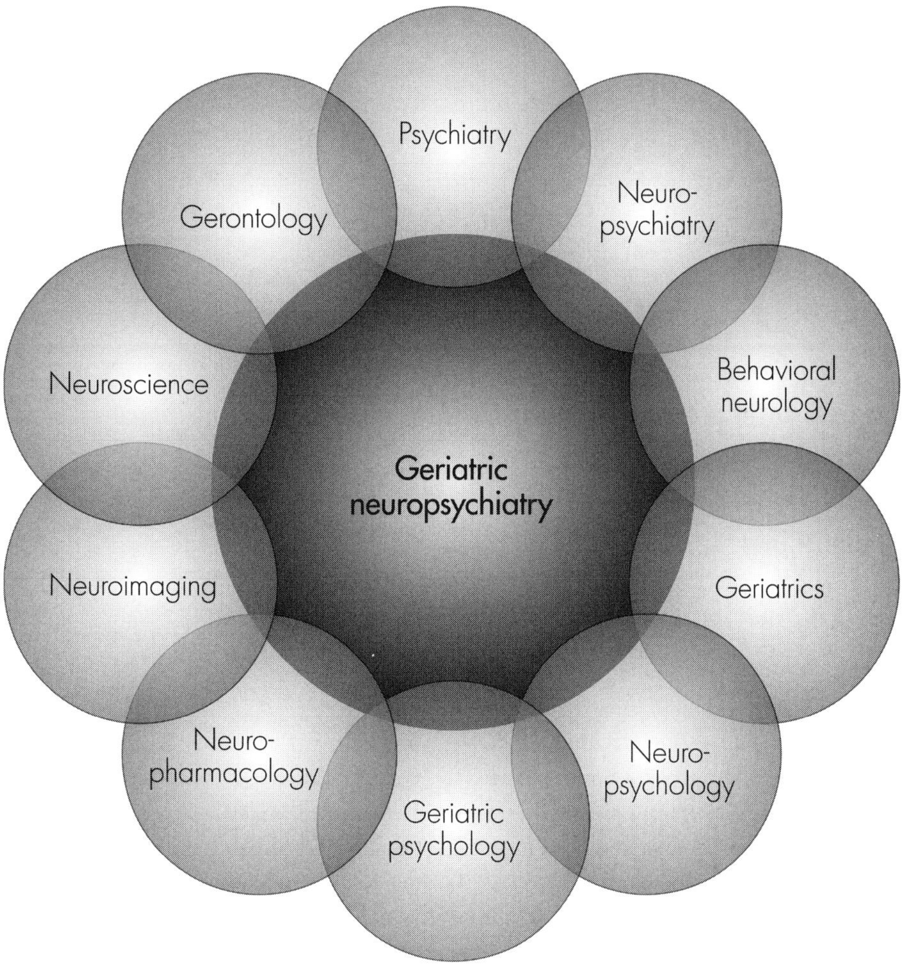

FIGURE 1–1. Disciplines comprising geriatric neuropsychiatry.

similar concepts to relate abnormal behavior to brain dysfunction. Furthermore, individual patients often manifest both deficit and productive disorders, making it imperative that clinicians have knowledge of both neuropsychiatry and behavioral neurology. This knowledge is particularly important in geriatric neuropsychiatry, because the prevalence of acquired brain disease as a cause of altered behavior is high.

A corollary of the absence of boundaries between behavioral neurology and neuropsychiatry is the transcendence of traditional restrictive definitions of individual diseases as "neurological" or "psychiatric." Alzheimer's disease and Parkinson's disease are examples of disorders traditionally considered to be "neurological," whereas depression and obsessive-compulsive disorder have historically been thought of as "psychiatric." Neither of these assumptions proves to be true from the perspective of geriatric neuropsychiatry. Alzheimer's disease and Parkinson's disease both have major behavioral manifestations, whereas depression and obsessive-compulsive disorder are increasingly well understood as brain disorders. It is ever more evident that designating disorders as neurological or psychiatric—although convenient for some historical and administrative purposes—is arbitrary and misleading. These designations are clinically unhelpful and may hinder the evolution of a behavioral neuroscience commensurate with optimum patient care. As Martin (2002) noted, the interests of neurology and psychiatry converge within the framework of modern neuroscience, and progress in understanding the brain basis of behavior will both demand and facilitate more collaboration and integration of these fields.

Geriatric Neuropsychiatry and Clinical Training

There is a marked lack of availability of individuals with expertise in geriatric neuropsychiatry, as well as a dearth of training programs to provide experience in this area. This deficiency reflects the widespread lack of training in clinical care and research regarding both behavioral neuroscience and the care of elderly patients (Cummings et al. 1998). Few neurology residency programs in the United States provide formal research training. Geriatric psychiatry and geriatric medicine are decidedly understaffed (Medicare Payment Advisory Commission 2003). Development of a cadre of individuals with expertise in the assessment and management of geriatric neuropsychiatric abnormalities is an essential response to the expanding elderly population. Currently available training programs are inadequate to meet the growing need. Although there is no board certification in the United States for geriatric neuropsychiatry, the United Council for Neurologic Specialties offers a board program in behavioral neurology and neuropsychiatry, available to both neurologists and psychiatrists with appropriate training (Silver 2006).

Converging Information in Geriatric Neuropsychiatry

The two principal dimensions in geriatric neuropsychiatry are the psychiatric manifestations of neurological disorders and the neurobiological basis of psychiatric illnesses. One exciting aspect of neuropsychiatry is the convergence of conclusions emanating from these two avenues of research. For example, Robinson and Starkstein (1990) demonstrated that depression is most common among stroke patients when the cerebrovascular lesion involves the anterior structures of the left hemisphere (see Chapter 25, "Cerebrovascular Disease"), whereas studies of idiopathic depression have found evidence of reduced frontal lobe volume (Coffey et al. 1993) and altered metabolism in related corticolimbic structures (Drevets 2007; Fujimoto et al. 2008) (see Chapter 19, "Mood Disorders"). Thus, both avenues of investigation lead to similar anatomical implications.

Neuropathological investigations in schizophrenia have revealed abnormalities in the cellular architectonics in the temporal lobe (Zaidel et al. 1997), and studies of neurological disease with psychosis demonstrated that the temporal lobe is a common site of pathological changes (Cummings 1992b) (see Chapter 21, "Psychosis"). Again, studies of psychiatric and neurological disorders with similar symptoms suggest shared pathophysiologies.

In studies of idiopathic obsessive-compulsive disorders, Saxena et al. (2004) found increased metabolism in the orbitofrontal cortex and related circuitry, and Cummings (1993) observed that obsessions and compulsions occur in neurological disease when there is involvement of structures participating in the frontal-subcortical circuit originating in medial frontal and orbitofrontal cortical regions (see Chapter 20, "Anxiety Disorders"). Preliminary studies with positron emission tomography (PET) have suggested that altered regional metabolic activity occurs in anxiety disorders (Evans et al. 2009), and anxiety symptoms have been associated with structural lesions of related cortical areas in neurological diseases (Anderson et al. 2006) (see Chapter 20).

The convergence of information from the neurological and psychiatric approaches to neuropsychiatry has many implications. When clinical neuropsychiatric symptoms are similar, even in seemingly different disorders, there may be involvement of the same underlying neuroanatomical structures and common pathobiological mechanisms. These observations also support the use of the same therapeutic agents for symptom control in patients with diverse underlying diseases but similar neuropsychiatric symptoms.

These convergent data in neuropsychiatric research justify the working assumptions of geriatric neuropsychiatry that the relationship between brain dysfunction and behavioral disturbances is rule governed, that the axioms relating structure and function are discoverable, and that the rules will apply regardless of the etiology of the underlying disorder (Cummings 1999).

Aging, the Brain, and Geriatric Neuropsychiatry

The brain undergoes a variety of neurochemical, structural, and neurophysiological alterations in the course of normal aging (Galluzzi et al. 2008) (see Chapter 2, "Neurobiology of Aging"). Grossly, a small decrease in brain weight occurs in the course of normal aging with widening of cerebral cortical sulci and enlargement of the lateral ventricles (see Chapter 6, "Imaging the Structure of the Aging Human Brain").

Microscopically, neuronal loss occurs in specific cortical and subcortical structures. In addition, lipofuscin, granulovacuolar changes, and neurofibrillary tangles accumulate in the course of aging, and there is a progressive shrinkage of the dendritic domain of some cortical and subcortical neurons (Dickstein et al. 2007).

Neurochemical changes also accompany aging. Decreased activity of catecholamine-synthesizing enzymes and increased activity of monoamine oxidase (an enzyme involved in catecholamine catabolism) have been documented (Dreher et al. 2008). These biochemical and structural changes may underlie the psychomotor retardation of elderly individuals, as well as the mild parkinsonian habitus associated with aging, and they may contribute to the occurrence of depression in elderly people. Neurochemical alterations may have a role in age-associated memory impairment observed in elderly individuals (Taylor et al. 2008).

The underlying mechanisms of aging remain mysterious, but strides are being made in understanding some of the processes that contribute to age-related changes in function. Oxidative metabolism catalyzed by oxygen free radicals damages enzymes, and this in turn leads to a reduced synthetic ability and compromise of the aged organism's ability to respond to changing biological contingencies (Stadtman 1992). Trophic factors may be responsible for maintaining cellular connectivity, and changes in tropism with aging may contribute to some age-related brain alterations (Serrano and Klann 2004). Finally, some cells have genetically determined life spans, whereas other cell populations manifest few, if any, changes in the course of aging (Finch 1990). Deciphering the molecular mechanisms responsible for programmed aging is critical to a comprehensive understanding of the neurobiology of aging.

The brain is continuously changing from its fetal developmental period through senescence. The changes associated with aging are not global, and they affect specific cellular populations, structures, and transmitters more than others. The temporal sequence of aging varies among different structures. The neurobiological changes of aging, as well as the differential involvement of functional systems, may influence the types of neuropsychiatric disorders to which elderly people are vulnerable.

Aging, Brain Diseases, and Geriatric Neuropsychiatry

The emergence and growth of geriatric neuropsychiatry are driven by four circumstances: 1) the growth of the size of the elderly population, 2) the increased prevalence of brain diseases among elderly persons, 3) a high frequency of psychiatric disorders among elderly people, and 4) the recognition that behavioral disturbances often are manifestations of brain dysfunction.

Demography of Aging

In 1900, there were 3.1 million elderly people in the United States, representing 4% of the population. By 1950, there were 12.3 million elderly people, representing 8.1% of the U.S. population. This group had grown to 35 million and 12.4% by 2000. With the aging of the baby boomer population, a marked shift will occur in the structure of the U.S. population such that by 2030 there will be 70 million people over age 65; of those, 8.9 million persons will be over age 85, the age group most likely to exhibit Alzheimer's disease (Rice and Fineman 2004).

Aging and the diseases of elderly people present a global challenge. The world's elderly population is growing at a rate of 2.4% per year, faster than the rest of the population. Twenty-three countries had 2 million or more elderly individuals in 1985, whereas 50 countries will have this number by 2025. The growth of the world's elderly population will occur disproportionately in economically developed countries; 69% of the world's elderly people will live in developing nations by the year 2025 (Forti et al. 2000). In contrast, by 2030 China will be home to only 24.6% of the world's population ages 65 and older and to 21.9% of the population ages 80 and older (Kincannon et al. 2005).

Neurological Diseases With Behavioral Manifestations

The three neurological conditions most responsible for neuropsychiatric morbidity in elderly individuals are 1) Alzheimer's disease and other dementing disorders, 2) Parkinson's disease, and 3) stroke. The prevalence of dementia increases dramatically with age (see Chapter 16, "Alzheimer's Disease and the Frontotemporal Dementia Syndromes"). A demographic study of dementia in Stockholm, Sweden (Fratiglioni et al. 1991), found that 5.7% of individuals ages 75–79 years had mental status changes indicative of dementia, and 9.6% of those ages 80–84 years had dementia; the proportion rose to 20.4% in those ages 85–89 years and to 32% in those ages 90 and older. Epidemiological studies demonstrate that the rate of Alzheimer's disease among elderly persons in the United States is ~3% in those ages 65–74 years, 17% in those ages 75–84 years, and 40%–50% in those ages 84 and older. Parkinson's disease also exhibits an age-related prevalence (see Chapter 24, "Parkinson's Disease and Movement Disorders"). The reported frequency varies among studies, but representative investigations reveal the following prevalence rates: 1% among people ages 55–59 years; 4%, ages 60–64 years; 6%, ages 65–69 years; 12%, ages 70–74 years; 20%, ages 75–79 years; and 10%, ages 80–84 years. The prevalence of stroke and vascular dementia likewise increases with age (see Chapter 25, "Cerebrovascular Disease"). The prevalence of cerebrovascular disease rises from 4% in those ages 65–74 to 8% in those ages 75–84, and to 10% in those over age 85 (Ziegler-Graham et al. 2008). The cumulative prevalence of neurological disease among elderly persons and the chronic nature of many neurological illnesses make brain diseases a major source of morbidity and mortality among elderly individuals.

Neurological diseases of elderly people are often manifested by alterations in behavior. The dementia syndromes are defined by loss of cognitive abilities, but many patients with dementia also exhibit delusions, depression, anxiety, agitation, and aggressiveness (Cummings and Benson 1992; Mega et al. 1996). Dementia occurs in 41% of patients with Parkinson's disease (Mayeux et al. 1992), and 40%–60% of patients with Parkinson's disease have depressive disorders, anxiety, and apathy (Cummings 1992a). With treatment, hallucinations and delusions may emerge in previously asymptomatic individuals. Eighty percent of strokes involve the cerebral hemispheres, where they produce neurobehavioral and neuropsychiatric syndromes such as aphasia, amnesia, visuospatial disturbances, depression, or psychosis (Beckson and Cummings 1991). Up to three-fourths of all patients hospitalized with stroke have evidence of cognitive impairment (Nys et al. 2007). Thus, behavioral disturbances are the principal clinical manifestations of many brain diseases of elderly people. Recognition and management of geriatric neuropsychiatric disorders are critical in an aging society.

Psychiatric Illness

Psychiatric disorders are common in elderly persons. Some are late-persisting disorders that began in earlier life and continue, whereas others occur for the first time with aging. Schizophrenia, bipolar disorder, anxiety, and obsessive-compulsive disorder are most likely to be late-persisting conditions, whereas depression may occur for the first time in older persons (see Chapter 19, "Mood Disorders"). Paraphrenia is an uncommon late-onset psychotic disorder (see Chapter 26, "Traumatic Brain Injury"). Substance abuse, particularly alcoholism, is also present in the elderly population, and prescription drug abuse involving pain medications or other agents is not uncommon among older persons (see Chapter 17, "Addiction"). The first appearance of a new behavioral change in an older person should always lead to consideration of an evolving brain disorder, such as Alzheimer's disease. Depression may be the first sign of the presence of Alzheimer's disease, and mild cognitive impairment as a prodrome to Alzheimer's disease is often accompanied by neuropsychiatric symptoms including depression and apathy (Geda et al. 2008; Teng et al. 2007).

Dementia, alcoholism, anxiety, and mood disorders are the most common psychiatric conditions among elderly people. Each of these diseases has an important neurobiological dimension. Dementia is an overt brain disorder produced by Alzheimer's disease, cerebrovascular disease, or other encephalopathic processes (Cummings and Benson 1992). In individuals with alcohol abuse, PET reveals diminished brain glucose metabolism (Volkow et al. 1992), and dysfunction of basal ganglia-limbic circuits is implicated in alcohol craving (Modell et al. 1990). Patients with anxiety disorder have an increased frequency of structural alterations of the right temporal lobe (Fontaine et al. 1990), exhibit regional alterations in metabolism (Evans et al. 2009), and evidence functional disturbances involving a variety of neurotransmitter systems.

Depression occupies a particularly important place in geriatric neuropsychiatry (see Chapter 19, "Mood Disorders"). This disorder is disabling and treatable and may occur for the first time in elderly individuals. If not detected and treated, depression may be fatal; men ages 65–74 years have the highest suicide rate of any age group in the United States (Erlangsen et al. 2003; Shah 2007). Imaging studies suggest that depression is associated with alterations in brain structure and function, particularly in elderly people. Reported structural abnormalities include cortical atrophy (especially of the frontal lobes), ventricular enlargement, and subcortical encephalomalacia (Coffey 1996; Coffey et al. 1993; Duffy and Coffey 1997). These findings may be related to the onset of mental disorders in late life (Coffey 1991), and they are associated with a poor long-term prognosis. Functional imaging studies reveal evidence of altered regional cerebral blood flow and metabolism in depressive disorders; the frontal lobes are most prominently affected (Drevets 2007; Fujimoto et al. 2008). Although relatively few studies have examined elderly subjects, data suggest that functional and molecular brain imaging may be useful in distinguishing the neurodegenerative dementias from the dementia of depression. Together, these observations indicate that alterations of brain structure and function may interact with the aging process to facilitate the emergence of affective disorders in late life.

Late-onset psychoses may occur, although they are considerably rarer than late-occurring depression or anxiety (see Chapter 21, "Psychosis"). Investigations reveal that about half of patients with late-onset delusional disorders have an identifiable underlying brain disease (Webster and Grossberg 1998). Thus, delusions may be the heralding feature of a neurological disease.

Together, these studies indicate that mental disorders are an important aspect of geriatric care, that there is an emerging understanding of the neurobiology of these psychiatric conditions, and that brain abnormalities are associated with many late-onset psychiatric disturbances. Geriatric neuropsychiatry addresses both the neurobiology of idiopathic psychiatric disorders and the psychiatric disturbances associated with neurological conditions.

Cost of Brain Disorders

The total cost of brain disorders in Europe is estimated at £386 billion (2004 value) (Pugliatti et al. 2008). The annual cost of brain diseases in the United States has been calculated, and the yearly expense is staggering. The Alzheimer's Study Group (2009) estimated that the cost of caring for patients with Alzheimer's disease alone was more than $100 billion annually. Fifteen percent of the average annual income of workers in the United States is devoted to brain diseases. Although the costs of diseases of elderly persons were not separately calculated, dementia accounted for the largest share (45%) of the cost of all neurological illnesses, and a substantial share of the funds expended on brain disorders concerns diseases of elderly patients.

Medical Illness, Drugs, and Geriatric Neuropsychiatry

The rise of geriatric neuropsychiatry is fueled by the marked rise in medical illness in the elderly population and the increased frequency of associated behavioral disturbances. Medical disorders become increasingly common among elderly people, medications are more frequently administered, and changes in drug metabolism occur with aging. These alterations create a neurobiological setting that is conducive to brain dysfunction and behavioral abnormalities (Figure 1–2).

Medical illnesses are common in elderly people, and many of these affect brain function and produce behavioral alterations (see Chapter 29, "Neuropsychiatric Disorders Associated With General Medical Therapies"). Among the 10 most common nonneurological diseases of elderly people are hypertension, diabetes, and arteriosclerosis (McNabney et al. 2008). These diseases may involve the brain through direct mechanisms, such as stroke, or through indirect mechanisms, including hypoxia and renal failure. Epidemiological studies have revealed that ~20% of patients with medical illness have significant depressive symptoms and 5%–20% experience major depressive episodes; 10%–15% of patients with medical illness manifest anxiety disorders. The coexistence of medical and psychiatric illnesses increases the length of stay of hospitalized patients and is associated with poorer postdischarge prognosis (Mayou et al. 1991; Saravay et al. 1991). Conversely, ~50% of elderly patients with psychiatric illness have significant medical illnesses. Nearly 60% of these conditions are undiagnosed before psychiatric admission, and in 10%–20% of these patients, the behavioral changes are directly attributable to the physical pathology (Mayou et al. 1991; Saravay et al. 1991).

The high prevalence of medical illness among elderly people results in an increase in the number of medications prescribed. Elderly people take more prescribed and over-the-counter medications than any other age group. They make up 12% of the population and take 25%–30% of all prescribed drugs. The average older U.S. citizen receives 4.5 prescribed medications, and two-thirds also take at least one over-the-counter agent (Beers 1992). Forty percent of the elderly individuals who take medications receive prescriptions from more than one physician, and 12% take drugs prescribed for someone else. These practices are further complicated by intentional or accidental noncompliance with prescribing instructions. Up to 30% of elderly patients make serious errors in the way they take their medications, and up to 50% default on one or more prescribed agents (Qato et al. 2008).

Drug metabolism is altered in elderly patients, and the changes may have marked consequences for brain function and the treatment of behavioral abnormalities (see Chapter 9, "Geriatric Neuropsychopharmacology"). An increased sensitivity of receptors for most classes of drugs occurs in the course of aging, making lower levels more effective and "standard" doses more likely to induce toxicity (Hilmer 2008; Perucca 2006). Changes also occur in drug distribution with aging. A relative increase in body fat and decrease in muscle produce a greater volume of distribution for fat-soluble drugs (e.g., benzodiazepines) and a smaller volume of distribution for drugs absorbed primarily in lean body mass (e.g., lithium). Reduced liver blood flow and impaired oxidative metabolism by hepatic enzymes occur in the course of normal aging, leading to reduced hepatic metabolism of many pharmacological agents. Renal function also declines with age; glomerular filtration rate is reduced by approximately one-third in elderly individuals (Hilmer 2008). These changes all tend to increase the risk of toxicity when medications are administered to elderly patients. Adverse drug reactions account for ~12%–17% of all hospital admissions of elderly patients, and 20% of all elderly patients experience adverse side effects while in the hospital (Hajjar et al. 2007; Qato 2008).

The higher frequency of medical illness in the elderly population and the concomitant need for more drug administration place elderly patients at a substantially increased risk of toxic metabolic neuropsychiatric disturbances. Delirium, dementia, depression, mania, psychosis, and anxiety have all been observed in patients with brain dysfunction secondary to systemic illnesses and drug toxicity (Cummings 1985).

Geriatric Neuropsychiatry and Neuroscience

Neuroimaging

The increase in diagnostic technologies has accelerated the development of geriatric neuropsychiatry. Among these, neuroimaging has had a great impact. Neuroimaging plays an increasingly large role in the diagnosis, differential diagnosis, and treatment monitoring of behavioral disturbances in elderly persons. Structural, functional, and molecular imaging has provided new insights into brain function, the pathophysiology of brain disorders, and the neurobiology of normal aging (see Chapter 6, "Imaging the Structure of the Aging Human Brain," and Chapter 7, "Molecular Imaging in Neuropsychiatry").

Imaging of brain structure, metabolism, and chemical composition is now possible (Apostolova and Thompson 2007; Klunk et al. 2004). In addition, specialized techniques allow visualization of arterial and venous blood flow. Images of brain structure are generated by computed tomography (CT) and magnetic resonance imaging (MRI). These techniques reveal the structure of the brain and ventricular system. Tumors, large strokes, subdural hematomas, large demyelinating lesions, arteriovenous malformations, and hydrocephalus are demonstrated by both techniques. MRI is more sensitive than CT to changes in white matter of the central nervous system and is superior in revealing evidence of ischemic and inflammatory disease.

MRI has been shown to have a potential role in predicting adverse responses to therapy. Patients with depression who have basal ganglia lesions and increased white matter abnor-

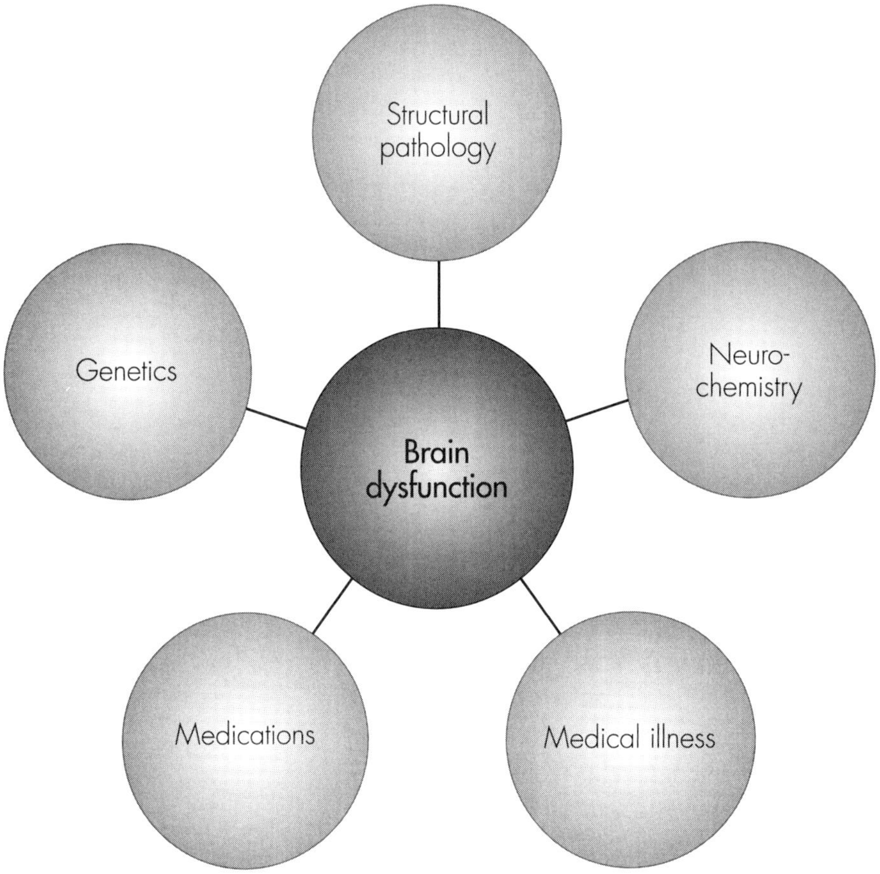

FIGURE 1–2. Influences on brain formation capable of influencing neuropsychiatric symptoms in elderly persons.

malities are more likely to exhibit prolonged interictal confusion during electroconvulsive therapy (ECT) and a higher frequency of antidepressant-induced deliria than are elderly patients with depression who have normal MRI results (Coffey 1996; Figiel et al. 1990; Herrmann et al. 2008). Elderly patients with depression who have enlarged ventricles and cortical atrophy may have a poorer prognosis for recovery than elderly patients with depression but without these structural changes (see Chapter 19, "Mood Disorders").

Magnetic resonance spectroscopy is a specialized application of magnetic resonance technology that allows the determination of the concentration of specific compounds (choline, *N*-acetyl aspartate, creatine, etc., depending on the assay methods) (Soares and Law 2009) in the brain, and advanced imaging techniques using magnetic resonance can be used to determine cerebral blood flow (Norris 2006). Diffusion tensor imaging allows visualization of white matter tracts in the brain and their disturbance in diseased states (Assaf and Pasternak 2008). The rapid advances in MRI technology suggest that this tool will be of increasing importance in neuropsychiatry (Prichard and Cummings 1997).

Except for the marked caudate nucleus atrophy associated with Huntington's disease, degenerative brain diseases (e.g., Alzheimer's disease and Parkinson's disease) produce no pathognomonic changes that are detectable on conventional structural imaging. In these disorders, structural imaging techniques such as CT and MRI provide little specific diagnostic information. Moreover, idiopathic neuropsychiatric disorders, such as depression, mania, psychosis, and anxiety, are not associated with diagnostic structural brain alterations. Functional brain imaging techniques, such as PET and single-photon emission computed tomography (SPECT), provide an informative approach to some of these neuropsychiatric disorders. PET may be used to study cerebral glucose metabolism (with radiolabeled glucose), cerebral blood flow (with radiolabeled oxygen), neurotransmitter function (with radiolabeled receptor, transporter, and transmitter ligands), and protein deposition (with radiolabeled protein ligands) (Klunk et al. 2004; Valotassiou et al. 2008). SPECT is typically used to measure cerebral blood flow but may also be applied to assessment of neurotransmitters, receptors, and transporters (Pimlott and Ebmeier 2007). Degenerative diseases and idiopathic neuropsychiatric illnesses may have distinctive alterations on metabolic, molecular, and perfusion imaging studies. For example, Alzheimer's disease typically causes reduced metabolism or perfusion in the temporoparieto-occipital junction region and posterior cingulate gyrus; frontal lobe degenerations cause decreased metabolism or perfusion of the frontal lobes; depression may be associated with diminished frontal lobe metabolism; and obsessive-compulsive disorder has been associated with increased metabolism of the orbitofrontal cortex (Drevets 2007; Fujimoto et al. 2008).

One brain imaging technique that is having high impact on geriatric neuropsychiatry and suggests advances to come is molecular imaging. Several ligands have been developed that label amyloid (Klunk et al. 2004) or amyloid and tau proteins (Small et al. 2006). Pittsburgh compound B (PiB) labels the amyloid protein, whereas 2-(1-{6-[(2-[F-18]fluoroethyl)(methyl)amino]-2-naphthyl}ethylidene)malononitrile (FDDNP) binds to amyloid and tau and possibly to other abnormal proteins in the brain (Ikonomovic et al. 2008; Small et al. 2006). Studies with these scans show that the protein accumulation begins in the brain while patients remain asymptomatic or do not yet manifest abnormal cognitive function (Aizenstein et al. 2008). Patients with mild cognitive impairment who have protein accumulation demonstrable on these scans progress to dementia, whereas those who do not exhibit protein abnormalities may not progress (Small et al. 2006). Scans of this type have also begun to inform investigators about the natural history of amyloid pathology; this protein appears to occur early and to plateau as the disease progresses (Klunk et al. 2006). This suggests that antiamyloid interventions might be most effective if they are provided early in the disease course. Treatments addressing other aspects of the pathophysiology of Alzheimer's disease may be required later in the disease process.

The success of amyloid imaging also suggests that molecular imaging of other diseases—such as imaging of α-synuclein in Parkinson's disease or dementia with Lewy bodies, as well as imaging of the TDP-43 protein present in some cases of frontotemporal dementia—may allow insights vital to determining the diagnosis of, understanding the pathophysiology of, and finding the optimal means of developing treatment for these disorders (Drzezga 2008).

These investigations demonstrate that reliable relationships exist between behavioral changes and brain imaging. Imaging research provides important insights into the pathophysiology of neuropsychiatric disorders and is likely to play an increasingly important role in geriatric neuropsychiatric practice and research.

Advances in Molecular Neurobiology

Spectacular advances have occurred in molecular neurobiology and the understanding of the molecular pathophysiology of Alzheimer's disease, Parkinson's disease, and other neurodegenerative neuropsychiatric illnesses. The metabolism of amyloid precursor protein by β-secretase and γ-secretase to form amyloid β-protein monomers, which aggregate into neurotoxic oligomers before fibrilizing and being deposited as less toxic insoluble amyloid plaque, has been well characterized at the molecular level (Cole and Vassar 2008). Similarly, the molecular pathophysiology of α-synuclein and its role in Parkinson's disease has been increasingly well delineated (Fasano and Lopiano 2008). The discovery of autosomal dominant forms of neurodegenerative neuropsychiatric illnesses has led to the ability to create transgenic animals that develop specific aspects of neurodegenerative disease, such as amyloid deposition in the brain, and to the opportunity to explore pathways contributing to the neurodegenerative disorder. Although these models are limited as simulacra of human disease, they provide a telescoped time course of some aspects of the disorder and allow testing of therapeutic interventions aimed at pathways recapitulated in the model. Improved understanding of pathophysiology, improved models of neurodegenerative and other forms of geriatric neuropsychiatric illness, and enhanced molecular genetic techniques promise to further advance understanding of the molecular neurobiology of geriatric neuropsychiatric illness and to inform attempts to intervene in these disease processes.

Advances in Treatment

The value of accurate diagnosis is enhanced when it proceeds in concert with advances in treatment. The recent past has seen an unparalleled increase in the availability of medications to treat neuropsychiatric disturbances (see Chapter 9, "Geriatric Neuropsychopharmacology"). Antidepressant agents have proliferated and have become highly differentiated, with relative selectivity for inhibition of reuptake of norepinephrine or serotonin. Conventional neuroleptic agents are now complemented by atypical antipsychotic drugs that produce fewer acute or chronic extrapyramidal side effects (Masand and Gupta 2003). With the evolution of these agents, patients experience less risk of dystonia, parkinsonism, or tardive dyskinesia as their psychiatric disorders are controlled. These advances must be balanced against evidence that antipsychotic agents, both typical and atypical, increase mortality when used in elderly patients with dementia, and some of these agents increase the risk of stroke (Salzman et al. 2008). This class of agents provides useful control of some types of behavior but must be used judiciously, and the adverse event profile indicates the need to continue to develop new agents with improved safety.

The discovery that carbamazepine, sodium valproate, and atypical antipsychotics have antimanic benefits has improved the treatment of mania while emphasizing that common neurophysiological processes are shared by some neurological and psychiatric illnesses (Yatham et al. 2005). The common use of specific drugs, such as carbamazepine, valproate, lamotrigine, or gabapentin, to control epilepsy, migraine, pain, and bipolar mania suggests that these disorders share a common pathophysiology and that channelopathy may be a common form of neuropsychiatric illness with a variety of clinical manifestations. The evolution of an understanding of shared mechanisms among neurological and psychiatric illnesses further serves to reify the tenet of neuropsychiatry that distinctions among these disorders are artificial and will be eroded by advances in scientific understanding of the pathophysiology of these disorders.

The rapid advances in neuropsychopharmacology provide the clinician with a varied and powerful armamentarium with which to meet the challenges of neuropsychiatric disease in the elderly patient. These developments also require that the clinician be familiar with the pharmacokinetics, side effects, and drug interactions of these new agents. Geriatric neuropsychiatry is the clinical discipline committed to implementation of these advances for the benefit of elderly individuals with behavioral disorders.

Geriatric neuropsychiatry appears to be on the verge of a new era of disease-modifying therapy (see Chapter 12, "Cognitive Impairment and Rehabilitation"). Neuropharmacological therapeutics have been devoted primarily to the control of symptoms, such as memory impairment in Alzheimer's disease, movement abnormalities in Parkinson's disease, psychosis in schizophrenia, mania in bipolar disorder, and so forth. With advances in understanding of the genetic and molecular pathology of neuropsychiatric illnesses (particularly neurodegenerative disorders), there are opportunities to intervene in the basic disease process and to advance disease-modifying therapies. These treatments will be distinguished from existing symptomatic therapies by intervening in the basic disease process and producing a concomitant effect on the progressive course of the disease (Cummings 2006). These agents are progressing through clinical trials that are being conducted by individuals experienced in geriatric neuropharmacology and interested in new drug development. New standards will be required from the U.S. Food and Drug Administration to determine the criteria that must be met to allow a drug to be approved for disease modification (Cummings 2006). Approval of these drugs and their implementation into geriatric neuropsychiatric practice will allow clinicians to prevent neurodegenerative disorders, delay the onset of symptoms, or slow the progression from mild to more severe forms of these diseases. Some types of disease-modifying therapies, such as intravenous therapy or subcutaneous administration, may have exceptional practice demands. Rigorous side-effect monitoring will be required, and substantial expertise in administering these agents may be necessary.

Therapeutics in geriatric neuropsychiatry is turning increasingly to the use of device-based procedures. ECT remains a safe and highly effective treatment for patients with certain severe neuropsychiatric disorders (see Chapter 10, "Electroconvulsive Therapy and Related Treatments"), and recent advances in the technique have dramatically improved its cognitive side effects. Vagal nerve stimulation is used for the treatment of epilepsy and is increasingly being explored as a treatment for specific types of depression (Daban et al. 2008) (see Chapter 11, "Brain Stimulation Therapies"). Repetitive transcranial magnetic stimulation was recently approved as a treatment for depression, and with its relatively benign side-effect profile, it will provide an important addition to the neuropsychiatric treatment armamentarium and may replace conventional ECT for some patients (Fregni et al. 2006) (see Chapter 11). Deep brain stimulation is widely applied to the treatment of Parkinson's disease with excessive on/off phenomena. This technique has substantial although temporary therapeutic benefit and occasionally produces adverse neuropsychiatric side effects (Wichmann and Delong 2006). An increasing role for device-related therapy in geriatric neuropsychiatry is anticipated.

Geriatric Neuropsychiatry and Ethical Issues

Ethical issues arise often in geriatric neuropsychiatry (see Chapter 14, "Ethical and Legal Issues"). The main challenges concern the ability of individuals to take responsibility for their own actions and the responsibility of society to preserve the rights of elderly citizens. The following are some of the ethical questions that are pondered: With regard to driving, at what point are the wishes of the patient to maintain independence and mobility in conflict with the safety of other drivers and pedestrians who might be endangered by the patient? At what point do patients relinquish their right to make decisions regarding disposition of property and wealth? When do they lose their right to decide when they can no longer live at home? When do they need a surrogate decision maker for questions of life support, treatment of infections, and postmortem autopsy? Who should make decisions for the patients when the patients themselves cannot? Should such decisions be based on family beliefs about what the patient would want, on advanced directives from the patient, or on an assessment of the apparent daily life satisfaction of the individual with dementia (Dresser 1992; Moody 1992)? Is euthanasia a viable societal response to severe dementia? These questions do not have categorical answers; they must be answered individually for each patient, taking into account the needs and abilities of the patient, the family context, other patient-specific contingencies, and the law.

Geriatric neuropsychiatric illnesses strike at the self and alter the individual's personal identity. For example, whereas a patient may "have" pneumonia, he or she "is" demented. How does and how should this change in identity affect decision making for the patient? How can the dignity of the patient be preserved when institutional caregivers know the person only after the onset of disease and are unacquainted with the unique biography of the individual under their care? For the individual with dementia, how can extended care become an extended meaningful life?

The majority of elderly people, as well as many of those in institutions, are competent, even if physically infirm. How can their autonomy, dignity, and quality of life be preserved? These ethical dilemmas must be given careful consideration as the elderly population grows, as more and more elderly individuals require institutional care, and as the resources available to care for them come steadily under greater pressure.

Agenda for Geriatric Neuropsychiatry

Patient Care

The growth of geriatric neuropsychiatry can improve the quality of patient care. Appropriate treatment of neuropsychiatric illness depends on accurate diagnosis, and diagnosis in elderly patients depends on a comprehensive understanding of brain-behavior relationships. In addition, diagnosis increasingly demands familiarity with neuroimaging, electrophysiology, and a variety of laboratory tests; geriatric neuropsychiatry incorporates data from these techniques into diagnostic formulations. New medications have been developed and are able to effectively ameliorate many behavioral disturbances and improve the quality of life of elderly patients with brain disorders. However, many of these agents have potentially serious side effects, and practitioners in this area must be familiar with both the effects and the adverse consequences of these new agents.

Education

The growth of the elderly population demands greater availability of practitioners of geriatric neuropsychiatry (Benjamin et al. 1995; Cummings and Hegarty 1994; Cummings et al. 1998). Because this field incorporates information from psychiatry, neurology, geriatrics, and neuroscience, training opportunities must be developed and expanded.

Research

Geriatric neuropsychiatry is a nascent field (Cummings et al. 1998). Its research agenda must include the application of advanced technologies to diagnosis in the elderly population: the usefulness of ^{18}fluoro-2-deoxyglucose PET, PiB, SPECT, and magnetic resonance spectroscopy has yet to be defined in detail. Complex behavioral changes, such as delusions and mood disorders, are unlikely to correspond to single specific lesions, and the shared characteristics of lesions and conditions producing similar syndromes demand investigation. New treatments are continuously emerging and must be integrated into clinical practice to provide the greatest benefit for elderly patients. The effects, side effects, and drug interactions of these new agents must be discovered. Effective nonpharmacological interventions must also be identified and perfected. Molecular underpinnings of aging must be identified and explored. The appropriate ethical responses of society to severe illness in elderly individuals must be carefully considered. Finally, a means of bridging the gap between neuroscience and human experience must be found. Geriatric neuropsychiatry will succeed to the extent that advances in the neurosciences can be related to the suffering of elderly people and its relief. We hold the conviction that research advances will translate directly into improved care and a higher quality of life for elderly individuals.

Key Points

- Brain diseases are common in the elderly.
- Brain disease often produces behavioral disturbances.
- Geriatric neuropsychiatry is a key clinical and research area addressing behavioral changes due to brain disorders in the elderly.
- Geriatric neuropsychiatry draws on information from a wide range of clinical and scientific disciplines.

- Imaging, genetics, and molecular biology have been particularly instrumental in advancing understanding of geriatric neuropsychiatric illnesses.
- Treatments are emerging that will revolutionize the care of the elderly with neuropsychiatric disorders.

References

Aizenstein HJ, Nebes RD, Saxton JA, et al: Frequent amyloid deposition without significant cognitive impairment among the elderly. Arch Neurol 65:1509–1517, 2008

Alzheimer's Study Group: A National Alzheimer's Strategic Plan: The Report of the Alzheimer's Study Group. Washington, DC, 2009. Available at: http://www.alz.org/documents/national/report_ASG_alzplan.pdf. Accessed November 1, 2010.

Anderson SW, Barrash J, Bechara A, et al: Impairments of emotion and real-world complex behavior following childhood- or adult-onset damage to ventromedial prefrontal cortex. J Int Neuropsychol Soc 12:224–235, 2006

Apostolova LG, Thompson PM: Brain mapping as a tool to study neurodegeneration. Neurotherapeutics 4:387–400, 2007

Assaf Y, Pasternak O: Diffusion tensor imaging (DTI)–based white matter mapping in brain research: a review. J Mol Neurosci 34:51–61, 2008

Beckson M, Cummings JL: Neuropsychiatric aspects of stroke. Int J Psychiatry Med 21:1–15, 1991

Beers MH: Medication use in the elderly, in Practice of Geriatrics. Edited by Calkins E, Ford AB, Katz PR. Philadelphia, WB Saunders, 1992, pp 33–49

Benjamin S, Cummings JL, Duffy JD, et al: Pathways to neuropsychiatry. J Neuropsychiatry Clin Neurosci 7:96–101, 1995

Coffey CE: Structural brain abnormalities in the depressed elderly, in Brain Imaging in Affective Disorders. Edited by Hauser P. Washington, DC, American Psychiatric Press, 1991, pp 89–111

Coffey CE: Brain morphology in primary mood disorders: implications for ECT. Psychiatr Ann 26:713–716, 1996

Coffey CE, Wilkinson WE, Weiner RD, et al: Quantitative cerebral anatomy in depression. Arch Gen Psychiatry 50:7–16, 1993

Cole SL, Vassar R: The role of amyloid precursor protein processing by BACE1, the beta-secretase, in Alzheimer disease pathophysiology. J Biol Chem 283:29621–29625, 2008

Cummings JL: Clinical Neuropsychiatry. Boston, MA, Allyn & Bacon, 1985

Cummings JL: Depression and Parkinson's disease: a review. Am J Psychiatry 149:443–454, 1992a

Cummings JL: Psychosis in neurologic disease: neurobiology and pathogenesis. Neuropsychiatry Neuropsychol Behav Neurol 5:144–150, 1992b

Cummings JL: Frontal-subcortical circuits and human behavior. Arch Neurol 50:873–880, 1993

Cummings JL: Principles of neuropsychiatry: towards a neuropsychiatric epistemology. Neurocase 5:181–188, 1999

Cummings JL: Challenges to demonstrating disease-modifying effects in Alzheimer's disease clinical trials. Alzheimers Dement 2:263–271, 2006

Cummings JL, Benson DF: Dementia: A Clinical Approach, 2nd Edition. Boston, MA, Butterworths, 1992

Cummings JL, Hegarty A: Neurology, psychiatry, and neuropsychiatry. Neurology 44:209–213, 1994

Cummings JL, Coffey CE, Duffy J, et al: The clinician-scientist in neuropsychiatry: a position statement from the Committee on Research of the American Neuropsychiatric Association. J Neuropsychiatry Clin Neurosci 10:1–9, 1998

Daban C, Martinez-Aran A, Cruz N, et al: Safety and efficacy of vagus nerve stimulation in treatment-resistant depression: a systematic review. J Affect Disord 110:1–15, 2008

Dickstein DL, Kabaso D, Rocher AB, et al: Changes in the structural complexity of the aged brain. Aging Cell 6:275–284, 2007

Dreher JC, Meyer-Lindenberg A, Kohn P, et al: Age-related changes in midbrain dopaminergic regulation of the human reward system. Proc Natl Acad Sci U S A 105:15106–15111, 2008

Dresser RH: Anatomy revisited: the limits of anticipatory choices, in Dementia and Aging: Ethics, Values, and Policy Choices. Edited by Binsock RH, Post SG, Whitehouse PJ. Baltimore, MD, Johns Hopkins University Press, 1992, pp 71–85

Drevets WC: Orbitofrontal cortex function and structure in depression. Ann N Y Acad Sci 1121:499–527, 2007

Drzezga A: Basic pathologies of neurodegenerative dementias and their relevance for state-of-the-art molecular imaging studies. Eur J Nucl Med Mol Imaging 35:S4–S11, 2008

Duffy JD, Coffey CE: The neurobiology of depression, in Contemporary Behavioral Neurology. Edited by Trimble MR, Cummings JL. Boston, MA, Butterworth-Heinemann, 1997, pp 275–288

Erlangsen A, Bille-Brahe U, Jeune B: Differences in suicide between the old and the oldest old. J Gerontol B Psychol Sci Soc Sci 58:S314–S322, 2003

Evans KC, Simon NM, Dougherty DD, et al: A PET study of tiagabine treatment implicates ventral medial prefrontal cortex in generalized social anxiety disorder. Neuropsychopharmacology 34:390–398, 2009

Fasano M, Lopiano L: Alpha-synuclein and Parkinson's disease: a proteomic view. Expert Rev Proteomics 5:239–248, 2008

Figiel GS, Coffey CE, Djang WT, et al: Brain magnetic resonance imaging findings in ECT-induced delirium. J Neuropsychiatry Clin Neurosci 2:53–58, 1990

Finch CE: Longevity, Senescence, and the Genome. Chicago: University of Chicago Press, 1990

Fontaine R, Breton G, Dery R, et al: Temporal lobe abnormalities in panic disorder: an MRI study. Biol Psychiatry 27:304–310, 1990

Forti EM, Johnson JA, Graber DR: Aging in America: challenges and strategies for health care delivery. J Health Hum Serv Adm 23: 203–213, 2000

Fratiglioni L, Grut M, Forsell Y, et al: Prevalence of Alzheimer's disease and other dementias in an elderly urban population: relationship with age, sex, and education. Neurology 41:1886–1892, 1991

Fregni F, Marcolin MA, Myczkowski M, et al: Predictors of antidepressant response in clinical trials of transcranial magnetic stimulation. Int J Neuropsychopharmacol 9:641–654, 2006

Fujimoto T, Takeuchi K, Matsumoto T, et al: Metabolic changes in the brain of patients with late-onset major depression. Psychiatry Res 164:48–57, 2008

Galluzzi S, Beltramello A, Filippi M, et al: Aging. Neurol Sci 29:S296–S300, 2008

Geda YE, Roberts RO, Knopman DS, et al: Prevalence of neuropsychiatric symptoms in mild cognitive impairment and normal cognitive aging: population-based study. Arch Gen Psychiatry 65:1193–1198, 2008

Hajjar ER, Cafiero AC, Hanlon JT: Polypharmacy in elderly patients. Am J Geriatr Pharmacother 5:345–351, 2007

Herrmann LL, Le Masurier M, Ebmeier KP: White matter hyperintensities in late life depression: a systematic review. J Neurol Neurosurg Psychiatry 79:619–624, 2008

Hilmer SN: ADME-tox issues for the elderly. Expert Opin Drug Metab Toxicol 4:1321–1331, 2008

Ikonomovic MD, Klunk WE, Abrahamson EE, et al: Post-mortem correlates of in vivo PiB-PET amyloid imaging in a typical case of Alzheimer's disease. Brain 131:1630–1645, 2008

Kincannon CL, He W, West LA: Demography of aging in China and the United States and the economic well-being of their older populations. J Cross Cult Gerontol 20:243–255, 2005

Klunk WE, Engler H, Nordberg A, et al: Imaging brain amyloid in Alzheimer's disease with Pittsburgh Compound-B. Ann Neurol 55:306–319, 2004

Klunk WE, Mathis CA, Price JC, et al: Two-year follow-up of amyloid deposition in patients with Alzheimer's disease. Brain 129:2805–2807, 2006

Lee TS, Ng BY, Lee WL: Neuropsychiatry—an emerging field. Ann Acad Med Singapore 37:601–605, 2008

Lishman WA: What is neuropsychiatry? J Neurol Neurosurg Psychiatry 55:983–985, 1992

Martin JB: The integration of neurology, psychiatry, and neuroscience in the 21st century. Am J Psychiatry 159:695–704, 2002

Masand PS, Gupta S: Long-acting injectable antipsychotics in the elderly: guidelines for effective use. Drugs Aging 20:1099–1110, 2003

Mayeux R, Denaro J, Hemenegildo N, et al: A population-based investigation of Parkinson's disease with and without dementia. Arch Neurol 49:492–497, 1992

Mayou R, Hawton K, Feldman E, et al: Psychiatric problems among medical admissions. Int J Psychiatry Med 21:71–84, 1991

McNabney MK, Samus QM, Lyketsos CG, et al: The spectrum of medical illness and medication use among residents of assisted living facilities in central Maryland. J Am Med Dir Assoc 9:558–564, 2008

Medicare Payment Advisory Commission: Report to the Congress: Impact of Resident Caps on the Supply of Geriatricians. Washington, DC, Medicare Payment Advisory Commission, 2003. Available at: http://www.medpac.gov/publications/congressional_reports/nov2003_Gtricians.pdf. Accessed April 26, 2010.

Mega MS, Cummings JL, Salloway S, et al: The limbic system: an anatomic, phylogenic, and clinical perspective. J Neuropsychiatry Clin Neurosci 9:315–330, 1996

Modell JG, Mountz JM, Beresford TP: Basal ganglia/limbic striatal and thalamocortical involvement in craving and loss of control in alcoholism. J Neuropsychiatry Clin Neurosci 2:123–144, 1990

Moody RH: A critical view of ethical dilemmas in dementia, in Dementia and Aging: Ethics, Values, and Policy Choices. Edited by Binsock RH, Post SG, Whitehouse PJ. Baltimore, MD, Johns Hopkins University Press, 1992, pp 86–100

Norris DG: Principles of magnetic resonance assessment of brain function. J Magn Reson Imaging 23:794–807, 2006

Northoff G: Neuropsychiatry: an old discipline in a new gestalt bridging biological psychiatry, neuropsychology, and cognitive neurology. Eur Arch Psychiatry Clin Neurosci 258:226–238, 2008

Nys GM, van Zandvoort MJ, de Kort PL, et al: Cognitive disorders in acute stroke: prevalence and clinical determinants. Cerebrovasc Dis 23:408–416, 2007

Perucca E: Clinical pharmacokinetics of new-generation antiepileptic drugs at the extremes of age. Clin Pharmacokinet 45:351–363, 2006

Pimlott SL, Ebmeier KP: SPECT imaging in dementia. Br J Radiol 80:S153–S159, 2007

Prichard JW, Cummings JL: The insistent call from functional MRI. Neurology 48:797–800, 1997

Pugliatti M, Sobocki P, Beghi E, et al: Cost of disorders of the brain in Italy. Neurol Sci 29:99–107, 2008

Qato DM, Alexander GC, Conti RM, et al: Use of prescription and over-the-counter medications and dietary supplements among older adults in the United States. JAMA 300:2867–2878, 2008

Rice DP, Fineman N: Economic implications of increased longevity in the United States. Annu Rev Public Health 25:457–473, 2004

Robinson RG, Starkstein SE: Current research in affective disorders following stroke. J Neuropsychiatry Clin Neurosci 2:1–14, 1990

Salzman C, Jeste DV, Meyer RE, et al: Elderly patients with dementia-related symptoms of severe agitation and aggression: consensus statement on treatment options, clinical trials methodology, and policy. J Clin Psychiatry 69:889–898, 2008

Saravay SM, Steinberg MD, Weinschel B, et al: Psychological comorbidity and length of stay in the general hospital. Am J Psychiatry 148:324–329, 1991

Saxena S, Brody AL, Maidment KM, et al: Cerebral glucose metabolism in obsessive-compulsive hoarding. Am J Psychiatry 161: 1038–1048, 2004

Serrano F, Klann E: Reactive oxygen species and synaptic plasticity in the aging hippocampus. Ageing Res Rev 3:431–443, 2004

Shah AS: The relationship between suicide rates and age: an analysis of multinational data from the World Health Organization. Int Psychogeriatr 19:1141–1152, 2007

Silver JM: Behavioral neurology and neuropsychiatry is a subspecialty. J Neuropsychiatry Clin Neurosci 18:146–148, 2006

Small GW, Kepe V, Ercoli LM, et al: PET of brain amyloid and tau in mild cognitive impairment. N Engl J Med 355:2652–2663, 2006

Soares DP, Law M: Magnetic resonance spectroscopy of the brain: review of metabolites and clinical applications. Clin Radiol 64:12–21, 2009

Stadtman ER: Protein oxidation and aging. Science 257:1220–1224, 1992

Taylor WD, Kuchibhatla M, Payne ME, et al: Frontal white matter anisotropy and antidepressant remission in late-life depression. PLoS One 3:e3267, 2008

Teng E, Lu PH, Cummings JL: Neuropsychiatric symptoms are associated with progression from mild cognitive impairment to Alzheimer's disease. Dement Geriatr Cogn Disord 24:253–259, 2007

Trimble MR: Neuropsychiatry or behavioral neurology. Neuropsychiatry Neuropsychol Behav Neurol 6:60–69, 1993

Valotassiou V, Wozniak G, Sifakis N, et al: Radiopharmaceuticals in neurological and psychiatric disorders. Curr Clin Pharmacol 3:99–107, 2008

Van Gorp WG, Mahler M: Subcortical features of normal aging, in Subcortical Dementia. Edited by Cummings JL. New York, Oxford University Press, 1990, pp 231–250

Volkow ND, Hitzemann R, Wang GJ, et al: Decreased brain metabolism in neurologically intact healthy alcoholics. Am J Psychiatry 149:1016–1022, 1992

Webster J, Grossberg GT: Late-life onset of psychotic symptoms. Am J Geriatr Psychiatry 6:196–202, 1998

Wichmann T, Delong MR: Deep brain stimulation for neurologic and neuropsychiatric disorders. Neuron 52:197–204, 2006

Yatham LN, Kennedy SH, O'Donovan C, et al: Canadian Network for Mood and Anxiety Treatments (CANMAT) guidelines for the management of patients with bipolar disorder: consensus and controversies. Bipolar Disord 7:5–69, 2005

Yudofsky SC, Hales RE: The reemergence of neuropsychiatry: definition and direction. J Neuropsychiatry Clin Neurosci 1:1–6, 1989a

Yudofsky SC, Hales RE: When patients ask...what is neuropsychiatry? J Neuropsychiatry Clin Neurosci 1:362–365, 1989b

Zaidel DW, Esiri MM, Harrison PJ: Size, shape, and orientation of neurons in the left and right hippocampus: investigation of normal asymmetries and alterations in schizophrenia. Am J Psychiatry 154:812–818, 1997

Ziegler-Graham K, Brookmeyer R, Johnson E, et al: Worldwide variation in the doubling time of Alzheimer's disease incidence rates. Alzheimers Dement 4:316–323, 2008

2

Neurobiology of Aging

Richard E. Powers, M.D.

The developmental stages of the normal human central nervous system (CNS) can be broadly divided into immaturity, maturity, and senescence. The definition of *normal senescent brain change* implies a discernible boundary between 1) stable maturity and expected age-related alterations and 2) disease. *Neurodegeneration* implies a pathological process that is distinct from senescent changes (Brayne 2007). The morphological substrates of human brain aging and neurodegeneration may be impacted by many variables, including an individual's age, gender, premorbid intellectual function, chronic health conditions, and so forth (Swerdlow 2007). Studies in nonhuman models suggest that life span can be manipulated by genetic, nutritional, and pharmacological interventions (Vijg and Campisi 2008).

Many studies contrast brains from young versus old subjects based on chronology versus neurobiology. *Old* is often defined by the life expectancy of the species, but this feature may depend on disease and environmental factors rather than biological brain aging. In this chapter, postadolescent maturity is divided into broad age groups to reflect a broad consensus of the neuropathological and neurobiological literature (Coleman 2004). The groupings account for cognitive function that plateaus between ages 20 and 30 years in humans and then exhibits a slow decline (Finch 2009; Salthouse 2009).

Brain aging can be defined at the macroscopic, microscopic, or molecular levels. The three major microscopic constituents of the human brain are neurons, glia, and blood vessels. Each constituent exhibits a heterochronological age-related developmental timetable in which neuronal development and remodeling occur up to adolescence, whereas white matter maturation extends into the fourth decade of life (Bartzokis 2004). Other mammals, including most nonhuman primates, do not exhibit this type of prolonged, dyssynchronous brain development during either immaturity or senescence, thus limiting the application of nonhuman animal models of aging or age-related disease to the human neurodegenerative disorders. Selected populations of neurons and glia retain the capacity for regeneration or plasticity in the mature adult human brain, further complicating the distinction between normal and disease.

Neurons, glia, and blood vessels exhibit age-related changes that are unique to the cell line, location within the brain, and cellular function. Some neurodegenerative diseases may preferentially affect neuronal and glial constituents (e.g., manifesting in senile plaques and neurofibrillary degeneration) in regions that mature later in life, including the frontal and temporal lobes, whereas other brain regions that mature early in development, such as the primary motor and primary sensory cortices, appear relatively resistant to such damage. Defining the line between normal aging and age-related disease must be interpreted in the context of normal human neurodevelopment, microscopic constituents of the brain, selective vulnerability of specific brain regions to age-related changes, and the function and synaptic connectivity of involved areas. The technical method of measurement, such as brain imaging versus postmortem examination, may yield conflicting data. The large number of potentially confounding variables in human brain development and aging may explain the wide subject-to-subject variation of age-related pathology seen in human senescence, as well as the limited applicability of nonhuman models of neurodegeneration to human diseases (Kelly et al. 2006).

The human brain reaches full maturity in the second or third decade of life, and senescent microscopic neuropathological alterations may become apparent after age 40. Each human brain has a unique mixture of age-related alterations that vary according to the type, location, and severity of the pathology. The rates of progression of age-related changes can range from linear to parabolic; however, the aging process is progressive in most instances. Genetic and environmental influences on the neurobiology of brain aging may begin in utero, and age-related pathology such as vascular disease may begin to appear during adolescence.

Neuroscientists do not know whether human brain aging follows Gompertz's law, which states that mortality rates increase exponentially with age. Newer theories suggest that death rates may level off for the oldest old (Barinaga 1992). Biodemographic longevity studies suggest deceleration of mortality rates after age 80 (Vaupel et al. 1998). Studies in centenarians suggest that these individuals may possess a unique mixture of genetic and environmental strengths that allows them to survive past age 90 (Perls et al. 2002).

Scientists have studied those individuals with extraordinary longevity, especially centenarians, to identify unique features that might provide insight into aging. Marked human longevity is not limited to the twentieth century: Titian lived to 90 and Michelangelo to 91, and the Greek philosopher Sophocles lived to past 90 (Perls et al. 2002). Centenarians are rare in the general population, occurring at 10–20 per 100,000; however, certain populations have extraordinary longevity—for example, the centenarian population in Okinawa is 40–50 per 100,000 (Willcox et al. 2006). At least 20% of centenarians are cognitively intact, and in one study about 90% were functioning independently at age 90 (Hitt et al. 1999). The oldest documented person, Madame Jeanne Calment, died at age 122 in 1999. Siblings of centenarians live longer than the general populations, with female siblings having a 3.6-fold and male siblings a 3.4-fold improved likelihood of living to age 65 compared with the general population. Compared with age-matched comparison groups, the offspring of long-lived parents have significantly reduced prevalence of hypertension, diabetes, and stroke.

In this chapter, I summarize many of the important scientific observations of gross, microscopic, and molecular changes seen in the aging human and nonhuman CNS. However, the distinction between so-called normal human brain aging and age-related disease remains controversial (Brayne 2007; Swerdlow 2007).

Theories of Aging

Aging is distinct from age-related diseases, and aging can occur either from a purposeful program that is genetically controlled or from random events. Aging occurs in most animals that reach a fixed size and often commences at the age of reproductive maturity. The increased molecular disorder that occurs during aging reduces the cellular capacity to maintain molecular fidelity or repair mechanisms (Hayflick 2007). Many theories attempt to explain the age-related degeneration that occurs across mammalian species. Aging theories can be divided into organ-based, physiological, and genomic hypotheses (Hayflick 1985). Organ-based theories hypothesize that human aging results from incremental loss of organ function driven by the immune system or alterations in endocrine function of the CNS. Physiological theories suggest that toxic levels of cellular waste products accumulate over time, resulting from free-radical damage, incapacitation of neuroprotective mechanisms, or cross-linkage of vital molecules, such as collagen, DNA, and vital proteins. Genomic theories hypothesize that aging is the consequence of somatic mutations, multiple genetic errors, or programmed cell death. Lifespan studies suggest that heritability accounts for less than 35% of variance in human survival duration. Human twin studies show that nonshared environmental factors account for over 65% of variance in survivals (Finch and Tanzi 1997).

Aging and Genomic Function

The role of genetics in aging is illustrated by life spans that vary from 1 day for mayflies to 150 years for some turtles. The human genome contains 3 billion base pairs arrayed in 24 distinct chromosomes that range in length from 50 million to 250 million base pairs. The human genome is estimated to contain 20,000–30,000 genes that code for proteins; these genes occupy only 2% of the human genome. The remaining "noncoding" regions of the human genome have structural or regulatory functions. Individual humans share many genetic similarities (99.9%), and as few as 3 million single polymorphisms may distinguish one human from another. Genetic profiles of young versus old human subjects (Table 2–1) revealed a difference in gene expression for 6.3% of sampled genes, while 91% of genes were identical (Kyng et al. 2003).

Acceleration of the human aging process occurs in several common complex genetic disorders, such as Turner's and Down's syndromes; however, accelerated aging is the primary manifestation in several disorders termed *progeria* (Table 2–2), such as Hutchinson-Gilford and Werner's syndromes (Brown 1990). Progeria is a rare syndrome occurring in 1 per 8 million individuals, and affected patients survive about 12 years from birth. Most patients (80%) die from myocardial infarctions produced by disseminated atherosclerosis. These children retain normal intellect but manifest many age-related physical changes (e.g., cataracts, balding, osteoporosis, neoplasms). Progeroid syndromes can be divided into three categories: 1) those arising from defects in genes that encode DNA repair factors, such as Werner's syndrome and Cockayne syndrome; 2) those related to genes that alter the structure or posttranslational maturation of lamin A, such as Hutchinson-Gilford progeria syndrome; and 3) syndromes of undetermined causes, such as Hallermann-Streiff syndrome (Navarro et al. 2006). Several animal models of accelerated aging involve defects of signaling between the nucleus and mitochondria. DNA is damaged by a range of insults, and DNA repair mechanisms are essential to cell survival (see Table 2–2).

Candidate genes for longevity may produce results that mimic calorie restriction (Vijg and Campisi 2008). Some can-

TABLE 2–1. Age-related changes in genetic expression attributed to human gene aging

Study	Ages (years)	*N*	Number of examined genetic loci	Tissue sampled	Significant findings from study
Kyng et al. 2003	22.5 vs. 90	15	6,912	Fibroblast cell lines	6.3% of analyzed genes changed with aging In changed genes, gene function was affected as follows: 27% DNA and RNA metabolism, 11% signal transduction, 11% stress response
Geigl et al. 2004	8–92	6	14,500	Fibroblast cell lines	2.8% of genes exhibited age-related differences, multiple alterations of genes controlling cell cycle and proliferation
Lu et al. 2004	26–106	30	11,000	CNS	4% of genes were altered in frontal lobe samples; associated with synaptic plasticity, vesicular transport, and mitochondrial function
Erraji-Benchekroun et al. 2005	13–79	39	22,000	CNS	7.5% of transcripts showed progressive age-related changes Upregulated transcripts: glia enriched, related to inflammation and cellular defenses; downregulated transcripts: neuron enriched, related to cellular communication and signaling
Berchtold et al. 2008	20–99	55	5,029	CNS	Significant sexually dimorphic changes in 6th to 7th decade; number of changes varied by brain region, gender, and age

Note. CNS=central nervous system (i.e., aged human brain tissue).

didate genes alter insulin signaling (insulin-like growth factor 1; IGF-1), inflammatory responses, stress resistance, and cardiovascular function.

Integrity of genomic function depends on accuracy of base-pair sequences, as well as on histone content, three-dimensional molecular conformation, methylation states, and multiple other biochemical variables that affect the accuracy and speed of genetic transcription. Studies in rodents and primates suggest that aging may simultaneously alter DNA base-pair sequence, genetic repair mechanisms, messenger ribonucleic acid (mRNA) metabolism, posttranslational modification, protein biochemistry, and axonal transport.

Telomere loss may control senescence and might constitute a "mitotic clock" (Ehrenstein 1998). Telomeres are tandem, G-rich repeat sequences of noncoding DNA with lengths that depend on a range of variables, including the chromosome, the person, the individual's age, the tissue of origin, and environmental factors. Telomeric length is shortened in liver, spleen, and kidney at the rate of 29–60 base pairs per year, but neural tissue does not normally exhibit this same rate of shortening. The telomere is synthesized by the ribonucleoprotein enzyme telomerase (Fossel 1998), and this segment of amino acid repeats is located at the ends of each eukaryotic chromosome (Edo and Andres 2005). Every human chromosome must have telomeres of sufficient length to ensure replicative function. A threshold level of telomerase activity may be necessary to sustain sufficient telomere length to protect the replicative ability. Telomeric length is associated with a range of age-related chronic diseases, such as diabetes, atherosclerosis, and other vascular disease (Edo and Andres 2005). Human brain telomere length in postmitotic cells has been measured at 12.3 kilobase pairs for gray matter and 11.4 for white matter. The telomere length declines throughout life until the late 70s, but very old individuals appear to have longer lengths (Nakamura et al. 2007). Data suggest that individuals with longer baseline telomere length may survive longer than individuals with shorter length.

Other genetic theories suggest that aging results from multiple genomic errors accumulated over time. Experimental models involving animals exposed to radiation or mutagens failed to show accelerated aging (Hayflick 1985). Age-related reactivation of X-linked genes may increase the expression in females of steroid sulfatase and monoamine oxidase A (MAO-A) (Wareham et al. 1987). Age-related de-

TABLE 2–2. Human DNA repair deficiency syndromes that may cause accelerated aging or neurological disorders, based on type of molecular lesion

Type	Disease	Possible neurological disorder
DNA double-strand break repair deficiency	Ataxia Telangiectasia	Neurodegenerative disorder
DNA single-strand break repair deficiency	Spinocerebellar ataxia with axonal neuropathy	Neurodegenerative disorder
Nucleotide excision repair deficiency	Cockayne's syndrome	Progeria
DNA cross-link repair deficiency	Fanconi's anemia	Microcephaly
Helicase/exonuclease deficiency	Werner's syndrome	Progeria

Source. Katyal and McKinnon 2007.

methylation of 5-methyldeoxycitidine can also occur in aging. Aged rodent DNA shows age-dependent change of capacity for excision repair and reduction of single-strand break repair (Niedermuller et al. 1985). A variety of human diseases are associated with impaired ability to repair common forms of DNA damage, including single-strand breaks, double-strand breaks, nucleotide excision repair deficiency, DNA cross-link repair deficiency, and helicase deficiency (see Table 2–2).

Gene expression can change in the aging brain, based on gender and anatomical region (Berchtold et al. 2008; see Table 2–1). Microarray analysis of multiple cortical regions can detect changes that begin in adulthood and may become more prominent in the sixth to seventh decades of life. A pattern of sexually dimorphic genetic expression occurs for both upregulation and downregulation in multiple cortical regions. Males show up to three times more gene changes than females with aging. Males exhibit changes in the sixth decade, whereas females demonstrate changes later in life. About two-thirds of male genes altered during aging are downregulated, in contrast to only one-half of female genes. Genes that alter cellular metabolism, immune response, synaptic plasticity, and vesicular transport are heavily represented in chromosomes altered during aging (Berchtold et al. 2008; Erraji-Benchekroun et al. 2005).

Mitochondria are double-membrane-bound, tubular-shaped cellular organelles that perform aerobic respiration utilizing the Krebs cycle, glycolysis, and the electron transport chain. These tubular organelles, which may have evolved from free-standing organisms, routinely cycle through fission or fusion with other mitochondria, or the organelle is recycled within the cell. Each human neuron contains hundreds of mitochondria with multiple copies of mitochondrial DNA (mtDNA). Human mitochondrial DNA spans 16,500 base pairs and contains 37 genes. The mitochondrial genome codes for 13 polypeptides that are critical to the respiratory chain, as well as two ribosomal RNAs (rRNAs) and 22 transfer RNAs (tRNAs) that are essential for protein synthesis. In the mid-30s, many human mtDNA mutations, including point mutations, major deletions, and duplications, begin to accumulate (Lee and Wei 2007). Defective repair mechanisms for mtDNA may also contribute to neuronal dysfunction or apoptosis (Katyal and McKinnon 2008). Nongenomic mtDNA lacks intrinsic repair mechanisms. Specific biomarkers for oxidative damage are increased 10-fold in human mtDNA over nuclear DNA and 15-fold in neuronal DNA from individuals over age 70. Although mtDNA exhibits high rates of age-related defects, mtDNA damage is not clearly linked to neuronal death (Tomei and Umansky 1998). The quantity of mutated mtDNA may be small in comparison to the size of available genetic material. Mitochondrial mutations may need to exceed 50%–80% of the mitochondrial genomic pool for clinical expression (Johnson et al. 1999). The significance of cumulative age-related oxidative damage to DNA remains unclear (Johnson et al. 1999), although many investigators believe these changes contribute to oxidative burden and neurodegeneration (Droge and Schipper 2007; Lee and Wei 2007).

Multiple families of genes are implicated in age-associated mitochondrial molecular pathology or neurodegeneration, including those for the *Sortilin receptor*, which is a "traffic-cop" protein that may move β-amyloid through the endocytic pathway, and a class of proteins termed *Sirtuins protein deacetylases*, which may control transcriptional repression. The complex mitochondrial biology produces a myriad of potential genes and transcription products that may be altered in aging and disease (Guarente 2009).

The mammalian RNA repertoire is not drastically altered with aging; however, selected RNAs may be increased or decreased (Finch and Morgan 1990). For instance, the abundance of pro-opiomelanocortin mRNA decreases by 30% in aging rodents, whereas luteinizing hormone–releasing hormone production remains constant (Finch and Morgan 1990). Total RNA content and poly(A) RNA do not significantly change in aging rodent or primate brain, but selected human RNA, such as tachykinin message in hypothalamus, is increased (Rance and Young 1991). Reductions of nuclear or nucleolar size in the same neurons of elderly humans suggest diminished gene or RNA activity. Selected human neuronal populations have reductions in nuclear and nucleolar volumes that reflect perikaryal atrophy. Nucleolar shrinkage may result from decreased transcription of rRNA cistrons and diminished assembly of ribosomes. Neuron populations that are damaged by neurofibrillary tangles (NFTs) have reduced RNA metabolism as well (Doebler et al. 1987).

Studies in aging rodents show slowing of protein synthesis and axonal transport. Increased amounts of conformationally altered, inactive enzymes accumulate in aging rodents (Finch and Morgan 1990). Some proteins are produced simultaneously by astrocytes and neurons. The interpretation of neuronal protein content is complicated by age- or disease-related increases in the numbers of astrocytes (Frederickson 1992). For example, stability in the number of adrenergic receptors in aging rodents may reflect diminished numbers of neuronal receptors counterbalanced by increased numbers of astrocytes with this molecule. The increased number of astrocytes in aging human brain may obscure similar alterations (Finch and Morgan 1990).

Age-related changes in posttranslational modification of proteins can produce accumulations of advanced glycation end products in pyramidal neurons. The production of these complex molecules is increased by oxidative stress and inhibited by free-radical scavengers or thiol antioxidants (Munch et al. 1997, 1998). This family of glycosylated proteins may contribute to free-radical damage, amyloid deposition, and neurofibrillary degeneration (Munch et al. 1997).

Most research shows that genomic function, transcription, translation, and posttranslational modification of some proteins may be altered in human brain aging. Disease models of accelerated aging, such as progeria, produce complex changes, including lethal vascular disease. Age-related alterations of both mitochondrial and eukaryotic DNA or protein synthesis are likely to promote aging, age-related diseases, and neurodegeneration.

Aging and Oxidative Stress

Oxidative stress results from an imbalance between the production and detoxification of reactive oxygen species and may contribute to aging and neurodegenerative diseases (Perry et al. 2007). Research on reactive oxygen species in mammalian systems is complicated by the instability of these molecules. These molecules can damage both proteins and lipids. Oxidative damage can be produced by extrametabolic insults, such as pollution and radiation, or intrinsic metabolic sources. Approximately 2%–3% of oxygen consumed by cells will be reduced to oxygen free radicals. Electron transport systems within mitochondrial membranes produce oxygen-derived superoxide in response to free radicals as well as multiple other toxic products, such as hydrogen peroxide and hydroxyl radicals. The levels of highly unstable reactive oxygen species in human brain are difficult to measure; however, scientists can measure stable end products of reactive oxygen species' interactions, including isoprostanes, neuroprostanes, and adrenoprostanes.

Nitric oxide (NO) is another reactive oxygen species that plays an active role in neurodevelopment, neural transmission, and gene expression. NO is a small, easily diffusible free radical controlled by NO synthetase that can produce neurotoxicity by a variety of mechanisms (Perry et al. 2007). Damage produced by reactive oxygen species is mediated by a variety of mechanisms, including lipid peroxidation, downregulation of essential protein mediators such as Sirtuins, disruption of insulin signaling, and multiple other pathways (Anekonda and Reddy 2006).

Mammalian aging is often described in the rodent models, where metabolic rates may influence the rate of aging. A 40% reduction of caloric intake will extend rodents' life span by 40%–60%. Diminished feeding of rodents will slow aging and prolong reproductive life span while increasing neurogenesis. Such dietary restriction may lower oxidative stress by slowing metabolism, and similar nutritional limitations may contribute to exceptional longevity in human populations such as the Okinawans. Studies in humans suggest that specific markers for accelerated aging are reduced after 6 months of calorie restrictions in overweight persons (Heilbronn et al. 2006). Elevated body mass index in conjunction with central obesity in humans is a significant risk factor for accelerated brain aging and dementia (Whitmer et al. 2008). Insulin resistance produced by obesity contributes to adverse effects on brain and cognition in older adults. The gene encoding insulin-degrading enzyme may influence human life span, and this enzyme is linked to amyloid metabolism. Thus, obesity and excess caloric intake may add to the oxidative load while altering other mechanisms linked to aging and neurodegeneration.

Multiple antioxidant defenses, including superoxide dismutase catalase and multiple peroxidases, remove excess superoxides and hydrogen peroxide. Glutathione, vitamin E, and ascorbic acid also function as antioxidants. Severe long-term calorie restriction is not endorsed as an antiaging intervention.

Healthy aging may require a proper balance of free-radical production and detoxification. Oxidative stress may result from increased sensitivity to free-radical damage, decreased antioxidant protection, altered calcium homeostasis, or impaired ability to repair damage.

Neuropathological Features of Normal Brain Aging Versus Age-Related Disease

The neuropathological distinctions between "normal" aging and age-related disease are frequently obscure, and conclusions drawn from human postmortem studies may differ from those drawn by investigators conducting in vivo studies such as brain imaging or neuropsychological measurements. Senile plaques, amyloid deposits, and cholinergic deficits were previously considered disease markers until studies demonstrated similar alterations in the brains of some cognitively intact elderly humans (Braak and Braak 1997).

Subtle anoxic neuronal injury can be extremely difficult to identify, and considerable ischemic damage may escape detection by standard histopathological methods (Garcia 1992). Some neuropathologists propose a continuum from normal aging through pathological aging to disease states (Dickson 1997). These unresolved clinical and pathological distinctions between normal senescent changes and age-related disease will continue until more sophisticated markers of disease are available.

Neurons, astrocytes, oligodendrocytes, microglia, and endothelial cells are the major cellular constituents of the human CNS (Figure 2–1). Each cell line may develop age-related changes, and the variable mixture of cellular pathology within each cellular population may contribute to the age-related burden in the brain. The neuropil is the woven fabric of the cortex that includes neuronal and astrocytic processes. A normal neuron has a large nucleus, prominent nucleolus, conspicuous dendrites, and straight, thin axons that are difficult to visualize in routine preparations (see Figure 2–1). Neuronal atrophy is defined by a decrease in size of the cell body (perikaryon), nucleus, and nucleolus and by retraction or loss of dendritic arborization. Senescent changes of glia and vascular tissue may contribute to neural dysfunction or neurodegenerative disorders, as well as to atrophy or death of neurons.

Structural Brain Alterations in Aging

Changes in Gross Anatomy

Based on 12 studies from 1892 to 1997, postmortem brain weights increased over the century. For example, the mean male and female brain weights in studies published in 1892 were 1,343 g and 1,239 g, respectively, for persons ages 20–30 years, but mean weights published in 1997 had increased to 1,607 g and 1,360 g, respectively, for males and females in the same age group (Svennerholm et al. 1997). For males and females, the average human brain exhibits a 36% decrease in dry solids from age 20 to age 100 (Svennerholm et al. 1994). The male brain is typically 150 g heavier than the female brain. Numerous brain imaging volumetric studies have determined brain volume changes by examining large groups of normal subjects arranged by decade or by performing serial studies on the same individuals. Cross-sectional studies (Table 2–3) demonstrate peak volumes during adolescence, followed by a slow steady decline in volume and compensatory expansion of cerebrospinal fluid (CSF).

The dura mater contains the meningeal artery and venous sinus systems that include arachnoid granulations. This fibrous covering can thicken and ossify during aging. Cortical atrophy expands the arachnoid space, increases the length of bridging veins spanning from the cerebral hemisphere to the sagittal sinus, and may account for the higher rate of subdural hematomas in elderly people (Adams and Duchen 1992).

Human postmortem brain volume peaks in the second or third decade and begins a gradual decline that is readily apparent after age 60 (Haug and Eggers 1991). The volume of the frontal lobes decreases approximately 10% with aging, and white matter is reduced 11% when brain volumes from younger subjects (20–40 years) are compared with those of elderly subjects (75–85 years). Volumetric brain imaging and postmortem brain weight studies agree that cortical volume peaks in mid-adolescence and begins a consistent decline during the third decade of life (see Table 2–3). The slope of that decline varies by population and measurement techniques, but most authors describe peak volume during adolescence when human reproductive life begins and maximum stature is achieved.

Atrophy is defined as widening of sulci and narrowing of gyri. Atrophy in frontal, parasagittal, and temporal lobes is present in both aging and Alzheimer's disease (Tomlinson et al. 1970) (Figures 2–2 and 2–3). Severe cortical atrophy is rare in individuals whose cognition is intact; however, mild to moderate ventriculomegaly is sometimes present (Blessed et al. 1968; Tomlinson et al. 1970) (see Figure 2–2). The volumes of basal ganglia and thalamus are reduced by up to 20% in aging (Murphy et al. 1992). The volume of the parieto-occipital region is found to be constant (Eggers et al. 1984) when autopsy specimens from young individuals (20–40 years) are compared with those from subjects over age 75.

Cellular Changes in Aging

The major cellular constituents of the human brain include neurons, glia, and blood vessels. The glial cell line includes astrocytes, oligodendrocytes, ependymal cells, and microglia (see Figure 2–1).

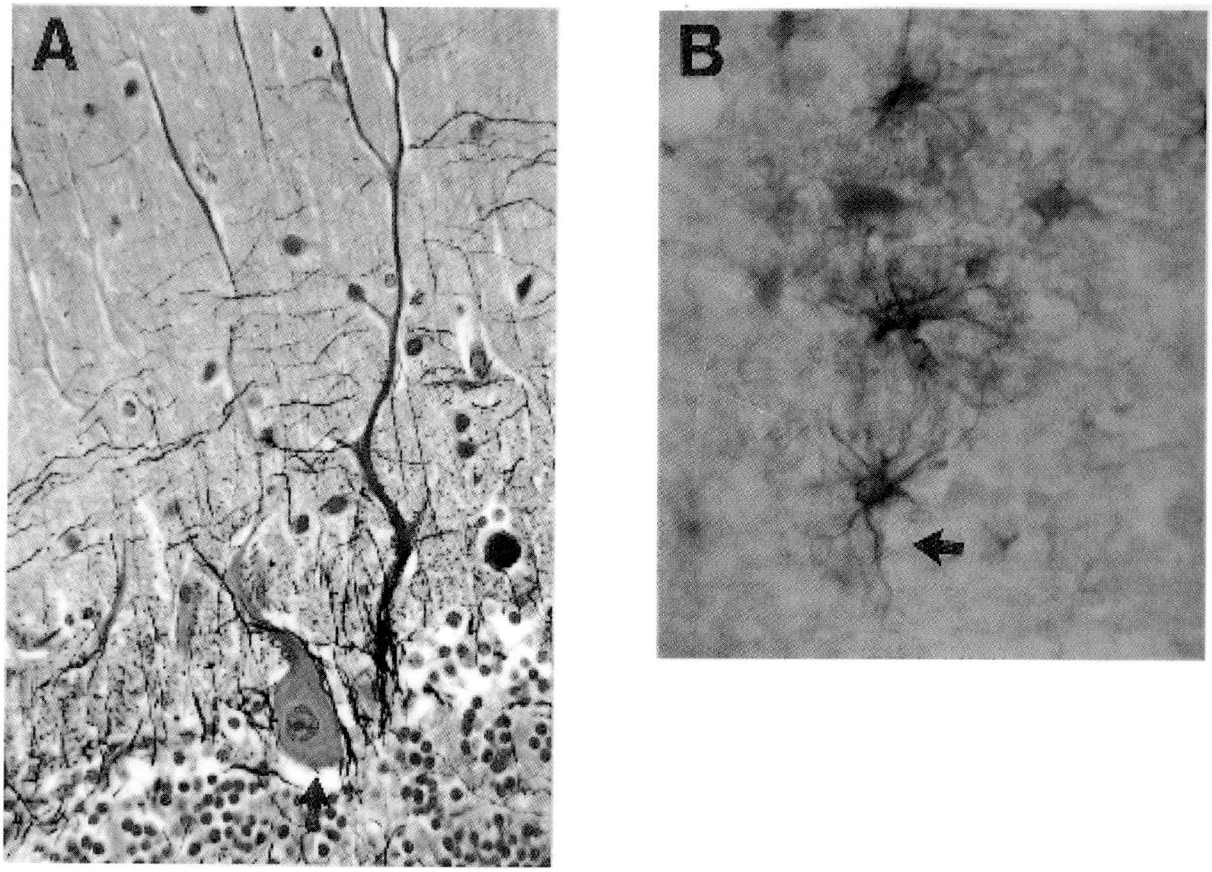

FIGURE 2–1. Normal neurons and reactive astrocytes.

Panel A: A silver preparation of human cerebellum demonstrating Purkinje cell *(arrow)* with a prominent nucleus and nucleolus. Many straight, thin axons are seen. **Panel B:** An immunocytochemical stain of reactive astrocytes using antibodies to glial fibrillary acidic protein. These astrocytes have many long, thin processes and variable amounts of cytoplasm *(arrow).*

Microscopic Neuronal Changes in Aging

A historical review of the publications that describe the effect of aging on the microscopic anatomy of human CNS neurons reveals a confusing and contradictory literature (Hof and Morrison 2004; Uylings and de Brabander 2002). Publications from 1950 to 1990 suggest that neurons, especially large-diameter neurons, are depleted from the neocortex with aging. The use of computer-assisted stereological methodologies after 1990 has produced different conclusions and suggested minimal loss of neurons in individuals through the ninth decade of life. Few quantitative studies include adequate numbers of normal human subjects over age 80 to draw firm conclusions on changes in the very old (i.e., age 85 and older) or the ultra-old (i.e., age 100 and older). The increased numbers of neurons in male versus female brains are attributed to gender differences in brain size (Pakkenberg and Gundersen 1997). Other changes, such as myelin integrity, synaptic density, and vascular permeability, may play an equally important role in age-related functional decline. An age-related shift in neuronal size hypothesized to result from atrophy of larger-diameter neurons has been discussed and disputed (Stark et al. 2007).

The cellular substrate of the progressive brain volume reduction that commences in the third decade of life is unclear (see Table 2–3). Cerebral atrophy may result from a net loss of neurons, neuronal perikaryal volume, dendrites, glia, and synapses. The reported number of neurons in the human brain ranges from 13.9 billion in both sexes (Haug and Eggers 1991) to 19 billion in females and 23 billion in males (Pakkenberg and Gundersen 1997). Stereological methods demonstrate about a 10% reduction in neuronal numbers through age 90 (Morrison and Hof 1997). The estimated loss of 9.5% of neurons with aging would result in a depletion rate of 85,000 neurons per day or one neuron per second (Pakkenberg et al. 2003). Selected populations of hippocampal and subcortical neurons are depleted in subjects over age 65. Some discrepancies may result from methodological problems, such as variations of sampling, and shrinkage artifact. Several authors (Haug and Eggers 1991;

TABLE 2–3. Cerebral gray and white matter volume alterations in magnetic resonance imaging of normal individuals from adolescence to old age

Study	Subjects	Age range (years)	Cortical volume	White matter volume
Raz et al. 1997	148	18–77	↓ 4.9% per decade prefrontal ↓ 4.3% per decade superior parietal ↓ 2.0% per decade hippocampus	Slight ↓ prefrontal white matter in older subjects
Courchesne et al. 2000	116	1.5–80	↑ volume to age 15 years ↓ 26% from age 16 to 80 years Volume at age 80 years similar to that at age 3 years ↓ 5% per decade after 15 years	↑ 74% infant to adolescent ↓ 13% over age 70 years
Bartzokis et al. 2001	70	19–76	Linear ↓ GM volume in FL and TL in adults	↑ FL to age 44 years ↑ TL to age 47 years then ↓ volume
Good et al. 2001	465	18–79	↓ volume over age 18 ↓ superior parietal, insula, frontal operculum	↓ bilateral FL, optic radiations posterior IC
Jernigan et al. 2001	78	30–99	↓ 14% cortical volume ↓ 35% hippocampal volume	↓ 26%
Ge et al. 2002	54	20–86	↓ 4.9% for older vs. younger (under 50 years) Linear decline from age 50	↑ from age 20 to 40 years ↓ over 40 years ↓ quadratic curve
Allen et al. 2005	87	22–88	Linear ↓ 9.1%–9.8% from age 30 to 70 years ↓ 11.3%–12% from age 70 to 80 years	↑ to age 50 years ↓ 21.6%–25% by age 80 years

Note. FL=frontal lobes; GM=gray matter; IC=internal capsule; TL=temporal lobe.

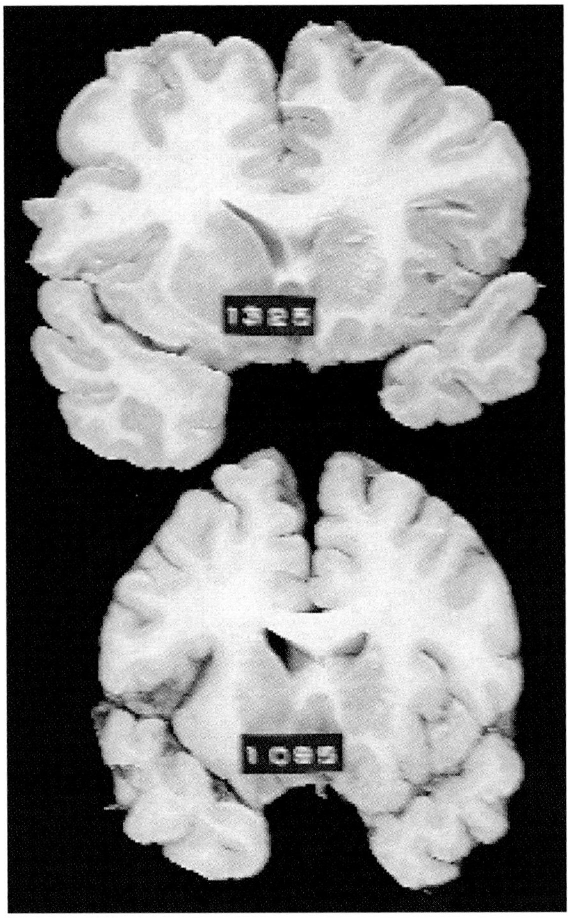

FIGURE 2–2. Normal age-related atrophy.

Coronal brain sections of frontal and temporal lobe contrast brain atrophy in an 85-year-old patient with nonspecific age-related atrophy (**bottom**) and in a 15-year-old with a brain weight of 1,325 g (**top**). Volume loss occurs in frontal, parasagittal, and temporal cortices.

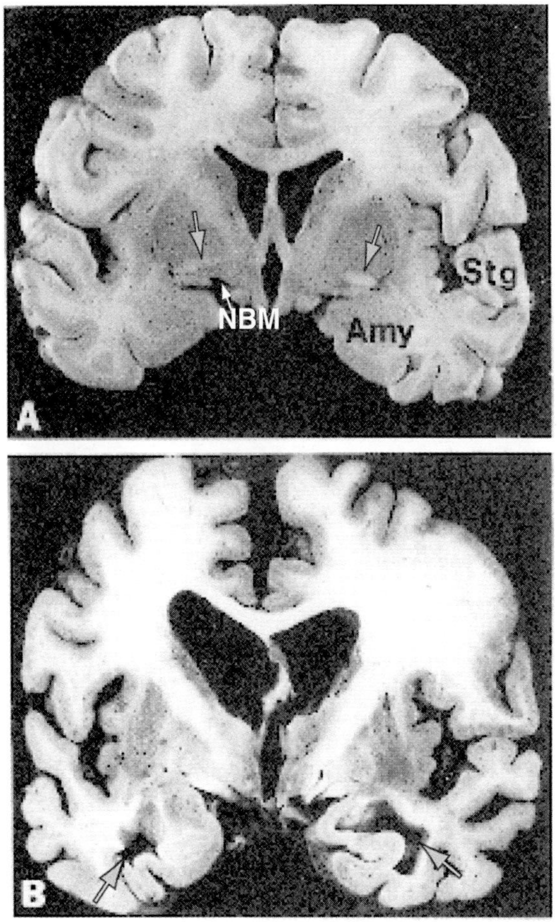

FIGURE 2–3. The coronal sections of normal (Panel A) and atrophic (Panel B) brain.

Panel A: The brain from a 67-year-old control subject with minimal atrophy and normal ventricle size. The anterior commissure is highlighted by *gray arrows,* and the nucleus basalis of Meynert (NBM) is seen immediately beneath the anterior commissure *(white arrow).* Normal-appearing amygdala (Amy) and superior temporal gyrus (Stg) are present. The third ventricle is normal in size, and hypothalamic nuclei are located immediately adjacent to the third ventricle. Histological examination of this brain showed occasional senile plaques. **Panel B:** A coronal brain section from a 70-year-old subject with Alzheimer's disease demonstrating atrophy, ventriculomegaly, and dilation of the lateral sulci. The inferior horns of the lateral ventricles *(gray arrows)* and lateral ventricles are dilated. The hippocampus, entorhinal cortex, and amygdala are reduced in volume. The third ventricle is moderately dilated. Histological examination of this brain showed high densities of senile plaques, neurofibrillary tangles, and neuronal loss (see Figure 2–5).

Haug et al. 1984) have reported stable numbers of cortical neurons with age-related reduction of neuronal perikaryal diameter and diminished cortical thickness. This neuronal atrophy begins around age 60 and may be region and layer specific. For example, in subjects over age 65, neurons in layer 3 of gyrus rectus are shrunken, but those in layer 5 remain constant (Haug et al. 1984). Neuronal atrophy is reported after age 40 in a few cortical regions, such as area 6 (Haug and Eggers 1991). Neuronal shrinkage may explain a reported net increase in the numbers of small neurons with aging (i.e., shrunken large neurons are counted with small neurons) (Finch 1993).

The average human brain is estimated to contain 12 million kilometers of dendrites and 100,000 kilometers of axons.

Each dendrite is studded by outcroppings called *dendritic spines* that range in size from 0.01 to 0.8 μm^3 and exhibit dendritic densities that range from 1 to 10 spines per micrometer (Dickstein et al. 2007). Only about 1% of neurons communicate with the external environment. Age-related dendritic changes are reported in a variety of species (Table 2–4). Dendritic atrophy begins with loss of dendritic spines, followed by alterations of horizontal branches and the ultimate loss of the dendritic shaft in selected neuronal populations. Quantitative studies using Golgi stains of cortical areas 10 and 18 from aged human brains demonstrate an 11% reduction of dendritic length but a 50% reduction in numbers of dendrite spines when compared with subjects under age 50 (Jacobs et al. 1997).

Synapses are the specialized contacts between neurons where neurotransmitter neuromodulators, trophic factors, and other molecules are physically translocated from one neuron to another. Synapses are highly dynamic structures that can rapidly form or disassemble in response to the level of electrical activity, trophic factors, and a variety of other stimuli or inhibitors. Synaptic numbers are difficult to calculate in human brain tissue because measurements are performed with electron microscopic methodologies that require well-preserved tissue with a short postmortem interval and little tissue damage, such as hypoxia, in the period before death. A wide range of synaptic sizes, shapes, and locations exist in the human brain that significantly impact the effect of transmission. The density of synapses in human cortex is projected at 1,100 million synapses per mm^3, whereas that of rats is 1,397 million. The density of synapses does not seem to differ greatly among mammals and would not explain cognitive differences (Oberheim et al. 2006). Synaptogenesis, the formation of synapses, begins in the third prenatal trimester and continues until about 2 years of age, resulting in an overproduction of synapses. Following the completion of synaptogenesis, significant pruning occurs, with about a 60% reduction in the total number of contacts in mature brains (Huttenlocher and Dabholkar 1997). Synaptic biology and development may be region specific. For example, synaptic pruning appears complete by age 12 in auditory cortex but continues into mid-adolescence in the middle frontal gyrus. The typical adult neuron has between 5,000 and 10,000 synapses of various types. In adult males, the typical number of synapses in the human brain is 164×10^{12}, which is equivalent to the number of stars in 1,400 Milky Way galaxies (Pakkenberg et al. 2003; Pelvig et al. 2003; Tang et al. 1997).

Synaptic density declines with aging in selected regions, and some studies suggest that presynaptic terminals are reduced by 20% in adults over age 60 (Masliah et al. 1993). Synaptic proteins associated with dendritic or axonal structural plasticity that control remodeling are reduced with aging (Hatanpaa et al. 1999). Brains from individuals with Alzheimer's disease have substantial synaptic loss, and tangle-bearing neurons contribute to this reduction (Callahan and Coleman 1995; Dickson et al. 1995). Senescent reduction of synaptic numbers varies by brain region. Synaptic damage may better predict functional loss than neuronal depletion in older individuals. Rodents with hippocampal learning deficits and normal numbers of hippocampal neurons (Rapp and Gallagher 1996) demonstrate that clinical deficits may be produced by synaptic loss rather than neuronal depletion. The age-related regression of synaptic density predicts synaptic numbers similar to those in patients with dementia by age 120 (Katzman 1997). Aged monkeys demonstrate age-related loss of apical dendrites (−28% to −37%) and reduction of synaptic numbers (−40% to −50%) (Dickstein et al. 2007). For instance, aged primates demonstrate a 30% loss of synapses in layers 2 and 3 of frontal cortex from age 5 to age 30 years (Peters et al. 2008a).

The role of β-amyloid in synaptic biology remains unclear. Some data suggest a toxic effect via reduction of spines and signaling (Knobloch and Mansuy 2008), whereas other research suggests that the protein may be a compensatory response to other synaptic injuries (Lee et al. 2004).

Microscopic Alterations of Glia During Aging

The human brain contains approximately 36 billion glia, of which 75% are oligodendrocytes, 19% are astrocytes, and 6% are microglial cells (Pelvig et al. 2003). The numbers of ependymal cells that line the ventricles and the choroid plexus have not been estimated. Each glial cell line has a distinct morphology, molecular biology, and function in the brain. Oligodendrocytes and vascular tissue are the major cellular constituents of white matter within the cerebral hemisphere. A population of small bipolar neurons is present in white matter that exhibits age-related histological alterations or Alzheimer-type changes (van de Nes et al. 2002).

The volume and development of white matter are anatomical features that are unique to the human brain. Human white matter develops in a heterochronological timeline, meaning that different white matter pathways mature at different speeds across the first four decades of life. Hemispheric white matter in humans accounts for about 20% more brain volume than in the closest species, the great apes. Myelin composes about 35% of dry brain weight, which is almost one-third greater than the proportional myelin content of rodent brain (Bartzokis 2004). Myelin sheath is produced and sustained by the oligodendroglial cell, the most common glial cell in the human brain. Oligodendrocytes synthesize cholesterol, which accounts for 28% of the brain's lipid weight. In human brain, beginning at age 20 years, total solids, phospholipids, cholesterol, cerebrosides, and sulfatides show a curvilinear reduction in the frontal and temporal white matter but a linear decline in the cortex. Gangliosides increase in frontal lobe until age 50, when they become stable and do not decline until

TABLE 2–4. Overview of age-related dendritic changes in various species

Length	Human	Primate	Dogs	Mice
Arbors	↓ (9%–11%)	↓	↓	↓
Spines	↓ (50%)	↓ (25%)	↓	↓
Synapses	↓	↓ (40%–50%)	NR	↓

Note. NR=not reported; ↓=decreased number or density.
Source. Dickstein et al. 2007.

age 70 years (Svennerholm et al. 1997). The membrane lipid data seem to parallel brain imaging data that depict steady decline of cortical volume after adolescence but a complicated quadratic trajectory for white matter with decline after age 50.

Myelin is an essential component to saltatory conduction along axons, and this form of action potential propagation can increase speed by 10-fold compared to unmyelinated fibers while reducing the refractory period. Saltatory conduction is essential to integration of information through the integrated neural networks of the cerebral cortex. Myelinated axons are more energy efficient and therefore reduce oxidative load for the neuron. Conduction delays or temporal dispersion of impulses caused by damage to myelin from ischemia or inflammation may reduce synchronization of impulses from dispersed systems that mediate tasks such as retrieval of information or management of executive function. Numerous fiber pathways in the human frontal and temporal lobes possess the thinnest myelin sheath because they are the last to myelinate during adolescence and early adulthood. For example, motor fibers from the precentral gyrus and sensory fibers from the visual cortex are thickly myelinated with a single oligodendrocyte ensheathing a single axon, whereas late-developing neurons, such as those in the frontal lobe, are ensheathed by oligodendrocytes that produce a thin myelin covering for up to 50 axons. Cortical motor fibers are myelinated early in the immature brain, whereas fibers from the prefrontal cortex myelinate in the fourth decade of life. In the corpus callosum, 20%–30% of fibers in the genu, compared with 7% of fibers in the splenium, are unmyelinated (Bartzokis 2004).

Some oligodendrocytes retain the ability to regenerate into later life (Zhang et al. 1999). The precise location and biology of these oligodendroglial stem cells is undetermined in the human brain. Oligodendrocytes contain over half the brain iron in association with myelin. Iron is typically stored on the protein ferritin; however, injury to the oligodendrocyte by conditions such as ischemia can release the iron from the cellular compartment and enhance toxicity of the microenvironment.

Although the age-related loss of neurons varies according to brain region, the age-related loss of white matter appears more diffuse (see Table 2–3). Several types of histopathology can be detected in white matter, including loss of myelin sheath, loss of axons, damage to existing myelin, and inflammation within the white matter (Bartzokis 2004; Piguet et al. 2009). Age-related reduction of white matter can be detected with standard magnetic resonance imaging (MRI) as well as reduction of fractional anisotropy. Several investigators have described an age-related decline in white matter ranging from 15% to 45% of total volume, with a decrease of about 10% per decade in older individuals, based on in vivo imaging (Tang et al. 1997). The age-to-volume curve in humans is parabolic, with the peak volume in the fourth decade.

Autopsy studies revealed an 11% reduction in total white matter volume in elderly subjects (Haug and Eggers 1991). Stereological methods defined a 15% age-related reduction in white matter and a 17% reduction in total volume of myelinated fibers, although individual variations were so great that these alterations were not statistically significant (Tang et al. 1997). The estimated total length of myelinated fibers in white matter was 118,000 kilometers in young versus 86,000 kilometers in old subjects. The 27% loss of myelinated fibers may explain diminished white matter volume (Tang et al. 1997). Other postmortem studies demonstrated age-related loss of white matter volume up to 28% (Pakkenberg and Gundersen 1997; Stark et al. 2007), with estimates of white matter loss of 2 mL per year over age 60 (Double et al. 1996).

Studies of occipital cortex from humans ranging in age from 30 through 90 years revealed a linear, age-dependent myelin loss in the stripe of Gennari (Lintl and Braak 1983). The optic nerve loses more than 5,600 axons per year (Lintl and Braak 1983) from childhood through senescence. Morphological data on white matter are limited by methodological problems with measuring the volume of myelin or packing densities of axis cylinders in postmortem material. Studies in aging monkeys demonstrated that some oligodendrocytes develop bulbous inclusions and myelin degeneration (Peters et al. 1996). Primate studies suggested that active remyelination may occur in aged animals, producing shorter, more frequent intermodal segments along the myelination axon. Few studies have examined the morphological changes of aging myelin sheaths or the biological activity of oligodendrocytes in aging human brain, especially in the old-old and the ultra-old.

Astrocytes are the second most abundant type of glial cell in the human brain and compose about 19% of all glial cells (see Figure 2–1, Panel B). Astrocytes are involved with structural, metabolic, vascular, and metabotropic regulation (Oberheim et al. 2006). The astrocytic process may contribute to neurotransmission by directly supporting synaptic stability. Protoplasmic astrocytes have an average of 40 processes that are arrayed in specific topographies, and each cell can support about 2 million synapses. These long thin processes are woven into the neuropil and manage ion or water homeostasis. Astrocytes participate in the blood-brain barrier through foot processes on blood vessels that occupy a highly ordered territory. This pattern of unique overlapping spatial domains allows the cell to precisely regulate vascular tone in response to neural activity (Iadecola and Nedergaard 2007). Rodent models demonstrate a highly flexible astrocyte-synapse relationship that allows morphological changes of astrocytic processes within minutes (Volterra and Meldolesi 2005). Astrocytic excitation allows these glial cells to deliver specific chemically encoded messages to target cells through a process termed *gliotransmission*. However, astrocytes cannot propagate an action potential. The repertoire of gliotransmitters includes glutamate, adenosine triphosphate, adenosine, and others (Volterra and Meldolesi 2005). Astrocytes help regulate the structural integrity of synapses and modulate stem cell proliferation. Astrocytic function and gliotransmission can be affected by a range of common, age-related insults, including ischemia, epilepsy, and trauma. The age-related changes in human astrocytic function are poorly defined despite the crucial role of these cells in managing the microenvironment and facilitating transmission. Astrocytes are present in senile plaques, and these cells are involved with both normal and pathological processing of amyloid. Astrocytic proliferation is triggered by many types of brain injuries, including ischemia and metabolic encephalopathy.

Glial gene expression may be altered during aging or in response to injury (see Table 2–1). Genetic analysis of human white matter from areas of ischemia demonstrates changes in eight major molecular pathways for cell cycle, apoptosis, and other critical molecular systems (Simpson et al. 2009).

Studies in aged rodents and older humans have demonstrated increased glial fibrillary acidic protein, an intermediate filament specific for astrocytes, as well as increased glial markers such as glutamine synthetase (Finch and Morgan 1990; Frederickson 1992). However, some authors have described a minimal increase in astrocytic numbers in aging (Haug and Eggers 1991; Haug et al. 1984). A distinct population of astrocytes in the hippocampus, striatum, and periventricular zones of normal aged subjects accumulates cytoplasmic inclusions that may result from oxidative stress (Schipper 1996).

Microglial cells are thin, rod-shaped cells that constitute the smallest percentage of intrinsic glia (6%). These cells retain mitotic capacity into late life; however, they exhibit replicative senescence with aging (Streit 2006). Microglia can hypertrophy, divide, or become dystrophic. Microglial cells from older human brains are more likely to exhibit morphological differences from those in younger brains, including deramification, spheroid formation, and fragmentation of processes (Streit 2006). The turnover rate of microglial cells in healthy brain is probably low; however, these cells can become activated in areas of white matter damage (Ekdahl et al. 2009). Microglial cells can release brain-derived neurotrophic factor and glial-derived neurotrophic factor, and they can remove synapses or diminish excitotoxic damage. Microglial cells are activated in subcortical or periventricular white matter lesions, where these cells may respond to disruption of the blood-brain barrier or exhibit innate amoeboid activity in deep subcortical white matter (Simpson et al. 2007a; Streit 2006). More activated microglia may be present in periventricular lesions than in deep white matter lesions because the periventricular lesions are more likely to disrupt the blood-brain barrier (Simpson et al. 2007b).

Molecular Neuropathology of Aging

Aging neurons and glia undergo a series of histological, ultrastructural, and molecular biological changes that may appear as collections of intracellular extraneous materials or abnormal collections of intrinsic cytoskeletal elements. Lipofuscin, a brown wear-and-tear pigment, begins to accumulate within neuronal perikarya (Figure 2–4, Panel A). Neuromelanin, a dark pigment common to catecholamine-producing neurons, becomes visible in the brains of adolescent humans and progressively accumulates over years (Graham 1979) (Figure 2–4, Panel F). Neuronal inclusions, such as Hirano bodies, and granulovacuolar degeneration begin to appear in hippocampal pyramidal neurons (Figure 2–4, Panels C and D). Lewy bodies are seen usually in catecholamine-producing neurons of older subjects (Figure 2–4, Panel E).

Corpora amylacea, dense spherical glycoprotein inclusions, appear around the ventricles and in the neuropil, where they are numerous in aging and neurodegenerative disorders (Adams and Duchen 1992). These 5- to 50-μm inclusions are commonly present in astrocytic processes and may result from oxidative stress, iron imbalance, or mitochondrial damage (Keller 2006).

Neuromelanin and lipofuscin are pigments commonly found in neurons and some glia. Neuromelanin deposits are usually visible to light microscopy, and these amorphous collections of brown-black material are found in catecholamine-

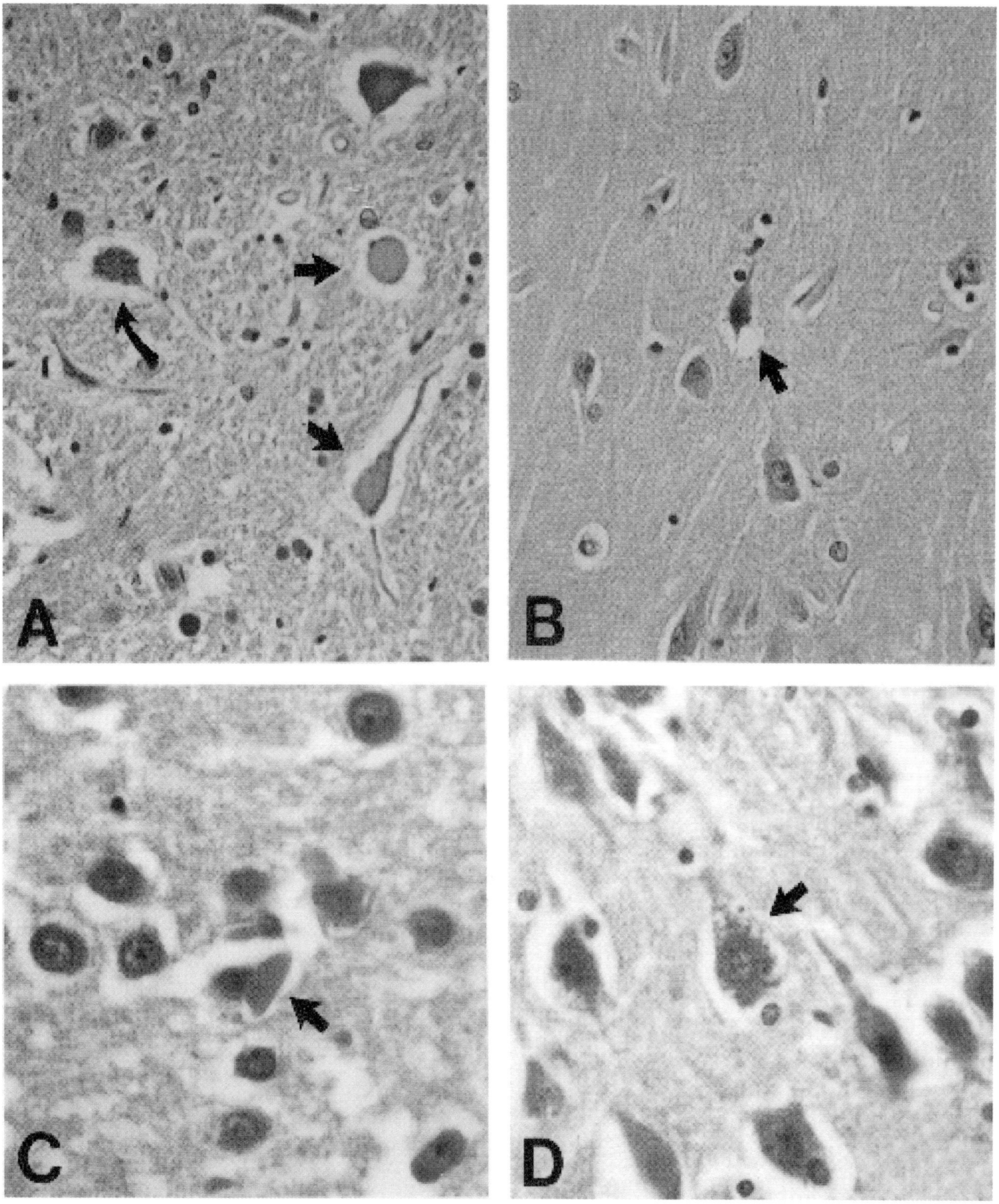

Figure 2-4 and legend continue on next pages.

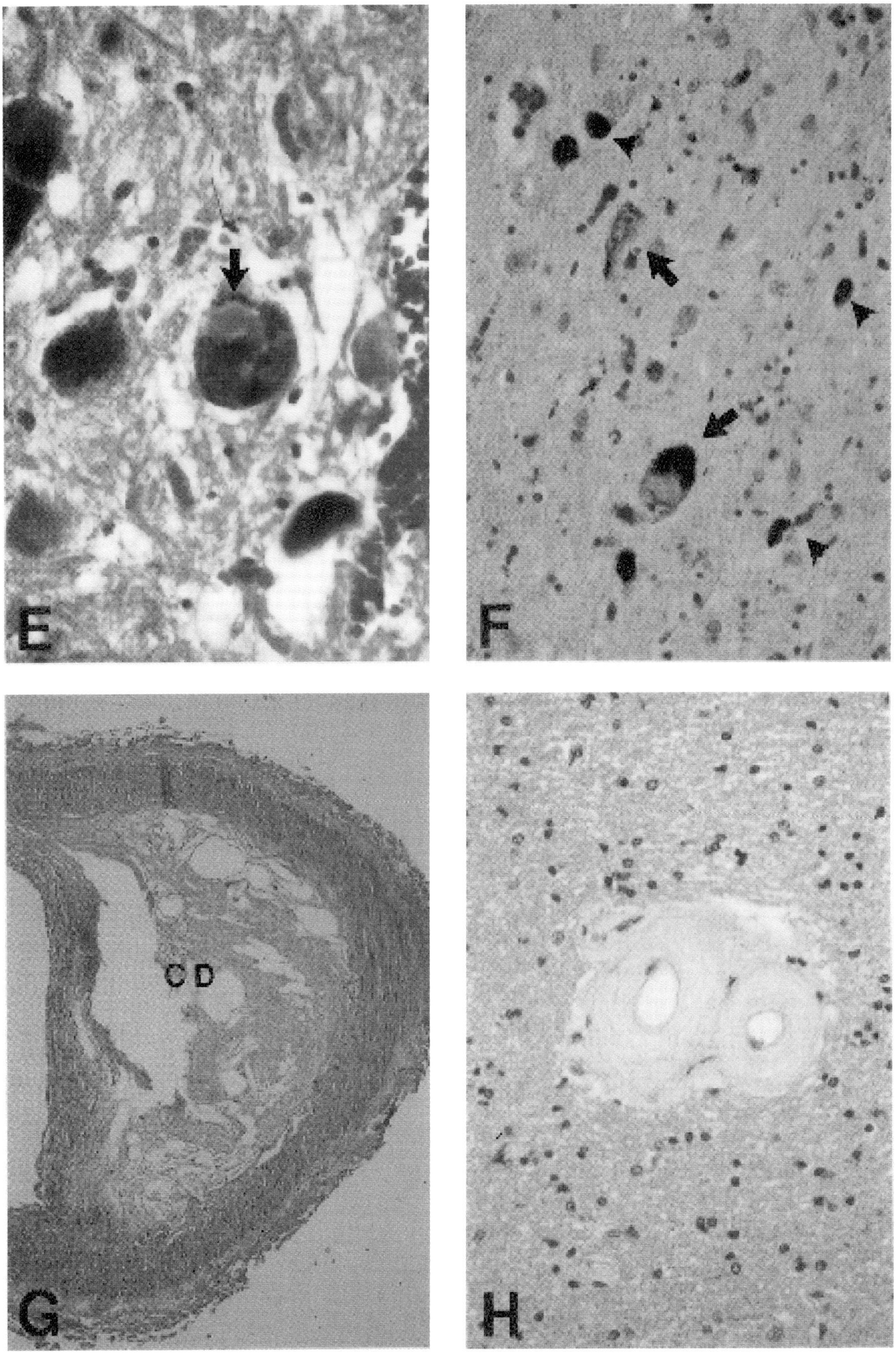
E
F
CD
G
H

FIGURE 2–4. Eight hematoxylin and eosin preparations showing microscopic alterations frequently observed in the brains of elderly humans, including lipofuscin (Panel A), ischemic neuronal injury (Panel B), Hirano bodies (Panel C), granulovacuolar degenerations (Panel D), Lewy bodies (Panel E), loss of neuromelanin-containing neurons (Panel F), atherosclerosis (Panel G), and arteriosclerosis (Panel H).

Panel A: Several neurons are shown. Two *(straight arrows)* contain abundant lipofuscin, a light-brown pigment. A normal neuron with abundant Nissl substance is present *(curved arrow).* **Panel B:** Photomicrograph of human hippocampus from a 68-year-old cognitively intact individual who had experienced brief cerebral hypoxia. Normal neurons surround a single shrunken pyramidal neuron in the center of the field with ischemic, eosinophilic degeneration *(arrow).* **Panel C:** Hirano bodies in hippocampal neurons from CA1 region. A Hirano body, the cigar-shaped eosinophilic rod immediately adjacent to the nucleus, is seen in the center of the field *(arrow).* **Panel D:** Granulovacuolar degenerations in the pyramidal neurons of CA3 region. In the cytoplasm of the neuron in the center of the field, there are multiple round, clear spaces with a central, slightly basophilic core *(arrow).* **Panel E:** Lewy bodies, circular eosinophilic masses with a thin, peripheral clear space *(arrow)* that displaces the neuromelanin, in the cytoplasm of substantia nigra neurons. Neurons that contain neuromelanin are also present. **Panel F:** Age-related damage of substantia nigra. Two normal-appearing pigmented neurons are shown *(arrows);* however, most neuromelanin is present in macrophages or in the neuropil *(arrowheads).* **Panel G:** Atherosclerotic damage in a branch of the posterior cerebral artery. The intima is detached and badly damaged with cholesterol deposition (CD), but the media is intact. **Panel H:** Lipohyalinosis in basal ganglia from a 74-year-old hypertensive individual. A small penetrating blood vessel in the center of the field contains pink hyalinized material in the media and adventitia.

producing neurons of the hypothalamus, brain stem, and spinal cord. Lipofuscin is a light brown material commonly found in neurons of the cerebral cortex and subcortical neurons, including those of the spinal cord. Neuromelanin is an organic polymer of catecholaminergic metabolic products that includes proteins and lipids. Lipofuscin contains aldehyde-linked protein residues, lipids, and some carbohydrates. Lipofuscin metabolism may affect the general aging of neurons, whereas neuromelanin may impact the aging of dopaminergic and noradrenergic neurons (Double et al. 2008). Similar melanic pigments are located within neurons of the putamen, cortex, and cerebellum (Zecca et al. 2008). Neuroscientists are unsure whether these substances are toxic or protective to human neurons.

Iron and other metals play an important role in cell respiration and cytotoxicity. Neuromelanin and ferritin form stable complexes with iron, which provide stable iron storage in pigmented neurons. Free iron can be highly toxic in neurons and oligodendrocytes. Iron content in neuromelanin is 30,000 ng/mg, which is 10 times higher than in the cytoplasm of neurons (Zecca et al. 1994). Neuromelanin also contains zinc and other trace elements in higher concentrations than are present in the cytoplasm. Iron and other metals may accumulate in senescent cells, and disruption of iron homeostasis may cause mitochondrial dysfunction and cell death (Atamna 2004; Zecca et al. 2001).

The neuronal cytoskeleton is the delicate meshwork of microtubules, neurofilaments, and other proteins (e.g., microtubule-associated proteins) present in all neurons. This matrix is barely visualized with the electron microscope. This meshwork provides structure to neurons and organizes neuronal transport. The cytoskeleton is a dynamic system, constantly cycling through production, transport, and degradation (Peng et al. 1986). Age-related alteration of axonal transport in human neurons is poorly defined, but slow transport is decreased by 30% in aging rodent brain (Finch and Morgan 1990). The production of antibodies to specific cytoskeletal antigenic sites (i.e., epitopes) allows the identification of molecular constituents within neurons. Immunocytochemical methods demonstrate the appearance of abnormal collections of cytoskeletal constituents in neurons of human neocortex and allocortex in the fifth or sixth decade before developing NFTs (Figure 2–5, Panel A). For example, phosphorylated neurofilament epitope is normally present in the axon but not in the neuronal perikarya (Goldman and Yen 1986). Immunocytochemical methods demonstrate accumulation of phosphorylated neurofilament epitope in the body of aging neurons.

Microtubules serve as an intracellular ladder with microtubule-associated proteins as the rungs. Kinesins are specific motor proteins that pull materials, such as vesicles, down the ladder through the axon (Mandelkow et al. 1995). Hyperphosphorylation of tau is integral to the production of paired helical filaments, which are major constituents in NFTs (Morishima-Kawashima et al. 1995). Tau, a low-molecular-weight, microtubule-associated protein, is present in most forms of age- and disease-related microscopic pathology. Tau gene mutations are implicated in several neurodegenerative diseases such as frontotemporal dementia.

Cytoskeleton is a major constituent of many age- and disease-related cellular histopathologies. Hirano bodies (see Figure 2–4, Panel C) contain actin, granulovacuolar degenerations (see Figure 2–4, Panel D) contain tubulin, Lewy bodies (see Figure 2–4, Panel E) contain filaments (Goldman et al. 1983), dystrophic neurites contain paired helical filament and tau, and NFTs (see

Figure 2–5, Panel A) contain multiple cytoskeletal constituents (Maurer et al. 1990). NFTs consist of masses of all six hyperphosphorylated isoforms of phosphorylated tau (p-Tau). p-Tau is increased fourfold to eightfold in brains of patients with Alzheimer's disease; however, no change occurs in normal tau or tau mRNA levels. Much of tau (40%) is soluble within the cytosol, and this molecule will sequester microtubule-associated proteins MAP1A and MAP1B, as well as MAP2. This process will disassemble existing healthy microtubules and facilitate self-assembly of p-Tau into NFTs (Pittman et al. 2006). Consequently, age-related disruption of tau metabolism may contribute to histopathology associated with multiple neurodegenerative diseases, including Alzheimer's disease, Pick's disease, and progressive supranuclear palsy (Iqbal et al. 2009).

α-Synuclein was cloned from the neuromuscular junction of the electric eel. Antibodies that recognize this protein labeled both synapses and nuclei, and the protein was thus called synuclein. The normal function for this protein is poorly understood, and the molecule is associated with presynaptic vesicles. Synuclein is found in numerous tissues, and lymphocyte levels increase with age and are higher in males (Brighina et al. 2010). This molecule is present in the "classic" brain stem Lewy bodies, the cortical Lewy bodies, and the dystrophic neurites seen in Parkinson's disease and diffuse Lewy body disease (Figure 2–6). The precise mechanism for the neurotoxic effect of α-synuclein is not understood, and some theories suggest that accumulation of the molecule may be evidence of self-protection by the neuron (Cookson 2009). The synuclein-based alterations in aging partially involve protein misfolding that cannot be reversed by chaperone refolding or degradation by proteasomes. The resistance of misfolded proteins, such as synuclein or amyloid, to protective molecular processing results in oligomerization and cytotoxicity (Kazantsev and Kolchinsky 2008).

The age-related accumulation of synuclein, which may begin in the peripheral nervous system, progresses centrally toward the cerebral cortex. α-Synuclein pathology begins in many affected older individuals within the peripheral autonomic system, medulla, and olfactory nerves, with gradual progression up the brain stem toward the substantia nigra. Involvement of the neocortex and mesial temporal structures occurs late in the disease (Braak et al. 2003). The clinical significance and progression of neuropathology is unclear because 30%–55% of individuals with widespread Lewy body pathology report no neuropsychiatric symptoms (Jellinger 2008; Zaccai et al. 2008).

Vascular Alterations in Aging

Cerebrovascular aging may reflect the cumulative vascular burden of damage caused by age-related changes of the heart, extracranial arteries, intracranial arteries, arterioles, capillaries, venous system, and the neural mechanisms that control vascular tone, as well as integrity of the blood-brain barrier. Most older persons have some form of age-related cerebrovascular change or pathology that may include luminal dilation, medial or intimal thickening without atherosclerosis, atherosclerosis, increased vessel wall stiffness, reduced vascular compliance, dysfunction of endothelial cells or pericytes, or impaired angiogenesis or impaired endovascular repair such as replacement of damaged endothelial cells (Lakatta 2008). These age-related changes are not unique to the human brain and affect other well-vascularized organs, such as kidney. The presence of end-organ damage, such as retinopathy, cardiomyopathy, or nephropathy, increases the likelihood of cognitive decline (Thompson and Hakim 2009).

Five major types of cerebrovascular pathology occur in aging human brain: atherosclerosis, arteriosclerosis, congo-

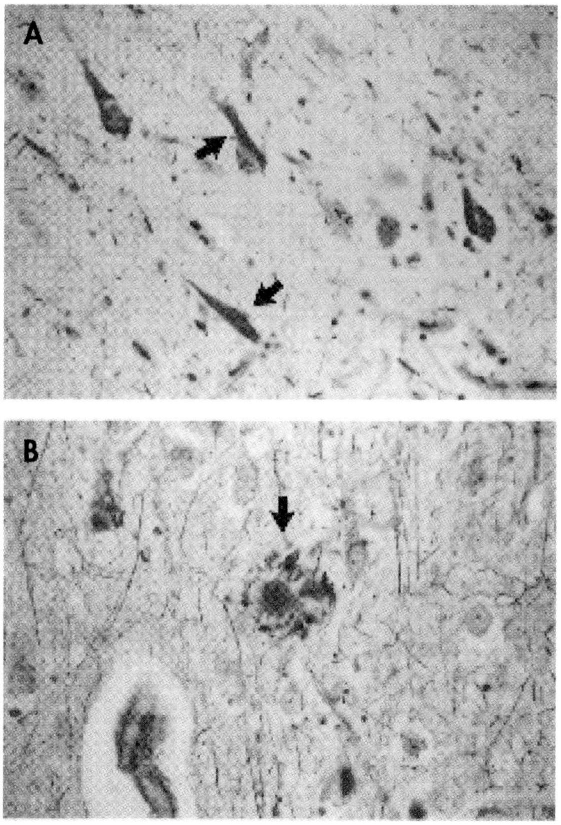

FIGURE 2–5. Photomicrographs showing the appearance of neurofibrillary tangles (Panel A) and senile plaques (Panel B) in a 100-year-old subject.

Panel A: Four hippocampal pyramidal neurons with neurofibrillary tangles (i.e., flame-shaped masses of filamentous material *[arrows]*). Tangles were not present in neocortex. **Panel B:** A silver preparation of neocortex. A senile plaque *(arrow)* contains swollen neurites, an amyloid core, glia, and microglia. Insufficient numbers were present in neocortex to warrant diagnosis of Alzheimer's disease.

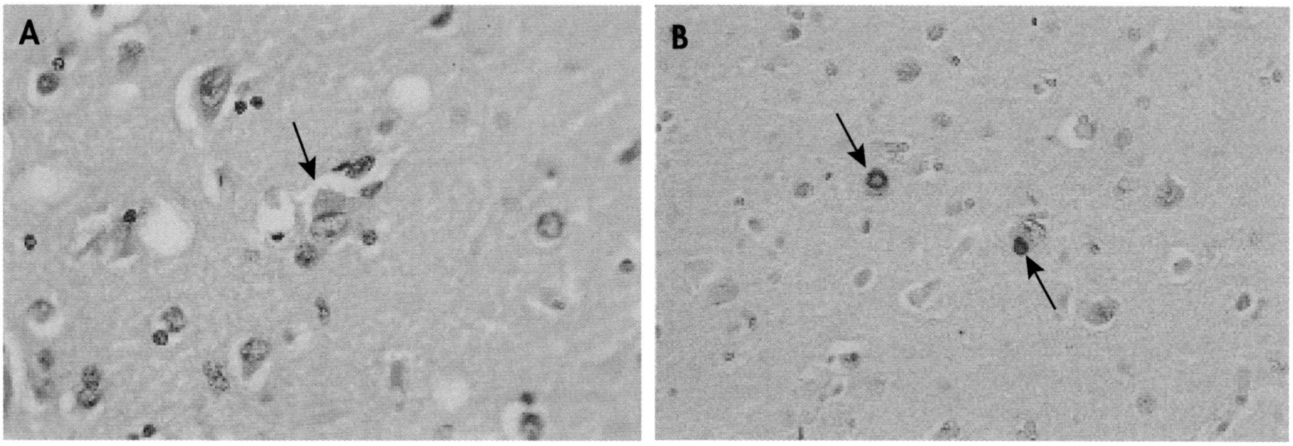

FIGURE 2–6. The appearance of cortical Lewy bodies.

Panel A: Hematoxylin and eosin-stained preparation through parahippocampal cortex from a patient with diffuse Lewy body disease. The indistinct eosinophilic cytoplasmic inclusion in the neuron in the middle of the field is the Lewy body *(arrow)*. **Panel B:** Antibodies to ubiquitin intensely stain two circular Lewy bodies (i.e., brown spheres in neurons in center of field) *(arrows)*.

philic angiopathy, hypoperfusion, and disruption of vascular permeability (Table 2–5). Atherosclerosis is damage to the intima of large-caliber vessels, in contrast to arteriosclerosis, which is damage to the media of small-caliber vessels. Congophilic angiopathy is the deposition of amyloid around small vessels in the arachnoid, pia, or brain parenchyma or within the vessel wall. Disruption of vascular permeability may result from injury to endothelial cells, pericytes, or other elements of the blood-brain barrier. Hypoperfusion results from hypoxia or poor cardiac function. Cumulative brain damage may occur from a combination of each type of brain pathology, and the risk varies according to the age, gender, ethnicity, and systemic medical conditions unique to the individual.

Appropriate neuronal function depends on the provision of adequate nutrients, such as oxygen and glucose, via cerebral blood flow, as well as removal of toxic by-products of metabolism. Vascular pathology, autoregulatory dysfunction, or cardiac disease can produce focal or diffuse abnormalities of cerebral perfusion. Brain imaging studies demonstrate a gradual reduction of cerebral blood flow with aging (Choi et al. 1998).

Autoregulation controls the response of cerebral blood vessels based on systemic blood pressure, oxygen tension, carbon dioxide tension, and cerebral metabolism. Cerebral vascular autoregulation may be affected by age-related diseases such as atherosclerosis, hypertension, and diabetes (Choi et al. 1998).

The brain represents only 2% of body weight but receives 17% of cardiac output and requires 20% of the body's oxygen to maintain normal function. The circle of Willis meets the brain's metabolic demand via an extensive anastomotic network that sustains adequate cerebral perfusion despite occlusion of major vessels, such as the internal carotid artery (Figure 2–7). The tapering of blood vessel diameters in distal branches of major arteries dampens the effect of blood pressure on penetrating vessels. Vessels that branch directly from large-diameter arteries, such as the lenticulostriate arteries of the basal ganglia, may lack this protective dampening effect, and these small penetrating vessels frequently demonstrate hypertensive damage.

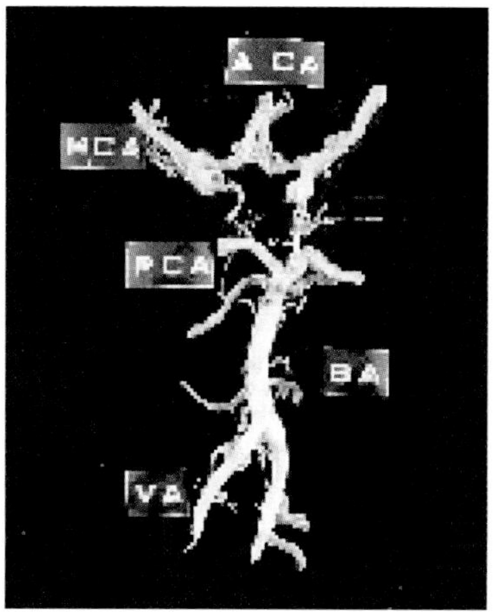

FIGURE 2–7. The circle of Willis as dissected from the base of the brain.

The internal carotid artery divides to form the anterior cerebral artery (ACA) and middle cerebral arteries (MCA). Anterior and posterior communicating arteries are not labeled. The vertebral arteries (VA) fuse to form the basilar artery (BA), which then divides to form the posterior cerebral arteries (PCA). This anastomotic network ensures adequate brain perfusion despite occlusion of single major vessels. See Figure 2–9A for in situ appearance.

TABLE 2–5. Common causes of age-related vascular brain damage in human brain

Type of damage	Typical anatomical distribution of damage	Typical location of lesion	Figures that depict change	Potential etiology of lesion	Commonly associated complications from damage
Atherosclerosis	Large-caliber extracerebral vessels	Intima	2–4G 2–7 2–9	Hyperlipidemia Diabetes Hypertension	Stroke
Arteriosclerosis	Penetrating vessels of white matter	Media	2–13 2–8	Hypertension	Lacunes (?) Hemorrhages (?)
Congophilic angiopathy	Arachnoidal and parenchymal vessels	Adventitia	2–15	Aβ-amyloid production	Unclear
Hypoperfusion	Watershed zone	Cardiovascular dysfunction	2–12 2–16	Low systemic blood pressure	Pale or red infarcts
Vascular permeability	White matter	Endothelium	2–4H 2–13	Damage to endothelium	Retraction of neuropil; promotion of inflammatory cascade

Note. (?)=inadequate data.

The brain is ensheathed by three layers of connective tissue: dura, arachnoid, and pia. The cerebral arteries course through the arachnoid and then penetrate the brain parenchyma ensheathed by the pia. The potential gap between the penetrating vessel and the pia is termed the *Virchow-Robin space* (VRS). Dilation of this space is common in older persons and younger individuals with specific brain diseases such as mucopolysaccharidosis. Some studies suggest a correlation between VRS volume and cognition in older subjects (Maclullich et al. 2004). Microscopic pathology within the VRS can include dilation, inflammatory infiltrates, hemorrhage, and evidence of disruption of the blood-brain barrier.

The large cerebral white matter structures such as the centrum semiovale are perfused by long, penetrating vessels that arise at right angles from arteries within the arachnoid space and radiate inward (Figure 2–8). Deep white matter is perfused by branches that originate from vessels located beneath the ventricular surface and radiate outward. The outer vessels are termed *centripetal* and the inner are termed *ventriculofugal.* White matter vessels, sometimes termed *medullary vessels,* do not arborize, but perpendicular side branches, termed *distributing vessels,* perfuse adjacent white matter (Pantoni and Garcia 1997). This overlapping system is vulnerable to changes produced by hypertension. Subcortical U-fibers are perfused by short branches of cortical vessels. The U-fibers are association bands immediately beneath the cortical ribbon, and this distinct perfusion reduces vulnerability to ischemia (Pantoni and Garcia 1997).

Arteries contain three layers: intima, media, and adventitia. The intima includes endothelial lining cells, pericytes, and a connective tissue stroma that prevent thrombosis and control movement of molecules into adjacent brain parenchyma. The media contains smooth muscle that regulates the luminal diameter and accommodates to blood pressure. The adventitia contains a loose connective tissue stroma that is adjacent to the VRS, and this space may act as a conduit for inflammatory cells. Arterioles, capillaries, and veins lack the distinctive thick muscular media present in arteries.

Atherosclerosis results in damage to the intima of large- or medium-diameter vessels and contributes to most strokes in elderly individuals (see Figures 2–7 and 2–9). The frequency or severity of this vascular pathology varies by age, gender, and ethnic background. Atherosclerotic changes, which have been found even in vessels of Egyptian mummies, first appear as discrete areas of white or yellow discoloration within thickened segments of blood vessel wall that subsequently provoke an inflammatory response in reaction to the damage. The microscopic changes progress to include loss or fibrosis of intima, lipid or cholesterol deposits beneath endothelial cells, narrowing of vessel lumen, and thrombosis on the plaques (see Figure 2–4, Panel G; Figure 2–9B). Concentric thickening can ultimately lead to slow occlusion of the vessel. Hemorrhage within a plaque can also produce a thrombus that occludes the vessel lumen. Small but significant reductions in atheroma volumes can be achieved in some adults through reductions of cholesterol or raising of the HDL value. Statins can also reduce the macrophage and lymphocytic contents in a plaque, as well as lipid content and collagen (Insull 2009). Systemic atherosclerosis may begin in the second decade of life in a small portion of the general population and accelerates after the third decade. Only 4% of individuals over age 90

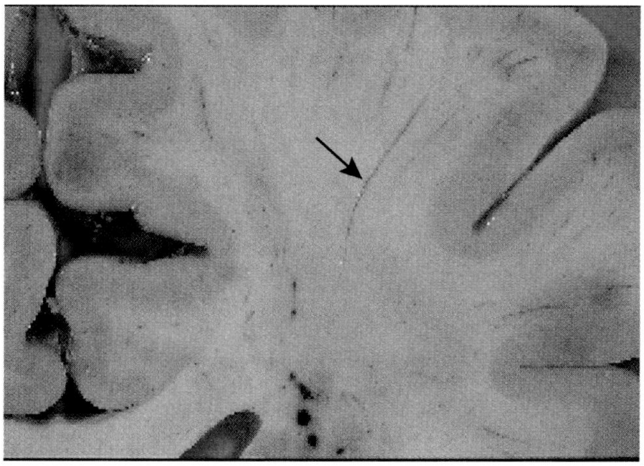

FIGURE 2–8. White matter vessels.

The thin dark lines are long, penetrating vessels that pass through the cortical ribbon, traverse into the centrum semiovale, and perfuse a cylinder of white matter adjacent to the vessel *(arrow)*. Deeper white matter is perfused by branches originating from beneath the lateral ventricle *(lower left)*. White matter structures are sensitive to certain types of anoxic injury, and these vessels sustain hypertensive vascular damage.

avoid atherosclerotic damage (Gorelich 1993). Fatty streaks occur within the aortic walls in the first decade of life, followed by fatty streaks in coronary arteries or extracranial carotid vessels in the second. Fibrous plaques appear in vertebral arteries in subjects over age 30 (Moossy 1993).

The development of vascular damage and risk factors for atherosclerosis may begin in utero for some individuals. Reduced birth weight is associated with multiple chronic health problems in later life that increase the risk for age-related disease, including hypertension, diabetes, and cardiovascular disease (Palinski and Napoli 2008). Fatty streaks are present in the aortas of some infants at autopsy, a finding that correlates to maternal hyperlipidemia (Napoli et al. 1997). Postmortem studies in subjects ages 15–35 years demonstrate inflammatory response to atherogenic lesions of the intima, including macrophages and T lymphocytes (Millonig et al. 2002). Postmortem studies from the Bogalusa Heart Study show coronary atherosclerosis in 90% of young decedents (Berenson and Srinivasan 2005).

Rodent and rabbit studies demonstrate a relationship between maternal cardiovascular disease and severity of arterial disease or changes of vascular gene expression in offspring (Napoli et al. 2002). Treatment of animal models with lipid-lowering medications reduced fetal and postnatal atherogenesis (Palinski and Napoli 2002).

Childhood health behaviors such as exercise, smoking, obesity, and diet may affect systemic vascular risk factors (Napoli and Palinski 2005). The pathogenesis of early-onset carotid vascular disease as defined by intimal-medial thickness may be affected by multiple childhood health factors associated with metabolic syndrome, including obesity, pulse pressure (Raitakari et al. 2009), dyslipidemia (Magnussen et al. 2009), body mass, and other factors such as levels of apolipoprotein B and A1 (Raitakari et al. 2003) and levels of physical exercise (Hopkins et al. 2009). These insights gained from animal models and human postmortem studies of early life vascular pathology suggest that the cascade of vascular changes may begin very early in life.

Age-related alterations of the brain microvascular system may be important for both gray and white matter. Cortical microvasculature studies show intertwining of small arterial branches, convoluted vessels, and mild perivascular glial proliferation (Ravens 1978). Veins demonstrate fibrous thickening with aging that may slow venous return and increase edema in white matter. This periventricular venous collagenosis occurs in 65% of individuals over age 60 and may promote leukoaraiosis—that is, white matter thinning (Moody et al. 1995). Microscopic examination of age-related cerebral microvascular damage reveals thickening of basement membrane of arterioles and capillaries as well as perivascular deposits of collagen. Smooth muscle can be replaced by fibrohyalinized material. Microvascular damage may trigger a chain of events, including localized ischemia and reduction of nutrient transport. The resulting oxidative stress may promote the release of cytokines that stimulate astrocytes and microglia as well as recruitment of circulating fibroblasts (Thompson and Hakim 2009).

At least six studies have examined capillary density in aging human neocortex, hippocampus, and hypothalamus. The density of hippocampal capillary clusters decreases in older subjects, but the mean diameter of capillaries and arterioles increases (Bell and Ball 1981). Most recent studies have demonstrated a 15%–20% decline in capillary density to age 90 (Riddle et al. 2003). The density of capillaries is generally greatest in regions with high densities of synapses, lower in regions with neuronal cell bodies, and lowest in fiber tracts. Sensory and association areas tend to have higher capillary densities than motor regions. Some data suggest that microvascular decline with aging parallels decline of IGF-1 and neurogenesis. The effect of age-related microvascular changes on the blood-brain barrier has been studied using biochemical and neuroimaging methodologies. Findings from a meta-analysis of 31 published studies suggest that permeability of the blood-brain barrier increases with normal aging and further increases in persons with dementia or white matter lesions (Farrall and Wardlaw 2009).

Few animal models exist for age-related microvascular disease. A small number of models can produce microinfarcts that resemble lacunar infarcts (see Figure 2–13D), but these models cannot replicate the unique pathological features of human brain microvascular aging (Bailey et al. 2009).

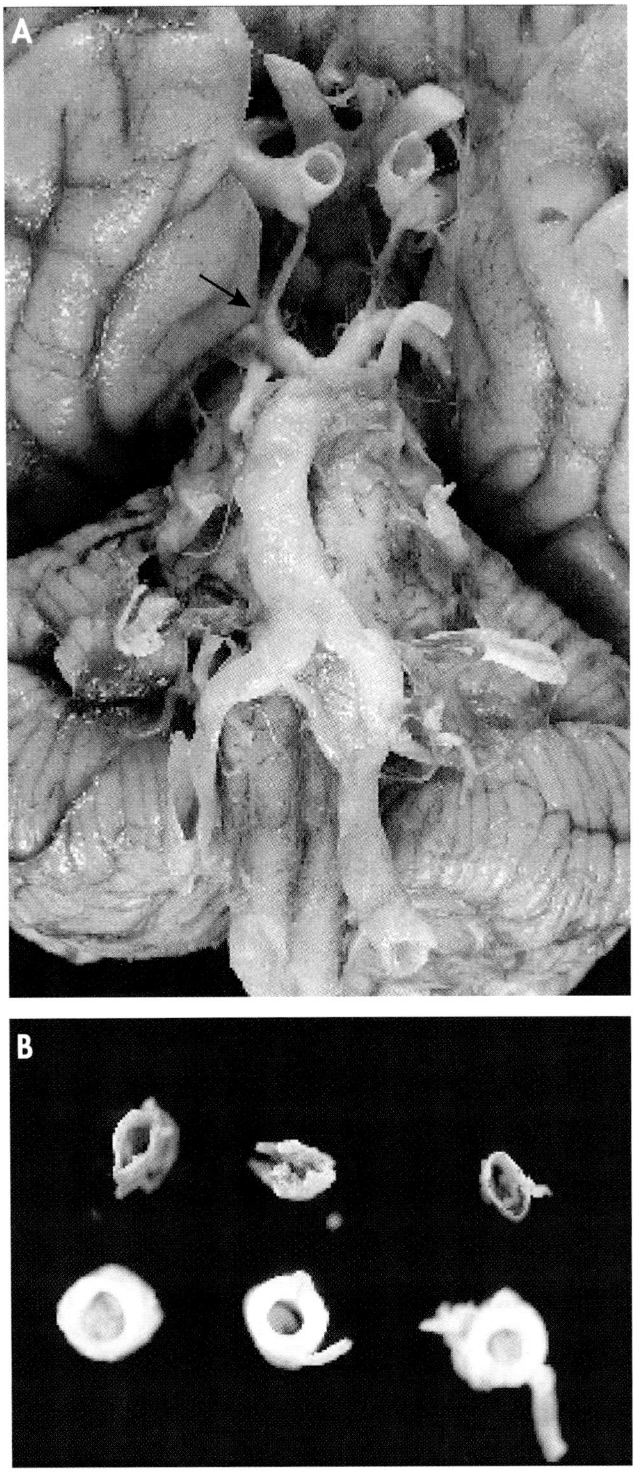

FIGURE 2–9. Atherosclerosis of the circle of Willis.

Panel A: Typical atherosclerosis in a basilar artery from a 68-year-old subject. Normal basilar artery has a translucent appearance, whereas this atherosclerotic artery *(arrow)* has a thickened tortuous wall and an opaque white appearance. Thin posterior communicating arteries connect posterior cerebral to internal carotid arteries. **Panel B:** Cross sections of normal and atherosclerotic arteries. The *top field* demonstrates normal paper-thin muscular arteries, whereas the *lower field* contains serial sections through the thickened, narrowed atherosclerotic vessel.

Atherosclerosis has a complex pathogenesis, with risk factors that include hyperlipidemia, homocystine deficiency, hypertension, elevated platelet numbers, and a myriad of other factors. Intimal damage from atherosclerosis can lead to thrombotic occlusion of vessels or embolization into distal arteries, with resulting cerebral infarction. Extracranial vascular pathology frequently produces cerebral damage. Embolization also results from either atrial fibrillation or myocardial infarction when a mural thrombus forms in either the atrium or the left ventricle (Ott et al. 1997) (Figure 2–10). Liquefaction necrosis and discrete loss of brain parenchyma, termed *encephalomalacia,* are apparent to gross inspection within weeks or months following brain infarction (Figure 2–11). Abrupt revascularization may convert a pale or ischemic infarct into a red or hemorrhagic infarct (Figure 2–12, Panel A). Smaller emboli lodged in arterioles produce small discrete infarction within segments of cortical ribbon (Figure 2–12, Panel B). Tiny emboli produce microinfarctions, which are difficult to visualize with in vivo imaging and require microscopic examination for identification.

Hypertension produces a variety of brain lesions via arteriolosclerosis and damage to medium- and small-caliber arteries and arterioles (see Table 2–5). Arteriolosclerosis is characterized by damage to the muscular media of small penetrating arteries or arterioles that occurs commonly in small, nonarborizing branches from large-caliber arteries, for example, the lenticulostriate system. Vessels with arteriolosclerosis have hyalinization or necrosis of the media that may lead to thrombosis or leakage (see Figure 2–4, Panel H). Hypertensive brain lesions include loss of neuropil around small penetrating arteries, disruption of the blood-brain barrier, arteriolar sclerosis, lacunar infarcts, and intracerebral hemorrhages (Figure 2–13).

Lacunar infarcts are slitlike lesions measuring 1–10 mm in the cerebral hemisphere (Figure 2–13, Panel C) and 1–5 mm in the brain stem (Figure 2–13, Panel D). These punched-out lesions are common in deep nuclei, hemispheric white matter, brain stem, and cerebellar peduncles. Lacunar infarcts are present in up to 49% of autopsy brains, with lesions most commonly found in hemispheric white matter and subcortical nuclei (Dozono et al. 1991). Lacunar infarcts are associated with older age, increased diastolic blood pressure, heavy smoking, internal carotid artery stenosis exceeding 50%, and diabetes mellitus (Longstreth et al. 1998).

Lacunar infarcts are associated with significant cognitive morbidity related to dementia (15%–20%), dependency (38%), and second strokes (25%) over the ensuing 5 years (Futrell 2004). The lacunar infarction may be an epiphenomenon for more serious vascular pathology; however, the etiology of these common age-related lesions remains controversial. The original studies published by Fisher et al. in the 1960s formed the scientific basis of ascribing this type of brain pathology to hypertension. More recent clinical and pathological studies found hypertension in 24%–73% of persons with lacunar infarction, a rate similar to that in other strokes (Futrell 2004). An unresolved de-

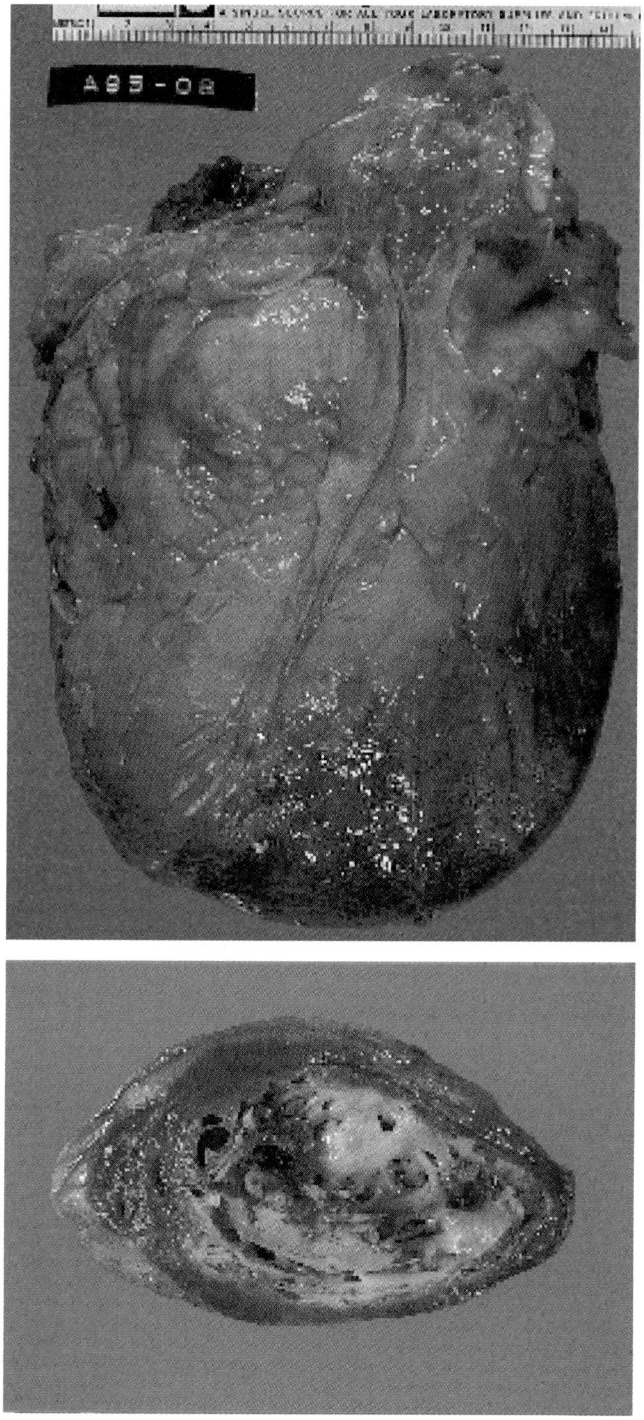

FIGURE 2–10. Cerebrovascular damage from heart disease.

Cardiac disease produces arrhythmias and emboli that damage brain. This patient had hypotensive and embolic infarcts caused by atherosclerotic cardiomyopathy (**top**) with a 15% ejection fraction and an apical thrombus in the left ventricle (**bottom**).

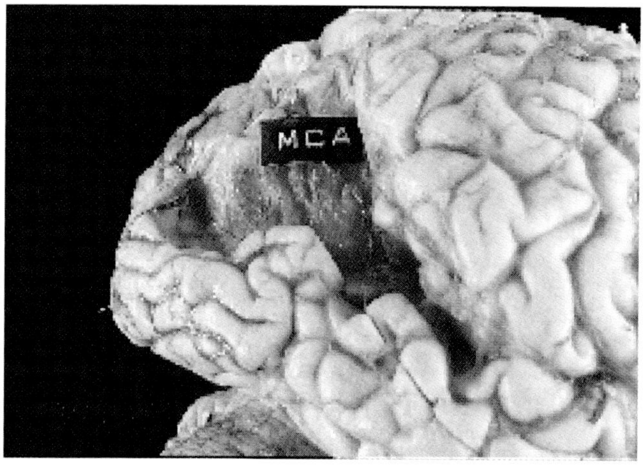

FIGURE 2–11. A stroke in the distribution of the middle cerebral artery (MCA).

Encephalomalacia of the inferior parietal, anterior occipital, and superior temporal gyrus regions produces a cavity after a stroke.

bate focuses on whether lacunes result from microembolic disease or primary occlusion of penetrating vessels. Other potential etiologies include embolic events, stenosis, occlusion, or disruption of blood-brain barrier. Minimal differences occur in risk factors for other strokes and lacunar infarcts, including atrial fibrillation, diabetes, hypertension, and carotid stenosis (Jackson and Sudlow 2005; Wardlaw 2005). Hypertensive vascular pathology can also produce extensive damage via intracerebral hemorrhage (Figure 2–14) and associated complications such as bleeding into the ventricles or subarachnoid space. Lacunar infarcts are associated with subtle, diffuse dysfunction of the blood-brain barrier, which is proposed as a pathogenetic mechanism in leukoaraiosis (Wardlaw et al. 2008, 2009).

Congophilic angiopathy is common in patients over age 90. Proteinaceous material is deposited in the media or adventitia of small arachnoidal or cortical arterioles (see Table 2–5). Although amyloid angiopathy increases the risk for intracerebral hemorrhage, its effect on cerebral perfusion is unclear. Congophilic deposits probably alter blood-brain barrier function in aging (Figure 2–15); however, there is no documented relationship with cognitive function.

Low perfusion from systemic hypotension can damage brain parenchyma while providing few observable alterations (see Table 2–5). Watershed or boundary zones are cortical regions that are located between distal vascular perfusion areas of the cerebral arteries. For example, cortex adjacent to the superior frontal sulcus is vulnerable to hypoperfusion during episodes of systemic hypotension because this region is perfused by distal branches of the anterior and middle cerebral arteries (see Figure 2–12, Panel A). Neuronal vulnerability to anoxia

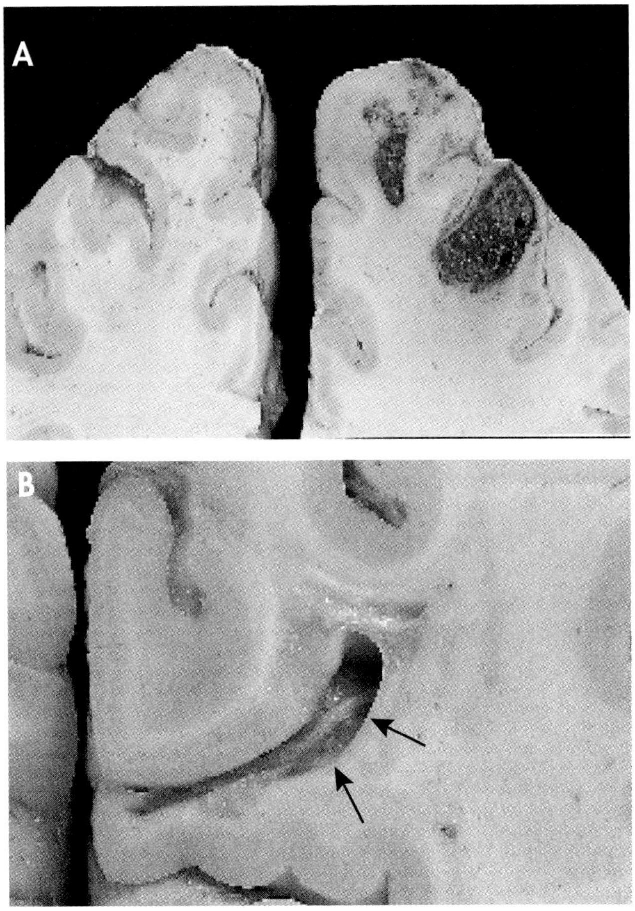

FIGURE 2–12. Reperfusion and embolic infarctions.

Panel A: Coronal sections of frontal lobe from an individual who sustained hypotensive brain injury after a cardiac arrest (see Figure 2–10). Hemorrhage occurs in necrotic brain tissue located between the superior and middle frontal gyri, a common boundary zone location. Hemorrhagic or red infarcts are produced by reperfusion of infarcted brain parenchyma or lysis of thrombi within occluded blood vessels. **Panel B:** A small infarction in the occipital parietal cortex. A discrete strip of cortical ribbon in the center of the field is absent, but adjacent cortex is intact. This discrete loss of cortical ribbon results from embolic occlusion of small arteries *(arrows).*

may increase with aging. Specific regions such as hippocampus have selective vulnerability to anoxia and excitotoxic damage. Poor cardiac pump function (i.e., cardiac arrhythmias), systemic hypotension (Sulkava and Erkinjuntti 1987), and cardiac left ventricular ejection fraction less than 30% (Zuccala et al. 1997) may cause low flow to vulnerable brain regions that contributes to cognitive loss in older subjects (Figure 2–16).

Age-Related Changes of the Blood-Brain Barrier

The blood-brain barrier has two major functions: transport of essential materials and protection of brain homeostasis. Although nutrients can reach the brain via spinal fluid, the volume of the blood-brain barrier is 5,000 times greater than the CSF-brain boundary (de la Torre 1997). The blood-brain barrier is located in the brain's microvasculature and consists of tight junctions and fenestration of brain capillary endothelium that use selective pinocytosis to control movement of molecules. Unlike capillaries of non-CNS organs, brain capillary pores do not allow free movement of substances. Carrier-mediated transports in the brain capillaries select specific substances for entrance into the CNS. This barrier function is mediated by tight junctions between endothelial cells. The blood-brain barrier is the locus of three essential functions: 1) transport for critical nutrients, hormones, or drugs; 2) export of metabolic waste products; and 3) protection against influx of toxins and osmotically damaging agents (Mooradian 1988). Disruption of the VRS may contribute to the breakdown of the blood-brain barrier, as can occur in multiple sclerosis (Wuerfel et al. 2008). Specific proteins, such as the P-glycoprotein, manage cellular efflux to prevent the accumulation of toxic metabolic by-products. Brain imaging detects a loss of P-glycoprotein function in aging brain, especially in white matter such as the corona radiata. Age-related reduction in such systems might contribute to age-related brain dysfunction (Bartels et al. 2009).

Histochemical studies of brains from human subjects over age 45 show alterations in the biochemical composition of arterioles, capillaries, and venules (Sobin et al. 1992). Aging of brain microvasculature may result in minor leakage through the blood-brain barrier. Human serum proteins, such as IgG, IgA, IgM, and α_2-macroglobulin, leak into cortical tissue of elderly subjects and are found in some neurons (Mooradian 1988). Common systemic diseases in the elderly, such as hypertension and diabetes mellitus, damage the blood-brain barrier. Hypertension and mild ischemia increase transport of high-molecular-weight proteins through accelerated transendothelial transport and transcytosis. Leakage across blood-brain barriers increases proportionally to severity of ischemia—damage that loosens the tight junctions of endothelium.

Pericytes and endothelial cells are intimately involved with blood-brain barrier and vascular function. Blood vessels are lined by a monolayer of flattened endothelial cells that originate from circulating endothelial progenitor cells (EPCs). EPCs are derived from the bone marrow and contribute to re-endothelialization of damaged vessels or neovascularization of damaged brain. Pericytes are stellate-shaped cells that are located immediately adjacent to the endothelial cell and encircle ~22%–32% of the capillary surface (Fisher 2009). Both pericytes and endothelial cells have stem potential and modulate brain homeosta-

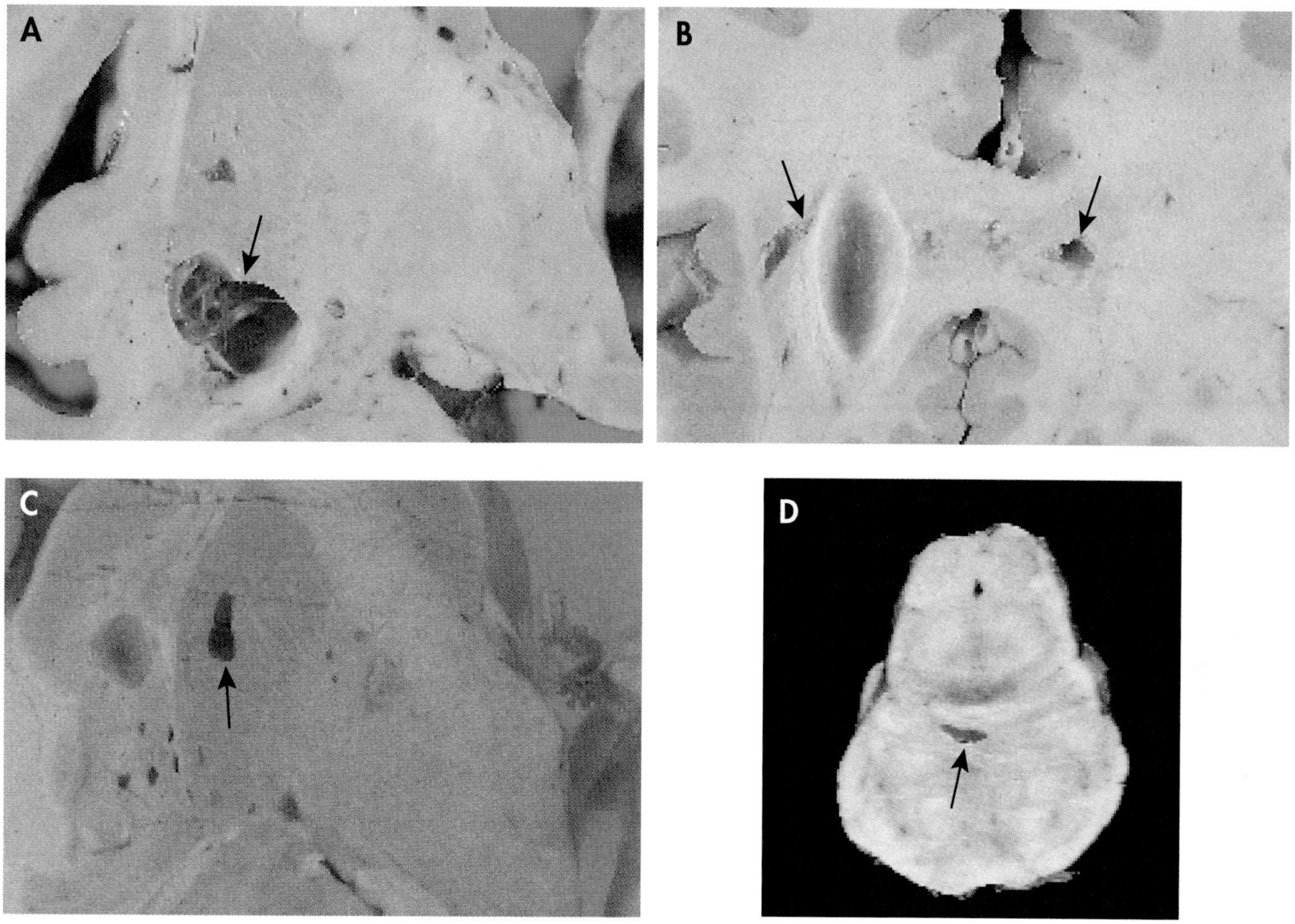

FIGURE 2–13. Hypertensive brain damage.

Panel A: Demonstrates loss of neuropil around penetrating vessels in basal ganglia *(arrow)*. The intact vessel remains within the cavity. **Panel B:** Demonstrates periventricular leukomalacia. Computed tomography scan showed that this patient had extensive white matter thinning. The neuropil about the frontal horn of the lateral ventricle is thin and demonstrates a granular appearance *(arrows)*. Extensive atherosclerosis is present in the anterior cerebral arteries bending around the genu of the corpus callosum. **Panel C:** A lacunar infarction in the putamen. This slitlike lesion is well demarcated *(arrow)*. Hemorrhage from such lesions causes intracerebral hematoma (see Figure 2–14). **Panel D:** Lacunar infarct in the pons. This slitlike lesion in the basis pontis can produce nonlateralizing neurological symptoms *(arrow)*.

sis. EPCs are impacted by age-related diseases and aging. The length of telomeres in the EPCs declines with age, especially after age 55 (Kushner et al. 2009). Aging, hypertension, and cardiovascular risk factors are associated with reduced numbers of EPCs (Umemura et al. 2008). Low EPC levels may also be associated with cerebrovascular disease (Ghani et al. 2005).

Cerebrospinal Fluid and Aging

CSF is clear liquid produced by the choroid plexus within the ventricles and reabsorbed via the arachnoidal granulations located along the sagittal sinus. CSF was first described by the Egyptians as brain water about 2,700 years ago. The cuboidal epithelium that lines the choroid plexus functions to transport and clear endogenous molecules and xenobiotics as well as participate in drug metabolism (Redzic et al. 2005). CSF, produced at 0.3–0.4 mL/min, contains electrolytes, protein, sugar, and a small number of cells. The rate of CSF production is reduced in aging, and CSF protein content is increased (May et al. 1990). The number or type of inflammatory cells in CSF is unchanged with aging. Ventricular CSF volume increases by up to 25% or 30% through age 80 compared with that of young adults. The CSF volume begins to expand after the second decade of life, when the fluid comprises ~7%–9% of intracranial volume and expands to 20%–33% of volume by age 80 (Redzic et al. 2005). There is evidence for subtle increased resistance to CSF drainage with aging. The physiology of CSF reabsorption is poorly defined, and obstruction of return flow

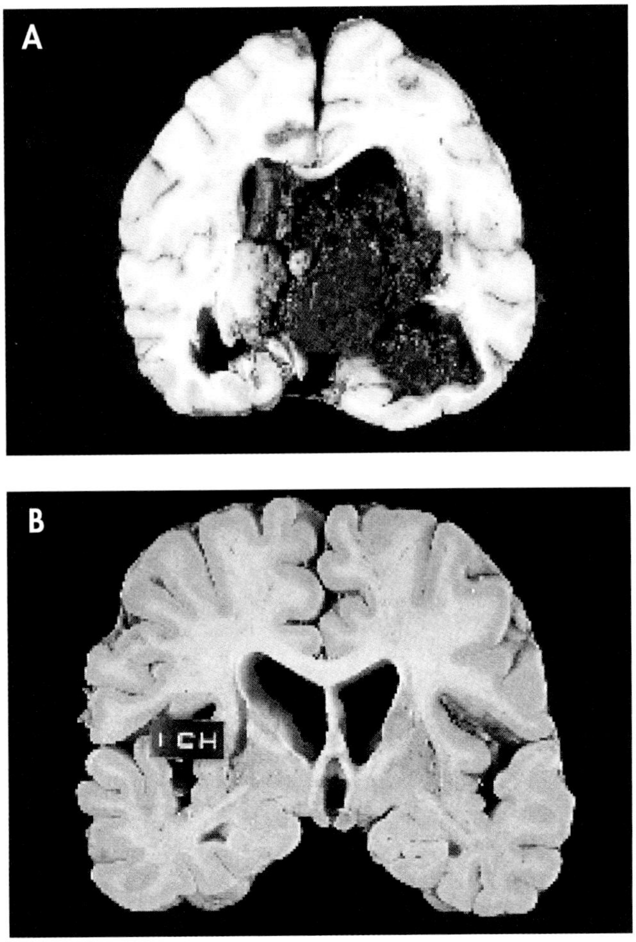

FIGURE 2–14. Hypertensive vascular disease.

Coronal sections from different brains that demonstrate acute and long-term consequences of hypertensive damage. **Panel A:** An acute hemorrhage into basal ganglia and thalamus produces cerebral edema and death. **Panel B:** An old healed intracerebral hemorrhage causes a lens-shaped lesion *(labeled ICH)* in the putamen and internal capsule that produced a spastic hemiparesis. This lesion would also damage ascending catecholaminergic fibers.

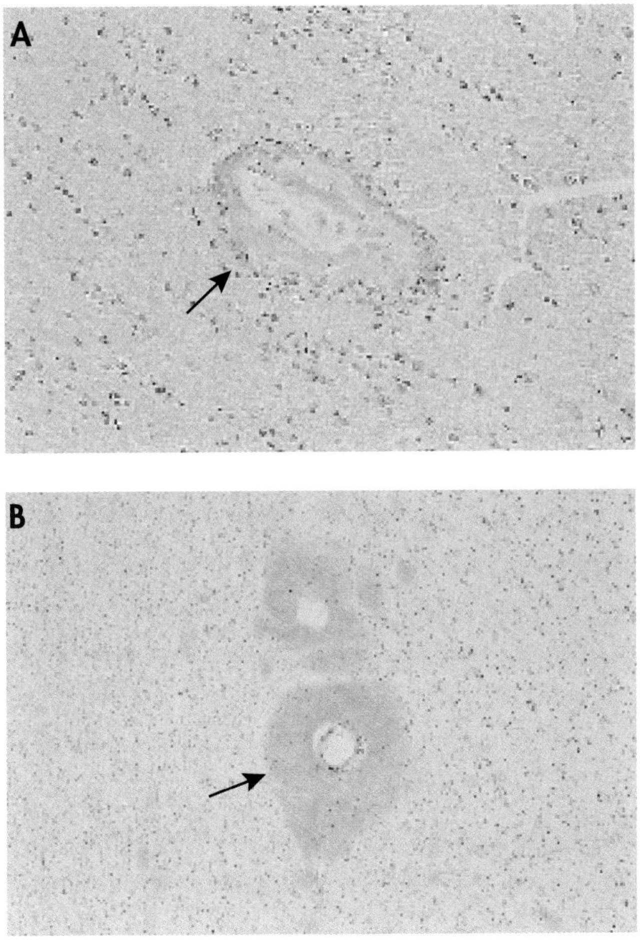

FIGURE 2–15. Perivascular amyloid visualized by Congo red and immunoperoxidase stains in the brain of a 91-year-old subject.

Panel A: The faint-red discoloration of amyloid deposition within adventitia blood vessel stained by Congo red *(arrow)*. Polarizing light confirmed the amyloid. **Panel B:** Immunoperoxidase stains of blood vessel, with anti-amyloid antibody demonstrating pale brown amyloid deposits *(arrow)* around small cortical blood vessels.

into the arachnoidal granulations may produce normal-pressure hydrocephalus. Transmitter metabolic content of CSF changes in aging.

Alterations of Neurotransmitter Systems in Aging

The impact of aging on specific transmitter systems can be measured at the presynaptic or postsynaptic level. Presynaptic levels of chemical transmitters can be reduced by death or dysfunction of neurons that produce the transmitter, diminished release, and alterations of reuptake. Postsynaptic effects include alteration of postsynaptic receptor density, alterations of the receptor, and changes in signal transduction mechanisms that translate the receptor activation into cellular or membrane events. Signal transmission may be altered at several levels, confusing the interpretation of human data. Although many human brain transmitter markers are altered in aging, in this chapter I focus on systems of most importance to the geriatric neuropsychiatrist.

Cholinergic Systems

Acetylcholine innervation is widely present throughout the mammalian CNS (Hedreen et al. 1984). The anatomy of the

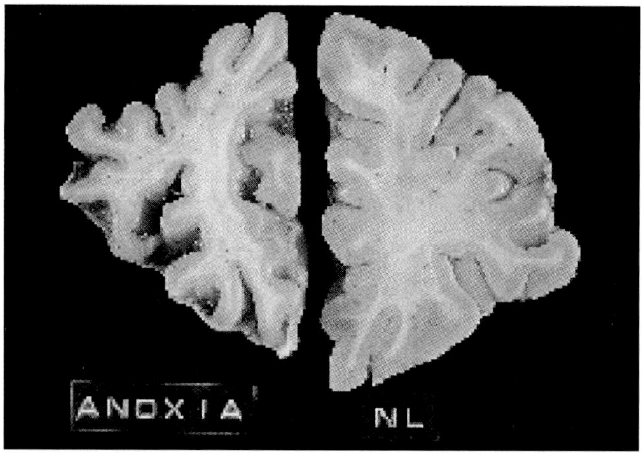

FIGURE 2–16. Diffuse anoxic injury.

A normal (NL) frontal lobe (**right**) is contrasted with a coronal section from an individual with prolonged anoxia (**left**). The sulcal gyral pattern remains intact; however, the cortical ribbon is markedly reduced. Microscopic examination revealed severe neuronal loss and gliosis.

cortical cholinergic system includes neuronal perikarya situated along the base of the forebrain that project to cortical neurons via ascending fibers that traverse deep white matter structures such as the centrum semiovale (Table 2–6). Most cortical cholinergic fibers originate from neurons in the nucleus basalis of Meynert (NBM), a band of large-diameter neurons, termed *magnocellular*, in the basal forebrain that is most conspicuous beneath the anterior commissure (Mesulam et al. 1983) (see Figure 2–3). The cholinergic innervation of the neocortex and limbic structures is provided by an estimated 210,000 neurons in each hemisphere located within the NBM (Gilmor et al. 1999). A second cholinergic system exists in the pontine reticular area. Acetylcholine esterase and the sister molecule, butyrylcholinesterase, are present throughout the neocortex and share similar roles in controlling cerebral blood flow, cortical activation, and the sleep-wake cycle (Schleibs and Arendt 2006).

When viewed in the axial plane, the NBM is a diamond-shaped group of large-diameter neurons located in the base of the brain beneath the basal ganglia and stretches in the rostral-caudal plane from the level of the caudate nucleus to the level of the lateral geniculate nucleus. The NBM cells are divided into four areas (see Table 2–6) and contain mixed populations of variably sized neurons that express cholinergic, peptidergic, and other transmitter markers. A mixture of smaller diameter neurons contains the M_2 muscarinic acetylcholine receptor as well as nicotinamide adenine dinucleotide phosphate (NADPH)–diaphorase, γ-aminobutyric acid (GABA), and calcium-binding proteins. The boundary for this diffuse band of neurons is difficult to precisely localize on brain imaging, and age-related volumetric changes are unclear, although atrophy is likely present in patients with Alzheimer's disease (Hanyu et al. 2007).

In postmortem specimens, age-related neuronal loss in the NBM is minimal, but significant changes in molecular biology occur after the sixth decade of life, suggesting the molecular dysfunction of morphologically intact neurons (Mufson et al. 2003). Markers for tau-related neuronal pathology begin to appear in the brains of normal older subjects and of individuals with mild cognitive impairment (MCI) despite otherwise normal cortical markers for cholinergic activity (Mesulam et al. 2004). Markers for TrkA, the high-affinity receptor for nerve growth factor (NGF), are diminished in MCI, but the overall number of neurons in the nucleus remains relatively constant. Although choline acetyltransferase activity may not be diminished until early or mid-stage Alzheimer's disease, the cholinergic forebrain is not normal during the transition from normal aging to MCI (Sarter and Bruno 2004). Cholinergic loss in Alzheimer's disease appears asynchronous with clinical symptoms, because decline of cholinergic activity does not parallel the decline in synaptic numbers. Choline acetyltransferase activity is upregulated in the hippocampus of persons with MCI, and nicotinic receptors are not reduced until the clinical transition into dementia (Sabbagh et al. 2006). Age-related cholinergic axonal pathology first appears in normal subjects during middle age, although receptor studies show little effect during the time period (Geula et al. 2008; Sarter and Bruno 2004). Although acetylcholine transferase, the synthetic enzyme for acetylcholine, is reduced in Alzheimer's disease, the conflicting data in normal aging (Giaquinto 1988; Muller et al. 1991) demonstrate minimal reductions or relative stability. This minor senescent cholinergic loss may reflect complex alterations in the number and size of neurons in the NBM with aging (see Figure 2–3). The perikaryal diameters of some human forebrain cholinergic neurons may increase until age 60. NBM neurons in humans over age 60 begin to atrophy, and neuronal loss varies according to region sampled (e.g., 0% in the anterior portion and up to 65% in posterior subdivisions) (de Lacalle et al. 1991; Finch 1993). A similar sequence of changes is seen in rodent and monkey. These "magnocellular" neurons may contain occasional NFTs or Lewy bodies in older human subjects, and their loss accounts for cholinergic deficits in Alzheimer's disease. Aging has a minimal effect on high-affinity choline uptake, the rate-limiting step in the production of acetylcholine. Levels of acetylcholinesterase are increased in CSF of elderly subjects (Hartikainen et al. 1991; Muller et al. 1991). The significant variation of 17% in the number of neurons in the NBM of normal elders may obscure subtle losses in Alzheimer's disease that average 15% in older subjects. Younger patients with Alzheimer's disease have greater

TABLE 2–6. Summary of age-related changes to the cholinergic (CH) system of the forebrain

CH area	Regional nomenclature	% ACH neurons	Projection target	Age-related changes	MCI
1	Medial septal	10%	Hippocampus	?	NC
2	Diagonal band of Broca, vertical limb	70%	Limbic Anterior Cingulate	?	NC
3	Diagonal band of Broca, horizontal limb	1%–2%	Olfactory bulb Limbic	?	NC
4	a) NBM b) Anterior NBM, intermediate c) NBM, posterior	90%	Amygdala Neocortex	NC	NC

Note. ?=inadequate data; ACH=acetylcholine; MCI=mild cognitive impairment; NBM=nucleus basalis of Meynert; NC=adequate data to suggest no change.
Source. Mufson et al. 2003; Sarter and Bruno 2004; Schleibs and Arendt 2006.

loss; however, neuron numbers in MCI and early dementia often overlap with normal numbers (Gilmor et al. 1999).

A plexus of cholinergic fibers is seen in the cerebral cortex (Mesulam et al. 1983), and immunocytochemical methodologies with antisera directed against nicotinic receptors demonstrate postsynaptic densities over neurons in layers 2, 3, and 5 of neocortex (Schroder et al. 1991). Cholinergic fibers are altered in elderly humans and old primates (Decker 1987), and cholinergic deficits in rodents, primates, and humans are correlated with cognitive impairment (Olton et al. 1991). The density of cholinergic receptors may change with aging; however, imaging and postmortem studies have yielded conflicting results. Most postmortem and imaging studies suggest an age-related reduction in the level of choline acetyltransferase.

Alterations may occur in both muscarinic and nicotinic receptor systems. Postmortem brain specimens from aging subjects demonstrate a 10%–30% reduction of muscarinic receptors in samples of cortex, hippocampus, and striatum, whereas other studies show little reduction (Norbury et al. 2005) (Table 2–7). Some variations in study results may relate to variability of ligands. Measurement of M_2 receptor avidity via distribution volume suggests an increase that may result from a lower concentration of acetylcholine in the synapse (Podruchny et al. 2003). The presence of *APOE*E4* genotype may further increase the likelihood of lower distribution volume (Cohen et al. 2003). In the thalamus, the density of nicotinic receptors decreases, but density of muscarinic receptors increases (Giacobini 1990, 1991). Nicotinic receptor binding is mildly reduced in neocortex with aging, but significant reductions occur in entorhinal cortex and presubiculum over age 40 (Court et al. 1997). In normal elderly subjects, the α_4 nicotinic receptor subunit appears stable, but the α_2 subunit is diminished (Tohgi et al. 1998b).

Noradrenergic Systems

Noradrenergic systems in human brain include an extensive network of fibers and receptors in neocortex, allocortex, selected diencephalic structures, and brain stem (Fallon and Loughlin 1987). In the human forebrain, noradrenaline is produced by the locus coeruleus, bilateral bands of neurons located immediately beneath the fourth ventricle in the pons that range in number from 11,000 to 25,000 (Ohm et al. 1997) (Figure 2–17). A variable mixture of α- and β-adrenergic receptors is present throughout the cerebral cortices (Mendelsohn and Paxinos 1991). Older conventional counting methodologies demonstrated a progressive loss of noradrenergic neurons throughout the aging human brain stem, commencing between ages 30 and 40 and progressing with a linear relationship to age (Mann et al. 1983, 1984) (see Table 2–7). In the locus coeruleus, conventional counting methods demonstrate that 40% of pigmented neurons are lost by age 90, and similar losses are sustained by the A-2 cell groups in the medulla (i.e., the dorsal motor nucleus of the vagus). More recent stereological estimates suggest smaller age-related loss of pigmented neurons (Ohm et al. 1997) in the locus coeruleus. These neurons contain occasional NFTs or abnormal collections of hyperphosphorylated tau, and such pathology is reported in 2%–5.6% of normal older subjects as opposed to 6.9%–18% of individuals with cognitive impairment (Grudzien et al. 2007). Noradrenergic neurites (i.e., abnormal, swollen processes that contain dopamine β-hydroxylase) are present in the neuropil and within senile plaques of elderly subjects (Powers et al. 1988), as well as

TABLE 2–7. Senescent changes of selected cholinergic and catecholaminergic markers usually present in aging human brain

Transmitter	Location of neurons producing transmitter age-related changes	Neuronal numbers	Receptor location	Alterations of receptor densities with aging
Acetylcholine	Nucleus basalis of Meynert	No change or decrease	Neocortex	Decrease in M_1 and M_2 Decrease in N
	Medial septal region	?	Hippocampus	Decrease in M_1, M_3, and M_4 Decrease in N
Serotonin	Raphe	?	Neocortex	Decrease in 5-HT_1 Decrease in 5-HT_2
Noradrenaline	Locus coeruleus	Decrease	Neocortex	Decrease in α-adrenergic Decrease in β-adrenergic
Dopamine	Substantia nigra	Decrease	Basal ganglia	Increase in postsynaptic D_1 Decrease in postsynaptic D_2

Note. ?=definitive data unavailable; 5-HT_1=serotonin subtype 1; 5-HT_2=serotonin, subtype 2; D_1=dopamine, subtype 1; D_2=dopamine, subtype 2; M_1=muscarinic, subtype 1; M_2=muscarinic, subtype 2; M_3=muscarinic, subtype 3; M_4=muscarinic, subtype 4; N=nicotinic.
Source. Court et al. 1997; Gottfries 1990; Hubble 1998; Mendelsohn and Paxinos 1991; Muller et al. 1991.

within the pineal gland (Jengeleski et al. 1989). Enzymatic activities are reduced for tyrosine hydroxylase, the rate-limiting enzyme in the production of dopamine and noradrenaline, as well as dopamine β-hydroxylase, the committed enzyme for the production of noradrenaline. Brain concentrations of methoxyhydroxylphenylglycol may remain constant in aging (Gottfries 1990), but CSF levels are increased.

Age-related loss of β-adrenergic receptors is region dependent. Receptor numbers remain constant in the frontal cortex (Kalaria et al. 1989); however, cingulate, precentral, temporal, and occipitotemporal regions demonstrate a linear age-dependent loss (Mendelsohn and Paxinos 1991).

Adrenergic receptors demonstrate a substantial decline in aging human brain (Pascual et al. 1992). Rodent studies also demonstrate age-related loss of adrenergic receptors in all regions except cortex, a phenomenon that is possibly a result of diminished receptor synthesis (Miller and Zahniser 1988; Scarpace and Abrass 1988). Pharmacological studies in rodent show a progressive age-dependent loss of postsynaptic response to noradrenaline and serotonin (Bickford-Wimer et al. 1988). This cumulative evidence suggests a gradual senescent loss of noradrenergic production and region-dependent loss of adrenergic receptors in human brain.

Serotonergic Systems

Serotonin is produced in the raphe nuclei, clusters of indistinct neurons in the midline of the midbrain and pons (Fallon and Loughlin 1987) (see Figure 2–17). Methodological problems limit quantitation of nonpigmented serotonergic neurons in human brain stem. Extensive serotonergic innervation is found in human neocortex, allocortex, and some diencephalic structures. Serotonin content is reduced in selected neocortical and allocortical regions of aging human brain (Gottfries 1990). Concentrations of 5-hydroxyindoleacetic acid, the primary metabolite of serotonin, are not reduced in brain or CSF in healthy elders. However, imipramine binding, a putative marker for serotonin reuptake, is reduced in aging. Activity of tryptophan hydroxylase, the synthetic enzyme for the production of serotonin, is reduced in the brains of aging rodents.

Multiple subtypes of serotonin (5-HT) receptors are described using autoradiographic or in situ hybridization methodology (Burnet et al. 1995), and the densities of 5-HT_1 and 5-HT_2 are reduced in brains of elderly humans. Postmortem autoradiograph studies suggest that 5-HT_{1B} is more abundant than 5-HT_{1D} (Varnas et al. 2001). The mRNAs for 5-HT_{1A} and 5-HT_{2A} are widely distributed in neocortex, but age-related changes are unclear. In aged brains, the density of 5-HT_2 receptors is reduced by 20%–50% of normal, and 5-HT_1 declines up to 70% (Mendelsohn and Paxinos 1991). In a study by Sheline et al. (2002), the age-related decline of 5-HT_{2A} binding was not linear and exhibited an average 17% loss from the third decade of life until the fifth decade, when the decline flattened. The density of 5-HT_{1A} receptors is diminished in aging (Dillon et al. 1991). Serotonin transporter ligand binding is reduced by 9.6% per decade in the thalamus and 10.5% in midbrain of aged humans (Yamamoto et al. 2002).

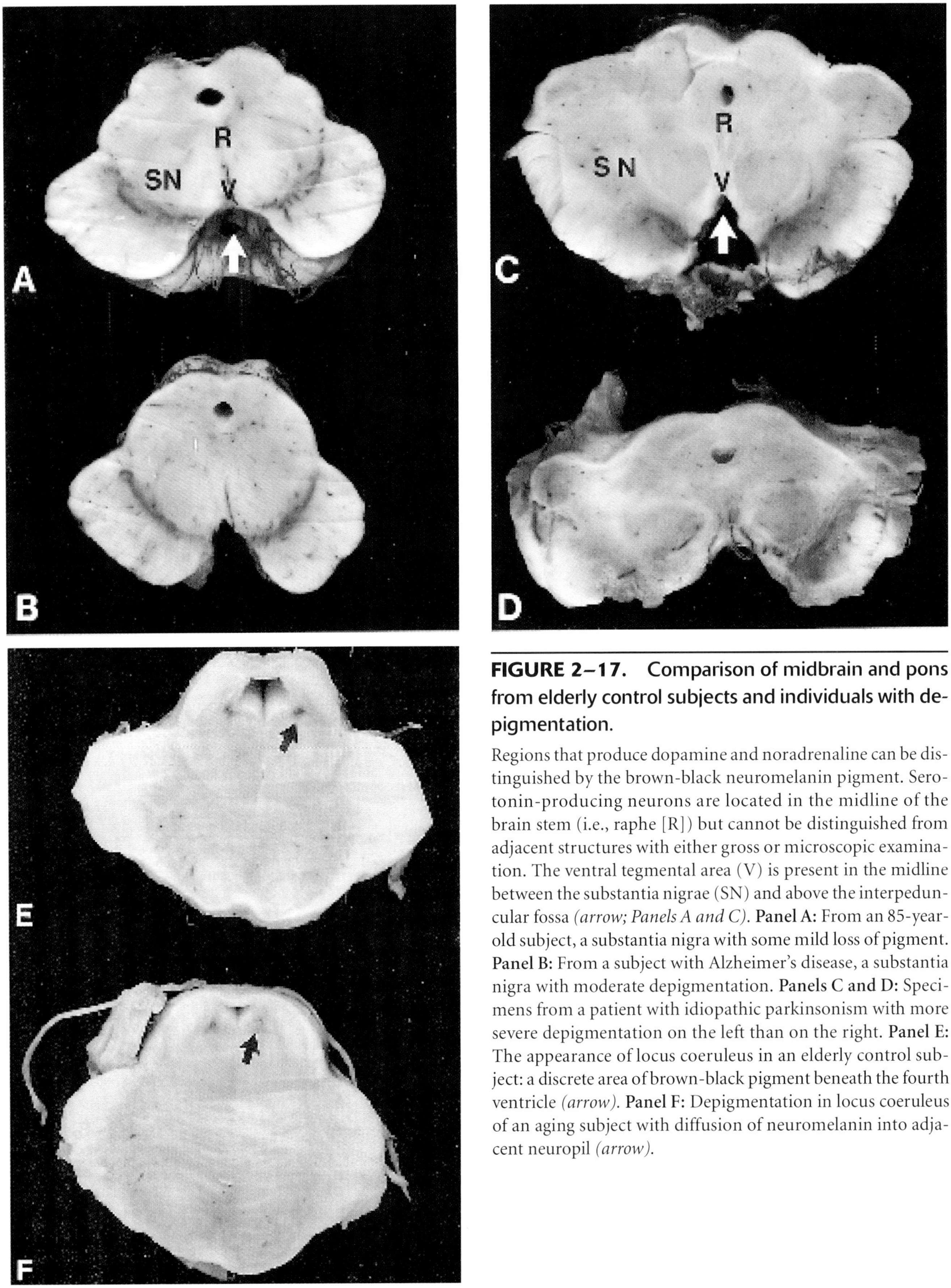

FIGURE 2–17. Comparison of midbrain and pons from elderly control subjects and individuals with depigmentation.

Regions that produce dopamine and noradrenaline can be distinguished by the brown-black neuromelanin pigment. Serotonin-producing neurons are located in the midline of the brain stem (i.e., raphe [R]) but cannot be distinguished from adjacent structures with either gross or microscopic examination. The ventral tegmental area (V) is present in the midline between the substantia nigrae (SN) and above the interpeduncular fossa *(arrow; Panels A and C)*. **Panel A:** From an 85-year-old subject, a substantia nigra with some mild loss of pigment. **Panel B:** From a subject with Alzheimer's disease, a substantia nigra with moderate depigmentation. **Panels C and D:** Specimens from a patient with idiopathic parkinsonism with more severe depigmentation on the left than on the right. **Panel E:** The appearance of locus coeruleus in an elderly control subject: a discrete area of brown-black pigment beneath the fourth ventricle *(arrow)*. **Panel F:** Depigmentation in locus coeruleus of an aging subject with diffusion of neuromelanin into adjacent neuropil *(arrow)*.

Depletion of neurons in the raphe nuclei would explain the decreased serotonin content but not the decreased serotonin receptor density. These limited data on serotonergic systems in human aging suggest a gradual loss of serotonin production and receptor densities, but the physiological effect of these changes is unclear.

Dopaminergic Systems

Dopamine is produced by neurons in the hypothalamus, brain stem, and spinal cord. Dopamine is the end product of a multistep enzymatic pathway for which tyrosine hydroxylase is the final step, although other catecholaminergic cells, such as those in the locus coeruleus, may also contain this enzyme. Dopaminergic axons project widely through cortex and basal ganglia. Dopaminergic innervation undergoes a complex sequence of events during development. Striatal dopamine as well as tyrosine hydroxylase levels increase by twofold to threefold in the postnatal through adolescent phases of brain development, after which time these markers begin to decline. Striatal dopamine transporter exhibits a similar increase but not a decline with aging (Haycock et al. 2003). These paradoxical findings suggest a senescent decrease in dopamine production rather than loss of the dopamine fiber plexus.

Dopaminergic systems are altered during aging and in many neurodegenerative disorders, including Alzheimer's disease, Parkinson's disease, and progressive supranuclear palsy. The brain stem neurons of the mesocortical and nigrostriatal dopaminergic pathways are well defined in human brain (see Figure 2–17). Although dopaminergic neurons are present in the human septal and hypothalamic regions (Gaspar et al. 1985), the tuberoinfundibular system is poorly defined in humans. The substantia nigra is a band of neurons that extend in the rostrocaudal axis from the hypothalamic-mesencephalic junction to the ponto-mesencephalic junction. This W-shaped tract of large, pigmented neurons sits astride the cerebral peduncles and contains the pars compacta and pars reticulata. The substantia nigrae contain a modest population of neurons that range in number from 400,000 pigmented cells in young individuals (Table 2–8) to estimates of about 32,000 pigmented neurons and 64,000 without neuromelanin (Cabello et al. 2002). Some pigmented neurons may not produce dopamine. The long, thinly myelinated axons from this mesencephalic structure project to frontal and temporal cortices, as well as diencephalic structures, via deep white matter pathways. The estimation of neuronal counts in the substantia nigra depends on whether the measurement includes 1) all neurons, 2) neuromelanin-containing neurons, or 3) tyrosine hydroxylase–labeled neurons. The outcome of cell counts depends on the methodology for measurement, the level at which brain stem counts were performed, and the neuronal labeling technique. At least eight human studies have been published using stereological techniques that minimize sampling errors. The significant subject-to-subject variation in the numbers of pigmented neurons reduces the ability to detect subtle age-related changes. The historic estimate of neuronal loss in the substantia nigra has been about 10% per decade after age 20, suggesting a very severe loss with advanced aging, but more recent studies report less decline (Stark and Pakkenberg 2004). Other markers, such as the concentration of dopamine transporter protein and some dopaminergic receptors, have averaged about 6%–8% decline per decade in the same time frame. Microglial proliferation in this region is well documented, suggesting reaction to age-related cell loss. Other reports suggest a more subtle neuronal loss than previously described, and several studies suggest that remaining neurons exhibit evidence of hypertrophy (Cabello et al. 2002). The estimates for cortical and subcortical dopamine loss with aging range from 0% to 10% per decade, and this projected loss would predict motor symptoms in persons over age 110 regardless of disease state (Rollo 2009). The age-related decline in numbers of pigmented cells in middle-age or older individuals versus younger subjects is depicted in Table 2–8. Contrasting numbers for individuals with Parkinson's disease that was symptomatic for 7–20 years demonstrate the dramatic loss associated with disease (Rudow et al. 2008). The age-related decline of dopamine presynaptic and postsynaptic markers ranges from 4% to 10% in persons over age 20. Nucleolar volume of substantia nigra neurons is reduced after age 65, and NFTs or Lewy bodies begin to appear in small numbers in older subjects (Mann et al. 1984). Cytochrome *c* oxidase defects indicate an alteration of the respiratory chain function within nigral neurons (Itoh et al. 1996). Relatively few extrapyramidal symptoms are produced by senescent decline because 80% of nigral neurons are usually lost before the onset of symptoms of parkinsonism.

Age-related loss of neurons in the ventral tegmental area has not been determined. Surviving catecholaminergic neurons progressively accumulate neuromelanin (Graham 1979), which displaces perikaryal RNA and reduces nucleolar volume (McGeer et al. 1977). Senescent alterations of dopamine-producing neurons in hypothalamus are unknown. Concentrations of dopamine are reduced in the striatum of individuals over age 65; however, homovanillic acid, the primary dopamine metabolite, remains constant in tissue and CSF (Gottfries 1990; Hartikainen et al. 1991).

Immunocytochemical and receptor autoradiographic studies show an extensive plexus of dopaminergic fibers, terminals, and receptors in frontal, temporal, hippocampal, and parahippocampal cortices as well as basal ganglia. In aging, the density of the dopamine D_2 receptor that binds haloperidol in caudate nucleus declines about 1% per year after age 18 (Wong et al. 1997) and 0.6% per year over age 30 for ^{11}C-raclopride binding in putamen (Antonio et al. 1993). The level of dopa-

TABLE 2–8. Changes in brain weight and neuronal numbers in substantia nigra in postmortem specimens from neurologically intact subjects compared with subjects with clinical manifestations of Parkinson's disease

Group	Mean age (years)	Brain weight (g)	Pigmented neurons (number)
Normal			
Young	19.9	1,571	423,796
Middle age	50.1	1,430	378,313
Old	87.6	1,323	304,540
Parkinson's disease	74.8	1,249	83,158

Source. Rudow et al. 2008.

mine transporter content also declines in basal ganglia during normal aging (Volkow et al. 1994). D_1 receptor binding declines 6.9% per decade in the caudate and 7.4% per decade in the putamen (Wong et al. 1997). Similar D_1 reductions are also described in the frontal and occipital cortex (Hubble 1998). Women exhibit a decline of D_2 receptors similar to that of males, with a 12% decline per decade in the frontal lobe, 9% per decade in the temporal lobe, and 6% per decade in the thalamus. Decline in the frontal lobe may plateau in midlife, and the changes appear unrelated to estrogen and progesterone levels (Kaasinen et al. 2002).

Postmortem studies demonstrate diminished expression of mRNA for D_2 receptors in putamen with no alteration of D_1 mRNA levels (Tohgi et al. 1998a); these alterations might result from senescent loss of neurons in the basal ganglia. This decline of striatal dopaminergic activity is associated with loss of fine motor functions and impaired neuropsychological performance, for example, in the Wisconsin Card Sorting Test (Heaton 1985) or Stroop Color-Word Test (Stroop 1935; Volkow et al. 1998).

Monoamine oxidase (MAO) activity is significantly altered in the aging human brain. MAO-A, which facilitates the oxidative deamination of noradrenaline, serotonin, and partially dopamine, is not drastically altered in aging. MAO-B, which catalyzes the oxidative deamination of several amines and partially dopamine, increases with age (Fowler et al. 1997; Gottfries 1990). The importance of these age-related alterations is unclear, although increased quantities of this catabolic enzyme may result in depletion of dopamine and other catecholamines.

Dopaminergic neurons in the substantia nigra of normal older individuals begin to exhibit synuclein pathology in late middle age. The data on neuronal loss, receptor changes, and histopathology suggest a slow incremental decline of dopaminergic systems in aged human brain, with the slow accumulation of neuronal micropathology and secondary inflammatory response.

Aging primates demonstrate neuronal loss in the substantia nigra, where the number of tyrosine hydroxylase–labeled neurons dropped from 110,000 in rhesus monkeys ages 3–5 to 55,000 in aged animals (Stark and Pakkenberg 2004). Compared with humans, aged primates do not seem to develop the range of histopathology seen in dopaminergic neuronal systems, such as Lewy bodies.

Glutamatergic Systems

Glutamate is a major excitatory neurotransmitter in the human brain. Glutamate interacts with a range of neurotrophic factors to regulate neurogenesis, neurite growth, synaptogenesis, and synaptic plasticity. The human brain contains two major types of ionotropic glutamate receptors that are widely distributed in the CNS. These receptors can alter sodium or calcium fluxes as well as signal transduction. These systems can produce rapid dendritic changes in membrane excitability, cytoskeletal architecture, and transcriptional changes for genes involved with neural plasticity (Mattsson 2008). Age-related reductions of glutamate have been reported in motor cortex, parietal cortex, and basal ganglia; however, glutamate levels may be increased in white matter (Kaiser et al. 2005).

Other Transmitter Systems

Histamine 2-(4-imidazole) ethylamine is produced by a range of cell lines, including gastric, immune, and neural. Histaminergic innervation originates from hypothalamic neurons that project to neocortex and limbic structures (Higuchi et al. 2000). CNS histamine is involved with wakefulness, appetite control, emotion, memory, and learning. Some differences exist between receptor distributions based on positron emission tomographic imaging versus postmortem histaminic H_1 densities (Mochizuki et al. 2004). Histamine release affects blood vessel tone and is implicated in atherosclerosis (Tanimoto et al. 2006). Limited human data suggest reduced brain binding in aging and Alzheimer's disease. Although the histaminergic system is extensively distributed in human brain, relatively little is known about the neurobiology and neuropathology of aging histaminergic systems.

Wide arrays of neuropeptides function as neuromodulators and colocalize with other classical transmitters such as noradrenaline and serotonin. Corticotropin-releasing factor is diminished in aging; however, other more abundant peptides, such as somatostatin and neuropeptide Y, are not reduced (Giaquinto 1988; Gottfries 1990). Age-related alterations of precursor proteins for substance P and enkephalin suggest a preferential loss of neurons in putamen that produce GABA and substance P (Tohgi et al. 1997). The binding protein for the neurokinin-1 receptor that binds substance P is reduced an average of 7% per decade in cortex and mesial temporal lobe in normal older subjects (Nyman et al. 2007). The neuronal levels of mRNA for prodynorphin and proenkephalin are reduced in putamen during aging; however, the level of mRNA for the 67-kDa isoform of glutamic acid decarboxylase (GAD67) is unchanged with aging (Backman et al. 2007).

Hypocretin, which comes from the combination of hypothalamus and secretin, regulates sleep, alertness, energy, and pleasure. This peptide, also called orexin, modulates multiple endocrine systems and may be deficient in narcolepsy (Ganjavi and Shapiro 2007). Serum levels may increase with aging, but morphological changes are not described in human brain.

Various neuropeptides are present in dystrophic neurites and senile plaques of elderly subjects; these neuropeptides include somatostatin, neuropeptide Y, and corticotropin-releasing factor (Struble et al. 1987). CSF contents of somatostatin and endorphin are not changed in elderly humans (Hartikainen et al. 1991). Studies in aging rodents show no loss of enkephalinergic receptors or diminished receptor affinity (Ueno et al. 1988). The density of orexin fibers in locus coeruleus is reduced in aged macaques and cats (Downs et al. 2007; Zhang et al. 2002).

Trophic Factors

Trophic factors are substances produced by neurons or glia that maintain or promote the growth and integrity of cell populations. Neurotrophins are molecular mediators that may significantly control brain plasticity and mediate brain repair of specific types of neuronal injuries. NGF was one of the first neurotrophins to be discovered. These molecules bind to two classes of receptors, the common p75NTR, which is a member of the tumor necrosis factor receptor family, and the tropomyosin-related kinase receptor family (Trk), which includes at least three receptors. Most neurotrophins can bind to the p75NTR receptor family, but Trk receptor binding is more selective. In mammalian brain, TrkA is expressed by cholinergic neurons in the basal forebrain, and TrkB and TrkC are present in hippocampus. Synthesis of these substances can be regulated by specific transmitter systems such as glutamate (Thoenen et al. 1991). Many molecules qualify as neurotrophins, including NGF, brain-derived neurotrophic factor (BDNF), neurotrophin-3, and neurotrophin-4 (Fuxe and Agnati 1992). Glial cell line–derived neurotrophic factor (GDNF) is produced from glial cells and affects neurons (Gash et al. 1998).

NGF comprises three subunits: alpha, beta, and gamma. Biological activity appears to be present in the beta subunit. This peptide promotes neurite extension and stimulates the activity of tyrosine hydroxylase and dopamine β-hydroxylase (Fuxe and Agnati 1992). NGF is essential to the normal development and maintenance of cholinergic neurons. Administration of NGF to aging rodents was found to reverse the age-related dendritic spine loss of cortical pyramidal neurons (Mervis et al. 1991).

At the cellular level, NGF may increase the degradation of superoxide radicals and hydrogen peroxides. Human data suggest an age-related reduction in the synthesis of NGF (Hefti and Mash 1989). NGF protects damaged cholinergic forebrain neurons in monkeys, and a similar protective role is postulated for human neurons.

IGF-1, which has a structure and amino acid identity similar to that of insulin, is a second important trophic factor. IGF-1 is secreted primarily by the liver under the control of pituitary growth hormone. The brain can also secrete this protein, but this production may not be controlled by growth hormone. The level of circulating IGF-1 may decrease with aging; however, brain IGF-1 remains constant or may increase slightly (Puglielli 2008). IGF-1 can mimic insulin in the brain and exert a broad range of cellular influences through signal transduction. This pathway may be involved with the pathogenesis of Alzheimer's disease and aging. IGF-1, platelet-derived growth factor, and fibroblast growth factor affect the production of neurites, development of glia, and regulation of nigrostriatal neurons in nonhuman models.

GDNF is one of many molecules that promote recovery of damaged neurons. GDNF has distinct neuronal receptors and activity on dopaminergic neurons. Infusion of GDNF into rhesus monkey increases dopaminergic neuronal size and neurite extent (Gash et al. 1998). Growth factors such as GDNF can arrest or reverse some of the atrophic changes in aging rodent brain and are a focus of pharmacological research for neurodegenerative diseases such as Alzheimer's disease or Parkinson's disease.

BDNF is an important neurotrophin, and its receptor TrkB is highly expressed in regions with high levels of plasticity such as the cortex, hypothalamus, and hippocampus (Tapia-Arancibia et al. 2008). Circulating BDNF is mostly derived from platelets. Serum BDNF and NGF levels are not evenly distributed in the population, with some individuals exhibiting quite high levels. At low nanomolar concentrations, BDNF may excite some neurons as a "classic" excitatory transmitter such as glutamate through activation of the sodium channels when expressed with the TrkB receptor. BDNF can also act as a classic neuromodulator and a promoter of neurogenesis. BDNF may affect long-term potentiation through regulation of dendritic mRNA production. In rodent models, dietary restriction and exercise may promote release of this molecule.

Age-related changes in humans have been described for serum and brain levels of neurotrophins. BDNF and TrkB mRNA probably decline with age, as does NGF, but studies show substantial person-to-person variability in serum levels (Tapia-Arancibia et al. 2008).

Numerous trophic factors are described in the human brain. The central and peripheral levels of some of these molecules are reduced in human aging and in Alzheimer's disease (Tapia-Arancibia et al. 2008). Some trophins such as BDNF may exert a protective influence against β-amyloid, and loss of the neurotrophin may enhance the toxicity of amyloid. This class of molecules provides a valuable pharmacological target for future therapeutic interventions for aging and age-related diseases.

Neuroendocrinology of Aging

Senescent endocrinological changes of the pancreas, thyroid, and ovary produce significant direct or secondary brain alterations (Epelbaum 2008) (Table 2–9). Multiple other endocrine systems develop important age-related alterations mediated by changes in the hypothalamic-pituitary axis. The human hypothalamus consists of multiple nuclei adjacent to the third ventricle (see Figure 2–3). The hypothalamus receives noradrenergic, serotonergic, and cholinergic innervation (Mendelsohn and Paxinos 1991), affecting control of many pituitary-releasing factors. These small clusters of neurons control the pituitary gland via direct neuronal input or via factors released into the hypophyseal portal system. The pituitary gland is a small collection of cells in the sella turcica and is divided into anterior and posterior lobes. The anterior pituitary secretes multiple hormones, such as growth hormone and thyroid-stimulating hormone (TSH), whereas the posterior pituitary secretes oxytocin and vasopressin. Hypothalamic control of neuroendocrine functions is regulated by catecholaminergic inputs that influence the release of inhibiting factors.

Aging humans undergo a series of senescent sexual and neuroendocrinological alterations (Rance et al. 1993). Circulating gonadotropins and hypothalamic nuclei manifest age-dependent, gender-specific alterations. Senescent hypothalamic neurons can atrophy, hypertrophy, or remain constant.

The sexually dimorphic nucleus and the preoptic area of the human hypothalamus contain neurons whose density and size are gender specific (Hofman and Swaab 1989). These neurons undergo a series of orderly, predictable changes with age. Sexually dimorphic structures have a sex-dependent pattern of growth and decay (Hofman and Swaab 1989). In old subjects (ages 70–90 years) compared with young control subjects (ages 20–30 years), males have a 43% reduction and females have a 62% reduction of the volume of the sexually dimorphic nucleus-preoptic area.

Menopause occurs in most women around age 50 and includes many physiological and psychological alterations. Menopause is caused by disruption of the gonadal-hypothalamic-pituitary cycle through loss of cyclical ovarian estrogen production (Lamberts et al. 1997; Rance 1992). The number of human ova peaks in utero at mid-gestation (7 million) and is 1 million at birth. This number falls to 400,000 at menarche. This gradual ovarian attrition from ages 20 to 50 ends in ovarian follicles being unresponsive to gonadotropins. Levels of serum follicle-stimulating hormone and luteinizing hormone rise as levels of serum estrogens fall (Evans and Williams 1992; Hazzard et al. 1990). Estrogen probably retards atherosclerotic heart disease and osteoporosis. Estrogen withdrawal during menopause occurs concurrently with other age-related changes that produce a net reduction of 5%–15% of bone mass, with 80% coming from trabecular bone (Chahal and Drake 2007).

The potential neural protective mechanisms of estrogen are unclear, although this hormone may interact with NGF and may be neuroprotective for hippocampal neurons. Rodents retain a more "youthful" hippocampal synaptic phenotype when fed estrogen following oophorectomy (Adams and Morrison 2003). Gene expression during menopause for "proneurotoxic" markers, such as estrogen, glucocorticoid, and interleukin-6 receptors, suggests a potential shift in the "biological milieu" that might increase risk for neurodegeneration (Bonomo et al. 2009). Estrogen replacement for postmenopausal women may increase risk for breast or endometrial cancer. Selected populations of postmenopausal women may be considered for estrogen replacement, weighing the modest risk of thrombotic disease, malignancy, or hysterectomy against risk of heart disease, osteoporosis, and dementia.

The cyclical nature of the menstrual cycle may be partially driven by neurons in the anterior hypothalamus, which receive a variety of catecholaminergic inputs (Wise et al. 1987). Rodent studies have indicated that the release of luteinizing hormone is influenced by noradrenergic, serotonergic, dopaminergic, and peptidergic inputs. In postmenopausal senescent women, some hypothalamic nuclei hypertrophy to include marked increase in the diameter of infundibular neurons expressing estrogen receptors (Rance et al. 1990) and increased tachykinin message in selected hypothalamic nuclei (Rance and Young 1991). Infundibular neurons expressing kisspeptin transcripts in postmenopausal women increase in

TABLE 2–9. Endocrinology of aging

System	Primary abnormality	Clinical consequence	Effective therapy
Pituitary gland			
Pituopause	↓ GH ↓ LH ↓ FSH	↑ Frailty	Unclear
Thyroid gland			
Thyropause	↓ T_3/T_4	↑ TSH Subclinical hypothyroidism	Yes
Male gonad			
Andropause	↓ Testosterone	Unclear	Unclear
Female gonad			
Menopause	↓ Estrogen	Osteoporosis Atherosclerosis	Yes
Adrenal gland			
Adrenopause	↓ DHEA ↓ DHEAS ↓↑ Cortisol	↑ Frailty	Unclear
Pancreas			
Pancreopause	↓ Insulin	Diabetes mellitus	Yes

Note. Values represent consensus opinions from multiple sources. Therapy indicates treatments that are available, effective, and cost efficient. DHEA=dehydroepiandrosterone; DHEAS=dehydroepiandrosterone sulfate; FSH=follicle-stimulating hormone; GH=growth hormone; LH=luteinizing hormone; T_3/T_4=triiodothyronine/tetraiodothyronine; TSH=thyroid-stimulating hormone.

size (Rometo et al. 2007). The intensity of neuropeptide Y gene expression in retrochiasmatic and infundibular neurons increases while those expressing pro-opiomelanocortin are reduced (Escobar et al. 2004). Vasomotor symptoms of menopause may result from shifts in the hypothalamic thermoregulatory system produced by dysregulation of serotonin and 5-HT_{2A} receptors that result from loss of estrogen (Chahal and Drake 2007). Animal models suggest that some of these changes are directly linked to hormonal alterations, whereas others seem unrelated to neuroendocrine influences.

The senescent changes of gonadotropic nuclei that provoke the decline of sexual function in elderly men are poorly defined. The male sexually dimorphic nucleus is reduced in size with aging. Testosterone levels fall after age 50, and more than 60% of older men have levels below those of younger men (Lamberts et al. 1997), thus producing "andropause." Unlike menopause in women, older males demonstrate significant variability in the age at onset, severity of loss, and effect of reduced testosterone (Chahal and Drake 2007). The number of testicular Leydig cells is reduced in older men, and the age-related reduction of testosterone levels appears to be the result of reduced production of the hormone. The physiological significance of low testosterone on sexual function, muscle bulk, and mood is unclear. Peripheral levels of sex hormones may be related to the number of NFTs and vascular brain pathology but not to amyloid deposition, as measured in a postmortem study of a community sample of older men (Strozyk et al. 2007). The preventive use of exogenous testosterone by healthy older men is limited by questions of efficacy and by concerns over the hormone's potential hypertrophic effect on the prostate gland (Rowe and Kahn 1998).

The function of the hypothalamic-pituitary-adrenal (HPA) axis has been extensively described in elderly patients, producing the concept of "adrenopause" (Lamberts et al. 1997) (see Table 2–9). Basal levels of plasma cortisol may increase with age, but the reactivity of the axis as determined by suppression with oral dexamethasone is unchanged (Hazzard et al. 1990; Veith and Raskind 1988). The pattern of cortisol secretion varies significantly in elders, but the secretion of adrenocorticotropic hormone remains relatively stable (Lupien et al. 1996). Between ages 20 and 80 years, there may be a 20%–50% increase in 24-hour mean cortisol levels, and the evening nadir may be higher and occur earlier (Chahal and Drake 2007).

The role of stress and dysregulation of the HPA axis on the neurobiology of aging is unclear. Glucocorticoids are important to brain maturation through action on dendrites and axons. Stress provoked by a perceived threat can initiate autonomic, neuroendocrinic, metabolic, and immune responses that may affect development, function, and neuronal survival (Lupien et al. 2009). Glucocorticoid receptors are located in the hippocampus and frontal cortex as well as other cortical regions. Postmortem studies in tissue from human frontal cortex demonstrate an inverted U-shaped effect of glucocorticoids on axonal transport (Lupien et al. 2009). Glucocorticoids and their receptors in the brain change during development. High levels of receptor mRNA are present during adolescence, with reduction in older humans (Perlman et al. 2007). Excess steroid is associated with reduction of hippocampal volume in humans, as well as with reduction of neurogenesis in rodents and primates. The impact of perinatal and early life stress on the aging trajectory is unknown; however, physiological stressors are known to increase risk for age-associated diseases such as diabetes and hypertension (Kajantie 2008). Gender-specific impact is unknown, although some studies suggest a greater risk for women (Wolf and Kudielka 2008).

Another important adrenal hormone is dehydroepiandrosterone (DHEA) and its sulfate, DHEAS. This steroid is 10 times more abundant than cortisol, and the age-related decline of DHEA/DHEAS levels is associated with loss of physical and functional ability. These precursor steroids are transformed into active androgens or estrogens in peripheral target tissue. Plasma DHEA levels peak at age 20 and decline with age, resulting in levels at 70% of normal around age 60 and 20% of normal at age 85. In older men, lower DHEA levels are associated with higher mortality rates at 2 and 4 years following assessment (Berr et al. 1996). A series of studies on the benefit of DHEA replacement for age-related disorders has yielded little compelling data to recommend the use of replacement therapy (Chahal and Drake 2007). The effect of calorie restriction on DHEA secretion in humans is unclear, although restrictions in monkeys will diminish the expected age-related loss from 30% to 3% (Redman and Ravussin 2009).

Growth hormone is released from the pituitary gland in pulses that remain constant during aging; however, the pulse amplitude and hormone secretion are diminished (see Table 2–9). The somatotropic system performs anabolic and lipolytic functions. The age-related fall in circulating growth hormone causes the liver and other organs to reduce production of IGF-1. Noradrenaline affects the release of growth hormone via control of growth hormone–releasing factor and somatostatin. Growth hormone secretion is increased by adrenergic and dopaminergic receptor activation and inhibited by adrenergic stimulation. The peak of growth hormone secretion occurs in adolescence, followed by a progressive decline over years. Growth hormone production and circulating IGF-1 secretion may be reduced by more than 50% in healthy older individuals (Wise et al. 1987).

Studies have shown that growth hormone injection in older humans produces a short-term increase of lean body mass (8.8%), skin thickness (7.1%), and bone density, while lowering adipose tissue mass (14.4%) (Rudman et al. 1990); however, these improvements may diminish after 12 months. Growth hormone replacement is expensive, and its potential side effects limit the usefulness of this therapeutic modality (Schoen 1991). Functional ability may not improve for older individuals with growth hormone supplements, and replacement therapy is not recommended for elderly patients (Feller et al. 1997; Papadakis et al. 1996; Rowe and Kahn 1998). Calorie restriction does not appear to alter secretion or levels of either growth hormone or IGF-1 despite weight loss, reduction of visceral fat, and improvement of insulin sensitivity (Redman and Ravussin 2009).

Abnormalities of thyroid function are common in elderly patients (see Table 2–9). Between 4% and 12% of individuals over age 60 may have chemical hypothyroidism. Progressive but subtle age-related changes occur in levels of thyroxine (T_4) and TSH, but the net effect is considered minimal in the majority of older individuals. Reductions in the levels of thyroid hormone secretion are counterbalanced by reduction in the hormone's clearance. Serum total and free triiodothyronine (T_3) concentrations are reduced in aging, but this alteration may result from peripheral conversion of T_4 to T_3 (Chahal and Drake 2007). Calorie restriction appears to reduce serum T_3 levels, but T_4 and TSH may remain unchanged (Redman and Ravussin 2009).

Models of Aging: Hippocampal Alterations and Synucleinopathies in Ascending Pathways

Age-related changes in two important brain systems define the complex changes seen with senescence and the problems with defining normal aging from age-related disease. The hippocampus is a discrete neural system that is critical to memory. The function of this mesial temporal structure is affected by multiple age-related pathologies, and this system is susceptible to tau-, amyloid-, and synuclein-based pathology. The ascending catecholaminergic system is important to motor and cognitive function. These neurons are susceptible to pathologies produced by alterations in the metabolic pathways for tau or synuclein and provide an excellent model for alteration in projection systems. The hippocampus receives inputs from the locus coeruleus and the raphe that are critical to proper function. Hence, these functionally and anatomically distinct circuits are interrelated and interdependent.

Normal Intrinsic Hippocampal Connections

The hippocampus is frequently studied because most mammalian species have hippocampi with well-defined neuronal population, consistent morphology, and similar connectivity (Rosene and Van Hoesen 1986). The hippocampus is the center of a series of interconnected structures and neural circuits often referred to as the *limbic lobes* (Figure 2–18).

The hippocampus is an allocortical structure (i.e., three-layered cortex), and adjacent parahippocampal cortex is neocortex (i.e., six-layered cortex). The entorhinal cortex is a five-layered transitional cortex situated between these two cortical regions. These structures are usually altered in human aging and damaged in neurodevelopmental as well as neurodegenerative diseases (Braak and Braak 1991; Powers 1999).

The hippocampus, entorhinal cortex, and associated parahippocampal cortices form a jelly roll–shaped structure that spans 3.5 cm of the bilateral mesial temporal lobes (Figures 2–18 and 2–19). The hippocampal formation is important for short-term memory, and transmission through this allocortical structure proceeds in an orderly fashion. Afferent inputs originate from layer II of entorhinal cortex and synapse on dendrites of granule cells in the molecular layer of the dentate gyrus. Transmission proceeds to the CA4–CA3 region via mossy fibers and then to the CA1 subiculum via axons termed the *Schaffer collaterals.* Information is relayed out to the deeper layers of the entorhinal cortex (i.e., layer IV) and to neocortical regions such as the temporal lobe. Important basal forebrain cholinergic inputs project to the dentate gyrus (Decker 1987) and synapse on the dendrites of granule cells in the molecular layer (Rosene and Van Hoesen 1986). Noradrenergic and serotonergic fibers project onto dendrites of neurons located in the CA4–CA1 region (Powers et al. 1988; Rosene and Van Hoesen 1986). Adrenergic and serotonergic receptors are present in hippocampus, and rodent studies show that these catecholamines will facilitate or synchronize hippocampal transmission (Rosene and Van Hoesen 1986). A pool of neuronal progenitor cells is located along the margin between the dentate gyrus and the CA4 region; however, these neurons are morphologically indistinguishable from other granule cells. Molecular markers are required to identify those neurons with stem cell potential.

GABAergic and peptidergic neurons are present in CA4 and provide inhibitory transmission. Proper hippocampal

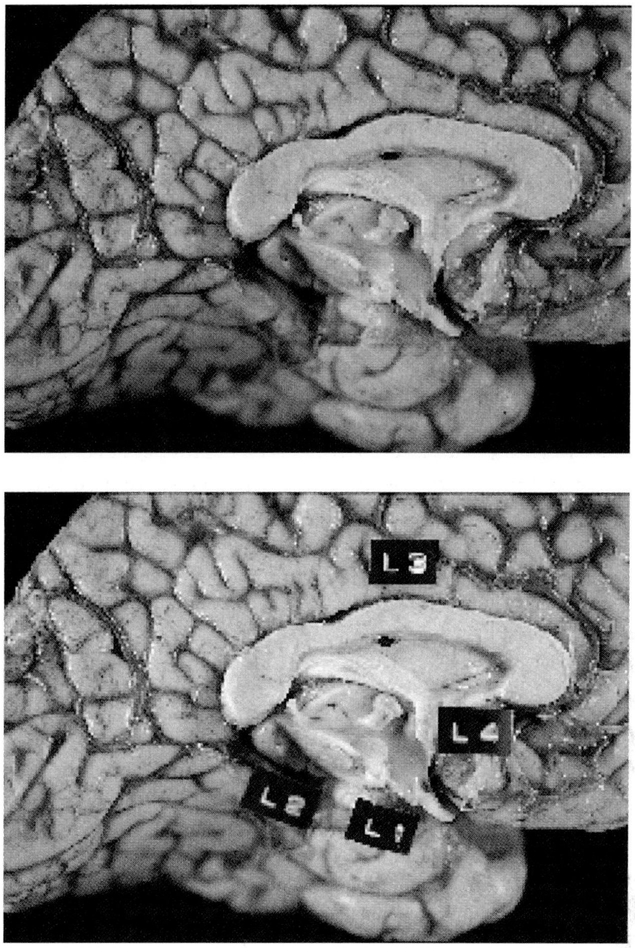

FIGURE 2–18. The limbic lobe is a system of interconnected structures including temporal lobe (L1 and L2), cingulate gyrus (L3), and basal forebrain (L4). This midsagittal section of brain demonstrates corpus callosum and mesial temporal lobe structures visualized after removal of brain stem. Four major components of the limbic system include amygdala and associated uncinate cortices, hippocampus and parahippocampal cortices, cingulate gyrus, and hypothalamus where the fornix enters the mammillary bodies. The hippocampus courses lateral to the mesial temporal cortex (L1 and L2), spanning approximately 3.5 cm of the temporal lobe, and swings around the splenium of the corpus callosum. Entorhinal cortex spreads over the uncinate gyrus at the level of rostral hippocampus (L1) and tapers down to a narrow band of cells in mid-level hippocampus (L2).

function depends on a balance of these excitatory, inhibitory, and neuromodulatory transmitters. Pharmacological and environmental factors may influence neuronal reproduction and synaptic plasticity.

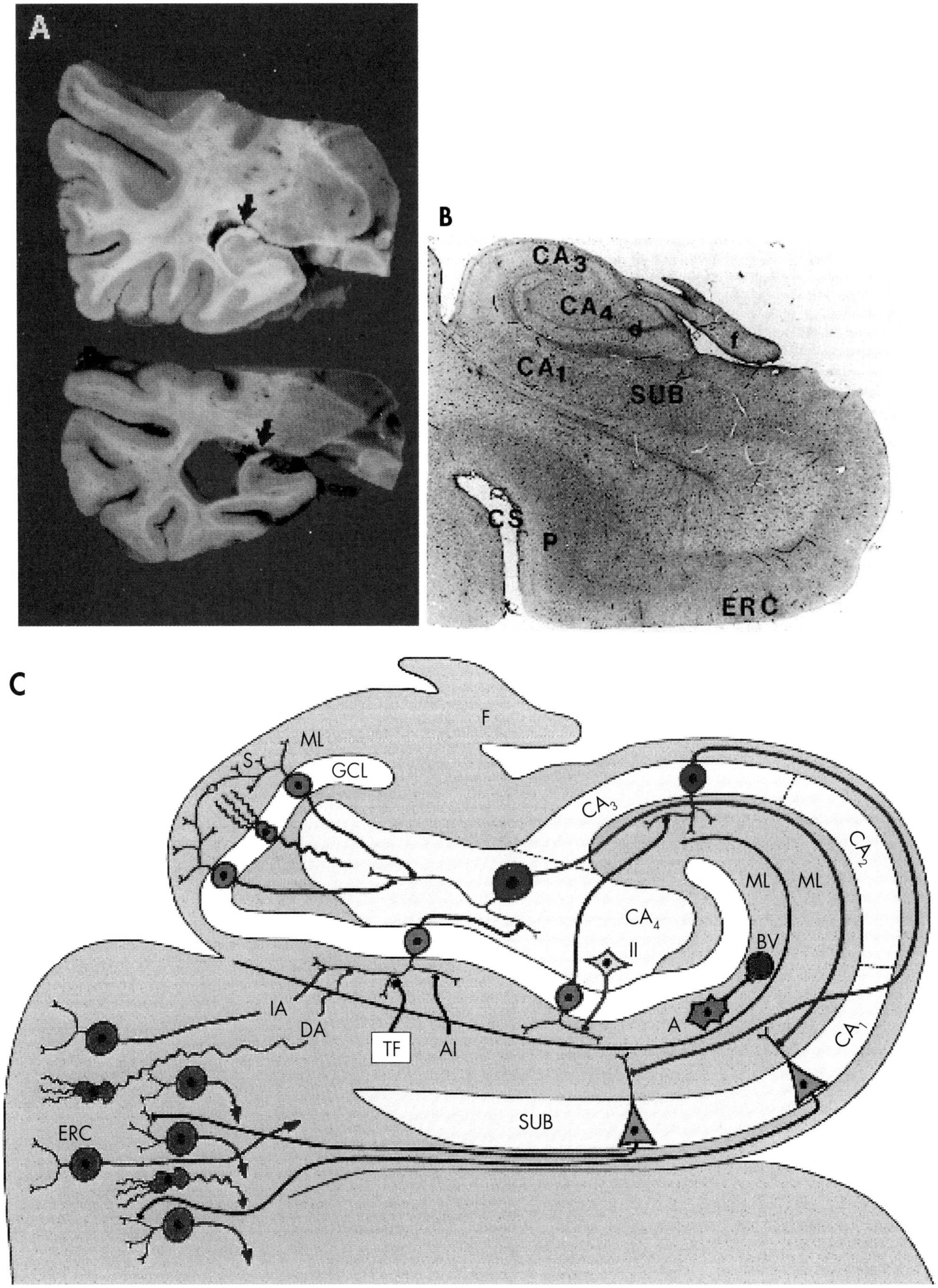
A
B
CA_3
CA_4
d
f
CA_1
SUB
CS
P
ERC
C
F
ML
S
GCL
CA_3
CA_2
ML
ML
CA_4
II
BV
A
CA_1
IA
DA
TF
AI
SUB
ERC

FIGURE 2–19. Gross and microscopic appearance of hippocampus from elderly control subjects and an individual with Alzheimer's disease.

A schematic drawing depicts hippocampal neuronal pathways. **Panel A:** Coronal hippocampal sections are dissected from the midsegment of mesial temporal lobe. Comparison of temporal lobes and hippocampi *(arrows)* from an elderly control subject (**upper**) and a subject with Alzheimer's disease (**lower**). A normal hippocampus and inferior horn of lateral ventricle are seen in the control subject. The subject with Alzheimer's disease has atrophy of the hippocampus, widening of the collateral sulcus, and ventriculomegaly. **Panel B:** A low-magnification photomicrograph of a normal hippocampus stained with cresyl violet. Important anatomical regions include dentate gyrus (d), cornu ammonis (Ammon's horn [CA4 through CA1]), subiculum (SUB), entorhinal cortex (ERC), parahippocampal cortex (P) beside the collateral sulcus (CS), and fimbria (F). This hippocampus is depicted in *Panel C.* The granule cell layer is part of the dentate gyrus. Boundaries between the four fields CA4 through CA1 are determined by microscopic examination. **Panel C:** Schematic drawing of hippocampus depicting the complicated neuronal interactions in a typical 65-year-old human. Inputs from ERC neurons synapse on granule cell dendrites in the molecular layer (ML) of the dentate (intact afferents). Axons (mossy fibers) from the granule cells (GCL) synapse on CA4 and CA3 neurons that project to CAl-subicular neurons via Schaffer collateral axons. Neurons in CA1 subiculum complete the loop with axons that synapse on neurons in ERC or temporal cortex. Each granule cell neuron is receiving many types of inputs from intact afferents (IA), damaged afferents (DA), and temporal cortices (e.g., from neurons in ERC); aminergic inputs (AI) from noradrenaline- or serotonin-producing neurons in brain stem; cholinergic inputs from basal forebrain neurons; trophic factors (TF) such as nerve growth factor; and inhibitory inputs (II) such as γ-aminobutyric acid. Age-related decrease or loss of each type of input can affect granule cell firing and synaptic density. The vacant dendritic fields of some damaged granule cells may be partially occupied by dendritic sprouting (S) from adjacent healthy granule cells. Age-related loss of neurons in CA1 region or subiculum (SUB) will eliminate targets for axons from CA3 neurons. Loss of neurons in deep layers of ERC will disrupt outflow from CA1-subicular neurons. Hippocampal neurons and astrocytes (A) also respond to alterations of blood-brain barrier resulting from vascular damage (BV) such as arteriolosclerosis.

Cellular Hippocampal Alterations During Normal Aging

The hippocampus provides an excellent system of interconnected neural circuits to illustrate the complexity of age-related changes. A range of neuronal alterations occurs in hippocampus of aging human brains. The Braak system of staging the histopathology of Alzheimer's disease conceptualizes the hippocampus as the starting point for amyloid- and tau-based pathologies (Braak and Braak 1991). Neuropathology appears first in the mesial temporal cortex and spreads into other limbic structures as well as sophisticated association cortices located in the frontal and temporal lobes. Neuronal damage in the entorhinal cortex correlates to symptoms of MCI, whereas hippocampal damage appears related to the amnestic symptoms of several types of dementia.

An age-related decline in volume and numbers of hippocampal neurons, particularly in CA1 and subiculum, has been confirmed by stereological techniques, which provide the most accurate assessments (West 1993). Early studies showed that the number of granule cell neurons in the dentate gyrus is reduced by 15% when comparing young with old subjects (Dam 1979). These small neurons provide a useful model for age-related changes. The dendritic tree of granule cells increases in humans ages 50–70 and declines in the very old (those over age 90) or those with Alzheimer's disease (Flood and Coleman 1988). This proliferation may reflect attempts by intact granule cell neurons to compensate for the senescent loss of neighboring neurons (Flood et al. 1985). Loss of inputs from neurons in entorhinal cortex results in sprouting by axons from other afferent neurons to fill the vacant synaptic fields. The release of neurotrophic factors may enhance dendritic growth and synaptogenesis (Mattsson et al. 2008). Collateral axons can develop from cholinergic neurons, intrinsic hippocampal neurons, and neurons of other temporal lobe areas (Geddes and Cotman 1991). Dendritic extent in the neighboring CA3–CA2 region shows no change with aging (see Figure 2–19, Panels B and C). Dendritic length of CA1 neurons also remains constant in normal aging but is significantly shortened in Alzheimer's disease (Hanks and Flood 1991). Loss of neurons may provoke gliosis (i.e., increased numbers of astrocytes with more conspicuous amounts of cytoplasm). Hippocampal neurons are sensitive to a range of metabolic insults, including hypoxia, hypoglycemia, and excitotoxic damage. For example, the hippocampus contains high densities of corticosteroid receptors. Elevation of adrenal steroids causes dendritic regression in rodents as well as suppression of neurogenesis and may damage hippocampal circuits in humans (McEwen 1998). Steroid sensitivity may provide a link between stress and structural brain alterations in some individuals. Hippocampal volume can be dependent on reproductive hormonal levels, as hippocampal gray matter can increase in postmenstrual women (Protopopescu et al. 2008).

The entorhinal cortex contains about 13 million neurons, about 1 million of which are located in layer II (West and Slomianka 1998). The number of these neurons remains stable with aging; however, some neurons begin to exhibit NFTs or argyrophilic grains after age 65. Stereological counts show that a loss of 40%–60% of neurons in the entorhinal cortex is required to produce the clinical symptoms of MCI, as opposed to 90% depletion required for severe dementia (Gomez-Isla et al. 1996). Selective injury to one group of neurons in the hippocampal circuit can disconnect the hippocampus and is one mechanism proposed in Alzheimer's disease (Hyman et al. 1984).

Theoretically, some damaged or apoptotic hippocampal neurons could be replaced through neurogenesis, although this process is not confirmed outside the dentate gyrus. Sophisticated molecular markers are required to identify progenitor cells in the human hippocampus, because these neurons lack distinctive microscopic features. The numbers of reproducing hippocampal neurons are reduced in aged rodents and primates. The migrational pattern of postmitotic neurons in aged primates appears to differ from that of younger animals. However, the phenotype of aging rodent progenitor cells appears stable (Aizawa et al. 2009; Hattiangady and Shetty 2008). Neuroproliferation does persist in Alzheimer's disease; however, generated neurons do not appear to mature (Li et al. 2008). BDNF may function as a mediator of environmental effects on neurogenesis, such as the increases produced by exercise, calorie restriction, and cognitive enhancement (Mattsson et al. 2008).

Cholinergic, serotonergic, and noradrenergic inputs can be lost as a result of damage to neurons in the basal forebrain (Decker 1987), raphe, or locus coeruleus. Intrinsic hippocampal neurons that employ excitatory amino acids can be damaged by NFTs, ischemic injury, or other disease processes. These processes, disturbing the inherent balance of excitatory and inhibitory transmission, also damage intrinsic inhibitory GABAergic and peptidergic neurons. While the process of neuronal injury and death proceeds, undamaged hippocampal neurons attempt reinnervation and reorganization.

Animal models have been helpful in defining therapeutic interventions that may alter age-related changes in the hippocampal circuit. Aged canines demonstrate a 30% reduction in the number of hilar neurons, but this loss can be improved by 18% with antioxidant therapy and environmental stimulation (Siwak-Tapp et al. 2008). A similar effect may be seen in humans, as demonstrated by findings that aerobic fitness is related to larger hippocampal volumes (Erickson et al. 2009).

In conclusion, the aging human hippocampus can be conceptualized as a dynamic structure that exhibits age-associated neuronal loss, neuronal plasticity, and limited regeneration. Dysfunction occurs when this dynamic balance is disrupted, neural reserve has been exhausted, or these events occur in conjunction with loss of critical innervations from ascending catecholaminergic, indolaminergic, or cholinergic systems.

Age-Related Changes of the Ascending Catecholaminergic Systems

Age-related changes occur in the ascending catecholaminergic and indolaminergic systems whose cell bodies are located in the brain stem and whose axons travel via discrete neural pathways through deep white matter structures to project onto cortical neurons. These brain stem neurons are susceptible to perikaryal damage that may produce abnormal collections of synuclein or tau, as well as to axonal damage caused by white matter ischemia. Parkinson's disease is a model of catecholaminergic and indolaminergic neural system degeneration that produces motor, cognitive, and psychiatric symptoms. As discussed earlier in "Dopaminergic Systems," catecholaminergic neurons undergo senescent changes that may contribute to some motor symptoms of aging.

Parkinson's disease can be defined as a synucleinopathy where synuclein accumulates in selected central and autonomic neuronal populations as classic Lewy bodies, cortical Lewy bodies, cytoplasmic aggregates, or dystrophic neuritis. The synuclein-based neuropathology of Parkinson's disease was proposed as a progression of disease that begins in distal neurons of the peripheral nervous system and spinal cord and progresses in a rostral direction toward the neocortex (Braak and Del Tredici 2008; Braak et al. 2003). The evolution of clinical symptoms parallels the pathological manifestations within the peripheral and central nervous systems. Early symptoms of bowel dysfunction, orthostasis, and reduced olfactory recognition mirror damage to the autonomic and olfactory centers. The Braak histopathological classification system for synucleinopathies incorporates clinical manifestations that range from subsyndromal changes through severe disability (Table 2–10). As for many proposed clinicopathological classification systems, other published research questions the universality of disease progression described by Braak. Some publications demonstrate that about half of Parkinson's disease cases conform to the Braak progression, whereas others have pathology limited to limbic and neocortical regions (Zaccai et al. 2008). Other studies showed that microscopic examination of brains from 30%–55% of elderly subjects in large unselected retrospective autopsy series exhibited changes consistent with Braak stage V or VI disease despite minimal neuropsychiatric symptoms (Jellinger 2008). The frequency of incidental Lewy bodies is rare in the brains of young subjects postmortem but rises in frequency to over one-third of individuals over age 90.

TABLE 2–10. Summary of clinicopathological correlations to synuclein-based changes in central nervous system of older human subjects according to the Braak system for staging Parkinson's disease

Braak pathology stage	Clinical phase	Commonly damaged brain regions	Typical MMSE scores	Common clinical symptoms	Potential transmitter alterations
I	Preclinical or early	Olfactory DMNV	NL	↓ Olfaction ↓ Constipation	Dopamine VIP (Auerbach neurons)
II		Medullary raphe Reticular system	NL	(?) Mood (?) Sleep	Serotonin
III	Midclinical	Pons NBM	25–30	Motor Variable cognitive	Acetylcholine Norepinephrine
IV			21–24		Dopamine Norepinephrine
V	Late or advanced symptoms	Prefrontal Limbic	11–20	Severe motor Variable cognitive Variable neuropsychiatric	Multiple
VI		↓ Neocortex	6–10		Multiple

Note. The Braak classification system for Parkinson's disease is distinct from the Braak system for Alzheimer's disease.
(?) = inadequate data; DMNV = dorsal motor nucleus of the vagus; MMSE = Mini-Mental State Examination; NBM = nucleus basalis of Meynert; NL = normal (26–30); VIP = vasoactive intentional polypeptide.
Source. Braak and Del Tredici 2008; Braak et al. 2006.

The nigrostriatal system has a substantial synaptic reserve, because greater than 50% of striatal innervation and 60% of dopamine transporter must be depleted to produce motor symptoms. This neuronal reserve may explain the long preclinical phase that could span up to 20 years between the appearance of microscopic brain pathology and the manifestation of symptoms (Jellinger 2008). Akinesia and rigidity are linked to loss of neurons in the substantia nigra pars compacta, but Lewy body numbers do not correlate to severity of motor symptoms. The mean survival time for a neuron containing a Lewy body is estimated at 6.2 months, with 71% neuron loss in substantia nigra over 20 years of neurodegeneration.

The catecholaminergic system displays important similarities to other neural systems that undergo neurodegeneration. First, vulnerable neurons possess long, small-caliber axons that are disproportionately thin in comparison to the cell body. Second, axons originating from catecholaminergic neurons in the brain stem are thinly myelinated, which causes the neuron to expend higher energy for signal propagation. The thickly myelinated fibers, such as those in the pyramidal motor pathways, are more energy efficient, less likely to exhibit sprouting, and perhaps less vulnerable to oxidative stress (Braak et al. 2006).

Thin or protracted myelination during brain development is cited as a risk factor for neuronal populations to develop Alzheimer's disease as well as Parkinson's disease (Braak et al. 2003). The differences between early and late-maturing oligodendrocytes are cited as a risk factor rather than the type of transmitter produced by the neuron population. Projection neurons with short axons seem more resistant to age-related damage. Prefrontal and high-level association cortices such as temporal lobe neurons are vulnerable to injury in the early stage of the disease process, and this pattern of vulnerability is a reversal of the normal neurodevelopmental sequence. The molecular biology of vulnerable neurons differs from that of primary motor or sensory cortical neurons, which exhibit suppression of plasticity. For example, primary auditory cortex within the transverse temporal gyrus is relatively spared from Alzheimer-type damage, while the immediately adjacent superior temporal gyrus is often heavily damaged. This selective vulnerability may produce unique challenges to crafting therapeutic interventions that specifically target at-risk neuronal populations while not adversely impacting less vulnerable populations of neurons. Moreover, the role of oligodendroglial cells in the pathogenesis of these neurodegenerative disorders is largely unknown.

Age-Related Alterations of the Special Senses

Aging may affect all five of the special senses. Increased sensory thresholds for touch-pressure, vibration, and cooling are present in aging. Age-related deficits of olfaction, sight, and hearing are immensely important to neuropsychiatrists because they may affect psychological testing and clinical management of patients.

Taste

Taste is perceived by a chemosensory mechanism located in tongue, cheek margin, soft palate, and other oral structures. Taste is mediated by specialized taste cells that detect specific chemicals. These gustatory receptor cells are present within taste buds located in the papillae. Each circumvallate papilla includes about 250 buds. Taste cells have regenerative capacity, with a life cycle of 10–20 days, and these specialized cells can perceive multiple tastes. The facial nerve (cranial nerve 7, or CN7) innervates the anterior two-thirds of the tongue, the glossopharyngeal nerve (CN9) innervates the posterior one-third, and the vagus (CN10) carries taste information from the back of the mouth (Heckmann et al. 2003). Impaired taste perception is common in older patients. More than 250 medications alter taste, and dentures that cover the soft palate diminish taste perception. Taste impairment is classified as *ageusia* (absence of taste) and *hypogeusia* (diminished taste sensitivity). Taste thresholds for both detection and recognition are elevated in aging. Detection thresholds in elders are 2.7 times higher for sweets and 11.6 times higher for salts, and such taste alteration may cause elderly people with diabetes to use more sugar and those with hypertension to use more salt (Schiffman 1997). The neuropsychiatric sequelae of diminished taste include weight loss, poor compliance with dietary restrictions, and loss in quality of life.

Olfaction

Aging humans lose multiple olfactory abilities (Kesslak et al. 1988), including the ability to perceive, discriminate, recognize, and remember odors (Giaquinto 1988). Alteration of nasal mucosa, cribriform plate stenosis, upper airway pathology, and other factors contribute to olfactory loss (Doty 1991). Age-related olfactory histopathology, such as NFTs or synuclein pathology, begins to occur in individuals over age 50 (Doty 1991). Olfaction association areas such as amygdala and uncal cortices are frequently damaged in age-related diseases. Patients with Alzheimer's disease may demonstrate clinical olfaction deficits, and neuropathology is often detected in all components of the olfactory pathway at autopsy. The loss of taste and smell can reduce the drive to eat, a problem corrected with simple dietary or behavioral intervention, such as by enhancing the flavors and odors of foods.

Vision

Senescent visual loss results from environmental, genetic, metabolic, and vascular etiologies (Evans and Williams 1992; Hazzard et al. 1990). The central visual fields, termed Brodmann area 17, include 140 million neurons in human adult brain. A minimal number of neurons are lost with aging, and age-related reduction of visual cortical surface area may result from loss of neuropil, for example, a reduction in the number of synapses (Leuba and Kraftsik 1994).

Primate studies show that visual information is processed along two pathways involving temporal and parietal cortices. A striate-inferior temporal circuit processes information about form and color distinction (Morrison et al. 1991). A striate-parietal pathway processes visuospatial and motor data. The effect of aging on these interconnected, high-level association cortices is not known; however, these brain regions are damaged in Alzheimer's disease (Hof and Morrison 1990) and other dementias.

Visual impairment is common in elderly individuals. Frequent causes of visual impairment include opacification of the lens (cataracts), increased intraocular pressure (glaucoma), retinal damage (diabetic retinopathy), deterioration of the macula (macular degeneration), or disturbance of ocular optics (presbyopia) (Table 2–11). Visual functional changes often begin in the third decade with predominantly myopia. Acuity begins to decline in the sixth decade of life in studies of subjects from industrialized nations, and a significant blurring of vision often occurs after age 60 (Ferrer-Blasco et al. 2008). Cataracts occur in about half the population over age 65 and result in about 1.5 million surgical procedures per year (Solomon and Donnenfeld 2003). Risk factors for cataracts include female gender, smoking, and age. Several types of cataract lesions occur, including nuclear cataracts with opacification in the center of the lens, cortical cataracts with opacification throughout the lens, and posterior subcapsular cataracts with the lesion on the back of the lens (Jager et al. 2008). Surgical extraction and insertion of implant produces excellent improvement of vision.

Glaucomas are common causes of blindness in older persons. Glaucoma may damage the optic nerve via several mechanisms, including increased intraocular pressure that com-

TABLE 2–11. Common causes and treatment of low vision in the elderly

Type	Location of lesion	Etiology	Clinical symptoms	Therapy
Cataract	Lens	Age-related lens degeneration	Like a blurry film over the eye	Lens extraction
Glaucoma	Anterior chamber	Increased intraocular pressure Open angle 80% Angle-closure 10%	Progressive insidious loss of peripheral vision	Medication Laser surgery
Macular degeneration	Retinal area for central vision	Primary retinal degeneration Wet type 10% Dry type 90%	Patient cannot focus clearly on an object as a result of loss of central vision	Laser therapy VEGF therapy
Diabetic retinopathy	Multiple foci on retina	Diabetic vascular disease and retinal hemorrhages	Multifocal, variable loss of vision—described as looking through the top of a salt shaker	Prevention Laser therapy

Note. VEGF=vascular endothelial growth factor.

monly results from diminished drainage of aqueous fluid through the trabecular meshwork (Weinreb and Khaw 2004). Intraocular pressure of 20–30 mmHg can cause damage over several years, whereas pressures of 40–50 mmHg can produce rapid visual loss (Khaw et al. 2004). Increasing age, ethnicity, thin corneal thickness, and myopia may increase risk, and possible genetic loci for glaucoma may colocalize with loci for hypertension (Duggal et al. 2007).

The loss of retinal ganglion cells in glaucoma may produce neurodegeneration in the lateral geniculate nucleus and the central visual fields located in the occipital lobes (Gupta and Yucel 2007). Retinal ganglion cells originate about 1.2 million axons, and disruption of this axonal pathway may alter segments of the visual pathway by disruption of axonal transport, loss of neurotrophins, and other secondary effects (Vrabec and Levin 2007).

Diabetic retinopathy is likely in older individuals who have type 1 diabetes and about 80% of persons with type 2 who survive for 20 years. The common pathological features are microaneurysms and intraretinal hemorrhages. New vessels that extend into the vitreous cavity can hemorrhage, producing blindness. Therapy focuses on limiting the abnormal vascular proliferation (Frank 2004).

Macular degeneration causes vision loss in 54% of older white Americans, affecting 8 million older persons through all stages of the disease. The risk for any stage of macular lesion is about two-fifths for individuals ages 65–74, two-thirds for those ages 75–84, and three-quarters for those over age 85 (Coleman et al. 2008). Multiple candidate genetic loci for macular degeneration are reported, and these linkages impart about 23% of risk for developing macular degeneration in older individuals. The essential lesion for macular degeneration is the drusen, which are focal deposits of acellular debris between the retinal pigment epithelium and Bruch's membrane. Many older individuals may have a few small lesions without symptoms, but multiple or large lesions produce atrophy of the retinal pigmented epithelium through inflammatory responses that promote pathological vascularity and hemorrhages. Treatment of macular degeneration provides limited results. Laser therapies have limited benefit, while vascular endothelial growth factor inhibitors can provide some stabilization of visual acuity.

Low vision can worsen neuropsychiatric symptoms and complicate clinical management of older patients. Recognition of low vision, correction of refractive error, and maximal use of environmental light are important in management of the geriatric population.

Auditory Functions

Hearing impairment is a chronic condition that affects 30% of individuals over age 65. Auditory impairment worsens with age and affects 60% of individuals ages 71–80 (Davis et al. 1990). Causes of hearing loss in elderly people include disorders of the outer, middle, and inner ear. High-frequency hearing loss increases with aging and is usually caused by mechanical failure of the inner ear. Cerumen impaction is a common problem of the outer ear. Hearing loss from damage to the inner ear has four primary causes: sensory presbycusis, neural presbycusis, strial presbycusis, and cochlear conductive presbycusis. Precise epidemiological data are limited because correlative histopathological studies of the auditory apparatus are few, and many conditions have mixed pathology. Most age-related hearing loss is mechanical, and age-related histopathology (e.g., senile plaques or NFTs) is not reported in the peripheral auditory system. Conductive or sensorineural hearing loss can be improved with appropriate hearing amplification. The auditory cortex can be severely damaged in Alzheimer's disease (Esiri et al. 1986).

Subtle auditory impairment may be difficult to detect in the elderly patient who has developed accessory methods such as lip and face reading. Even a mild (10-dB) hearing loss can significantly lower the quality of life for an older individual (Bess et al. 1989). Hearing loss can remain undetected by caregivers, and this communication problem can be misinterpreted by caregivers as patient obstinacy. Unrecognized hearing loss can produce neuropsychiatric symptoms that are preventable or reversible, such as confusion or irritability.

Aging and the Immune System

The human immune system incorporates innate and adaptive components that may determine the course of aging. The innate system is composed of proinflammatory cytokines and an array of other peptides that can provoke a low-grade, chronic inflammatory response. Adaptive immunity consists of T cell and B cell systems that develop recognition for specific antigens. The term *inflammaging* has been proposed to describe the low-grade upregulation of selected proinflammatory responses resulting from excess cytokines, including interleukin-1, interleukin-6, and others (Giunta et al. 2008). The term *immunosenescence* refers to the age-associated decrease in immune competence that increases the older person's susceptibility to disease (Ostan et al. 2008). Age-related alterations of adaptive immunity during aging may reflect involutional changes in the thymus that result in the loss of thymic epithelial cells and thymopoiesis, substantially reducing the output of circulating antigen-naive T cells. The replacement of thymus gland by adipose tissue progresses until age 50; however, total loss of the thymic tissue is projected to occur after age 100 (Ostan et al. 2008). The age-related increase in the number of antigen-experienced T cells accelerates the accumulation of incompetent memory lymphocytes (Giunta et al. 2008). The B cell–mediated response exhibits age-related reductions of immunoglobulin production and specificity. The proinflammatory state of older persons is associated with many age-related diseases or conditions that impact brain function, including atherosclerosis, metabolic syndrome, neurodegeneration, and depression. The interaction of brain aging and the immune system can be viewed in two ways, as either the effect of aging brain on immune function or the effect of an aging immune system on the brain. Components of the immune system, such as spleen, thymus, and lymph nodes, receive direct noradrenergic innervations and respond to substances (e.g., cortisol) produced by the neuroendocrine system. Numerous cytokine receptors have been identified on neurons that can modulate the hypothalamicopituitary axis. Age-related alterations of cortisol secretion may play an important role in counterbalancing changes that occur in the immune response during senescence.

The brain does not have a system of lymphatics or lymphoid tissue as other organs do (e.g., lung, gastrointestinal tract) (Adams and Duchen 1992), although some lymphocyte migration may occur through the VRSs. Microglia, the immune cells of the brain, are either hematogenous or CNS constituents. Intrinsic brain microglial cells most likely are derived from myeloid lineage and populate the CNS during early development. These cells manifest a phagocytic function but also facilitate the reorganization of circuits in response to injury (Neumann et al. 2009). Subjects without neurological disease who are over age 60 have increased numbers of activated microglial cells that express the cytokine interleukin-1, and the number of enlarged or phagocytic microglial cells is increased, whereas quiescent cells are unchanged (Mrak et al. 1997; Thomas 1992).

Interleukin-1, a cytokine that mediates acute phase reaction, innervates key endocrine and autonomic neurons in human hypothalamus that affect many components of the acute phase immune reaction (Breder et al. 1988). Interleukin-2 is centrally active and affects firing of locus coeruleus neurons (Nistico and De Sarro 1991). Interleukin-1 mRNA content is increased in aging brain.

Many systemic diseases of the elderly population, such as arthritis, are immune mediated. The intact blood-brain barrier provides some protection against autoimmunity; however, age- and disease-related changes increase its permeability for selected immunoglobulins. Astrocytes and microglial cells participate in the immune response of the brain by presenting antigen to T cells. Microglial cells are present in senile plaques and are associated with intracellular and extracellular NFTs (Giunta et al. 2008). Activated microglial cells are also present within white matter lesions as detected by MRI in both periventricular and deep white matter regions. Inflammation may also impact aging through vascular pathology. The proinflammatory properties of *APOE*E4* coupled with enhanced age-related inflammation that alters vascular integrity may contribute to the vascular component of neurodegeneration (Finch 2005).

The human immune system undergoes a series of complex age-related changes that vary based on an individual's age, health condition, and genotype. The balance between proinflammatory factors and inflammatory modulators may impact many age-related diseases, including those of the brain.

Animal Models for the Neurobiology of Aging

A wide range of vertebrate and invertebrate genetic models (e.g., round worm, fruit fly, mouse) have been used to study aging and age-related diseases (Gotz and Ittner 2008). In the study of brain aging and neurodegenerative and other age-related diseases, rodents are most frequently used. They are genetically manipulated to produce specific behavioral, neuropathological, or molecular biological outcomes, but even these sophisticated animal systems are inadequate to reproduce the full range of alterations that occur in human brain aging or Alzheimer's disease (Duyckaerts et al. 2008).

The mouse is the primary animal system for genetic research. The mouse models can be produced by either selective inbreeding for phenotypic selection, as seen with the senescence-accelerated mice (SAM), or genetic manipulations, as seen with the transgenic mice (Takeda 2009). Two SAM strains were developed for comparison purposes: those that were prone to phenotypic changes of aging (SAMP) and those that appeared resistant to such changes (SAMR). Specific subtypes of strains may manifest distinct age-related changes, such as the cognitive or neuropathological features of dementia (SAMP8 and 10) or systemic vascular pathology (SAMP8). The SAMP strains also demonstrated age-related behavioral phenotypes such as cognitive dysfunction, behavioral patterns suggestive of depression, and alterations of circadian rhythms. Behavioral changes were also accompanied by brain neurochemical alterations in the noradrenergic, cholinergic, and serotonergic systems. Some age-related neuronal loss was seen in the locus coeruleus and the substantia nigra as compared to the SAMR control brains (Tomobe and Nomura 2009). The very old SAMP mouse (16 months) can recapitulate some molecular neuropathology seen in human age-related disease or dementia, such as β-amyloid deposition or tau hyperphosphorylation within neurons. Although amyloid precursor protein (APP) mRNA and protein product were elevated in the hippocampus of aged SAMP8 mice, this model demonstrated minimal neuronal loss. Mitochondrial damage, oxidative stress, alterations of the blood-brain barrier, and dysregulation of the receptor for advanced glycation end product were also identified (Wu et al. 2009). Other systemic alterations have been described in the SAMP model, such as endothelial dysfunction and greater smooth muscle contractility in the aorta, altered immunity, and osteoporosis (Chen et al. 2009; Forman et al. 2010; Llorens et al. 2007). Age-related alterations of hippocampal neuronal reproduction have been identified in other mouse models, such as the C57 mice in which the ratio of dying and proliferating cells changed during the point when the animal achieved reproductive capacity and again at the end of normal life expectancy (Ben Abdallah et al. 2010).

Transgenic and trisomic mice can be produced to express a wide range of neurological disorders. The three isoforms of human APP have been used as transgenic agents to produce amyloid deposits in mouse models as well as genes associated with human tauopathies. Crucial enzymes in the amyloid cascade, such as the β-secretase enzyme (BACE), can be knocked out of the murine genome, and mice with multiple genetic manipulations can partially mimic the mixtures of pathologies seen with aging and dementia. In triple-transgenic Alzheimer's disease mice, select proteins exhibit significant dysregulation; one-third of these are related to mitochondrial functions (Rhein et al. 2009). APP transgenic mice develop amyloid deposits in the brain that are associated with many of the important features for human disease, including synaptic loss in adjacent neuropil, dystrophic neurites in the vicinity of the deposits, glial activation, and adjacent free-radical generation (Spires et al. 2005). Alterations or loss of dendritic spines appear reversible over time, suggesting a dynamic process that may be a target for future preventive or therapeutic interventions (Smith et al. 2009). The adjacent dystrophic neurites exhibit tau-based pathology. Compared with nonenriched mice, environmentally enriched transgenic mice for APP showed improved neural reproduction and plasticity (Herring et al. 2009).

The molecular differences between the mouse and human tau protein limit the interpretation of this genetic model. Mouse brain typically contains four-repeat (4R) tau exclusively, whereas human brain contains a variable mixture of 4R and 3-repeat (3R) isoforms. Mouse and human tau sequences differ by 14 amino acids at the N-terminal region. The mouse model for overexpression of human tau protein will produce the insoluble tau aggregates within neurons and astrocytes that are integral to the NFT. Discrete NFTs can be produced within neurons of the murine hippocampus or amygdala (Gotz et al. 2001). This process is accelerated in rodents with streptozotocin-induced diabetes (Ke et al. 2009; Planel et al. 2007). In some transgenic mouse models for expression of mutant tau, suppression of tau production can improve memory function and stabilize neuronal pathology (Santacruz et al. 2005). Such observations suggest that deficits may partially result from reversible neuronal dysfunction or improve through systems remodeling. The neuropathology in these transgenic mice does not replicate the spread of neurofibrillary degeneration seen in brains of aging humans or individuals with Alzheimer's disease.

Genetic manipulation of other molecules, such as apolipoprotein E, has provided additional insights into genetic interactions that produce neurodegeneration. Transgenic mice for APP that are also engineered to produce *APOE*4* and to suppress *APOE*3* have more brain amyloid than rodents that lack one of the genes. High levels of physical exercise seem to improve cognition and hippocampal plasticity in mice engineered to produce *APOE*4* (Nichol et al. 2009).

Transgenic models for synuclein dysregulation produce many microscopic changes seen in human aging and disease, including neuronal perikarya, dendrites, and dystrophic neurites stained with antibodies to α-synuclein as well as a smaller number of neurons that stain for ubiquitin (van der Putten et al. 2000).

The neurodevelopmental impact of a transgenic molecular manipulation on the neurobiology of an immature mouse brain may limit the interpretation of the pathology produced in the adult animal. Human aging and age-related diseases usually occur in brains that have experienced normal development. The transgenic manipulation may alter that normal developmental process, or the animals may develop early compensatory mechanisms to changes caused by the engineered genetic mutation (Duyckaerts et al. 2008). The neuronal loss in aged, transgenic animals has been mild compared with that in humans, in whom disease-related loss is severe over time. The topographic progression of neuropathology in rodents frequently differs from the order of damage in human aging or disease-related changes as described elsewhere in this chapter. The transgenic rodent models cannot fully recapitulate the neurological impact of environmental variables such as education, chronic health problems such as hypertension, and health behaviors such as exercise, as experienced by humans with much longer life expectancies. Despite these clear limitations, the SAM and transgenic mouse models provide valuable insight into the molecular pathways impacted by crucial molecules such as β-amyloid and tau.

Larger mammals used as models in aging research include sheep, monkey, bear, dog, and others (Cork et al. 1988; Maurer et al. 1990). Postmortem brain weights of aging monkeys remain relatively constant over time (Herndon et al. 1998). Dystrophic neurites and senile plaques are described in many animal models, and substantial numbers of NFTs are described in the brains of aging bears and sheep (Cork et al. 1988). Other age-related changes such as granulovacuolar degeneration, Hirano bodies, and Lewy bodies (see Figure 2–4) are not commonly described. Hypertensive rodents demonstrate some cerebrovascular brain alterations (Wyss and van Groen 1992; Wyss et al. 1992). Monkeys with surgically induced hypertension will manifest cognitive deficits and multiple cortical infarctions.

Aging primates demonstrate subtle cognitive decline similar to that of elderly humans (Price et al. 1991). Senescent cognitive deficits in aging rhesus monkeys correlate with alterations in prefrontal cortex and brain stem nuclei that project to neocortex, as well as damage to central myelin (Peters 1996). However, MRI volumetric studies of aged rhesus monkeys found subtle declines in forebrain volume (−5.01%) and in forebrain white matter volume (−11.53%) (Wisco et al. 2008), changes that are not correlated to functional data for the animals. Similar reductions are described in the bilateral, dorsolateral, and ventrolateral prefrontal cortices and the orbitofrontal region (Alexander et al. 2008). Unlike aging humans, aged monkeys demonstrate neither severe cortical atrophy nor severe hippocampal damage (Herndon et al. 1998). Aged monkeys exhibit preservation of prefrontal and hippocampal neurons in aging (Keuker et al. 2003); however, synaptic density is decreased in selected regions. Electron microscopic analysis of primate prefrontal cortex shows a 30% reduction of synaptic numbers in layers 2 and 3 of neocortex (Peters et al. 2008b).

Minimal synaptic loss is present in the dentate gyrus of monkey hippocampus (Tigges et al. 1996), and neurons in layer 2 of entorhinal cortex are spared in aging macaques (Gazzaley et al. 1997). Aging monkey brain can develop senile plaques, dystrophic neurites, and congophilic angiopathy closely resembling those of aging humans. Apolipoprotein E is present in senile plaques of aging orangutans (Gearing et al. 1997). The β-amyloid peptide $A\beta_{40}$ length predominates in aging monkeys, as opposed to the $A\beta_{42}$ length in humans with Alzheimer's disease.

Aged dogs have become an important model for dementia and amyloid deposition. For example, the beagle has a life span of 18 years. Those dogs that survive past age 15 years are considered to be "successful agers" and may be a useful model for very old and ultra-old humans. These animals exhibit oxidative damage, loss of discrete neuronal populations such as in the hippocampus or raphe nuclei, diminished neurogenesis, and β-amyloid pathology (Bernedo et al. 2009; Pekcec et al. 2008). Chronic antioxidant therapy may reduce neuronal damage (Head 2009; Siwak-Tapp et al. 2008). β-Amyloid immunization did not alter the cognitive symptoms of aged dogs (Head et al. 2008).

NFTs are seen in aging bears, aging sheep, and very old primates with advanced disease (Cork et al. 1988; Nelson and Saper 1995). Individual bear and monkey neurons will atrophy, accumulate abnormal cytoskeletal proteins, and express amyloid precursor protein. Markers for cholinergic, noradrenergic, serotonergic, and peptidergic systems are decreased in brains of aging primates, suggesting that age-related pathology is not species specific but rather reflects the longevity of the animal (Price et al. 1991).

The applicability of animal models to human diseases has numerous limitations. The brain development and longevity of other mammalian species can differ dramatically from those of the human species. Thinly myelinated axons that develop later in human life are not a significant developmental feature of the canine or primate nervous system. Environmental effects, such as intellectual stimulation, physical activity, and diet, may differ significantly in humans and other animals. Many dietary issues of importance to humans, such as polyunsaturated fatty acids or dietary aluminum, may not affect other animals. Chronic diseases such as hypertension, diabetes, and hyperlipidemia are more common in older humans than in other aged animals. The co-occurrence of human pathologies, such as amyloid deposition in the brain of an older person who has hypertension and some synuclein deposition, is difficult to model. Despite these limitations, the animal models provide invaluable insight into the molecular pathways of individual age-related diseases.

Conclusion

The secret of successful aging is unknown; however, the aging process may begin while in utero. The distinction between "normal" senescent phenomena and age-related disease remains unclear. Human neuronal aging includes a complex mixture of atrophy, hypertrophy, synaptic reorganization, and cell death. Genetic, environmental, systemic, and immunological factors may influence human brain aging. Smoking, exercise, and body mass in middle to late life predict both survival and disability. Elderly individuals with good health habits may survive longer and compress end-of-life disability into fewer years.

Key Points

- Human brain aging probably begins in the fourth decade of life.
- Aging affects all cellular brain components including neurons, glia, and vascular tissues.
- Selected populations of neurons are susceptible to age-related changes.
- Vascular aging and age-related diseases are common contributors to age-related brain damage.
- Animal models only partially replicate human age-related changes and disease.
- The clinical manifestations of neurodegenerative disorders like Alzheimer's disease may reflect the cumulative burden of age-related and disease-specific damage.

Recommended Readings

Bartzokis G: Age-related myelin breakdown: a developmental model of cognitive decline and Alzheimer's disease. Neurobiol Aging 25:5–18, 2004

Dickstein DL, Kabaso D, Rocher AB, et al: Changes in the structural complexity of the aged brain. Aging Cell 6:275–284, 2007

Pakkenberg B, Pelvig D, Marner L, et al: Aging and the human neocortex. Exp Gerontol 38:95–99, 2003

Salthouse TA: When does age-related cognitive decline begin? Neurobiol Aging 30:507–514, 2009

References

Adams JH, Duchen LW: Greenfield's Neuropathology, 5th Edition. New York, Oxford University Press, 1992

Adams MM, Morrison JH: Estrogen and the aging hippocampal synapse. Cereb Cortex 13:1271–1275, 2003

Aizawa K, Ageyama N, Terao K, et al: Primate-specific alterations in neural stem/progenitor cells in the aged hippocampus. Neurobiol Aging Feb 5, 2009 [Epub ahead of print]

Alexander GE, Chen K, Aschenbrenner M, et al: Age-related regional network of magnetic resonance imaging gray matter in the rhesus macaque. J Neurosci 28:2710–2718, 2008

Allen JS, Bruss J, Brown CK, et al: Normal neuroanatomical variation due to age: the major lobes and a parcellation of the temporal region. Neurobiol Aging 26:1245–1260, 2005

Anekonda TS, Reddy PH: Neuronal protection by sirtuins in Alzheimer's disease. J Neurochem 96:305–313, 2006

Antonio A, Leenders KL, Reist H, et al: Effect of age on D_2 dopamine receptors in normal human brain measured by positron emission tomography and ^{11}C-raclopride. Arch Neurol 50:474–480, 1993

Atamna H: Heme, iron, and the mitochondrial decay of ageing. Ageing Res Rev 3:303–318, 2004

Backman CM, Shan L, Zhang Y, et al: Alterations in prodynorphin, proenkephalin, and GAD67 mRNA levels in the aged human putamen: correlation with Parkinson's disease. J Neurosci Res 85:798–804, 2007

Bailey EL, McCulloch J, Sudlow C, et al: Potential animal models of lacunar stroke: a systematic review. Stroke 40:e451–e458, 2009

Barinaga M: Mortality: overturning received wisdom. Science 258: 398–399, 1992

Bartels AL, Kortekaas R, Bart J, et al: Blood-brain barrier P-glycoprotein function decreases in specific brain regions with aging: a possible role in progressive neurodegeneration. Neurobiol Aging 30:1818–1824, 2009

Bartzokis G: Age-related myelin breakdown: a developmental model of cognitive decline and Alzheimer's disease. Neurobiol Aging 25:5–18, 2004

Bartzokis G, Beckson M, Lu PH, et al: Age-related changes in frontal and temporal lobe volumes in men: a magnetic resonance imaging study. Arch Gen Psychiatry 58:461–465, 2001

Bell MA, Ball MJ: Morphometric comparison of hippocampal microvasculature in ageing and demented people: diameters and densities. Acta Neuropathol 53:299–318, 1981

Ben Abdallah NM, Slomianka L, Vyssotski AL, et al: Early age-related changes in adult hippocampal neurogenesis in C57 mice. Neurobiol Aging 31:151–161, 2010

Berchtold NC, Cribbs DH, Coleman PD, et al: Gene expression changes in the course of normal brain aging are sexually dimorphic. Proc Natl Acad Sci U S A 105:15605–15610, 2008

Berenson GS, Srinivasan SR: Cardiovascular risk factors in youth with implications for aging: the Bogalusa Heart Study. Neurobiol Aging 26:303–307, 2005

Bernedo V, Insua D, Suarez ML, et al: Beta-amyloid cortical deposits are accompanied by the loss of serotonergic neurons in the dog. J Comp Neurol 513:417–429, 2009

Berr C, Lafont S, Debuire B, et al: Relationships of dehydroepiandrosterone sulfate in the elderly with functional, psychological, and mental status, and short-term mortality: a French community-based study. Proc Natl Acad Sci U S A 93:13410–13415, 1996

Bess FH, Lichtenstein MJ, Logan SA, et al: Hearing impairment as a determinant of function in the elderly. J Am Geriatr Soc 37:123–128, 1989

Bickford-Wimer PC, Granholm A-CH, Gerhardt GA: Cerebellar noradrenergic systems in aging: studies in situ and in oculo grafts. Neurobiol Aging 9:591–599, 1988

Blessed G, Tomlinson BE, Roth M: The association between quantitative measures of dementia and of senile change in the cerebral grey matter of elderly subjects. Br J Psychiatry 114:797–811, 1968

Bonomo SM, Rigamonti AE, Giunta M, et al: Menopausal transition: a possible risk factor for brain pathologic events. Neurobiol Aging 30:71–80, 2009

Braak H, Braak E: Neuropathological staging of Alzheimer's-related changes. Acta Neuropathol (Berl) 82:239–259, 1991

Braak H, Braak E: Frequency of stages of Alzheimer-related lesions in different age categories. Neurobiol Aging 18:351–357, 1997

Braak H, Del Tredici K: Invited article: nervous system pathology in sporadic Parkinson disease. Neurology 70:1916–1925, 2008

Braak H, Del Tredici K, Rub U, et al: Staging of brain pathology related to sporadic Parkinson's disease. Neurobiol Aging 24:197–211, 2003

Braak H, Rub U, Del Tredici K: Cognitive decline correlates with neuropathological stage in Parkinson's disease. J Neurol Sci 248:255–258, 2006

Brayne C: The elephant in the room: healthy brains in later life, epidemiology and public health. Nat Rev Neurosci 8:233–239, 2007

Breder CD, Dinarello CA, Saper CB: Interleukin-1 immunoreactive innervation of the human hypothalamus. Science 240:321–324, 1988

Brighina L, Prigione A, Begni B, et al: Lymphomonocyte alpha-synuclein levels in aging and in Parkinson disease. Neurobiol Aging 31:884–885, 2010

Brown WT: Genetic diseases of premature aging as models of senescence. Annu Rev Gerontol Geriatr 10:23–42, 1990

Burnet PW, Eastwood SL, Lacey K, et al: The distribution of 5-HT1A and 5-HT2A receptor mRNA in human brain. Brain Res 676: 157–168, 1995

Cabello CR, Thune JJ, Pakkenberg H, et al: Ageing of substantia nigra in humans: cell loss may be compensated by hypertrophy. Neuropathol Appl Neurobiol 28:283–291, 2002

Callahan LM, Coleman PD: Neurons bearing neurofibrillary tangles are responsible for selected synaptic deficits in Alzheimer's disease. Neurobiol Aging 16:311–314, 1995

Chahal HS, Drake WM: The endocrine system and ageing. J Pathol 211:173–180, 2007

Chen H, Zhou X, Emura S, et al: Site-specific bone loss in senescence-accelerated mouse (SAMP6): a murine model for senile osteoporosis. Exp Gerontol 44:792–798, 2009

Choi JY, Morris JC, Hsu CY: Aging and cerebrovascular disease. Neurol Clin 16:687–711, 1998

Cohen RM, Podruchny TA, Bokde AL, et al: Higher in vivo muscarinic-2 receptor distribution volumes in aging subjects with an apolipoprotein E-epsilon4 allele. Synapse 49:150–156, 2003

Coleman HR, Chan CC, Ferris FL III, et al: Age-related macular degeneration. Lancet 372:1835–1845, 2008

Coleman PD: How old is old? Neurobiol Aging 25:1, 2004

Cookson MR: Alpha-synuclein and neuronal cell death. Mol Neurodegener 4:9, 2009

Cork LC, Powers RE, Selkoe DJ, et al: Neurofibrillary tangles and senile plaques in aged bears. J Neuropathol Exp Neurol 47:629–641, 1988

Courchesne E, Chisum HJ, Townsend J, et al: Normal brain development and aging: quantitative analysis at in vivo MR imaging in healthy volunteers. Radiology 216:672–682, 2000

Court JA, Lloyd S, Johnson M, et al: Nicotinic and muscarinic cholinergic receptor binding in the human hippocampal formation during development and aging. Brain Res Dev Brain Res 101:93–105, 1997

Dam AM: The density of neurons in the human hippocampus. Neuropathol Appl Neurobiol 5:249–264, 1979

Davis AC, Ostri B, Parving A: Longitudinal study of hearing. Acta Otolaryngol Suppl 476:12–22, 1990

de la Torre JC: Cerebromicrovascular pathology in Alzheimer's disease compared to normal aging. Gerontology 43:26–43, 1997

de Lacalle S, Iraizoz I, Ma GL: Differential changes in cell size and number in topographic subdivisions of human basal nucleus in normal aging. Neuroscience 43:445–456, 1991

Decker MW: The effects of aging on hippocampal and cortical projections of the forebrain cholinergic system. Brain Res 434:423–438, 1987
Dickson DW: Neuropathological diagnosis of Alzheimer's disease: a perspective from longitudinal clinicopathological studies. Neurobiol Aging 18:S21–S26, 1997
Dickson DW, Crystal HA, Bevona C, et al: Correlations of synaptic and pathological markers with cognition of the elderly. Neurobiol Aging 16:285–298, 1995
Dickstein DL, Kabaso D, Rocher AB, et al: Changes in the structural complexity of the aged brain. Aging Cell 6:275–284, 2007
Dillon KA, Gross-Isseroff R, Israeli M, et al: Autoradiographic analysis of serotonin 5-HT1A receptor binding in the human brain postmortem: effects of age and alcohol. Brain Res 554:56–64, 1991
Doebler JA, Markesbery WR, Anthony A, et al: Neuronal RNA in relation to neuronal loss and neurofibrillary pathology in the hippocampus in Alzheimer's disease. J Neuropathol Exp Neurol 46:28–39, 1987
Doty RL: Olfactory capacities in aging and Alzheimer's disease: Psychophysical and anatomic considerations. Ann N Y Acad Sci 640:20–27, 1991
Double KL, Halliday GM, Kril JJ, et al: Topography of brain atrophy during normal aging and Alzheimer's disease. Neurobiol Aging 17:513–521, 1996
Double KL, Dedov VN, Fedorow H, et al: The comparative biology of neuromelanin and lipofuscin in the human brain. Cell Mol Life Sci 65:1669–1682, 2008
Downs JL, Dunn MR, Borok E, et al: Orexin neuronal changes in the locus coeruleus of the aging rhesus macaque. Neurobiol Aging 28:1286–1295, 2007
Dozono K, Ishii N, Nishihara Y, et al: An autopsy study of the incidence of lacunes in relation to age, hypertension, and arteriosclerosis. Stroke 22:993–996, 1991
Droge W, Schipper HM: Oxidative stress and aberrant signaling in aging and cognitive decline. Aging Cell 6:361–370, 2007
Duggal P, Klein AP, Lee KE, et al: Identification of novel genetic loci for intraocular pressure: a genomewide scan of the Beaver Dam Eye Study. Arch Ophthalmol 125:74–79, 2007
Duyckaerts C, Potier MC, Delatour B: Alzheimer disease models and human neuropathology: similarities and differences. Acta Neuropathol 115:5–38, 2008
Edo MD, Andres V: Aging, telomeres, and atherosclerosis. Cardiovasc Res 66:213–221, 2005
Eggers R, Haug H, Fischer D: Preliminary report on macroscopic age changes in the human prosencephalon: a stereologic investigation. J Hirnforsch 25:129–139, 1984
Ehrenstein D: Immortality gene discovered. Science 279:177, 1998
Ekdahl CT, Kokaia Z, Lindvall O: Brain inflammation and adult neurogenesis: the dual role of microglia. Neuroscience 158:1021–1029, 2009
Epelbaum J: Neuroendocrinology and aging. J Neuroendocrinol 20:808–811, 2008
Erickson KI, Prakash RS, Voss MW, et al: Aerobic fitness is associated with hippocampal volume in elderly humans. Hippocampus 19:1030–1039, 2009
Erraji-Benchekroun L, Underwood MD, Arango V, et al: Molecular aging in human prefrontal cortex is selective and continuous throughout adult life. Biol Psychiatry 57:549–558, 2005
Escobar CM, Krajewski SJ, Sandoval-Guzman T, et al: Neuropeptide Y gene expression is increased in the hypothalamus of older women. J Clin Endocrinol Metab 89:2338–2343, 2004
Esiri MM, Pearson RC, Powell TP: The cortex of the primary auditory area in Alzheimer's disease. Brain Res 366:385–387, 1986
Evans J, Williams T (eds): Oxford Textbook of Geriatric Medicine. New York, Oxford University Press, 1992
Fallon JH, Loughlin S: Monoamine innervation of cerebral cortex and a theory of the role of monoamines in cerebral cortex and basal ganglia, in Cortex. Edited by Jones EG. New York, Plenum, 1987, pp 41–127
Farrall AJ, Wardlaw JM: Blood-brain barrier: ageing and microvascular disease—systematic review and meta-analysis. Neurobiol Aging 30:337–352, 2009
Feller AG, Cohn L, Rudman IW: Growth hormone and function in elderly persons. Ann Intern Med 126:583–584, 1997
Ferrer-Blasco T, Gonzalez-Meijome JM, Montes-Mico R: Age-related changes in the human visual system and prevalence of refractive conditions in patients attending an eye clinic. J Cataract Refract Surg 34:424–432, 2008
Finch CE: Neuron atrophy during aging: programmed or sporadic? Trends Neurosci 16:104–110, 1993
Finch CE: Developmental origins of aging in brain and blood vessels: an overview. Neurobiol Aging 26:281–291, 2005
Finch CE: The neurobiology of middle-age has arrived. Neurobiol Aging 30:515–520, 2009
Finch CE, Morgan DG: RNA and protein metabolism in the aging brain. Annu Rev Neurosci 13:75–88, 1990
Finch CE, Tanzi RE: Genetics of aging. Science 278:407–411, 1997
Fisher M: Pericyte signaling in the neurovascular unit. Stroke 40:S13–S15, 2009
Flood DG, Coleman PD: Neuron numbers and sizes in aging brain: comparisons of human, monkey, and rodent data. Neurobiol Aging 9:453–463, 1988
Flood DG, Buell SJ, Defiore CH, et al: Age-related dendritic growth in dentate gyrus of human brain is followed by regression in the "oldest old." Brain Res 345:366–368, 1985
Forman K, Vara E, Garcia C, et al: Cardiological aging in SAM model: effect of chronic treatment with growth hormone. Biogerontology 11:275–286, 2010
Fossel M: Telomerase and the aging cell: implications for human health. JAMA 279:1732–1735, 1998
Fowler JS, Volkow ND, Wang GJ, et al: Age-related increases in brain monoamine oxidase B in living healthy human subjects. Neurobiol Aging 18:431–435, 1997
Frank RN: Diabetic retinopathy. N Engl J Med 350:48–58, 2004
Frederickson RCA: Astroglia in Alzheimer's disease. Neurobiol Aging 13:239–253, 1992
Futrell N: Lacunar infarction: embolism is the key. Stroke 35:1778–1779, 2004
Fuxe K, Agnati LF: Neurotrophic factors and central dopamine neurons. Neuroscience Facts 3:81, 1992

Ganjavi H, Shapiro CM: Hypocretin/Orexin: a molecular link between sleep, energy regulation, and pleasure. J Neuropsychiatry Clin Neurosci 19:413–419, 2007

Garcia JH: The evolution of brain infarcts: a review. J Neuropathol Exp Neurol 51:387–393, 1992

Gash DM, Zang Z, Gerhardt G: Neuroprotective and neurorestorative properties of GDNF. Ann Neurol 44:S121–S125, 1998

Gaspar P, Berger B, Alvarez C, et al: Catecholaminergic innervation of the septal area in man: immunocytochemical study using TH and DBH antibodies. J Comp Neurol 241:12–33, 1985

Gazzaley AH, Thakker MM, Hof PR, et al: Preserved number of entorhinal cortex layer II neurons in aged macaque monkeys. Neurobiol Aging 18:549–553, 1997

Ge Y, Grossman RI, Babb JS, et al: Age-related total gray matter and white matter changes in normal adult brain, part I: volumetric MR imaging analysis. Am J Neuroradiol 23:1327–1333, 2002

Gearing M, Tigges J, Mori H, et al: Beta-amyloid (A beta) deposition in the brains of aged orangutans. Neurobiol Aging 18:139–146, 1997

Geddes JW, Cotman CW: Plasticity in Alzheimer's disease: too much or not enough? Neurobiol Aging 12:330–333, 1991

Geigl JB, Langer S, Barwisch S, et al: Analysis of gene expression patterns and chromosomal changes associated with aging. Cancer Res 64:8550–8557, 2004

Geula C, Nagykery N, Nicholas A, et al: Cholinergic neuronal and axonal abnormalities are present early in aging and in Alzheimer disease. J Neuropathol Exp Neurol 67:309–318, 2008

Ghani U, Shuaib A, Salam A, et al: Endothelial progenitor cells during cerebrovascular disease. Stroke 36:151–153, 2005

Giacobini E: Cholinergic receptors in human brain: effects of aging and Alzheimer disease. J Neurosci Res 27:548–560, 1990

Giacobini E: Nicotinic cholinergic receptors in human brain: effects of aging and Alzheimer's disease. Adv Exp Med Biol 296:303–315, 1991

Giaquinto S: Aging and the Nervous System. New York, Wiley, 1988

Gilmor ML, Erickson JD, Varoqui H, et al: Preservation of nucleus basalis neurons containing choline acetyltransferase and the vesicular acetylcholine transporter in the elderly with mild cognitive impairment and early Alzheimer's disease. J Comp Neurol 411:693–704, 1999

Giunta B, Fernandez F, Nikolic WV, et al: Inflammaging as a prodrome to Alzheimer's disease. J Neuroinflammation 5:51, 2008

Goldman JE, Yen SH: Cytoskeletal protein abnormalities in neurodegenerative diseases. Ann Neurol 19:209–223, 1986

Goldman JE, Yen SH, Chiu FC, et al: Lewy bodies of Parkinson's disease contain neurofilament antigens. Science 221:1082–1084, 1983

Gomez-Isla T, Price JL, McKeel DW Jr, et al: Profound loss of layer II entorhinal cortex neurons occurs in very mild Alzheimer's disease. J Neurosci 16:4491–4500, 1996

Good CD, Johnsrude IS, Ashburner J, et al: A voxel-based morphometric study of ageing in 465 normal adult human brains. Neuroimage 14:21–36, 2001

Gorelich P: Distribution of atherosclerotic vascular lesions: effects of age, race, and sex. Stroke 24:116–121, 1993

Gottfries CG: Neurochemical aspects on aging and diseases with cognitive impairment. J Neurosci Res 27:541–547, 1990

Gotz J, Ittner LM: Animal models of Alzheimer's disease and frontotemporal dementia. Nat Rev Neurosci 9:532–544, 2008

Gotz J, Chen F, van Dorpe J, et al: Formation of neurofibrillary tangles in P301l tau transgenic mice induced by Abeta 42 fibrils. Science 293:1491–1495, 2001

Graham DG: On the origin and significance of neuromelanin. Arch Pathol Lab Med 103:359–362, 1979

Grudzien A, Shaw P, Weintraub S, et al: Locus coeruleus neurofibrillary degeneration in aging, mild cognitive impairment and early Alzheimer's disease. Neurobiol Aging 28:327–335, 2007

Guarente L: Cell biology: hypoxic hookup. Science 324:1281–1282, 2009

Gupta N, Yucel YH: Glaucoma as a neurodegenerative disease. Curr Opin Ophthalmol 18:110–114, 2007

Hanks SD, Flood DG: Region-specific stability of dendritic extent in normal human aging and regression in Alzheimer's disease, I: CA1 of hippocampus. Brain Res 540:63–82, 1991

Hanyu H, Shimizu S, Tanaka Y, et al: MR features of the substantia innominata and therapeutic implications in dementias. Neurobiol Aging 28:548–554, 2007

Hartikainen P, Soininen H, Reinikainen KJ, et al: Neurotransmitter markers in the cerebrospinal fluid of normal subjects: effects of aging and other confounding factors. J Neural Transm Gen Sect 84:103–117, 1991

Hatanpaa K, Isaacs KR, Shirao T, et al: Loss of proteins regulating synaptic plasticity in normal aging of the human brain and in Alzheimer disease. J Neuropathol Exp Neurol 58:637–643, 1999

Hattiangady B, Shetty AK: Aging does not alter the number or phenotype of putative stem/progenitor cells in the neurogenic region of the hippocampus. Neurobiol Aging 29:129–147, 2008

Haug H, Eggers R: Morphometry of the human cortex cerebri and corpus striatum during aging. Neurobiol Aging 12:336–338, 1991

Haug H, Kuhl S, Mecke E, et al: The significance of morphometric procedures in the investigation of age changes in cytoarchitectonic structures of human brain. J Hirnforsch 25:353–374, 1984

Haycock JW, Becker L, Ang L, et al: Marked disparity between age-related changes in dopamine and other presynaptic dopaminergic markers in human striatum. J Neurochem 87:574–585, 2003

Hayflick L: Theories of biological aging. Exp Gerontol 20:145–159, 1985

Hayflick L: Biological aging is no longer an unsolved problem. Ann N Y Acad Sci 1100:1–13, 2007

Hazzard W, Andres R, Bierman E, et al: Principles of Geriatric Medicine and Gerontology. New York, McGraw-Hill, 1990

Head E: Oxidative damage and cognitive dysfunction: antioxidant treatments to promote healthy brain aging. Neurochem Res 34:670–678, 2009

Head E, Pop V, Vasilevko V, et al: A two-year study with fibrillar beta-amyloid (Abeta) immunization in aged canines: effects on cognitive function and brain Abeta. J Neurosci 28:3555–3566, 2008

Heaton RK: Wisconsin Card Sorting Test. Odessa, FL, Psychological Assessment Resources, 1985

Heckmann JG, Heckmann SM, Lang CJ, et al: Neurological aspects of taste disorders. Arch Neurol 60:667–671, 2003

Hedreen JC, Struble RG, Whitehouse PJ, et al: Topography of the magnocellular basal forebrain system in human brain. J Neuropathol Exp Neurol 43:1–21, 1984

Hefti F, Mash DC: Localization of nerve growth factor receptors in the normal human brain and in Alzheimer's disease. Neurobiol Aging 10:75–87, 1989

Heilbronn LK, de Jonge L, Frisard MI, et al: Effect of 6-month calorie restriction on biomarkers of longevity, metabolic adaptation, and oxidative stress in overweight individuals: a randomized controlled trial. JAMA 295:1539–1548, 2006

Herndon JG, Tigges J, Klumpp SA, et al: Brain weight does not decrease with age in adult rhesus monkeys. Neurobiol Aging 19: 267–272, 1998

Herring A, Ambree O, Tomm M, et al: Environmental enrichment enhances cellular plasticity in transgenic mice with Alzheimer-like pathology. Exp Neurol 216:184–192, 2009

Higuchi M, Yanai K, Okamura N, et al: Histamine H(1) receptors in patients with Alzheimer's disease assessed by positron emission tomography. Neuroscience 99:721–729, 2000

Hitt R, Young-Xu Y, Silver M, et al: Centenarians: the older you get, the healthier you have been. Lancet 354:652, 1999

Hof PR, Morrison JH: Quantitative analysis of a vulnerable subset of pyramidal neurons in Alzheimer's disease, II: primary and secondary visual cortex. J Comp Neurol 301:55–64, 1990

Hof PR, Morrison JH: The aging brain: morphomolecular senescence of cortical circuits. Trends Neurosci 27:607–613, 2004

Hofman MA, Swaab DF: The sexually dimorphic nucleus of the preoptic area in the human brain: a comparative morphometric study. J Anat 164:55–72, 1989

Hopkins ND, Stratton G, Tinken TM, et al: Relationships between measures of fitness, physical activity, body composition and vascular function in children. Atherosclerosis 204:244–249, 2009

Hubble JP: Aging and the basal ganglia. Neurol Clin 16:649–657, 1998

Huttenlocher PR, Dabholkar AS: Regional differences in synaptogenesis in human cerebral cortex. J Comp Neurol 387:167–178, 1997

Hyman BT, Van Hoesen GW, Damasio AR, et al: Alzheimer's disease: cell-specific pathology isolates the hippocampal formation. Science 225:1168–1170, 1984

Iadecola C, Nedergaard M: Glial regulation of the cerebral microvasculature. Nat Neurosci 10:1369–1376, 2007

Insull W Jr: The pathology of atherosclerosis: plaque development and plaque responses to medical treatment. Am J Med 122:S3–S14, 2009

Iqbal K, Liu F, Gong CX, et al: Mechanisms of tau-induced neurodegeneration. Acta Neuropathol 118:53–69, 2009

Itoh K, Weis S, Mehraein P, et al: Cytochrome c oxidase defects of the human substantia nigra in normal aging. Neurobiol Aging 17: 843–848, 1996

Jackson C, Sudlow C: Are lacunar strokes really different? A systematic review of differences in risk factor profiles between lacunar and nonlacunar infarcts. Stroke 36:891–901, 2005

Jacobs B, Driscoll L, Schall M: Life-span dendritic and spine changes in areas 10 and 18 of human cortex: a quantitative Golgi study. J Comp Neurol 386:661–680, 1997

Jager RD, Mieler WF, Miller JW: Age-related macular degeneration. N Engl J Med 358:2606–2617, 2008

Jellinger KA: A critical reappraisal of current staging of Lewy-related pathology in human brain. Acta Neuropathol 116:1–16, 2008

Jengeleski CA, Powers RE, O'Connor DT, et al: Noradrenergic innervation of human pineal gland: abnormalities in aging and Alzheimer's disease. Brain Res 481:378–382, 1989

Jernigan TL, Archibald SL, Fennema-Notestine C, et al: Effects of age on tissues and regions of the cerebrum and cerebellum. Neurobiol Aging 22:581–594, 2001

Johnson BF, Sinclair DA, Guarente L: Molecular biology of aging. Cell Press 96:291–302, 1999

Kaasinen V, Kemppainen N, Nagren K, et al: Age-related loss of extrastriatal dopamine D(2) -like receptors in women. J Neurochem 81:1005–1010, 2002

Kaiser LG, Schuff N, Cashdollar N, et al: Age-related glutamate and glutamine concentration changes in normal human brain: 1H MR spectroscopy study at 4 T. Neurobiol Aging 26:665–672, 2005

Kajantie E: Early life events: effects on aging. Hormones (Athens) 7:101–113, 2008

Kalaria RN, Andorn AC, Tabaton M, et al: Adrenergic receptors in aging and Alzheimer's disease: increased beta 2-receptors in prefrontal cortex and hippocampus. J Neurochem 53:1772–1781, 1989

Katyal S, McKinnon PJ: DNA repair deficiency and neurodegeneration. Cell Cycle 6:2360–2365, 2007

Katyal S, McKinnon PJ: DNA strand breaks, neurodegeneration and aging in the brain. Mech Ageing Dev 129:483–491, 2008

Katzman R: The aging brain: limitations in our knowledge and future approaches. Arch Neurol 54:1201–1205, 1997

Kazantsev AG, Kolchinsky AM: Central role of alpha-synuclein oligomers in neurodegeneration in Parkinson disease. Arch Neurol 65:1577–1581, 2008

Ke YD, Delerue F, Gladbach A, et al: Experimental diabetes mellitus exacerbates tau pathology in a transgenic mouse model of Alzheimer's disease. PLoS One 4:e7917, 2009

Keller JN: Age-related neuropathology, cognitive decline, and Alzheimer's disease. Ageing Res Rev 5:1–13, 2006

Kelly KM, Nadon NL, Morrison JH, et al: The neurobiology of aging. Epilepsy Res 68(suppl):S5–S20, 2006

Kesslak JP, Cotman CW, Chui HC, et al: Olfactory tests as possible probes for detecting and monitoring Alzheimer's disease. Neurobiol Aging 9:399–403, 1988

Keuker JI, Luiten PG, Fuchs E: Preservation of hippocampal neuron numbers in aged rhesus monkeys. Neurobiol Aging 24:157–165, 2003

Khaw PT, Shah P, Elkington AR: Glaucoma—1: diagnosis. BMJ 328:97–99, 2004

Knobloch M, Mansuy IM: Dendritic spine loss and synaptic alterations in Alzheimer's disease. Mol Neurobiol 37:73–82, 2008

Kushner EJ, Van Guilder GP, Maceneaney OJ, et al: Aging and endothelial progenitor cell telomere length in healthy men. Clin Chem Lab Med 47:47–50, 2009

Kyng KJ, May A, Kolvraa S, et al: Gene expression profiling in Werner syndrome closely resembles that of normal aging. Proc Natl Acad Sci U S A 100:12259–12264, 2003

Lakatta EG: Arterial aging is risky. J Appl Physiol 105:1321–1322, 2008

Lamberts SW, van den Beld AW, van der Lely AJ: The endocrinology of aging. Science 278:419–424, 1997

Lee HC, Wei YH: Oxidative stress, mitochondrial DNA mutation, and apoptosis in aging. Exp Biol Med (Maywood) 232:592–606, 2007

Lee HG, Moreira PI, Zhu X, et al: Staying connected: synapses in Alzheimer disease. Am J Pathol 165:1461–1464, 2004

Leuba G, Kraftsik R: Changes in volume, surface estimate, three-dimensional shape and total number of neurons of the human primary visual cortex from midgestation until old age. Anat Embryol (Berl) 190:351–366, 1994

Li B, Yamamori H, Tatebayashi Y, et al: Failure of neuronal maturation in Alzheimer disease dentate gyrus. J Neuropathol Exp Neurol 67:78–84, 2008

Lintl P, Braak H: Loss of intracortical myelinated fibers: a distinctive age-related alteration in the human striate area. Acta Neuropathol 61:178–182, 1983

Llorens S, de Mera RM, Pascual A, et al: The senescence-accelerated mouse (SAM-P8) as a model for the study of vascular functional alterations during aging. Biogerontology 8:663–672, 2007

Longstreth WT Jr, Bernick C, Manolio TA, et al: Lacunar infarcts defined by magnetic resonance imaging of 3660 elderly people: the Cardiovascular Health Study. Arch Neurol 55:1217–1225, 1998

Lu T, Pan Y, Kao SY, et al: Gene regulation and DNA damage in the ageing human brain. Nature 429:883–891, 2004

Lupien S, Lecours AR, Schwartz G, et al: Longitudinal study of basal cortisol levels in healthy elderly subjects: evidence for subgroups. Neurobiol Aging 17:95–105, 1996

Lupien SJ, McEwen BS, Gunnar MR, et al: Effects of stress throughout the lifespan on the brain, behaviour and cognition. Nat Rev Neurosci 10:434–445, 2009

Maclullich AM, Wardlaw JM, Ferguson KJ, et al: Enlarged perivascular spaces are associated with cognitive function in healthy elderly men. J Neurol Neurosurg Psychiatry 75:1519–1523, 2004

Magnussen CG, Venn A, Thomson R, et al: The association of pediatric low- and high-density lipoprotein cholesterol dyslipidemia classifications and change in dyslipidemia status with carotid intima-media thickness in adulthood evidence from the cardiovascular risk in Young Finns study, the Bogalusa Heart study, and the CDAH (Childhood Determinants of Adult Health) study. J Am Coll Cardiol 53:860–869, 2009

Mandelkow E, Song YH, Schweers O, et al: On the structure of microtubules, tau, and paired helical filaments. Neurobiol Aging 16:347–354, 1995

Mann DM, Yates PO, Hawkes J: The pathology of the human locus ceruleus. Clin Neuropathol 2:1–7, 1983

Mann DM, Yates PO, Marcyniuk B: Monoaminergic neurotransmitter systems in presenile Alzheimer's disease and in senile dementia of Alzheimer type. Clin Neuropathol 3:199–205, 1984

Masliah E, Mallory M, Hansen L, et al: Quantitative synaptic alterations in the human neocortex during normal aging. Neurology 43:192–197, 1993

Mattsson N, Ronnemaa T, Juonala M, et al: Arterial structure and function in young adults with the metabolic syndrome: the Cardiovascular Risk in Young Finns Study. Eur Heart J 29:784–791, 2008

Maurer K, Riederer P, Beckman J: Alzheimer's Disease: Epidemiology, Neuropathology, Neurochemistry, and Clinics. New York, Springer-Verlag, 1990

May C, Kaye JA, Atack JR, et al: Cerebrospinal fluid production is reduced in healthy aging. Neurology 40:500–503, 1990

McEwen BS: Stress, adaptation, and disease: allostasis and allostatic load. Ann N Y Acad Sci 840:33–44, 1998

McGeer PL, McGeer EG, Suzuki JS: Aging and extrapyramidal function. Arch Neurol 34:33–35, 1977

Mendelsohn F, Paxinos G: Receptors in the Human Nervous System. San Diego, CA, Academic Press, 1991

Mervis RF, Pope D, Lewis R, et al: Exogenous nerve growth factor reverses age-related structural changes in neocortical neurons in the aging rat: a quantitative Golgi study. Ann N Y Acad Sci 640:95–101, 1991

Mesulam MM, Mufson EJ, Levey AI, et al: Cholinergic innervation of cortex by the basal forebrain: cytochemistry and cortical connections of the septal area, diagonal band nuclei, nucleus basalis (substantia innominata), and hypothalamus in the rhesus monkey. J Comp Neurol 214:170–197, 1983

Mesulam M, Shaw P, Mash D, et al: Cholinergic nucleus basalis tauopathy emerges early in the aging-MCI-AD continuum. Ann Neurol 55:815–828, 2004

Miller JA, Zahniser NR: Quantitative autoradiographic analysis of 125I-pindolol binding in Fischer 344 rat brain: changes in beta-adrenergic receptor density with aging. Neurobiol Aging 9:267–272, 1988

Millonig G, Malcom GT, Wick G: Early inflammatory-immunological lesions in juvenile atherosclerosis from the Pathobiological Determinants of Atherosclerosis in Youth (PDAY) study. Atherosclerosis 160:441–448, 2002

Mochizuki H, Kimura Y, Ishii K, et al: Quantitative measurement of histamine H(1) receptors in human brains by PET and [11C]doxepin. Nucl Med Biol 31:165–171, 2004

Moody DM, Brown WR, Challa VR, et al: Periventricular venous collagenosis: association with leukoaraiosis. Radiology 194:469–476, 1995

Mooradian AD: Effect of aging on the blood-brain barrier. Neurobiol Aging 9:31–39, 1988

Moossy J: Pathology of cerebral atherosclerosis: influence of age, race, and gender. Stroke 24:I22–I23, 1993

Morishima-Kawashima M, Hasegawa M, Takio K, et al: Hyperphosphorylation of tau in PHF. Neurobiol Aging 16:365–371, 1995

Morrison JH, Hof PR: Life and death of neurons in the aging brain. Science 278:412–419, 1997

Morrison JH, Hof PR, Bouras C: An anatomic substrate for visual disconnection in Alzheimer's disease. Ann N Y Acad Sci 640:36–43, 1991

Mrak RE, Griffin WST, Graham DI: Aging-associated changes in human brain. J Neuropathol Exp Neurol 56:1269–1275, 1997

Mufson EJ, Ginsberg SD, Ikonomovic MD, et al: Human cholinergic basal forebrain: chemoanatomy and neurologic dysfunction. J Chem Neuroanat 26:233–242, 2003

Muller WE, Stoll L, Schubert T, et al: Central cholinergic functioning and aging. Acta Psychiatr Scand Suppl 366:34–39, 1991

Munch G, Thome J, Foley P, et al: Advanced glycation endproducts in ageing and Alzheimer's disease. Brain Res Brain Res Rev 23:134–143, 1997

Munch G, Gerlach M, Sian J, et al: Advanced glycation end products in neurodegeneration: more than early markers of oxidative stress? Ann Neurol 44:S85–S88, 1998

Murphy DG, DeCarli C, Schapiro MB, et al: Age-related differences in volumes of subcortical nuclei, brain matter, and cerebrospinal fluid in healthy men as measured with magnetic resonance imaging. Arch Neurol 49:839–845, 1992

Nakamura K, Takubo K, Izumiyama-Shimomura N, et al: Telomeric DNA length in cerebral gray and white matter is associated with longevity in individuals aged 70 years or older. Exp Gerontol 42:944–950, 2007

Napoli C, Palinski W: Neurodegenerative diseases: insights into pathogenic mechanisms from atherosclerosis. Neurobiol Aging 26:293–302, 2005

Napoli C, D'Armiento FP, Mancini FP, et al: Fatty streak formation occurs in human fetal aortas and is greatly enhanced by maternal hypercholesterolemia: intimal accumulation of low density lipoprotein and its oxidation precede monocyte recruitment into early atherosclerotic lesions. J Clin Invest 100:2680–2690, 1997

Napoli C, de Nigris F, Welch JS, et al: Maternal hypercholesterolemia during pregnancy promotes early atherogenesis in LDL receptor-deficient mice and alters aortic gene expression determined by microarray. Circulation 105:1360–1367, 2002

Navarro C, Cau P, Levy N: Molecular bases of progeroid syndromes. Hum Mol Genet 15:R151–R161, 2006

Nelson PT, Saper CB: Ultrastructure of neurofibrillary tangles in the cerebral cortex of sheep. Neurobiol Aging 16:315–323, 1995

Neumann H, Kotter MR, Franklin RJ: Debris clearance by microglia: an essential link between degeneration and regeneration. Brain 132:288–295, 2009

Nichol K, Deeny SP, Seif J, et al: Exercise improves cognition and hippocampal plasticity in APOE epsilon4 mice. Alzheimers Dement 5:287–294, 2009

Niedermuller H, Hofecker G, Skalicky M: Changes of DNA repair mechanisms during the aging of the rat. Mech Ageing Dev 29:221–238, 1985

Nistico G, De Sarro G: Is interleukin 2 a neuromodulator in the brain? Trends Neurosci 14:146–150, 1991

Norbury R, Travis MJ, Erlandsson K, et al: In vivo imaging of muscarinic receptors in the aging female brain with (R,R)[123I]-I-QNB and single photon emission tomography. Exp Gerontol 40:137–145, 2005

Nyman MJ, Eskola O, Kajander J, et al: Gender and age affect NK1 receptors in the human brain: a positron emission tomography study with [18F]SPA-RQ. Int J Neuropsychopharmacol 10:219–229, 2007

Oberheim NA, Wang X, Goldman S, et al: Astrocytic complexity distinguishes the human brain. Trends Neurosci 29:547–553, 2006

Ohm TG, Busch C, Bohl J: Unbiased estimation of neuronal numbers in the human nucleus coeruleus during aging. Neurobiol Aging 18:393–399, 1997

Olton D, Markowska A, Voytko ML, et al: Basal forebrain cholinergic system: a functional analysis. Adv Exp Med Biol 295:353–372, 1991

Ostan R, Bucci L, Capri M, et al: Immunosenescence and immunogenetics of human longevity. Neuroimmunomodulation 15: 224–240, 2008

Ott A, Breteler MM, de Bruyne MC, et al: Atrial fibrillation and dementia in a population-based study. The Rotterdam Study. Stroke 28:316–321, 1997

Pakkenberg B, Gundersen HJ: Neocortical neuron number in humans: effect of sex and age. J Comp Neurol 384:312–320, 1997

Pakkenberg B, Pelvig D, Marner L, et al: Aging and the human neocortex. Exp Gerontol 38:95–99, 2003

Palinski W, Napoli C: The fetal origins of atherosclerosis: maternal hypercholesterolemia, and cholesterol-lowering or antioxidant treatment during pregnancy influence in utero programming and postnatal susceptibility to atherogenesis. FASEB J 16:1348–1360, 2002

Palinski W, Napoli C: Impaired fetal growth, cardiovascular disease, and the need to move on. Circulation 117:341–343, 2008

Pantoni L, Garcia JH: Cognitive impairment and cellular/vascular changes in the cerebral white matter. Ann N Y Acad Sci 826:92–102, 1997

Papadakis MA, Grady D, Black D, et al: Growth hormone replacement in healthy older men improves body composition but not functional ability. Ann Intern Med 124:708–716, 1996

Pascual J, del Arco C, Gonzalez AM, et al: Quantitative light microscopic autoradiographic localization of alpha 2-adrenoceptors in the human brain. Brain Res 585:116–127, 1992

Pekcec A, Baumgartner W, Bankstahl JP, et al: Effect of aging on neurogenesis in the canine brain. Aging Cell 7:368–374, 2008

Pelvig DP, Pakkenberg H, Regeur L, et al: Neocortical glial cell numbers in Alzheimer's disease: a stereological study. Dement Geriatr Cogn Disord 16:212–219, 2003

Peng I, Binder LI, Black MM: Biochemical and immunological analyses of cytoskeletal domains of neurons. J Cell Biol 102:252–262, 1986

Perlman WR, Webster MJ, Herman MM, et al: Age-related differences in glucocorticoid receptor mRNA levels in the human brain. Neurobiol Aging 28:447–458, 2007

Perls T, Kunkel LM, Puca AA: The genetics of exceptional human longevity. J Am Geriatr Soc 50:359–368, 2002

Perry JJ, Fan L, Tainer JA: Developing master keys to brain pathology, cancer and aging from the structural biology of proteins controlling reactive oxygen species and DNA repair. Neuroscience 145:1280–1299, 2007

Peters A: Age-related changes in oligodendrocytes in monkey cerebral cortex. J Comp Neurol 371:153–163, 1996

Peters A, Rosene DL, Moss MB, et al: Neurobiological bases of age-related cognitive decline in the rhesus monkey. J Neuropathol Exp Neurol 55:861–874, 1996

Peters A, Sethares C, Luebke JI: Synapses are lost during aging in the primate prefrontal cortex. Neuroscience 152:970–981, 2008a

Peters A, Verderosa A, Sethares C: The neuroglial population in the primary visual cortex of the aging rhesus monkey. Glia 56:1151–1161, 2008b

Piguet O, Double KL, Kril JJ, et al: White matter loss in healthy ageing: a postmortem analysis. Neurobiol Aging 30:1288–1295, 2009

Pittman AM, Fung HC, de Silva R: Untangling the tau gene association with neurodegenerative disorders. Hum Mol Genet 15: R188–R195, 2006

Planel E, Tatebayashi Y, Miyasaka T, et al: Insulin dysfunction induces in vivo tau hyperphosphorylation through distinct mechanisms. J Neurosci 27:13635–13648, 2007

Podruchny TA, Connolly C, Bokde A, et al: In vivo muscarinic 2 receptor imaging in cognitively normal young and older volunteers. Synapse 48:39–44, 2003

Powers RE: The neuropathology of schizophrenia. J Neuropathol Exp Neurol 58:679–690, 1999

Powers RE, Struble RG, Casanova MF, et al: Innervation of human hippocampus by noradrenergic systems: normal anatomy and structural abnormalities in aging and in Alzheimer's disease. Neuroscience 25:401–417, 1988

Price DL, Martin LJ, Sisodia SS, et al: Aged non-human primates: an animal model of age-associated neurodegenerative disease. Brain Pathol 1:287–296, 1991

Protopopescu X, Butler T, Pan H, et al: Hippocampal structural changes across the menstrual cycle. Hippocampus 18:985–988, 2008

Puglielli L: Aging of the brain, neurotrophin signaling, and Alzheimer's disease: is IGF1-R the common culprit? Neurobiol Aging 29:795–811, 2008

Raitakari OT, Juonala M, Kahonen M, et al: Cardiovascular risk factors in childhood and carotid artery intima-media thickness in adulthood: the Cardiovascular Risk in Young Finns Study. JAMA 290:2277–2283, 2003

Raitakari OT, Juonala M, Taittonen L, et al: Pulse pressure in youth and carotid intima-media thickness in adulthood. The Cardiovascular Risk in Young Finns Study. Stroke 40:1519–1521, 2009

Rance NE: Hormonal influences on morphology and neuropeptide gene expression in the infundibular nucleus of postmenopausal women. Prog Brain Res 93:221–235, 1992

Rance NE, Young WS III: Hypertrophy and increased gene expression of neurons containing neurokinin-B and substance-P messenger ribonucleic acids in the hypothalami of postmenopausal women. Endocrinology 128:2239–2247, 1991

Rance NE, McMullen NT, Smialek JE, et al: Postmenopausal hypertrophy of neurons expressing the estrogen receptor gene in the human hypothalamus. J Clin Endocrinol Metab 71:79–85, 1990

Rance NE, Uswandi SV, McMullen NT: Neuronal hypertrophy in the hypothalamus of older men. Neurobiol Aging 14:337–342, 1993

Rapp PR, Gallagher M: Preserved neuron number in the hippocampus of aged rats with spatial learning deficits. Proc Natl Acad Sci U S A 93:9926–9930, 1996

Ravens JR: Vascular changes in the human senile brain. Adv Neurol 20:487–501, 1978

Raz N, Gunning FM, Head D, et al: Selective aging of the human cerebral cortex observed in vivo: differential vulnerability of the prefrontal gray matter. Cereb Cortex 7:268–282, 1997

Redman LM, Ravussin E: Endocrine alterations in response to calorie restriction in humans. Mol Cell Endocrinol 299:129–136, 2009

Redzic ZB, Preston JE, Duncan JA, et al: The choroid plexus-cerebrospinal fluid system: from development to aging. Curr Top Dev Biol 71:1–52, 2005

Rhein V, Song X, Wiesner A, et al: Amyloid-beta and tau synergistically impair the oxidative phosphorylation system in triple transgenic Alzheimer's disease mice. Proc Natl Acad Sci U S A 106: 20057–20062, 2009

Riddle DR, Sonntag WE, Lichtenwalner RJ: Microvascular plasticity in aging. Ageing Res Rev 2:149–168, 2003

Rollo CD: Dopamine and aging: intersecting facets. Neurochem Res 34:601–629, 2009

Rometo AM, Krajewski SJ, Voytko ML, et al: Hypertrophy and increased kisspeptin gene expression in the hypothalamic infundibular nucleus of postmenopausal women and ovariectomized monkeys. J Clin Endocrinol Metab 92:2744–2750, 2007

Rosene DL, Van Hoesen GW: The hippocampal formation of the primate brain: a review of some comparative aspects of cytoarchitecture and connections, in Cerebral Cortex. Edited by Jones EG, Peters A. New York, Plenum, 1986, pp 345–456

Rowe JW, Kahn RL: Successful aging. Gerontologist 37:433–440, 1998

Rudman D, Feller AG, Nagraj HS, et al: Effects of human growth hormone in men over 60 years old. N Engl J Med 323:1–6, 1990

Rudow G, O'Brien R, Savonenko AV, et al: Morphometry of the human substantia nigra in ageing and Parkinson's disease. Acta Neuropathol 115:461–470, 2008

Sabbagh MN, Shah F, Reid RT, et al: Pathologic and nicotinic receptor binding differences between mild cognitive impairment, Alzheimer disease, and normal aging. Arch Neurol 63:1771–1776, 2006

Salthouse TA: When does age-related cognitive decline begin? Neurobiol Aging 30:507–514, 2009

Santacruz K, Lewis J, Spires T, et al: Tau suppression in a neurodegenerative mouse model improves memory function. Science 309:476–481, 2005

Sarter M, Bruno JP: Developmental origins of the age-related decline in cortical cholinergic function and associated cognitive abilities. Neurobiol Aging 25:1127–1139, 2004

Scarpace PJ, Abrass IB: Alpha- and beta-adrenergic receptor function in the brain during senescence. Neurobiol Aging 9:53–58, 1988

Schiffman SS: Taste and smell losses in normal aging and disease. JAMA 278:1357–1362, 1997

Schipper H: Astrocytes, brain aging and neurodegeneration. Neurobiol Aging 17:467–480, 1996

Schleibs R, Arendt T: The significance of the cholinergic system in the brain during aging and in Alzheimer's disease. J Neural Transm 113:1625–1644, 2006

Schoen EJ: Growth hormone in youth and old age (the old and new deja vu). J Am Geriatr Soc 39:839, 1991

Schroder H, Giacobini E, Struble RG, et al: Cellular distribution and expression of cortical acetylcholine receptors in aging and Alzheimer's disease. Ann N Y Acad Sci 640:189–192, 1991

Sheline YI, Mintun MA, Moerlein SM, et al: Greater loss of 5-HT(2A) receptors in midlife than in late life. Am J Psychiatry 159:430–435, 2002

Simpson JE, Fernando MS, Clark L, et al: White matter lesions in an unselected cohort of the elderly: astrocytic, microglial and oligodendrocyte precursor cell responses. Neuropathol Appl Neurobiol 33:410–419, 2007a

Simpson JE, Ince PG, Higham CE, et al: Microglial activation in white matter lesions and nonlesional white matter of ageing brains. Neuropathol Appl Neurobiol 33:670–683, 2007b

Simpson JE, Hosny O, Wharton SB, et al: Microarray RNA expression analysis of cerebral white matter lesions reveals changes in multiple functional pathways. Stroke 40:369–375, 2009

Siwak-Tapp CT, Head E, Muggenburg BA, et al: Region specific neuron loss in the aged canine hippocampus is reduced by enrichment. Neurobiol Aging 29:39–50, 2008

Smith DL, Pozueta J, Gong B, et al: Reversal of long-term dendritic spine alterations in Alzheimer disease models. Proc Natl Acad Sci U S A 106:16877–16882, 2009

Sobin SS, Bernick S, Ballard KW: Histochemical characterization of the aging microvasculature in the human and other mammalian and non-mammalian vertebrates by the periodic acid-Schiff reaction. Mech Ageing Dev 63:183–192, 1992

Solomon R, Donnenfeld ED: Recent advances and future frontiers in treating age-related cataracts. JAMA 290:248–251, 2003

Spires TL, Meyer-Luehmann M, Stern EA, et al: Dendritic spine abnormalities in amyloid precursor protein transgenic mice demonstrated by gene transfer and intravital multiphoton microscopy. J Neurosci 25:7278–7287, 2005

Stark AK, Pakkenberg B: Histological changes of the dopaminergic nigrostriatal system in aging. Cell Tissue Res 318:81–92, 2004

Stark AK, Toft MH, Pakkenberg H, et al: The effect of age and gender on the volume and size distribution of neocortical neurons. Neuroscience 150:121–130, 2007

Streit WJ: Microglial senescence: does the brain's immune system have an expiration date? Trends Neurosci 29:506–510, 2006

Stroop JR: Studies of interference of serial verbal reaction. J Exp Psychol 18:643–662, 1935

Strozyk D, White LR, Petrovitch H, et al: Sex hormones and neuropathology in elderly men: the HAAS. Neurobiol Aging 28:62–68, 2007

Struble RG, Powers RE, Casanova MF, et al: Neuropeptidergic systems in plaques of Alzheimer's disease. J Neuropathol Exp Neurol 46:567–584, 1987

Sulkava R, Erkinjuntti T: Vascular dementia due to cardiac arrhythmias and systemic hypotension. Acta Neurol Scand 76:123–128, 1987

Svennerholm L, Bostrom K, Jungbjer B, et al: Membrane lipids of adult human brain: lipid composition of frontal and temporal lobe in subjects of age 20 to 100 years. J Neurochem 63:1802–1811, 1994

Svennerholm L, Bostrom K, Jungbjer B: Changes in weight and compositions of major membrane components of human brain during the span of adult human life of Swedes. Acta Neuropathol 94:345–352, 1997

Swerdlow RH: Is aging part of Alzheimer's disease, or is Alzheimer's disease part of aging? Neurobiol Aging 28:1465–1480, 2007

Takeda T: Senescence-accelerated mouse (SAM) with special references to neurodegeneration models, SAMP8 and SAMP10 mice. Neurochem Res 34:639–659, 2009

Tang Y, Nyengaard JR, Pakkenberg B, et al: Age-induced white matter changes in the human brain: a stereological investigation. Neurobiol Aging 18:609–615, 1997

Tanimoto A, Sasaguri Y, Ohtsu H: Histamine network in atherosclerosis. Trends Cardiovasc Med 16:280–284, 2006

Tapia-Arancibia L, Aliaga E, Silhol M, et al: New insights into brain BDNF function in normal aging and Alzheimer disease. Brain Res Rev 59:201–220, 2008

Thoenen H, Zafra F, Hengerer B, et al: The synthesis of nerve growth factor and brain-derived neurotrophic factor in hippocampal and cortical neurons is regulated by specific transmitter systems. Ann N Y Acad Sci 640:86–90, 1991

Thomas WE: Brain macrophages: evaluation of microglia and their functions. Brain Res Brain Res Rev 17:61–74, 1992

Thompson CS, Hakim AM: Living beyond our physiological means: small vessel disease of the brain is an expression of a systemic failure in arteriolar function: a unifying hypothesis. Stroke 40:e322–e330, 2009

Tigges J, Herndon JG, Rosene DL: Preservation into old age of synaptic number and size in the supragranular layer of the dentate gyrus in rhesus monkeys. Acta Anat (Basel) 157:63–72, 1996

Tohgi H, Utsugisawa K, Yoshimura M, et al: Reduction in the ratio of beta-preprotachykinin to preproenkephalin messenger RNA expression in postmortem human putamen during aging and in patients with status lacunaris: implications for the susceptibility to parkinsonism. Brain Res 768:86–90, 1997

Tohgi H, Utsugisawa K, Yoshimura M, et al: Age-related changes in D1 and D2 receptor mRNA expression in postmortem human putamen with and without multiple small infarcts. Neurosci Lett 243:37–40, 1998a

Tohgi H, Utsugisawa K, Yoshimura M, et al: Alterations with aging and ischemia in nicotinic acetylcholine receptor subunits alpha4 and beta2 messenger RNA expression in postmortem human putamen: implications for susceptibility to parkinsonism. Brain Res 791:186–190, 1998b

Tomei LD, Umansky SR: Aging and apoptosis control. Neurol Clin 16:735–745, 1998

Tomlinson BE, Blessed G, Roth M: Observations on the brains of demented old people. J Neurol Sci 11:205–242, 1970

Tomobe K, Nomura Y: Neurochemistry, neuropathology, and heredity in SAMP8: a mouse model of senescence. Neurochem Res 34:660–669, 2009

Ueno E, Liu DD, Ho IK, et al: Opiate receptor characteristics in brains from young, mature and aged mice. Neurobiol Aging 9:279–283, 1988

Umemura T, Soga J, Hidaka T, et al: Aging and hypertension are independent risk factors for reduced number of circulating endothelial progenitor cells. Am J Hypertens 21:1203–1209, 2008

Uylings HB, de Brabander JM: Neuronal changes in normal human aging and Alzheimer's disease. Brain Cogn 49:268–276, 2002

van de Nes JA, Sandmann-Keil D, Braak H: Interstitial cells subjacent to the entorhinal region expressing somatostatin-28 immunoreactivity are susceptible to development of Alzheimer's disease-related cytoskeletal changes. Acta Neuropathol 104:351–356, 2002

van der Putten H, Wiederhold KH, Probst A, et al: Neuropathology in mice expressing human alpha-synuclein. J Neurosci 20:6021–6029, 2000

Varnas K, Hall H, Bonaventure P, et al: Autoradiographic mapping of 5-HT(1B) and 5-HT(1D) receptors in the post mortem human brain using [3H]GR 125743. Brain Res 915:47–57, 2001

Vaupel JW, Carey JR, Christensen K, et al: Biodemographic trajectories of longevity. Science 280:855–860, 1998

Veith RC, Raskind MA: The neurobiology of aging: does it predispose to depression? Neurobiol Aging 9:101–117, 1988

Vijg J, Campisi J: Puzzles, promises and a cure for ageing. Nature 454:1065–1071, 2008

Volkow ND, Fowler JS, Wang GJ, et al: Decreased dopamine transporters with age in health human subjects. Ann Neurol 36:237–239, 1994

Volkow ND, Gur RC, Wang GJ, et al: Association between decline in brain dopamine activity with age and cognitive and motor impairment in healthy individuals. Am J Psychiatry 155:344–349, 1998

Volterra A, Meldolesi J: Astrocytes, from brain glue to communication elements: the revolution continues. Nat Rev Neurosci 6: 626–640, 2005

Vrabec JP, Levin LA: The neurobiology of cell death in glaucoma. Eye 21(suppl):S11–S14, 2007

Wardlaw JM: What causes lacunar stroke? J Neurol Neurosurg Psychiatry 76:617–619, 2005

Wardlaw JM, Farrall A, Armitage PA, et al: Changes in background blood-brain barrier integrity between lacunar and cortical ischemic stroke subtypes. Stroke 39:1327–1332, 2008

Wardlaw JM, Doubal F, Armitage P, et al: Lacunar stroke is associated with diffuse blood-brain barrier dysfunction. Ann Neurol 65: 194–202, 2009

Wareham KA, Lyon MF, Glenister PH, et al: Age-related reactivation of an X-linked gene. Nature 327:725–727, 1987

Weinreb RN, Khaw PT: Primary open-angle glaucoma. Lancet 363:1711–1720, 2004

West MJ: New stereological methods for counting neurons. Neurobiol Aging 14:275–285, 1993

West MJ, Slomianka L: Total number of neurons in the layers of the human entorhinal cortex. Hippocampus 8:69–82, 1998

Whitmer RA, Gustafson DR, Barrett-Connor E, et al: Central obesity and increased risk of dementia more than three decades later. Neurology 71:1057–1064, 2008

Willcox D Craig, Willcox Bradley J, et al: Genetic determinants of exceptional human longevity: insights from the Okinawa Centenarian Study. Age 28:313–332, 2006

Wisco JJ, Killiany RJ, Guttmann CR, et al: An MRI study of age-related white and gray matter volume changes in the rhesus monkey. Neurobiol Aging 29:1563–1575, 2008

Wise PM, Cohen IR, Weiland NG: Hypothalamic monoamine function during aging: its role in the onset of reproductive infertility, in Molecular Neuropathology of Aging. Edited by Davies P, Finch CE. New York, Cold Spring Harbor Laboratory, 1987, pp 159–164

Wolf OT, Kudielka BM: Stress, health and ageing: a focus on postmenopausal women. Menopause Int 14:129–133, 2008

Wong DF, Young D, Wilson PD, et al: Quantification of neuroreceptors in the living human brain, III: D2-like dopamine receptors: theory, validation, and changes during normal aging. J Cereb Blood Flow Metab 17:316–330, 1997

Wu B, Ueno M, Onodera M, et al: RAGE, LDL receptor, and LRP1 expression in the brains of SAMP8. Neurosci Lett 461:100–105, 2009

Wuerfel J, Haertle M, Waiczies H, et al: Perivascular spaces: MRI marker of inflammatory activity in the brain? Brain 131:2332–2340, 2008

Wyss JM, van Groen T: Early breakdown of dendritic bundles in the retrosplenial granular cortex of hypertensive rats: prevention by antihypertensive therapy. Cereb Cortex 2:468–476, 1992

Wyss JM, Fisk G, van Groen T: Impaired learning and memory in mature spontaneously hypertensive rats. Brain Res 592:135–140, 1992

Yamamoto M, Suhara T, Okubo Y, et al: Age-related decline of serotonin transporters in living human brain of healthy males. Life Sci 71:751–757, 2002

Zaccai J, Brayne C, McKeith I, et al: Patterns and stages of alpha-synucleinopathy: relevance in a population-based cohort. Neurology 70:1042–1048, 2008

Zecca L, Pietra R, Goj C, et al: Iron and other metals in neuromelanin, substantia nigra, and putamen of human brain. J Neurochem 62:1097–1101, 1994

Zecca L, Tampellini D, Gerlach M, et al: Substantia nigra neuromelanin: structure, synthesis, and molecular behaviour. Mol Pathol 54:414–418, 2001

Zecca L, Bellei C, Costi P, et al: New melanic pigments in the human brain that accumulate in aging and block environmental toxic metals. Proc Natl Acad Sci U S A 105:17567–17572, 2008

Zhang JH, Sampogna S, Morales FR, et al: Age-related changes in hypocretin (orexin) immunoreactivity in the cat brainstem. Brain Res 930:206–211, 2002

Zhang SC, Ge B, Duncan ID: Adult brain retains the potential to generate oligodendroglial progenitors with extensive myelination capacity. Proc Natl Acad Sci U S A 96:4089–4094, 1999

Zuccala G, Cattel C, Manes-Gravina E, et al: Left ventricular dysfunction: a clue to cognitive impairment in older patients with heart failure. J Neurol Neurosurg Psychiatry 63:509–512, 1997

3

Neurobiological Basis of Behavior

David B. Arciniegas, M.D., F.A.N.P.A., C.B.I.S.T.
C. Edward Coffey, M.D.
Jeffrey L. Cummings, M.D.

All behaviors and experiences are mediated by the brain. No behavior, thought, or emotion lacks a corresponding cerebral event, and abnormalities of human behavior are frequently a reflection of abnormal brain structure and are accompanied by aberrant brain function. This premise does not deny the influence of learning, life events, education, or the sociocultural dimension of human existence; these factors create the context of human behavior and exert powerful biological, developmental, and situational influences. In all cases, however, psychological and sociocultural effects are mediated through brain function. Thus, a comprehensive approach to human behavior demands an understanding of the neurological basis of human cognition, emotion, and psychopathology.

A life-span, or neurodevelopmental, perspective adds another dimension to understanding behavior: brain structure and function change dramatically with age—from fetal development through infancy, childhood, adolescence, adulthood, and old age. Physiological functions vary more widely in elderly people than in young people, tolerance of injury and potential for recovery are diminished in elderly patients, and the neurobehavioral consequences of brain dysfunction often differ as a function of the patient's age.

In this chapter, we provide a review of the neuroanatomical and neurochemical bases of human behavior. First, we present a synoptic model of behavioral neuroanatomy as a framework for the remaining discussion. The model divides the nervous system into three behaviorally relevant zones: an inner zone surrounding the ventricular system, a middle zone encompassing the basal ganglia and limbic system, and an outer zone comprised primarily of the neocortex. We present the anatomy of each zone and describe the behavioral consequences of injury to each. Next, we describe two distributed systems; these cross the three zones to allow information to enter the brain (thalamocortical system) and to allow impulses mediating action to exit the brain (frontal-subcortical circuits). We also present neuropsychiatric syndromes associated with abnormalities of these systems. Finally, we integrate the biochemical basis of behavior with this anatomical approach.

Model of Behavioral Neuroanatomy

Paul Yakovlev developed a comprehensive model of the nervous system in terms relevant to behavior (Yakovlev 1948, 1968; Yakovlev and Lecours 1967). He adopted an evolutionary perspective and noted that the brain consists of three general regions: a median zone surrounding the ventricular system, containing the hypothalamus and related structures; a paramedian-limbic zone consisting primarily of limbic system structures, basal ganglia, and parts of the thalamus; and a supralimbic zone containing the neocortex (Figure 3–1).

In this chapter, we present the Yakovlev approach—updated with information from more recent anatomical studies (Benarroch 1997; Mesulam 2000)—as a foundation for understanding brain-behavior relationships. The *median zone* is immediately adjacent to the central canal, is poorly myelinated, and has neurons with short axons that synapse on nearby cells, as well as on cells with longer axons that project to more distant nuclei. The median zone contains the hypothalamus, medial thalamus, and periventricular gray matter of the brain stem, as well as functionally related areas of the amygdala and insular cortex. The system mediates energy metabolism, homeostasis, peristalsis, respiration, and circulation. The median zone contains the reticular activating system and the nonspecific thalamocortical projections that maintain consciousness and arousal in the awake state and participate in sleep mechanisms. No lateral specialization is evident

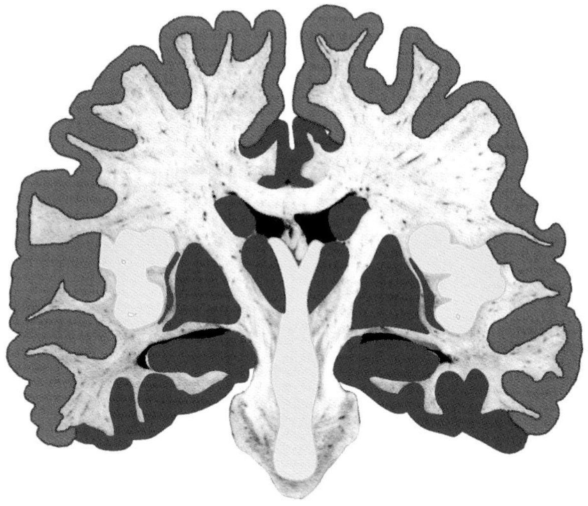

FIGURE 3–1. Updated version of Yakovlev's model of the nervous system demonstrating the median zone (*yellow*), paramedian-limbic zone (*blue*), and supralimbic zone (*red*).

Source. Adapted with permission from Yakovlev PI, Lecours A-R: "The Myelogenetic Cycles of Regional Maturation of the Brain," in *Regional Development of the Brain in Early Life.* Edited by Minkowski A. Oxford, UK, Wiley-Blackwell, 1967, pp. 3–65.

in the median zone. This system is fully functional at birth and is responsible for the early survival of the infant.

The *paramedian-limbic zone* contains neurons that are more fully myelinated than those of the median zone. Neurons here are grouped in nuclear structures that are connected in series. Many of the thalamic nuclei, the basal ganglia, cingulate gyrus, insula, orbitofrontal region, hippocampus, and parahippocampal gyri are included in this zone. The paramedian-limbic zone includes the structures composing the limbic system (Papez 1937). Structures of this zone mediate posture, are essential for the experiential aspects of emotional states, and contribute to the outward expression of emotion (i.e., vocalization, gestures, and facial display). There is little lateral specialization of the paramedian structures. Phylogenetically, this level of brain development is present in reptiles (MacLean 1990). The paramedian-limbic zone is partially functional at birth, and its emerging integrity becomes evident in smiling and crawling. Disorders of motivation, mood, and emotion are associated with paramedian-limbic dysfunction, and this zone is the anatomical site of structures involved in many neuropsychiatric disorders. Parkinson's disease, with its depression, apathy, akinesia, masked face, hypophonic voice, and marked postural changes, is an example of a common disease of elderly people affecting the paramedian-limbic zone.

The *supralimbic zone* is outermost in the brain and includes the neocortex and the lateral thalamic nuclei. The neurons of this zone have long, well-myelinated axons that project via white matter tracts to more distant targets. The supralimbic neocortex contains the neurons mediating higher cortical (association) functions, as well as the pyramidal neurons projecting to limbs, lips, and tongue. It mediates highly skilled, fine motor movements evident in human speech and hand control. Ontogenetically, this zone first finds expression in the pincer grasp and articulate speech. Phylogenetically, the supralimbic zone first appears in mammals and is most well developed in humans (MacLean 1990). The supralimbic zone is expressed in human cultural achievements, including art, manufacture, speech, and writing. The supralimbic zone exhibits lateral specialization with marked differences between the functions of the neocortex within the two hemispheres.

The supralimbic zone is vulnerable to some of the most common neurological disorders associated with aging, including stroke and Alzheimer's disease. For example, the expansion of the neocortex has been at the expense of a secure vasculature. The enlarged association areas have created border zone areas between the territories of the major intracranial blood vessels that are at risk of stroke because of limited interconnections and poor collateral flow; reduced cerebral perfusion with carotid artery disease or cardiopulmonary arrest regularly results in border zone infarctions at the margins between these vascular territories. In addition, penetrating branches form arterial end zones that have no collateral supply as they project through the white matter to the borders of the ventricles. This vascular anatomy creates an area of vulnerability to ischemia at the margins of the lateral ventricles. Periventricular brain injury has been associated with depression (Coffey et al. 1988; Sneed et al. 2008); vascular cognitive impairment, no dementia (Stephan et al. 2009); vascular dementia (Kirshner 2009); and Binswanger's disease. Along with the hippocampus, the supralimbic zone is the major site of pathological changes in Alzheimer's disease (Savoiz et al. 2009). Focal lesions of the neocortex also result in deficits restricted to the neurobehavioral domain, such as aphasia (language), apraxia (skilled purposeful movements, termed *praxis*), and agnosia (recognition).

This model of behavioral neuroanatomy provides an ontogenetic life-span perspective showing the emerging function of these structures in early life and their disease-related vulnerability in later life. The model reflects an evolutionary perspective of the brain, emphasizing its development through time and its increasing complexity in response to evolutionary pressures. From a clinical point of view, most neuropsychological deficit syndromes, such as disorders of language, praxis, and recognition, are associated with dysfunction of the supralimbic neocortex. By contrast, disorders of mood, psychosis, and personality alterations are more likely to occur with abnormalities in the paramedian-limbic zone or disturbed interactions between this zone and the median and supralimbic zones (Gardini et al. 2009; Javitt 2007; Mayberg 2003). The median zone is responsible for more basic life-sustaining functions, and disturbances there are reflected in disorders of consciousness and abnormalities of metabolism, respiration, and circulation. Thus, the patterns of neuropsychiatric disturbance occurring with brain disorders are highly organized events that reflect the history, structure, and function of the nervous system.

Neocortex (Supralimbic Zone)

Histological Organization of the Cortex and Behavior

Brodmann's maps remain the classic guide to the histological organization of the cerebral mantle. Within Brodmann's areas (abbreviated BA followed by the number of the area), three types of cortex relevant to understanding behavior have been identified: a three-layered allocortex, a six-layered neocortex, and an intermediate paralimbic cortex. The limbic system cortex such as the hippocampus has a three-layered allocortical structure, whereas the sensory, motor, and association cortices of the hemispheres have a six-layered organization (Mesulam 2000). In the neocortex, layer I is outermost and consists primarily of axons connecting local cortical areas; layers II and III have a predominance of small pyramidal cells and serve to connect one region of cortex with another; layer IV has mostly nonpyramidal cells, receives most of the cortical input from the thalamus, and is greatly expanded in primary sensory cortex; layer V is most prominent in motor cortex and has large pyramidal cells that have long axons descending to subcortical structures, brain stem, and spinal cord; and layer VI is adjacent to the hemispheric white matter and contains pyramidal cells, many of which project to thalamus (Mesulam 2000) (Figure 3–2). Layers II and IV have the greatest cell density and the smallest cells; conversely, layers III and V have the lowest density and the largest cells. Cell size correlates with the extent of dendritic ramification, implying that cells of the layers III and V projecting to other cortical regions have the largest dendritic domains (Schade and Groeningen 1961).

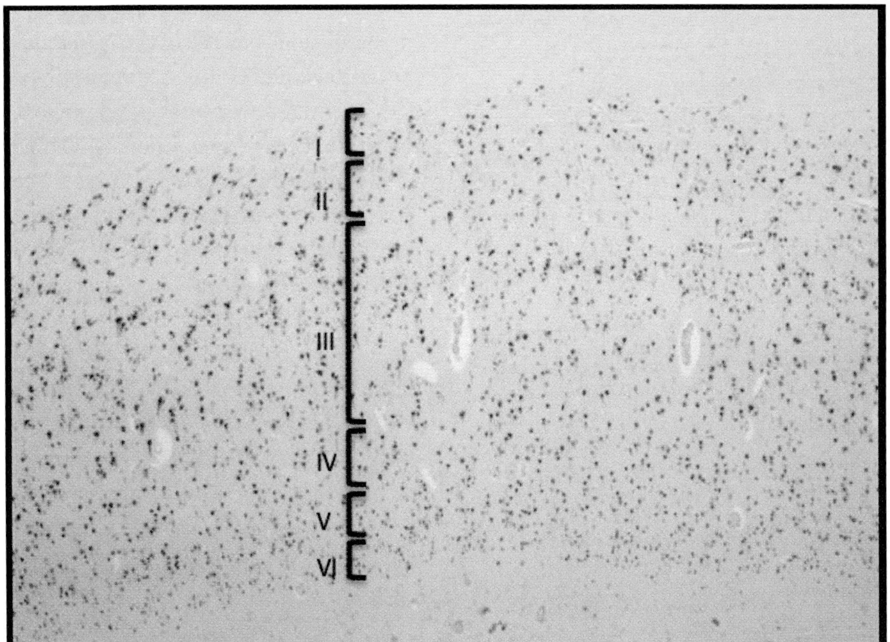

FIGURE 3–2. Histological structure of six-layered neocortex in a 5-year-old male (NeuN immunostain).

Roman numerals along each band correspond to the following layers: I–plexiform (molecular); II–external granular; III–pyramidal; IV–internal granular; V–ganglionic; VI–multiform (polymorphous).

Source. Micrograph courtesy of Bette K Kleinschmidt-DeMasters, M.D., University of Colorado School of Medicine.

Functional Organization of the Neocortex

The *neocortex* is highly differentiated into primary motor and sensory areas and unimodal and heteromodal association regions (Mesulam 2000) (Table 3–1). Association cortex occupies 84% of the human neocortex, whereas primary motor and sensory areas account for only 16%; this indicates the marked importance of association cortex in human brain function (Rapoport 1990). The neocortex is organized in a mosaic of cortical columns, and local circuit neurons (confined to the cortex) compose ~25% of the cellular population (Rapoport 1990). Cortical regions receive and send information via white matter tracts.

Primary motor cortex occupies the motor strip in the posterior frontal lobe and serves as the origin of the pyramidal motor system. Lesions of the motor cortex produce contralateral weakness, particularly of the leg flexors and arm extensors; hyperreflexia; and an extensor plantar response. *Primary somatosensory cortex* is located in the postcentral gyrus in the anterior parietal lobe, *primary auditory cortex* occupies Heschl's gyrus in the superior temporal lobe anterior to Wernicke's area, and *primary visual cortex* is situated in the calcarine region of the occipital lobe (Figure 3–3). Lesions of these regions typically result in contralateral hemisensory deficits (the auditory system is an exception).

Unimodal association areas mediate the second level of information processing in the cerebral cortex after the primary sensory cortex. Unimodal somatosensory association cortex is located in the superior parietal lobule; unimodal auditory association cortex is situated in the superior temporal gyrus immediately anterior to Wernicke's region in the left hemisphere and the equivalent area of the posterior superior temporal cortex of the right hemisphere; and unimodal visual cortex occupies peristriate, midtemporal, and inferotemporal cortical regions (Figure 3–4). Lesions of these regions produce deficits confined to a single sensory modality; the syndromes associated with dysfunction of these regions reflect the higher level of information processing. Lesions of the auditory association cortex (not involving Wernicke's area or its nondominant hemisphere homologue) produce auditory agnosia (inability to recognize sounds), pure word deafness (dominant hemisphere), or various forms of amusia (inability to recognize music). Lesions of the unimodal visual association cortex produce visual agnosias (e.g., visual object agnosia, prosopagnosia, and environmental agnosia) (Kirshner 1986; Mesulam 2000).

The highest level of information processing in the cerebral hemispheres occurs in the *heteromodal association cortices*. It is also primarily in these regions that sensory information from primary sensory and unimodal association cortex is integrated with limbic and paralimbic input (Mesulam 2000). Wernicke's area (BA22, adjacent areas of heteromodal cortex in BA39–40, and perhaps parts of the middle temporal gyrus) is a particularly interesting example of heteromodal cortex: it serves as a temporoparietal transmodal (heteromodal) gateway for lexical/semantic processing of language (Mesulam 2000). Wernicke's area lesions produce fluent aphasia (fluent output with impaired comprehension, repetition, and naming). Lesions of right-sided homologue of Wernicke's area produce the inability to understand the linguistic and emotional prosodic elements of spoken language (Wildgruber et al. 2006). Two other well-recognized regions of heteromodal association cortex include the inferior parietal lobule and the prefrontal cortex (Figure 3–5). Dysfunction of these areas produces complex behavioral deficits that transcend single modalities. Lesions of the left inferior parietal lobule produce the angular gyrus syndrome with alexia, agraphia, acalculia, right-left disorientation, finger agnosia, anomia, and constructional disturbances (Benson et al. 1982). Right-sided inferior parietal lesions produce visuospatial deficits affecting constructions, spatial attention, and body-environment orientation. Prefrontal cortical dysfunction produces deficits in motor programming, memory retrieval, abstraction, and judgment (Stuss and Benson 1986; Tekin and Cummings 2002). Posterior heteromodal association cortex dysfunction observed with inferior parietal lobe lesions reflects abnormalities of the highest level of processing of incoming sensory information; anterior heteromodal association cortex dysfunction in conjunction with prefrontal disturbances produces deficits in active organizational or executive behaviors.

Thus, a behavioral neuroanatomy can be discerned in the organization of the cerebral cortex. Information processing proceeds through progressively more complicated levels of analysis and integration and is then translated into action through a series of executive processes (using anterior heteromodal cortex) and finally through supplementary and primary motor cortices. Each cortical region carries on specific types of information processing activities, and regional injury or dysfunction produces a signature syndrome. From a clinical perspective, neurobehavioral and neuropsychological abnormalities such as aphasia, aprosodia, and agnosia are products of dysfunction of neocortical association cortex or connecting pathways. Although each region has unique functions, each also contributes to more complex integrative processes required for human experience and behavior.

White Matter Connections

The cerebral white matter links cortical areas with each other and with subcortical structures through multiple discrete bundles of myelinated axons, or fiber pathways. These pathways are essential for the function of the distributed neural networks that subserve sensorimotor function, cognition, emotion, and behavior. Within these neural networks are five general types of white matter fiber pathways that emanate from every neo-

TABLE 3–1. Structure and function of different types of cerebral cortex

Cortex	Layer number	Brain regions	Relevant behaviors
Neocortex			
Primary cortex			
Koniocortex	6	Primary sensory cortex (parietal)	Vision, hearing, somatic sensation
Macropyramidal cortex	6	Primary motor cortex (motor cortex)	Movement
Unimodal association cortex	6	Secondary association (parietal, temporal, occipital cortex)	Modality-specific processing of vision, hearing, and somatic sensation
Heteromodal association cortex	6	Multimodal association (inferior parietal lobule, prefrontal cortex)	Higher-order association
Allocortex			
Archicortex	3	Hippocampus	Memory
Paleocortex	3	Piriform cortex	Olfaction
Paralimbic cortex (mesocortex)	4, 5	Orbitofrontal cortex, insula, temporal pole, parahippocampal gyrus, cingulate gyrus	Emotional behavior

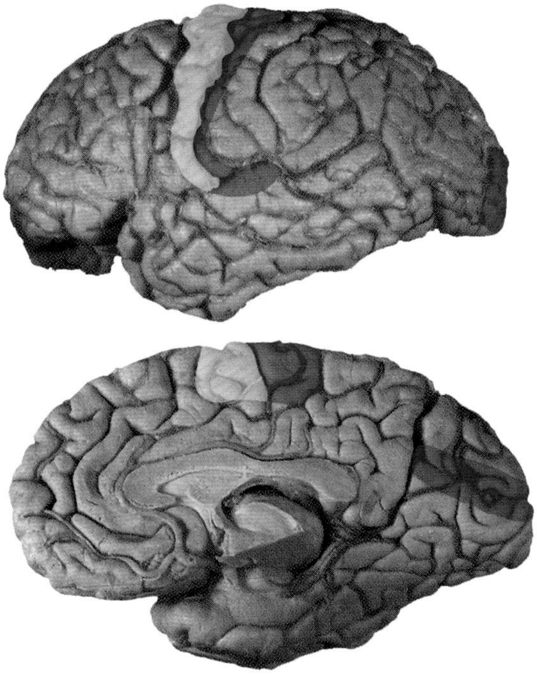

FIGURE 3–3. Primary motor (*green*) and sensory (*blue*) cortex.

Source. Image courtesy of M. Mega and the UCLA Laboratory of Neuroimaging.

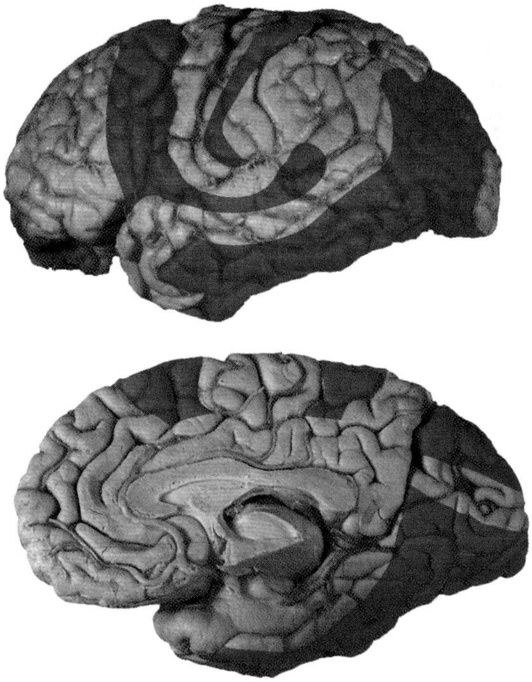

FIGURE 3–4. Unimodal association cortex (*red*).

Source. Image courtesy of M. Mega and the UCLA Laboratory of Neuroimaging.

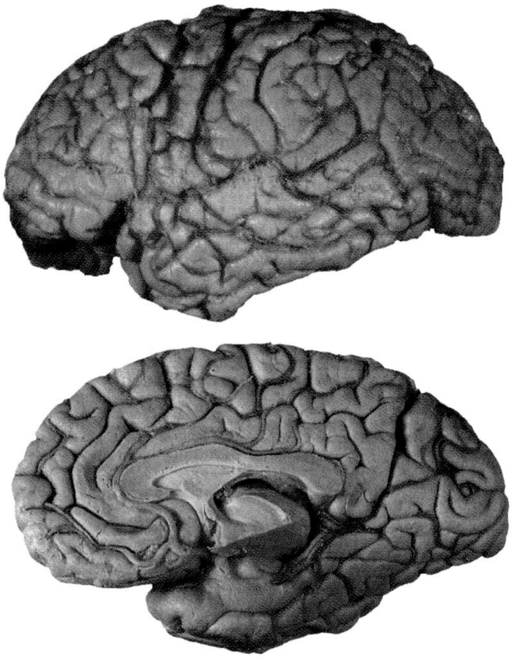

FIGURE 3–5. Heteromodal association cortex (*pink*).

Source. Image courtesy of M. Mega and the UCLA Laboratory of Neuroimaging.

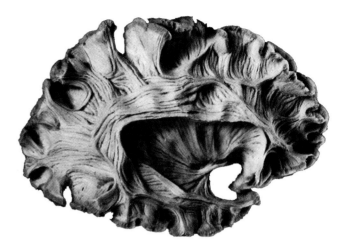

FIGURE 3–6. Brain dissection shows short cortico-cortical connections and intrahemispheric connections.

Source. Image courtesy of M. Mega and the UCLA Laboratory of Neuroimaging.

cortical area: 1) cortico-cortical association fibers; 2) corticostriatal fibers; 3) commissural fibers connecting the cerebral hemispheres; and cortico-subcortical pathways that project to 4) the thalamus and 5) the pontocerebellar system, brain stem, and/or spinal cord (Schmahmann et al. 2008). The principal *projection tracts* include the efferent corticostriatal projections; corticothalamic connections; corticobulbar, corticopontine, and corticospinal fibers; and the afferent thalamocortical radiations. There are also short and long *association fibers*. The short association or "U" fibers connect adjacent sulci; the long association fibers form large tracts connecting more distant regions within each hemisphere (Figure 3–6).

The main long association tracts are listed as follows (Schmahmann et al. 2007):

- The uncinate fasciculus, connecting the orbital and medial prefrontal region with the rostral temporal region, enabling interactions between emotion and cognition, self-regulation, and visual learning
- The arcuate fasciculus and also the extreme capsule, which project between superior temporal areas and the superior and dorsal prefrontal cortex and which are involved in linking posterior and anterior language areas as well as integrating sound localization with spatial attention
- The first superior longitudinal fasciculus, linking the superior parietal lobule, which is involved in appreciating limb and trunk location in space, with premotor areas engaged in higher aspects of motor behavior and the supplementary motor area for intention and initiation of motor activity
- The second superior longitudinal fasciculus, which connects the caudal inferior parietal lobule and posterior prefrontal cortices in the service of spatial attention
- The third superior longitudinal fasciculus, which links the rostral inferior parietal lobule with the supramarginal gyrus, ventral premotor area, and ventral prefrontal areas, which collectively support gestural aspects of language as well as orofacial working memory
- The frontal-occipital fasciculus, which supports visuospatial processing
- The middle longitudinal fasciculus, which courses rostrocaudally in the white matter of the superior temporal gyrus and which links associative and paralimbic cortices in the parietal, cingulate, parahippocampal, and prefrontal regions with the heteromodal cortices of the superior temporal region
- The inferior longitudinal fasciculus connecting the occipital and temporal lobes, which supports object recognition, discrimination, and memory, as well as face recognition
- The cingulum bundle, linking the caudal cingulate gyrus with the hippocampus and parahippocampus (for memory) as well as with the dorsolateral prefrontal cortices (BA9 and BA46) for executive function and working memory, and the rostral (anterior) cingulate gyrus for motivation and drive

The *commissural fibers* are situated in the massive corpus callosum interconnecting all lobes of one hemisphere with areas of the contralateral hemisphere. Commissural fibers are also located in the more diminutive anterior commissure interconnecting the olfactory regions and the middle and inferior temporal gyri of the hemispheres.

Intact cerebral function depends on the integrity of the axons of the white matter, as well as on the activity of the neurons of the gray matter. White matter diseases with diffuse or multifocal demyelination produce memory abnormalities, dementia, depression, mania, delusions, and personality alterations. Focal lesions of white matter tracts produce a number of *disconnection syndromes* that arise when critical neuronal areas are uncoupled by an intervening lesion (Geschwind 1965; Kirshner 1986; Schmahmann et al. 2007, 2008). Table 3–2 summarizes the principal disconnection syndromes.

Disruption of *commissural fibers* by stroke, surgery, or trauma disconnects the left and right hemispheres, and several commissural or callosal syndromes are recognized clinically. With an anterior callosal lesion, the right hemisphere controlling the left hand becomes disconnected from the left hemisphere; thus, the left hand no longer has access to the verbal and motor skills of the left hemisphere, resulting in callosal apraxia, left-hand tactile anomia, and left-hand agraphia. When the splenium of the corpus callosum is damaged in association with injury to the left occipital cortex (usually from a left posterior cerebral artery occlusion), the visual information available to the right hemisphere cannot be transferred to the left for semantic decoding, and alexia without agraphia ensues.

Disconnection syndromes also occur with lesions of association fiber tracts. Lesions of the right inferior longitudinal fasciculus produce prosopagnosia and environmental agnosia, whereas bilateral inferior longitudinal fasciculus damage causes visual object agnosia. Hemisensory deficits and homonymous hemianopsia result from lesions affecting the thalamocortical projections, and hemimotor syndromes occur with lesions of the descending corticospinal projections. The locked-in syndrome occurs with bilateral lesions of descending corticobulbar and corticospinal projection tracts at the pontine level.

The complex histological organization of the cerebral cortex, with its different cytoarchitectonic areas subsuming different processing tasks (as described above), is reflected in the complex connectivity of the cerebral white matter. White matter tracts connect specialized cortical regions, and neuropsychological syndromes may reflect focal cortical injury or disconnection of the cortical regions through injury to the white matter connections. Disconnection syndromes occur with lesions of commissural, long association, or projection fibers. Discrete neurobehavioral syndromes have been identified and occur primarily when lesions of callosal or association fibers disconnect unimodal association areas (e.g., interruption of visual processing in the agnosias or motor activities in the apraxias).

Hemispheric Specialization, Laterality, and Dominance

Anatomical Asymmetries

The two cerebral hemispheres, although grossly symmetrical, differ in some aspects of development, structure, and biochemical composition. Differences between the right and left hemispheres have been shown in both the upper surface of the temporal lobes and the inferolateral surface of the frontal lobe. The temporal lobe area corresponding to Wernicke's area and the frontal region corresponding to Broca's area are both larger than the corresponding right-brain regions (in 65% of cases and 83% of cases, respectively) (Falzi et al. 1982; Galaburda et al. 1978). The superior temporal surface is longer and the total area is approximately one-third larger in the left hemisphere. The sylvian fissure is longer and more horizontal on the left, whereas it is curved upward on the right (Galaburda et al. 1978). Cytoarchitectonic differences correspond to these morphological asymmetries: there is a larger region corresponding to Wernicke's area on the left compared to that on the right.

Other gross asymmetries of the human brain include a wider and longer left occipital lobe, wider right frontal lobe, larger left occipital horn of the lateral ventricular system, and a tendency for the left descending pyramidal tract to decussate before the right in the medulla (Galaburda et al. 1978). Asymmetries of neurotransmitter concentrations also have been identified. Cortical choline acetyltransferase activity is greater in the left than in the right temporal lobe (Amaducci et al. 1981).

Cerebral asymmetries do not occur in the brains of nonprimates but are present in gorillas, chimpanzees, and orangutans, as well as in humans (LeMay 1976). Studies of endocasts of fossil skulls reveal that brain asymmetries similar to those of modern humans were evident in the brains of Neanderthal people 40,000 years ago and may have been present as early as 400,000 years ago in Peking man (Galaburda et al. 1978).

Investigations of asymmetries between the two hemispheres have identified differences at the gross morphological level in the cytoarchitectonic structure of the hemispheres, in the shape of the brain, in the shape of specific aspects of the ventricular system, and in the concentrations of neurotransmitters. The magnitude of these differences is relatively small and does not correspond to the marked differences in hemispheric function. The means by which the dramatic differences in function of the two hemispheres are achieved remain enigmatic. The advantage of hemispheric specialization and lateralized development of functional capacities is that the

TABLE 3–2. Fiber tracts and related disconnection syndromes of the cerebral hemispheres

Fiber type	Tract	Symptoms
Commissural	Corpus callosum	Left-hand tactile anomia, left-hand agraphia, left-hand apraxia, inability to match hand postures or tactile stimuli of the two hands, reduced constructional skills in the right hand
	Splenium	Alexia without agraphia (this syndrome occurs when there is a left occipital injury and right homonymous hemianopsia in addition to the splenial lesion)
Association	Arcuate fasciculus	Conduction aphasia
	Arcuate fasciculus	Parietal apraxia
	Inferior longitudinal fasciculus (right)	Prosopagnosia, environmental agnosia
	Inferior longitudinal fasciculus (bilateral)	Visual object agnosia
Projection	Corticospinal tract	Locked-in syndrome

capacity of the human brain is nearly doubled (Levy 1977). The principal disadvantage is that reduced redundancy exaggerates the effects of lateralized cerebral injury; in humans, a unilateral lesion often has devastating behavioral consequences because of the limited compensatory capability of the contralateral hemisphere.

Asymmetric Cognitive Function of the Hemispheres

Hemispheric specialization refers to the differential functions of the two hemispheres. Nearly all human behavior has contributions from both hemispheres, and complex behavior requires the integrated action of both halves of the brain. Almost no skills are completely unique to one hemisphere. Nevertheless, the two hemispheres differ substantially in their potential for many skills and are differentially engaged in most tasks. Numerous attempts have been made to identify antinomies of function that characterize the right and left hemispheres (i.e., verbal vs. nonverbal, propositional vs. appositional, holistic vs. analytic); none of these has been entirely successful, and it is unlikely that the brain is organized along such polar dimensions. A more accurate approach is to acknowledge that the two hemispheres perform different but not necessarily correlated or complementary roles. Table 3–3 lists capacities mediated to a significantly different extent by the two hemispheres.

Language is the best known example of a lateralized function. The right hemisphere mediates the prosodic aspects of linguistic communication; the left brain mediates propositional aspects of language. The left hemisphere is specialized for symbol usage, including words (spoken, written, heard, and read), mathematical symbols, symbolic gesture, and verbal memory. The left brain is language dominant in nearly all right-handed individuals and in most left-handed people. The lateralization of language functions is not complete, and rudimentary language skills are present in the right brain.

Praxis refers to the ability to execute learned movements on command. This ability is mediated by the left hemisphere, and most instances of apraxia occur in patients with left-sided brain injury (Leiguarda and Marsden 2000).

The right hemisphere is dominant for *visuospatial functions*, but the left hemisphere has considerable visuospatial ability and injuries to the left hemisphere frequently produce at least minor visuospatial deficits. The most marked and enduring visuospatial abnormalities occur with lesions of the posterior right hemisphere. Elementary visuoperceptual skills (e.g., judging line orientation, depth perception), complex visual discrimination and recognition abilities (e.g., discriminating between two unfamiliar faces, recognizing familiar faces), and visuomotor skills (e.g., drawing, copying, dressing) are mediated primarily by the right hemisphere (Kimura and Durnford 1974).

Cortically mediated processes are well lateralized, and neurobehavioral phenomena such as aphasia, alexia, agraphia, abnormalities of visual discrimination and recognition, and altered affective expression occur with local damage to the left or right hemisphere. The cortex is composed of regionally specialized modules that can be rendered dysfunctional by local cortical injury or by disconnection from other regions by white matter lesions.

TABLE 3–3. Abilities mediated primarily by the right or left hemisphere and corresponding clinical deficits resulting from lateralized lesions

Hemispheric function	Correlated clinical deficit
Left hemisphere	
Language	Aphasia
Execution	Nonfluent aphasia
Comprehension	Comprehension defect
Reading	Alexia
Writing	Agraphia
Verbal memory	Verbal amnesia
Verbal fluency (word list generation)	Reduced verbal fluency
Mathematical abilities	Anarithmetia
Praxis	Apraxia
Musical rhythm (execution)	Impaired rhythm in singing
Contralateral spatial attention	Right-sided neglect
Contralateral motor function	Right hemiparesis
Contralateral sensory function	Right hemisensory loss
Contralateral visual field perception	Right homonymous hemianopia
Right hemisphere	
Speech prosody	Aprosodia
Executive prosody	Executive aprosodia
Receptive prosody	Receptive aprosodia
Nonverbal memory	Nonverbal amnesia
Design fluency (novel figure generation)	Reduced design fluency
Elementary visuospatial skills	
Depth perception	Reduced depth perception
Angle discrimination	Reduced angle discrimination
Complex visuospatial skills	
Familiar face recognition	Prosopagnosia
Familiar place recognition	Environmental agnosia
Unfamiliar face discrimination	Impaired facial discrimination
Visuomotor abilities	
Constructional ability	Constructional disturbance
Dressing (body-garment orientation)	Dressing disturbance
Musical melody (perception and execution)	Amusia
Contralateral spatial attention	Left-sided neglect
Contralateral motor function	Left hemiparesis
Contralateral sensory function	Left hemisensory loss
Contralateral visual field perception	Left homonymous hemianopia
Miscellaneous	
Familiar voice recognition	Phonagnosia

Limbic System (Paramedian Zone)

Limbic system structures comprise a critical neuroanatomical substrate for the mediation of mood, emotion, and motivation. Limbic dysfunction contributes to a variety of neuropsychiatric syndromes including psychosis, depression, mania, personality alterations, and obsessive-compulsive disorder.

Limbus means "edge," "fringe," or "border," and *limbic* was first used in an anatomical context by Broca, the French anatomist, to describe the structures that lie beneath the neocortex and that surround the brain stem (Isaacson 1974). In 1937, Papez authored the landmark article "A Proposed Mechanism of Emotion," in which he hypothesized that these structures surrounding the upper brain stem formed a functional system mediating human emotion. Since then, research and clinical observations have largely confirmed the idea that limbic structures are involved in the mediation of behaviors and experiences that share the common feature of having an emotional component.

As currently conceived, the limbic system—composed of limbic and paralimbic structures—includes the entorhinal-hippocampal complex, fornix, mammillary body, olfactory bulb and piriform cortex, caudal orbitofrontal cortex, insula, temporal pole, parahippocampal gyrus, cingulate gyrus, amygdala, orbitofrontal cortex, septal nuclei, nucleus accumbens, hypothalamus, and selected thalamic nuclei (Carpenter 1991; Mesulam 2000) (Figure 3–7). The limbic system is poised between the hypothalamus, with its neuroendocrine control systems of the internal milieu, and the neocortex, mediating action on the external environment. Within this system, the entorhinal-hippocampal complex, as well as its outflow through the forniceal-mammillo-thalamic tract, is an essential component of the brain networks involved in declarative new learning and memory consolidation. Localized injury to the hippocampus or its outflow tract produces an amnestic disorder with deficient storage of new information. This syndrome has been described with hippocampal damage secondary to stroke, anoxia, trauma, early Alzheimer's disease, and herpes encephalitis. The paralimbic elements of the limbic system include brain regions critical to emotional control, social judgment, civility, and motivated behavior. Lesions of the orbitofrontal cortex produce marked personality changes with disinhibition, impulsiveness, loss of tact, and coarsened behavior. Cingulate dysfunction results in marked apathy with disinterest and loss of motivation (Cummings 1993).

Portions of the basal ganglia also are included in the limbic system, at least from a functional perspective. The head of the caudate nucleus consists of ventromedial and dorsolateral portions. The ventromedial section has major limbic system connections and receives projections from the hippocampus, amygdala, cingulate cortex, and the orbitofrontal cortex. The dorsolateral portion, in contrast, receives projections from the lateral prefrontal cortex and has little limbic input (Nauta 1986). The globus pallidus is divided similarly into dorsal-nonlimbic portions and ventral-limbic portions. As predicted by these anatomical observations, basal ganglia diseases are commonly accompanied by emotional dysfunction and psychopathology.

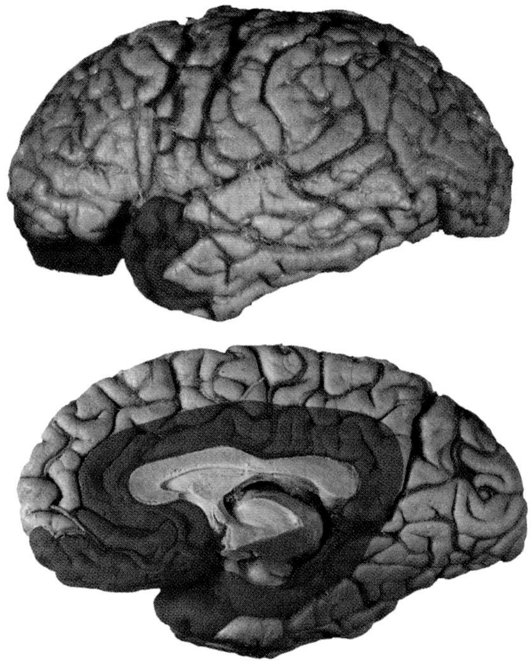

FIGURE 3–7. Limbic and paralimbic cortex (*purple*).

Source. Image courtesy of M. Mega and the UCLA Laboratory of Neuroimaging.

Various clinical neuropsychiatric disorders are associated with limbic system dysfunction (Cummings 1985; Doane 1986) (Table 3–4). The limbic system serves no single unifying function, and the only common feature shared by disorders involving the limbic system is that they frequently involve some manner of altered emotional or social function. For example, psychosis, mood disorders, obsessive-compulsive behavior, personality alterations, and disturbances of sexual behavior have all been linked to limbic system dysfunction. By contrast, limbic system lesions produce relatively little intellectual deficit, notwithstanding impairments of declarative new learning produced by lesions of the entorhinal-hippocampal-forniceal-mammillo-thalamic pathway.

Psychosis occurs with lesions of the temporal lobes and subcortical limbic system structures, as well as with abnormal interactions between limbic and other cortical and brain stem

TABLE 3–4. Neuropsychiatric disorders with evidence of limbic system dysfunction

Neuropsychiatric disorder	Limbic and paralimbic structures implicated	Diseases affecting structure
Amnesia	Hippocampus, hypothalamus	Stroke, anoxia, trauma, tumors, herpes encephalitis
Psychosis	Temporal cortex	Epilepsy, stroke, tumors, herpes encephalitis, Alzheimer's disease
	Striatum	Huntington's disease, idiopathic basal ganglia calcification, lacunar state, schizophrenia
Depression	Striatum, thalamus, insula, medial orbitofrontal cortex	Stroke, Huntington's disease, Parkinson's disease, idiopathic basal ganglia calcification, idiopathic depression
Mania	Striatum	Huntington's disease, idiopathic basal ganglia calcification
	Thalamus	Stroke
	Right basotemporal cortex	Stroke, trauma
OCD	Lateral orbitofrontal cortex, nucleus accumbens, basal ganglia, thalamus	Idiopathic OCD
	Striatum, globus pallidus	Huntington's disease, Sydenham's chorea, PEPD, manganese intoxication, carbon monoxide intoxication
Personality alterations	Orbitofrontal cortex	Trauma, tumors, degenerative disorders
	Temporal cortex	Epilepsy
	Amygdala	Herpes encephalitis, trauma
Anxiety	Amygdala	PTSD, social phobia, specific phobia
	Insula	Idiopathic anxiety
	Rostral anterior cingulate, ventral medial prefrontal cortex	PTSD
	Temporal cortex, basal ganglia	Alzheimer's disease, Parkinson's disease, stroke, trauma
Apathy	Anterior cingulate, ventral striatum, nucleus accumbens, thalamus	Stroke, trauma, tumors, degenerative disorders
Hyposexuality	Temporal cortex	Epilepsy (interictal)
	Hypothalamus	Trauma (surgical)
Hypersexuality	Orbitofrontal cortex	Tumors, trauma
	Temporal cortex	Epilepsy (ictal)
	Amygdala	Herpes encephalitis, trauma
	Septal nuclei	Trauma
Paraphilias	Hypothalamus	Tumors, trauma, encephalitis
Addictions	Septal nuclei, anterior cingulate, orbitofrontal cortex, nucleus accumbens, hypothalamus	Idiopathic addictive behavior

Note. OCD=obsessive-compulsive disorder; PEPD=postencephalitic Parkinson's disease; PTSD=posttraumatic stress disorder.

systems (Javitt 2007). The schizophrenia-like disorder of epilepsy occurs almost exclusively in patients with seizure foci in the temporolimbic cortex (Perez et al. 1985). Stroke, tumors, herpes encephalitis, and Alzheimer's disease are other disorders that affect the temporal cortex and produce psychotic features in elderly individuals. At the subcortical limbic level, Huntington's disease, idiopathic basal ganglia calcification, and lacunar state are examples of conditions with pathology of the limbic system and increased frequencies of psychosis.

Mood disorders also have been related to limbic system dysfunction (Duffy and Coffey 1997), although current models of depression incorporate a large set of limbic-cortical interactions (Mayberg 2003). Depression occurs with basal ganglia dysfunction in stroke, movement disorders, and idiopathic depressive disorders (Baxter et al. 1985; Cummings 1992; Starkstein et al. 1987, 1988b). Manic behavior has been associated with disorders affecting the caudate nuclei, thalamus, and basotemporal areas (Bogousslavsky et al. 1988; Cummings and Mendez 1984; Folstein 1989; Oster et al. 2007; Starkstein et al. 1988a).

Investigation of idiopathic *obsessive-compulsive behavior* has revealed aberrant regulation of limbic and paralimbic structures involved in reward (orbitofrontal cortex and nucleus accumbens), error detection (anterior cingulate), activation of motor and behavioral programs (basal ganglia), and storing information regarding behavioral sequences (prefrontal cortices) (Huey et al. 2008). Imaging, surgical, and lesion studies suggest that the orbitofrontal and anterior cingulate cortices, in particular, as well as the basal ganglia and thalamus, are involved in the genesis of obsessive-compulsive disorder (Baxter et al. 1987; Huey et al. 2008), and that focal lesions and neurological disorders producing obsessive-compulsive behavior frequently involve the caudate nucleus or globus pallidus (Cummings and Cunningham 1992).

A variety of *personality alterations* have been correlated with limbic system lesions. Orbitofrontal or orbitofrontal-subcortical circuit lesions produce disinhibited, impulsive, and tactless behavior; temporolimbic epilepsy has been associated with a rigid, viscous demeanor with hypergraphia, circumstantiality, hyposexuality, and hyperreligiosity (Brandt et al. 1985); and bilateral amygdala lesions produce behavioral placidity as part of the Klüver-Bucy syndrome (Lilly et al. 1983).

Anxiety is a core feature of many psychiatric conditions and a common consequence of brain disorders. Relatively heightened amygdala activation is observed in response to disorder-relevant stimuli in posttraumatic stress disorder, social phobia, and specific phobia, and activation in the insular cortex appears to be heightened in many of the anxiety disorders (Shin and Liberzon 2010). Unlike other anxiety disorders, posttraumatic stress disorder also features diminished responsivity in the rostral anterior cingulate cortex and adjacent ventral medial prefrontal cortex (Shin and Liberzon 2010). Anxiety has been associated with temporal lobe and basal ganglia disorders, including Parkinson's disease and Alzheimer's disease (Reisberg et al. 1989; Stein et al. 1990), and is a common but less conclusively localized problem following stroke or trauma (Carota et al. 2002; Jorge et al. 2004).

Apathy is recognized increasingly as a common behavioral change in patients with brain disorders. The core features of the syndrome of apathy are reductions in goal-directed cognition, emotion, and behavior (Marin 1991). This syndrome varies in severity from mild loss of interest and reduced involvement in previous affairs (i.e., diminished motivation) to an akinetic mute state with markedly reduced movement, speech, and intellectual content (Marin and Wilkosz 2005). The syndrome most commonly results from lesions of the anterior cingulate cortex or related structures of the cingulate-subcortical circuit, including nucleus accumbens, globus pallidus, and thalamus (Cummings 1993; Lavretsky et al. 2007).

Disorders of sexual function also may reflect limbic system disturbances. Diminished libido has been associated with hypothalamic injury and with the interictal state of patients with temporal lobe seizure foci. Hypersexuality, including new-onset pedophilic hypersexual behavior, has been observed in patients with orbitofrontal injury (Burns and Swerdlow 2003) or trauma to the septal region and also as an ictal manifestation in the course of temporal lobe seizures (Gorman and Cummings 1992). Paraphilic behavior, including pedophilia, transvestism, sadomasochistic behavior, and exhibitionism, has been observed in patients with temporal lobe injury and epilepsy, basal ganglia disorders, and brain tumors involving limbic (including orbitofrontal) structures (Burns and Swerdlow 2003; Cummings 1985; Mendez et al. 2000; Miller et al. 1986). Drug *addictions* appear to be mediated in part by alterations of reward circuitry, including anterior cingulate and orbitofrontal interactions with the nucleus accumbens (Kalivas and Volkow 2005).

Disorders involving limbic and paralimbic structures produce a wide range of disturbance in thought, emotion, and behavior. Importantly, conditions with isolated involvement of the "traditional" limbic system described by Papez (1937) tend to produce little intellectual impairment, except impairments in declarative new learning. Instead, these conditions are more often associated with "productive" disorders of emotional function with the new appearance of positive neuropsychiatric symptoms.

Limbic System Asymmetries and Lateralized Neuropsychiatric Syndromes

Anatomical and Biochemical Asymmetries of the Limbic System

Asymmetries of subcortical structures are less marked than are asymmetries of cortical regions, but the left globus pallidus, right medial geniculate nucleus of the thalamus, and left lateral posterior nucleus of the thalamus have been found to be larger than the corresponding nuclei of the contralateral hemisphere (Eidelberg and Galaburda 1982; Kooistra and Heilman 1988). Asymmetries of neurotransmitter concentrations in limbic system structures have been identified. The content of dopamine and choline acetyltransferase (a marker of cholinergic function) is increased in the left globus pallidus compared with their content in the right (Glick et al. 1982); norepinephrine concentrations are greater in the left pulvinar and in the right somatosensory nuclei of the thalamus (Oke et al. 1978); and choline acetyltransferase activity is greater in the left than in the right temporal lobe (Amaducci et al. 1981). Transmitter asymmetries may underlie the differential occurrence of mood disorders and anxiety with lesions of the left and right hemispheres.

Lateralized Neuropsychiatric Syndromes

Some aspects of emotional function may be lateralized, with greater representation in one hemisphere than in the other (Coffey 1987; Sackeim et al. 1982). Emotional functions include the perception of emotional stimuli in the environment (e.g., apprehending facial expression, comprehending voice inflection, and interpreting postural adjustments), the expression of emotion (e.g., facial display and inflection of voice), and the subjective experience of emotion.

With respect to the lateralization of emotional processing, two hypotheses dominate the literature: the right-hemisphere hypothesis and the valence-specific hypothesis. The right-hemisphere hypothesis proposes that the right half of the brain is specialized for processing all emotions irrespective of their valence. By contrast, the valence-specific hypothesis proposes that both hemispheres process emotion, but each hemisphere is specialized for emotions of particular valences. There are two variations of the valence-specific hypothesis: one suggests that the left hemisphere is dominant for positive emotions and the right hemisphere is dominant for negative emotions, whereas the other suggests that lateralization of emotion is linked more strongly to approach (left anterior) and avoidance (right anterior) behaviors than to valence per se. Despite their conceptual differences, the only major point of disagreement between them is their hemispheric assignment of anger; although colloquially regarded as a "negative" emotion, anger is often, even if sometimes maladaptively, associated with approach behaviors.

A meta-analysis of 105 neuroimaging studies using the emotional faces paradigm (or variants thereof) in a total of 1,600 healthy subjects (Fusar-Poli et al. 2009) failed to support the hypothesis of overall right-lateralization of emotional processing of faces, although it could not preclude preferential right hemisphere activation for emotions provoked by stimuli other than human faces (e.g., animals, figures). The authors observed that all emotional conditions, irrespective of stimulus valence, produced bilateral activations of the parahippocampal gyrus and amygdala, posterior cingulate, middle temporal gyrus, inferior frontal and superior frontal gyri, fusiform gyrus, lingual gyrus, precuneus, and inferior and middle occipital gyri. A valence-specific lateralization to the left amygdala during processing of negative emotions was observed, as was a "left/approach" and "right/withdrawal" pattern of imaging activation to emotional faces. This neuroimaging-based meta-analysis of emotional processing favors the valence-specific hypothesis, but suggests that emotional processing is a complex phenomenon that may be understood most usefully by integrating elements of a laterality hypothesis and both variations of the valence-specific hypothesis.

Experiential aspects of emotion are more difficult to study, and the underlying neurobiology is less securely established. Information has been derived from depth electrode investigations, from emotional changes reported in association with epileptic seizures, and from lesion studies. Stimulating depth electrodes located in and around the amygdala produces the sense of déjà vu, anxiety, visceral sensations, hallucinations (Halgren et al. 1978), and occasionally intense fear or anger (Girgis 1981), irrespective of which hemisphere is stimulated. Fear is the most common affect experienced in the course of spontaneous epileptic seizures. Some studies have found a predominance of right-sided foci (Hermann et al. 1992), but fear is also observed in patients with left-sided lesions, suggesting that this experience is not consistently lateralized (Strauss et al. 1982). Sadness is the second most common ictal affect and occurs with both left- and right-sided foci (Williams 1956). A small number of patients have positive emotional experiences as ictal manifestations, and laughter as an ictal behavior may be more common with left- than with right-sided seizure foci (Sackeim et al. 1982). However, consensus is lacking regarding interpretation of this observation (Coffey 1987). Damasio et al. (2000), using [15O] positron emission tomography, studied the neural correlates of happiness, sadness, fear, and anger using a personal life–episodes recall paradigm in 41 healthy individuals; although there were individual variations in the specific brain regions activated during subjects' experiences of these emotions, all involved activation of bilateral structures in limbic, paralimbic, somatosensory, prefrontal, brain stem, and cerebellar areas. Taken together with the emotional processing of faces literature, these observations suggest that many experiential aspects of emotion are mediated by complex, typically bilateral, limbic-cortical and limbic–brain stem systems.

Studies of patients with unilateral lesions tend to favor a relative lateralization of emotional disturbance after neurological injury. Patients with left hemisphere lesions are more likely to experience pathological crying, catastrophic reactions, depression, and anxiety, whereas patients with right hemisphere lesions evidence more indifference and tend to joke about, minimize, or deny their disability (Gainotti 1972; Sackeim et al. 1982). Investigations of stroke patients have found that those with left frontal lobe lesions have a higher prevalence of severe depression, whereas patients with right-brain lesions exhibit more undue cheerfulness or, occasionally, frank mania (Jorge et al. 2004; Oster et al. 2007; Robinson 2006). Van Lancker (1991) observed that many functions of the right hemisphere subserve determination of the personal relevance of environmental stimuli. Weintraub and Mesulam (1983) reported that children who sustained right-brain injury characteristically had interpersonal difficulties, shyness, and impaired prosody and gesture. An impaired ability to comprehend personally relevant information or to execute interpersonal cues appropriately may lead to difficulties in establishing interpersonal relationships and to subsequent social isolation. In elderly individuals, right hemisphere dysfunction may contribute to the disengagement and interpersonal abnormalities evident in many patients with right-brain strokes and dementia syndromes. Table 3–5 summarizes the neuropsychiatric syndromes associated with lateralized brain dysfunction.

Another avenue for investigating the hemisphericity of emotion is to search for evidence of lateral brain dysfunction in idiopathic psychiatric disorders. Early neuroimaging studies, generally employing measures of regional cerebral blood flow, sometimes identified lateralized dysfunction in association with mood disorders (Baxter et al. 1985; Delvenne et al. 1990; Dolan et al. 1992; Drevets et al. 1992; George et al. 1996; Sackeim et al. 1990). Consistent with the findings of Fusar-Poli et al. (2009), however, current models of the neurology of emotion and emotional regulation (in healthy individuals and also those with idiopathic depression) favor a ventral-dorsal dichotomy for emotional generation and regulation and do not rest on a lateralized view of emotion (Mayberg 2003; Seminowicz et al. 2004). Meta-analysis of the neuroimaging data used to construct these models reveals that the function of right and left BA9 (an element of the dorsolateral prefrontal cortex and of these models of idiopathic depression) is highly intercorrelated, and their replacement by one another in these models produces similarly robust results (Seminowicz et al. 2004). Similarly, in deep brain stimulation of the subgenual cingulate gyrus among patients with refractory depression, treatment effect does not differ as a function of laterality of stimulation (Hamani et al. 2009). Collectively, clinically derived models of emotional generation and regulation suggest that these are bilaterally mediated functions of limbic-cortical and limbic–brain stem systems.

In a single case report, Marshall et al. (1997) reported excessive activity of the right anterior cingulate and right orbitofrontal cortex in a patient with conversion disorder involving unilateral limb paralysis ("hysterical paralysis"). Spence et al. (2000) observed hypofunction of the left dorsolateral prefrontal cortex in three individuals with unilateral hysterical paralysis regardless of the side of their conversion symptoms. A subsequent study (Vuilleumier et al. 2001) involving a group of seven subjects failed to find a lateralized association with conversion paralysis; instead, deficient activation of striatothalamocortical circuits subserving sensory motor function and voluntary motor behavior contralateral to the side of conversion paralysis was observed. Contrary to

TABLE 3–5. Neuropsychiatric disorders associated with lateralized brain dysfunction

Neuropsychiatric disorder	Predominant laterality of associated lesion
Disorders of personal relevance	
Unilateral hemispatial neglect	Right
Prosopagnosia (inability to recognize familiar faces)	Right
Environmental agnosia (inability to recognize familiar places)	Right
Phonagnosia (inability to recognize familiar voices)	Right
Affective aprosodia (inability to inflect one's language to communicate emotion or to comprehend the emotion communicated in the inflections of others)	Right
Emotional disorders	
Secondary depression	Left
Catastrophic reaction	Left
Pathological crying	Left
Secondary mania	Right
Secondary euphoria	Right
Eutonia	Right
Pathological laughing	Right

earlier views on the laterality of conversion symptoms, and in accord with the more recent studies on the anatomy of emotion and emotional disturbances, current evidence suggests that conversion disorder involving limb paralysis is associated with aberrant function of and/or interactions between paralimbic-subcortical circuits and sensorimotor systems in a manner that is not predictably lateralized.

In contrast to the lateralization of neuropsychiatric syndromes are the consequences of anomalous (or neurodevelopmentally diminished) cerebral asymmetry. This aberrancy of interhemispheric asymmetry has been observed in a number of psychiatric disorders, including schizophrenia (Crow 2008; Gregorio et al. 2009; Kawasaki et al. 2008; Wilson et al. 2007), in which it is a well-replicated finding, as well as bipolar disorder (Reite et al. 2009; Wilson et al. 2007), autism (Chiron et al. 1995), dyslexia (Leonard and Eckert 2008; Zadina et al. 2006), eating disorders in women (Eviatar et al. 2008), and psychopathy (Mayer and Kosson 2000), among others. These observations suggest the possibility that failure to develop (or a subsequent neurodevelopmental loss of) normal cerebral asymmetry may play a role in the development of neuropsychiatric disorders featuring prominent impairments of limbically dependent neurobehavioral functions.

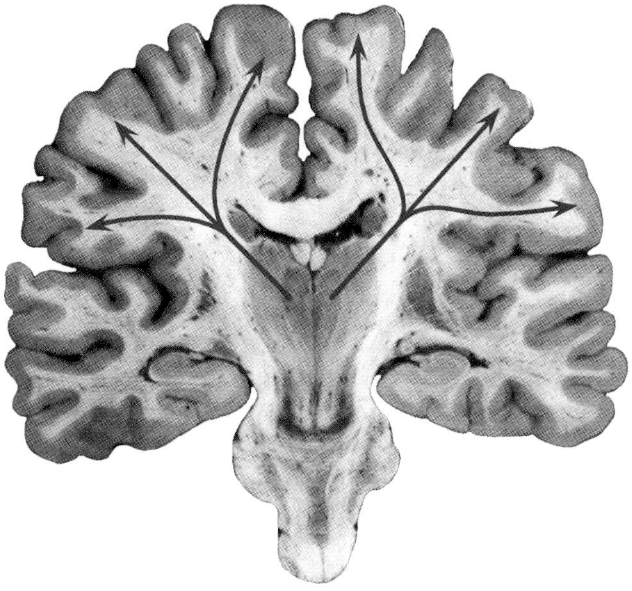

FIGURE 3–8. Cortical projections from the thalamus (*blue*).

Source. Image courtesy of M. Mega and the UCLA Laboratory of Neuroimaging.

Reticular Formation (Median Zone)

The median zone contains the reticular formation, including the ascending reticular activating system, the vasopressor and respiratory mechanisms, and the central components of the sympathetic and parasympathetic nervous systems (Carpenter 1991). The reticular formation is a dense network of neurons with short and long axons that form nuclei in the periventricular gray areas surrounding the cerebral aqueduct in the midbrain, is adjacent to the floor of the fourth ventricle in the pons, and extends into the medulla. The ascending reticular activating system projects to the intralaminar nuclei of the thalamus, and these in turn project to the cerebral cortex. The intralaminar nuclei project primarily to layer I of the cortex, the layer comprising parallel fibers whose stimulation results in local cortical activation (Figure 3–8).

The thalamic reticular nucleus is a unique structure that forms a thin shell around the anterior aspects of the thalamus and governs cortical arousal. It receives projections from the cerebral cortex, dorsal intralaminar nucleus, and dorsal specific sensory nuclei. It has no projections to the cerebral cortex but projects back to the dorsal thalamic nuclei. It is positioned to serve as a gate, modifying and censoring information projected from thalamus to cortex, and its principal effect is to inhibit cortical activity (Carpenter and Sutin 1983; Plum and Posner 1980).

Increased input from the brain stem reticular activating system reduces the tonic inhibition of the reticular nucleus and activates the cortex by disinhibiting the cortical projections of other thalamic nuclei (Plum and Posner 1980). The ascending reticular activating system is responsible for the maintenance of consciousness, and disturbances of the system result in impaired arousal varying from drowsiness to obtundation, stupor, and coma.

Nuclei of the reticular formation also are involved in control of heart rate, blood pressure, and respiratory rhythms (Carpenter 1991). Dysfunction of these nuclei results in alterations in blood pressure, cardiac arrhythmias, and respiratory irregularities. The hypothalamus is contained in the median zone, and abnormalities of basic life functions (e.g., appetite, libido, sleep) may occur in individuals who sustain hypothalamic injury. The hypothalamus influences endocrine function via its connections with the pituitary gland, and endocrine abnormalities are produced by hypothalamic lesions.

Connections Between the Cerebral Cortex and Subcortical Structures

Information enters the nervous system one principal way, and there is one principal exit pathway by which humans act on their environment. The entry pathway is via thalamocortical afferents that receive sensory information from peripheral sensory receptors and convey the data to the cortex. The principal exit pathway is via the descending corticospinal tracts, particularly the pyramidal system. Thus, the flow of information is from the thalamus to the primary sensory cortex, unimodal association cortex, and then heteromodal association cortex. From there, the long association fibers connect the posterior heteromodal cortex to the anterior (frontal lobe) heteromodal cortex that in turn connects to the subcortical nuclei. After processing through frontal-subcortical circuits, executive commands flow to the primary motor cortex and then to bulbar and spinal effector mechanisms. The thalamocortical afferents and frontal-subcortical efferents are distributed systems that include portions of both the paramedian (limbic) and supralimbic (neocortical) zones. Activation of brain structures is not limited to the sequence described above; there is simultaneous activation of many brain regions, as well as feedback mechanisms from ongoing activity.

Thalamocortical Relationships

The thalamus plays several crucial roles in human brain function. Specific thalamic nuclei receive input from a relatively restricted number of sources and project to layers III and IV of the cortex.

The specific nuclei include sensory nuclei that process all incoming sensory information except olfaction (ventral posterior, medial geniculate, and lateral geniculate); nuclei that participate in the motor pathways (ventroanterior and ventrolateral); association nuclei that have major connections with frontal (medial dorsal nuclei) or temporoparietal (lateral nuclei) association cortex; and nuclei that are included in the limbic circuits (anterior and medial nuclei) (Carpenter and Sutin 1983; Mesulam 2000; Nauta and Feirtag 1986; Shipp 2003). Table 3–6 presents a functional classification of thalamic nuclei with their principal afferents and efferents.

A number of distinctive behavioral disorders have been associated with dysfunction of the associative and sensory thalamic nuclei. Disorders of the associative medial dorsal nuclei produce amnesia and a "frontal lobe"–type syndrome (Cummings 1993; Stuss et al. 1988). Apathy also is common after dorsal medial nuclear injury. Lesions of the specific thalamic sensory nuclei cause deficits in primary sensation. Ventral posterior nuclear lesions disrupt all sensory abilities of the contralateral limbs, trunk, and face. In some cases, spontaneous disabling pain of the affected side occurs (Dejerine-Roussy syndrome) (Adams and Victor 1981). Lesions of the lateral geniculate bodies produce a contralateral visual field defect. Mania has been observed in several patients with right-sided thalamic lesions involving the paramedian thalamic nuclei (Bogousslavsky et al. 1988; Cummings and Mendez 1984; Starkstein et al. 1988a).

Frontal-Subcortical Circuits

The frontal lobe is the origin of executive processes that guide action. The output from the frontal lobe is through subcortical circuits that eventually reach motor pathways. Five circuits connecting the frontal lobes and subcortical structures are currently recognized: a motor circuit originating in the supplementary motor area, an oculomotor circuit with origins in the frontal eye fields, and three circuits originating in prefrontal cortex (dorsolateral prefrontal cortex, lateral orbital cortex, and anterior cingulate cortex) (Alexander and Crutcher 1990; Alexander et al. 1986, 1990; Lichter and Cummings 2001). The prototypic structure of all circuits is an origin in the frontal lobes, projection to striatal structures (caudate, putamen, or nucleus accumbens), connections from striatum to globus pallidus and substantia nigra, projections from these two structures to specific thalamic nuclei, and a final link back to the frontal lobe (Figure 3–9).

The *motor circuit* originates from neurons in the supplementary motor area, premotor cortex, motor cortex, and somatosensory cortex (Alexander and Crutcher 1990; Alexander et al. 1986; Lichter and Cummings 2001). Throughout the circuit, the discrete somatotopic organization of movement-related neurons is maintained. Distinct types of motor disturbances are associated with lesions at different sites in the motor circuit. Motor initiation abnormalities (akinesia) are associated with supplementary motor area lesions; parkinsonism and dystonia are observed with putaminal dysfunction; and choreiform movements occur with caudate and subthalamic nucleus damage.

The *oculomotor circuit* originates in the frontal eye fields, as well as in the prefrontal and posterior parietal cortex. Acute lesions of the cortical eye fields produce ipsilateral eye deviation, whereas more chronic lesions produce ipsilateral gaze impersistence. Lesions in other areas of the circuit produce supranuclear gaze palsies such as those seen in Parkinson's disease, progressive supranuclear palsy, and Huntington's disease.

Three distinct frontal lobe neurobehavioral syndromes are recognized, and each corresponds to a region of origin of one of the three prefrontal-subcortical circuits. Dysfunction of any of the member structures of the circuits results in similar circuit-specific behavioral complexes, and these frontal-subcortical circuits compose major anatomical axes governing behavior (Cummings 1993; Lichter and Cummings 2001). The *dorsolateral prefrontal circuit* originates in the convexity of the frontal lobe and projects primarily to the dorsolateral head of the caudate nucleus (Alexander and Crutcher 1990; Alexander et al. 1986; Lichter and Cummings 2001) (Figure 3–10). This caudate region connects to globus pallidus and substantia nigra, and pallidal and nigral neurons of the circuit project to the medial dorsal thalamic nuclei that in turn project back to the dorsolateral prefrontal region. The dorsolateral pre-

TABLE 3–6. Function and anatomical relationships of the thalamic nuclei

Nuclei	Input	Output	Function
Limbic nuclei			
Anterior and laterodorsal	Mammillary body	Posterior cingulate, retrosplenial area, entorhinal-hippocampal complex	Learning and memory
Motor nuclei			
Ventroanterior	Globus pallidus	Frontal cortex	Modulation of motor function
Ventrolateral	Cerebellum	Frontal cortex	Modulation, coordination, and learning of movement
Sensory nuclei			
Ventral posterolateral	Sensory tracts from body	Parietal sensory cortex	Somatosensory function
Ventral posteromedial	Sensory tracts from face	Parietal sensory cortex	Facial sensation
	Solitary tract	Cortical gustatory area and anterior insula	Taste
Lateral geniculate	Optic tracts	Occipital cortex	Vision
Medial geniculate	Inferior colliculi	Temporal cortex	Hearing
Association nuclei			
Medial dorsal	Globus pallidus, amygdala, temporal and frontal cortex	Prefrontal cortex	Executive function, memory, social cognition, emotion
Lateral nuclear group (pulvinar)	Frontal, parietal, temporal, and occipital cortex	Frontal, parietal, temporal, and occipital cortex	Coordinates intra- and cross-modal cortical information processing
Nonspecific nuclei			
Midline	Hypothalamus	Amygdala, cingulate, hypothalamus	Visceral function
Intralaminar	Reticular formation, precentral and premotor cortex	Striatum, cortex	Activation
Reticular	Thalamic nucleus and cortex	Dorsal thalamic nuclei	Samples, gates, and focuses thalamocortical output

frontal syndrome is characterized primarily by executive function deficits. Abnormalities include developing poor strategies for solving visuospatial problems or learning new information and reduced ability to shift sets. Such behavioral changes are observed in patients with dorsolateral prefrontal lesions, as well as in those with caudate, globus pallidus, and thalamic dysfunction.

The *lateral orbitofrontal circuit* contains primarily limbic system structures. It begins in the inferolateral prefrontal cortex and projects to the ventromedial caudate nucleus (Alexander and Crutcher 1990; Alexander et al. 1986; Lichter and Cummings 2001) (see Figure 3–10). This caudate region projects to the pallidum and substantia nigra. Pallidum and nigra connect to medial portions of the ventroanterior and medial dorsal thalamic nuclei that project back to the orbitofrontal cortex. Disorders involving cortical or subcortical structures of the orbitofrontal circuit feature marked changes in personality, including a tendency to be more outspoken, more irritable, and more tactless and to worry less and have an elevated mood.

The *anterior cingulate circuit* begins in the cortex of the anterior cingulate gyrus (BA24) and projects to the ventral striatum (also known as the *limbic striatum*), which includes the

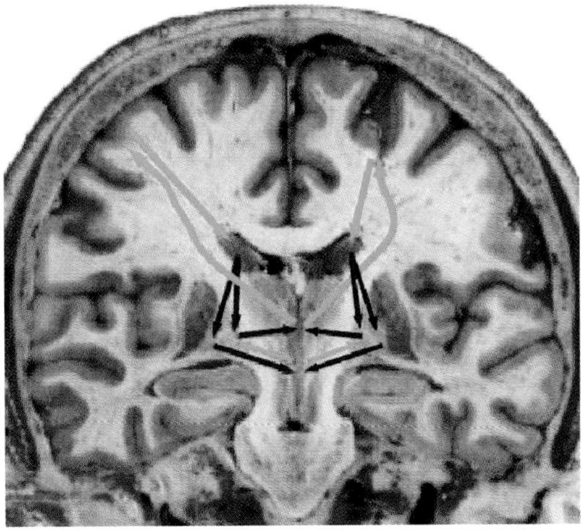

FIGURE 3–9. Organization of the prefrontal-subcortical circuits.

The prefrontal cortical regions (dorsolateral prefrontal, lateral orbitofrontal, and anterior cingulate) project to specific striatal regions *(green)* that in turn project to globus pallidus and substantia nigra *(blue)*. These structures project to the thalamic nuclei (in *blue*, projections from globus pallidus interna to thalamus and from globus pallidus externa to subthalamic nucleus; in *green*, from subthalamic nucleus to globus pallidus interna) that subsequently connect to the frontal lobe *(green)*, completing the circuit.

Source. Image adapted from M. Mega and the UCLA Laboratory of Neuroimaging.

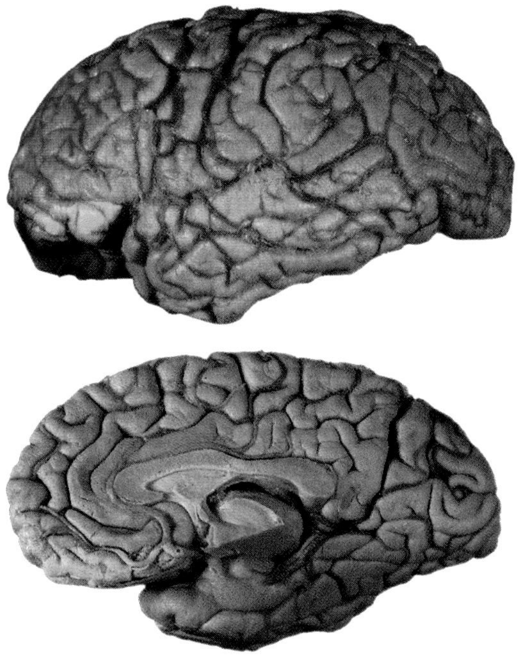

FIGURE 3–10. Prefrontal cortical origins of the dorsolateral (*blue*), anterior cingulate (*pink*), and lateral orbitofrontal (*green*) circuits.

Source. Image courtesy of M. Mega and the UCLA Laboratory of Neuroimaging.

nucleus accumbens and the ventromedial portions of the caudate and putamen (Alexander and Crutcher 1990; Alexander et al. 1986; Lichter and Cummings 2001) (see Figure 3–10). The most dramatic cases of anterior cingulate injury exhibit akinetic mutism. The patients are profoundly apathetic: they typically have their eyes open, do not speak spontaneously, answer questions in monosyllables if at all, and are profoundly indifferent. Apathy also has been associated with lesions of nucleus accumbens, globus pallidus, and thalamus, the principal subcortical members of the anterior cingulate circuit. Table 3–7 summarizes the behaviorally relevant frontal-subcortical circuits, including the anatomical structures involved, the behavioral disturbances observed with circuit dysfunction, and the common diseases affecting each circuit.

Frontal-subcortical circuits are involved in several neuropsychiatric disorders. In addition to personality alterations (e.g., apathy and disinhibition), mood changes and obsessive-compulsive behaviors are associated with focal brain lesions affecting these circuits. Depression occurs with lesions of the dorsolateral prefrontal cortex and the head of the caudate nucleus, particularly when the left hemisphere is affected (Jorge et al. 2004; Robinson 2006; Robinson et al. 1984; Starkstein et al. 1987, 1988b). Current models of the neurocircuitry of depression (Mayberg 2003; Seminowicz et al. 2004) identify roles for all three of these circuits in idiopathic major depression, as well as secondary depressive disorders. Lesions producing secondary mania also involve nuclei and connections of frontal-subcortical circuits. Mania has been observed with lesions of the medial orbitofrontal cortex, diseases of the caudate nuclei such as Huntington's disease, and injury to the right thalamus (Bogousslavsky et al. 1988; Cummings and Mendez 1984; Folstein 1989; Oster et al. 2007; Starkstein et al. 1988a).

Both acquired and idiopathic obsessive-compulsive disorders have been related to dysfunction of frontal-subcortical circuits. Obsessive-compulsive behavior has been observed in patients with caudate dysfunction in Huntington's disease and after Sydenham's chorea (Cummings and Cunningham 1992; Swedo et al. 1989), as well as with globus pallidus lesions in postencephalitic Parkinson's disease, in progressive supranuclear palsy, in manganese-induced parkinsonism, and after anoxic injury (Laplane et al. 1989; Mena et al. 1967; Schilder 1938). Idiopathic obsessive-compulsive disorder involves disturbances across the three neurobehaviorally salient frontal-subcortical circuits, with current models (Huey et al. 2008) identifying roles for the orbitofrontal cortex (in reward), the anterior cingulate cortex (in error detection), the basal ganglia

TABLE 3–7. Behavioral abnormalities associated with frontal-subcortical circuit disorders

Disease	Personality change	Mania	Depression	Obsessive-compulsive disorder	Neuropsychological impairment
Prefrontal cortical disorders					
Dorsolateral prefrontal syndrome	No	No	Yes	Yes	Yes
Lateral orbitofrontal syndrome	Yes	Yes	Yes	Yes	No
Anterior cingulate syndrome	Yes	Yes	Yes	Yes	Yes
Caudate disorders					
Parkinson's disease	Yes	No	Yes	No	Yes
Progressive supranuclear palsy	Yes	No	Yes	Yes	Yes
Huntington's disease	Yes	Yes	Yes	Yes	Yes
Sydenham's chorea	Yes	No	No	Yes	Yes
Wilson's disease	Yes	Yes	Yes	No	Yes
Neuroacanthocytosis	Yes	Yes	Yes	Yes	Yes
Fahr disease	UD	Yes	Yes	No	Yes
Infarction	Yes	No	Yes	Yes	Yes
Globus pallidus disorders					
Postencephalitic Parkinson's disease	Yes	Yes	Yes	Yes	Yes
Manganese toxicity	Yes	UD	UD	Yes	Yes
Carbon monoxide toxicity	Yes	No	No	Yes	Yes
Infarction	Yes	UD	UD	No	Yes
Thalamic disorders					
Infarction	Yes	Yes	No	No	Yes
Degeneration	Yes	UD	UD	UD	Yes

Note. UD=undetermined.

(in threshold setting for motor and behavioral program activation), and the dorsolateral prefrontal cortex (in storing memories of behavioral sequences).

Frontal-subcortical circuits are affected in patients who have diseases of the basal ganglia. The high frequency of neuropsychological alterations, the increased prevalence of personality and mood disturbances, the occurrence of obsessive-compulsive disorder, and the similarity between behaviors of patients with basal ganglia diseases and patients with frontal lobe injury are attributable to dysfunction of multiple frontal-subcortical circuits in basal ganglia disorders.

Neurochemistry and Behavior

The anatomical organization of the brain is complemented by an equally complex neurochemical organization. Many behavioral disorders reflect biochemical dysfunction, and the most effective interventions available are neurochemical in nature. Neurobehavioral deficits stemming from focal cortical lesions (e.g., aphasia and apraxia) have limited available remediable neurochemical treatments; neuropsychiatric disorders associated with limbic system dysfunction are frequently modifiable through neurochemical interventions.

There are two types of cerebral transmitters: 1) projection or extrinsic transmitters that originate in subcortical and brain stem nuclei and project to brain targets and 2) local or intrinsic transmitters that originate in neurons of the brain and project locally to adjacent or nearby cells. Projection transmitters or their synthetic enzymes must be transported within neurons for long distances from subcortical nuclei to distant regions and are vulnerable to disruption by stroke, tumors, and other processes. Transmitters are highly conserved from an evolutionary point of view, and many function locally in some neuronal systems and function as projection transmitters in others. The classic neurotransmitters have served neuronal communication for 600 million years of evolution (Rapoport 1990). Table 3–8 summarizes the origins and destinations of the extrinsic transmitters.

The effects of neurotransmitters are mediated by receptors to which the transmitter binds after it has been released into the synaptic cleft. Receptors may be located on the presynaptic or postsynaptic terminal. Presynaptic receptors (autoreceptors) regulate neurotransmitter synthesis or release. Postsynaptic receptors mediate the effects of the neurotransmitter on the postsynaptic cell. Heteroreceptors (receptors for neurotransmitters other than those produced by the neuron) also regulate synaptic activity. Binding of a neurotransmitter to a receptor results either in opening of an ion channel (ionotropic receptors) or initiation of second messenger cascades via guanosine triphosphate-binding proteins (metabotropic receptors). The neurotransmitter is removed from the synapse (either before or after binding to a receptor) by enzymatic degradation or by active reuptake into the presynaptic terminal by a high-affinity transporter protein. Behavioral effects can rarely be assigned to alterations in a single transmitter, but some aberrant behaviors are associated with changes that affect predominantly one type of transmitter. Table 3–9 presents the principal transmitter-behavior relationships currently identified.

Several discrete *cholinergic nuclei* project from subcortical sites to the brain. In the brain stem, the laterodorsal tegmental and pedunculopontine nuclei originate in the reticular formation and project via the dorsal tegmental pathway to the thalamus. This pathway is the essential component of the ascending reticular activating system (Nieuwenhuys 1985; Salmond et al. 2005). The cholinergic cell groups of the basal forebrain are the principal sources of cerebral acetylcholine (Perry et al. 1999; Salmond et al. 2005; Selden et al. 1998). Cholinergic projections in the septal nucleus and the vertical limb of the diagonal band of Broca project via the fornix to the hippocampus. The cells of the horizontal limb of the diagonal band of Broca supply the olfactory bulb. The neurons composing the nucleus basalis of Meynert project in several discrete bundles to the amygdala, to the cingulate and orbitofrontal cortices, to the insula and opercular cortices, and also to the rest of the neocortex (Figure 3–11). The afferents to the nucleus basalis are primarily from cortical and subcortical

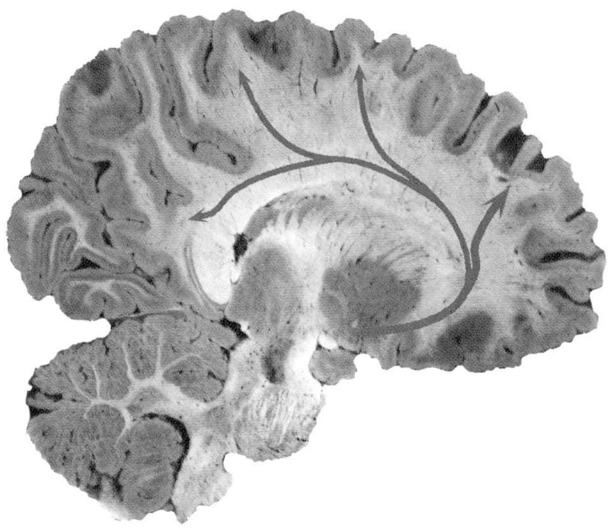

FIGURE 3–11. Cholinergic projections from the nucleus basalis (*red*).

Source. Image courtesy of M. Mega and the UCLA Laboratory of Neuroimaging.

limbic system structures, establishing the nucleus basalis as a relay between the limbic system afferents and efferents to the neocortex (Mesulam and Mufson 1984).

Cholinergic function is mediated by either nicotinic (ionotropic) or muscarinic (metabotropic) receptors. The muscarinic receptors are classified pharmacologically as M_1 (located postsynaptic) or M_2 (located presynaptic) and have different distributions throughout the brain. Cholinergic systems mediate a wide range of behaviors. Disruption of central cholinergic function (e.g., through the administration of cholinergic receptor blocking agents such as scopolamine) produces amnesia (Bartus et al. 1982), and intoxication with anticholinergic compounds produces delirium and delusions. Alzheimer's disease is one major disorder associated with cholinergic deficiency. This disease produces atrophy of the nucleus basalis, with consequent reduction in the synthesis of choline acetyltransferase, the enzyme that synthesizes acetylcholine; loss of synthetic activity leads to interruption of cortical cholinergic function (Katzman and Thal 1989). Increasing evidence indicates that some of the neuropsychiatric disturbances of Alzheimer's disease—hallucinations, apathy, disinhibition, and purposeless behavior—are produced by the cholinergic deficit (Cummings and Kaufer 1996). Cholinergic hyperactivity has been posited to play a role in the genesis of depression (Dilsaver and Coffman 1989), and in some species cholinergic stimulation of limbic system structures produces aggression (Valzelli 1981).

There are three main *dopaminergic projections* from the brain stem to the cerebral hemispheres: 1) a nigrostriatal projection arising from the compact portion of the substantia nigra

TABLE 3–8. Origins and destinations of the major extrinsic transmitter projections

Neurotransmitter	Origin	Destination
Acetylcholine		
Basal forebrain system	Nucleus basalis and nucleus of diagonal band of Broca	Neocortex, hippocampus, hypothalamus, and amygdala
Reticular system	Reticular formation	Thalamus
Dopamine		
Nigrostriatal system	Substantia nigra	Putamen and caudate nucleus
Mesolimbic system	Ventral tegmental area	Nucleus accumbens, septal nucleus, and amygdala
Mesocortical system	Ventral tegmental area	Medial temporal and frontal lobes and anterior cingulate cortex
Histamine	Posterior hypothalamus	Entire brain
GABA	Zona incerta	Neocortex, basal ganglia, and brain stem
	Caudate and putamen	Globus pallidus and substantia nigra
	Globus pallidus and substantia nigra	Thalamus
Glutamate	Neocortex	Caudate, putamen, thalamus, and nucleus accumbens
	Subthalamic nucleus	Globus pallidus
	Thalamus	Neocortex
	Hippocampus and subiculum	Septal region
	Entorhinal cortex	Hippocampus
Norepinephrine		
Dorsal pathway	Locus coeruleus	Thalamus, amygdala, basal forebrain, hippocampus, and neocortex
Ventral pathway	Locus coeruleus	Hypothalamus and midbrain reticular formation
Serotonin	Raphe nuclei	Entire brain

Note. GABA=γ-aminobutyric acid.

and projecting to the putamen and caudate, 2) a mesolimbic projection originating in the ventral tegmental area and projecting to limbic system structures, and 3) a mesocortical system beginning in the ventral tegmental area and projecting to frontal and temporal areas (Nieuwenhuys 1985) (Figure 3–12). Targets of the mesolimbic dopaminergic projection include the nucleus accumbens, septal nucleus, and amygdala. The mesocortical projections terminate primarily in the medial frontal lobe, medial temporal lobe, and the anterior cingulate region. Less robust projections are distributed to the neocortex.

Dopaminergic function is mediated by metabotropic receptors that can be classified pharmacologically as D_1-like (stimulate cAMP) or D_2-like (inhibit cAMP). These receptors have different distributions throughout the brain. The D_2 receptors are blocked by the neuroleptics, and it is possible that subtypes of the D_2 receptor differentially mediate the motor and mental effects of dopaminergic drugs.

Dopamine plays a key role in motoric functions and behavior. Dopamine deficiency or blockade leads to parkinsonism; dopamine excess produces chorea, dyskinesia, or tics. Behaviorally, dopamine deficiency causes at least mild cognitive impairment and may contribute to the depression that commonly accompanies Parkinson's disease and other parkinsonian syndromes. Dopamine excess leads to psychosis, elation or hypomania, and confusion. Dopamine hyperactivity may contribute to the pathophysiology of schizophrenia,

TABLE 3–9. Behavioral alterations associated with transmitter disturbances

Neurotransmitter	Reduced function	Increased function
Acetylcholine	Memory impairment, apathy, delirium, delusions	Depression, aggression
Dopamine		
Motor function	Parkinsonism	Chorea, tics
Behavior	Cognitive impairment (especially inattention), apathy, depression	Hallucinations, delusions, elation, obsessive-compulsive behavior, paraphilias
GABA	Seizures, anxiety	Amnesia, incoordination, sedation
Glutamate	Cognitive impairment (especially amnesia), psychosis, apathy	Seizures, excitotoxicity
Norepinephrine	Cognitive impairment (especially inattention), depression, dementia	Anxiety
Serotonin	Depression, anxiety, suicide, aggression	Confusion, hypomania, agitation, myoclonus

Note. GABA=γ-aminobutyric acid.

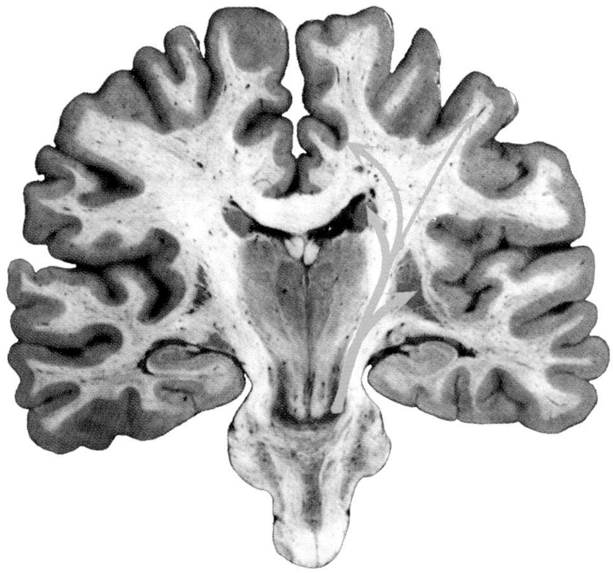

FIGURE 3–12. Nigrostriatal and mesocortical dopaminergic projections arising from the substantia nigra and ventral tegmental area, respectively (*green*).

Source. Image courtesy of M. Mega and the UCLA Laboratory of Neuroimaging.

obsessive-compulsive behavior, anxiety, and some paraphilic behaviors (Cummings 1985, 1991).

The locus coeruleus and adjacent nuclei comprise the origin of the *noradrenergic projection system.* A dorsal noradrenergic bundle courses in the dorsal brain stem to the septum, thalamus, amygdala, basal forebrain, hippocampus, and neocortex (Nieuwenhuys 1985) (Figure 3–13). A ventral noradrenergic bundle projects to the hypothalamus and midbrain reticular formation. Adrenergic function is mediated by metabotropic receptors that can be classified pharmacologically as α (inhibit cAMP) or β (stimulate cAMP) receptors. The α-adrenergic receptors can be further subtyped as α_1 or α_2; the former are located postsynaptically, and the latter presynaptically and postsynaptically. These receptors have different distributions throughout the brain. Effective treatment for depression is associated with decreased numbers (downregulation) of β-adrenergic receptors. Noradrenergic hypofunction has been linked to depression, dementia, and diminished alertness and concentration (Agid et al. 1987). Increased noradrenergic activity has been linked to anxiety (Lechin et al. 1989).

Serotonergic neurons are located almost exclusively in the median and paramedian raphe nuclei of the medulla, pons, and midbrain (Figure 3–14). The projection system of these serotonergic neurons is a complex, highly branched fiber system that embraces virtually the entire central nervous system (Nieuwenhuys 1985). Serotonergic function is mediated by multiple metabotropic receptors (5-HT_1, 5-HT_2, 5-HT_4) and to a lesser extent by ionotropic receptors (5-HT_3). These receptors have different distributions throughout the brain. Serotonin deficiency has been hypothesized to play a major role in suicide, depression, anxiety, and aggression (Agid et al. 1987), and excesses of cerebral serotonin may produce confusion, hypomania, agitation, and myoclonus (Isbister and Buckley 2005).

γ-Aminobutyric acid (GABA) is an inhibitory neurotransmitter present in both projection systems and local neuronal circuits. The principal GABA projection system begins in the

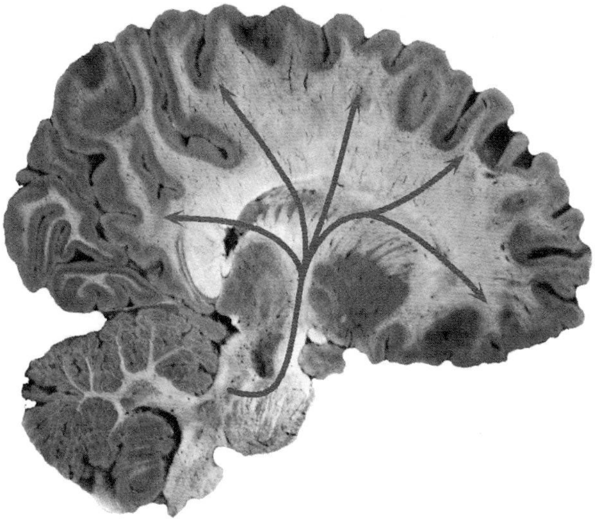

FIGURE 3–13. Noradrenergic projections from the locus coeruleus (*pink*).

Source. Image courtesy of M. Mega and the UCLA Laboratory of Neuroimaging.

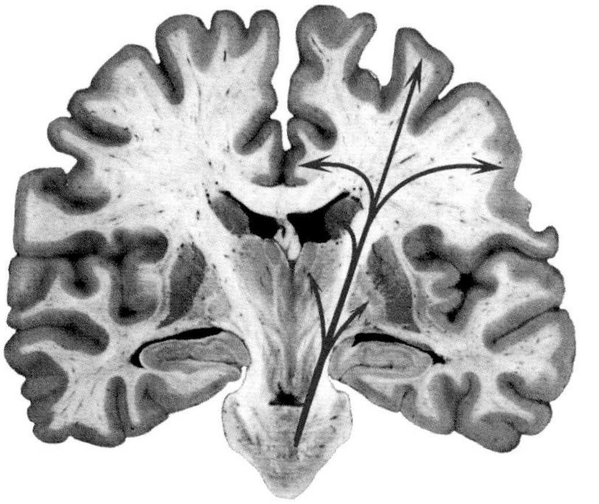

FIGURE 3–14. Serotonergic projections (*blue*).

Source. Image courtesy of M. Mega and the UCLA Laboratory of Neuroimaging.

zona incerta and projects bilaterally to the entire neocortex, basal ganglia, and brain stem (Lin et al. 1990). In subcortical regions, one projection system originates in the caudate and putamen and projects to the globus pallidus and substantia nigra, and another begins in the globus pallidus and substantia nigra with projections to the thalamus (Alexander and Crutcher 1990; Nieuwenhuys 1985). Local circuit neurons using GABA are found in the raphe nuclei, reticular nucleus of the thalamus, and basal ganglia. Local circuit neurons of the cerebral cortex also use GABA as their principal neurotransmitter (Rapoport 1990). GABA function is mediated by ionotropic ($GABA_A$) and metabotropic ($GABA_B$) receptors, the former being of special interest to neuropsychiatry because they contain the binding sites for alcohol, anticonvulsants, and benzodiazepines. These receptors have different distributions throughout the brain. GABA concentrations are decreased in the basal ganglia of patients with Huntington's disease, and the GABA deficiency may contribute to dementia, mood disorder, obsessive-compulsive disorder, and psychosis in this condition (Morris 1991).

Glutamate is an excitatory neurotransmitter that is used in the massive projection from the neocortex to the ipsilateral caudate, putamen, and nucleus accumbens. Glutamate is the principal neurotransmitter of projections from cortex to thalamus, from thalamus to cortex, and from one region of cortex to another. Glutamatergic neurons also project from subthalamic nucleus to globus pallidus. Glutamate functions in several hippocampus-related projections, including the perforant pathway projecting from entorhinal cortex to hippocampus and the pathways originating in hippocampus and adjacent subiculum and projecting to the septal region (Alexander and Crutcher 1990; Nieuwenhuys 1985). Glutamatergic function is mediated by ionotropic and metabotropic receptors, with subtypes of the former (e.g., *N*-methyl-D-aspartate, or NMDA, receptor) having been implicated in learning, excitotoxicity, and the psychotomimetic effects of phencyclidine (PCP). These receptors have different distributions throughout the brain. Glutamate release is inhibited by several drugs used in clinical practice. These include lamotrigine (anticonvulsant) and riluzole (amyotrophic lateral sclerosis). The behavioral consequences of alterations in glutamate function are substantial. Antagonism of NMDA receptors induced by PCP or ketamine is a useful pharmacological model for schizophrenia in that it results in the positive symptoms (hallucination, delusion, behavioral dyscontrol), negative symptoms (alogia, anhedonia, inanition), and cognitive impairments of this condition (Javitt 2007). Conversely, glutamatergic excesses are implicated in the ictogenesis (development of seizures) in general and particularly in mesial temporal lobe epilepsy (Eid et al. 2008).

Several other transmitters occur in behaviorally relevant areas, but their role in human behavior remains to be determined. *Histaminergic* neurons are situated in the posterior hypothalamus and project diffusely to most brain structures, including the neocortex, amygdala, septum, caudate, and putamen (Nieuwenhuys 1985). *Glycine* is an inhibitory transmitter that may function in local circuit neurons in the substantia nigra, caudate, and putamen. *Substance P* is present in the projection from caudate and putamen to the substantia nigra, and *enkephalin*-containing neurons project from caudate and putamen to the globus pallidus (Alexander and

Crutcher 1990; Nieuwenhuys 1985). *Vasoactive intestinal peptide* neurons are intrinsic to the cortex and participate in local neuronal circuits (Nieuwenhuys 1985).

Conclusion

The brain consists of a median zone mediating arousal and basic life-sustaining functions, such as respiration, digestion, circulation, and neuroendocrine function; a paramedian-limbic zone mediating extrapyramidal function and many aspects of emotional experience; and a supralimbic-neocortical zone mediating instrumental cognitive functions, such as language and praxis (Table 3–10). Injury of the supralimbic-neocortical zone is associated with neurobehavioral deficit syndromes, such as aphasia and apraxia; dysfunction of the paramedian-limbic zone correlates with neuropsychiatric disorders, including mood disorders, psychoses, anxiety, and obsessive-compulsive disorder. Within each zone, behavioral deficits can be related to dysfunction of specific neurotransmitters. This approach provides a comprehensive framework for understanding brain-behavior relationships.

TABLE 3–10. Summary of the anatomy, functions, and syndromes of the median, paramedian-limbic, and supralimbic-neocortical zones of the brain

Zone	Myelination	Neuronal connectivity/ anatomy	Ontogeny	Function	Behavioral syndromes
Median	Poor	Feltwork; reticular	Functional at birth	Arousal	Disturbances of arousal, neuroendocrine control, respiration, circulation
Paramedian-limbic	Intermediate	Series; limbic system and basal ganglia	Functional within first few months	Emotion; extrapyramidal function	Neuropsychiatric disorders; movement disorders
Supralimbic-neocortical	Complete	Parallel; neocortex	Functional in adulthood	Sensory cortex, motor cortex, association cortex	Neurobehavioral disorders

Key Points

- All behaviors and experiences are mediated by the brain. No behavior, thought, or emotion lacks a corresponding cerebral event, and abnormalities of human behavior are frequently a reflection of abnormal brain structure and are accompanied by aberrant brain function.
- The brain comprises three general regions: a median zone surrounding the ventricular system, containing the hypothalamus and related structures; a paramedian-limbic zone consisting primarily of limbic system structures, basal ganglia, and parts of the thalamus; and a supralimbic zone containing the neocortex.
- The median zone subserves arousal and basic life-sustaining functions, such as respiration, digestion, circulation, and neuroendocrine function.
- The paramedian-limbic zone mediates extrapyramidal function and many aspects of emotional experience. Dysfunction of the paramedian-limbic zone correlates with neuropsychiatric disorders, including anxiety and mood disorders, psychoses, and obsessive-compulsive disorder.

- The supralimbic-neocortical zone mediates instrumental cognitive functions. Injury of the supralimbic-neocortical zone is associated with specific, and often lateralized, neurobehavioral syndromes (see Table 3-3).
- Within each zone, behavioral deficits can be related to dysfunction of specific neurotransmitters.

References

Adams RD, Victor M: Principles of Neurology, 2nd Edition. New York, McGraw-Hill, 1981

Agid Y, Ruberg M, Dubois B, et al: Anatomoclinical and biochemical concepts of subcortical dementia, in Cognitive Neurochemistry. Edited by Stahl SM, Iversen SD, Goodman EC. New York, Oxford University Press, 1987, pp 248–271

Alexander GE, Crutcher MD: Functional architecture of basal ganglia circuits: neural substrates of parallel processing. Trends Neurosci 13:266–271, 1990

Alexander GE, DeLong MR, Strick PL: Parallel organization of functionally segregated circuits linking basal ganglia and cortex. Annu Rev Neurosci 9:357–381, 1986

Alexander GE, Crutcher MD, DeLong MR: Basal ganglia–thalamocortical circuits: parallel substrates for motor, oculomotor, "prefrontal" and "limbic" functions. Prog Brain Res 85:119–146, 1990

Amaducci L, Sorbi S, Albanese A, et al: Choline acetyltransferase (ChAT) activity differs in right and left human temporal lobes. Neurology 31:799–805, 1981

Bartus RT, Dean RL III, Beer B, et al: The cholinergic hypothesis of geriatric memory dysfunction. Science 217:408–417, 1982

Baxter LR Jr, Phelps ME, Mazziotta JC, et al: Cerebral metabolic rates for glucose in mood disorders. Arch Gen Psychiatry 42:441–447, 1985

Baxter LR Jr, Phelps ME, Mazziotta JC, et al: Local cerebral glucose metabolic rates in obsessive-compulsive disorder. Arch Gen Psychiatry 44:211–218, 1987

Benarroch EE: Central Autonomic Network: Functional Organization and Clinical Correlations. Armonk, NY, Futura, 1997

Benson DF, Cummings JL, Tsai SY: Angular gyrus syndrome simulating Alzheimer disease. Arch Neurol 39:616–620, 1982

Bogousslavsky J, Ferrazzini M, Regli F, et al: Manic delirium and frontal-like syndrome with paramedian infarction of the right thalamus. J Neurol Neurosurg Psychiatry 51:116–119, 1988

Brandt J, Seidman LJ, Kohl D: Personality characteristics of epileptic patients: a controlled study of generalized and temporal lobe cases. J Clin Exp Neuropsychol 7:25–38, 1985

Burns JM, Swerdlow RH: Right orbitofrontal tumor with pedophilia symptom and constructional apraxia sign. Arch Neurol 60:437–440, 2003

Carota A, Staub F, Bogousslavsky J: Emotions, behaviors and mood changes in stroke. Curr Opin Neurol 15:57–69, 2002

Carpenter MB: Core Text of Neuroanatomy, 4th Edition. Baltimore, MD, Williams & Wilkins, 1991

Carpenter MB, Sutin J: Human Neuroanatomy, 8th Edition. Baltimore, MD, Williams & Wilkins, 1983

Chiron C, Leboyer M, Leon F, et al: SPECT of the brain in childhood autism: evidence for lack of normal hemispheric asymmetry. Dev Med Child Neurol 37:849–860, 1995

Coffey CE: Cerebral laterality and emotion: the neurology of depression. Compr Psychiatry 28:197–219, 1987

Coffey CE, Figiel GS, Djang WT, et al: Leukoencephalopathy in elderly depressed patients referred for ECT. Biol Psychiatry 24:143–161, 1988

Crow TJ: The "big bang" theory of the origin of psychosis and the faculty of language. Schizophr Res 102:31–52, 2008

Cummings JL: Clinical Neuropsychiatry. New York, Grune & Stratton, 1985

Cummings JL: Behavioral complications of drug treatment of Parkinson's disease. J Am Geriatr Soc 39:708–716, 1991

Cummings JL: Depression and Parkinson's disease: a review. Am J Psychiatry 149:443–454, 1992

Cummings JL: Frontal-subcortical circuits and human behavior. Arch Neurol 50:873–880, 1993

Cummings JL, Cunningham K: Obsessive-compulsive disorder in Huntington's disease. Biol Psychiatry 31:263–270, 1992

Cummings JL, Kaufer DI: Neuropsychiatric aspects of Alzheimer's disease: the cholinergic hypothesis revisited. Neurology 47:876–883, 1996

Cummings JL, Mendez MF: Secondary mania with focal cerebrovascular lesions. Am J Psychiatry 141:1084–1087, 1984

Damasio AR, Grabowski TJ, Bechara A, et al: Subcortical and cortical brain activity during the feeling of self-generated emotions. Nat Neurosci 3:1049–1056, 2000

Delvenne V, Delecluse F, Hubain PP, et al: Regional cerebral blood flow in patients with affective disorders. Br J Psychiatry 157:359–365, 1990

Dilsaver SC, Coffman JA: Cholinergic hypothesis of depression: a reappraisal. J Clin Psychopharmacol 9:173–179, 1989

Doane BK: Clinical psychiatry and the physiodynamics of the limbic system, in The Limbic System: Functional Organization and Clinical Disorders. Edited by Doane BK, Livingston KE. New York, Raven, 1986, pp 285–315

Dolan RJ, Bench CJ, Brown RG, et al: Regional cerebral blood flow abnormalities in depressed patients with cognitive impairment. J Neurol Neurosurg Psychiatry 55:768–773, 1992

Drevets WC, Videen TO, Price JL, et al: A functional anatomical study of unipolar depression. J Neurosci 12:3628–3641, 1992

Duffy JD, Coffey CE: The neurobiology of depression, in Contemporary Behavioral Neurology. Edited by Trimble MR, Cummings JL. Boston, MA, Butterworth-Heinemann, 1997, pp 275–288

Eid T, Williamsom A, Lee TS, et al: Glutamate and astrocytes—key players in human mesial temporal lobe epilepsy? Epilepsia 49 (suppl 2):42–52, 2008
Eidelberg D, Galaburda AM: Symmetry and asymmetry in the posterior thalamus. Arch Neurol 39:325–332, 1982
Eviatar Z, Latzer Y, Vicksman P: Anomalous lateral dominance patterns in women with eating disorders: clues to neurobiological bases. Int J Neurosci 118:1425–1442, 2008
Falzi G, Perrone P, Vignolog LA: Right-left asymmetry in anterior speech region. Arch Neurol 39:239–240, 1982
Folstein SE: Huntington's Disease: A Disorder of Families. Baltimore, MD, Johns Hopkins University Press, 1989
Fusar-Poli P, Placentino A, Carletti F, et al: Laterality effect on emotional faces processing: ALE meta-analysis of evidence. Neurosci Lett 452:262–267, 2009
Gainotti G: Emotional behavior and hemispheric side of lesion. Cortex 8:41–55, 1972
Galaburda AM, LeMay M, Kemper TL, et al: Right-left asymmetries in the brain. Science 199:852–856, 1978
Gardini S, Cloninger CR, Venneri A: Individual differences in personality traits reflect structural variance in specific brain regions. Brain Res Bull 79:265–270, 2009
George MS, Ketter TA, Kimbrell TA, et al: What functional imaging has revealed about the brain basis of mood and emotion. Advances in Biological Psychiatry 2:63–113, 1996
Geschwind N: Disconnection syndromes in animals and man. Brain 88:237–294, 585–644, 1965
Girgis M: Neural Substrates of Limbic Epilepsy. St. Louis, MO, Warren H. Green, 1981
Glick SD, Ross DA, Hough LB: Lateral asymmetry of neurotransmitters in human brain. Brain Res 234:53–63, 1982
Gregorio SP, Sallet PC, Do KA, et al: Polymorphisms in genes involved in neurodevelopment may be associated with altered brain morphology in schizophrenia: preliminary evidence. Psychiatry Res 156:1–9, 2009
Gorman DG, Cummings JL: Hypersexuality following septal injury. Arch Neurol 49:308–310, 1992
Halgren E, Walter RD, Cherlow DG, et al: Mental phenomena evoked by electrical stimulation of the human hippocampal formation and amygdala. Brain 101:83–117, 1978
Hamani C, Mayberg H, Snyder B, et al: Deep brain stimulation of the subcallosal cingulate gyrus for depression: anatomical location of active contacts in clinical responders and a suggested guideline for targeting. J Neurosurg 111:1209–1215, 2009
Hermann BP, Wyler AR, Blumer D, et al: Ictal fear: lateralizing significance and implications for understanding the neurobiology of pathological fear states. Neuropsychiatry Neuropsychol Behav Neurol 5:205–210, 1992
Huey ED, Zahn R, Krueger F, et al: A psychological and neuroanatomical model of obsessive-compulsive disorder. J Neuropsychiatry Clin Neurosci 20:390–408, 2008
Isaacson RL: The Limbic System. New York, Plenum, 1974
Isbister GK, Buckley NA: The pathophysiology of serotonin toxicity in animals and humans: implications for diagnosis and treatment. Clin Neuropharmacol 28:205–214, 2005
Javitt DC: Glutamate and schizophrenia: phencyclidine, *N*-methyl-D-aspartate receptors, and dopamine-glutamate interactions. Int Rev Neurobiol 78:69–108, 2007
Jorge RE, Robinson RG, Moser D, et al: Major depression following traumatic brain injury. Arch Gen Psychiatry 61:42–50, 2004
Kalivas PW, Volkow ND: The neural basis of addiction: a pathology of motivation and choice. Am J Psychiatry 162:1403–1413, 2005
Katzman R, Thal L: Neurochemistry of Alzheimer's disease, in Basic Neurochemistry, 4th Edition. Edited by Siegel GJ, Agranoff BW, Albers RW, et al. New York, Raven, 1989, pp 827–838
Kawasaki Y, Suzuki M, Takahashi T, et al: Anomalous cerebral asymmetry in patients with schizophrenia demonstrated by voxel-based morphometry. Biol Psychiatry 63:793–800, 2008
Kimura D, Durnford M: Normal studies on the function of the right hemisphere in vision, in Hemisphere Function in the Human Brain. Edited by Dimond SJ, Beaumont JG. London, Elek Science, 1974, pp 25–47
Kirshner HS: Behavioral Neurology: A Practical Approach. New York, Churchill Livingstone, 1986
Kirshner HS: Vascular dementia: a review of recent evidence for prevention and treatment. Curr Neurol Neurosci Rep 9:437–442, 2009
Kooistra CA, Heilman KM: Motor dominance and lateral asymmetry of the globus pallidus. Neurology 38:388–390, 1988
Laplane D, Levasseur M, Pillon B, et al: Obsessive-compulsive and other behavioral changes with bilateral basal ganglia lesions. Brain 112:699–725, 1989
Lavretsky J, Ballmaier M, Pham D, et al: Neuroanatomical characteristics of geriatric apathy and depression: a magnetic resonance imaging study. Am J Geriatr Psychiatry 15:386–394, 2007
Lechin F, van der Dijs B, Amat J, et al: Central neuronal pathways involved in anxiety behavior: experimental findings, in Neurochemistry and Clinical Disorders: Circuitry of Some Psychiatric and Psychosomatic Syndromes. Edited by Lechin F, van der Dijs B. Boca Raton, FL, CRC Press, 1989, pp 49–64
Leiguarda RC, Marsden CD: Limb apraxias: higher-order disorders of sensorimotor integration. Brain 123:860–879, 2000
LeMay M: Morphological cerebral asymmetries of modern man, fossil man, and nonhuman primate. Ann N Y Acad Sci 280:349–366, 1976
Leonard CM, Eckert MA: Asymmetry and dyslexia. Dev Neuropsychol 33:663–681, 2008
Levy J: The mammalian brain and the adaptive advantage of cerebral asymmetry. Ann N Y Acad Sci 299:264–272, 1977
Lichter DC, Cummings JL: Introduction and overview, in Frontal-Subcortical Circuits in Psychiatric and Neurological Disorders. Edited by Lichter DG, Cummings JL. New York, Guilford Press, 2001, pp 1–43
Lilly R, Cummings JL, Benson DF, et al: The human Klüver-Bucy syndrome. Neurology 33:1141–1145, 1983
Lin C-S, Nicolelis MAL, Schneider JS, et al: A major direct GABAergic pathway from zona incerta to neocortex. Science 248:1553–1556, 1990
MacLean PD: The Triune Brain in Evolution. New York, Plenum, 1990

Marin RS: Apathy: a neuropsychiatric syndrome. J Neuropsychiatry Clin Neurosci 3:243–254, 1991
Marin RS, Wilkosz PA: Disorders of diminished motivation. J Head Trauma Rehabil 20:377–388, 2005
Marshall JC, Halligan PW, Fink GR, et al: The functional anatomy of a hysterical paralysis. Cognition 61:B1–B8, 1997
Mayberg HS: Modulating dysfunctional limbic-cortical circuits in depression: towards development of brain-based algorithms for diagnosis and optimised treatment. Br Med Bull 65:193–207, 2003
Mayer AR, Kosson DS: Handedness and psychopathy. Neuropsychiatry Neuropsychol Behav Neurol 13:233–238, 2000
Mena I, Marin O, Fuenzalida S, et al: Chronic manganese poisoning. Neurology 17:128–136, 1967
Mendez MF, Chow T, Ringman J, et al: Pedophilia and temporal lobe disturbances. J Neuropsychiatry Clin Neurosci 12:71–76, 2000
Mesulam M-M: Behavioral Neuroanatomy: Large-scale networks, association cortex, frontal syndromes, the limbic system, and hemispheric specializations, in Principles of Cognitive and Behavioral Neurology. Edited by Mesulam M-M. Oxford, UK, Oxford University Press, 2000, pp 1–120
Mesulam M-M, Mufson EJ: Neural inputs into the nucleus basalis of the substantia innominata (Ch4) in the rhesus monkey. Brain 107:253–274, 1984
Miller BL, Cummings JL, McIntyre H, et al: Hypersexuality or altered sexual preference following brain injury. J Neurol Neurosurg Psychiatry 49:867–873, 1986
Morris M: Psychiatric aspects of Huntington's disease, in Huntington's Disease. Edited by Harper PS. Philadelphia, PA, WB Saunders, 1991, pp 81–126
Nauta WJH: Circuitous connections linking cerebral cortex, limbic system, and corpus striatum, in The Limbic System: Functional Organization and Clinical Disorders. Edited by Doane BK, Livingston KE. New York, Raven, 1986, pp 43–54
Nauta WJH, Feirtag M: Fundamental Neuroanatomy. New York, WH Freeman, 1986
Nieuwenhuys R: Chemoarchitecture of the Brain. New York, Springer-Verlag, 1985
Oke A, Keller R, Mefford I, et al: Lateralization of norepinephrine in human thalamus. Science 200:1411–1413, 1978
Oster TJ, Anderson CA, Filley CM, et al: Quetiapine for mania due to traumatic brain injury. CNS Spectr 12:764–769, 2007
Papez JW: A proposed mechanism of emotion. Arch Neurol Psychiatry 38:725–743, 1937
Perez MM, Trimble MR, Murray NMF, et al: Epileptic psychosis: an evaluation of PSE profiles. Br J Psychiatry 146:155–163, 1985
Perry E, Walker M, Grace J, et al: Acetylcholine in mind: a neurotransmitter correlate of consciousness? Trends Neurosci 22: 273–280, 1999
Plum F, Posner JB: The Diagnosis of Stupor and Coma. Philadelphia, PA, FA Davis, 1980
Rapoport SI: Integrated phylogeny of the primate brain, with special reference to humans and their diseases. Brain Res Rev 15:267–294, 1990
Reisberg B, Franssen E, Sclan SG, et al: Stage specific incidence of potentially remediable behavioral symptoms in aging and Alzheimer's disease. Bull Clin Neurosci 54:95–112, 1989
Reite M, Teale P, Rojas DC, et al: MEG auditory evoked fields suggest altered structural/functional asymmetry in primary but not secondary auditory cortex in bipolar disorder. Bipolar Disord 22: 371–381, 2009
Robinson RG: The Clinical Neuropsychiatry of Stroke, 2nd Edition. Cambridge, UK, Cambridge University Press, 2006
Robinson RG, Kubos KL, Starr LB, et al: Mood disorders in stroke patients: importance of location of lesion. Brain 107:81–93, 1984
Sackeim HA, Greenburg MS, Weiman AL, et al: Hemispheric asymmetry in the expression of positive and negative emotions. Arch Neurol 39:210–218, 1982
Sackeim HA, Prohovnik I, Moeller JR, et al: Regional cerebral blood flow in mood disorders. Arch Gen Psychiatry 47:60–70, 1990
Salmond CH, Chatflied DA, Menon DK, et al: Cognitive sequelae of head injury: involvement of basal forebrain and associated structure. Brain 128:189–200, 2005
Savoiz A, Leuba G, Vallet PG, et al: Contribution of neural networks to Alzheimer's disease progression. Brain Res Bull 80:309–312, 2009
Schade JP, Groeningen VV: Structural organization of the human cerebral cortex. Acta Anat (Basel) 47:79–111, 1961
Schilder P: The organic background of obsessions and compulsions. Am J Psychiatry 94:1397–1416, 1938
Schmahmann JD, Pandya DN, Wang R, et al: Association fibre pathways of the brain: parallel observations from diffusion spectrum imaging and autoradiography. Brain 130:630–653, 2007
Schmahmann JD, Smith EE, Eichler FS, et al: Cerebral white matter: neuroanatomy, clinical neurology, and neurobehavioral correlates. Ann N Y Acad Sci 1142:266–309, 2008
Selden NR, Gitelman DR, Salamon-Murayama N, et al: Trajectories of cholinergic pathways within the cerebral hemispheres of the human brain. Brain 121:2249–2257, 1998
Seminowicz DA, Mayberg HS, McIntosh AR, et al: Limbic-frontal circuitry in major depression: a path modeling metanalysis. Neuroimage 22:409–418, 2004
Shin LM, Liberzon I: The neurocircuitry of fear, stress, and anxiety disorders. Neuropsychopharmacology 35:169–191, 2010
Shipp S: The functional logic of cortico-pulvinar connections. Philos Trans R Soc Lond B Biol Sci 358:1605–1624, 2003
Sneed JR, Rindskopf D, Steffens DC, et al: The vascular depression subtype: evidence of internal validity. Biol Psychiatry 64:491–497, 2008
Spence SA, Crimlisk HL, Cope H, et al: Discrete neurophysiologic correlates in prefrontal cortex during hysterical and feigned disorder of movement. Lancet 356:162–163, 2000
Starkstein SE, Robinson RG, Price TR: Comparison of cortical and subcortical lesions in the production of post-stroke mood disorders. Brain 110:1045–1059, 1987
Starkstein SE, Boston JD, Robinson RG: Mechanisms of mania after brain injury: twelve case reports and review of the literature. J Nerv Ment Dis 176:87–100, 1988a

Starkstein SE, Robinson RG, Berthier ML, et al: Differential mood changes following basal ganglia vs. thalamic lesions. Arch Neurol 45:725–730, 1988b

Stein MB, Heuser IJ, Juncos JL, et al: Anxiety disorders in patients with Parkinson's disease. Am J Psychiatry 147: 217–220, 1990

Stephan BC, Matthews FE, Khaw KT, et al: Beyond mild cognitive impairment: vascular cognitive impairment, no dementia (VCIND). Alzheimers Res Ther 1:4, 2009

Strauss E, Risser A, Jones MW: Fear responses in patients with epilepsy. Arch Neurol 39:626–630, 1982

Stuss DT, Benson DF: The Frontal Lobes. New York, Raven, 1986

Stuss DT, Guberman A, Nelson R, et al: The neuropsychology of paramedian thalamic infarction. Brain Cogn 8:348–378, 1988

Swedo SE, Rapoport JL, Cheslow DL, et al: High prevalence of obsessive-compulsive symptoms in patients with Sydenham's chorea. Am J Psychiatry 146:246–249, 1989

Tekin S, Cummings JL: Frontal-subcortical neuronal circuits and clinical neuropsychiatry: an update. J Psychosom Res 53:648–654, 2002

Valzelli L: Psychobiology of Aggression and Violence. New York, Raven, 1981

Van Lancker D: Personal relevance and the human right hemisphere. Brain Cogn 17:64–92, 1991

Vuilleumier P, Chicherio C, Assal F, et al: Functional neuroanatomical correlates of hysterical sensorimotor loss. Brain 124:1077–1090, 2001

Weintraub S, Mesulam M-M: Developmental learning disabilities of the right hemisphere. Arch Neurol 40:463–468, 1983

Wildgruber D, Ackermann H, Kreifelts B, et al: Cerebral processing of linguistic and emotional prosody: fMRI studies. Prog Brain Res 156:249–268, 2006

Williams D: The structure of emotions reflected in epileptic experiences. Brain 79:29–67, 1956

Wilson TW, Rojas DC, Teale PD, et al: Aberrant functional organization and maturation in early onset psychosis: evidence from magnetoencephalography. Psychiatry Res 156:59–67, 2007

Yakovlev PI: Motility, behavior and the brain. J Nerv Ment Dis 107: 313–335, 1948

Yakovlev PI: Telencephalon "impar," "semipar," and "totopar." Int J Neurol 6:245–265, 1968

Yakovlev PI, Lecours A-R: The myelogenetic cycles of regional maturation of the brain, in Regional Development of the Brain in Early Life. Edited by Minkowski A. Oxford, UK, Blackwell Scientific, 1967, pp 3–65

Zadina JN, Corey DM, Casbergue RM, et al: Lobar asymmetries in subtypes of dyslexic and control subjects. J Child Neurol 21:922–931, 2006

PART II

Neuropsychiatric Assessment

4

Neuropsychiatric Assessment

John J. Campbell III, M.D.

Neuropsychiatry is an ambiguous construct. Its precise definition remains elusive (Cummings and Hegarty 1994; Lishman 1992; Trimble 1993). In practice, however, a neuropsychiatric approach permits a broad conceptualization of a particular clinical problem that transcends the basic neurological or psychiatric paradigm. This approach is of particular relevance for the geriatric patient, in whom the interplay between biology and psychology is complex and pervasive. A thorough neuropsychiatric examination can reconcile this dichotomy and form the basis for a comprehensive treatment plan. Several outstanding reviews have detailed the areas relevant to a proper assessment (Cummings 1985a; Ovsiew 2007; Schiffer and Najara-Lanson 2003; Strub and Black 2000; Weintraub 2000).

Schiffer and Najara-Lanson (2003) have elaborated on the neuropsychiatric gestalt. The approach represents a fundamental departure from traditional psychiatry and neurology in several ways. Collateral confirmation of historical details is emphasized. Because neuropsychiatric syndromes often affect recall and insight, the examiner often needs supplementary history from those who know the patient. The reciprocal influences of psychology and cerebral dysfunction are appreciated. Although both processes are brain related, each has its own unique and significant influence on behavior. Localization of signs and symptoms in the brain takes precedence over standard psychiatric diagnoses. Therefore, a more comprehensive and flexible assessment of mental status is undertaken.

The neuropsychiatric assessment is data driven. The collection of the data and their synthesis into a coherent formulation serve to establish neuropsychiatry as a unique clinical discipline. In this chapter, I provide an overview of the neuropsychiatric assessment of the geriatric patient, emphasizing the relationship between functional neuroanatomy and neuropathology. The basic framework of this assessment includes taking a history, doing a mental status examination, performing a physical examination, and making a formulation.

Clinical Interview

The geriatric neuropsychiatry clinical interview has unique aspects. Patients commonly experience hearing impairment, diminished cognitive efficiency, attentional impairments, lack of insight, impaired memory, and dysphasias, all of which challenge the skills of the interviewer. In addition, the caregiver must be an integral source of historical information. Caregivers play an increasingly important role as the patient experiences functional declines and requires increasing assistance. The presence of impaired memory and insight may interfere with the gathering of the history to such an extent that the caregiver provides the essential collateral information.

Furthermore, the ongoing responsibility of taking care of an impaired individual can lead to demoralization, isolation, and depression, which serve to diminish the effectiveness of the caregiver. This diminished effectiveness can result in a possibly preventable patient accident, such as falling and fracturing a hip; a nursing home placement; or even elder abuse. Thus, inquiring as to how the caregivers are dealing with their own stresses is part of the geriatric neuropsychiatric assessment.

The neuropsychiatric history explores two interrelated realms of human existence—the development of a central nervous system and the development of a person. Therefore, this exploration begins before conception, with the *genetic history of the parents*, through gestation and birth, up to the day of the examination. The clinical interview described below has been organized along a time line, to address issues of psychological development along with the typical starting points for important behavioral and neurological considerations, such as the occurrence of depression or the onset of Parkinson's disease. The interview emphasizes that the patients are products of their past experiences regardless of the manifesting complaint. The completed history will establish a qualitative functional baseline, along with an appreciation of inherited and acquired influences on development, their impact, and the role of biological and psychological attempts at compensation. Table 4–1 lists the elements of the neuropsychiatric clinical interview.

Gestation and Birth

The central nervous system develops in an orderly sequence notable for the germination, migration, and differentiation of neurons and glia throughout gestation. During this period, cerebral and somatic development is vulnerable to numerous perturbations from many causes. Maternal drug use, infection, and injury can negatively influence the developmental process. Labor and delivery impose additional stresses on the neonatal brain. Maternal hemorrhage or circulatory impairment can result in hypoxic brain injury, and cranial trauma to the neonate during delivery can cause cerebral contusions and intracerebral hemorrhage, all of which may negatively affect neurodevelopment.

The *gestational and birth history* is not generally accessible with geriatric patients. Ideally, higher-functioning patients or caregivers can provide this information. Otherwise, several clues in the history and physical examination may raise the index of suspicion. Early hemispheric damage often leads to subtle contralateral hemiatrophy. Careful observation of the face or comparison of the hands can reveal somatic asymmetry and developmental anomaly. For example, manifestations of fetal alcohol syndrome include facial changes with epicanthic eye folds, poorly formed concha, small teeth with faulty enamel, and microcephaly with mental retardation (Streissguth and Landesman-Dwyer 1980). Delays in the timely *achievement of developmental milestones* may signal inherited or acquired dysfunction. Scholastic difficulties with speech, language, or arithmetic may reflect left-hemispheric anomaly. In addition, Rourke (1989) described a syndrome of social impairment and dysprosodia localized to the right hemisphere.

Ovsiew (2007) listed several additional signs that may suggest developmental abnormality. These include an abnormal head circumference, fine "electric" hair, more than one hair whorl, abnormal epicanthic folds of the eyes, abnormal interorbital distance, low-set or malformed ears, high palate, and furrowed tongue. Peripheral signs include curved fifth finger, single palmar crease, wide gap between first and second toes, partial fusion of the toes, and third toe longer than second toe.

Handedness may reflect anomalous cerebral development. Geschwind and Galaburda (1985a, 1985b, 1985c) proposed a model of handedness based on intrauterine influences on development. They described a continuum of handedness ranging from strongly right-handed to ambidextrous to strongly left-handed and suggest that the degree of left-handedness may reflect compensation for negative intrauterine influences on left hemisphere development.

TABLE 4–1. Elements of the neuropsychiatric clinical interview

Gestational and birth history
Achievements of developmental milestones
Handedness
Genetic history of the parents and siblings
School history: academic and disciplinary
History of violence or criminal behavior
History of head injury
Psychiatric history
Substance abuse history
Behavioral and cognitive baseline
Occupational history
Medical and surgical history
Medication history
Review of systems
Survey of the vegetative functions
Assessment of activities of daily living
History of recent changes in behavior and cognition

Childhood

The challenges of childhood include refining social and scholastic skills. School represents an intellectual and behavioral laboratory in which deficits may be revealed, and the *school history* requires thorough probing. It is important to obtain information about any remedial classes or a history of being held back. Often, formal testing was done, and a report may be available. Such testing is a relatively recent development in U.S. education, however, and such information may not be obtainable for elderly persons.

A *history of disciplinary troubles* may reflect the presence of attention-deficit/hyperactivity disorder or disruptive behavior disorder. Asking patients to describe their behavior in the classroom is a helpful probe, if recall is sufficient. Signs of inattention in the classroom include making careless mistakes, failing to finish schoolwork, easy distractibility, and forgetfulness in daily activities. Signs of hyperactivity and impulsivity include fidgeting, frequently leaving the seat, intrusiveness, and running about excessively. Attention-deficit/hyperactivity disorder is believed to continue into adulthood in some cases (Wender 1981; Zametkin et al. 1990). The presentation in adults is somewhat different, however, and includes difficulty being organized, low frustration tolerance, impulsivity, restlessness, and mood swings (Woods 1986). It is not known whether residual attention-deficit/hyperactivity disorder extends into senescence.

Behavioral patterns are typically established in childhood. A repetitive pattern of aggression to people and animals, destruction of property, deceitfulness or theft, and serious violations of social norms is evidence for a conduct disorder (American Psychiatric Association 2000). Conduct disorder may represent the presence of developmental anomaly (Nachson 1991). The interviewer must inquire about any *history of violence or criminal behavior* beginning in childhood and adolescence. Violent behaviors can also appear as sequelae to numerous central nervous system disorders (Elliott 1992).

Many neurological disorders that may be relevant later in life occur during childhood, including Tourette's syndrome, epilepsy, meningitides, and closed head injury. These conditions are often associated with cognitive and behavioral sequelae that may persist into senescence. Older individuals may have contracted many neurological diseases now considered to be rare, such as poliomyelitis, dementia paralytica, or encephalitis lethargica.

Adolescence

During adolescence, individuals develop a social identity and begin to form strong attachments outside the family. They may also join the workforce. Maladaptive patterns of behavior established during childhood can continue into adolescence. Adolescents may also begin to experiment with drugs, occasionally resulting in substance abuse and dependence. Risk-taking behaviors, such as reckless driving, are not uncommon. Injury is a common cause of morbidity in adolescence. A *history of head injury* should be elicited. Many head injuries do not result in gross cerebral trauma. Asking patients if their ability to think was affected by an injury can often elicit evidence of subtle cerebral pathology. Lishman (1987) reported that the degree of anterograde and retrograde amnesia after a head injury is a predictor of postinjury cognitive sequelae. The history should define the window of amnesia preceding and subsequent to the injury.

A thorough review of *past psychiatric history* is an essential part of the neuropsychiatric history. Numerous psychiatric illnesses, including anxiety, mood, and thought disorders, have their onset during adolescence. Psychiatric illness can reflect neurobiological anomaly and certainly affects psychological development. Schizophrenia is hypothesized to result from abnormal migration of hippocampal neurons during gestation (Roberts 1990). Other investigations have focused on pathology of the prefrontal and temporal heteromodal association cortex, rendering an individual vulnerable to hallucinations and psychosis (Shenton et al. 1992; Weinberger 1988). Mood disorders are associated with diminished metabolism in prefrontal and subcortical regions (Johansen-Berg et al. 2008; Ketter et al. 1996) (see Chapter 19, "Mood Disorders").

The *substance abuse history* must be thoroughly explored. Substance abuse can lead to acquired neurological insult and chronic symptoms. Intoxication with alcohol or other substances increases the risk for accidents and head injury. Alcohol abuse and prescription drug abuse in elderly patients are often missed by clinicians (see Chapter 17, "Addiction"). Use of cocaine can precipitate stroke (Levine et al. 1990). The use of the designer drug 1-methyl-4-phenyl-1,2,3,6-tetrahydropyridine (MPTP) has been reported to lead to an acute parkinsonian syndrome (Tetrud et al. 1989). Lysergic acid diethylamide (LSD) use is occasionally associated with recurrent visual hallucinatory experiences, known as hallucinogen persisting perception disorder (American Psychiatric Association 2000). Sharing hypodermic needles exposes individuals to numerous infectious agents, including human immunodeficiency virus, which can cross the blood-brain barrier and affect cognition (Gibbs et al. 1990; Tross and Hirsch 1988) while also predisposing the user to opportunistic central nervous system infections.

Adulthood

Adulthood heralds the establishment of a stable *pattern of behavior and cognitive performance*, representing an important baseline. Elderly individuals typically present for neuropsychiatric evaluation after a decline from these prior levels of functioning, so this baseline must be clearly identified in the history. Patients establish an *occupational history* during adulthood that should be explored for continuity, stability, and possible exposure to toxic substances or brain injury.

The persistence of maladaptive behaviors from adolescence into adulthood introduces an element of chronicity that may have relevance for the neuropsychiatric evaluation. Chronic use of alcohol can sometimes result in an alcoholic dementia (Charness et al. 1989; Lishman 1990). Malnutrition associated with heavy alcohol use can precipitate thiamine deficiency and the Wernicke-Korsakoff syndrome (Greenberg and Diamond 1986). A pattern of poorly managed aggression and violence can lead to traumatic brain injury, creating a downward spiral of further maladaptive behaviors and cognitive impairment.

Neurological problems that have particular relevance to the neuropsychiatric evaluation and typically arise before age 65 include brain tumors, Huntington's disease, and inflammatory disorders such as lupus erythematosus and multiple sclerosis. Health habits such as nicotine dependence that place an individual at risk for cerebrovascular disease, along with the onset of medical conditions such as hypertension, diabetes mellitus, and hypercholesterolemia, are noted during adulthood.

Senescence

The elder person presenting for neuropsychiatric evaluation has a wealth of life experiences that contribute to current functioning. Erikson et al. (1994) described the primary challenge of this life epoch as consolidating these experiences into a cohesive sense of integrity. The alternative is a feeling of despair that goals have not been accomplished, dreams have not been realized, and time is running out. Neuropsychiatric disorders represent a significant threat to this sense of integrity. Important neurological conditions that arise in senescence, in addition to those previously listed, include Parkinson's disease and the various cortical degenerative disorders, such as amyloidopathies, tauopathies, α-synucleinopathies, and prionopathies, along with normal-pressure hydrocephalus, and subdural hematoma.

Elderly persons are far more likely to have chronic medical problems and to be prescribed multiple medications (see Chapter 29, "Neuropsychiatric Disorders Associated With General Medical Therapies"). The examiner should include a complete *medication history* that includes both prescribed and over-the-counter medications. A *comprehensive medical and surgical history* should be accomplished, along with a thorough *review of systems* to screen for any current medical conditions, such as urinary tract infections, endocrine disorders, acute neurological deficits, cardiac symptoms, or respiratory conditions, that may lower the threshold for an acute confusional state. The presence of bowel or bladder incontinence should be determined. Elderly patients often report somatic and cognitive symptoms in the context of major depressive disorder. The review of systems should include a *survey of the vegetative functions* affected by mood disorder, including sleep, appetite, and libido. At times, an alteration in the vegetative functions may be the only way to differentiate primary psychiatric diagnosis, such as depression, from a neuropsychiatric syndrome, such as acquired apathy. Individuals with depression commonly have sleep and appetite changes, whereas patients with apathy syndromes, also known as pseudodepression, will eat when presented with food and do not experience significant sleep disruption. Recent changes in a patient's medication regimen can precipitate a confusional state or cause unsteady gait and should be documented. Any medication capable of crossing the blood-brain barrier has the potential to cause myriad central nervous system side effects in elderly individuals.

Many elderly patients are functioning relatively well with a "preclinical" dementia but lose their functional reserve and appear to have frank dementia or a depressive disorder in the context of acute general medical conditions. The aging brain, with a limited cortical reserve and an often tenuous blood supply, is quite vulnerable to acute dysfunction from systemic illness and is more susceptible to the cognitive and behavioral toxicity of many commonly prescribed medications. Recovery from these confusional states is often slow to proceed. The "acute dementia" or "acute depression" will slowly resolve upon adequate treatment of the underlying general medical condition.

The clinical interview of the geriatric patient should also include an *assessment of activities of daily living* to explore functional status. These activities include cooking, dressing, performing household chores, shopping, driving, maintaining personal hygiene, and paying bills. Several instruments have been developed to assess functional status in elderly persons (Applegate et al. 1990). They provide the clinician with useful measures to document and monitor a person's level of independence. The degree of autonomy and effectiveness at functioning in one's environment is a crucial historical domain that must be thoroughly assessed.

Historical information, particularly a *history of recent changes in behavior and cognition*, must be organized to direct the focus of the mental status and physical examinations. The various neural systems in the brain are associated with rather discrete behavioral and cognitive functions. The signs of neuropsychiatric illness reflect dysfunction in these neuronal networks. The neuropsychiatric examination must, therefore, have localizing value. Through an understanding of functional neuroanatomy and neuropathology, the neuropsychiatrist will be able to clarify problems identified in the history and expand on them through strategic use of bedside testing to arrive at a more complete understanding of the clinical problem.

Major Neuropsychiatric Syndromes of the Elderly

Elderly patients frequently present for neuropsychiatric evaluation with chief complaints of forgetfulness, personality change, or mental status change. The differential diagnoses for these symptoms include virtually all medical conditions prevalent in the elderly population. Careful neuropsychiatric evaluation can assist the clinician by discriminating among a depressive disorder, a confusional state, a benign condition of age-related cognitive decline, and intellectual impairment caused by significant cerebral or somatic dysfunction. Major neuropsychiatric syndromes affecting cognition will typically involve, in addition to memory, other cognitive domains, as well as the executive, motor, and limbic systems. These syndromes are described in the following sections to assist in the focus of the clinical interview and to begin to structure the approach to the mental status examination.

Clinical Characteristics of Age-Related Cognitive Changes

Cognitive decline is not an inevitable consequence of aging; however, numerous studies have demonstrated intellectual impairment of mild to moderate severity in a significant proportion of elderly individuals not diagnosed with a dementia (Ebly et al. 1995; Petersen et al. 1992; Rapp and Amaral 1992). The cognitive domain that is most commonly affected appears to be memory and, in particular, acquisition or learning (Petersen et al. 1992). Elderly individuals appear to acquire less information than younger adults but retain the ability to store and recall the learned material.

The issue of when aging ends and disease begins remains to be resolved. A longitudinal study of healthy, independent seniors with an isolated mild memory impairment showed that ~10%–15% of these individuals experienced progression to clinically diagnosable dementia of the Alzheimer's type each year (Petersen et al. 1997). Age-associated memory impairment is discussed in Chapter 16, "Alzheimer's Disease and the Frontotemporal Dementia Syndromes."

Clinical Characteristics of Prefrontal Systems Dysfunction

Prefrontal systems dysfunction is recognized as a condition that can cause gross disruption of behavior while sparing basic motor, sensory, and cognitive functions. The metacognitive functions subserved by prefrontal systems are essential for ongoing adaptive functioning in one's ever-changing environment. Despite their vital role in human behavior, the so-called executive cognitive functions are not routinely tested with common cognitive screening instruments, such as the Mini-Mental State Examination (Folstein et al. 1975) or the Short Portable Mental Status Questionnaire (Pfeiffer 1975). However, an understanding of their contributions to adaptive behavior, together with an appreciation of the cardinal signs of prefrontal dysfunction, can lead to a proper diagnosis and treatment plan. Signs of prefrontal systems dysfunction range from the dramatic personality changes associated with orbitofrontal and mesial frontal dysfunction to a perplexing inability to function well in the presence of only mild motor, sensory, or cognitive impairment, as is often seen with dysfunction of the dorsolateral convexity network (Table 4–2).

TABLE 4–2. Regional prefrontal syndromes

Region	Cardinal signs
Orbitofrontal system	Behavioral disinhibition; environmental dependency
Dorsolateral convexity system	Cognitive disorganization
Mesial frontal system	Apathy syndrome

Dorsal Convexity Dysexecutive Syndrome

The high-level cognitive functions mediated by the dorsolateral prefrontal lobe and its connections include cognitive flexibility, temporal ordering of recent events, planning ahead, regulating actions based on environmental stimuli, and learning from experience (Goldman-Rakic 1993). Patients exhibiting dysfunction in these cognitive domains become concrete and perseverative and show impairment in reasoning and flexibility that impairs coping with life events. The examiner should probe the ability to pay bills on time; organize daily activities, such as going to the bank or market; keep a tidy house; and cook balanced meals. The "tea and toast diet" frequently results from loss of the organizational capacity to purchase diverse groceries in response to dwindling home supplies and then plan and prepare a meal consisting of several items. In addition, such patients are characterized by a paucity of spontaneous behavior. They often appear apathetic and may become irritable during mental status testing when fatigue easily ensues. They typically struggle with adjusting emotionally to being placed in assisted living or a nursing home.

Orbitofrontal Disinhibition Syndrome

The orbitofrontal cortex has discrete connections with the paralimbic cortex and thus plays a role in the elaboration and integration of limbic drives. This area receives highly processed information concerning the individual's experience of an environmental stimulus and the anticipated consequences of various behavioral responses to it (Malloy and Duffy 1992). This process allows a person to maintain consistent behavior in keeping with his or her self-concept. Patients with orbitofrontal damage often exhibit poor impulse control, explosive aggressive outbursts, inappropriate verbal lewdness, jocularity, and lack of interpersonal sensitivity. The fatuous behaviors observed with orbitofrontal system dysfunction are known as moria or witzelsucht. The stimulus-bound behaviors noted with this syndrome are commonly observed in nursing homes, where residents frequently wander and happen upon numerous stimuli: a doorknob will be turned and a room entered, a sleeve hanging from a drawer is an invitation to disrobe and put on the newly discovered clothes, and a shower stall is an open invitation for a shower. The patients often become agitated and aggressive when someone interferes with them. The diagnosis of the orbitofrontal disinhibition syndrome is primarily clinical. Such gross disruption of behavior often leads to misdiagnosis of mania. Careful review of the history will not, however, demonstrate associated symptoms, such as diminished need for sleep, pressured speech, religiosity, or grandiose delusions.

Mesial Frontal Apathetic Syndrome

Mesial frontal pathology affects the functional balance between the cingulum and the supplementary motor area. Disruption of this network leads to a dysmotivational syndrome ranging from apathy to akinetic mutism (Duffy and Campbell 1994). Patients with this pathology often appear depressed, yet they lack the dysphoria, negative cognitions, and neurovegetative signs of major depression. The diagnosis of a mesial frontal apathy syndrome is entirely clinical. One patient, after a gunshot wound to the frontal lobes, lapsed onto a state of inertia when left alone. When questioned, he related an awareness of a personality change. He denied boredom and described his change as a "loss of motivation" in that he entertained numerous ideas for activities but felt no impetus to act on them. His facial expression was one of casual indifference, and he would often respond with simple gestures instead of speaking. Caregivers for patients with apathy syndromes are commonly frustrated with what they incorrectly perceive as willful indifference to the home environment.

Clinical Characteristics of Generalized Cortical Systems Disorders

The neurodegenerative disorders that compose the classic dementias typically affect the cerebral cortex in regional patterns. Dementia of the Alzheimer's type appears to preferentially involve the heteromodal association cortex and the limbic system (Hyman et al. 1984; Pearson et al. 1985). Mesencephalic projection nuclei, including dopaminergic, cholinergic, serotonergic, and noradrenergic systems, are variably involved (Jellinger 1987). Common "cortical" clinical findings include *amnesia*, *aphasia*, *apraxia*, *agnosia*, *acalculia*, and *visuospatial impairment*. The degree of involvement of these cognitive domains is quite variable across patients. Dementia with Lewy bodies may represent a clinicopathological variant of Alzheimer's disease. Patients present with a mixed picture of cortical and subcortical pathology, characterized by cortical cognitive impairment, along with fluctuating attention, visual hallucinations, and spontaneous motor features of parkinsonism (McKeith et al. 1996). Frontotemporal dementia syndromes include gross disruption of social comportment with an eventual transition to an apathetic state (Chui 1989).

Clinical Characteristics of Focal Cortical Dementia Syndromes

Focal cortical degeneration syndromes can manifest in a slowly progressive manner and are regularly noted. Their etiology is not well understood, but autopsy findings in many cases reveal the neuropathology of generalized cortical dementias, including neuritic plaques (amyloidopathy), neurofibrillary tangles (tauopathy), and Lewy bodies (α-synucleinopathies) (Benson and Zaras 1991; Brun 1987; Hof et al. 1989; Morris et al. 1984). Thus, these syndromes may represent uncommon manifestations of more common disorders. Caselli (1995) identified four general syndromes, including progressive frontal systems dysfunction, progressive aphasias, progressive perceptual-motor syndromes, and progressive bitemporal syndromes. The progressive frontal syndromes are described earlier in this chapter in the section "Clinical Characteristics of Prefrontal Systems Dysfunction."

Progressive Aphasias

The progressive aphasias include fluent and nonfluent types, as well as anomic and mixed types. They progress slowly, and the primary deficit for at least 2 years is limited to language function. Fluent aphasia—alternatively known as Wernicke's aphasia, receptive aphasia, and posterior aphasia—is characterized by effortless yet incomprehensible speech, together with difficulty comprehending the speech of others. This aphasia is most commonly caused by damage to unimodal association cortex in area 22 of the left hemisphere (Damasio 1992). This area is located in the superior temporal gyrus in the posterior regions adjacent to the supramarginal gyrus.

Nonfluent aphasia is also known as Broca's aphasia, expressive aphasia, and anterior aphasia. This aphasia is notable for effortful, agrammatic or telegraphic speech in which the patient has great difficulty using words such as *if*, *and*, *or*, *but*, *to*, *from*, and so on. Anterior aphasia results from damage to the inferior left frontal gyrus in the left hemisphere. Deficits in anomic aphasias are limited to word finding and naming. Anomic aphasia can result from damage to numerous sites in the left hemisphere. The mixed aphasia syndrome appears to involve numerous aspects of language function and is associated with degeneration in the left temporal and perisylvian regions. Other commonly noted aphasia syndromes, such as global aphasia, conduction aphasia, transcortical aphasias, and pure word deafness, are typically vascular in origin and are not commonly the product of progressive cortical degeneration (Damasio 1989).

Progressive Perceptual-Motor Syndromes

The progressive perceptual-motor syndromes are divided into visual syndromes and motor syndromes. The progressive visual syndromes involve occipitoparietal and occipitotemporal networks and include progressive simultanagnosia, Balint's syndrome, and visual agnosia. Focal pathology in the occipitoparietal system bilaterally affects higher-order processing of visual information into a coherent whole. Consequently, simultanagnosia is the inability to adequately integrate important aspects of a visual scene, a problem known as visual disorientation. Patients can describe certain details but cannot integrate the entirety of the information (Damasio 2000). Balint's syndrome consists of simultanagnosia along with oculomotor apraxia, an impairment of voluntary gaze, and optic ataxia, an inability to point accurately to a target under visual guidance (Balint 1909). Bilateral dysfunction in the occipitotemporal system results in visual agnosia, an inability to name visualized objects. Prosopagnosia is a particular type of visual agnosia with a circumscribed deficit of facial recognition (Damasio et al. 1982).

Two progressive motor syndromes have been described that involve the parietofrontal junction (Caselli 1995). The syndromes are not specifically named. The first consists of hemispasticity, hemiparesis, and hemisensory impairments in the form of astereognosis or agraphesthesia and myoclonus. The second motor syndrome is defined by a mixed apraxia, or disorder of higher-order motor integration, consisting of limb apraxia, gestural apraxia, dressing apraxia, constructional apraxia, and writing apraxia. Limb apraxia is characterized by difficulty executing simple motor tasks, such as combing the hair or brushing the teeth. Gestural apraxia is a form of limb apraxia in which the patient has great difficulty imitating symbolic movements. Dressing apraxia is the inability to dress despite absence of significant sensorimotor disturbance. Constructional and writing apraxias involve impaired ability to draw and write, respectively.

Progressive Bitemporal Syndromes

The progressive bitemporal syndromes include progressive amnesia and progressive prosopagnosia, described previously, and Klüver-Bucy syndrome. Klüver-Bucy syndrome results from bilateral destruction of the amygdalae and is characterized by hyperorality; emotional placidity; hypersexuality; compulsive exploration of the environment, known as hypermetamorphosis; and psychic blindness (Klüver and Bucy 1939; Lilly et al. 1983).

Clinical Characteristics of Subcortical Systems Disorders

Basal Ganglia Dysfunction

The basal ganglia have a significant anatomical and thus functional relationship with specific regions of frontal cortex. Alexander and Crutcher (1990) identified five independent neural loop circuits uniting striatum, globus pallidus, dorsomedial thalamus, and frontal cortex. The physical integrity of these loops appears to be critical to optimal functioning of the behaviors modulated by each circuit. The supplementary motor area participates in a circuit responsible for integration of motor function. Similarly, a circuit involving the frontal eye fields subserves oculomotor function. The dorsolateral prefrontal, lateral orbitofrontal, and anterior cingulate areas participate in discrete circuits subserving cognitive organization, social comportment, and motivation, respectively (Duffy and Campbell 1994). The cardinal signs of basal ganglia pathology represent impaired participation of the striatum in these networks, resulting in cognitive impairment, motor dysfunction, and mood disorders.

The motor signs of basal ganglia dysfunction may be readily apparent during the clinical interview. The classic triad of movement disorders includes tremor, rigidity, and akinesia. It is helpful to observe the gait when the patient first arrives. A shuffling gait with diminished arm swing may represent an early clue. Other signs include a bland expression with infrequent blinking, difficulty sitting down with ease, and a paucity of movement. "Striatal hand" may be evident, which is characterized by an ulnar deviation with flexion of the fingers at the metacarpal phalangeal joints. A "pill rolling" tremor of 4–7 Hz involving the thumb and forefinger is frequently noted. When these signs are evident, the examiner should probe further for progressive symptoms of stiffness, loss of agility, involuntary movements, or difficulty walking. Chorea may be observed with other striatal disorders, such as Huntington's disease. Patients often attempt to mask these embarrassing involuntary movements by quickly stroking their hair or adjusting an article of clothing.

Controversy exists over the presence of cognitive impairment associated with basal ganglia pathology (McHugh 1989). Carefully conducted studies, however, have identified the presence of a pattern of deficits that appears to reflect derangement of the frontal-subcortical contribution to cognition (Brown and Marsden 1990). Albert et al. (1974) and McHugh and Folstein (1975) described a "subcortical dementia" consisting of mental torpor, cognitive dilapidation, apathy, and depression, without impairment of learning, speech and language, or other "cortical" functions such as praxis or mathematical calculating. The ability to retrieve stored material is often impaired (Brown and Marsden 1990). Patients will require prompts to produce historical information, such as the names of recent presidents. The number of prompts required to recall material is a good indicator of the degree of the retrieval deficit. Other signs of subcortical dementia notable during the mental status examination include impersistence and slowed completion of tasks. These patients usually require much encouragement to complete the cognitive screening tasks. Pathological conditions that involve the basal ganglia include α-synucleinopathies, tauopathies, and genetic disorders, such as Parkinson's disease, corticobasal degeneration, progressive supranuclear palsy, multisystem atrophy, and Huntington's disease, along with Wilson's disease, état lacunaire, and tumors.

Vascular dementias are a heterogeneous group resulting from cerebral infarctions of any etiology. Wallin et al. (2003) organized the vascular dementias into the following subtypes:

- Poststroke dementia (strategic infarct, multi-infarct, and intracerebral hemorrhage–associated)
- Subcortical vascular dementia (lacunar infarcts and ischemic white matter lesions)
- Alzheimer's disease plus cerebrovascular disease

They found a reliable clinicopathological correlation between subcortical white matter ischemia and a subcortical dementia pattern. The clinical presentation of multi-infarct and strategic-infarct subtypes of dementias varies widely in accordance with extent of involvement and lesion location. Campbell and Coffey (2001) reviewed the relationship between white matter ischemia and cognition and noted surprisingly modest levels of cognitive impairment in the setting of white matter ischemia. The concept of vascular dementia requires revision, with the hope of refining clinicopathological relationships (Erkinjuntti and Hachinski 1993). Postmortem examinations of elderly patients with cerebrovascular disease identify a high prevalence of co-occurring cortical degenerative disorders in the form of a "mixed" etiology dementia, which makes confident diagnosis of a primarily vascular etiology suspect (Londos et al. 2002).

Clinical Characteristics of Cerebellar Disorders

Cerebellar Syndromes

The cerebellum has traditionally been considered as participating in motor function by coordinating the rate, rhythm, and force of contraction of the muscles and permitting smooth movement. The syndrome of the cerebellar vermis is characterized by gross postural and ambulatory disturbances in the form of truncal ataxia. Dysarthria is often present. Degeneration of the anterior lobe of the cerebellum can also cause gross disturbances of equilibrium and coordination. The syndrome of the cerebellar hemispheres spares axial systems but involves unilateral impairments in skilled movements of the arm, hand, leg, and foot associated with dysmetria and dysdiadochokinesis.

Cerebellar Cognitive Affective Syndrome

Cerebellar disorders are often associated with affective and cognitive disorders (Schmahmann 2004). As a result, the role of the cerebellum has been expanded to include neuropsychiatric syndromes. The cerebellar cognitive affective syndrome occurs in the setting of motor signs of cerebellar dysfunction. In addition, affective dysregulation in the form of mood disorders (primarily depression) and cognitive impairment in the form of dysexecutive syndromes are noted. Patients presenting with signs of cerebellar dysfunction should be carefully screened for evidence of mood disorders or executive cognitive impairment, which can significantly extend the morbidity of the obvious movement disorder.

Mental Status Examination

The mental status examination is an assessment of brain function. A proper assessment should enable the examiner to estimate a patient's cognitive capacities in terms of domains of relative strength and impairment. Several general cognitive screening instruments are commonly used by clinicians to investigate intellectual impairment. These include the Mini-Mental State Examination (Folstein et al. 1975), Cognitive Capacities Screening Examination (Jacobs et al. 1977), and Short Portable Mental Status Questionnaire (Pfeiffer 1975). Screening instruments developed to assess dementing processes include the Dementia Rating Scale (Mattis 1973), Blessed Dementia Scale (Blessed et al. 1968), and Alzheimer's Disease Assessment Scale (Devenny et al. 1992). The Executive Interview (Royall et al. 1992) and the Frontal-Subcortical Assessment Battery (Rothlind and Brandt 1993) have been developed to more specifically assess frontal systems dysfunction.

Malloy et al. (1997) reviewed the merits of these instruments as cognitive screens. Importantly, however, the geriatric patient presenting for neuropsychiatric evaluation requires a flexible and comprehensive cognitive assessment, which is not permitted by these standard instruments. Furthermore, no single instrument adequately surveys the commonly assessed cognitive and metacognitive domains. The principal drawbacks include substantial false-negative rates, indicating a lack of sensitivity for mild dementia, and inadequate evaluation of right hemisphere and frontal system function (Nelson et al. 1986).

The clinical assessment of cognition is an area of neglect. In a survey of neuropsychiatric clinicians, only 57% of respondents reported the use of formal assessment of cognitive status (Coffey et al. 1994). Many respondents routinely requested formal neuropsychological testing as their primary means for assessing cognition. This routine approach is neither clinically nor economically acceptable. Bedside mental status testing has been demonstrated to be a reasonable clinical indicator of cognitive impairment as a result of cerebral dysfunction of many etiologies (Malloy et al. 1997).

Neuropsychological assessment should be considered as an adjunct in the geriatric neuropsychiatric assessment (see Chapter 5, "Neuropsychological Assessment"). Formal neuropsychological testing is an expensive and time-consuming process that can be very helpful for certain indications. When not indicated, however, neuropsychological testing frequently does not provide any additional information to assist in treatment planning. Proper indications include the establishment of a quantitative cognitive baseline to track over time, clarification of confusing or variable findings at the bedside, more thorough assessment of specific cognitive domains, or addressing a question of malingering or conversion disorder. It is helpful to compare closely the bedside cognitive findings with findings from the neuropsychological testing, because they should concur. A common cause of discrepancy is suboptimal bedside technique or misinterpretation of the bedside findings. In these situations, the neuropsychologist can assist the bedside examiner by reviewing the technique or recommending other more reliable tests to add to the bedside armamentarium.

Cognitive Assessment

Discussion of bedside cognitive testing is provided throughout Chapter 12, "Cognitive Impairment and Rehabilitation." Throughout the administration of the cognitive tasks, the examiner should consider the patient's performance in terms of quality, localizing value, and functional status. The popular cognitive screening instruments provide numerical scores as a reflection of cognitive capacity; however, cognitive performance falls on a qualitative continuum. All results must be considered in terms of expected level of performance. Simply relying on a numerical descriptor may result in a false-negative assessment for many patients, particularly those with significant cognitive strengths, who are left with ample reserve despite cognitive decline.

Furthermore, the diagnosis of most dementing disorders is primarily clinical. No laboratory assays exist to confidently differentiate Alzheimer's disease from most other dementias, and brain biopsy is not part of a general workup of progressive cognitive dysfunction. Neuropsychiatric syndromes in elderly people typically involve either widespread pathology or more focal lesions. The pattern of deficits can thus differentiate between a generalized process, such as typical Alzheimer's disease, and a focal process, such as a left parietal lobe infarction. Organizing the cognitive examination to assess regional functions can assist with this process.

I perform a simple office or bedside examination of cognition that is sensitive to dysfunction in various cognitive domains (Table 4–3). This examination is not validated but serves to identify areas of relative deficit and strength that can be investigated further, if necessary, with additional bedside cognitive testing or formal neuropsychological testing.

The results of this cognitive examination can assist the examiner in developing an accurate differential diagnosis of dementia syndromes (Table 4–4).

The findings of the neuropsychiatric evaluation should fit with the person's functional status in his or her usual setting and help to explain and understand current difficulties. In some instances, the findings may conflict with the history. A common scenario is finding a patient who appears to be cognitively intact but who reports an obvious decline in ability to function effectively at home. This outcome is likely the result of a so-called dysexecutive syndrome. The structure of the office provides an artificially optimal environment for the cognitive assessment. Patients having executive dysfunction will benefit from this external structure and may appear much less impaired on mental status testing unless frontal systems are carefully assessed. In addition, the tasks that make up the mental status examination are rather arbitrary and do not necessarily assess the neural networks relied upon for daily living, which have evolved over millions of years without being shaped by the environmental stressor of mental status testing.

Formal assessment of cognition includes screening for amnesias, aphasias, apraxias, and agnosias. Common "cortical" cognitive domains (and their particular syndromes) include memory (amnesia), speaking (aphasia), manual dexterity (apraxia), visual naming (agnosia), calculating (acalculia), and spatial relations (visuospatial impairment).

Neurobehavioral Assessment

Formal assessment of mental status includes a review of pertinent domains of psychiatric functioning, including mood and affect, anxiety, compulsive and repetitive behaviors, personality changes, thought process and content, and perceptions. Upon completion of the clinical interview, the examiner will have acquired numerous clues to guide more thorough exploration of these areas.

Assessment of Mood and Affect

Depressive symptoms are more commonly encountered in elderly persons than in individuals under age 65. Despite this, major depressive disorder, as defined by DSM-IV-TR (American Psychiatric Association 2000), has a lower prevalence among elderly persons. In addition, common neuropsychiatric disorders such as stroke (Robinson and Price 1982) and Parkinson's disease (Starkstein et al. 1990) are associated with a higher incidence of depressive illness. Bipolar disorder in the form of mania is occasionally encountered after stroke and traumatic brain injury (Robinson et al. 1988).

In neurologically intact individuals, affect remains congruent with the mood state. Neuropsychiatric disorders can disconnect affect from mood and thus disrupt a person's ability to effectively and accurately communicate his or her prevailing mood. Right hemisphere pathology can produce an expressive dysprosodia through which facial expression, gesticulation, and speech inflection become limited. Such per-

TABLE 4–3. Office examination of cognition

Domain	Task
High-level attention	"Begin with Sunday and say the days of the week backwards." (*This task requires intact executive function but eliminates mathematical issues associated with serial subtraction.*)
Declarative memory (encoding)	"I am going to give you 4 words that I want you to remember. Listen carefully, and when I'm done, repeat the words back to me." (*Ask patient to repeat the word list twice. Repeat the entire list if patient does not encode all 4 words after a trial.*) "Now hold on to them, and I'll ask for them later." (*This should normally be done in one or two trials.*)
Executive cognition	"I want you to copy what I'm doing with my hands." (*Alternating motor sequence simultaneously and alternately opening and closing both fists.*) "When I touch my nose, you raise your finger. When I raise my finger, you touch your nose, so you do the opposite of what I'm doing." (*Look for copying of examiner's movements.*) "Say as many different words as you can in 1 minute that begin with the letter 'A.' Don't include names of people, like 'Adam,' or names of places, like 'Alaska.' (*Look for ~15 words without repetition or loss of set.*) "I have drawn a circle for you. Please make it into a clock by adding the numbers.... Now make the clock say '10 past 11.'" (*Look for proper spacing of the numbers and proper placement of the hands.*) "Copy this design (alternating squares and triangles)." (*Look for perseveration of the square or the triangle.*)
Declarative memory (retrieval and storage)	"Now tell me the 4 words I asked you to remember." (*If the words aren't recalled, give first a* category *prompt—e.g., "Fruit" for "lemon"—then a* forced choice*—e.g., "It was either a lemon, an orange, or an apple." If the word is then recalled, the patient is demonstrating a retrieval, but not a storage, deficit. Note the number recalled spontaneously, the number recalled with prompts, and the number not recognized despite a forced choice.*)
Aphasia	"Are we in a hospital? A library? A supermarket?" "Repeat this sentence: 'Pry the tin can's lid off.'" "Name several objects." "Write me a sentence about you."
Calculations	"How much is 5+3?" "How much is 17+5?" "How much is 31−8?" "How much is 36/3?"
Praxis	"Make a salute." "Show me how you would use a toothbrush." "Beckon a friend over with each hand."
Visuoconstruction	"Copy this (transparent) cube."
Judgment	"What would you do if you saw a young child wandering alone at the supermarket?"

sons often appear depressed despite denying feelings of dysphoria (Ross 2005). Frontal systems dysfunction resulting in apathy syndromes and Parkinson's disease are also associated with limited affective expression of internal mood states. Pseudobulbar palsy manifests with excessive displays of affect in response to minimal emotional stimuli and results from bilateral damage to corticobulbar tracts, generally in the setting of cerebrovascular disease. I find the Cornell Depression Scale (Alexopolous et al. 1988) or the Geriatric Depression Scale–15 (Yesavage et al. 1982–1983) to be useful clinical aids in screening for depression in elderly patients.

Assessment of Anxiety

Anxiety is often evoked during the neuropsychiatric evaluation and can affect a person's ability to concentrate and perform optimally on cognitive examination. The examiner should promptly identify signs of anxiety and make efforts to moderate the patient's distress. Gentle reassurances are usu-

TABLE 4–4. Differential diagnosis of dementia

	Area of impairment				
	Memory				
Syndrome	Executive (encoding/retrieval)	Cortical (storage)	Executive	Parietal[a]	EPS
Dementia of the Alzheimer's type (NP+NFT)	Yes	Yes	Yes	Yes	No
Frontotemporal dementia (NFT, NP+NFT)	Yes	No	Yes	No	No Yes later
Dementia with Lewy bodies[b] (LB)	Yes	Yes	Yes	Yes	Yes
Subcortical dementia (LB, NFT)[c]	Yes	No	Yes	No	Yes
Vascular dementia	Yes	No	Yes	No	Yes
Alzheimer's plus Parkinson's disease[d] dementia (LB+NP+NFT)	Yes	Yes	Yes	Yes	Yes

Note. EPS=extrapyramidal side effects; LB=Lewy bodies; NFT=neurofibrillary tangles; NP=neuritic plaques.
[a]Language, calculations, praxis, visuoconstructional.
[b]Visual hallucinations, systematized delusions, frequent falls, syncope, waxing and waning attentional and cognitive symptoms, neuroleptic sensitivity; onset of all symptoms temporally related.
[c]Parkinson's disease, Huntington's disease, progressive supranuclear palsy.
[d]Parkinson's disease precedes the Alzheimer's-type dementia by at least 1 year.

ally all that are required for the patient to continue with the examination. The examiner should also inquire about the presence of any specific or recurrent worries or fears that the patient experiences. Anxiety disorders are among the most common psychiatric syndromes in elderly persons. Blazer et al. (1991) reported a 6-month prevalence of 19.7% for any anxiety disorder in the elderly population.

Assessment of Compulsions and Repetitive Behavior

Obsessive-compulsive symptoms are occasionally sequelae of neuropsychiatric illness. Positron emission tomographic studies of symptomatic individuals have shown disturbances in orbitofrontal–basal ganglia networks (Baxter et al. 1988). Disorders affecting the basal ganglia can be associated with symptoms of obsessive-compulsive disorder, including intrusive thoughts, repetition, preoccupation with cleanliness, and ruminations (Tomer et al. 1993). The examiner should determine if the patient has been experiencing any troubles with intrusive thoughts or the need to perform rituals such as checking, counting, or cleaning. I also ask the family if the patient has any tendencies to hoard items in the home.

Assessment of Personality Changes

Personality changes are commonly encountered in the setting of frontal systems dysfunction of any etiology (Campbell 2007). Affected individuals often lack awareness of any change in their social comportment. The inquiry into pertinent personality changes should therefore include the caregiver's perception of change. The examiner should specifically ask about silliness, vulgarity, hostility, loss of empathy, or apathy. Ott et al. (1996) found that right hemisphere pathology is associated with a reduction in insight.

Assessment of Thought

Disordered thinking is a common symptom in elderly persons. Both thought process and thought content are vulnerable to derangement by numerous neuropsychiatric conditions (Cummings 1985b). The influence of primary psychiatric diagnoses such as mania and schizophrenia on thought process is well known; however, frontal systems dysfunction can mimic these presentations by disrupting the ability to screen out irrelevant stimuli and maintain a given behavioral set. Consequently, stimulus-bound individuals may reveal tangential thinking or flight of ideas. Patients with apathy syndromes may appear to have a poverty of thoughts. Their paucity of speech precludes confident assessment of the thought process. Damage to the posterior language areas can manifest as rambling, incoherent speech, which may be misdiagnosed as thought derailment.

Disorders of thought content are known to arise late in life. Monosymptomatic or content-specific delusions, in particular, have been reported as sequelae of a number of generalized and focal neurological conditions affecting the brain (Malloy and Richardson 1994). The delusional themes include the duplication of person (Capgras syndrome) or place (reduplicative paramnesia), sexual themes of infidelity (Othello syndrome) or love (de Clerambault's syndrome), or physical changes such as being infested with parasites (Ekbom's syndrome) or being dead (Cotard's syndrome). Lesions affecting the heteromodal association cortex of the right hemisphere appear to be especially likely to result in the occurrence of monosymptomatic delusions (Cutting 1991).

Assessment of Perceptions

Disordered perception in elderly persons typically manifests as illusions or hallucinations. Illusions are a misperception of a sensory stimulus, such as mistaking a shoe for a cat, and are often experienced by cognitively impaired individuals with diminished vision or hearing, especially at night. These problems are readily treated with correction of the visual problem, use of a hearing aid, or improved lighting. Hallucinations, the experience of a sensory perception in the absence of a stimulus, may indicate the presence of encephalopathy and can occur with any sensory modality. Charles Bonnet syndrome is a unique type of visual hallucination often misdiagnosed and mistreated as a primary psychosis. Charles Bonnet described individuals with anterior visual pathology as reporting well-formed visual hallucinations consisting of "Lilliputians" or small animals (Terao and Collinson 2000). The hallucinations are nonthreatening and often arouse curiosity or pleasure.

Sensorimotor Examination

Sensorimotor impairments significantly affect functional status in elderly individuals and require thorough assessment. The major neuropsychiatric syndromes described earlier in this chapter are often associated with sensorimotor findings. Careful identification of sensorimotor impairments is necessary to provide remedial interventions. Elderly individuals with gait impairment are at increased risk for falls, which may be prevented by using some form of ambulatory assistance such as a cane or walker, by avoiding doses of medication known to cause ataxia, or by optimizing treatment of the underlying cause, such as Parkinson's disease. In addition, in situations where the cognitive examination reveals a focal or unilateral pattern of deficits, sensorimotor signs can further refine the bedside localization of cerebral pathology. For an outstanding review of the neurological examination, the reader is referred to Campbell (2005). The examination discussed below is limited to information that is more directly applicable to the neuropsychiatric assessment.

Observation

A great deal of information can be gleaned from the patient through simple observation. The gait can be scrutinized as the patient walks to the examiner's office. The posture may reveal the simian stance of Parkinson's disease or spinal abnormalities such as kyphosis, lordosis, or scoliosis brought on by osteoporosis. Diminished arm swing and shuffling may be a sign of Parkinson's disease. Frontal systems disease is often associated with a gait apraxia in which the patient's feet appear to stick to the floor like magnets. Circumduction of one leg may be caused by spasticity resulting from an upper motor neuron lesion. Ataxia is frequently noted as a side effect of many psychotropic medications with anticholinergic or antidopaminergic properties. Walking heel to toe can elicit dystonic posturing of a hand and arm, suggesting contralateral hemispheric injury. Impaired tandem gait can also be a result of peripheral sensory loss, pain, or focal weakness.

Observation of the face during the neuropsychiatric examination may reveal a Horner's syndrome resulting from ipsilateral carotid atherosclerosis. The full Horner's syndrome includes unilateral ptosis, meiosis, and anhidrosis. A flattened nasolabial fold can indicate a facial plegia from a contralateral lesion such as a stroke. A masked, bland facies with diminished blinking is a common sequela of Parkinson's disease. Exophthalmos may be a sign of hyperthyroidism.

Failure to shave or apply cosmetics to the left side of the face is often seen with left hemineglect as a result of right hemisphere lesion.

Vision and Hearing

Vision and hearing should be assessed. Elderly patients may not be fully aware of a gradual decline in these sensory modalities and often present with significant impairment. Providing elderly patients with proper eyeglasses and hearing aids can immediately improve functional status and diminish risk of accidents. Ocular and ear diseases are also associated with increased risk for modality-specific release hallucinations (Hammeke et al. 1983; White 1980). Anterior visual pathology can lead to the Charles Bonnet syndrome, characterized by well-formed visual hallucinations (Berrios and Brook 1984; Terao and Collinson 2000). Diminished ability to discriminate others' speech may exacerbate a tendency toward paranoia in susceptible individuals (Cooper and Curry 1976).

Oculomotion

Examining eye movement provides a wealth of information with localizing value. Patients who cannot track the examiner's moving finger without also moving their head may be stimulus bound from frontal systems disease. A unilateral lesion of the frontal eye fields will lead to ipsilateral gaze preference. The pupils will not cross the midline with voluntary gaze to the contralateral hemispace. Difficulty with voluntary saccades can be an early sign of Huntington's disease in susceptible individuals (Grafton et al. 1990). Internuclear ophthalmoplegia reflects brain stem pathology, commonly a result of multiple sclerosis. Damage to the right medial longitudinal fasciculus will cause failure of the left eye to cross the midline to the right, while the right eye will track normally but exhibit monocular nystagmus. Inability to track a downward moving finger below the midline may be a sign of progressive supranuclear palsy. Lid lag with downward gaze may be a sign of hypothyroidism.

Examination of the visual fields by confrontation can help to localize temporal, parietal, and occipital lesions from damage to the optic radiations. Visual information from the superior quadrants is carried by the inferior aspect of the optic radiations, known as Meyer's loop. Temporal lobe lesions will produce a contralateral superior quadrantanopia. Inferior parietal lesions can cause a contralateral inferior quadrantanopia. Patients with left hemineglect caused by a right hemisphere lesion may appear to have a complete contralateral hemianopia. However, testing of visual fields in this situation is very difficult because of the strong tendency to neglect left-sided stimuli.

Extrapyramidal Motor Examination

Diseases of the basal ganglia are commonly encountered in geriatric neuropsychiatric practice and manifest with parkinsonian signs and symptoms and subcortical dementia syndrome. The clinical assessment of extrapyramidal motor function is an essential element of proper diagnosis and treatment. The typical gait and tremor of a patient with Parkinson's disease have been described earlier in the section "Clinical Characteristics of Subcortical Systems Disorders." In addition to the shuffling quality of the gait, festination is noted, whereby the patient will tend to increase speed and fall forward. Patients cannot turn around easily and tend to turn slowly by shuffling in place. Extrapyramidal muscular rigidity is present throughout the entire range of motion of the neck, trunk, and extremities. A jerky yielding of resistance known as cogwheeling is often noted when examining nuchal, truncal, or limb flexor tone. Repeated rapid opening and closing of the hands will demonstrate a gradual reduction in speed and amplitude. Diffuse increases in tone are noted with lacunar states but are not associated with cogwheeling unless a parkinsonian tremor is also present.

An additional sign of upper motor neuron and extrapyramidal pathology is gegenhalten, a direct resistance to passive changes in position and posture. Gegenhalten is often associated with apraxia (Tyrrell and Rossor 1988). Patients who actively move a limb with the examiner despite requests to remain passive demonstrate mitgehen, a finding often noted with frontal systems dysfunction. The pronator drift test can often elicit subtle changes in motor tone as a result of hemispheric dysfunction. A slow pronation of the contralateral wrist with slight flexion of the elbow and fingers along with downward and lateral drift of the hand is noted. After the pronator drift test, the patient can be examined for propulsion and retropulsion by giving the patient a sudden push in either direction. Patients with Parkinson's disease cannot rapidly execute counteractive muscle groups and will stumble in the direction of the push.

Reflexes

Examination of muscle stretch reflexes—in particular, the biceps, triceps, brachioradialis, patellar, and Achilles reflexes—not only assesses the integrity of the sensory and motor systems but also has localizing value. Focal lesions involving upper motor neurons originating in the precentral gyrus or the axonal tracts coursing caudally through the internal capsule to form the corticospinal tract can cause a contralateral increase in reflex response. The presence of a Babinski sign (i.e., dorsiflexion and fanning of the toes in response to stimulating the sole of the foot) is an additional important lateralizing sign of corticospinal pathology. Geriatric patients with dementia are often variably cooperative with neuropsychiatric testing. However, the reflexes can be reliably tested despite a lack of complete cooperation by the patient.

The value of frontal release signs in neuropsychiatry tends to be overstated. The integrity of the frontal systems is reflected by the quality of the person's behavior over time. A clinical history of behavioral change, along with impaired performance on bedside tests of frontal functions, is sufficient to offer a diagnosis of executive impairment. The absence of snout, glabellar, and palmomental reflexes in this situation would not exclude the diagnosis. Further, the presence of these reflexes in the absence of behavioral changes or impairment with frontal tests does not suggest the presence of frontal systems dysfunction.

Further Investigations

A complete neuropsychiatric evaluation usually includes laboratory and radiological investigations. These are undertaken to assist in identifying primary or secondary physical conditions that may be causing or contributing to the manifesting complaint. At times, patients with medical conditions may present primarily with neuropsychiatric symptoms, and physical signs may be minimal or absent. The differential diagnoses for neuropsychiatric presentations can include a very long list of physical conditions. It is beyond the scope of this chapter to provide an all-inclusive list of investigations, but more specific recommendations can be found elsewhere in this text.

A reasonable set of general laboratory orders for the geriatric patient should include serum electrolytes, glucose, liver function tests, renal tests, serum calcium, and serum globulins. At many institutions, these are often bundled together as a comprehensive metabolic panel. In addition, a complete blood cell count should be ordered. Other important tests include erythrocyte sedimentation rate, thyroid stimulating hormone, syphilis serology such as rapid plasma reagin (RPR) or venereal disease research laboratory (VDRL), vitamin B_{12} level, and folate level. Additional laboratory studies would be guided by physical findings.

In general, neuroimaging studies will be primarily structural imaging in the form of computed tomography (CT) or magnetic resonance imaging (MRI) (see Chapter 6, "Imaging the Structure of the Aging Human Brain"). For most presentations, noncontrast CT scans of the brain are sufficient to identify atrophy or strokes. If neoplasia is suspected based on an unusual presentation or a focal neurological examination, intravenous contrast agents can be ordered. However, elderly patients are at risk for contrast-induced nephropathy, particularly in the setting of diabetes mellitus or preexisting renal impairment, and the routine use of intravenous contrast is not recommended (Wong and Irwin 2007).

MRI provides high-resolution information on brain structure and, in particular, the white matter and cerebellum. MRI is also an ideal choice in the diagnosis of acute stroke. Many elderly patients do not tolerate the physical discomfort of remaining motionless in the scanner for extended periods and can report claustrophobia; however, newer MRI sequences have drastically reduced the time needed for scanning and can accommodate modest motion from the patient.

Although not part of the standard neuropsychiatric evaluation, functional imaging in the form of functional MRI, magnetic resonance spectroscopy, single-photon emission computed tomography, or positron emission tomography can be considered to assist with diagnosis for patients experiencing neuropsychiatric dysfunction in the setting of normal or abnormal structural neuroimaging (see Chapter 7, "Molecular Imaging in Neuropsychiatry"). Knopman et al. (2001) wrote an excellent, evidence-based review of diagnosing dementia that includes recommendations for laboratory tests and imaging studies.

Electroencephalography is especially useful when epilepsy, sleep disorders, or delirium are diagnostic considerations. Many neuropsychiatric syndromes arise in the setting of epilepsy, most notably, partial seizures. There are limitations to electrodiagnosis (Pedley 1980). If the examiner is sufficiently suspicious about the possibility of a seizure disorder, a normal electroencephalogram (EEG) should be repeated once or even twice to better rule in or exclude epilepsy. For cases of impaired attention, the EEG can detect generalized or diffuse slowing in cases where the presence of delirium cannot be clearly established clinically.

Formulation: Localizing the Findings

An important aspect of the biological domain of the formulation is to place the findings in the brain. The diagnostic necessity for this is discussed earlier in the context of widespread impairments in the cortical dementias. However, patterns of deficits are commonly noted. These patterns often reflect regional impairments caused by localized pathology, such as a stroke or a tumor. The data from the clinical interview, mental status examination, and sensorimotor examination can be organized in a regional fashion. Table 4–5 is intended to assist the reader with neuropsychiatric localization. The table illustrates the relationship among the three areas of inquiry and can serve as a rough guideline for the cardinal signs and symptoms of regional cerebral dysfunction.

Conclusion

The neuropsychiatric formulation is the synthesis of the collected data into a cohesive clinical picture. The data are best organized in terms of the biopsychosocial model (Engel 1980). Biological deficits always elicit some psychological response. Furthermore, the patient's support persons will have a response of their own to the patient, which influences the effectiveness of the patient's attempts at adaptation. A case example follows.

An elderly woman presented to the neuropsychiatry clinic with the complaint of progressive memory impairment. She noted a significant decrease in her ability to manage the household. Her husband had taken up many chores formerly done by the patient. She believed that the need for assistance meant that she was "a failure" and that she was "a burden on her husband." He tended to downplay the patient's memory problem and believed she was being "lazy." Her sleep and appetite were diminished, and she experienced less interest in pleasurable activities. She had a history of poorly controlled hypertension.

Mental status testing demonstrated difficulty with alternating motor sequences as described by Luria (1980), mirroring the examiner's movements on a go/no-go task, and perseveration when copying an alternating design. She also had diminished storage and retrieval of new verbal informa-

TABLE 4–5. Localizing neuropsychiatric findings

Region	History	Mental status	Sensorimotor
Frontal	Disorganization	High-level attention deficit	Gait apraxia
	Disinhibition	Luria motor sequences deficit	Mitgehen
			Ipsilateral gaze preference
		Go/no-go task deficit	Primitive reflexes
		Decrease in verbal fluency	
		Perseveration	
		Losses of set	
		Confabulation	
		Witzelsucht	
	Apathy	Dilapidation	Hypokinesis
Subcortical	Motor impairment	Dilapidation	Hypokinesis
	Social withdrawal	Mental torpor	Masked facies
	Cognitive impairment	Retrieval deficit	Simian stance
			Festinating gait
			Adventitious movement
			Muscular rigidity
			Cogwheeling
			Gegenhalten
			Downward gaze palsy
Right hemisphere	Confusional state	Dysprosodia	Left hypertonus
	Delusions	Visuoconstructive deficit	Left Babinski sign
	Spatial disorientation	Spatial analysis deficit	Left astereognosis
	Neglect	Left hemineglect	Left dysgraphesthesia
	Denial of deficit	Visual memory deficit	Double simultaneous extinction
	Dressing difficulties	Dressing apraxia	Posturing of left hand/arm with tandem gait
	Left-sided motor impairment		Left pronator drift
			Left quadrantanopia
Left hemisphere	Confusional state	Ideomotor apraxia	Right hypertonus
	Language impairment	Dysphasia	Right Babinski sign
	Match impairment	Dyslexia	Right astereognosis
		Dyscalculia	Right dysgraphesthesia
		Dysgraphia	Posturing of right hand/arm with tandem gait
		Right/left disorientation	Right pronator drift
		Finger agnosia	Right quadrantanopia
Bitemporal	Placidity	Amnesia	Superior quadrantanopia
	Hyperorality	Agnosia	
	Hypersexuality	Visual right	
		Auditory left	
		Anomia	
		Prosopagnosia	
Biparietal	Spatial disorientation	Asimultanagnosia	Inferior quadrantanopia
			Ocular apraxia
			Optic ataxia

tion and required prompting to complete a chronological list of recent presidents. The sensorimotor examination revealed a mild bilateral increase in muscular tone and reflexes, greater on the right side. Computed tomography of the brain showed mild to moderate generalized cortical atrophy along with several lacunar infarcts in the basal ganglia bilaterally.

Without going into further clinical detail, biologically, the patient had acquired a syndrome of impaired cognition and depressed mood. Her cognitive and neuroimaging findings suggested frontotemporal systems dysfunction of a possibly mixed cortical degenerative and subcortical vascular pattern, exacerbated by the depressive syndrome.

Psychologically, she equated being an effective household manager with being a good and useful person. The executive deficits threatened her fragile sense of self-esteem. She also experienced a significant psychological threat from the diminished autonomy associated with her deficits and the need to rely on her seemingly unempathic husband. Her husband appeared to deny the possibility of a progressive dementing syndrome, which may have protected him from acknowledging the potential loss of his partner through dementia.

Socially, her husband struggled with assisting her, which compounded her dysphoria by making her feel like a burden. Her depressive syndrome made her anergic and even less able to meet the demands of household management. The couple had become less active and withdrawn from their usual social activities.

Once a case is summarized in this fashion, the clinician can construct a treatment plan to address the patient's depression, dementia, and issues with her spouse; the spouse's issues with the patient's deteriorating condition; and the couple's suboptimal communication.

Key Points

- Geriatric neuropsychiatry provides clinicians with a comprehensive approach for understanding and helping elderly persons with cerebral dysfunction of any etiology.
- The progressive increase in longevity of the U.S. population means that an increasing proportion of the populace will be at risk for acquiring a neuropsychiatric syndrome.
- The ability to diagnose these varied conditions in their early stages and institute aggressive therapeutic and remedial measures will prolong the independent functioning of patients, improve the quality of their lives, and diminish the significant expense of caring for elderly persons unable to function autonomously.
- Recent advances in understanding brain function in healthy and pathological states will provide opportunities to offer more effective treatments in the future.
- The time-honored skills of inquiry, listening, and physical examination will remain the cornerstones of the practice of neuropsychiatry.

Recommended Readings and Web Sites

Coffey CE, McAllister TW, Silver JM (eds): Guide to Neuropsychiatric Therapeutics. Philadelphia, Lippincott Williams & Wilkins, 2007

Cummings JL: Clinical Neuropsychiatry. Orlando, FL, Grune & Stratton, 1985

Mesulam MM: Principles of Behavioral and Cognitive Neurology, 2nd Edition. New York, Oxford University Press, 2000

Ovsiew F: Bedside neuropsychiatry: eliciting the clinical phenomena of neuropsychiatric illness, in The American Psychiatric Publishing Textbook of Neuropsychiatry and Behavioral Neurosciences, 5th Edition. Edited by Yudofsky SC, Hales RE. Washington, DC, American Psychiatric Publishing, 2007, pp 137–187

Strub RL, Black FW: The Mental Status Examination in Neurology, 4th Edition. Philadelphia, FA Davis, 2000

Alliance for Aging Research: The Silver Book. 2010. Available at: http://www.silverbook.org. Accessed April 28, 2010. An almanac of facts, statistics, graphs, and data from more than 200 agencies, organizations, and experts. This searchable database is constantly updated and expanded to highlight the latest research and data on the burden of chronic disease.

Merck Manual of Geriatrics. Available at: http://www.merck.com/mkgr/mmg/contents.jsp. Accessed April 28, 2010. An online clinical manual providing up-to-date information about clinical issues associated with aging. It includes useful links to related Web sites.

References

Albert ML, Feldman RG, Willis AL: The "subcortical dementia" of progressive supranuclear palsy. J Neurol Nerosurg Psychiatry 37:121–130, 1974

Alexander GE, Crutcher MD: Functional architecture of basal ganglia circuits: neural substrates of parallel processing. Trends Neurosci 13:266–271, 1990

Alexopolous GS, Abrams RC, Young RC: Cornell Scale for Depression in Dementia. Biol Psychiatry 23:271–284, 1988

American Psychiatric Association: Diagnostic and Statistical Manual of Mental Disorders, 4th Edition, Text Revision. Washington, DC, American Psychiatric Association, 2000

Applegate WB, Blass JD, Williams TF: Instruments for the functional assessment of older patients. N Engl J Med 322:1207–1214, 1990

Balint R: Seelenahmung des "schauens," optische ataxie, raumliche storung der autmerksamkeit. Monatsschr Psychiat Neurol 25: 51–81, 1909

Baxter LR Jr, Schwartz JM, Mazziotta JC, et al: Local cerebral glucose metabolic rates in non-depressed patients with obsessive-compulsive disorder. Am J Psychiatry 145:1650–1563, 1988

Benson DF, Zaras BW: Progressive aphasia: a case with post-mortem correlation. Neuropsychiatry Neuropsychol Behav Neurol 4: 215–223, 1991

Berrios GE, Brook P: Visual hallucinations and sensory delusions in the elderly. Br J Psychiatry 144:662–664, 1984

Blazer D, George LK, Hughes D: The epidemiology of anxiety disorders: an age comparison, in Anxiety in the Elderly. Edited by Salzman C, Lebowitz BD. New York, Springer, 1991, pp 17–30

Blessed G, Tomlinson BE, Roth M: The association between quantitative measures of dementia and of senile change in the cerebral grey matter of elderly subjects. Br J Psychiatry 114:797–810, 1968

Brown RG, Marsden CD: Cognitive function in Parkinson's disease: from description to theory. Trends Neurosci 13:21–28, 1990

Brun A: Frontal lobe degeneration of the non-Alzheimer type, I: neuropathology. Arch Gerontol Geriatr 6:193–208, 1987

Campbell JJ: Changes in personality, in Guide to Neuropsychiatric Therapeutics. Edited by Coffey CE, McAllister TW, Silver JM. Philadelphia, PA, Lippincott Williams & Wilkins, 2007, pp 267–286

Campbell JJ, Coffey CE: Neuropsychiatric significance of subcortical hyperintensity. J Neuropsychiatry Clin Neurosci 13:261–288, 2001

Campbell W (ed): DeJong's The Neurologic Examination, 6th Edition. Philadelphia, PA, Lippincott Williams & Wilkins, 2005

Caselli RJ: Focal and asymmetric cortical degeneration syndromes. Neurologist 1:1–19, 1995

Charness ME, Simon RP, Greenberg DA: Ethanol and the nervous system. N Engl J Med 321:442–453, 1989

Chui H: Dementia a review emphasizing clinicopathologic correlation and brain-behavior relationships. Arch Neurol 46:806–814, 1989

Coffey CE, Cummings JL, Duffy JD, et al: Assessment of treatment outcomes in neuropsychiatry: a report from the Committee on Research of the American Neuropsychiatric Association. J Neuropsychiatry Clin Neurosci 7:287–289, 1994

Cooper AF, Curry AR: The pathology of deafness in the paranoid and affective psychoses of later life. J Psychosom Res 20:97–105, 1976

Cummings JL (ed): The neuropsychiatric interview and mental status examination, in Clinical Neuropsychiatry. Orlando, FL, Grune & Stratton, 1985a, pp 5–16

Cummings JL (ed): Secondary psychoses, delusions, and schizophrenia, in Clinical Neuropsychiatry. Orlando, FL, Grune & Stratton, 1985b, pp 163–182

Cummings JL, Hegarty A: Neurology, psychiatry, and neuropsychiatry. Neurology 44:209–213, 1994

Cutting J: Delusional misidentification and the role of the right hemisphere in the appreciation of identity. Br J Psychiatry 14 (suppl):70–75, 1991

Damasio AR: Aphasia. N Engl J Med 326:531–539, 1992

Damasio AR: Disorders of complex visual processing, in Principles of Behavioral and Cognitive Neurology, 2nd Edition. Edited by Mesulam M-M. New York, Oxford University Press, 2000, pp 332–372

Damasio AR, Damasio H, Van Hoesen GW: Prosopagnosia: anatomic basis and behavioral mechanisms. Neurology 32:331–341, 1982

Damasio H: Neuroimaging contributions to the understanding of aphasia, in Handbook of Neuropsychology, Vol 2. Edited by Boller F, Grafman J. Amsterdam, Elsevier, 1989, pp 3–46

Devenny DA, Hill AL, Patxot O, et al: The Alzheimer's Disease Assessment Scale: useful for both early detection and staging of dementia of the Alzheimer type. Alzheimer Dis Assoc Disord 6:89–102, 1992

Duffy JD, Campbell JJ: The regional prefrontal syndromes: a theoretical and clinical overview. J Neuropsychiatry Clin Neurosci 6: 379–387, 1994

Ebly EM, Hogan DB, Parhad IM: Cognitive impairment in the nondemented elderly. Arch Neurol 52:612–619, 1995

Elliott FA: Violence: the neurologic contribution: an overview. Arch Neurol 49:595–603, 1992

Engel GL: The clinical application of the biopsychosocial model. Am J Psychiatry 137:535–544, 1980

Erikson EH, Erikson JM, Kivnich HG: Vital Involvement in Old Age. New York, WW Norton, 1994

Erkinjuntti T, Hachinski VC: Rethinking vascular dementia. Cerebrovasc Dis 3:3–23, 1993

Folstein MF, Folstein SE, McHugh PR: "Mini-Mental State": a practical method for grading the cognitive state of patients for the clinician. J Psychiatr Res 12:189–198, 1975

Geschwind N, Galaburda AM: Cerebral lateralization: biological mechanisms, associations, and pathology, I: a hypothesis and a program for research. Arch Neurol 42:428–459, 1985a

Geschwind N, Galaburda AM: Cerebral lateralization: biological mechanisms, associations, and pathology, II: a hypothesis and a program for research. Arch Neurol 42:521–552, 1985b

Geschwind N, Galaburda AM: Cerebral lateralization: biological mechanisms, associations, and pathology, III: a hypothesis and a program for research. Arch Neurol 42:634–654, 1985c

Gibbs A, Andrewes DG, Szmukler G, et al: Early HIV-related neuropsychological impairment: relationship to stage of viral infection. J Clin Exp Neuropsychol 12:766–780, 1990

Goldman-Rakic PS: Specification of higher cortical functions. J Head Trauma Rehabil 8:15–23, 1993

Grafton ST, Mazziota JC, Pahl JJ, et al: A comparison of neurological, metabolic, structural, and genetic evaluations in persons at risk for Huntington's disease. Ann Neurol 28:614–621, 1990

Greenberg DA, Diamond I: Wernicke-Korsakoff syndrome, in Alcohol and the Brain: Chronic Effects. Edited by Tarter RE, Van Thiel DH. New York, Plenum, 1986, pp 295–314

Hammeke TA, McQuillen MP, Cohen BA: Musical hallucinations associated with acquired deafness. J Neurol Neurosurg Psychiatry 46:570–572, 1983

Hof PR, Bouras C, Constantinidis J, et al: Balint's syndrome in Alzheimer's disease: specific disruption of the occipito-parietal visual pathway. Brain Res 49:368–375, 1989

Hyman BT, Van Hoesen GW, Damasio AR, et al: Alzheimer's disease: cell-specific pathology isolates the hippocampal formation. Science 225:1168–1170, 1984

Jacobs JW, Bernard MR, Delgado A, et al: Screening for organic mental syndromes in the medically ill. Ann Intern Med 86:40–47, 1977

Jellinger K: Neuropathological substrates of Alzheimer's disease and Parkinson's disease. J Neural Transm 24(suppl):109–129, 1987

Johansen-Berg H, Gutman DA, Behrens TE, et al: Anatomical connectivity of the subgenual cingulate region targeted with deep brain stimulation for treatment-resistant depression. Cereb Cortex 18:1374–1383, 2008

Ketter TA, George MS, Kimbrell TA, et al: Functional brain imaging, limbic function, and affective disorders. Neuroscientist 2:55–65, 1996

Klüver H, Bucy PC: Preliminary analysis of functions of temporal lobes in monkeys. Arch Neurol Psychiatry 42:979–1000, 1939

Knopman DS, Dekosky ST, Cummings JL, et al: Practice parameter: diagnosis of dementia (an evidence-based review). Neurology 56:1143–1153, 2001

Levine SR, Brust JCM, Futrell N, et al: Cerebrovascular complications of the use of the "crack" form of alkaloidal cocaine. N Engl J Med 323:699–704, 1990

Lilly R, Cummings JL, Benson DF, et al: The human Klüver-Bucy syndrome. Neurology 33:1141–1145, 1983

Lishman WA (ed): Head injury, in Organic Psychiatry: The Psychological Consequences of Cerebral Disorder, 2nd Edition. Oxford, UK, Blackwell Scientific, 1987, pp 137–181

Lishman WA: Alcohol and the brain. Br J Psychiatry 156:635–644, 1990

Lishman WA: What is neuropsychiatry? J Neurol Neurosurg Psychiatry 55:983–985, 1992

Londos E, Passant U, Gustafson L, et al: Contributions of other brain pathologies in dementia. Dement Geriatr Cogn Disord 13:130–148, 2002

Luria AR: Higher Cortical Function in Man. New York, Basic Books, 1980

Malloy PF, Duffy JD: The frontal lobes in neuropsychiatric disorders, in Handbook of Neuropsychology, Vol 8. Edited by Boller F, Spinnler H. New York, Elsevier, 1992, pp 203–232

Malloy PF, Richardson ED: The frontal lobes and content-specific delusions. J Neuropsychiatry Clin Neurosci 6:455–466, 1994

Malloy PF, Cummings JL, Coffey CE, et al: Cognitive screening instruments in neuropsychiatry: a report of the Committee on Research of the American Neuropsychiatric Association. J Neuropsychiatry Clin Neurosci 9:189–197, 1997

Mattis S: Dementia Rating Scale Professional Manual. Odessa, FL, Psychological Assessment Resources, 1973

McHugh PR: The neuropsychiatry of basal ganglia disorders: a triadic syndrome and its explanation. Neuropsychiatry Neuropsychol Behav Neurol 2:239–247, 1989

McHugh PR, Folstein MF: Psychiatric syndromes of Huntington's chorea: a clinical and phenomenologic study, in Psychiatric Aspects of Neurologic Disease. Edited by Benson DR, Blumer D. New York, Grune & Stratton, 1975, pp 267–286

McKeith IG, Galasko D, Kosaka K, et al: Consensus guidelines for the clinical and pathologic diagnosis of dementia with Lewy bodies (DLB). Neurology 47:1113–1124, 1996

Morris JC, Cole M, Banker BQ, et al: Hereditary dysphasic dementia and the Pick/Alzheimer spectrum. Ann Neurol 16:455–466, 1984

Nachson I: Neuropsychology of violent behavior controversial issues and new developments in the study of hemispheric function, in Neuropsychology of Aggression. Edited by Miller JS. Boston, MA, Kluwer Academic, 1991, pp 93–116

Nelson A, Fogel BS, Faust D: Bedside cognitive screening instruments: a critical assessment. J Nerv Ment Dis 174:73–83, 1986

Ott BR, Noto RB, Fogel BS: Apathy and loss of insight in Alzheimer's disease: a SPECT imaging study. J Neuropsychiatry Clin Neurosci 8:41–46, 1996

Ovsiew F: Bedside neuropsychiatry: eliciting the clinical phenomena of neuropsychiatric illness, in The American Psychiatric Press Textbook of Neuropsychiatry, 5th Edition. Edited by Yudofsky SC, Hales RE. Washington, DC, American Psychiatric Publishing, 2007, pp 137–187

Pearson RCA, Esiri MM, Hiorns RW, et al: Anatomical correlate of the distribution of the pathologic changes in the neocortex in Alzheimer's disease. Proc Natl Acad Sci U S A 82:4531–4534, 1985

Pedley TA: Interictal epileptiform discharges: discriminating characteristics and clinical correlations. Am J EEG Technol 20:101–119, 1980

Petersen RC, Smith G, Kokmen E, et al: Memory function in normal aging. Neurology 42:396–401, 1992

Petersen RC, Smith GE, Waring SC, et al: Aging, memory and mild cognitive impairment. Int Psychogeriatr 9 (suppl 1):65–69, 1997

Pfeiffer E: A short portable mental status questionnaire for the assessment of organic brain deficit in elderly patients. J Am Geriatr Soc 23:433–441, 1975

Rapp PR, Amaral DG: Individual differences in the cognitive and neurobiological consequences in normal aging. Trends Neurosci 15:340–345, 1992

Roberts GW: Schizophrenia: the cellular biology of a functional psychosis. Trends Neurosci 13:207–211, 1990

Robinson RG, Price TR: Post-stroke depressive disorders: a follow up study of 103 patients. Stroke 13:635–641, 1982

Robinson RG, Boston JD, Starkstein SE, et al: Comparison of mania with depression following brain injury. Am J Psychiatry 145: 172–178, 1988

Ross ED: Affective prosody and the aprosodias, in Principles of Behavioral and Cognitive Neurology, 2nd edition. Edited by Mesulam M-M. New York, Oxford, 2005, pp 316–331

Rothlind JC, Brandt J: A brief assessment of frontal and subcortical functions in dementia. J Neuropsychiatry Clin Neurosci 5:73–77, 1993

Rourke BP: Nonverbal Learning Disabilities: The Syndrome and the Model. New York, Guilford, 1989

Royall DR, Mahurin RK, Gray KF: Bedside assessment of executive cognitive impairment: the Executive Interview. J Am Geriatr Soc 40:1221–1226, 1992

Schiffer R, Najara-Lanson W: Neuropsychiatric examination, in Neuropsychiatry, 2nd Edition. Edited by Schiffer RB, Rao SM, Fogel BS. Baltimore, MD, Lippincott Williams & Wilkins, 2003, pp 3–19

Schmahmann JD: Disorders of the cerebellum: ataxia, dysmetria of thought, and the cerebellar cognitive affective syndrome. J Neuropsychiatry Clin Neurosci 16:367–378, 2004

Shenton ME, Kikinis R, Jolesz FA: Abnormalities of the left temporal lobe and thought disorder in schizophrenia: a quantitative magnetic resonance imaging study. N Engl J Med 327:605–612, 1992

Starkstein SE, Bolduc PL, Mayberg HS, et al: Cognitive impairment and depression in Parkinson's disease: a follow up study. J Neurol Neurosurg Psychiatry 53:597–602, 1990

Streissguth AP, Landesman-Dwyer S: Teratogenic effects of alcohol in humans and laboratory animals. Science 209:353, 1980

Strub RL, Black FW: The Mental Status Examination in Neurology, 4th Edition. Philadelphia, PA, FA Davis, 2000

Terao T, Collinson S: Charles Bonnet syndrome and dementia. Lancet 355:2168, 2000

Tetrud JW, Langston JW, Garbe PL, et al: Mild parkinsonism in persons exposed to 1-methyl-4-phenyl-1,2,3,6-tetrahydropyridine (MPTP). Neurology 39:1483–1487, 1989

Tomer R, Levin BE, Weiner WJ: Obsessive-compulsive symptom and motor asymmetries in Parkinson's disease. Neuropsychiatry Neuropsychol Behav Neurol 6:26–30, 1993

Trimble MR: Neuropsychiatry or behavioral neurology. Neuropsychiatry Neuropsychol Behav Neurol 6:60–69, 1993

Tross S, Hirsch DA: Psychological distress and neuropsychological complications of HIV infection and AIDS. Am Psychol 43:929–934, 1988

Tyrrell P, Rossor M: The association of gegenhalten in the upper limbs with dyspraxia. J Neurol Neurosurg Psychiatry 51:995–997, 1988

Wallin A, Milos V, Sjögren M, et al: Classification and subtypes of vascular dementia. Int Psychogeriatr 15 (suppl 1):27–37, 2003

Weinberger DR: Schizophrenia and the frontal lobe. Trends Neurosci 11:367–370, 1988

Weintraub S: Neurological assessment of mental state, in Principles of Behavioral Neurology, 2nd Edition. Edited by Mesulam M-M. New York, Oxford University Press, 2000

Wender PH: Attention deficit disorder ("Minimal brain dysfunction") in adults. Arch Gen Psychiatry 38:449–456, 1981

White NJ: Complex visual hallucinations in partial blindness due to eye disease. Br J Psychiatry 136:284–286, 1980

Wong GTC, Irwin MG. Contrast-induced nephropathy. Br J Anaesth 99:474–483, 2007

Woods D: The diagnosis and treatment of attention deficit disorder, residual type. Psychiatr Ann 16:23–28, 1986

Yesavage JA, Brink TL, Rose TL, et al: Development and validation of a geriatric depression screening scale: a preliminary report. J Psychiatr Res 17:37–49, 1982–1983

Zametkin AJ, Nordahl TE, Gross M, et al: Cerebral glucose metabolism in adults with hyperactivity of childhood onset. N Engl J Med 323:1361–1366, 1990

5

Neuropsychological Assessment

Kenneth Podell, Ph.D.
Jennifer M. Keller, Psy.D.

The neuropsychological evaluation of older adults has become increasingly important as a component of the neuropsychiatric evaluation. Neuropsychological assessment can be considered a more in-depth extension and quantification of the mental status examination and, as such, focuses on the psychometric assessment of cognitive processes. A thorough neuropsychological evaluation can add much to the clinical diagnostic process and neuropsychiatric assessment (see Chapter 4, "Neuropsychiatric Assessment") and can complement information gathered through electrophysiological, neuroanatomical, and functional neuroimaging technologies (see Chapter 6, "Imaging the Structure of the Aging Human Brain," and Chapter 7, "Molecular Imaging in Neuropsychiatry").

In this chapter, we review the applications of neuropsychological assessment to geriatric patients and discuss relevant issues regarding the establishment of appropriate normative databases for this population. The selection and use of neuropsychological tests, the interpretation of test results, and the use of these results in the treatment planning process are specifically discussed. We also discuss and contrast fixed battery and flexible approaches of neuropsychological testing in the assessment of elderly patients.

Goals of the Geriatric Neuropsychological Evaluation

Neuropsychological test results are used in various ways depending on the training of the neuropsychologist, the setting, the referral question, and the treatment program. Despite differing approaches to assessment, the three primary goals of neuropsychological assessment are generally the same: 1) to establish an individual's cognitive and behavioral strengths and weaknesses, 2) to interpret findings from a diagnostic viewpoint (i.e., differential diagnosis), and 3) to support recommendations for treatment and rehabilitation (La Rue 1992).

Indications for Neuropsychological Testing

For the geriatric population, neuropsychological testing is commonly used as one of the diagnostic procedures in a dementia workup. Unique among the armament of neurodiagnostic tests used in the assessment of dementia, only neuropsychological testing can determine comprehensively the patient's cognitive functioning, which in turn is the only way to determine his or her functional abilities—which drives the most common questions of the families confronting a loved one with dementia.

Physicians commonly request a neuropsychological evaluation to determine the presence of cognitive impairment, which is required for a diagnosis of dementia, as well as to help with dementia typing. Although neuropsychological testing is considered critical in diagnosing dementia, it is not independently capable of determining etiology, and therefore various neuroimaging techniques (electroencephalography, computed tomography, magnetic resonance imaging, single-photon emission computed tomography, or positron emission tomography), blood work, and genetic testing supplement neuropsychological testing in a comprehensive dementia workup.

The most common reason to request neuropsychological testing is when the patient or a family member reports changes in the patient's behavior or cognition. Memory is the most common complaint, but other complaints are attention problems, speech problems, and behavioral changes. The behavioral changes can be wide ranging and include depression, anxiety, apathy, lack of initiation or disinhibition, hallucinations, inappropriate behavior, and lack of insight. In addition, any reports of functional difficulties by the patient or significant other can trigger the need for neuropsychological testing. For example, complaints that the patient has been getting lost while driving, forgetting to take medications (or taking too much), or forgetting to pay bills can all be subtle signs that dementia is evolving.

Another important reason for neuropsychological testing is to determine functional capacity. Even if a diagnosis of dementia has been made, neuropsychological testing is quite useful in determining the individual's functional capacity, such as whether he or she has the ability to live (level of supportive living required) or drive independently, can manage personal finances, can make independent medical decisions, or has testamentary capacity. Also, serial neuropsychological testing can be used to monitor changes in cognition and behavior, observe medication effects, and adjust treatment recommendations and options.

Normal Aging

The aging process affects the brain, as it does all other organs. Although the aging process affects cognitive abilities in specific patterns, several misconceptions still abound. Many assume or believe that memory problems are a normal part of the aging process. This attitude causes a delay in diagnosis and treatment, resulting in cognitive deficits that are quite prominent and cause impairment in the patient's daily functioning. Recent research of the aging processes shows that individuals are not bound to across-the-board cognitive decline as they age. Rather, certain cognitive skills actually grow stronger in normal aging (Goldberg 2005), and the aging brain sprouts new neuronal connections. In contrast, research indicates that the adage of "use it or lose it" may apply to cognitive skills as well as motor skills in elderly individuals. This has become an important topic as baby boomers are reaching their 60s and wanting to maintain their cognitive health. Several authors have shown either maintenance or enhancement of cognitive skills with practice in healthy elderly subjects (Loewenstein and Acevedo 2006; Unverzagt et al. 2009; Zehnder et al. 2009). These findings have led to an explosion of scientific and commercial programs designed to keep individuals cognitively fit as they grow older. However, as the old adage states, "Buyer beware." Most of the available programs are not scientifically based and have not been proven to be effective. It is difficult for the consumer to know the difference, and it is up to our profession to help guide them in using evidence-based programs.

The understanding of cognitive changes in normal aging is evolving given the more recent studies examining this issue (Clark et al. 2009; Johnson et al. 2008; Zanto et al. 2009). Although older adults experience cognitive, structural, and chemical brain changes, these changes are not necessarily the result of a neurodegenerative process and occur in healthy individuals as part of the normal aging process. Functional neuroimaging studies reveal more lateralized activation in younger adults and bilateral and diffuse activation in older adults who performed the same visual memory and episodic memory tasks. These studies suggest that older adults may use different brain pathways and processing strategies for the same task (Cabeza 2002; Goldberg 2005; Langley and Madden 2000).

Aging affects cognitive domains differently and in varying degrees. The most common change is an increase in so-called crystallized intelligence. More routinized knowledge remains relatively stable, whereas "fluid" abilities, such as reasoning, abstraction, and processing speed, tend to diminish progressively with age, beginning as early as the mid-30s (Compton et al. 2000; Singer et al. 2003). Motor, cognitive, and perceptual speeds are slowed in elderly individuals and considered the hallmark of normal aging (Pickholtz and Malamut 2008; Smith and Bondi 2008). In a study comparing younger and older adults' performance on an immediate task, the older adults completed it with similar accuracy to younger subjects but required more time to do so (Multhaup et al. 1996).

Older adults are prone to increased distractibility or can exhibit diminished selective attention. They also have more trouble with divided and sustained attention as task complexity increases. Diminished attention and processing speed may give the appearance of a decline in memory, in combination with slower learning and reduced acquisition (Smith and Bondi 2008). Many individuals may not simply have short-term memory problems or forgetfulness. Instead, it is common for elderly persons to experience decreased, less efficient encoding abilities rather than an amnesia or inability to retain information. They may require repetition or rehearsal to learn and recall new information and to remember it over time. These individuals may have difficulty accessing or independently retrieving information, but their ability to recognize or recall it with cues will be intact.

Lexical retrieval is the most common type of language complaint in the older population. Individuals often experience a tip-of-the-tongue phenomenon in which they know the name of a person, object, or place but have difficulty coming up with it quickly (Bowles and Poon 1985; Burke and Laver 1990). Rate of speech and fluency may become slower and comprehension may be adversely affected at much later ages (i.e., 70s and 80s, respectively).

Executive dysfunction underlies many other age-related cognitive changes. Cognitive processes associated with prefrontal cortical functioning, such as cognitive flexibility and temporal sequencing, can be disrupted and prevent an individual from being able to rapidly switch between rules or to judge an order of events. This dysfunction can manifest as source memory impairment, in that the individual can recognize information as something previously learned but is unable to place its origin. Abstract reasoning ability can be diminished. Older adults are less likely to use organizational strategies spontaneously when learning new information, and they approach verbal learning tasks in a manner similar to patients with frontal lobe dysfunction (Stuss et al. 1996a). Working memory, an individual's ability to hold information in immediate memory while manipulating it, declines with age. Changes in working memory are believed to be due to disrupted executive abilities as well as reduced encoding and retrieval systems (Keefover 1998).

However, all is not doom and gloom in aging. Emerging evidence shows that specific cognitive skills can actually increase or improve with normal aging. For example, older subjects, although less efficient at speed of information processing and integration, are better than younger individuals at using past experiences and knowledge to draw inferences and new ideas (Goldberg 2005).

Methodological Issues in Geriatric Neuropsychology

The clinical neuropsychological evaluation is highly dependent on appropriate comparison groups that allow the cognitive dysfunction related to pathological processes to be separated from normal age-related changes. The normative sample provides the basis for this comparison of individual patient performance to established standards for a given age group and is an important prerequisite to the assessment process. However, to date, the usefulness of neuropsychological testing with older adults has been limited by a relative dearth of normative data. The development of valid and realistic normative data for geriatric patients continues to be a major challenge for geriatric neuropsychology, particularly with the psychometric assessment of patients over age 75. Demographic characteristics have a substantial impact on normative values. Research has shown that age, education, literacy, and ethnicity affect performance in various cognitive domains differentially in urban- and rural-dwelling patients (Hohl et al. 1999; Lichtenberg et al. 1998; Manly et al. 1999; Marcopulos et al. 1997; Strick et al. 1998).

Substantial limitations exist in age-based normative data, including limited heterogeneity of education and health variables among normative samples (La Rue 1992), as well as poor reliability, validity, and normative data relevant to "old-old" patient groups (i.e., those ages 75 and older) (Kaszniak 1989). This lack of an adequate normative base has at times fostered a reliance on norms obtained from younger subject groups—a practice that can lead to an overdiagnosis of pathological cognitive impairment in geriatric patients.

In the absence of current age-appropriate normative data, some clinicians have tended to rely on data that were collected many years earlier and from samples of geriatric subjects who may have differed significantly from the individual patient whose performance is being evaluated. Given generational differences in the availability of medical treatment, education, nutrition, and a host of other factors that can influence performance on neuropsychological tests, it may not be valid to compare the test performance of an elderly patient in the 2010s to normative data gathered during the 1970s or before. This cohort effect (Schaie and Schaie 1977) limits the usefulness of previously established normative data to current samples of patients; it is akin to the Flynn effect, the phenomenon wherein performance (e.g., intelligence episodic memory) improves across successive generations. Thus, using outdated tests may yield an artificially higher score that can mask the presence of a mild deficit.

One additional concern with using age-appropriate normative data in a geriatric population is making sure that the normative data have adequate psychometric properties, even if they have large sample sizes with appropriate age and education ranges. Potential flooring effects are extremely problematic for more difficult tests of memory and executive control, which are particularly important cognitive domains in assessing geriatric populations. For example, normative data are available for performance on the Wisconsin Card Sorting Test extending through the eighth decade (Heaton et al. 1993). This test, which is difficult even for younger, more educated individuals, is extremely difficult for older, less educated patients. The flooring effect has very real implications in terms of test interpretation and translation to real-world activities or ecological validity. We believe not only that a test's developers need to ensure adequate norming in terms of demographic variables, but also that the test must accurately reflect the range of abilities in the age group and must have appropriate psychometric properties (e.g., minimized ceiling or flooring effects).

In neuropsychology, because predisease or baseline data are often unavailable for patients, professionals tend to use level of education (among other variables) as a marker of premorbid cognitive abilities. They use this to compare current performance to determine if a meaningful decline has occurred. However, level of education for geriatric patients most likely does not have the same meaning as the educational level of people in their 30s, for example. In our experience, level of education, unless very high or very low, may not have the same predictive abilities as assumed with a younger population. Therefore, in our clinic, to help predict lifelong cognitive abilities, we also rely on measures considered highly resilient to any type of central nervous system dysfunction. One such measure is single-word reading recognition and vocabulary skills (Bayles et al. 1985).

Another methodological issue that has affected the neuropsychological evaluation of elderly patients involves differing definitions of what constitutes the expected cognitive pattern of "normal aging." For example, some researchers have distinguished between usual aging, in which the effects of the aging process are influenced by extrinsic factors such as nutrition and psychosocial factors, and successful aging, in which these factors play a neutral or positive role (Rowe and Kahn 1987). Still others have studied unusually healthy groups of geriatric subjects, documenting cognitive functioning in patients who are uncharacteristically free of the general medical problems that often afflict elderly persons (MacInnes et al. 1983). Obviously, the comparison of a patient's performance to norms gathered from these disparate samples could lead to markedly different conclusions regarding pathological cognitive decline in a given patient. Comparison of the typical elderly patient with norms derived from a sample of unusually healthy individuals may result in an overdiagnosis of pathological cognitive dysfunction (Albert 1981).

Despite past limitations in the development of normative data on cognitive functioning in geriatric patients, significant improvement has occurred in the development of neuropsychological tests that provide geriatric norms. More recent tests have been developed that include normative data extending into the eighth decade. Regardless, one needs to evaluate carefully if critical variables such as gender, education, and ethnicity were reported or incorporated into the grouping.

Medication side effects on cognitive abilities are another factor that may influence both neuropsychological assessment and treatment. Commonly prescribed medications, such as cimetidine, can produce alterations in cognition. Similarly, the use of anticholinergic and antidopaminergic medications (both over-the-counter and prescribed) must be taken into consideration because of their known deleterious effects on memory (Drachman and Leavitt 1974; Fick et al. 2003) and executive control skills, respectively (see Fuster 1989).

When determining the cause of possible decline in neuropsychological abilities, one may be tempted to assume it is a neurodegenerative effect. However, one must be highly cognizant of more subtle causes, some of which are reversible—for example, vitamin deficiencies (B_{12} and D). Autoimmune disorders (Sjögren's syndrome) and even genetic factors (fragile X tremor and ataxia syndrome) should be considered as potential causes.

Finally, a distinction between age-appropriate cognitive abilities, as defined by performance relative to normative data, and functional abilities needed for the individual's given situation must be clearly defined and addressed in a neuropsychological evaluation. What may be age-appropriate cognitive functioning (e.g., for an 85-year-old individual) may not be sufficient for the level of independent functioning required in the individual's living situation. For example, the same individual may be sufficiently cognitively intact relative to age-appropriate normative data to return to live in an assisted living apartment building where he or she has some increased supervision, but he or she may not be sufficiently cognitively intact to live alone and be independently responsible for instrumental activities of daily living and medical management.

Neuropsychological Evaluation Process

The neuropsychological assessment is a complex process requiring the integration of knowledge from several different areas of medicine (including neurology, psychiatry, neurobiology), clinical psychology and aging, psychometrics, and, of course, neuropsychology (Kaszniak 1989). The evaluation typically consists of a comprehensive clinical interview, test selection, scoring and interpretation of test results (e.g., functional level, brain systems involved, possible etiologies), diagnosis, and treatment and rehabilitation recommendations.

The primary goal of the clinical interview should be to develop hypotheses regarding the patient's overall cognitive status, current problems and symptoms, and capacity to engage in further neuropsychological evaluation, as well as potential etiology of any disturbance. In addition, the clinical interview provides an opportunity for the examiner to develop rapport with the patient, explain the nature of the evaluation, and answer any of the patient's questions, which may help to alleviate initial anxiety.

Because some elderly patients are not capable of giving a precise and thorough history, in our clinic we request that a significant other accompany each patient. After obtaining permission from the patient, we routinely interview the significant other to verify and/or obtain appropriate history. Additionally, functionality questionnaires completed by the significant other can be used to add information about functional status. A thorough interview should yield relevant demographic background information (e.g., age, education, occupational history, handedness), a review of medical and psychiatric history (including past and present medication use), substance use or abuse, familial (both medical and psychiatric) and developmental information, current living situation, support network, and an exhaustive review of symptomatology. We also do a complete review of sensory and motor systems, sleep homeostasis (querying about parasomnias) and autonomic functioning, and changes in cognition and affect, emphasizing recent changes in language, memory, thinking, and affect. We also review for any recent stressors (e.g., death of spouse or loss of driving license); information pertaining to activity level and hobbies; motivation; and the patient's understanding of why he or she was referred for neuropsychological evaluation.

Throughout the clinical interview and direct interaction with the patient, the neuropsychologist gathers important qualitative information regarding cognitive functioning. This information includes a general sense of the patient's orientation, attentional capacity, motivation, awareness of impairment, willingness to engage in neuropsychological testing, and social appropriateness. Integrity of gross language and motor function, memory capacity, and stamina can be assessed, as well. The older patient's performance during the neuropsychological evaluation may be affected by limitations, including tremors, fatigue, reduced vision and hearing, and the effects of overmedication (Goreczny and Nussbaum 1994; Russell 1984), that are detectable in the clinical interview and adjusted for during testing.

Similarly, the method of test administration must sometimes be altered to conform to a patient's sensorial limitations. For example, a subject with poor hearing but intact vision may have to read a word list presented on cue cards rather than listen to the list being presented. Although this approach clearly violates standard administration, it allows for a "qualitative" analysis and can yield useful information for an experienced neuropsychologist. In addition, the patient should be encouraged to continue working on tasks even after reaching specified time limits. This testing-the-limits approach can help to establish the patient's capacity to perform a cognitive task when motor abnormalities, as in Parkinson's disease, and sensory deficits might limit the patient's ability to complete the testing within specified time boundaries.

The administration of neuropsychological tests usually begins directly after the clinical interview. Test selection is based on the following five factors: 1) the referral question, 2) the patient's level of functioning as ascertained during the clinical interview, 3) hypotheses regarding the differential diagnosis, 4) the patient's physical limitations, and 5) the need to document cognitive deficiencies and relative strengths. The latter point has relevance to the patient's ability to function in everyday life.

The selection of tests may differ based on individual patient needs. For example, older patients with severe cognitive or medical disturbances may lack the stamina or attentional capacity to undergo a comprehensive neuropsychological evaluation. For these patients, the selection of tests that tap specific domains of cognitive functioning in combination with the use of a more broad-based screening instrument may be the most useful approach. In contrast, a patient with relatively preserved cognitive abilities and without serious medical complications may be engaged in a more thorough cognitive assessment involving the in-depth assessment of multiple domains of neuropsychological functioning (Russell 1984). Regardless of the estimated level of cognitive functioning or the hypothesized nature of the cognitive impairment, we recommend the use of a brief cognitive screen as part of the interview process with the older patient. This not only permits an initial assessment of the patient's general cognitive capacity but also provides direction for the selection of instruments to be used in the neuropsychological evaluation. The use of cognitive screening instruments within the more general context of the neuropsychological evaluation also promotes the comparison of test results across different testing sessions, even when the patient has deteriorated to a degree that precludes a more comprehensive evaluation.

Although brief screening instruments are extremely useful in detecting (i.e., diagnosing) the presence of dementia (Stuss et al. 1996b), they do not provide information regarding functional abilities, placement and competency issues, etiology, or recommendations. These limitations should be considered when interpreting results based solely on a brief screening instrument.

Various demographic variables can influence performance scores on brief screening instruments. For example, advanced age and lower education can produce an overestimate of cognitive impairments on the Mini-Mental State Examination (MMSE) (Malloy et al. 1997; Naugle and Kawczak 1989). Some existing screening tests have been renormed to take age and education into account (e.g., Dementia Rating Scale [Lucas et al. 1998]; St. Louis University Mental Status examination [Tariq et al. 2006]) and to obtain better sensitivity (van Gorp et al. 1999). Highly focused, very brief screening instruments to assess memory loss in dementia have also been developed (e.g., Memory Impairment Screen; Buschke et al. 1999). Additionally, researchers have found that brief screening instruments can be somewhat insensitive to mild forms of dementia (particularly the memory component), thus increasing type II errors (false negatives) (Benedict and Brandt 1992; Pfeffer et al. 1981). Other screening instruments, such as the Cognistat (Kiernan et al. 1987; formerly known as the Neurobehavioral Cognitive Status Examination), offer better delineation of the patient's cognitive deficits but may not offer good discrimination for dementia type (van Gorp et al. 1999). Depending on the history and referral question, the use of a brief cognitive screening instrument solely to determine the need for further testing may cause an inaccurate assessment in either direction.

Approaches to the Neuropsychological Evaluation of Geriatric Patients

As a discipline, clinical neuropsychology is generally concerned with the study of brain-behavior relationships. However, clinical approaches to the assessment of these relationships vary widely (Kane 1991; Podell 2009). Currently well-accepted strategies for neuropsychological assessment include the use of fixed batteries of neuropsychological tests, flexible evaluation strategies, and a combination of these approaches. With the need to better define cognitive and behavioral deficits and changes associated with different dementia types, appropriately choosing tests to suit the individual assessment may be the most productive method (Benton 1985; Costa 1983). In this section, we review the application of these different approaches with adults ages 65 and older (for more detailed discussions on using fixed vs. flexible battery approaches, see Lezak 2004; Russell 1998).

Fixed Test Battery Approaches

In a fixed battery approach, the same test instruments are administered to every patient in a standard manner regardless of the patient's presenting illness or referral question (Kane 1991; Kaszniak 1989). The two most popular neuropsychological batteries are the Halstead-Reitan Neuropsychological Test Battery (HRNB; Reitan and Wolfson 1985) and the Luria-Nebraska Neuropsychological Battery (Golden et al. 1980; see also Incagnoli et al. 1986; Lezak 2004).[1] Advantages of the fixed battery approach to neuropsychological assessment include that it provides a comprehensive assessment of multiple cognitive domains and that because of its standardized format, the test data can be incorporated into databases for clinical and scientific analysis. Disadvantages of the fixed battery approach include time and labor intensiveness and a lack of flexibility in different clinical situations.

A large literature exists on the psychometric properties of fixed batteries such as HRNB (Anthony et al. 1980; Heaton and Pendleton 1981; Kane 1991; Parsons 1986; Reitan 1976; Reitan and Davison 1974; Reitan and Wolfson 1985). However, relatively little empirical research exists regarding the psychometric properties of flexible or fixed battery approaches with the elderly population (Kaszniak 1989).

Halstead-Reitan Neuropsychological Test Battery

The HRNB represents one of the most popular battery approaches to neuropsychological assessment (Table 5–1). This battery measures cognitive functioning across a number of cognitive domains but is often too difficult for elderly individuals with more than mild cognitive impairment. Despite its widespread use in nongeriatric patients, the use of this battery with elderly patients (as well as with younger patients) has been criticized (Fastenau and Adams 1996). Several studies have established age and education as important moderator variables for several of the battery's subtests (Heaton et al. 1986, 1991). Older or more poorly educated subjects were misclassified on the HRNB Impairment Index (a summary score based on seven different measures) as having brain damage more often than two other matched groups. Finally, the sample sizes for individual groups were not given in the published normative data, and evidence suggests that some of the normative groups had very few subjects in them (Fastenau and Adams 1996) and that use of a regression model produced a higher rate of missed diagnoses (Fastenau 1998).

TABLE 5–1. Halstead-Reitan Neuropsychological Test Battery (HRNB) with measures of general intellect and memory

HRNB
Tactual Performance Test
Total time[a]
Localization[a]
Memory[a]
Finger Oscillation Test (dominant hand)[a]
Seashore Rhythm Test[a]
Speech Sounds Perception Test[a]
Aphasia Screening Test
Sensory-Perceptual Examination
Grip Strength Test
Tactile Form Recognition Test
General intelligence
Wechsler Adult Intelligence Scale–III (Wechsler 1997a)
Memory
Wechsler Memory Scale–III (Wechsler 1997b)

Note. Some of the tests have published normative data, independent of the HRNB normative data.
[a]These scores make up the Impairment Index.
Source. Adapted from Heaton et al. 1991.

[1]The Luria-Nebraska Neuropsychological Battery (Golden and Maruish 1986; Golden et al. 1980; Kane 1991; Purisch and Sbordone 1986) is not discussed in this chapter because its administration and scoring parameters place the geriatric patient at a disadvantage and potentially increase the chance of misdiagnosis (Lezak 2004).

The principal concerns with reliance on the HRNB in assessment of older adults are that 1) the HRNB may overestimate brain impairment in otherwise nonneurologically impaired older adults; 2) the amount of time and effort required to complete the HRNB is likely inappropriate for elderly patients who are prone to fatigue easily; 3) the HRNB may not adequately assess both the strengths and the weaknesses of the elderly patient because it uses subtests that measure primarily fluid abilities (e.g., novel problem-solving, reasoning, and spatial processes) that are known to decline with normal aging; and 4) the HRNB potentially has poor psychometric properties, especially for older groups. For these reasons, some have argued against the use of the HRNB with the elderly population (La Rue 1992).

Despite these concerns, some HRNB subtests are useful and commonly included in neuropsychological evaluations (e.g., Trail Making and Finger Oscillation Tests). Additionally, efforts have been made to develop HRNB age and education corrections for older adults (see Heaton et al. 1991), and a short form of the HRNB has been developed (Storrie and Doerr 1980).

Flexible Approach to Neuropsychological Assessment

In a flexible approach to neuropsychological testing, individual tests are chosen on the basis of the patient's presenting illness or referral question (Goodglass 1986; Kane 1991; Kaszniak 1989; Lezak 2004; Schear 1984). Primary advantages of the flexible approach to neuropsychological evaluation include a potentially shorter administration time, economic favorability, and adaptability to differing patient situations and needs. Some (Goodglass 1986; Russell 1984) have argued that the flexible approach permits better specification of the deficits within a given cognitive domain as well as their underlying neural systems, rather than simply documentation of the presence or absence of brain damage. Others use the flexible approach because it permits easy evaluation of qualitative features such as the patient's use of problem-solving strategies (Kaplan 1983). Finally, test modification inherent in the flexible approach makes it adaptable to a wide variety of clinical situations (Kane 1991).

Disadvantages of the flexible approach include the need for greater clinical experience; a lack of standardization of administration rules for some tests, as well as of the tests administered; a potential lack of comprehensiveness; and limitations in establishing systematic databases (Kane 1991; Tarter and Edwards 1986). An understanding of developmentally normal aging, age-related cognitive decline, neuropsychological principles, neuropathological conditions in elderly patients, and other issues pertinent to differential diagnosis are particularly important when using the flexible neuropsychological assessment approach with elderly patients.

The flexible approach does not lend itself well to empirical investigation because of the individualized nature of the tasks and the difficulty comparing results across institutions or centers. However, this individualized approach to neuropsychological assessment remains popular with many neuropsychologists because of its adaptability, flexibility, clinical usefulness of qualitative information, efficiency with severely impaired patients, and applicability with patients who are vulnerable to fatigue, distress, or sensory limitations (Kane 1991; La Rue 1992). For these reasons, the flexible neuropsychological evaluation is a useful, and possibly the best, approach for the clinical assessment of older adults (Benton 1985; Costa 1983).

Tests of Cognitive Functioning

Screening Instruments

Cognitive screening instruments can be used at either an individual or a community level. Individually, they serve to quickly and inexpensively identify those persons who need further diagnostic assessment or treatment for dementia. At the community level, they identify those individuals who would benefit from additional medical intervention or assessment or those in need of further community-based services (Mitrushina 2009).

Timely detection of cognitive decline or dementia is critical in the geriatric setting because it serves to identify those in need of treatment or assistance in daily functioning and community services. Rapid and early detection allows for quick intervention, both medically and functionally, and helps to ensure the best quality of life for a longer period.

Cognitive screenings are useful, particularly for older patients who would have difficulty completing longer protocols due to their age, fatigability, physical limitations, impaired cognition, or medical condition. Table 5–2 gives a brief listing of some of the more commonly used screening instruments. For more detailed descriptions of these and additional measures, see Lezak (2004), Mitrushina (2009), and Strauss et al. (2006).

In theory the perfect screening instrument is brief, easy to administer, easily tolerated by the patient, and reliable, with excellent sensitivity and specificity. In reality, however, no instrument meets all of those requirements. They all have limitations, and the professional needs to be cognizant of the pros and cons of the screening instrument being used. Different situations and requirements will determine which screening instrument would be best. It appears that the length of a screening instrument tends to be proportionate to its sensitivity for milder forms of cognitive impairment. Those screening instruments that have more in-depth tests and that assess a greater variety of neuropsychological domains tend to have greater sensitivity to mild cognitive impairment (Mitrushina 2009). Perhaps the

TABLE 5–2. Commonly used dementia screening tests

Screening instruments for dementia	Typical administration time, minutes	Comments
Consortium to Establish a Registry for Alzheimer's Disease (Morris et al. 1989)	20–30	Includes standardized tests with extensive research (some longitudinal with autopsy data).
Dementia Rating Scale (Mattis 1988)	15–25	Assesses broad range of cognitive domains; well normed with some culturally adjusted norms.
Mini-Mental State Examination (MMSE; Folstein et al. 1975)	5–10	Well-established instrument with limited normative data and poor sensitivity (positive predictive values) to earlier stages of dementia.
Montreal Cognitive Assessment (Nasreddine 2003)	10–15	Extends MMSE with limited assessment of language, memory, and normative data.
Repeatable Battery for the Assessment of Neuropsychological Status (Randolph 1998)	20–30	Assesses broad range of cognitive domains, based on standard neuropsychological measures. Looks at cortical and subcortical patterns. Provides good memory assessment. Well normed across the age spectrum.
St. Louis University Mental Status examination (Tariq et al. 2006)	10–15	Extended MMSE with limited language and executive measures. Norms are corrected for high school education.

most critical issue that is most often missed and poorly understood relates to the sensitivity of the screening instrument for the context for which it is being used. Clinicians are often unaware of an instrument's sensitivity (if sensitivity was even empirically determined during test development), and therefore patients might be exposed to a meaningless test. Probably the best example of this would be MMSE (Folstein et al. 1975). The MMSE is the best known and probably most commonly used screening instrument for neuropsychological impairment, yet very few clinicians who use it know anything about its psychometric properties, let alone its sensitivity. For example, the MMSE is highly sensitive to the effects of education, and the cutoff used to determine impairment differs drastically based on demographic factors (Ostrosky-Solis et al. 2000). Therefore, when adjusted for age and education, the MMSE's specificity and sensitivity improve greatly in a patient population over age 65 (Harvan and Cotter 2006), but only in at least moderately impaired patients because it tends to have poorer sensitivity with more mildly impaired patients (Tombaugh and McIntyre 1992).

Specific Neuropsychological Domains

Even when a flexible approach to neuropsychological assessment is adopted, a broad range of cognitive processes should be evaluated. The major domains of cognitive functioning that should be assessed include attention and concentration, general intelligence, memory and learning, conceptual processes and executive functioning, visuospatial skills, language, fine motor speed, coordination, strength, and emotional status (see Albert and Moss 1988; Russell 1984). In addition, we like to include the assessment of functional abilities, in terms of completing activities of daily living, and to obtain ratings by relatives or significant others. We find that by including these last two areas in our comprehensive geriatric neuropsychological assessment, we are better able to address issues of competency, improve our ecological validity, address a patient's ability to live alone, and obtain a more accurate picture of the individual's current functioning. Table 5–3 lists individual neuropsychological tests that are commonly used in evaluating the major domains of cognitive functioning in older adults. A complete review of these cognitive domains and the instruments that measure them is beyond the scope of this chapter; for excellent reviews on this topic, see Albert and Moss (1988), La Rue (1992), La Rue and Swanda (1997), and Lezak (2004).

Attentional Processes

After the informal assessment of the patient's basic level of arousal, alertness, and orientation, the examiner should evaluate the patient's attentional capacity. Assessment of attention is necessary because it is a prerequisite for successful performance in other cognitive domains (Albert 1981). If the patient appears to fatigue in the course of testing, the examiner may

TABLE 5–3. Cognitive domains and representative neuropsychological tests

Attention	Cancellation tests (number, letter, or figure)	
	Continuous Performance Test	Loong 1988; Rosvold and Mirsky 1956
	Digit Span (Wechsler Adult Intelligence Scale–III and WMS-III)	Wechsler 1997a, 1997b
	Stroop Color and Word Test	Golden 1978
	Trail Making Test	Reitan and Wolfson 1985
	Spatial Span (WMS-III)	Wechsler 1997b
Memory	California Verbal Learning Test–II	Delis et al. 2000
	Hopkins Verbal Learning Test	Brandt 1991
	Rey Auditory-Verbal Learning Test	Rey 1964
	Rey-Osterrieth Complex Figure	Meyers and Meyers 1995; Osterrieth 1944
	WMS-III	Wechsler 1997b
Executive functions	Category Test	Reitan and Wolfson 1985
	Delis-Kaplan Executive Function System	Delis et al. 2001
	Executive Control Battery	Goldberg et al. 2000
	Stroop Color and Word Test	Golden 1978
	Tower of London	Shallice 1982
	Trail Making Test	Reitan and Wolfson 1985
	Wisconsin Card Sorting Test	Berg 1948; Heaton 1981
Language	Boston Diagnostic Aphasia Examination	Goodglass and Kaplan 1972
	Multilingual Aphasia Examination	Benton and Hamsher 1978
	Reitan-Indiana Aphasia Screening Test	Reitan and Wolfson 1985
	Wepman Auditory Discrimination Test	Wepman and Jones 1961
Visuospatial and visuomotor processes	The Revised Visual Retention Test, 4th Edition	Benton 1974
	Facial Recognition Test	Benton et al. 1983
	Judgment of Line Orientation	Benton et al. 1983
	Rey-Osterrieth Complex Figure (copy)	Osterrieth 1944
	Visual Form Discrimination Test	Benton et al. 1983
Motor processes	Finger Oscillation Test	Reitan and Wolfson 1985
	Grip Strength Test	Reitan and Wolfson 1985
	Grooved Pegboard Test	Matthews and Kløve 1964
	Purdue Pegboard Test	Purdue Research Foundation 1948

Note. WMS-III=Wechsler Memory Scale–III.

need to reassess attention to determine the effect of exhaustion on test performance.

Attention is not a unitary phenomenon; it is a multifactorial and complex cognitive activity. Attentional processes can be impaired in patients with delirium or dementing disorders but may also be significantly impaired in geriatric patients with depression and in patients with focal brain lesions. For the purposes of the clinical evaluation of the geriatric patient, it is useful to evaluate both verbal and nonverbal aspects of attention, because these components of attention can be variably impaired depending on the etiology of the neuropsychological impairment.

Auditory attentional processes are most readily assessed by the use of span procedures. The Wechsler Memory Scale—Third Edition (WMS-III; Wechsler 1997b) has span procedures that are both auditorily and visually based. The verbally based procedure, called Digit Span, asks the patient to repeat auditorily presented strings of numbers of increasing length in both forward and backward order. The nonverbal, spatially analogous version, called Spatial Span, requires the patient to repeat the tapping order of progressively longer sequences of colored boxes attached to a board after watching the test administrator do so. Again, the patient's ability to perform this task in both forward and backward order is evaluated. Letter and number cancellation tasks (Talland and Schwab 1964) can be used to assess visual attentional processes and require the patient to cross off designated stimuli on a sheet of paper within a short period of time. Visual cancellation tests are particularly useful for patients with hearing loss but are contraindicated in patients with decreased visual acuity. Several other techniques can be used to assess attention in elderly patients, such as cancellation tasks, the Stroop Color and Word Test (Golden 1978), or Trail Making Test Part A. With other domains, however, the examiner must be certain that the geriatric patient's visual and auditory acuity are intact and do not account for any poor performance. In our clinic we often do brief visual acuity and hearing assessment prior to testing and/or use enlarged stimuli or provide hearing amplifiers to help conduct our evaluations.

Once the patient's ability to focus and sustain attention has been evaluated, the patient's level of cognitive functioning in other domains can be evaluated. If the patient's ability to attend is judged to be severely impaired, further neuropsychological assessment beyond a brief cognitive screen may not be useful.

Intellectual Processes

Intellectual processes are differentially affected by the aging process and by dementing disorders. Overlearned crystallized intellectual functions (Cattell 1963), such as fund of general information and vocabulary development, are often preserved, whereas the ability to use abstract reasoning and cognitive flexibility (fluid intelligence) usually declines both with normal aging and with disease-associated processes. Complete batteries of intellectual abilities, such as the Wechsler Adult Intelligence Scale—Third Edition (WAIS-III; Wechsler 1997a), are the most commonly used tests of general intelligence but can take more than 1–2 hours to administer to an elderly patient, making this testing impractical in many cases. When the complete administration of these batteries is not possible because of lack of time, limitations in the patient's stamina, or severity of cognitive impairment, the administration of selected subtests can be useful. In particular, measures of vocabulary and general knowledge (e.g., the Vocabulary and Information subtests on WAIS-III) are relatively good indicators of the patient's premorbid level of functioning. The Wechsler Abbreviated Scale of Intelligence (Psychological Corporation 1999) is a two- or four-subtest version of the WAIS-III with normative data extending into the eighth decade. Also, reading recognition measures are resistant to dementia and are commonly used as measures of lifelong level of abilities.

Memory

The evaluation of memory represents an extremely critical component of the neuropsychological assessment of the geriatric patient and yields important diagnostic information. The patient's performance can help discriminate the effects of brain impairment from normal aging and can also help in the differential diagnosis of pseudodementia and various dementia types. For example, one dissociation of memory performance includes the difference between impaired free recall and recognition of recent information versus impaired free recall but relatively preserved recognition of recent information. Impaired free recall and recognition performance may be classified as a "pure amnesia" with concomitant dysfunction of encoding and storage. This type of memory loss is typically associated with medial-temporal lobe damage, particularly to the hippocampus, and is characteristic of Alzheimer's disease. Impaired free recall with relatively preserved recognition performance suggests a retrieval deficit consistent with dysfunction of the frontal-subcortical circuitry and is characteristic of subcortical dementias (Cummings 1992; Delis et al. 1991). However, some evidence shows that after controlling for dementia severity, there may not be any difference in memory performance between patients with Alzheimer's disease and those with multi-infarct dementia (La Rue 1989).

Both verbal and visuospatial memory should be assessed and may have relevance for the localization of brain dysfunction to the left hemisphere (verbal memory) or right hemisphere (visuospatial memory). Verbal memory processes are most often assessed through the use of word lists that are presented a specified number of times or through the presentation of brief "stories" that the patient is asked to recall at some later time (e.g., immediately after presentation and after a 30-minute delay, as in the WMS-III). The Rey Auditory-Verbal Learning Test (Rey 1964) and the California Verbal Learning Test—Second Edition (Delis et al. 2000) are commonly used list-learning tasks, although these tests are challenging because of the length of the lists (15 and 16 words, respectively) and the five required repetitions of the lists. These tests may be too difficult for geriatric patients who have more than a mild level of dementia or who have reduced stamina. The Hopkins Verbal Learning Test (Benedict et al. 1998; Brandt 1991) and the Short Form of the California Verbal Learning Test—Second Edition (Delis et al. 2000) may be preferable because they use shorter word lists and, in the case of the Hopkins Verbal Learning Test, fewer repetitions.

Evaluation of the patient's ability to learn and remember abstract spatial information is also an important component of the neuropsychological assessment process, and disruption of spatial memory relative to other test results may suggest right hemisphere dysfunction. Testing most often involves the reproduction and subsequent recall of abstract designs, such as in the Visual Reproduction subtest from the WMS-III; the Rey-Osterrieth Complex Figure (Osterrieth 1944), which is prone to floor effects with the elderly population; and the Brief Visuospatial Memory Test—Revised (Benedict 1997). The latter test is unique among published visuospatial memory tests in that it has multiple trials and thus allows study of the subject's visuospatial learning and comparison with the subject's learning curve on a verbal word list–learning test.

In the evaluation of spatial memory, it is particularly important to dissociate the patient's ability to reproduce the designs (constructional disturbance) from memory, per se. One way of conveniently accomplishing this is by asking the patient to copy the design before the memory component of the evaluation is completed, such as in the administration of the Rey-Osterrieth Complex Figure. Figure 5–1 provides an example of severe constructional disturbance in a 77-year-old patient with suspected Alzheimer's disease. In addition, other assessment procedures such as the Benton Visual Retention Test—Fifth Edition (Benton 1992) and the Brief Visuospatial Memory Test—Revised allow separation of constructional disturbance from impairment of spatial memory by providing separate normative data for the reproduction (i.e., copy) and retention of figural information. Finally, nonverbal memory can be assessed by using a recognition paradigm. In this type of test, the subject is exposed to a series of geometric stimuli. This is followed by a long series of geometric designs. Although some designs repeat those shown initially, most are new (i.e., are not part of the initial stimuli shown to the subject). The subject is asked to say "yes" if the stimulus looks familiar and "no" if it does not. This type of paradigm has absolutely no graphomotor component, but it also has no free recall component (Paolo et al. 1998).

Remote memory, also referred to as tertiary memory, refers to the recall of events that occurred during the early years of one's life (La Rue 1992). Interestingly, older adults typically report the ability to recall events from remote memory (e.g., names of grade school teachers) while complaining of anterograde memory loss for recent events (e.g., what they had for lunch that day). Traditional measures of remote memory include the Famous Faces Test and Famous Events Test (see Lezak 2004), which assess the individual's ability to recall famous faces or events during different decades of the twentieth century. In addition, from a qualitative perspective, the clinician can ask the geriatric patient various autobiographical questions that can be verified by a significant other. It is important to sample a wide range of questions that span decades in order to assess for a temporal gradient found in retrograde amnesias.

As found with measures of new learning (e.g., word list learning), performance on tests of remote memory can differentiate between cortical (e.g., Alzheimer's disease) and subcortical (e.g., Huntington's disease) dementias. The former tends to show the typical temporal gradient in recall of past events (better recall of older events), whereas the latter tends to show equal impairment across decades. A similar explanation of poor consolidation (cortical) versus retrieval (subcortical) has been proposed (see Salmon and Bondi 1997). The assessment of remote memory is difficult because the examiner is usually uncertain about the amount of the subject's initial exposure to the stimuli or subsequent rehearsal of this information (Craik 1977). In other words, what may appear as remote memory failure in a given patient may actually be a lack of exposure to the event in question or even possibly an anterograde amnesia that developed at an earlier time. Research documents significant age differences in a comparison of remote memory (public events) between young middle-aged and older adults (Howes and Katz 1988). Specifically, the elderly group demonstrated significantly poorer performance in recall of remote events during the time periods when both groups had lived. However, the elderly group demonstrated consistent recall across the five decades.

The issue of whether older subjects demonstrate consistent recall across decades remains a controversial issue (Squire 1974; Warrington and Sanders 1971). Overall, remote memory appears to be affected by age, but this finding should continue to be interpreted with caution because methodological differences remain across studies (La Rue 1992).

In summary, assessment of memory in the geriatric patient should be thorough, encompassing aspects of learning, retention, and recognition as well as remote memory. This is important because it aids in differential diagnosis and because various components of memory differentially decline with age (see Lezak 2004).

Executive Functioning

Along with memory, executive control skills show significant decline with normal aging (Libon et al. 1994; see La Rue 1992). In fact, some investigators have postulated that the cognitive changes in normal aging are most pronounced in executive control functioning (Mittenberg et al. 1989), which is due to greater cortical (Terry et al. 1987) and neurotransmitter (Carlsson 1981; Goldman-Rakic and Brown 1981) loss in the frontal lobe, as well as a greater decline in metabolic activity (Shaw et al. 1984; Smith 1984). Thus, age-appropriate normative data on measures of executive control are highly relevant to an older population (Mahurin et al. 1993) to account

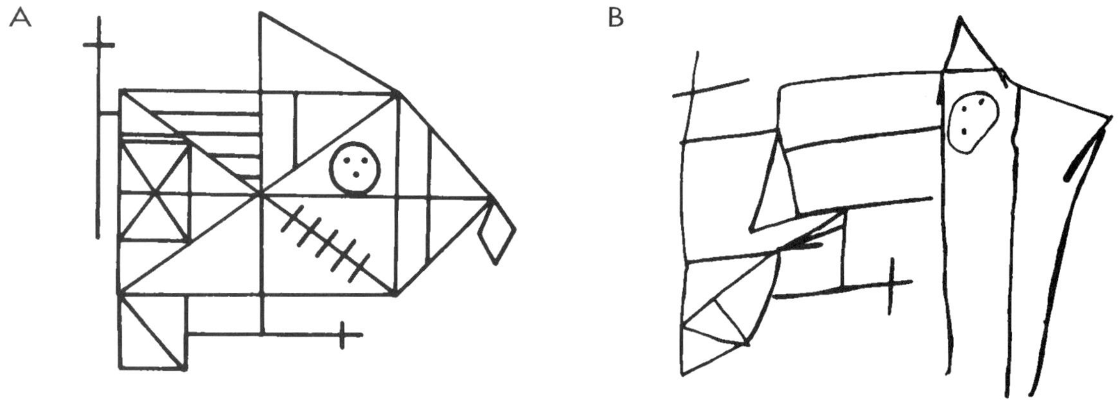

FIGURE 5–1. Rey-Osterrieth Complex Figure (Panel A; Osterrieth 1944) and reproduction of this figure by a 77-year-old man with suspected Alzheimer's disease (Panel B).

The patient's copy of the figure demonstrates severe impairment of visuoconstructional processes often associated with parietal lobe damage.

for the general decline seen on these tests and suggest that simply "renorming" an existing test of executive control may be somewhat problematic. Renorming the test for older patients who are known to decline on that measure increases the chance of that test's having poor psychometric properties for the older population. For example, the Wisconsin Card Sorting Test (Heaton et al. 1993) is used to assess executive control skills; however, it is particularly prone to floor effects in older populations and thus loses its clinical utility (i.e., sensitivity).

Executive control functioning is a constellation of multicompartmental cognitive skills that encompasses mental planning and organization, novel problem solving (e.g., cognitive flexibility), set development and shifting, and error monitoring. These components can be assessed individually or in combination. The Wisconsin Card Sorting Test is used to assess cognitive flexibility (e.g., novel problem solving) and set shifting. However, as mentioned previously, it may have poor clinical utility in older patients. Tests such as Trail Making Test Part B can be used to assess sequencing and visual search skills, although these skills also decline sharply with advancing age.

Two additional measures of executive control functioning that are showing promising results in the clinical assessment of elderly patients are the Executive Control Battery (ECB; Goldberg et al. 2000; Podell 2009) and Cognitive Bias Test (Goldberg et al. 1994). The ECB was designed to quantify the qualitative features of executive dyscontrol as developed by A.R. Luria and E. Goldberg. The ECB consists of four relatively simple subtests: Competing Programs, Manual Postures, Graphical Sequences, and Motor Programming. The subtests are quick and easy to administer and can be given individually. The battery measures perseveration, field dependency, impulsivity, and sequencing errors. The battery is sensitive to prefrontal lesions (Podell et al. 1992a, 1992b; Zimmerman et al. 1994), the decline in executive control associated with advanced normal aging (Libon et al. 1994), and the differential effects of Alzheimer's versus cerebrovascular dementia on graphomotor perseverations (Lamar et al. 1997). See Figure 5–2 for examples of graphomotor perseverations elicited on the ECB Graphical Sequences subtest.

The Cognitive Bias Test is an innovative computerized test that assesses the subject's response preference along a continuum of context-dependent/independent responding. For example, after being presented with a stimulus, does the subject use it as a context for which to make a subsequent judgment (context dependent), or does the subject make all choices independent of any context (i.e., context independent)? Performance on the Cognitive Bias Test is sensitive to prefrontal functions with laterality and sexual dimorphic effects (Goldberg et al. 1994; Podell et al. 1995). Research in an elderly population has shown this test's sensitivity to the disease progression in Alzheimer's disease (Goldberg et al. 1997).

Visuospatial and Visuoconstructive Processes

Just as it is important to separate disorders of visual memory from difficulties secondary to impairment of constructional processes, it is also necessary to separate disorders of visuospatial analysis from those of visuoconstructive processes. This dissociation can have localizing value, aid in differential diagnosis, and address functional abilities. The separation of these different, but related, neuropsychological processes can be most effectively accomplished by comparing the results of constructional tasks such as Block Design from WAIS-III or copying of the Rey-Osterrieth Complex Figure to performance on motor-free spatial tasks such as the Visual Form Discrimina-

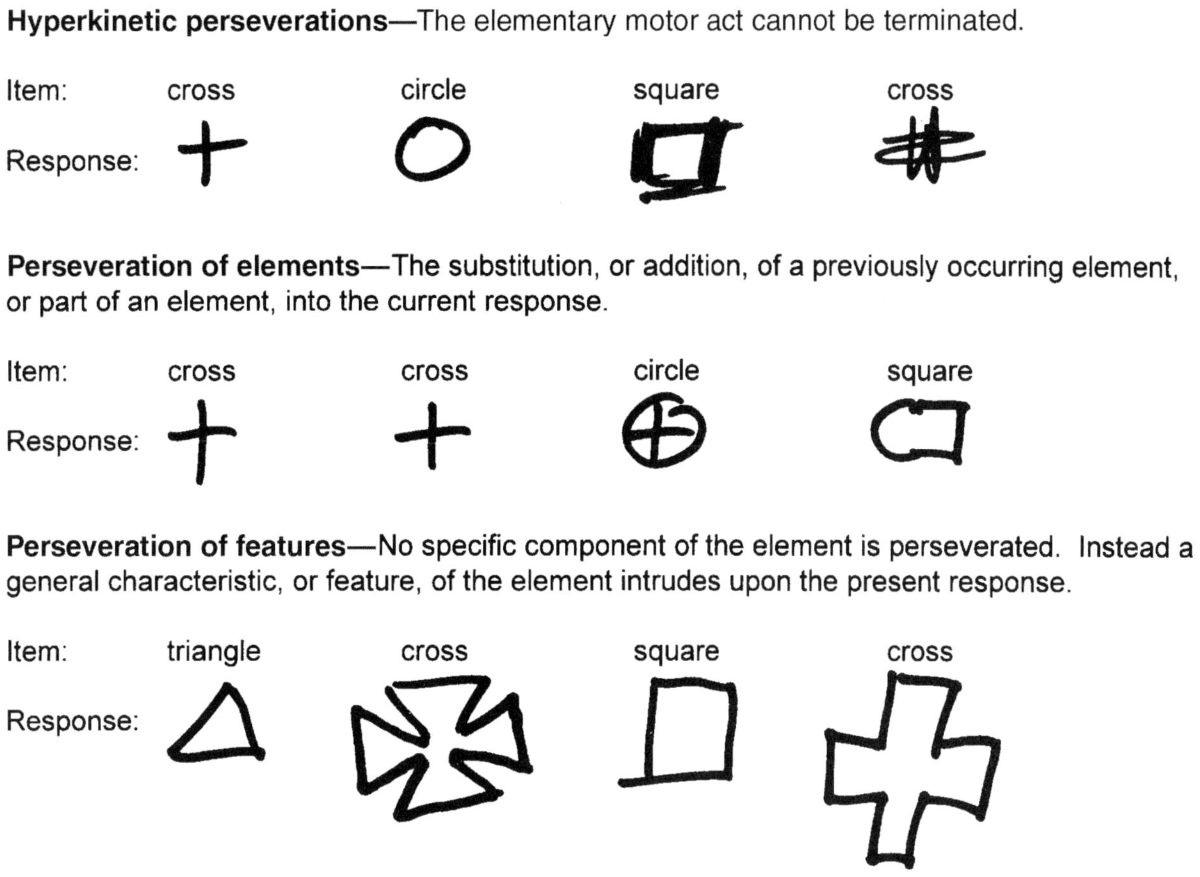
Hyperkinetic perseverations—The elementary motor act cannot be terminated.
Item: cross circle square cross
Response:
Perseveration of elements—The substitution, or addition, of a previously occurring element, or part of an element, into the current response.
Item: cross cross circle square
Response:
Perseveration of features—No specific component of the element is perseverated. Instead a general characteristic, or feature, of the element intrudes upon the present response.
Item: triangle cross square cross
Response:

FIGURE 5–2. Types of graphomotor perseverations from the Graphical Sequences subtest of the Executive Control Battery (Goldberg et al. 2000).

tion Test, Judgment of Line Orientation Test, and Facial Recognition Test developed by Benton et al. (1983). Poor performance in copying on the Rey-Osterrieth Complex Figure, for example, with better performance on motor-free tests, suggests a constructional rather than visuospatial disorder (see Figure 5–1). A Clock Drawing Test (command and copy trials) is useful in distinguishing among visuospatial, constructional, and executive control (planning) components in geriatric patients with moderate impairment. This test is relatively quick and easy to administer and has been extensively studied in patients with dementia (Freedman et al. 1994).

One caveat we would like to add concerns the issue of primary vision and assessment of visuospatial and constructional abilities. The examiner must be aware of, and sensitive to, the patient's primary visual acuity (e.g., effects from glaucoma, cataracts, and macular degeneration). We recommend a cursory visual acuity check (e.g., using a Snellen eye chart) for all geriatric patients undergoing any neuropsychological testing using visual stimuli. The examiner must consider the utility of administering these tasks, or the need for using enlarged stimuli, if the patient's primary visual acuity is poor.

Speech and Language

Clinical evaluation of speech and language processes is another necessary component in the neuropsychological evaluation of geriatric patients. Language processes in elderly individuals can be affected by the normal aging process (Albert and Moss 1988), depression (Speedie et al. 1990), and dementia (Hill et al. 1989), and a thorough evaluation of language can help differentiate these disorders clinically. In particular, disorders of object naming (tested by presenting the patient with pictures of common objects) are associated with dementing illness (Albert 1981; Hill et al. 1989) and, to a lesser degree, with cognitive impairment secondary to depression (Speedie et al. 1990).

Other aspects of language should also be assessed during the neuropsychological evaluation, including comprehension and verbal fluency, as well as reading and writing. Verbal fluency can be easily assessed via the Animal Naming subtest of the Boston Diagnostic Aphasia Examination (Goodglass and Kaplan 1972) and the Controlled Oral Word Association Test (Benton and Hamsher 1978) or the Verbal Fluency Test from the Delis-Kaplan Executive Function System (Delis et al. 2001). Comparison between the two fluency tasks can distinguish between a primary deficit in lexical-semantic accessing and an impairment in executive control functioning. For example, impaired performance on novel fluency (e.g., a specific letter) but intact semantic fluency indicates executive dyscontrol (e.g., poor novel generation). The converse, intact fluency for a novel cue but impaired animal naming, is indicative of impaired lexical-semantic accessing skills.

Motor Processes and Psychomotor Speed

Although motor speed and coordination decrease with normal aging, impairment of motor processes may signal underlying neuropathological processes. Decreased motor strength or speed can suggest a lateralized brain lesion, such as a stroke, tumor, or metastasis, or may occur as part of a dementing disorder. In addition, a disruption in the ability to produce complex motor acts (e.g., dressing and eating) may represent an apraxia and may point to dysfunction of specific brain systems. Finally, evidence indicates that tests of impairments in fine and complex motor skills are almost as sensitive as other cognitive measures in differentiating between healthy normal aging and the mild, early stages of dementia (Kluger et al. 1997). Peripheral, or non–central nervous system, diseases such as gout, arthritis, or peripheral neuropathies all affect motor performance and, if not taken into consideration, can lead to erroneous and incorrect interpretations.

Motor speed is most commonly evaluated through the use of the Finger Oscillation (Finger Tapping) Test from the HRNB (Reitan and Wolfson 1985), Grooved Pegboard Test (Matthews and Kløve 1964), or Purdue Pegboard Test (Purdue Research Foundation 1948). In general, better performance is expected of the dominant (usually right) hand relative to the nondominant hand, and the reversal of this pattern can help to localize a brain lesion to the contralateral hemisphere. The cautions concerning the use of age-appropriate norms are particularly germane to a discussion of the evaluation of motor processes. Comparison of an elderly patient's performance on a motor task to that of a younger normative group will result in spurious and misleading information. Finally, the examiner must be attuned to the contribution of peripheral factors on motor performance.

Daily Functional Abilities

Direct assessment of functional abilities (i.e., instrumental activities of daily living) has become increasingly more important in neuropsychological test batteries. Some clinicians advocate the assessment of functional capacity by using instruments specifically designed for this purpose (La Rue and Swanda 1997). Additionally, such instruments play an important role in determining cognitive capacity for addressing legal competency, which is a frequent referral question in neuropsychological assessments of older adults (Grisso 1994).

Functional abilities can be assessed through direct evaluation of the patient or through individual or collateral interviews or questionnaires, such as the Instrumental Activities of Daily Living Scale (Lawton and Brody 1969) and the Blessed Dementia Rating Scale (Blessed et al. 1968). Evidence indicates that individual or collateral reports do not correlate well with actual performance (see Grisso 1994). Having a patient actually perform the given tasks or the requisite skills needed for the task is a more accurate and valid assessment of his or her functional abilities.

In our clinic, we incorporate the direct assessment of functional abilities as part of our standard geriatric assessment. Specifically, we have used the Independent Living Scales (ILS; Loeb 1996). Through a series of verbal responses and actual task completion (e.g., writing a check, using a telephone), the ILS assesses several different areas—Memory/Orientation, Managing Money, Managing Home and Transportation, Health and Safety, and Social Adjustment—vital to independent functioning and competency. The instrument is well normed and has been extensively validated on several different populations. In fact, data from our clinic (Baird 2006; Baird et al. 2001) have shown a strong relationship between performance on the ILS and level of dementia as assessed on the Dementia Rating Scale.

Use of Neuropsychological Testing in Differential Diagnosis

As highlighted throughout this chapter, geriatric patients are at risk for a number of neuropathological disorders that affect cognitive functioning, which are often difficult to distinguish clinically. Although the neuropsychological evaluation can often be helpful in the differential diagnosis of neurological disorders, we emphasize that the results of neuropsychological testing should not be interpreted "in a vacuum," but should be integrated with other diagnostic information gathered within the broader context of the neuropsychiatric evaluation. Data should be obtained from a thorough medical, social, and psychiatric history; mental status examination; appropriate neuroimaging technologies; and appropriate laboratory studies. With these guidelines in mind, we briefly review the use of neuropsychological testing in the differential diagnostic process. (For a more detailed review, see La Rue 1992.)

Dementia

Dementing disorders are not a homogeneous group of conditions; they vary greatly with regard to etiology, neurological substrate, disease course, and treatment (see Chapter 16, "Alzheimer's Disease and the Frontotemporal Dementia Syndromes"). Therefore, the neuropsychological profiles (Table

5–4) and distinguishing behavioral features (Table 5–5) differ depending on the dementia type.

One of the more recent developments in the differential diagnosis of dementia is a newer classification of individuals who do not conform to a formal diagnosis of dementia (i.e., impairment in one or more cognitive domains affecting daily functioning) but who have circumscribed neuropsychological deficits greater than what can be expected for their age and background (i.e., −1.5 standard deviations) yet still have preserved daily functioning. This classification has been termed *mild cognitive impairment* (see Gauthier et al. 2006 for a comprehensive review; Petersen et al. 1999). There are various forms of mild cognitive impairment depending on the neuropsychological processes impaired, with the amnestic variant considered a precursor to dementia of the Alzheimer's type. However, there is debate whether all individuals diagnosed with mild cognitive impairment develop dementia.

The neuropsychological profile of *dementia of the Alzheimer's type* (see Bondi et al. 2008) is most often characterized by impairment of memory, executive control, visuospatial processes, intellectual processes, complex motor skills, and language, although impairment in all of these areas may not be present in every patient, particularly early in the disease. Memory impairment is usually the first sign of the disorder, although detailed neuropsychological evaluation may reveal subtle deficits in other areas (e.g., executive functioning). Dysnomia, decreased verbal fluency, and poor semantic processing are also common, even early in the disease process. The memory impairment is characterized by a relatively spared span of apprehension (as measured by the Digit Span procedure) but marked impairment in the retention of newly learned material. Intrusive errors (i.e., the inclusion of extraneous items, usually semantically related) are common both on list-learning (Delis et al. 1991) and story recall tasks.

Early in Alzheimer's disease, often subtle impairment of memory, mental flexibility, and executive functioning may be viewed by the patient (and by his or her family) as being part of the normal aging process. Language (word-finding) problems and visuospatial impairment may be evident in the patient's drawings and may range from mild distortions of designs to a complete inability to reproduce even simple two-dimensional copies. At later stages in the disease, more severe impairment of intellectual processes is observed, and agnosia and apraxia are often seen. Severe visuospatial impairment may take the form of an inability to tell time on an analogue clock or of spatial disorientation. This problem can become so severe that the patient is unable to find his or her room consistently. The memory and executive control deficits worsen. Personality and affective changes are common, especially in the later stages. Sundowning is often associated with Alzheimer's disease in the middle to late stages of the disease.

The term *frontotemporal dementia* is used to describe a number of disorders (e.g., Pick's disease, progressive subcortical gliosis, primary progressive aphasia, and what was previously referred to as dementia of the frontal lobe type) that primarily affect the prefrontal and anterior temporal regions (including hippocampi) of the brain. Frontotemporal dementia, which often develops before age 65 (often in the mid-40s or 50s), is most often characterized by a marked insidious personality change and impairment of executive functioning affecting all aspects of cognition (Cummings 1992; Moss et al. 1992). Although memory impairments can be present, they are usually associated with a preponderance of an executive control impairment (e.g., poor retrieval).

Unlike dementia of the Alzheimer's type, the first signs of frontotemporal dementia are usually neuropsychiatric rather than cognitive in nature. Personality changes can be characterized by two distinct behavioral syndromes: the dorsolateral syndrome, marked by apathy and behavioral inertia, or the orbitofrontal syndrome, marked by hypomanic-like, puerile, sometimes irritable disinhibition (Fuster 1989). Executive functioning impairment takes the form of perseveration, abulia (i.e., lack of initiation, stimulus boundedness (i.e., field dependency), impaired synthesis and planning, and poor error monitoring. In contrast to those with dementia of the Alzheimer's type, patients with frontotemporal dementia often have preserved visuospatial abilities and relatively better preserved memory functions, at least in the earlier parts of the disease (Neary and Snowden 1991). Although basic motor processes are usually intact, executive processes that involve a significant motor component are typically impaired. Language comprehension and expression are typically preserved, but echolalia and a progressive expressive aphasia can develop. The neuropsychiatric and cognitive difficulties seen in frontotemporal dementia can become so severe as to limit the patient's ability to complete a comprehensive evaluation. Short bedside procedures are often useful and should be part of the mental status examination.

Vascular dementia refers to a group of dementing disorders of a cerebrovascular nature consisting of an abrupt onset with a stepwise decline over time. Vascular dementia is characterized by "patchy" performance on neuropsychological measures with islands of preserved and impaired performance, depending on the site of the infarct(s) or ischemia. As the disease progresses, a stepwise decline in cognitive functioning is typically observed and can be documented through serial neuropsychological evaluations. Left hemisphere lesions often result in language and verbal memory impairment, whereas right hemisphere lesions result in greater impairment of visuospatial processes and visual memory. Small infarcts that do not affect motor or speech areas may go unnoticed by the patient or family but can be documented through neuroimaging and neuropsychological evaluation.

TABLE 5–4. Description and common characteristics of dementia types

Syndrome	Initial complaints	Neuropsychological profile	First to notice changes
Depression	Memory problems, poor focus	Fluctuating attention, slow learning curve, retrieval memory deficit with intact retention and recognition, fluctuating executive functioning, psychomotor slowing	Patient
Alzheimer's dementia	Repetition, forgetfulness, confusion	Slowly progressive anterograde memory deficit with poor learning, retention, and recognition; impaired naming, semantic fluency, and executive deficits; visuospatial processing deficits and apraxia, aphasia, and agnosia in advanced illness; functional decline	Patient/family
Frontotemporal dementia	Personality/behavioral change	Executive functioning deficits (perseveration, impulsivity, impaired planning, stimulus boundedness, impaired mental flexibility, impaired synthesis), impaired selective attention, relatively preserved memory in earlier stages	Family
Dementia with Lewy bodies	Good and bad days, confusion, delusions, hallucinations, parasomnias	Progressive insidious cognitive decline with pronounced attentional fluctuations and executive deficits; marked visuoperceptual errors; retrieval memory deficit initially followed by poor retention; autonomic dysfunction and falls; motor skills marked by parkinsonism; vivid, detailed visual hallucinations	Patient/family
Parkinson's dementia	Poor initiation, slowed thinking, perceptual problems	Fluctuating attention, intact learning curve, retrieval memory deficit with poor retention and intact recognition, mildly impaired naming, slow processing speed, visuospatial processing deficits, executive dysfunction, psychomotor slowing	Family

The *subcortical dementias* are a group of disorders that are characterized by primary dysfunction in subcortical brain areas. Unlike dementing conditions that primarily affect cortical areas, leading to aphasia, apraxia, agnosia, and anomia, subcortical dementia features motor dysfunction; speech impairment; memory dysfunction, characterized primarily by deficits in retrieval (Delis et al. 1991); executive disorders; and disturbances in mood and personality (Cummings 1985). Subcortical dementia occurs with extrapyramidal syndromes such as Parkinson's disease, Wilson's disease, progressive supranuclear palsy, multisystem atrophy, and Huntington's disease. Although a general decline in intellectual processes often occurs over time, this decline is usually much less severe than in other dementing disorders. Performance on neuropsychological testing varies across patients with Parkinson's disease, but deficits are often found on tests that require psychomotor speed, visuospatial processing, executive functioning, and memory (Pirozzolo et al. 1982). In addition, performance may be impaired on tests that measure concept formation and problem solving in new situations (Matthews and Haaland 1979), category fluency, and mental flexibility (Beatty et al. 1989).

Patients with Huntington's disease often exhibit executive functioning impairment that involves difficulty with mental flexibility and abstraction but with relatively preserved "overlearned" verbal skills (i.e., on the WAIS-III Information and Vocabulary subtests). Memory impairment also commonly occurs in patients with Huntington's disease and is characterized by impairment in the acquisition and retrieval of new information, as well as by impaired remote memory later in the disease process (Albert et al. 1981). In contrast with patients with Alzheimer's disease, who are characterized by dysnomia, patients with Huntington's disease can exhibit normal performance on confrontation naming tests (Butters et al. 1978).

Dementia with Lewy bodies (DLB) is a progressive, degenerative dementia that is often overlooked when making a differential diagnosis of dementia type, but one that has important implications for appropriate treatment (McKeith et al. 2005) and is now considered the second most common cortical

TABLE 5–5. Distinguishing manifestations of the dementias

Mood/behavior	AD: depression, anxiety, apathy DEP: vegetative symptoms FTD: marked personality/behavior changes, unawareness, disinhibition, apathy, fixations and compulsions, emotional blunting, poor hygiene, impulsivity DLB and PD: depression greater than in AD and may present before motor symptoms, apathy, impulsive/compulsive behavior from medication side effects in PD
Eating	AD: preference for salty and sweet foods DEP: increase or decrease in appetite FTD: specific food preferences, overeating DLB and PD: difficulties swallowing
Hallucinations/delusions	AD: hallucinations and delusions in advanced illness DEP: can be present in severe cases FTD: rare DLB: visual hallucinations early (often people and animals) PD: visual hallucinations late or related to medication side effects
Sleep	AD: disrupted circadian rhythms DEP: hypersomnia or insomnia FTD: disrupted circadian rhythms DLB and PD: parasomnias
Other	AD: motor skills mostly preserved, decreased smell/taste DEP: decreased libido, psychomotor retardation FTD: frontal release signs, slow eye movements, incontinence, increased interest in sex DLB: autonomic dysfunction, neuroleptic medication sensitivity, poor saccadic pursuit, bradyphrenia and bradykinesia. Cognitive difficulties develop before motor symptoms (within 1 year). PD: autonomic dysfunction in advanced illness, neuroleptic medication sensitivity, saccadic pursuit, cognitive difficulties develop at least 1 year after motor symptoms

Note. AD=Alzheimer's dementia; DEP=depression; FTD=frontotemporal dementia; DLB=dementia with Lewy bodies; PD=Parkinson's dementia.

dementia. As many as 20%–50% of patients undergoing autopsy may have diffuse or focal Lewy bodies present in the brain stem and cerebral cortex (see Lippa et al. 2007). The central cognitive features include progressive, insidious cognitive decline in executive control, attention, and visuospatial skills (memory deficits may not be evident early in the disease course but will progress over time). Other core features include fluctuations in arousal and alertness, parkinsonism, and visual hallucinations that are typically well formed and detailed (often in color and of animals or people—often tiny). Supportive features of DLB include rapid eye movement (REM) sleep disorders, severe neuroleptic sensitivity, syncope, falls, and severe autonomic dysfunction. Elderly patients who present with recent onset of a fixed delusional system with visual hallucinations should be considered for a diagnosis of DLB, and the use of a neuroleptic should be carefully considered (see McKeith et al. 2005). In fact, DLB, Parkinson's disease, and Parkinson's disease with dementia are all considered to fall under the "Lewy body disorder" umbrella as being the differential expression of an α-synuclein disorder (Lippa et al. 2007).

Depression-Related Cognitive Dysfunction

Of patients with depression, 10%–20% are estimated to have significant cognitive impairment (Reynolds and Hoch 1988) (see Chapter 19, "Mood Disorders"). In addition, depression frequently accompanies neurological disorders such as Alzheimer's disease (Kaszniak 1987), stroke (Robinson and Price 1982), and extrapyramidal diseases such as Parkinson's and Huntington's diseases (Cummings 1985). The labels *pseudodementia* (Kiloh 1961), *dementia syndrome of depression* (Folstein and McHugh 1978), *depression-induced organic mental disorder* (McAllister 1983), and *depression-related cognitive dysfunction* (Stoudemire et al. 1989) have been used to describe the reversible cognitive impairment in elderly patients with depression. Since Kiloh's (1961) initial characterization of pseudodementia, numerous articles have described the clinical features of cognitive impairment secondary to depression and its differentiation from progressive and irreversible conditions such as Alzheimer's disease (Bulbena and Berrios 1986; Cummings 1989; Jeste et al. 1990; Kaszniak 1987; for reviews, see Christensen et al. 1997 and Veiel 1997). Although the concept of depression-related cognitive impairment is well accepted and has had value in identifying potentially treatable forms of dementia, the term *pseudodementia* has come under criticism (Arie 1983; Lamberty and Bieliauskas 1993; Langenecker et al. 2009; Reifler 1982; Shraberg 1978, 1980). These criticisms have stemmed primarily from the implication that cognitive dysfunction secondary to depression does not represent a "real" or "organic" phenomenon. Additional criticisms have been based on the lack of diagnostic specificity of the term and from the lack of utility of the concept in predicting response to treatment.

Understanding of the complexity of cognitive dysfunction in elderly patients with depression has increased substantially since the 1990s, and an increasing number of systematic studies have been designed to assist in the separation of the potentially reversible (and treatable) dementia of depression from irreversible and often progressive conditions such as Alzheimer's disease and vascular dementia. Although no universally accepted neuropsychological template exists for the differentiation of depression-related cognitive dysfunction from cognitive impairment secondary to specific brain disease, research has suggested that neuropsychological test results may be useful in this regard. For example, several studies have pointed to the usefulness of confrontation naming tests, such as the Boston Naming Test (Kaplan et al. 1983), in the differential diagnostic process (Caine 1981; Hill et al. 1989; Petrick and Mittenberg 1992), although not all researchers have found this result (Speedie et al. 1990). Others have recommended that detailed historical information and behavioral features, along with qualitative aspects of neuropsychological performance, are helpful in making a differential diagnosis (Kaszniak and Christenson 1994). Further complicating the issue is research suggesting that depression might represent an early marker for later development of a progressive dementia (Kral and Emery 1989; Nussbaum et al. 1991; Reding et al. 1985). In fact, Bieliauskas (1993) has shown that more often the initial onset of depression in later life is associated with a neurological change than with primary depression and that new-onset depression in later life may be a harbinger to future cognitive decline (proportionate to severity of depression). The severity of depression does not clearly relate to the severity of neuropsychological impairment (across studies), although the expected trend—positive correlation—appears to be present (see Langenecker et al. 2009).

Christensen et al. (1997) performed a meta-analysis of studies looking at the cognitive effects of depression. Two types of comparisons were analyzed: patients with depression versus psychiatrically healthy control subjects and patients with depression versus patients with Alzheimer's disease. Essentially, patients with depression showed impaired performance across all cognitive domains with very few intact cognitive skills. One of the greatest effect sizes was in executive control skills. However, relative to psychiatrically healthy control subjects, patients with depression were mostly impaired on speeded tasks and vigilance tasks. No difference in effect size was found when comparing free recall to recognition memory, semantic processing, or use of verbal versus nonverbal material. Patients with depression were equivalent to those with Alzheimer's disease on recall compared with recognition and on verbal compared with nonverbal processing, and depressed patients were significantly better in all other cognitive domains. The notion that the difference between depression and dementia (especially that of the Alzheimer's type) is a result of effortful (including speeded tasks) versus noneffortful tasks received some support in the meta-analysis. Thus, the finding that patients with depression are impaired only on effortful (and speeded) tasks, but that patients with dementia are impaired on both effortful and noneffortful tasks (Hartlage et al. 1993), may have important use in the differential diagnosis between depression and dementia. However, not all noneffortful tasks discriminated well. Also, the notion that recognition versus recall distinguished depression from dementia was not supported by the meta-analysis. Christensen et al. (1997) proposed the possibility that speed of processing or attentional components might distinguish depression from dementia. This was also supported by another meta-analysis that compared younger patients with depression to psychiatrically healthy control subjects (Veiel 1997). The issue of cognitive dysfunction in elderly patients with depression is a complicated one that deserves further study.

Ecological Validity of Neuropsychological Tests

Because neuropsychologists are increasingly asked to render decisions about functional capacity and competency of elderly patients, the ecological validity of standard neuropsychological tests is a central and important issue. Indeed, the utility of neuropsychological assessment lies not only in its ability to aid in the diagnostic process but also in its capacity to provide information regarding a patient's ability to function in his or her natural environment. Neuropsychological test performance and outcome measures have only a moderate relationship (Acker 1990; Chelune and Moehle 1986) but have a greater predictive accuracy for functional skills demanding complex information processing, such as writing a check, than for basic functional capacity, such as performing a personal hygiene skill (Baird et al. 1999; Goldstein et al. 1992; Loeb 1996; McCue et al. 1990; Rogers et al. 1994).

Even with the good predictive validity that neuropsychological tests have for general functional abilities, little direct evidence indicates that neuropsychological test results can predict specific functional abilities, such as driving, or appropriate residential placement (see Blaustein et al. 1988; Kaszniak and Nussbaum 1990). Unfortunately, relatively few empirical data exist to support the predictive validity of neuropsychological test performance on these functional domains in older patients. The development of new neuropsychological tasks that more closely parallel activities of daily living is much needed (Zappala et al. 1989). Currently, decisions are more often based on estimates of the patient's performance on more traditional neuropsychological measures that have no direct corollary in "real life." In particular, decisions regarding the patient's ability to drive are often based on performance on visuospatial, attentional, memory, and executive functioning tasks, because these processes are generally thought to be requisite to the safe operation of an automobile. The development of ecologically valid neuropsychological tests to more directly assess the patient's ability to perform real-life activities requires continued attention and represents one of the biggest challenges for the field of geriatric neuropsychology. To this end, we see the direct assessment of functional abilities, such as by using the Independent Living Scales (Loeb 1996), as one method for trying to fill this void. We are better able to address the issues of functional capacity and level of competency by using standardized neuropsychological tests in conjunction with the direct assessment of functional abilities. Although not a perfect solution, this certainly is a step in the right direction.

Key Points

- The geriatric population has unique characteristics that influence neuropsychological assessments. Demographic factors and the variability of "normal" behavior influence interpretation of performance and affect tests' sensitivity.
- Different techniques are used in neuropsychological assessment, and it appears best to use the flexible approach, which involves selecting the individual neuropsychological tests required for the particular patient based on the patient's history, presenting problem, and needs.
- The assessment of geriatric patients presents unique challenges, and during a neuropsychological assessment, the examiner must consider sensorial acuity, fatigue, and other limitations.
- Neuropsychological deficit patterns can differentiate various dementia types. These patterns are part of a comprehensive method of determining dementia type that includes history, behavioral manifestations, and medical testing.
- Neuropsychological testing can help assess functional abilities and is critical in determining a patient's functional capacity. It is often used to determine the patient's ability to make his or her own medical and financial decisions, as well as the need for supervision and rehabilitation.

Recommended Readings

Attix DK, Welsh-Bohmer KA: Geriatric Neuropsychology: Assessment and Intervention. New York, Guilford, 2006

Bush SS, Martin TA: Geriatric Neuropsychology Practice Essentials. New York, Taylor & Francis, 2005

Mendez M, Cummings J: Dementia: A Clinical Approach, 3rd Edition. Oxford, UK, Butterworth-Heinemann, 2003

Miller BL, Boeve BL: The Behavioral Neurology of Dementia. Cambridge, UK, Cambridge University Press, 2009

References

Acker MB: A review of the ecological validity of neuropsychological tests, in The Neuropsychology of Everyday Life. Edited by Tupper DE, Cicerone KD. Boston, MA, Kluwer Academic, 1990, pp 19–55

Albert MS: Geriatric neuropsychology. J Consult Clin Psychol 49: 835–850, 1981

Albert MS, Moss MB: Geriatric Neuropsychology. New York, Guilford, 1988

Albert MS, Butters N, Brandt J: Development of remote memory loss in patients with Huntington's disease. J Clin Neuropsychol 3:1–12, 1981

Anthony WZ, Heaton RK, Lehman RAW: An attempt to cross-validate two actuarial systems for neuropsychological test interpretation. J Consult Clin Psychol 48:317–326, 1980

Arie T: Pseudodementia. BMJ 286:1301–1302, 1983

Baird AD: Fine tuning recommendations for older adults with memory complaints: using the Independent Living Scales with the Dementia Rating Scale. Clin Neuropsychol 20:649–661, 2006

Baird AD, Podell K, Lovell MR: Predicting functional status in older adults (abstract). Arch Clin Neuropsychol 14:44–45, 1999

Baird AD, Podell K, Lovell MR, et al: Complex real-world functioning and neuropsychological test performance in older adults. Clin Neuropsychol 15:369–379, 2001

Bayles KA, Tomoeda CK, Boone DR: A view of age-related changes in language function. Dev Neuropsychol 1:231–264, 1985

Beatty W, Staton RD, Weir WS, et al: Cognitive disturbances in Parkinson's disease. J Geriatr Psychiatry Neurol 2:22–23, 1989

Benedict RHB: Brief Visuospatial Memory Test—Revised. Odessa, FL, Psychological Assessment Resources, 1997

Benedict RHB, Brandt J: Limitations of the Mini-Mental State Examination for the detection of amnesia. J Geriatr Psychiatry Neurol 5:233–237, 1992

Benedict RHB, Schretlen D, Groninger L, et al: Hopkins Verbal Learning Test—Revised: normative data and analysis of interform and test-retest reliability. Clin Neuropsychol 12:43–55, 1998

Benton AL: The Revised Visual Retention Test, 4th Edition. New York, Psychological Corporation, 1974

Benton AL: Some problems associated with neuropsychological assessment. Bull Clin Neurosci 50:11–15, 1985

Benton AL: The Benton Visual Retention Test, 5th Edition. San Antonio, TX, Psychological Corporation, 1992

Benton AL, Hamsher K: Multilingual Aphasia Examination. Iowa City, University of Iowa Press, 1978

Benton AL, Hamsher K, Varney N, et al: Contributions to Neuropsychological Assessment: A Clinical Manual. New York, Oxford University Press, 1983

Berg GE: A simple objective test for measuring flexibility in thinking. J Gen Psychol 39:15–22, 1948

Bieliauskas LA: Depressed or not depressed? That is the question. J Clin Exp Neuropsychol 15:119–134, 1993

Blaustein MJL, Filipp CL, Dungan C, et al: Driving in patients with dementia. J Am Geriatr Soc 6:1087–1091, 1988

Blessed G, Tomlinson BE, Roth M: The association between quantitative measures of dementia and senile change in the cerebral gray matter of elderly subjects. Br J Psychiatry 114:797–811, 1968

Bondi M, Jak AJ, Delano-Wood L, et al: Neuropsychological contributions to the early identification of Alzheimer's disease. Neuropsychol Rev 18:17–93, 2008

Bowles NL, Poon LW: Aging and retrieval of words in semantic memory. J Gerontol 40:71–77, 1985

Brandt J: The Hopkins Verbal Learning Test: development of a new memory test with six equivalent forms. Clin Neuropsychol 5:125–142, 1991

Bulbena A, Berrios GE: Pseudodementia: facts and figures. Br J Psychiatry 148:87–94, 1986

Burke DM, Laver GD: Aging and word retrieval: selective age deficits in language, in Aging and Cognition: Mental Processes, Self-Awareness, and Interventions. Edited by Lovelace EA. Oxford, UK, North-Holland, 1990, pp 281–300

Buschke H, Kuslansky G, Katz M, et al: Screening for dementia with the Memory Impairment Screen. Neurology 52:231–238, 1999

Butters N, Sax D, Montgomery K, et al: Comparison of the neuropsychological deficits associated with early and advanced Huntington's disease. Arch Neurol 35:585–589, 1978

Cabeza R: Hemispheric asymmetry reduction in older adults: the HAROLD model. Psychol Aging 17:85–100, 2002

Caine ED: Pseudodementia: current concepts and future directions. Arch Gen Psychiatry 38:1359–1364, 1981

Carlsson A: Aging and brain neurotransmitters, in Strategies for the Development of an Effective Treatment for Senile Dementia. Edited by Crook T, Gershon S. New Canaan, CT, Mark Powley Associates, 1981, pp 93–104

Cattell RB: Theory of fluid and crystallized intelligence: a critical experiment. J Educ Psychol 54:1–22, 1963

Chelune GJ, Moehle KA: Neuropsychological assessment and everyday functioning, in The Neuropsychology Handbook: Behavioral and Clinical Perspectives. Edited by Wedding AM, Horton J, Webster J. New York, Springer, 1986, pp 489–525

Christensen H, Griffiths K, MacKinnon A: A quantitative review of cognitive deficits in depression and Alzheimer's-type dementia. J Int Neuropsychol Soc 3:631–651, 1997

Clark LJ, Gatz M, Zheng L, et al: Longitudinal verbal fluency in normal aging, preclinical, and prevalent Alzheimer's disease. Am J Alzheimers Dis Other Demen 24:461–468, 2009

Compton DM, Bachman LD, Brand D, et al: Age-associated changes in cognitive function in highly educated adults: emerging myths and realities. Int J Geriatr Psychiatry 15:75–85, 2000

Costa L: Clinical neuropsychology: a discipline in evolution. J Clin Neuropsychol 5:1–11, 1983

Craik FIM: Age differences in human memory, in Handbook of the Psychology of Aging. Edited by Birren JE, Schaie KW. New York, Van Nostrand Reinhold, 1977, pp 384–420

Cummings JL: Clinical Neuropsychiatry. Orlando, FL, Grune & Stratton, 1985

Cummings JL: Dementia and depression: an evolving enigma. J Neuropsychiatry Clin Neurosci 1:236–242, 1989

Cummings JL: Neuropsychiatric aspects of Alzheimer's disease and other dementing illnesses, in The American Psychiatric Press Textbook of Neuropsychiatry, 2nd Edition. Edited by Yudofsky SC, Hales RE. Washington, DC, American Psychiatric Press, 1992, pp 605–620

Delis DC, Massman PJ, Butters N, et al: Profiles of demented and amnesic patients on the California Verbal Learning Test: implications for the assessment of memory disorders. Psychol Assess 3:19–26, 1991

Delis D, Kramer JH, Kaplan E, et al: The California Verbal Learning Test, 2nd Edition. San Antonio, TX, Psychological Corporation, 2000

Delis, D, Kaplan E, Kramer JH: The Delis-Kaplan Executive Function System. San Antonio, TX, Pearson, 2001

Drachman DA, Leavitt J: Human memory and the cholinergic system: a relationship to aging? Arch Neurol 30:113–121, 1974

Fastenau PS: Validity of regression-based norms: an empirical test of the comprehensive norms with older adults. J Clin Exp Neuropsychol 20:906–916, 1998

Fastenau PS, Adams KM: Heaton, Grant and Matthews' Comprehensive Norms: an overzealous attempt. J Clin Exp Neuropsychol 18:444–448, 1996

Fick DM, Cooper JW, Wade WE, et al: Updating the Beers criteria for potentially inappropriate medication use in older adults: results of a U.S. consensus panel of experts. Arch Int Med 163:2716–2724, 2003

Folstein MF, Folstein SE, McHugh PR: "Mini-Mental State": a practical method for grading the cognitive state of patients for the clinician. J Psychiatr Res 12:189–198, 1975

Folstein MF, McHugh PR: Dementia syndrome of depression, in Alzheimer's Disease: Senile Dementia and Related Disorders. Edited by Katzman R, Terry RD, Bick KL. New York, Raven, 1978, pp 281–289

Freedman M, Leach L, Kaplan E, et al: Clock Drawing: A Neuropsychological Analysis. New York, Oxford University Press, 1994

Fuster JM: The Prefrontal Cortex: Anatomy, Physiology, and Neuropsychology of the Frontal Lobe, 2nd Edition. New York, Raven, 1989

Gauthier S, Reisberg B, Zaudig M, et al: International Psychogeriatric Association Expert Conference on Mild Cognitive Impairment: mild cognitive impairment. Lancet 367(9518):1262–1270, 2006

Goldberg E: The Wisdom Paradox: How Your Mind Can Grow Stronger as Your Brain Grows Older. New York, Gotham Books, 2005

Goldberg E, Podell K, Harner R, et al: Cognitive bias, functional cortical geometry, and the frontal lobes: laterality, sex and handedness. J Cogn Neurosci 6:276–296, 1994

Goldberg E, Kluger A, Malts L, et al: Assessment of early frontal-lobe dysfunction in dementia. Paper presented at the Eighth Congress of the International Psychogeriatric Association, Jerusalem, Israel, August 1997

Goldberg E, Podell K, Bilder R, et al: The Executive Control Battery. Melbourne, Australia, 2000

Golden CJ: The Stroop Color and Word Test: A Manual for Clinical and Experimental Use. Chicago, IL, Stoelting, 1978

Golden CJ, Maruish M: The Luria-Nebraska Neuropsychological Battery, in Neuropsychological Test Batteries. Edited by Incagnoli T, Goldstein G, Golden CJ. New York, Plenum, 1986, pp 193–227

Golden CJ, Hammeke TA, Purisch AD: The Luria-Nebraska Neuropsychological Battery Manual. Los Angeles, CA, Western Psychological Services, 1980

Goldman-Rakic PS, Brown RM: Regional changes of monoamines in cerebral cortex and subcortical structures of aging rhesus monkeys. Neuroscience 6:177–187, 1981

Goldstein G, McCue M, Roger J, et al: Diagnostic differences in memory test based predictions of functional capacity in the elderly. Neuropsychol Rehabil 2:307–317, 1992

Goodglass H: The flexible battery, in Neuropsychological Assessment. Edited by Incagnoli T, Goldstein G, Golden CJ. New York, Plenum, 1986, pp 121–131

Goodglass H, Kaplan E: Assessment of Aphasia and Related Disorders. Philadelphia, PA, Lea & Febiger, 1972

Goreczny AJ, Nussbaum PD: Behavioral medicine with military veterans, in Progress in Behavior Modification. Edited by Hersen M, Eisler RM, Miller PM. Sycamore, IL, Sycamore, 1994, pp 99–119

Grisso T: Clinical assessment for legal competence of older adults, in Neuropsychological Assessment of Dementia and Depression in Older Adults: A Clinician's Guide. Edited by Storandt M, VandenBos GR. Washington, DC, American Psychological Association, 1994, pp 119–140

Hartlage S, Alloy LB, Vazquez C, et al: Automatic and effortful processing in depression. Psychol Bull 113:247–278, 1993

Harvan JR, Cotter VT: An evaluation of dementia screening in the primary care setting. J Am Acad Nurse Pract 18:351–360, 2006

Heaton RK: The Wisconsin Card Sorting Test Manual. Odessa, FL, Psychological Assessment Resources, 1981

Heaton RK, Pendleton MG: Use of neuropsychological tests to predict adult patients' everyday functioning. J Consult Clin Psychol 49:807–821, 1981

Heaton RK, Grant I, Matthews CG: Differences in neuropsychological test performance associated with age, education, and sex, in Neuropsychological Assessment of Neuropsychiatric Disorders. Edited by Grant I, Adams KM. New York, Oxford University Press, 1986, pp 100–120

Heaton RK, Grant I, Matthews CG: Comprehensive Norms for an Expanded Halstead-Reitan Battery. Odessa, FL, Psychological Assessment Resources, 1991

Heaton RK, Chelune GJ, Talley JL, et al: The Wisconsin Card Sorting Test Manual Revised and Expanded. Odessa, FL, Psychological Assessment Resources, 1993

Hill C, Stoudemire A, Morris R, et al: Dysnomia in the differential diagnosis of major depression, depression-related cognitive dysfunction, and dementia. J Neuropsychiatry Clin Neurosci 4:64–69, 1989

Hohl U, Grundman M, Salmon DP, et al: Mini-Mental State Examination and Mattis Dementia Rating Scale performance differs in Hispanic and non-Hispanic Alzheimer's disease patients. J Int Neuropsychol Soc 4:301–307, 1999

Howes JL, Katz AN: Assessing remote memory with an improved public events questionnaire. Psychol Aging 3:142–150, 1988

Incagnoli T, Goldstein G, Golden CJ (eds): Neuropsychological Test Batteries. New York, Plenum, 1986

Jeste DV, Gierz M, Harris MJ: Pseudodementia: myths and realities. Psychiatr Ann 20:71–79, 1990

Johnson DK, Storandt M, Morris JC, et al: Cognitive profiles in dementia: Alzheimer disease vs. healthy brain aging. Neurology 71:1783–1789, 2008

Kane R: Standardized and flexible batteries in neuropsychology: an assessment update. Neuropsychol Rev 2:281–339, 1991

Kaplan E: Process and achievement revisited, in Towards a Holistic Developmental Psychology. Edited by Wapner S, Kaplan B. Hillsdale, NJ, Erlbaum, 1983, pp 143–156

Kaplan EF, Goodglass H, Weintraub S: The Boston Naming Test. Philadelphia, PA, Lea & Febiger, 1983

Kaszniak AW: Neuropsychological consultation to geriatricians: issues in the assessment of memory complaints. Clin Neuropsychol 1:35–46, 1987

Kaszniak AW: Psychological assessment of the aging individual, in Handbook of the Psychology of Aging. Edited by Birren JE, Schaie KW. San Diego, CA, Academic Press, 1989, pp 427–445

Kaszniak AW, Christenson GD: Differential diagnosis of dementia and depression, in Neuropsychological Assessment of Dementia and Depression. Edited by Storandt M, VandenBos GR. Washington, DC, American Psychological Press, 1994, pp 81–118

Kaszniak W, Nussbaum PD: Driving in older patients with dementia and depression. Paper presented at the annual meeting of the American Psychological Association, Boston, MA, August 1990

Keefover RW: Aging and cognition. Neurol Clin 16:635–648, 1998

Kiernan RJ, Mueller J, Langston JM, et al: The Neurobehavioral Cognitive Status Examination: a brief differentiated approach to cognitive assessment. Ann Intern Med 107:481–485, 1987

Kiloh LG: Pseudo-dementia. Acta Psychiatr Scand 37:336–351, 1961

Kluger A, Gianutsos JG, Golomb J, et al: Motor/psychomotor dysfunction in normal aging, mild cognitive decline, and early Alzheimer's disease: diagnostic and differential diagnostic features. Int Psychogeriatr 9 (suppl 1):307–316, 1997

Kral VA, Emery OB: Long-term follow-up of depressive pseudodementia of the aged. Can J Psychiatry 34:445–446, 1989

Lamar M, Podell K, Giovannetti T, et al: Perseverative behavior in Alzheimer's disease and subcortical ischemic vascular dementia. Neuropsychology 11:523–534, 1997

Lamberty CJ, Bieliauskas LA: Distinguishing between depression and dementia in the elderly: a review of neuropsychological findings. Arch Clin Neuropsychol 8:149–170, 1993

Langenecker SA, Jin Lee H, Bieliauskas LA: Neuropsychology of depression and related mood disorders, in Neuropsychological Assessment of Neuropsychiatric and Neuromedical Disorders, 3rd Edition. Edited by Grant I, Adams K. New York, Oxford University Press, 2009, pp 523–559

Langley LK, Madden DJ: Functional neuroimaging of memory: implications for cognitive aging. Microsc Res Tech 51:75–84, 2000

La Rue A: Patterns of performance on the Fuld Object Memory Evaluation in elderly inpatients with depression or dementia. J Clin Exp Neuropsychol 11:409–422, 1989

La Rue A: Aging and Neuropsychological Assessment. New York, Plenum, 1992

La Rue A, Swanda R: Neuropsychological assessment, in Handbook of Neuropsychology and Aging. Edited by Nussbaum PD. New York, Plenum, 1997, pp 360–384

Lawton MP, Brody EM: Assessment of older people: self-maintaining and instrumental activities of daily living. Gerontologist 9:179–186, 1969

Lezak M: Neuropsychological Assessment, 4th Edition. New York, Oxford University Press, 2004

Libon DJ, Glosser G, Malamut BL, et al: Age, executive functions, and visuo-spatial functioning in healthy older adults. Neuropsychology 8:38–43, 1994

Lichtenberg PA, Ross TP, Youngblade L, et al: Normative Studies Research Project Test Battery: detection of dementia in African American and European American elderly patients. Clin Neuropsychol 12:146–154, 1998

Lippa CF, Duda JE, Grossman M, et al: DLB and PDD boundary issues: diagnosis, treatment, molecular pathology, and biomarkers. Neurology 68:812–819, 2007

Loeb PA: The Independent Living Scales. San Antonio, TX, Psychological Corporation, 1996

Loewenstein D, Acevedo A: Training of cognitive and functionally relevant skills in mild Alzheimer's disease, in Geriatric Neuropsychology: Assessment and Intervention. Edited by Attix DK, Welsh-Bohmer KA. New York, Guilford, 2006, pp 261–274

Loong WK: The Continuing Performance Test. San Luis Obispo, CA, Wang Neuropsychological Laboratory, 1988

Lucas JA, Ivnik RJ, Smith GE, et al: Normative data for the Mattis Dementia Rating Scale. J Clin Exp Neuropsychol 20:536–547, 1998

MacInnes WD, Gillen RW, Golden CJ, et al: Aging and performance on the Luria-Nebraska Neuropsychological Battery. Int J Neurosci 19:179–190, 1983

Mahurin RK, Flanagan AM, Royall DR: Neuropsychological measures of executive function in frail elderly patients. Arch Clin Neuropsychol 7:356, 1993

Malloy PF, Cummings JL, Coffey CE, et al: Cognitive screening instruments in neuropsychiatry: a report of the Committee on Research of the American Neuropsychiatric Association. J Neuropsychiatry Clin Neurosci 9:189–197, 1997

Manly JJ, Jacobs DM, Sano M, et al: Effect of literacy on neuropsychological test performance in nondemented, education-matched elders. J Int Neuropsychol Soc 5:191–202, 1999

Marcopulos BA, McLain CA, Giuliano AJ: Cognitive impairment or inadequate norms? A study of healthy, rural, older adults with limited education. Clin Neuropsychol 11:111–131, 1997

Matthews CG, Haaland KY: The effect of symptom duration on cognitive and motor performance in parkinsonism. Neurology 29:951–956, 1979

Matthews CG, Kløve H: Instruction Manual for the Adult Neuropsychological Text Battery. Madison, University of Wisconsin Medical School Press, 1964

Mattis S: Dementia Rating Scale (DRS). Odessa, FL, Psychological Assessment Resources, 1988

McAllister TW: Overview: pseudodementia. Am J Psychiatry 140: 528–533, 1983

McCue M, Rogers J, Goldstein G: Relationships between neuropsychological and functional assessment in elderly neuropsychiatric patients. Rehabil Psychol 35:91–95, 1990

McKeith IG, Dickson DW, Lowe J, et al: Diagnosis and management of dementia with Lewy bodies: third report of the DLB Consortium. Neurology 65:1863–1872, 2005

Meyers JE, Meyers KR: Rey Complex Figure Test and Recognition Trial. Odessa, FL, Psychological Assessment Resources, 1995

Mitrushina M: Cognitive screening methods, in Neuropsychological Assessment of Neuropsychiatric and Neuromedical Disorders, 3rd Edition. Edited by Grant I, Adams K. New York, Oxford University Press, 2009, pp 101–126

Mittenberg W, Seidenberg M, O'Leary DS, et al: Changes in cerebral functioning associated with normal aging. J Clin Exp Neuropsychol 11:918–932, 1989

Morris JC, Heyman A, Mohs RC, et al: The Consortium to Establish a Registry for Alzheimer's Disease (CERAD), part I: clinical and neuropsychological assessment of Alzheimer's disease. Neurology 39:1159–1165, 1989

Moss MB, Albert MS, Kemper TL: Neuropsychology of frontal lobe dementia, in Clinical Syndromes in Adult Neuropsychology: The Practitioner's Handbook. Edited by White RF. Amsterdam, Elsevier, 1992, pp 287–304

Multhaup KS, Balota DA, Cowan N: Implications of aging, lexicality, and item length for the mechanisms underlying memory span. Psychon Bull Rev 3:112–120, 1996

Nasreddine Z: Montreal Cognitive Assessment. 2003. Available at: http://www.mocatest.org. Accessed May 4, 2010.

Naugle RI, Kawczak BA: Limitations of the Mini-Mental State Examination. Cleve Clin J Med 56:277–281, 1989

Neary D, Snowden JS: Dementia of the frontal lobe type, in Frontal Lobe Function and Dysfunction. Edited by Levin HS, Eisenberg HM, Benton AL. New York, Oxford University Press, 1991, pp 304–317

Nussbaum PD, Kaszniak AW, Allender J, et al: Cognitive deterioration in elderly depressed: a follow-up study. Paper presented at the annual meeting of the International Neuropsychological Society, San Antonio, TX, February 1991

Osterrieth PA: Le test de copie d'une figure complexe. Arch Psychol (Geneve) 30:306–356, 1944

Ostrosky-Solis F, Lopez-Arango G, Ardila A: Sensitivity and specificity of the Mini-Mental State Examination in a Spanish-speaking population. Appl Neuropsychol 7:25–31, 2000

Paolo AM, Troster AI, Ryan JJ: Continuous Visual Memory Test performance in healthy persons 60 to 94 years old. Arch Clin Neuropsychol 13:333–338, 1998

Parsons OA: Overview of the Halstead-Reitan Battery, in Clinical Applications of Neuropsychological Test Batteries. Edited by Incagnoli T, Goldstein G, Golden C. New York, Plenum, 1986, pp 155–189

Petersen RC, Smith GE, Waring SC, et al: Mild cognitive impairment: clinical characterization and outcome. Arch Neurol 56:303–308, 1999

Petrick JD, Mittenberg W: The course of naming dysfunction in dementia and depressive pseudodementia. Paper presented at the annual meeting of the National Academy of Neuropsychology, Pittsburgh, PA, November 1992

Pfeffer RI, Kurosaki TT, Harrah CH, et al: A survey diagnostic tool for senile dementia. Am J Epidemiol 114:515–527, 1981

Pickholtz JL, Malamut BL: Cognitive changes associated with normal aging, in Clinical Neurology of the Older Adult. Edited by Sirven JI, Malamut BL. Philadelphia, PA, Lippincott Williams & Wilkins, 2008, pp 64–76

Pirozzolo FJ, Hansch EC, Mortimer JA: Dementia in Parkinson's disease: a neuropsychological analysis. Brain Cogn 1:71–83, 1982

Podell K: When east meets west: systemizing Luria's approach to executive control assessment, in Luria's Legacy in the 21st Century. Edited by Christenson AL, Goldberg E, Bougakov D. New York, Oxford University Press, 2009, pp 122–145

Podell K, Zimmerman M, Rebeta JJ, et al: Assessing frontal lobe dysfunction. Poster presented at the 145th Annual Meeting of the American Psychiatric Association, Washington, DC, May 1992a

Podell K, Zimmerman M, Sovastion M, et al: The utility of the Graphical Sequence Test in assessing executive control deficits. Paper presented at the International Neuropsychological Society Annual Meeting, San Diego, CA, 1992b

Podell K, Lovell M, Zimmerman M, et al: The Cognitive Bias Task and lateralized frontal lobe functions in males. J Neuropsychiatry Clin Neurosci 7:491–501, 1995

Psychological Corporation: Wechsler Abbreviated Scale of Intelligence. San Antonio, TX, Psychological Corporation, 1999

Purdue Research Foundation: Examiner's Manual for the Purdue Pegboard. Chicago, IL, Science Research Associates, 1948

Purisch AD, Sbordone RJ: The Luria-Nebraska Neuropsychological Battery, in Advances in Clinical Neuropsychology. Edited by Goldstein G, Tarter RE. New York, Plenum, 1986, pp 291–316

Randolph C: Repeatable Battery for the Assessment of Neuropsychological Status. San Antonio, TX, Pearson, 1998

Reding M, Haycox J, Blass J: Depression in patients referred to a dementia clinic. Arch Neurol 42:894–896, 1985

Reifler BV: Arguments for abandoning the term pseudodementia. J Am Geriatr Soc 30:665–668, 1982

Reitan RM: Neurological and physiological bases of psychopathology. Annu Rev Psychol 27:189–216, 1976

Reitan RM, Davison LA: Clinical Neuropsychology: Current Status and Applications. New York, Winston-Wiley, 1974

Reitan RM, Wolfson D: The Halstead-Reitan Neuropsychological Test Battery. Tempe, AZ, Neuropsychology Press, 1985

Rey A: L'Examen Clinique en Psychologie. Paris, Press Universitaires de France, 1964

Reynolds CF, Hoch CC: Differential diagnosis of depressive pseudodementia and primary degenerative dementia. Psychiatr Ann 17:743–749, 1988

Robinson RG, Price TR: Poststroke depressive disorders: a follow-up study of 103 patients. Stroke 13:635–641, 1982

Rogers JC, Holm MB, Goldstein G, et al: Stability and change in functional assessment of patients with geropsychiatric disorders. Am J Occup Ther 48:914–918, 1994

Rosvold HE, Mirsky AF: A continuous performance test of brain damage. J Consult Psychol 20:343–350, 1956

Rowe JW, Kahn RL: Human aging: usual and unusual. Science 237: 143–149, 1987

Russell EW: Theory and development of pattern analysis methods related to the Halstead-Reitan battery, in Clinical Neuropsychology: A Multidisciplinary Approach. Edited by Logue PE, Schear JM. Springfield, IL, Charles C Thomas, 1984, pp 50–62

Russell EW: In defense of the Halstead-Reitan Battery: a critique of Lezak's review. Arch Clin Neuropsychol 13:365–382, 1998

Salmon DP, Bondi MW: The neuropsychology of Alzheimer's disease, in The Handbook of Neuropsychology and Aging. Edited by Nussbaum PD. New York, Plenum, 1997, pp 141–158

Schaie KW, Schaie J: Clinical assessment in aging, in Handbook of the Psychology of Aging. Edited by Birren J, Schaie KW. New York, Van Nostrand Reinhold, 1977, pp 692–723

Schear JM: Neuropsychological assessment of the elderly in clinical practice, in Clinical Neuropsychology: A Multidisciplinary Approach. Edited by Logue PE, Schear JM. Springfield, IL, Charles C Thomas, 1984, pp 199–236

Shallice T: Specific impairment of planning. Philos Trans R Soc Lond B Biol Sci 298:199–209, 1982

Shaw TG, Mortel KF, Meyer JS, et al: Cerebral blood flow changes in benign aging and cerebrovascular disease. Neurology 34:855–862, 1984

Shraberg D: The myth of pseudodementia: depression and the aging brain. Am J Psychiatry 135:601–603, 1978

Shraberg D: Questioning the concept of pseudodementia. Am J Psychiatry 137:260–261, 1980

Singer T, Verhaeghen P, Ghisletta P, et al: The fate of cognition in very old age: six-year longitudinal findings in the Berlin Aging Study (BASE). Psychol Aging 1:318–331, 2003

Smith CB: Aging and changes in cerebral energy metabolism. Trends Neurosci 7:203–208, 1984

Smith GE, Bondi MW: Normal aging, mild cognitive impairment, and Alzheimer's disease, in Textbook of Clinical Neuropsychology. Edited by Morgan JE, Ricker JH. New York, Psychology Press, 2008, pp 762–780

Speedie L, Rabins P, Pearlson G, et al: Confrontation naming deficit in dementia and depression. J Neuropsychiatry Clin Neurosci 2:59–63, 1990

Squire LR: Remote memory as affected by aging. Neuropsychologia 12:429–435, 1974

Storrie MC, Doerr HO: Characterization of Alzheimer's type dementia utilizing an abbreviated Halstead-Reitan Battery. Clin Neuropsychol 2:78–82, 1980

Stoudemire A, Hill C, Gulley LR, et al: Neuropsychological and biomedical assessment of depression-dementia syndromes. J Neuropsychiatry Clin Neurosci 1:347–361, 1989

Strauss E, Sherman EMS, Spreen O: A Compendium of Neuropsychological Tests: Administration, Norms and Commentary, 3rd Edition. New York, Oxford University Press, 2006

Strick L, Pittman J, Jacobs DM, et al: Normative data for a brief neuropsychological battery administered to English- and Spanish-speaking community-dwelling elders. J Int Neuropsychol Soc 4:311–318, 1998

Stuss DT, Craik FIM, Sayer L, et al: Comparison of older people and patients with frontal lesions: evidence from word list learning. Psych Aging 11:387–395, 1996a

Stuss DT, Meiran N, Guzman A, et al: Do long tests yield a more accurate diagnosis of dementia than short tests? Arch Neurol 53: 1033–1039, 1996b

Talland GA, Schwab RS: Performance with multiple sets in Parkinson's disease. Neuropsychologia 2:45–53, 1964

Tariq SH, Tumosa N, Chibnall JT, et al: Comparison of the Saint Louis University mental status examination and the mini-mental state examination for detecting dementia and mild neurocognitive disorder—a pilot study. Am J Geriatr Psychiatry 14:900–910, 2006

Tarter RE, Edwards KL: Neuropsychological batteries, in Clinical Application of Neuropsychological Test Batteries. Edited by Incagnoli T, Goldstein G, Golden CJ. New York, Plenum, 1986, pp 135–152

Terry RD, DeTeresa R, Hansen LA: Neocortical cell counts in normal human adult aging. Ann Neurol 21:530–539, 1987

Tombaugh TN, McIntyre NJ: The mini-mental state examination: a comprehensive review. J Am Geriatr Soc 40:922–935, 1992

Unverzagt FW, Smith DM, Rebok GW, et al: The Indiana Alzheimer Disease Center's Symposium on Mild Cognitive Impairment. Cognitive training in older adults: lessons from the ACTIVE Study. Curr Alzheimer Res 6:375–383, 2009

van Gorp WG, Marcotte TD, Sultzer D, et al: Screening for dementia: comparison of three commonly used instruments. J Clin Exp Neuropsychol 21:29–38, 1999

Veiel HOF: A preliminary profile of neuropsychological deficits associated with major depression. J Clin Exp Neuropsychol 19:587–603, 1997

Warrington EK, Sanders HI: The fate of old memories. Q J Exp Psychol 23:432–442, 1971

Wechsler D: Wechsler Adult Intelligence Scale, 3rd Edition. San Antonio, TX, Psychological Corporation, 1997a

Wechsler D: Wechsler Memory Scale, 3rd Edition. San Antonio, TX, Psychological Corporation, 1997b

Wepman J, Jones L: The Language Modalities Test for Aphasia. Chicago, IL, University of Chicago, 1961

Zanto TP, Toy B, Gazzaley A: Delays in neural processing during working memory encoding in normal aging. Neuropsychologia 48:13–25, 2009

Zappala G, Martini E, Crook T, et al: Ecological memory assessment in normal aging: a preliminary report on an Italian population. Clin Geriatr Med 5:583–594, 1989

Zehnder F, Martin M, Altgassen M, et al: Memory training effects in old age as markers of plasticity: a meta-analysis. Restor Neurol Neurosci 27:507–520, 2009

Zimmerman M, Poppen B, Podell K, et al: Lateralized frontal lobe dysfunction in males: the Wisconsin Card Sorting Test vs. the Graphical Sequences Test. Poster presented at The International Neuropsychological Society Annual Meeting, Cincinnati, OH, 1994

6

Imaging the Structure of the Aging Human Brain

C. Edward Coffey, M.D.
Anand Kumar, M.D.
Olusola Ajilore, M.D., Ph.D.

The evaluation of a patient with a neuropsychiatric disorder begins with a thorough history and physical examination (see Chapter 4, "Neuropsychiatric Assessment"). Laboratory studies, often including imaging, are then obtained if necessary to clarify the differential diagnosis, inform treatment, or estimate prognosis. With dramatic advances in imaging technologies, however, the role of brain imaging is beginning to move in some cases from that of supplementing the clinical evaluation to substituting for part of it.

The challenge to the neuropsychiatric clinician is determining the appropriate role for brain imaging for a given patient. For example, brain magnetic resonance imaging (MRI) is highly accurate for diagnosing tumors, but less clear is how to decide when a patient with psychosis needs a brain imaging study.

In this chapter, we review the techniques, indications, and utility of the main brain imaging modalities of importance to neuropsychiatric clinicians. We also discuss how structural imaging has provided information about the effects of aging on the human brain.

Clinical Imaging of Brain Structure in Neuropsychiatry

Structural Brain Imaging Techniques

Early imaging modalities provided only indirect visualization of the human brain by imaging the cranial bones (skull radiography), the cerebral vessels (arteriography), or the cerebrospinal fluid (CSF) spaces (pneumoencephalography). More recent developments in computer technology have made possible in vivo visualization of brain tissue with techniques such as computed tomography (CT) and MRI, which are the core methods for imaging brain structure in neuropsychiatry. These techniques differ in their safety, anatomical resolution, and sensitivity to tissue contrast. Historically, head CT imaging was viewed as faster and simpler than brain MRI, thereby lessening patient discomfort and motion artifact. Rapid imaging with MRI is now possible, however, with the advent of ultrafast methods, such as echo planar imaging, and MRI remains superior to CT with regard to its sensitivity to tissue physiology and biochemistry.

Head CT Scanning

An X-ray CT scanner (Figure 6–1) forms images when a fan beam of X rays is passed through the head from several different directions as the X-ray source rotates around the patient's head. Multiple detectors opposite the X-ray source also rotate around the patient's head and measure the extent to which passage of the X-ray beams has been attenuated by the intervening tissues. Computers relate this information to the density (typically in Hounsfield units) of the various structures (e.g., CSF, bone, gray matter, white matter) and then construct a series of tomographic images of the brain and cranium based on the average density within each pixel. The images are displayed on a computer monitor or printed onto X-ray film, and can be stored electronically.

The speed of CT scanning has been further increased with the introduction of helical (spiral) CT, in which multiple detectors rotate around the patient in a continuously overlapping spiral pattern. With multisection helical CT, the entire brain may be scanned in contiguous 2.5- to 5.0-mm sections, producing three-dimensional (3D) data sets in less than 1 minute. The shortened scanning time also dramatically reduces mo-

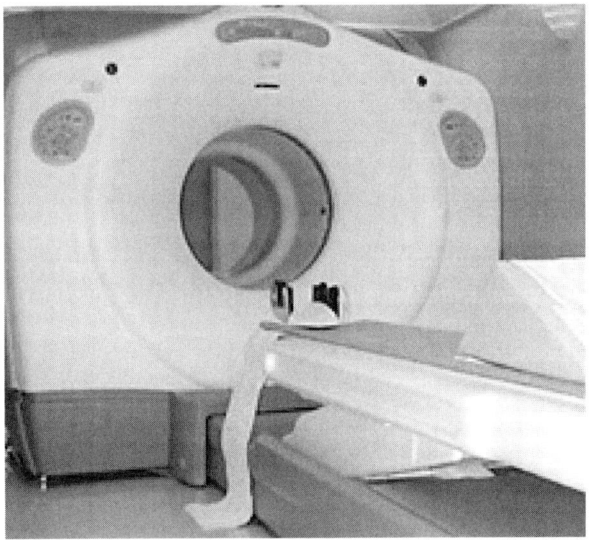

FIGURE 6–1. Contemporary computed tomography scanner.

tion artifact and makes possible imaging of dynamic processes such as cerebral blood flow (CT perfusion) and CT angiography (see Chapter 7, "Molecular Imaging in Neuropsychiatry").

X-ray CT is a relatively quick and inexpensive (as of this writing, charges generally in the range of $1,300) imaging modality, but it is limited by relatively low spatial and anatomical resolution, partial volume effects (averaging of tissue attenuation values within a voxel), and beam-hardening artifact (false elevation of brain CT values adjacent to the skull). This latter problem limits the precision with which boundaries can be determined for structures adjacent to bone (e.g., temporal lobes, apical cortex, inferior frontal lobes), regions of great interest to the neuropsychiatric clinician.

Head CT scanning carries a risk of radiation exposure of ~5 rads to the lens of the eye (a minimum of 200 rads is thought to be necessary to induce cataracts, although pediatric patients are more sensitive than adults). To avoid any radiation exposure to the eyes, some institutions set the orbitomeatal line as the inferior boundary of their scans. In addition, the dose of radiation to the brain is ~7 rads in adults and ~10 rads in infants. This exposure may be safe in adults, but there is controversy about whether it can cause long-term reduction in cognitive function in infants (Hall et al. 2004). There is no appreciable radiation exposure outside the head, but pregnant women are advised to wear lead aprons during the procedure.

Iodinated water-soluble contrast agents, which have high X-ray density, may be given intravenously immediately before CT imaging to illuminate vascular structures or reveal areas of breakdown in the blood-brain barrier. Under normal conditions these intravascular agents do not penetrate into the brain because they cannot pass through an intact blood-brain barrier. If that barrier is disrupted, such as by tumor or inflammation, the contrast agent leaks into the brain and changes its appearance on imaging. Contrast agents are associated with potentially dangerous immediate or delayed allergic reactions (both anaphylactoid and chemotoxic). These allergic reactions are less common with nonionic than ionic dyes, and guidelines exist to inform their usage (Cohan et al. 1998).

Brain MRI

An MRI scanner (Figure 6–2) forms images when the alignment of ions (in medical imaging, these are typically protons) in a strong magnetic field (typically 1.5–3.0 teslas) is disrupted by a brief radiofrequency (RF) pulse. When the pulse is terminated, RF energy is emitted as the protons become realigned within the magnetic field. This realignment of protons is characterized by two tissue-specific relaxation-time constants, T_1 and T_2 relaxation times, which describe different aspects of the reorientation—that is, interactions of the protons with surrounding nuclei (T_1) or with each other (T_2). Computers relate this emitted RF energy to various tissue (proton) characteristics, from which a series of planar or 3D images can be constructed. The spatial location of the proton is achieved by applying a magnetic field gradient across the magnet bore, which creates slight variations in proton resonance frequency across the object being imaged. For brain MRI, a close-fitting head coil is placed around the subject's head to improve the delivery and reception of the electromagnetic pulses and signals (Figure 6–3).

The unique information contained within the MRI is determined by the pulse sequence used to acquire the image (i.e., by the particular combination of RF and magnetic field pulses). Acquisition pulse sequences commonly employed in clinical practice include the fast spin echo (FSE) sequence, the gradient echo (GE or GRE) sequence, and diffusion-weighted (DW) imaging. With the FSE sequence, two factors are varied to emphasize different tissue properties: the repetition time or time to recovery (TR) and the echo time or time until echo (TE). By keeping both the TR and TE short, images are created that are heavily influenced by the T_1 relaxation times of the tissue. Such T_1-weighted images produce exceptional views of the anatomy and are thus preferred when detailed views of the structure are required. In contrast, images collected using relatively long TR and TE are more influenced by T_2 relaxation times. These T_2-weighted images are less anatomically distinct, but they have the advantage of being more sensitive to pathological tissue (the abnormality appears bright). To help distinguish this tissue abnormality from CSF (which also appears bright), a fluid-attenuated inversion recovery (FLAIR) sequence (a variant of the T_2-weighted scan) may be employed, which nullifies the CSF signal (CSF will appear dark) and makes it easier to visualize the abnormally increased T_2 signal.

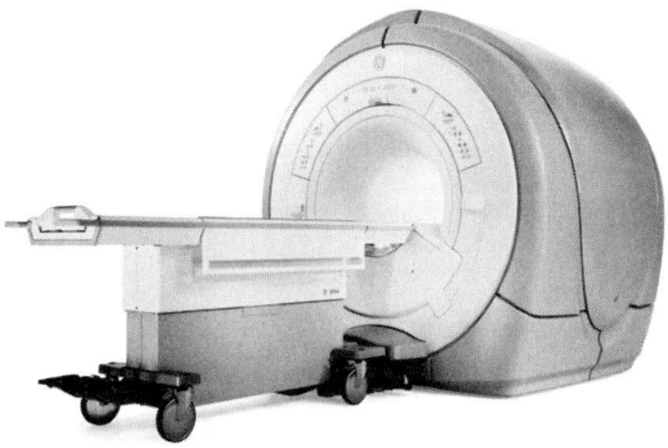

FIGURE 6–2. **Typical "closed" magnetic resonance imaging scanner.**

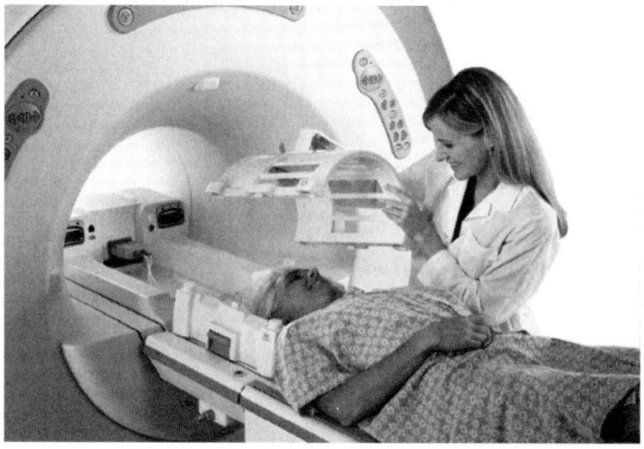

FIGURE 6–3. **Head coil used with brain magnetic resonance imaging. Openings in the coil help patients feel less claustrophobic.**

The GE sequence uses a gradient-reversing RF pulse to generate the echo, producing an image that is sensitive to tissue changes from calcium or hemorrhage, which cause magnetic field inhomogeneity. DW imaging is sensitive to the speed of water diffusion in tissue (areas of abnormally restricted water motion appear as high signal) and thus holds promise as a means of identifying ischemia within the first few hours of onset. A new and more complex variant of DW imaging is diffusion tensor imaging, which describes diffusional speed in a multidimensional matrix for every voxel in the image and which is thus very sensitive to processes that alter diffusion, including ischemia and gliosis (see "White Matter Integrity" later in this chapter). Finally, a new pulse sequence currently under study is magnetization transfer imaging, which is sensitive to interactions between bound protons (e.g., those in membranes) and unbound (free) protons (e.g., those in water) and which thus may provide insights into underlying pathological processes (see "White Matter Integrity" later in this chapter).

Relative to CT, MRI provides more accurate structural information because of clear differentiation of gray matter, white matter, and CSF; the absence of beam-hardening artifact; and the capability to image in multiple planes, thereby providing optimal views of regional cerebral structures with less volume-averaging artifact (see "Imaging Technique" later in this chapter). Additionally, MRI has greater sensitivity to detect pathological tissue, particularly hyperintense foci of the subcortical white matter and gray matter nuclei (subcortical hyperintensity) that occur with increasing frequency in elderly people (Campbell and Coffey 2001). Because MRI does not use ionizing radiation, serial studies in healthy subjects are possible. For these reasons, MRI appears to be uniquely suited to the study of age-related changes in brain morphology (see discussion "Methods of Image Analysis" later in this chapter).

It should be noted, however, that accurate assessment of brain structure with MRI may be affected by a number of technical factors, including choice of acquisition sequence parameters (affecting tissue contrast), slice section thickness (adjacent sections that are too thin may result in overlapping profiles and "crosstalk" artifact), and magnetic field homogeneity (inhomogeneous fields may result in spatial distortion of objects and object pixel nonuniformity). Movement artifact may also be induced by pulsation of blood and CSF, especially in the limbic system, where structures lie in close proximity to the ventricles and the carotid arteries; such artifact can be lessened with the use of cardiac-gating and flow-compensated pulse sequences. Careful consideration of these methodological issues is needed to ensure precision of measurement with MRI.

Compared with head CT, brain MRI is a more expensive (generally twice the price of head CT) and often more lengthy procedure, and some subjects may be unable to cooperate with the long imaging time, especially if they develop claustrophobia within the scanner. Recent advances in imaging technology have resulted in considerable shortening of scanning time with MRI, however, and the use of "open scanners" (Figure 6–4) has made the experience more tolerable for those patients with claustrophobia. Finally, MRI cannot be used for subjects who have a pacemaker or intracranial ferromagnetic objects such as surgical clips. The strong magnetic field can damage electrical, mechanical, or magnetic devices implanted in or attached to the patient, and it could cause movement of any implanted metallic object. Furthermore, such metallic objects may themselves distort the magnetic resonance image and lessen the quality of the examination. Pregnancy (especially the first trimester) is considered by some authorities a relative contraindication to MRI, primarily because safety data are incomplete. To date, however, no harmful effects of MRI have been demonstrated in either fetuses or pregnant women.

Intravenous water-soluble contrast agents are available for MRI, and most are chelates of gadolinium, a rare-earth heavy

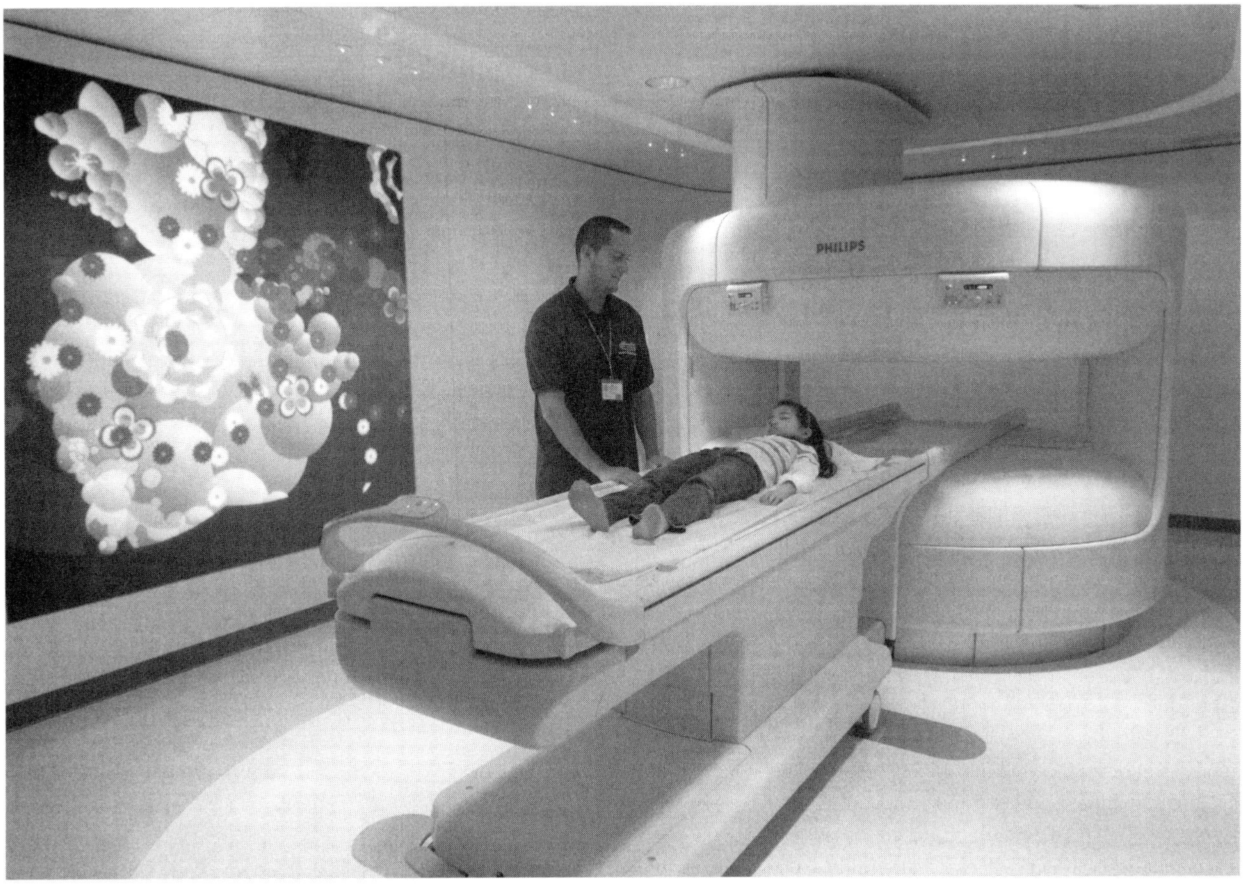

FIGURE 6–4. Newer "open" magnetic resonance imaging scanners make the procedure more tolerable for patients who experience claustrophobia.

metal. These agents cross the damaged blood-brain barrier, in a manner similar to that of the CT contrast agents discussed earlier, and shorten both T_1 and T_2 relaxation times, an effect best seen as high signal on T_1-weighted images. Such contrast-enhanced images are quite sensitive to neoplastic and inflammatory processes, including demyelination (e.g., multiple sclerosis plaques) and infection (e.g., meningitis, encephalitis, myelitis).

Relative Merits of Head CT Versus Brain MRI

MRI is the imaging method of choice for the majority of intracranial (and intraspinal) abnormalities, because of its greater anatomical specificity, a greater sensitivity to pathological tissue, the ability to image in multiple planes of orientation, the absence of beam-hardening artifact (permitting excellent visualization of parenchyma near bone), the lack of ionizing radiation, and a better safety profile with contrast enhancement than head CT. In addition, MRI produces a very rich and highly informative signal, which provides information on a variety of physiological processes such as blood flow, CSF motion, and biochemical makeup (see Chapter 7, "Molecular Imaging in Neuropsychiatry"). MRI is typically a longer and more expensive procedure than head CT, however, and is less widely available.

Relative to brain MRI, head CT imaging is widely considered the more reliable and unambiguous method for detecting acute brain parenchymal or extra-axial hemorrhage, especially subarachnoid hemorrhage. Head CT is also superior for examining bones of the cranium (although MRI is better for studying invasive processes of the bone marrow). For these reasons, and also for considerations of cost, speed, and availability, head CT is widely used for screening of patients with acute stroke or head injury. Finally, head CT is particularly useful for patients who are uncooperative or who cannot tolerate MRI (~5% experience claustrophobia) or who have contraindications to such imaging (e.g., pacemakers, metallic implants, or attached mechanical equipment such as respirators).

Indications for and Clinical Utility of Brain Imaging in Neuropsychiatry

The decision-making process for diagnosing and treating a patient with a neuropsychiatric disorder requires a blend of science and art. The clinician must collect and analyze data to determine the most likely outcomes for a variety of management options and harmonize these options with the individual patient's wants and needs. Because clinicians rarely have certainty with regard to any of these issues, their natural tendency is to obtain as much information as possible for making a decision. Such a "shotgun" approach, however, contains inherent dangers, both direct (e.g., financial costs and possible harmful effects of the test) and indirect (e.g., a false test result leading to inappropriate and potentially harmful care). In addition, the clinician has a responsibility to use all resources wisely so that such resources, some of which may be scarce, are available for those patients who truly need them.

These considerations raise two key questions for the neuropsychiatric diagnostician: Should I order a (another) test to improve my diagnostic or prognostic assessment? If so, which test is (tests are) best?

With regard to the first question, we recommend brain imaging to *confirm* the presence of focal pathology in a patient when findings from the history or physical examination suggest such pathology. The interpretation of a test result depends on what is already known about the patient. A test should be ordered only if it will provide additional information about the patient beyond what is available from a thorough and competent history and physical examination, and only if there is a reasonable chance that such information (positive or negative) will influence the patient's care. Some examples for which these criteria may pertain include the initial evaluation of patients with dementia (Knopman et al. 2001), psychosis (new onset or an atypical clinical presentation) (American Psychiatric Association 2004), brain injury, or other behavioral signs or symptoms (e.g., depression, mania, anxiety, delirium, confusion, agitation) in the setting of a focal neurological examination (American Psychiatric Association 2002). Routine use of brain imaging as a "screening" measure for patients with behavioral signs or symptoms would not meet these general criteria, despite some data suggesting that such screening might reveal unsuspected pathology that then alters treatment (Erhart et al. 2005). In our view, such studies raise questions of the thoroughness of the original clinical evaluation.

To answer the question about which test is best, we discussed the relative merits of head CT versus brain MRI in the previous subsection. Clearly, the choice of imaging modality requires that the clinician have a hypothesis about the nature of the brain pathological process for which the imaging study is being obtained.

Structural Imaging as a Window Into Human Brain Aging

In this section, we discuss the use of structural brain imaging as a tool to understand human brain aging. We focus on methodological issues and the effects of aging on human brain structure.

Methodological Issues

Study Design

Imaging studies of brain aging can be designed as either cross-sectional or longitudinal investigations. In cross-sectional studies, a single imaging evaluation is performed at roughly the same time on a group of subjects whose ages differ across a range of interest. Such studies allow for relatively rapid, efficient, and economical acquisition of large amounts of data (Jernigan et al. 2001; Longstreth et al. 2000). However, cross-sectional studies may be influenced by secular effects (e.g., the possibility that brain size exhibits systematic changes over successive birth cohorts in the general population). For example, successive generations may have, on average, larger parenchymal volumes and smaller ventricular volumes. If such trends actually exist in the population at large and if they are not secondary to secular trends associated with correlates of brain morphology, such as cranial size or years of education, then an assessment of the true effects of aging on brain size will require longitudinal investigation.

In longitudinal studies, imaging evaluations are repeated on the same group of subjects as they age over time. Such studies are thus free of secular effects, but they are labor intensive and may suffer from significant attrition effects (i.e., the characteristics of the sample may change dramatically or subjects drop out of the study over time). Longitudinal studies may also outlive their usefulness (the period effect); for example, an ongoing study of ventricular size that began in the era of pneumoencephalography would not be of great interest in today's world of high-resolution CT and MRI.

The interpretation of both cross-sectional and longitudinal investigations must also consider the possible influences of survivor effects and heterogeneity within the elderly population. *Survivor effect* refers to the overrepresentation in study samples of relatively healthy subjects (the survivors) because others with preexisting illnesses may have died before study entry. Relative to younger populations, elderly persons exhibit greater *heterogeneity* in a variety of physiological variables that could indirectly influence brain structure. In summary, both cross-sectional and longitudinal study designs have strengths and limitations; the choice of one approach over the other will depend on available resources and the specific aims of the investigation.

Subject Selection

Brain morphology may be affected by variables in the subject sample that are associated with the aging process (e.g., concomitant medical illnesses such as hypertension, diabetes mellitus), as well as by other variables that are relatively independent of it (e.g., gender, body or head size, handedness, education, socioeconomic status, psychiatric and drug-use history). These variables must be considered and appropriately controlled before conclusions can be reached about the effects of aging per se on brain anatomy. Also, the apparent effects of age on brain structure may vary depending on the age range of the sample studied. In general, aging effects have been less robust in samples with restricted age ranges.

Subject sample. Selection of an appropriate subject sample is a critically important first step in any investigation of aging effects on brain morphology. A sample of healthy volunteers from the community may differ markedly from a sample of medical or psychiatric patients with "normal" scans. Although the latter "patient" samples provide a convenient and economical source of readily available imaging data, such samples may include individuals with structural brain changes resulting from causes other than aging (Coffey et al. 1998). In addition, patient samples are generally less representative of the variability in brain morphology that exists within samples of healthy volunteers. As noted above, such heterogeneity is especially great among the elderly population, a finding that may be related in part to differences between "usual aging" (i.e., no clinically obvious brain disease) and "successful aging" (i.e., minimal decline in neurobiological function compared with that of younger subjects) (Coffey et al. 1998; DeCarli et al. 2005).

Thus, even within a sample of "healthy" community volunteers, considerable variability in brain morphology may exist depending on the relative mix of subjects with usual versus successful aging. Whenever possible, researchers should attempt to define the extent to which their study subjects fall within these two categories, based in part on thorough medical, neuropsychiatric, and neuropsychological evaluations, as well as on correlative imaging assessments of brain function (see Chapter 7, "Molecular Imaging in Neuropsychiatry"). Even these evaluations may fail to identify subjects with various other conditions (e.g., hypertension, diabetes mellitus, hyperlipidemia, alcohol use, cigarette smoking, elevated plasma homocysteine) that may affect brain morphology, including those with preclinical disease or with genetic predispositions to disease. In this chapter, we review those studies that have for the most part examined healthy volunteers from the community.

Sample size is also an important factor in interpreting results. Negative findings in studies with relatively small samples may be a result of low power.

Gender and body size. Women are smaller (i.e., shorter and lighter) on average than men are, and their heads and brains also tend to be smaller. Even within a single-gender study, however, differences in body or head size among subjects may confound apparent age-related differences. Although there is no generally accepted method of correcting for head or body size, this variable may be taken into account through subject matching (e.g., on height), statistical analysis (e.g., analysis of covariance), or ratio measures (e.g., intracranial or total brain size as the denominator).

Handedness. Differences exist in regional brain size or symmetry between right-handed and left-handed (or non-right-handed) individuals. Surprisingly, only a few investigations of the aging brain have specified the handedness of their subjects. This variable should be assessed with continuous quantitative measures (Coffey et al. 1992), and its effects on brain structure should be controlled statistically or through subject inclusion criteria (e.g., limiting the sample to those subjects with definite motoric lateralization).

Education and socioeconomic status. Imaging studies have reported a relationship between brain structure and educational level or socioeconomic class (Coffey et al. 1999). This relationship may be an indirect one, however, with both of these variables (and perhaps also IQ) serving as markers for body or head size. Studies of brain aging should assess the potential impact of these variables statistically (Coffey et al. 1992, 1999) or attempt to control them through subject matching procedures when appropriate (Pfefferbaum et al. 1998).

Psychiatric and drug-use history. Alterations of brain morphology have been described in patients with a variety of psychiatric disorders (Coffey et al. 1993; see also Part IV, "Neuropsychiatric Syndromes and Disorders," in this book). Although some earlier studies failed to specify the psychiatric histories of their subjects, more recent investigations have appropriately excluded patients with such histories. Alcohol and perhaps other drug use may also alter brain structure (see Chapter 17, "Addiction"), but again studies have varied in the extent to which these factors have been considered. Although more recent investigations of brain aging have generally excluded subjects with substance abuse or dependence, the effects of subclinical drug or alcohol consumption on structural brain aging have not been thoroughly assessed. One major impediment to such efforts has been the inability to obtain reliable and accurate data about the extent of lifetime drug use.

Imaging Technique

Imaging modality. Both CT and MRI have been used to study the effects of aging on brain structure. As discussed earlier, MRI appears to be uniquely suited to the study of age-related changes in brain morphology. However, accurate assessment of brain structure with MRI may be affected by a number of technical factors discussed earlier. Careful consideration of these methodological issues is needed to ensure precision of measurement with MRI.

Plane of imaging. The optimal orientation from which to visualize brain anatomy will vary depending on the structure of interest. For example, midsagittal images provide the best views of the corpus callosum and medial prefrontal cortex, axial images provide a good view of subcortical white matter and gray nuclei (e.g., thalamus and basal ganglia), and coronal sections are required for optimal views of the temporal lobes and limbic structures. With head CT, the plane of imaging is limited by the patient's position in the scanner; because the patient is typically supine, axial images are produced. With MRI, the plane of imaging can be determined simply by programming the magnetic gradients, making possible images in the coronal, axial, and sagittal planes, irrespective of patient positioning within the scanner.

Once the appropriate imaging plane has been selected, the images must be acquired in a standardized orientation so that valid comparisons across subjects are possible. Proper alignment of acquisition plane is especially critical for studies of brain asymmetry, because head tilt can result in artifactual right-left differences. External landmarks (e.g., the canthomeatal line) are relatively quick and easy to establish for orientation, but they may not be consistently related to brain structure. Such problems may be obviated by use of internal landmarks (e.g., the anterior commissure–posterior commissure line), but these can be more technically difficult to establish and thus may add to the length of the scanning procedure.

Slice thickness. Image resolution is affected by section thickness; each image data point (voxel) in the slice represents an average of slice thickness (millimeters) raised to the third power. Thus, the thinner the section is, the higher the resolution. However, with thin sections, a greater total scanning time is required to image a given volume, and thin sections are also associated with a reduced signal-to-noise ratio (less tissue is present to produce a signal). Furthermore, slice thickness with MRI is limited by certain technical factors, including gradient strength, quantity of RF energy used for excitation, and the phenomenon of cross-talk artifact. This latter problem can be partially obviated by leaving space between adjacent sections (interscan gap), but this method excludes a given portion of tissue from direct assessment, thereby reducing the accuracy of volume measurements (particularly of small or irregular structures). Section interleaving is another method for reducing cross-talk artifact, but this procedure doubles scanning time.

Phantom calibration. Verification of the accuracy of imaging data against a known standard (phantom) should be conducted on a regular basis to ensure stability of the imaging hardware. With MRI in particular, image data may be affected by variations in the main magnetic field, the magnetic field gradient systems, and the RF pulse system.

Head movement artifact. Involuntary head movement by subjects is another source of artifact that can degrade image quality. Head movement is more likely as the length of the scanning time increases, and it may be especially troublesome in certain clinical circumstances. For example, at least some elderly subjects with arthritic conditions may be unable to lie still for more than a few minutes, making comparisons with younger nonarthritic subjects problematic. Head movement may be reduced by physical restraints (e.g., Velcro straps or fitted plastic masks) or the use of sedative medications, but the latter are rarely appropriate for use in nonpatient volunteers.

Methods of Image Analysis

General considerations. The quality of imaging data is affected by several factors related to the methodology of image analysis. First, measurements can be made on a variety of different forms of imaging data, including radiographs, overhead projections of radiographs, photographs of the image, or displays of the original digital image data on computer consoles. Computerized digital data systems afford the greatest flexibility and permit standardization of window settings across images, thereby providing for greater consistency and accuracy of measurement than is possible from films, where window settings are fixed. Second, the interpretation of brain imaging data will be affected by the criteria used to define the structure of interest. For example, the measured size of the frontal lobes on MRI will vary depending on whether their posterior boundary has been defined by the optic chiasma, the genu of the corpus callosum, or the central sulcus (Coffey et al. 1992). Anatomical nonuniformity in these landmarks across subjects will also contribute to variability in regional brain measures. Third, the reliability of the measures of brain anatomy will vary with the skill of the rater. Both interrater and intrarater reliabilities should be reported for all raters, using either kappa statistics or intraclass correlation coefficients. Finally, because assessment of imaging data requires considerable subjective judgment on the part of the rater, all measurements should be performed by raters who are blind to subject data (e.g., age, gender, diagnostic group) or to study hypotheses that could bias such assessments.

Types of measures. The effects of aging on brain morphology have been assessed with both qualitative and quantitative measures. Qualitative measures consist of various scales to determine the presence and severity of parameters of interest, including, for example, cortical atrophy or ventricular enlargement. Qualitative measures are relatively inexpensive and easy to use, do not require sophisticated technological support, are frequently "clinically relevant," and may show good agreement with more quantitative assessments. Qualitative measures have limited resolution and sensitivity, however, and their accuracy is critically dependent on the skill of the particular rater. For this reason, comparing results from different studies is often difficult, especially when different rating scales have been used.

Quantitative measures of brain size may be linear (distance measurement), planimetric (area measurement), or volumetric (multisection planimetric). Linear and planimetric measures are relatively quick and inexpensive and are available to researchers who lack sophisticated computerized image processing capabilities. Such measures also correlate reasonably well with volumetric measures, at least for structures of regular shape. For more complicated structures with irregular shapes, however, volumetric measures are much more accurate, especially when the sections are relatively thin (<5 mm) and contiguous, and when they span the entire extent of the structure of interest. Volumetric measures are also more sensitive than linear and planimetric methods for detecting subtle group differences. Finally, volumetric measures are especially important for assessing left-right asymmetries because single-section measures are much more susceptible to the confounding effects of head tilt and patient positioning and because bilateral structures may not be aligned in a perfectly parallel position within the left and right hemispheres. In such situations, the left and right sides of a structure could differ with regard to the particular imaging section on which they appeared larger, in which case left-versus-right comparisons based on a single section clearly would not be representative of any asymmetry in the total volume of that structure.

Among the volumetric brain imaging studies, differences exist in the technique used to segment the cranial contents into bone, CSF, white matter, and gray matter compartments. Regions of interest may be outlined manually ("trace" technique) or with semiautomated guidance, and then volumes are approximated by numeric integration using a variety of algorithms. These volumetric (multislice) techniques are labor intensive, however, and because they are difficult to apply to regions where boundaries are poorly defined (e.g., insular cortex), they may be insensitive to change in such brain areas. These problems are minimized by more recently developed whole brain techniques, which employ sophisticated automated image segmentation and processing methods. These techniques involve registration of the image by aligning it with another image or with a stereotactic template using spatial normalization, then correction for various scan nonidealities, and finally construction of histogram or voxel-based maps of signal intensity (Good et al. 2001; Tisserand et al. 2004). Voxel-based morphometry is an example of a whole brain technique; it registers every brain at the voxel level to a template, and then after correction ("smoothing"), it compares the brains at every voxel. Because whole-brain techniques are less adept at segmenting regions with similar pixel intensity values (e.g., separating amygdala from hippocampus), more recent morphometric studies employ a combination of methods, including whole brain automated and manual or semiautomated volumetric techniques.

Effects of Aging on Human Brain Structure

Brain Atrophy

Consistent with postmortem data, CT and MRI investigations have consistently demonstrated shrinkage of the brain with age in humans, as measured by qualitative ratings of CSF spaces and by quantitative assessments of CSF spaces and brain parenchyma. Although the reported extent and trajectory of the atrophy vary depending on the study methodology, remarkably good agreement exists between cross-sectional studies (see reviews by Coffey 2000; Fotenos et al. 2005) and more recent longitudinal investigations (Appendix 6–1). Across the adult life span, whole brain volume (as a proportion of head size or intracranial volume) declines from ~85% at age 20 years to ~74% at age 80, or a rate of ~0.23% per year. This age-related shrinkage begins in early adult life but appears to accelerate beginning in late middle age, with rates approaching 0.5% per year in elderly samples. These age effects appear to be similar in men and women, and for the left and right hemispheres. In addition, increasing age is associated with a greater range in the measures of brain shrinkage, perhaps reflecting differences in usual versus successful aging. For most healthy subjects, the severity of such age-related atrophy is generally rated as clinically borderline or mild (Figure 6–5). Regional differences have been observed in many studies, with frontal regions typically showing greater age-related shrinkage (Coffey et al. 1992) (Appendix 6–1). In addition, some authors have found differences in the effects of age on cerebral gray and white matter, with the former showing an earlier age at onset of shrinkage (perhaps consistent with the latter's later age of full maturation). Some of the age-related regional brain changes may be related to changes in cognitive function with aging (see Chapter 5, "Neuropsychological Assessment," for a more complete review of this issue), and several studies have found that higher rates of age-related atrophy may predict the development of mild cognitive impairment or frank dementia (Appendix 6–1) (Weiner 2008). We (Coffey et al. 1999) and others (Fotenos et al. 2008) have found that such effects may be mitigated by factors (e.g., education level, socioeconomic status) that potentially contribute to cognitive "reserve."

Ventricular Enlargement

Cross-sectional (see reviews by Coffey 2000; Fotenos et al. 2005) and more recent longitudinal imaging investigations

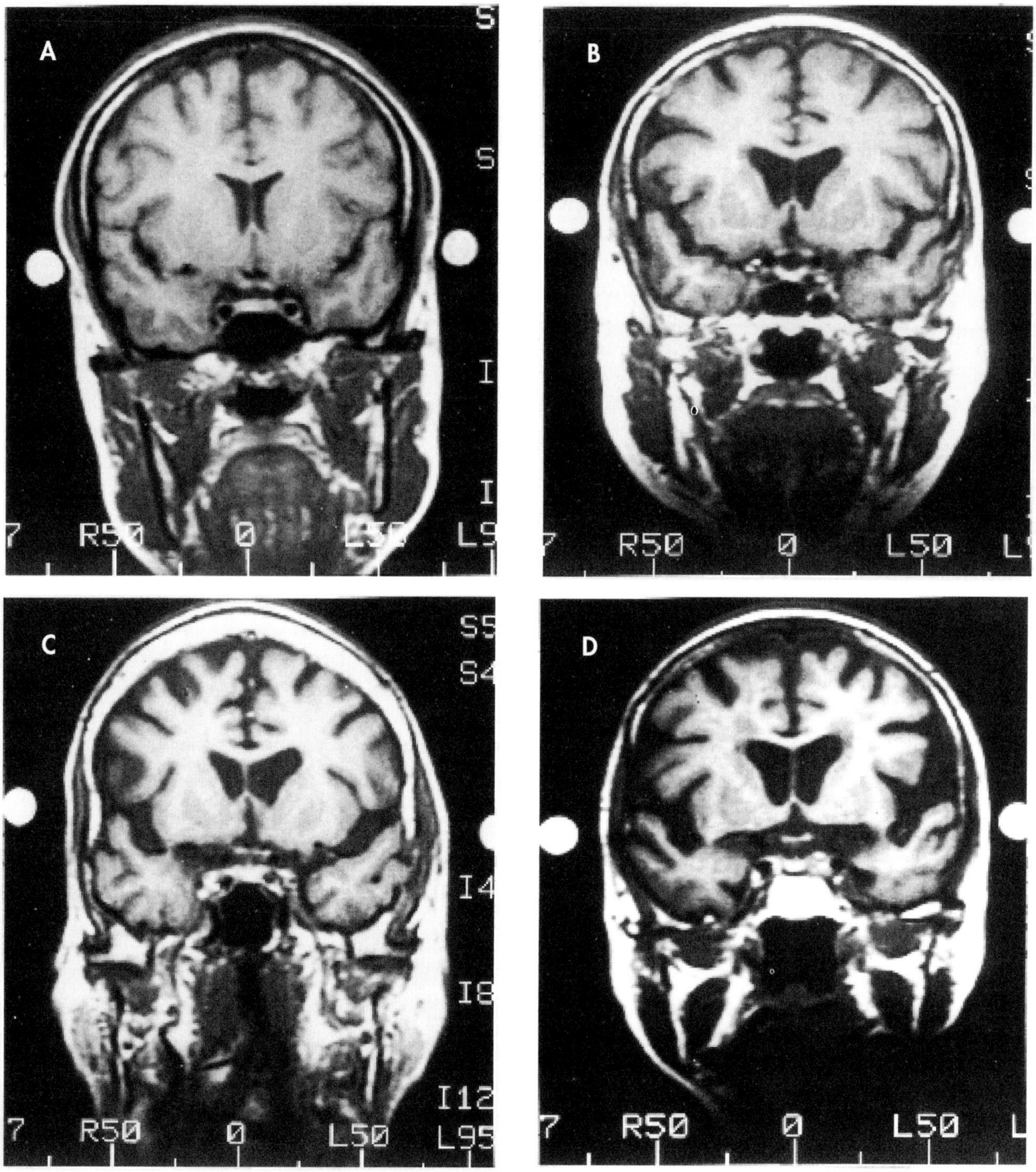

FIGURE 6–5. Visual standards for cortical atrophy score ratings on T_1-weighted coronal magnetic resonance images.

Repetition time=500 milliseconds; echo time=20 milliseconds. **Panel A:** Grade 0, 1=none, borderline. **Panel B:** Grade 2=mild cortical atrophy. **Panel C:** Grade 3=moderate cortical atrophy, with widening of the interhemispheric fissure. **Panel D:** Grade 4=severe cortical atrophy, with widening of almost all sulci. This scan also demonstrated moderately severe enlargement of the lateral ventricles.

Source. Reprinted from Coffey CE: "Structural Brain Abnormalities in the Depressed Elderly," in *Brain Imaging in Affective Disorders.* Edited by Hauser P. Washington, DC, American Psychiatric Press, 1991, pp. 92–93. Copyright © 1991 American Psychiatric Press. Used with permission.

(Appendix 6–1) confirm that age is associated with enlargement of the ventricular system. Over the first nine decades of life, the ventricular-brain ratio may increase nonlinearly from 2% to 17%, the proportion of ventricular fluid volume to brain volume may increase from 2%–4% to 4%–8%, and the proportion of ventricular fluid volume to cranial volume may increase from 1%–2% to 2%–4%. These age effects equate roughly to a ventricular enlargement rate of ~2%–4% per year, with an acceleration of that rate around middle age. These effects appear to be similar for the lateral and third ventricles. The fourth ventricle is rarely reported separately from the total ventricular system. Most studies find no gender or laterality effects. As noted above for brain parenchyma, increasing age is associated with a greater range in measures of ventricular size. For most healthy subjects, the severity of such ventricular enlargement is generally rated as clinically mild (see Figure 6–5). Ventricular enlargement with aging is presumed to occur as a result of shrinkage of periventricular brain matter, including the caudate and thalamus.

Subcortical Hyperintensity

Aging is associated with an increased prevalence and severity of subcortical hyperintensity (SH), or foci of increased signal on T_2-weighted MR images (Campbell and Coffey 2001; Coffey 2000; Malloy et al. 2007; Vernooij et al. 2007) in the subcortical white matter and gray matter nuclei (caudate, putamen, thalamus), as measured qualitatively (visual ratings of "severity"; see Figure 6–5) or quantitatively (manual tracing or computerized area and volume measures).

A growing body of neuropathological evidence has defined the pathophysiological significance of SH. Periventricular hyperintensities in the form of caps or halos/rims are common in healthy individuals and do not appear to constitute pathology (Figure 6–6, Panels A and B). Histological studies suggest that these changes likely reflect increased water content resulting from various factors, including a loose network of axons with low myelin content, a patchy loss of ependyma with astrocytic gliosis (so-called ependymitis granularis), and the normal convergence of flow of interstitial fluid within the periventricular region. Longitudinal imaging studies indicate that these SH changes are generally nonprogressive (Appendix 6–1).

The more severe changes of SH (e.g., confluent lesions) (Panel C in Figures 6–6 and 6–7), however, appear to be markers for tissue damage due to small-vessel cerebrovascular disease. In such lesions, a spectrum of histological changes may be present, which range from vascular ectasia and dilated perivascular spaces, to edema and demyelination, to frank lacunar infarctions (the latter typically also appear as areas of hypointense signal on T_1-weighted MRI). These more severe changes appear to be a consequence of chronic brain hypoperfusion stemming from some combination of advancing arteriosclerosis, hypertensive vascular disease, chronic recurrent hypotension, cerebral amyloid angiopathy, presence of "senile" arteriolar hyaline lesions, age-related thickening of meninges, and impaired autoregulation of cerebral circulation associated with aging. These confluent SH lesions show linear progression over time (volume increase of ~5%–13% per year), particularly among older individuals and those with hypertension or more severe SH at baseline (Appendix 6–1).

SH has important implications for the functional status of aging individuals. The severity or volume of SH is related to measures of ambulatory function (gait and balance) and cognitive function (e.g., psychomotor processing speed, executive functions, and visuoconstructional ability) (reviewed by Malloy et al. 2007), and is a predictor of later cognitive decline and frank dementia (Roman 2004; Vermeer et al. 2003). Severity of SH is related to risk of falls and depression (see Chapter 19, "Mood Disorders"), both of which are major impediments to successful aging (Campbell and Coffey 2001). Progression of SH is also related to gait and cognitive dysfunction (Appendix 6–1). The presumed mechanism for this association of SH and brain function is regional disconnection due to disruption in white matter networks. In addition, studies using MR magnetization transfer imaging (see "White Matter Integrity" later in this chapter) suggest that the pathophysiological changes associated with SH may extend beyond the subcortical white matter to include the gray matter (Mezzapesa et al. 2003), perhaps providing a partial explanation for the apparent relation between SH and cortical atrophy.

White Matter Integrity

Magnetization transfer imaging (MTI) and diffusion tensor imaging (DTI) are two advanced MRI techniques that have been applied to study age-related changes in white matter integrity.

Magnetization transfer imaging. MTI is a method to examine the biophysical properties of the brain parenchyma using MRI (Barbosa et al. 1994; Eng et al. 1991; Grossman 1994; Henkelman et al. 2001). MTI uses the two classes of water protons in biological tissues: water that is bound to macromolecules (bound water) and water that moves freely except for the constraints of biological compartmentation (free water). The free water signal is the main contributor to traditional structural MRI, wherein the bound water signal typically makes no contribution, due to its distribution across a very wide frequency band. In the MTI protocol, however, two images are acquired at every slice location within an organ. Acquisition of one image (the control) is preceded by an "off-resonance" RF pulse, which saturates the bound water protons and reduces to nearly zero their contribution to the overall proton signal. Another image is recorded, with parameters identical to the off-resonance image but with no preliminary off-resonance pulse.

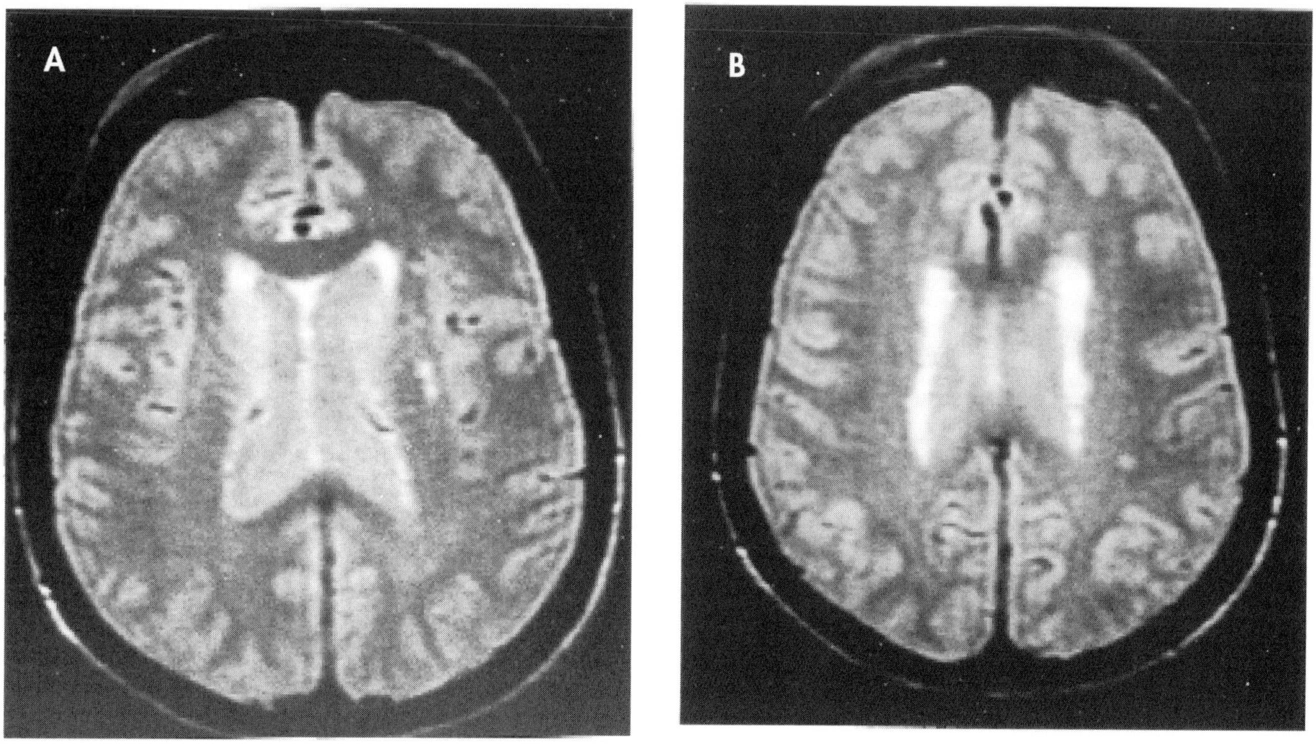

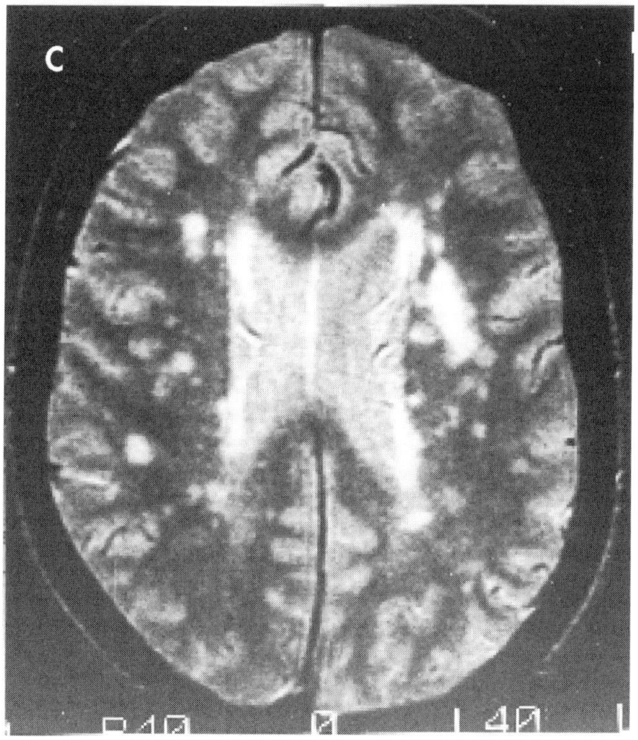

FIGURE 6–6. Visual standards for ratings of hyperintensity in the periventricular white matter on T_2-weighted magnetic resonance images.

Repetition time=2,500 milliseconds; echo time=80 milliseconds. **Panel A:** Grade 1="caps" at anterior tips of frontal horns. **Panel B:** Grade 2="halo" along border of lateral ventricles. **Panel C:** Grade 3=irregular extension of hyperintensity into the deep white matter.

Source. Reprinted from Coffey CE: "Structural Brain Abnormalities in the Depressed Elderly," in *Brain Imaging in Affective Disorders.* Edited by Hauser P. Washington, DC, American Psychiatric Press, 1991, pp. 94–95. Copyright © 1991 American Psychiatric Press. Used with permission.

The signal of this magnetization transfer acquisition is reduced compared to the control acquisition in every tissue region having water protons that exchange between the free and bound states. Therefore, a magnetization transfer ratio (MTR) image can then be created, reflecting the difference in signal intensity between the two images. In the white matter, myelin-related proteins are the primary macromolecules found to influence MTI, but its pathophysiological substrate in the gray matter is unclear.

MTR is a marker of myelin in the white matter and probably reflects increasing interactions between bound water and lipids and cholesterol found in myelin. MTR values increase in children during the first 2 years of life, probably because it reflects the increasing myelination that occurs during this stage of life. MTR is also greater in the white matter than in the gray matter and higher in the commissural and projection fibers than in the association fibers.

A small number of studies have focused on age-related changes in MTI. Spilt et al. (2006) demonstrated that the

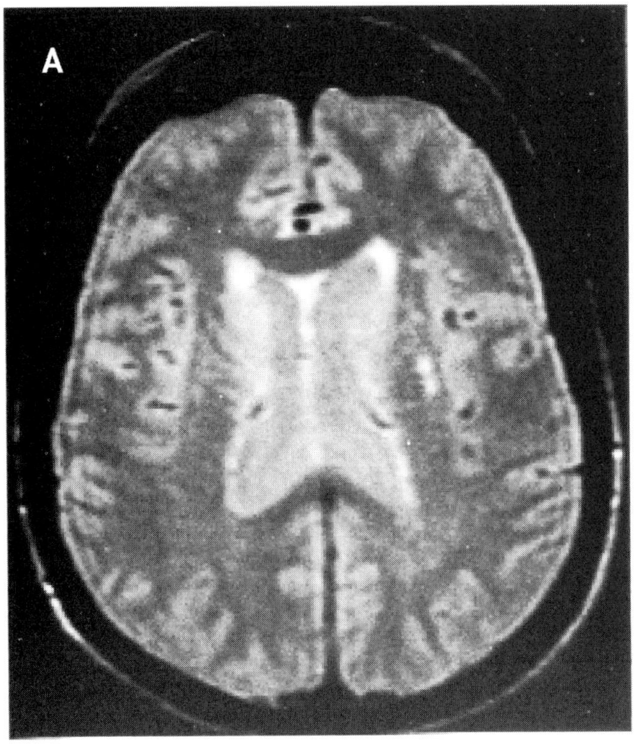

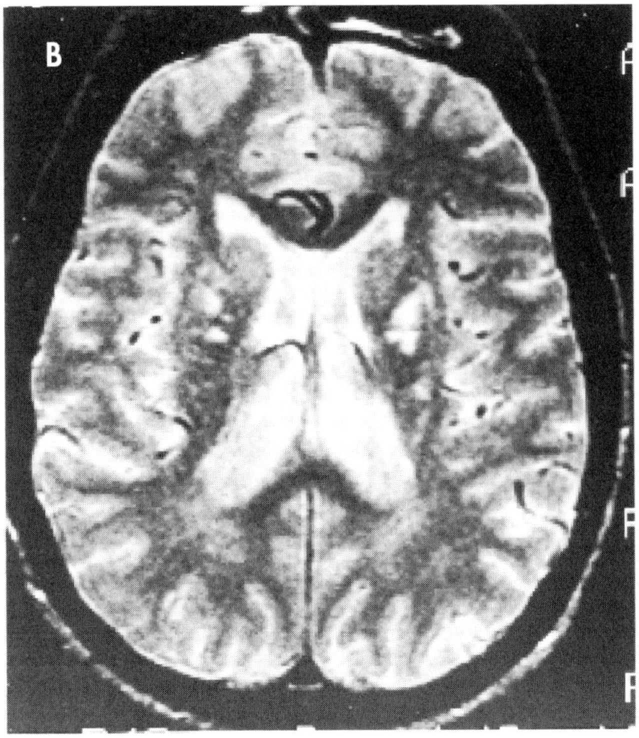

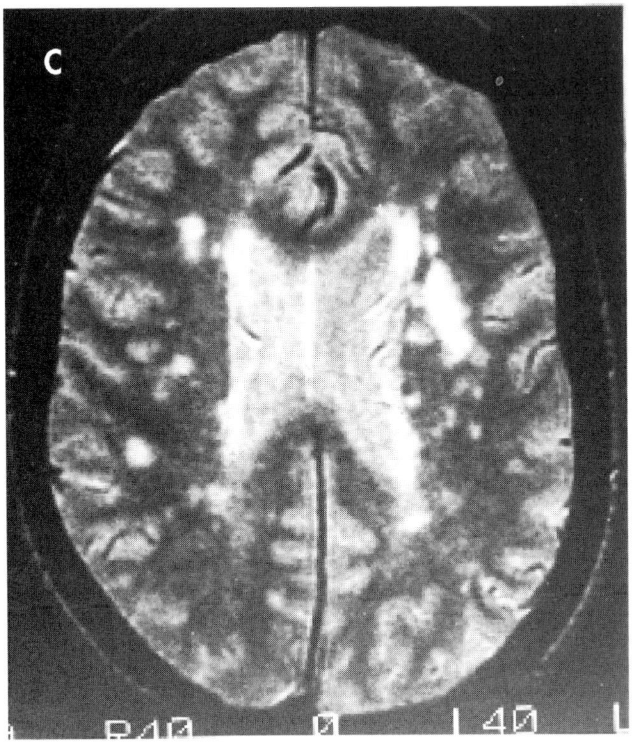

FIGURE 6–7. Visual standards for ratings of hyperintensity in the deep white matter on T_2-weighted magnetic resonance images.

Repetition time=2,500 m00illiseconds; echo time=80 milliseconds. **Panel A:** Grade 1=punctuate foci. **Panel B:** Grade 2=small confluence of foci. **Panel C:** Grade 3=large confluent areas of signal hyperintensity.

Source. Reprinted from Coffey CE: "Structural Brain Abnormalities in the Depressed Elderly," in *Brain Imaging in Affective Disorders.* Edited by Hauser P. Washington, DC, American Psychiatric Press, 1991, pp. 96–97. Copyright © 1991 American Psychiatric Press. Used with permission.

mean MTR of the white matter was lower in elderly subjects than in younger subjects. They also demonstrated that MTR values in the elderly subgroup with extensive white matter lesions were not significantly different from those in the subgroup with minimal white matter lesions. These findings were interpreted to demonstrate that high-intensity lesions and lower MTR values had different neurobiological underpinnings and correlates. Ge et al. (2002) demonstrated decreases in magnetization transfer histograms in both gray and white matter with age. Hofman et al. (1999) also reported decreases in MTR with age, in both men and women, although men had higher MTR values than women. These findings differ from those of Mehta et al. (1995), who did not find age-related differences in MTR values, and from Armstrong et al. (2004), who reported an increase in MTR with age in the cingulate and the cerebral white matter with trends in the occipital and temporal lobes. Such conflicting findings may reflect differences in the regions examined, the acquisition sequences employed, and the approaches to MTR image analysis (e.g., whole brain MTR estimates vs. MTR values from regions of interest).

Lee et al. (2004) demonstrated that brain parenchymal volumes, lesion volumes on T_2 images, and peak height MTR changed with aging and that all of these measures correlated with cognitive functions. MTR and parenchymal volumes showed a direct correlation with cognitive scores, whereas lesion volumes showed an inverse correlation. In other studies, diffusion tensor measures (discussed later in this section) were found to be more sensitive to age-related changes than was conventional MTR.

Postmortem MTI and biochemical studies demonstrate that in the white matter, lower MTRs are associated with demyelination and low axonal density (van Waesberghe et al. 1999). Reductions in MTR are consistently identified in multiple sclerosis, which is characterized by demyelination and underlying axonal transections (Bjartmar et al. 1999; Grossman 1994; van Waesberghe et al. 1999). Postmortem studies corroborate that low MTR is associated with myelin and/or axonal loss (Bjartmar et al. 1999; Grossman 1994; van Waesberghe et al. 1999). In patients with multiple sclerosis, abnormal MTR has been described both in specific lesions and in normal-appearing white matter in which no lesions are visualized using standard imaging sequences (Loevner et al. 1995). MTR is also low in cerebral pontine myelinolysis and wallerian degeneration, thereby establishing it as a relatively reliable marker of myelin injury in the white matter (Lexa et al. 1994; Mehta et al. 1996; Silver et al. 1996). Within the realm of behavioral disorders, MTR reductions have been identified in patients diagnosed with chronic schizophrenia, dementia of the Alzheimer's type, and mild cognitive impairment (Foong et al. 2001; Kabani et al. 2002). The precise pathological substrates responsible for the reduction in MTR in these conditions remain unknown at the present time. The biochemical correlates of low MTRs in the gray matter are less clear, although physiological impairments to cell membranes and proteins together with neuronal and synaptic loss are offered as plausible explanations (Audoin et al. 2007).

Diffusion tensor imaging. Another imaging technique that has been useful for the study of white matter integrity and brain microstructural changes is DTI. This technique works on the principle that water diffuses randomly in unrestricted environments, resulting in isotropic movement (or movement that is equivalent in all directions). This movement is restrained in white matter tracts; thus, water diffusion tends to move along the axis of axon sheath, leading to anisotropy. One of the ways DTI can be quantified is through fractional anisotropy (FA), which represents a measure of directional coherence and, in white matter tracts, the degree of structural alignment. Another quantification technique is the apparent diffusion coefficient, which measures the average diffusion of water in a voxel.

Several studies have used DTI to examine age-related microstructural changes in white matter, including white matter that appears normal using more conventional MRI techniques. Most DTI studies to date, both cross-sectional and longitudinal, have shown regional decreases in FA associated with normal aging (Nusbaum et al. 2001; Pfefferbaum et al. 2000; Virta et al. 1999). Abe et al. (2002) found significant decrease in FA in the genu of corpus callosum with advancing age. This finding was confirmed in later studies (Camara et al. 2007). Age-related changes detected by DTI appear to have regional specificity. For example, in a study by Pfefferbaum et al. (2005), lower FA in the older study sample was localized to frontal regions, while inferior and posterior regions were relatively spared from age effects. Based on these findings, it has been hypothesized that an anterior-posterior gradient is associated with age-related FA decreases. This is in contrast to pathological studies that found a greater degree of posterior FA changes in diseases such as Alzheimer's dementia (Head et al. 2004).

Few studies have correlated changes seen with DTI with actual histopathology. It has been speculated that lower FA is associated with axonal loss, demyelination, and expansion of extracellular space (Moseley 2002; Salat et al. 2005).

An important observation is that although DTI represents a promising advance in MR methodology, a number of limitations restrict its interpretation and use. The chief limitations mentioned in the literature are partial volume effects and crossing fibers within voxels (Pfefferbaum and Sullivan 2003). These artifacts can artificially lower FA and thus cause spurious results. Newer techniques, such as high angular resolution diffusion imaging, address some of these limitations and may allow for more detailed, accurate measurement of white matter integrity (Tuch et al. 2002).

The functional significance of DTI-detected microstructural changes has been explored in studies that demonstrate the relationship between cognition and FA. Because decreases in FA represent a likely disruption in critical circuits connecting important regions in cortex to subcortical and limbic systems, a wide variety of cognitive domains could be adversely affected. In an early study describing declines in FA associated with age, executive function (determined by the Trail Making Test) was significantly correlated with FA (O'Sullivan et al. 2001). Another study showed that processing speed and reasoning were significantly correlated with FA in frontal white matter (Stebbins et al. 2002). Response time was correlated with FA declines measured in the anterior limb of the internal capsule in a study comparing older and younger subjects (Madden et al. 2004). In addition, FA in the centrum semiovale was significantly correlated with performance on tasks of nonverbal reasoning, working memory, executive function, and information processing (Deary et al. 2006). Another study reinforced these findings, showing a significant relationship between working memory, information processing speed, executive function, and DTI measures in healthy middle-aged and elderly adults (Charlton et al. 2006).

Summary. Both MTI and DTI reveal that white matter integrity is compromised in the normal aging brain, even in brain tissue that appears normal on routine imaging. The neuropathological correlates of this disruption are thought to be related to demyelination and axonal loss. These findings from MTI and DTI are correlated with performance across a number of cognitive domains that involve frontal circuits.

Brain Biochemistry

In vivo magnetic resonance spectroscopy (MRS) is a noninvasive technique that provides a measure of biochemical metabolites in selected regions of the brain. MRS detects magnetic resonance signals from nuclei in molecules (except water) present in living tissues. In MRI, the image is generated from the signal derived from water hydrogen nuclei. MRS suppresses the water signal to measure metabolites in the tissue fluid. Magnetic field strengths are similar to those used in imaging studies, usually ranging from 1.5 to 4 teslas in human studies. Magnetic nuclear isotopes in a magnetic field produce a signal that can be represented by a characteristic spectrum (Figure 6–8). Each peak on the spectrum represents a metabolite of interest for a given nucleus.

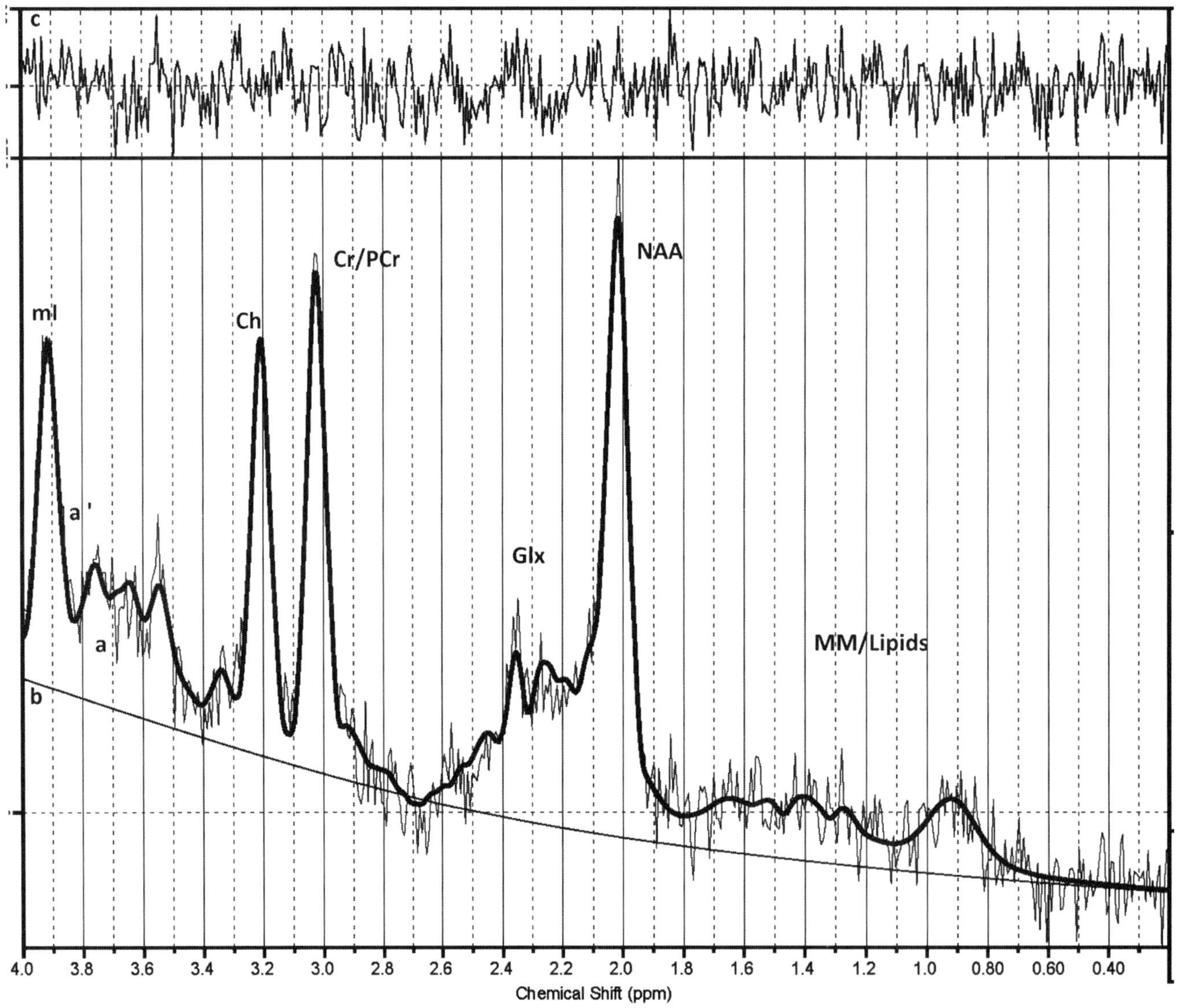

FIGURE 6–8. A sample water-suppressed 1H MR spectrum using a voxel size of 4 mL.

a′ = experimental and a = LC-Model fitted spectrum; b = baseline; c = noise predicted by the curve-fitting algorithm; Ch = choline; Cr/PCr = creatine/phosphocreatine; Glx = glutamate/glutamine; mI = myo-inositol; MM = macromolecules; NAA = *N*-acetylaspartate.

Several signal detection parameters determine the shape of a spectrum. One is the voxel size, which determines the region of tissue being studied and the concentration of metabolites measured. Another important parameter is relaxation time, which affects signal strength, because long T_1 and short T_2 are typically found in intracellular molecules with high molecular weights and thus can lead to weak signals. As a result of these factors, MRS is particularly useful for measuring small-molecular-weight molecules that are highly concentrated. Typical concentrations of metabolites detected by MRS are in the range of 4–10 mM. It is difficult to detect metabolites under 1 mM. These concentrations can be reported in absolute measures or as ratios to creatine concentrations, using creatine as an internal control (Thomas and Alger 1997).

Hydrogen or proton MRS is used to probe for the following neurochemicals: choline, creatine, *N*-acetylaspartate (NAA), myo-inositol, glutamate/glutamine, and γ-aminobutyric acid (GABA). The choline signal represents a composite of choline-containing metabolites such as phosphocholine, glycerophosphocholine, and phosphotidylcholine. These metabolites are involved in cell membrane integrity. NAA is generally viewed as a marker of neuronal viability and may represent a measure of neuronal volume, number, or function. Myo-inositol is seen as a marker of gliosis, and it is a storage form of the inositol phosphate second messenger system. Glutamate/glutamine and GABA are the most ubiquitous excitatory and inhibitory neurotransmitters, respectively.

Phosphorus MRS, or ^{31}P MRS, can be used to measure the following metabolites: adenosine triphosphate, phosphomonoesters (phosphorylcholine, phosphorylethanolamine, and glycerophosphate), phosphodiesters (glycerylphosphorylethanolamine, glycerylphosphorylserine, and glycerylphosphorylinositol), phosphocreatine, and inorganic phosphate. These metabolites may provide insight into the bioenergetics of neuronal processes. Other less commonly used nuclei for MRS include carbon, lithium, fluorine, and sodium.

Several studies have used MRS to study neurochemical changes associated with normal, healthy aging, with mixed results. Some early studies using MRS were generally negative, perhaps owing to methodological limitations (Chang et al. 1996; Saunders et al. 1999). However, in a study comparing brain uptake of choline using proton MRS in younger subjects (mean age 32) and older subjects (mean age 73), Cohen et al. (1995) found that older subjects had decreased choline uptake. Brooks et al. (2001) found a significant decline in frontal lobe NAA in a comparison of subjects from age 20 to age 70, with an overall decrease of 12%. This decline was interpreted as a decrease in neuronal volume, number, or function, because NAA is thought to be a marker of neuronal viability. These changes are not limited to frontal white matter, as demonstrated in a study that showed age-related decreases in NAA, NAA/choline, and NAA/creatine ratios across 30 different voxels (Angelie et al. 2001). In addition, decreases in hippocampal NAA associated with age have also been detected in a study using healthy subjects ranging in age from 36 to 85 years (Schuff et al. 1999). In a longitudinal study examining similar measures over a 3-year period, Ross et al. (2006) demonstrated that no significant changes occurred in brain metabolites, with the exception of myo-inositol, or cognitive function over the time period studied.

In a comprehensive review and meta-analysis of MRS studies in normal aging, Haga et al. (2009) found that although the majority of studies showed no significant change in metabolites with age, there was a trend toward an increase in frontal and parietal choline with increasing age, as well as a trend toward increases in parietal and occipital creatine with increasing age. Sailasuta et al. (2008) demonstrated that gender may differentiate age-related changes in brain metabolites; subcortical (particularly in basal ganglia) glutamate and parietal gray matter glutamate decreased with age in men but not in women.

The functional impact of age-related brain metabolic changes has also been studied. One of the first studies to show a relationship between brain metabolites and cognition in a healthy elderly population was done by Valenzuela et al. (2000). They showed that frontal white matter NAA concentrations were significantly correlated with performance on tests of executive function and attention. The association between frontal NAA and cognition has been replicated by Ross et al. (2005), showing correlation with a composite measure of information processing speed, attention, and visual memory. Other metabolites besides NAA have been correlated with cognitive function. In contrast to elderly depressed patients, in healthy elderly subjects, choline/creatine and myo-inositol/creatine levels were shown to be positively associated with performance on global cognition (Elderkin-Thompson et al. 2004). In a study of 82 adults ages 50–90 years, Charlton et al. (2007) found that total creatine increased with age and that creatine was significantly correlated with executive function, long-term memory, and fluid intelligence. The same study showed that although NAA levels were not correlated with age, NAA was significantly correlated with executive function.

In summary, the relationship between aging and changes in brain metabolites remains unclear, perhaps in part because of differences across studies in methodology (spatial location, study sample, acquisition parameters, etc.). However, there is a general trend toward an increase in membrane breakdown of products such as choline and myo-inositol and a decrease in neuronal measures such as glutamate and NAA associated with aging. These metabolite levels appear to be significantly correlated with global cognitive changes across several domains. Further study involving techniques to better resolve spectra, such as two-dimensional MRS, can lead to more accurate measurements of metabolites of interest (Thomas et al. 2001).

Key Points

- Brain imaging studies demonstrate that typical or normal aging is associated with a progressive decline in total and regional (particularly frontal) brain size, an increase in ventricular and cortical cerebrospinal fluid volume, an increase in the prevalence and severity of subcortical hyperintensities, alterations in white matter integrity, and possible disturbances in brain biochemistry. The rate of some of these changes appears to accelerate in late middle age.
- These findings vary considerably, depending on a plethora of methodological issues.
- Many of these age-related brain changes are associated with functional and neuropsychological decline.

Recommended Readings

Coffey CE: Anatomic imaging of the aging human brain: computed tomography and magnetic resonance imaging, in The American Psychiatric Press Textbook of Geriatric Neuropsychiatry, 2nd Edition. Edited by Coffey CE, Cummings JL. Washington, DC, American Psychiatric Press, 2000, pp 181–238

Fotenos AF, Mintun MA, Snyder AZ, et al: Brain volume decline in aging. Arch Neurol 65:113–120, 2008

Haga KK, Khor YP, Farrall A, et al: A systematic review of brain metabolite changes, measured with ^{1}H magnetic resonance spectroscopy, in healthy aging. Neurobiol Aging 30:353–363, 2009

Malloy P, Correia S, Stebbins G, et al: Neuroimaging of white matter in aging and dementia. Clinical Neuropsychol 21:73–109, 2007

References

Abe O, Aoki S, Hayashi N, et al: Normal aging in the central nervous system: quantitative MR diffusion-tensor analysis. Neurobiol Aging 23:433–441, 2002

American Psychiatric Association: Practice guideline for the treatment of patients with bipolar disorder (revision). Am J Psychiatry 159(suppl):1–50, 2002

American Psychiatric Association: Practice guideline for the treatment of patients with schizophrenia, second edition. Am J Psychiatry 161(suppl):1–56, 2004

Angelie E, Bonmartin A, Boudraa A, et al: Regional differences and metabolic changes in normal aging of the human brain: proton MR spectroscopic imaging study. AJNR Am J Neuroradiol 22: 119–127, 2001

Armstrong CL, Traipe E, Hunter JV, et al: Age-related, regional, hemispheric, and medial-lateral differences in myelin integrity in vivo in the normal adult brain. AJNR Am J Neuroradiol 25: 977–984, 2004

Audoin B, Davies G, Rashid W, et al: Voxel-based analysis of grey matter magnetization transfer ratio maps in early relapsing remitting multiple sclerosis. Mult Scler 13:483–489, 2007

Barbosa S, Blumhardt LD, Roberts N, et al: Magnetic resonance relaxation time mapping in multiple sclerosis: normal appearing white matter and the "invisible" lesion load. Magn Reson Imaging 12:33–42, 1994

Bjartmar C, Yin X, Trapp BD: Axonal pathology in myelin disorders. J Neurocytol 28:383–395, 1999

Brooks JC, Roberts N, Kemp GJ, et al: A proton magnetic resonance spectroscopy study of age-related changes in frontal lobe metabolite concentrations. Cereb Cortex 11:598–605, 2001

Camara E, Bodammer N, Rodriguez-Fornells A, et al: Age-related water diffusion changes in human brain: a voxel-based approach. Neuroimage 34:1588–1599, 2007

Campbell JJ, Coffey CE: Neuropsychiatric significance of subcortical hyperintensity. J Neuropsychiatry Clin Neurosci 13:261–288, 2001

Cardenas VA, Du AT, Hardin D, et al: Comparison of methods for measuring longitudinal brain change in cognitive impairment and dementia. Neurobiol Aging 24:537–544, 2003

Carlson NE, Moore MM, Dame A, et al: Trajectories of brain loss in aging and the development of cognitive impairment. Neurology 70:828–833, 2008

Carmichael O, Schwarz C, Drucker D, et al: Longitudinal changes in white matter disease and cognition in the first year of the Alzheimer Disease Neuroimaging Initiative. Arch Neurol 67:1370–1378, 2010

Chan D, Fox NC, Jenkins R, et al: Rates of global and regional cerebral atrophy in AD and frontotemporal dementia. Neurology 57:1756–1763, 2001

Chang L, Ernst T, Poland RE, et al: In vivo proton magnetic resonance spectroscopy of the normal aging human brain. Life Sci 58:2049–2056, 1996

Charlton RA, Barrick TR, McIntyre DJ, et al: White matter damage on diffusion tensor imaging correlates with age-related cognitive decline. Neurology 66:217–222, 2006

Charlton RA, McIntyre DJ, Howe FA, et al: The relationship between white matter brain metabolites and cognition in normal aging: the GENIE study. Brain Res 1164:108–116, 2007

Coffey CE: Anatomic imaging of the aging human brain: computed tomography and magnetic resonance imaging, in The American Psychiatric Press Textbook of Geriatric Neuropsychiatry, 2nd Edition. Edited by Coffey CE, Cummings JL. Washington DC, American Psychiatric Press, 2000, pp 181–238

Coffey CE, Wilkinson WE, Parashos IA, et al: Quantitative cerebral anatomy of the aging human brain: a cross-sectional study using magnetic resonance imaging. Neurology 42:527–536, 1992

Coffey CE, Wilkinson WE, Weiner RD, et al: Quantitative cerebral anatomy in depression: a controlled magnetic resonance imaging study. Arch Gen Psychiatry 50:7–16, 1993

Coffey CE, Lucke JF, Saxton JA, et al: Sex differences in brain aging: a quantitative magnetic resonance imaging study. Arch Neurol 55:169–179, 1998

Coffey CE, Saxton JA, Ratcliff G, et al: Relation of education to brain size in normal aging: implications for the reserve hypothesis. Neurology 53:189–196, 1999

Cohan RH, Matsumoto JS, Quaglianao PV: ACR Manual on Contrast Media, 4th Edition. Reston, VA, American College of Radiology, 1998

Cohen BM, Renshaw PF, Stoll AL, et al: Decreased brain choline uptake in older adults: an in vivo proton magnetic resonance spectroscopy study. JAMA 274:902–907, 1995

Cohen RM, Small C, Lalonde F, et al: Effect of apolipoprotein E genotype on hippocampal volume loss in aging healthy women. Neurology 57:2223–2228, 2001

Deary IJ, Bastin ME, Pattie A, et al: White matter integrity and cognition in childhood and old age. Neurology 66:505–512, 2006

DeCarli C, Massaro J, Harvey D, et al: Measures of brain morphology and infarction in the Framingham Heart Study: establishing what is normal. Neurobiol Aging 26:491–510, 2005

Driscoll I, Davatzikos C, An Y, et al: Longitudinal pattern of regional brain volume change differentiates normal aging from MCI. Neurology 72:1906–1913, 2009

Du AT, Schuff N, Zhu XP, et al: Atrophy rates of entorhinal cortex in AD and normal aging. Neurology 60:481–486, 2003

Elderkin-Thompson V, Thomas MA, Binesh N, et al: Brain metabolites and cognitive function among older depressed and healthy individuals using 2D MR spectroscopy. Neuropsychopharmacology 29:2251–2257, 2004

Eng J, Ceckler TL, Balaban RS: Quantitative ^{1}H magnetization transfer imaging in vivo. Magn Reson Med 17:304–314, 1991

Enzinger C, Fazekas F, Matthews PM, et al: Risk factors for progression of brain atrophy in aging: six-year follow-up of normal subjects. Neurology 64:1704–1711, 2005

Erhart SM, Young AS, Marder SR, et al: Clinical utility of magnetic resonance imaging radiographs for suspected organic syndromes in adult psychiatry. J Clin Psychiatry 66:968–973, 2005

Foong J, Symms MR, Barker GJ, et al: Neuropathological abnormalities in schizophrenia: evidence from magnetization transfer imaging. Brain 124:882–892, 2001

Fotenos AF, Snyder AZ, Girton LE, et al: Normative estimates of cross-sectional and longitudinal brain volume decline in aging and AD. Neurology 64:1032–1039, 2005

Fotenos AF, Mintun MA, Snyder AZ, et al: Brain volume decline in aging. Arch Neurol 65:113–120, 2008

Fox NC, Freeborough PA: Brain atrophy progression measured from registered serial MRI: validation and application to Alzheimer's disease. J Magn Reson Imaging 7:1069–1075, 1997

Gado M, Hughes CP, Danziger W, et al: Aging, dementia, and brain atrophy: a longitudinal computed tomography study. AJNR Am J Neuroradiol 4:699–973, 1983

Ge Y, Grossman RI, Babb JS, et al: Age-related total gray matter and white matter changes in normal adult brain, part II: quantitative magnetization transfer ratio histogram analysis. Am J Neuroradiol 23:1334–1341, 2002

Goldstein IB, Bartzokis G, Guthrie D, et al: Ambulatory blood pressure and the brain: a 5-year follow-up. Neurology 64:1846–1852, 2005

Good CD, Johnsrude IS, Ashburner J, et al: A voxel-based morphometric study of ageing in 465 normal adult human brains. Neuroimage 14:21–36, 2001

Grossman RI: Magnetization transfer in multiple sclerosis. Ann Neurol 36(suppl):S97–S99, 1994

Haga KK, Khor YP, Farrall A, et al: A systematic review of brain metabolite changes, measured with ^{1}H magnetic resonance spectroscopy, in healthy aging. Neurobiol Aging 30:353–363, 2009

Hall P, Adami HO, Trichopoulos D, et al: Effect of low doses of ionizing radiation in infancy on cognitive function in adulthood: Swedish population based cohort study. BMJ 328:19, 2004

Head D, Buckner RL, Shimony JS, et al: Differential vulnerability of anterior white matter in nondemented aging with minimal acceleration in dementia of the Alzheimer type: evidence from diffusion tensor imaging. Cereb Cortex 14:410–423, 2004

Henkelman RM, Stanisz GJ, Graham SJ: Magnetization transfer in MRI: a review. NMR Biomed 14:57–64, 2001

Hofman PA, Kemerink GJ, Jolles J, et al: Quantitative analysis of magnetization transfer images of the brain: effect of closed head injury, age and sex on white matter. Magn Reson Med 42:803–806, 1999

Jack CR Jr, Shiung MM, Gunter JL, et al: Comparison of different MRI brain atrophy rate measures with clinical disease progression in AD. Neurology 62:591–600, 2004

Jack CR Jr, Shiung MM, Weigand SD, et al: Brain atrophy rates predict subsequent clinical conversion in normal elderly and amnestic MCI. Neurology 65:1227–1231, 2005

Jack CR Jr, Weigand SD, Shiung MM, et al: Atrophy rates accelerate in amnestic mild cognitive impairment. Neurology 70:1740–1752, 2008

Jernigan TL, Archibald SL, Notestine CF, et al: Effects of age on tissues and regions of the cerebrum and cerebellum. Neurobiol Aging 22:581–594, 2001

Kabani NJ, Sled JG, Chertkow H: Magnetization transfer ratio in mild cognitive impairment and dementia of Alzheimer's type. Neuroimage 15:604–610, 2002

Knopman DS, DeKosky ST, Cummings JL, et al: Practice parameter: diagnosis of dementia. Neurology 56:1143–1153, 2001

Lee KY, Kim TK, Park M, et al: Age-related changes in conventional and magnetization transfer MR imaging in elderly people: comparison with neurocognitive performance. Korean J Radiol 5:96–101, 2004

Lexa FJ, Grossman RI, Rosenquist AC: Dyke Award paper. MR of wallerian degeneration in the feline visual system: characterization by magnetization transfer rate with histopathologic correlation. AJNR Am J Neuroradiol 15:201–212, 1994

Liu RS, Lemieux L, Bell GS, et al: A longitudinal study of brain morphometrics using quantitative magnetic resonance imaging and difference image analysis. Neuroimage 20:22–33, 2003

Loevner LA, Grossman RI, Cohen JA, et al: Microscopic disease in normal-appearing white matter on conventional MR images in patients with multiple sclerosis: assessment with magnetization-transfer measurements. Radiology 196:511–515, 1995

Longstreth WT Jr, Arnold AM, Manolio TA, et al: Clinical correlates of ventricular and sulcal size on cranial magnetic resonance imaging of 3,301 elderly people. The Cardiovascular Health Study. Collaborative Research Group. Neuroepidemiology 19:30–42, 2000

Madden DJ, Whiting WL, Huettel SA, et al: Diffusion tensor imaging of adult age differences in cerebral white matter: relation to response time. Neuroimage 21:1174–1181, 2004

Malloy P, Correia S, Stebbins G, et al: Neuroimaging of white matter in aging and dementia. Clin Neuropsychol 21:73–109, 2007

McDonald CR, McEvoy LK, Gharapetian L, et al: Regional rates of neocortical atrophy from normal aging to early Alzheimer disease. Neurology 73:457–465, 2009

Mehta RC, Pike GB, Enzmann DR: Magnetization transfer MR of the normal adult brain. AJNR Am J Neuroradiol 16:2085–2091, 1995

Mehta RC, Pike GB, Enzmann DR: Measure of magnetization transfer in multiple sclerosis demyelinating plaques, white matter ischemic lesions, and edema. AJNR Am J Neuroradiol 17:1051–1055, 1996

Mezzapesa DM, Rocca MA, Pagani E, et al: Evidence of subtle gray-matter pathologic changes in healthy elderly individuals with nonspecific white matter hyperintensities. Arch Neurol 60:1109–1112, 2003

Moseley M: Diffusion tensor imaging and aging: a review. NMR Biomed 15:553–560, 2002

Mueller EA, Moore MM, Kerr DCR, et al: Brain volume preserved in healthy elderly through the eleventh decade. Neurology 51: 1555–1562, 1998

Mungas D, Harvey D, Reed BR, et al: Longitudinal volumetric MRI change and rate of cognitive decline. Neurology 65:565–571, 2005

Nusbaum AO, Tang CY, Buchsbaum MS, et al: Regional and global changes in cerebral diffusion with normal aging. AJNR Am J Neuroradiol 22:136–142, 2001

O'Sullivan M, Jones DK, Summers PE, et al: Evidence for cortical "disconnection" as a mechanism of age-related cognitive decline. Neurology 57:632–638, 2001

Pfefferbaum A, Sullivan EV, Rosenbloom MJ, et al: A controlled study of cortical gray matter and ventricular changes in alcoholic men over a 5-year interval. Arch Gen Psychiatry 55:905–912, 1998

Pfefferbaum A, Sullivan EV, Hedehus M, et al: Age-related decline in brain white matter anisotropy measured with spatially corrected echo-planar diffusion tensor imaging. Magn Reson Med 44:259–268, 2000

Pfefferbaum A, Sullivan EV, Carmelli D: Morphological changes in aging brain structures are differentially affected by time-linked environmental influences despite strong genetic stability. Neurobiol Aging 25:175–183, 2004

Pfefferbaum A, Adalsteinsson E, Sullivan EV: Frontal circuitry degradation marks healthy adult aging: evidence from diffusion tensor imaging. Neuroimage 26:891–899, 2005

Podewils LJ, Guallar E, Beauchamp N, et al: Physical activity and white matter lesion progression: assessment using MRI. Neurology 68:1223–1226, 2007

Raz N, Rodrigue KM, Head D, et al: Differential aging of the medial temporal lobe: a study of a five-year change. Neurology 62:433–438, 2004

Raz N, Lindenberger U, Rodrigue KM, et al: Regional brain changes in aging health adults: general trends, individual differences and modifiers. Cereb Cortex 15:1676–1689, 2005

Resnick SM, Goldszal AF, Davatzikos C, et al: One-year age changes in MRI brain volumes in older adults. Cereb Cortex 10:464–472, 2000

Resnick SM, Pham DL, Kraut MA, et al: Longitudinal magnetic resonance imaging studies of older adults: a shrinking brain. J Neurosci 23:3295–3301, 2003

Roman GC: Age-associated white matter lesions and dementia. Arch Neurol 61:1503–1504, 2004

Ross AJ, Sachdev PS, Wen W, et al: Cognitive correlates of ^{1}H MRS measures in the healthy elderly brain. Brain Res Bull 66:9–16, 2005

Ross AJ, Sachdev PS, Wen W, et al: Longitudinal changes during aging using proton magnetic resonance spectroscopy. J Gerontol A Biol Sci Med Sci 61:291–298, 2006

Sachdev P, Wen W, Chen X, et al: Progression of white matter hyperintensities in elderly individuals over 3 years. Neurology 68:214–222, 2007

Sailasuta N, Ernst T, Chang L: Regional variations and the effects of age and gender on glutamate concentrations in the human brain. Magn Reson Imaging 26:667–675, 2008

Salat DH, Tuch DS, Greve DN, et al: Age-related alterations in white matter microstructure measured by diffusion tensor imaging. Neurobiol Aging 26:1215–1227, 2005

Saunders DE, Howe FA, van den Boogaart A, et al: Aging of the adult human brain: in vivo quantitation of metabolite content with proton magnetic resonance spectroscopy. J Magn Reson Imaging 9:711–716, 1999

Scahill RI, Frost C, Jenkins R, et al: A longitudinal study of brain volume changes in normal aging using serial registered magnetic resonance imaging. Arch Neurol 60:989–994, 2003

Schmidt R, Fazekas F, Kapeller P, et al: MRI white matter hyperintensities: three-year follow-up of the Austrian Stroke Prevention Study. Neurology 53:132–139, 1999

Schmidt R, Enzinger C, Ropele S, et al: Progression of cerebral white matter lesions: 6-year results of the Austrian Stroke Prevention Study. Lancet 361:2046–2048, 2003

Schmidt R, Scheltens PH, Erkinjuntti T, et al: White matter lesion progression: a surrogate endpoint for trials in cerebral small-vessel disease. Neurology 63:139–144, 2004

Schuff N, Amend DL, Knowlton R, et al: Age-related metabolite changes and volume loss in the hippocampus by magnetic resonance spectroscopy and imaging. Neurobiol Aging 20:279–285, 1999

Shear PK, Sullivan EV, Mathalon DH, et al: Longitudinal volumetric computed tomographic analysis of regional brain changes in normal aging and Alzheimer's disease. Arch Neurol 52:392–402, 1995

Silbert LC, Nelson C, Howieson DB, et al: Impact of white matter hyperintensity volume progression on rate of cognitive and motor decline. Neurology 71:108–113, 2008

Silbert LC, Howieson DB, Dodge H, et al: Cognitive impairment risk: white matter hyperintensity progression matters. Neurology 73: 120–125, 2009

Silver NC, Barker GJ, MacManus DG, et al: Decreased magnetisation transfer ratio due to demyelination: a case of central pontine myelinolysis. J Neurol Neurosurg Psychiatry 61:208–209, 1996

Spilt A, Goekoop R, Westendorp RG, et al: Not all age-related white matter hyperintensities are the same: a magnetization transfer imaging study. AJNR Am J Neuroradiol 27:1964–1968, 2006

Stebbins GT, Carrillo MC, Dorfman J, et al: Aging effects on memory encoding in the frontal lobes. Psychol Aging 17:44–55, 2002

Sullivan EV, Pfefferbaum A, Adalsteinsson E, et al: Differential rates of regional brain change in callosal and ventricular size: a 4-year longitudinal MRI study of elderly men. Cereb Cortex 12:438–445, 2002

Tang Y, Whitman GT, Lopez I, et al: Brain volume changes on longitudinal magnetic resonance imaging in normal older people. J Neuroimaging 11:393–400, 2001

Thomas MA, Alger J: Magnetic resonance spectroscopy of the brain, in Minimal Invasive Therapy of the Brain. Edited by Desalles AAF, Lufkin R. New York, Thime Medical, 1997, pp 63–77

Thomas MA, Yue K, Binesh N, et al: Localized two-dimensional shift correlated MR spectroscopy of human brain. Magn Reson Med 46:58–67, 2001

Tisserand DJ, van Boxtel MPJ, Pruessner MC, et al: A voxel-based morphometric study to determine individual differences in gray matter density associated with age and cognitive change over time. Cereb Cortex 14:966–973, 2004

Tuch DS, Reese TG, Wiegell MR, et al: High angular resolution diffusion imaging reveals intravoxel white matter fiber heterogeneity. Magn Reson Med 48:577–582, 2002

Valenzuela MJ, Sachdev PS, Wen W, et al: Dual voxel proton magnetic resonance spectroscopy in the healthy elderly: subcortical-frontal axonal *N*-acetylaspartate levels are correlated with fluid cognitive abilities independent of structural brain changes. Neuroimage 12:747–756, 2000

van Waesberghe JH, Kamphorst W, De Groot CJ, et al: Axonal loss in multiple sclerosis lesions: magnetic resonance imaging insights into substrates of disability. Ann Neurol 46:747–754, 1999

Vemuri P, Wiste HJ, Weigand SD, et al: Serial MRI and CSF biomarkers in normal aging, MCI, and AD. Neurology 75:143–151, 2010

Vermeer SE, Prins ND, den Heijer T, et al: Silent brain infarcts and the risk of dementia and cognitive decline. N Engl J Med 348:1215–1222, 2003

Vernooij MW, Ikram MA, Tanghe HL, et al: Incidental findings on brain MRI in the general population. N Engl J Med 357:1821–1828, 2007

Virta A, Barnett A, Pierpaoli C: Visualizing and characterizing white matter fiber structure and architecture in the human pyramidal tract using diffusion tensor MRI. Magn Reson Imaging 17:1121–1133, 1999

Wahlund LO, Almkvist O, Basun H, et al: MRI in successful aging, a 5-year follow-up study from the eighth to ninth decade of life. Magn Reson Imaging 14:601–608, 1996

Weiner MW: Expanding ventricles may detect preclinical Alzheimer disease. Neurology 70:824–825, 2008

Whitman GT, Tang Y, Lin A, et al: A prospective study of cerebral white matter abnormalities in older people with gait dysfunction. Neurology 57:990–994, 2001

APPENDIX 6–1. Representative longitudinal imaging studies of "normal" human brain aging

Study	Subjects	Imaging and measurement technique	Findings
Gado et al. 1983	24 elderly community-dwelling control subjects for a study of Alzheimer's disease Age 71±4.3 years 10 M; 14 W No history of neurological or psychiatric disorders (at baseline or follow-up), and no communicating hydrocephalus on baseline CT	CT Manual linear (n=24) and volume (subgroup, n=12) measurements from axial images Number of raters and rater reliabilities not specified Scan repeated at 12.9±2.9 months (different scanner for linear measures; same scanner for volume measures)	Ratio of ventricular volume to IV increased significantly by an average of 3.7%/year; no significant changes in linear measures of ventricular size (VBR, third ventricular ratio, frontal horn ratio). Ratio of sulcal CSF volume to IV increased significantly by an average of 13%/year. Interactions with gender or laterality were not reported.
Shear et al. 1995	35 healthy community-dwelling control subjects for a study of Alzheimer's disease Age 67.4±7.4 years 23 M; 12 W No history of major medical, neurological, or psychiatric illness (at baseline or follow-up)	CT (one of two identical scanners) Blinded volume measurements from six contiguous axial slices (10 mm thick) using computer-assisted pixel segmentation High rater reliabilities Scan repeated at 2.6±0.96 years	When the analysis controlled for a longitudinal method error in the scans, CSF volumes of frontal sulci increased by ~14%/year, sylvian fissure by ~58%/year, parieto-occipital sulci by ~9%/year, and ventricular system by ~4.9%/year; no regional differences in age-related rates of change. Interactions with gender were not reported.
Wahlund et al. 1996	13 "successfully aged" elderly community-dwelling volunteers Age 79 years (range 76–83 years) 4 M; 9 W Healthy with normal cognition at all assessments	MRI (0.02 tesla at baseline and time 2; 0.5 tesla at time 3); spin echo acquisition sequence Visual ratings (3-point scale) of ventricular size and of CSF spaces (6-point scale) from proton density and T_2-weighted axial images (12 sliced, 5 mm thick, 2 mm gap) Visual ratings (6-point scale) of SH from T_2-weighted images Scanning repeated at 2 years and 5 years	Ventricular size increased by ~7% of the maximum rating/year. Frontal CSF space increased by ~3% of the maximum rating/year; no change in temporal or parieto-occipital CSF spaces. "Mild" SH was present in 11 of 13 subjects at baseline; 9 subjects showed mild (~5.6% of the maximum rating/year) progression of the lesions at 5 years in deep white matter and basal ganglia, but not in the periventricular or infratentorial white matter.
Fox and Freeborough 1997	19 healthy control subjects for a study of Alzheimer's disease Age 50.3±7.9 years 11 M; 8 W No memory complaints, and no memory deficits on formal testing; mean MMSE=29	MRI (1.5 tesla); spoiled gradient echo acquisition sequence Volume measurements using computer-assisted brain boundary shift integral, of 124 contiguous coronal images (1.5 mm thick) Scanning repeated at 6–30 months	Mean whole brain volume decreased by 0.24%±0.32%/year.

APPENDIX 6–1. Representative longitudinal imaging studies of "normal" human brain aging *(continued)*

Study	Subjects	Imaging and measurement technique	Findings
Mueller et al. 1998	46 healthy elderly participants in the Oregon Brain Aging Study Ages 65–74 years (6 M; 5 W), 75–84 years (8 M; 7 W), and 85–95 years (9 M; 11 W) All functionally independent, MMSE≥24, and free of major medical and neurological illness, as well as depression (at baseline and follow-up) Handedness not specified	MRI (1.5 tesla); multislice spin echo acquisition sequence Volume measurements using computer-assisted pixel segmentation and manual tracing of contiguous T_1-weighted coronal images (4 mm thick) Excellent interrater reliabilities Scanning repeated annually or biannually over a mean of 5 years (range 3–9 years)	Significant increases were seen in lateral ventricular volume (~4%/year, M=W) for all three age groups. Significant volume decreases were seen in multiple regions depending on the age group, but primarily in hippocampus (~1%–2%/year) and parieto-occipital region.
Pfefferbaum et al. 1998	28 healthy M as control subjects for a study of alcoholism Age 51±13.8 years (21–68 years) No major medical, neurological, or psychiatric illness (at baseline or follow-up) Left-handers included (*n* not specified)	MRI (1.5 tesla); spin echo acquisition sequence Blinded volume measurements derived from semiautomated pixel segmentation of intermediate and T_2-weighted axial images (n=17–20, 5 mm thick, 2.5 mm interscan gap) Scanning repeated at 61.04 ± 1.36 months (range 55–62 months)	Volume of lateral ventricles increased ~4%/year; no increase in cortical sulcal CSF volume. Aging was associated with decreases in total cortical gray matter and in gray matter of prefrontal and posterior parieto-occipital regions.
Schmidt et al. 1999, 2003, 2004	296 community-dwelling asymptomatic adults in Austrian Stroke Prevention Study Age 50–75 years at baseline No history of neuropsychiatric disease, and normal neurological examination	MRI (1.5 tesla); multislice spin echo acquisition sequence Unblinded clinical ratings (3-point scale) and blinded volume measures using trace methodology, from contiguous T_2-weighted axial slices (5 mm thick) Scanning repeated at 3 years (Schmidt et al. 1999) and 6 years (Schmidt et al. 2003)	Subjects with mild SH at baseline showed minimal progression in SH rating or volume. Subjects with more extensive SH at baseline showed progression of lesion volume (0.45–1.55 mL/year); lesion progression associated with age and hypertension.

APPENDIX 6–1. Representative longitudinal imaging studies of "normal" human brain aging *(continued)*

Study	Subjects	Imaging and measurement technique	Findings
Resnick et al. 2000, 2003	92 older adults without dementia from Baltimore Longitudinal Study of Aging Age 59–85 years at baseline 50 M; 42 W Free of CNS disease, metastatic cancer, and severe cardiovascular or pulmonary disease	MRI (1.5 tesla) on two similarly configured scanners; multislice spoiled GRASS acquisition sequence Volume measurements using semiautomated pixel segmentation (RAVENS) of T_1-weighted reformatted axial images (1.5 mm thick), by raters with high test-retest correlations Scanning repeated at 2 years and 4 years after baseline	Rates of tissue loss were 0.5%/year for total brain volume, 0.002 mL/year for gray matter volume, and 0.003 mL/year for white matter volume. Tissue loss was greater for frontal (2.9%/year) and parietal (1.3%/year) lobe regions than for temporal (1.2%/year) and occipital (1%/year) regions. Ventricular volume increased by 4%/year, with higher rates in older individuals. No gender differences in age-related changes were found.
Chan et al. 2001	27 older adult control subjects for study of Alzheimer's disease Age 59.6±11.7 years at baseline Gender not specified No "subjective cognitive problems," MMSE≥28/30	MRI (1.5 tesla); multislice, spoiled gradient echo acquisition sequence Volume measurements using computer-assisted brain boundary shift integral, of contiguous T_1-weighted coronal images (1.5 mm thick), by blind raters with high reproducibility Scanning repeated at mean of 12.8 months (range 3.6–45.1 months) on same scanner, with same acquisition parameters	Annual volume loss was 0.5%±0.4% for whole brain, 0.3%±0.8% for left anterior quadrant, 0.5%±0.7% for left posterior quadrant, 0.2%±0.7% for right anterior quadrant, and 0.4%±0.5% for right posterior quadrant. There were no effects of age or gender on the rates of atrophy.
Cohen et al. 2001	25 healthy older W with normal cognition 9 *APOE*E4*-negative, age 60.6±10.2 years 16 *APOE*E4*-positive, age 55.1±6.0 years	MRI (1.5 tesla); T_1-weighted 3D gradient echo with RF spoiling acquisition sequence Volume measurements using interactive computer-assisted pixel segmentation (Medx) of cerebrum and hippocampus from contiguous sagittal images (1.5 mm thick), by single-blinded rater with high reliability Scanning repeated at 2 years	Annual hippocampal volume loss was greater in the allele-positive group (2.32%±1.75%) than the allele-negative group (0.77%±1.02%). No relation of hippocampal atrophy to neuropsychological test performance was found. The annual percentage of decline in total cerebral volume did not differ between the allele-positive group (1.02%±3.39%) and the allele-negative group (–.043%±1.02%).

APPENDIX 6–1. Representative longitudinal imaging studies of "normal" human brain aging *(continued)*

Study	Subjects	Imaging and measurement technique	Findings
Tang et al. 2001	66 healthy elderly community-dwelling control subjects in study of dementia Age 78.9±3.3 years (range 74–87 years) 34 M; 32 W At both baseline and follow-up, no history of cardiovascular, cerebrovascular, renal, or severe musculoskeletal disease; normal neurological examination; MMSE ≥26	MRI (1.5 tesla); spin echo acquisition sequence Volume measurements (Cavalieri stereological method) from T_2-weighted axial images (5 mm thick, 1.5 mm interscan gap) by raters with high reliability Scan repeated 3–5 years later on same scanners (but with upgraded hardware and software)	The annual rates of tissue loss were 2.1%±1.6% for cerebral volume and 1.2%±2.2% for cerebellar volume. The average annual increase in lateral ventricular volume was 5.6%±3.6%. No gender differences in age-related changes were found. Cross-sectional analysis of baseline and follow-up scans found no relation between age and brain volume.
Whitman et al. 2001	70 community-dwelling participants in a prospective study of gait and balance in the elderly Age 79±4 years (range 74–88 years)	MRI (1.5 tesla); fast spin echo acquisition sequence Blinded volume estimates of SH using the Cavalieri point grid technique, from 3 consecutive T_2-weighted axial slices (5 mm thick, 1.5 mm gap) Scanning repeated at 4–5 years	SH volume increased by ~8.9%/year; most subjects showed minimal change in SH volume; increase in SH volume was related to baseline SH volume, but not to gender or hypertension. Progression of SH volume was associated with gait and balance dysfunction.
Sullivan et al. 2002	215 community-dwelling elderly men Age 71.9±2.7 years (range 70–80 years) at baseline MMSE 27.5±2.2 201 were right-handed	MRI (1.5 tesla); spin echo acquisition sequence Semiautomated pixel segmentation (custom) used to measure corpus callosum area on T_1-weighted midsagittal slice (4 mm thick), and ventricular volume on three T_1-weighted coronal images (5 mm thick, contiguous), by raters with good reliabilities Scanning repeated at 4.0±0.4 years later	Aging was associated with callosal thinning (~0.9%/year; no regional variation) and lateral ventricular enlargement (2.9%/year; symmetrical). Thinning of splenium was related to decline in MMSE, and thinning of callosal body was related to decline in Stroop Test word reading. In a subsequent report (Pfefferbaum et al. 2004) of 142 of these subjects (34 monozygotic twin pairs, 37 dizygotic twin pairs), genetic factors were related to individual differences in brain structure, but not to age-related changes in the size of these structures.

APPENDIX 6–1. Representative longitudinal imaging studies of "normal" human brain aging *(continued)*

Study	Subjects	Imaging and measurement technique	Findings
Cardenas et al. 2003	16 cognitively normal elderly community-dwelling control subjects in study of Alzheimer's disease Age 76±5 years 10 M; 6 W	MRI (1.5 tesla); double spin echo and MPRAGE acquisition sequences Volume measurements of total brain size using several methods (computerized pixel segmentation, nonlinear warping, change in CSF/brain boundaries), hippocampal volume (semiautomated methods), and entorhinal cortex (manual) Scanning repeated 2.6±1.0 years (range 1–4 years) after baseline	Volume loss was 0.2%±0.1%/year for total brain, 0.9%±1.4%/year for cortical gray matter, 2.6%±2.2%/year for entorhinal cortex, and 1.8%±0.8%/year for hippocampus.
Du et al. 2003	23 elderly community-dwelling volunteers Age 76.5±7.9 years 16 M; 7 W Normal cognitive test scores, no psychiatric history	MRI (1.5 tesla); MPRAGE acquisition sequence Manual (trace) volume measurement of entorhinal cortex from contiguous T_1-weighted coronal sections (1.4 mm thick) Scanning repeated 1.8±0.6 years later	Aging was associated with an annual decline in volume of entorhinal cortex (normalized for total intracranial volume) of 1.4%±2.5% on left side and 1.4%±2.3% on right side; smaller baseline volume predicted greater atrophy.
Liu et al. 2003	90 healthy adult control subjects in longitudinal study of epilepsy Age 14–77 years 49 M; 41 W No history of substance abuse, significant CNS impairment, or head injury; no active neurological, psychiatric, or medical disorder that might affect the brain; no significant cerebral structural abnormalities on baseline MRI	MRI (1.5 tesla); 3D IR-SPGR acquisition sequence Volume measurements using a combination of manual and automated pixel segmentation (Exbrain, MRreg) of T_1-weighted contiguous coronal images (1.5 mm thick) Scanning repeated 3.5 years later, on same scanner	In cross-sectional analysis, age was associated with linear decrease in baseline total brain volume, total gray matter volume, and total cerebellar volume (all adjusted for total intracranial volume), but not hippocampal volume. Shrinkage was seen from age 35 to 54 in total brain volume (~0.2%/year) and white matter volume (~0.4%/year); and from age 55 in hippocampal volume (~0.7%/year); no changes in gray matter or cerebellar volume.

APPENDIX 6–1. Representative longitudinal imaging studies of "normal" human brain aging *(continued)*

Study	Subjects	Imaging and measurement technique	Findings
Scahill et al. 2003	39 healthy adults Age 31–84 years 18 M; 21 W No history of neurological problems or memory complaints or impairment; MMSE=29.6±0.7	MRI (1.5 tesla); volumetric multislice spin echo acquisition sequence Blinded volume measurements using a combination of semiautomated segmentation (MIDAS) and manual assessments of T_1-weighted contiguous coronal images (1.5 mm thick) Scanning repeated 356–754 days later on same scanner	When the analysis adjusted for IV, aging was associated with increased lateral ventricular volume; mean cross-sectional rates (0.5521 mL/year) were similar to longitudinal rates (0.650 mL/year). When the analysis adjusted for IV, aging was associated with decreased volume of whole brain (0.33%/year vs. 0.32%/year for cross-sectional vs. longitudinal studies), temporal lobes (0.35%/year vs. 0.68%/year), and hippocampus (0.35%/year vs. 0.82%/year).
Jack et al. 2004, 2005	91 cognitively healthy community-dwelling elderly from Mayo ADRC Age 81.9±7.5 years 36 M; 55 W	MRI (1.5 tesla); T_1-weighted volumetric SPGR acquisition sequence Computer-assisted volume measurement of whole brain and ventricles; manual tracing of hippocampal and entorhinal cortex volumes Scans repeated 1.4±0.3 years later (range 0.9–2.0 years)	Tissue loss was ~0.5%±0.7%/year for whole brain, ~5.0%±3.6%/year for entorhinal cortex, and ~1.7%±1.4%/year for hippocampus. Ventricular volume increased ~2.4%±2.0%/year. Higher rates of whole brain atrophy and ventricular enlargement were associated with a conversion to a more cognitively impaired state.
Raz et al. 2004, 2005	72 right-handed adult volunteers Age 52.6±14.1 years (range 20–77 years) at baseline 30 M; 42 W No "severe cardiovascular, neurological, or psychiatric conditions"; negative screen for dementia (MMSE≥26) and depression (GDQ≥15); all scans screened for "space-occupying lesions and significant cerebrovascular disease"	MRI (1.5 tesla); 3D spoiled gradient acquisition sequence Volume measurements from manual tracings of contiguous T_1-weighted axial images (1.3 mm thick), by blinded raters with good reliability Scanning repeated at mean of 5.27±0.3 years later (range 4.83–6.08 years), on same or two additional scanners	Aging was associated with shrinkage of volumes of caudate (0.75%/year), cerebellum (0.61%/year), hippocampus (0.79%/year), and association cortices (0.46%–0.91%/year); minimal change in entorhinal cortex (0.32%/year); and no change in primary visual cortex. Longitudinal measures of shrinkage exceeded cross-sectional estimates. Rate of shrinkage increased with age in some regions (hippocampus, prefrontal white matter). No sex differences in age effects were found, except for caudate (W>M). No relation of age effects to baseline brain volume, level of education, or change in cognitive status over follow-up interval were found. For the hippocampus, age effects were seen only in subjects with hypertension.

APPENDIX 6–1. Representative longitudinal imaging studies of "normal" human brain aging *(continued)*

Study	Subjects	Imaging and measurement technique	Findings
Enzinger et al. 2005	201 community-dwelling neurologically asymptomatic adults in Austrian Stroke Prevention Study Age 59.8±5.9 years 105 M; 96 W No history of neuropsychiatric disease, and normal neurological examination	MRI (1.5 tesla) on multiple scanners; multislice spin echo acquisition sequence Volume measurements using computer-assisted segmentation (SIENA) of T_2-weighted transverse images (5 mm thick) Visual global ratings (4-point scale) of WMH Scanning repeated 6 years later	Brain parenchymal fraction (parenchymal volume/parenchymal volume+CSF volume) decreased by 0.4%±0.29%/year (M=W); rate of brain atrophy accelerated with age. Rate of brain atrophy was related to hemoglobin A_{1C} and WMH score.
Fotenos et al. 2005, 2008	362 adults without dementia from Washington University ADRC Age 18–93 years 137 M; 225 W No stroke or depression	MRI (1.5 tesla); multislice MPRAGE acquisition sequence Volume measurements using computer segmentation of contiguous T_1-weighted axial slices (1.25 mm thick) 33 subjects received follow-up scanning (unclear if same scanner was used) an average of 3.1 times over an average of 4.3 years (range 3.1–6.5 years)	Cross-sectional data revealed a decline in whole brain volume (adjusted for total intracranial volume) of 0.22%/year between ages 20 and 80 years (0.24%/year for M; 0.2%/year for W). The rate of decline was greater (0.4%/year) in older subjects (ages 65–80 years) and in those with higher socioeconomic status. Rates in the longitudinal group were similar to those in the cross-sectional group.
Goldstein et al. 2005	121 healthy community-dwelling elderly volunteers Age 66.2±6 years at baseline 52 M; 69 W No serious current or prior illness	MRI (1.5 tesla); dual spin echo acquisition sequence Volume measurements using combination of manual and computer-assisted pixel segmentation, from contiguous T_2-weighted axial slices (3 mm thick); volumes expressed as a percentage of TIV. Scanning repeated at 4.9±0.63 years	On cross-sectional analysis at both baseline and follow-up, age was associated with higher percentage SH volume and smaller percentage total brain volume. On longitudinal analysis, percentage total brain volume decreased by ~0.62%/year. Percentage SH volume increased in white matter by ~35%/year and in insular cortex by ~10%/year. Volume changes were greater in older subjects and in those with higher blood pressure.

APPENDIX 6–1. Representative longitudinal imaging studies of "normal" human brain aging *(continued)*

Study	Subjects	Imaging and measurement technique	Findings
Mungas et al. 2005	58 older, cognitively normal community-dwelling adults Age 74.1±6.7 years 27 M; 31 W MMSE 29.0±1.4 (range 21–30); CDR score 0±2	MRI (1.5 tesla); spin echo acquisition sequence Computerized pixel segmentation followed by manual editing of axial segmented images (contiguous, 3 mm thick); manual tracing of lacunar and hippocampal volume; computerized regional analysis using the Talairach coordinate system Scanning repeated at 4 years (range 1.1–6.9 years)	Aging was associated with shrinkage of cortical gray matter (~0.6%/year) and hippocampus (~1.1%/year); decrease in lacunar volume (~0.002 mm^3/year); and increase in WMH volume (0.59 mm^3/year) (all volumes normalized for total intracranial volume). Decline in memory function was related to smaller baseline hippocampal volume and to greater decline in hippocampal volume. Decline in executive function was related to greater baseline cortical atrophy and to greater rates of cortical and hippocampal atrophy, as well as increasing lacunar volume.
Podewils et al. 2007	60 randomly selected elderly participants from the Cardiovascular Health Study Cognitive Cohort Age 77.3±5.8 years 23 M; 37 W Cognitively normal during median 5-year follow-up	MRI (1.0 tesla); double spin echo acquisition sequence Blinded visual ratings of periventricular and deep white matter SH from contiguous coronal T_2-weighted and proton density images, by single rater with good reliabilities Scanning repeated at median of 5 years.	Total periventricular SH score increased by ~9.6%/year, and total deep white matter SH score increased by ~18.9%/year. Physical activity (assessed with Minnesota Leisure Time Questionnaire) was not associated with less SH progression.
Sachdev et al. 2007	51 healthy elderly community-dwelling control subjects in the Sydney Stroke Study Mean age 71 years (range 58–85 years) 26 M; 25 W Living independently, with no history of neurological or psychiatric disorder	MRI (1.5 tesla) Volume measurement of periventricular and deep white matter SH, using semiautomated pixel segmentation of contiguous T_2-weighted coronal images (4 mm thick) Scanning repeated at 3 years	Aging was associated with increase in total SH volume (13%/year), periventricular SH volume (10%/year), and deep white matter SH volume (15%/year). SH progression was significant in frontal, temporal, and parietal regions, but not in occipital region or cerebellum. SH progression was related to baseline SH volume, but not to age, sex, or cardiovascular risk factors.

APPENDIX 6–1. Representative longitudinal imaging studies of "normal" human brain aging *(continued)*

Study	Subjects	Imaging and measurement technique	Findings
Carlson et al. 2008	79 healthy elderly participants in the Oregon Brain Aging Study (overlap with subjects in Mueller et al. 1998) Age 65–100 years at baseline Free of major medical illness; MMSE >23	MRI (1.5 tesla); multislice spin echo acquisition sequence Blinded volume measurements using semiautomated pixel segmentation of T_1-weighted sagittal images and T_2-weighted coronal images (4 mm thick, contiguous) Scanning repeated annually up to 15 years or until death (average 5.6±3.5 scans over an average of 6.4±3.4 years; range 1.9–14.1 years)	Among the 42 subjects (20 M, 22 W) who remained cognitively intact, trajectory of ventricular expansion decreased from ~4%/year (at age 75) to ~3%/year at age 95. No relation was found between trajectory of ventricular expansion and gender, body mass index, or *APOE*E4*.
Jack et al. 2008	46 community-dwelling "cognitively normal" elderly participants from Mayo ADRC Age 79.0 ± 5.7 years 23 M; 23 W Subjects remained cognitively normal over the follow-up period	MRI (1.5 tesla) and acquisition techniques as described above in Jack et al. 2004, 2005. Scanning repeated a median of 4 (range, 3 – 8) times, over a median follow-up period of 5.5 (range, 2.2–11) years.	Aging was associated with decreased whole brain volumes (by ~100 mL, or 8%) and increased ventricular volume (by ~30 mL, or 75%). The rates of brain shrinkage and ventricular expansion remained constant (i.e., were linear) over the follow-up period.
Silbert et al. 2008, 2009	104 healthy elderly participants in the Oregon Brain Aging Study Age 85.1±5.6 years (range 65–99 years) 41 M; 63 W MMSE >23	MRI (1.5 tesla); multiple spin echo acquisition sequence Blinded volume measurements of SH using semiautomated pixel segmentation of contiguous T_2-weighted coronal images (4 mm thick) Detailed neuropsychological testing, and evaluation of balance and motor function Subjects followed for 9.1±4.0 years (range 2–18 years), with 4.7±2.9 (range 3–13) scans obtained approximately annually	At baseline, age was associated with SH volume. During follow-up, most subjects (84%) had some increases in SH volume (~5%/year). Baseline SH and progression of SH were both associated with decreased gait performance; progression of SH also was associated with memory decline. In a subset of 49 subjects with at least 3 scans (Silbert et al. 2009), progression of total and periventricular SH was associated with persistent cognitive impairment, even after adjusting for baseline clinical and brain MRI volumes, and for rate of ventricular enlargement.
Driscoll et al. 2009	60 randomly selected elderly participants from the Cardiovascular Health Study Cognitive Cohort Age 77.3 ± 5.8 years 23 M; 37 W Cognitively normal during median 5-year follow up	MRI (1.0 tesla); double spin echo acquisition sequence Blinded visual ratings of periventricular and deep white matter SH from contiguous coronal T_2-weighted and proton density images, by single rater with good reliabilities Physical activity level	Total periventricular SH score increased by ~9.6%/year and total deep white matter SH score increased by ~18.9%/year. Physical activity (assessed with Minnesota Leisure Time Questionnaire) was not associated with less SH progression.

APPENDIX 6–1. Representative longitudinal imaging studies of "normal" human brain aging *(continued)*

Study	Subjects	Imaging and measurement technique	Findings
McDonald et al. 2009	51 healthy elderly community-dwelling controls in the Sydney Stroke Study Mean age 71 years (range 58–85 years) 26 M; 25 W Living independently, with no history of neurological or psychiatric disorder	MRI (1.5 tesla) Volume measurement of periventricular and deep white matter SH, using semiautomated pixel segmentation of contiguous T_2-weighted coronal images (4 mm thick) Scanning repeated at 3 years	Aging was associated with increase in total SH volume (13%/year), periventricular SH volume (10%/year), and deep white matter SH volume (15%/year). SH progression was significant in frontal, temporal, and parietal regions, but not in the occipital region or cerebellum. SH progression was related to baseline SH volume, but not to age, sex, or cardiovascular risk factors.
Carmichael et al. 2010	284 cognitively normal elderly control subjects in the Alzheimer's Disease Neuroimaging Initiative (ADNI) Age 76 ± 4.8 years 112 M; 112 W	MR imaging (1.5 tesla); T_1-weighted magnetization-prepared rapid gradient echo sequence and axial proton density/T_2-weighted fast spin echo sequence Volume measurements using boundary shift integral technique on spatially registered 3D image set Scanning repeated "in most subjects" at 6 and 12 months	At baseline, subjects had 0.51 ± 1.1 mL of SH. Age was associated with 0.082 ± 0.92 mL annual increase in SH volume.
Vemuri et al. 2010	92 cognitively normal elderly control subjects in the Alzheimer's Disease Neuroimaging Registry (ADNI) Median age 75 years (range 72–78 years) 48 M; 42 W	MR imaging (1.5 tesla); T_1-weighted magnetization-prepared rapid gradient echo acquisition sequence Volume measurements using boundary shift integral technique on spatially registered 3D image set Scanning repeated at 12 months	Ventricular volume increased by 1.4 mL (median; range 0.6–2.2 mL).

Note. 3D = three-dimensional; ADRC = Alzheimer's Disease Research Center; *APOE*E4* = apolipoprotein ε4 allele; CDR = Clinical Depression Rating; CNS = central nervous system; CSF = cerebrospinal fluid; CT = computed tomography; GDQ = Geriatric Depression Questionnaire; GRASS = gradient recalled acquisition in steady state; IR-SPGR = recovery prepared spoiled gradient echo; IV = intracranial volume; M = men; MIDAS = Medical Image Display and Analysis System; MMSE = Mini-Mental State Examination; MPRAGE = magnetization prepared rapid gradient echo; MRI = magnetic resonance imaging; RAVENS = regional analysis of volumes examined in normalized space; RF = radiofrequency; SH = subcortical hyperintensity; SIENA = structural image evaluation using normalization of atrophy; SPGR = spoiled gradient recalled; TIV = total intracranial volume; VBR = ventricular/brain ratio; VPR = ventricular/parenchymal ratio; W = women; WAIS–R = Wechsler Adult Intelligence Scale—Revised; WMH = white matter hyperintensities.

7

Molecular Imaging in Neuropsychiatry

Norman L. Foster, M.D.

Imaging has had a profound impact on medical practice. It has become essential for managing serious acute neurological illness. It also plays an expanding role in the chronic, often progressive disorders of geriatric neuropsychiatry. A broad range of disorders causes neurocognitive, behavioral, and motor symptoms. A careful history and examination are essential to identify clinical syndromes and narrow the range of diseases that must be considered. In support of the diagnostic evaluation, imaging can help confirm or refute a suspected diagnosis and sometimes provide irrefutable evidence. Later, imaging also may have a role when the clinical course deviates from expectations or there is a poor response to treatment. The case for using imaging in evaluating neurocognitive disturbance and dementia is particularly strong. Despite accumulated knowledge and the development of detailed clinical criteria, determining the cause of dementia remains difficult using current clinical methods alone. Different dementing diseases have similar symptoms and examination findings, and some of the diagnostic criteria overlap. Also, identifying the most salient features of a dementing illness can be difficult in complicated cases or when history is limited or unreliable. Neuroimaging has become an essential tool because it reveals without bias the pathological alterations of brain composition and structure. With minimal patient risk and discomfort, changes in the otherwise inaccessible brain can be visualized in detail. Even in rare situations when a brain biopsy is needed, neuroimaging provides essential information about the distribution and regional severity of pathological damage.

Neuroimaging can be challenging to use optimally. It is not a panacea for making diagnostic decisions and can answer only some of the many difficult questions that arise during neuropsychiatric care. Nevertheless, judicious use of imaging sometimes provides definitive information, sparing patients and their families the expense and frustration of unnecessary diagnostic odysseys.

In this chapter, I provide a rational approach for using neuroimaging in geriatric neuropsychiatry and for selecting the most appropriate brain imaging method given the clinical context and relevant clinical questions. Although neuroimaging, and particularly molecular imaging techniques, provides valuable information about the mechanisms of neuropsychiatric disorders, this chapter will focus on clinical applications. I critically review how current knowledge can be used to make everyday diagnostic and treatment decisions, and I preview emerging technologies. Although this chapter is not a primer on the technical aspects of imaging, adequate discussion is provided so the reader can be a knowledgeable user. Chapter 6, "Imaging the Structure of the Aging Human Brain," discusses the use of structural imaging methods of computed tomography (CT) and magnetic resonance imaging (MRI). This chapter will emphasize molecular imaging techniques using positron emission tomography (PET) and single-photon emission computed tomography (SPECT). Structural imaging will be discussed as having distinct and complementary uses whose findings also aid interpretation of molecular imaging. With both structural and molecular techniques taken

Supported in part by NIH grants RO1-AG22394 and U01-AG024904 (the Alzheimer's Disease Neuroimaging Initiative).

together, neuroimaging represents a significant addition to the neuropsychiatrist's armamentarium.

Rational Use of Neuroimaging in Neuropsychiatry

Evaluating a patient with neuropsychiatric symptoms is time-consuming, complex, and intellectually demanding. Diagnosis involves the formulation and resolution of a series of questions to determine the cause of symptoms and establish an appropriate plan for care. Questions arise incrementally and are modified as information accumulates from the available patient history and during a careful examination. Some of these questions can be answered by obtaining additional historical information or performing a more detailed and extensive examination; others are best approached with the aid of laboratory tests and imaging. In every case, results must be interpreted accurately and testing used appropriately. Ideal utilization of neuroimaging should answer questions that cannot otherwise be resolved. Neuroimaging should be used to test diagnostic hypotheses rather than to find a diagnosis. Imaging must be interpreted and take into account the clinical context. Only rarely is neuroimaging definitive. Indeed, if the radiologist does not know what to look for, abnormalities can be easy to overlook or dismiss as incidental. Neuroimaging does not simplify evaluations. In fact, by adding more information, it increases the complexity of clinical decision-making. On the other hand, the benefit is to increase diagnostic accuracy and diagnostic certainty by adding information that otherwise would be unavailable. The effort pays off in providing greater clarity to clinical problems and providing quantitative evidence of disease and treatment response.

Appropriate Clinical Context

Neuropsychiatric disorders can be classified as causing cognitive deficits, mood and behavioral disturbance, or progressive motor disability. Although a single disorder can account for two or even all three categories of symptoms, the primary diagnostic considerations and use of imaging differ depending on the symptom that is predominant at the patient's presentation (Table 7–1).

TABLE 7–1. Clinical contexts in which to consider neuroimaging in neuropsychiatry

Neurocognitive deficits
Objective evidence of neurocognitive deficit unexplained by medication or difficulty with attention
Suspected neurodegenerative disease
Rapid progression over weeks
Sudden worsening of symptoms
Mood and behavioral disturbance
Focal neurological deficit or history of stroke, head injury, or seizures
Worsening executive dysfunction in face of improving mood or psychotic symptoms
Late-life onset of psychosis
Progressive motor disability
History of stroke, head injury, or seizures
Family history of parkinsonism or dementia
Both action and resting tremor
Onset of cognitive deficits
Rapid progression of motor disability over weeks

Brain imaging is appropriate if there is objective evidence of otherwise unexplained neurocognitive deficit. A cognitive complaint is not sufficient. Memory complaints are common in the elderly and in patients with depression. Before a full evaluation is pursued, it is important to establish by mental status examination that there is objective evidence of impairment (see Chapter 4, "Neuropsychiatric Assessment"). Sometimes a bedside assessment is sufficient; in other situations, standardized neuropsychological testing that compares cognitive abilities with those in age- and education-appropriate populations may be required (see Chapter 5, "Neuropsychological Assessment"). A variety of simple explanations for cognitive problems also should be considered first. Medications with cognitive side effects, including sedatives, pain medication, and antiepileptic and anticholinergic drugs (including over-the-counter drugs), are common among the elderly and should be discontinued whenever possible (see Chapter 29, "Neuropsychiatric Disorders Associated With General Medical Therapies"). Standard lists of these medications are available (Fick et al. 2003; Zhang et al. 2010). Depression, psychosis, delirium, and chronic sleep disturbance all impair attention and may explain cognitive impairment. These should be addressed before the clinician embarks on an evaluation that includes imaging.

The evaluation of suspected dementing illness has two distinct and essential steps. The first is to recognize suspicious complaints and symptoms and to decide whether they indicate significant cognitive impairment. Brain imaging contributes little to this decision and cannot substitute for a careful clinical history and examination. Only a mental status examination provides the evidence necessary to determine whether cognitive deficits are sufficient to explain newly acquired impairment in everyday activities. Imaging abnormalities cannot be used to accurately infer the presence of cognitive disturbance. Individuals with dramatically abnormal scans may have normal cognition. Likewise, a normal imaging study does not rule out cognitive impairment.

If clinical evidence indicates significant cognitive impairment, the second essential step in evaluation is determining the cause. Once again, the patient's history, mental status, and physical examination are essential, but neuroimaging also plays a crucial role at this point. Brain imaging is always indicated in this phase of the evaluation (Knopman et al. 2001). Imaging provides important evidence of a dementing disease and may identify its cause by permitting the visual recognition of characteristic alterations in brain structure, chemistry, and function. Diagnosis cannot be based on brain imaging alone, but detecting specific abnormalities or documenting a lack of abnormality can be useful in supporting or refuting a particular diagnosis. Even after the cause of dementia has been determined, repeat imaging should be considered if there is rapid progression of symptoms from week to week (raising the possibility of another disease such as encephalitis or prion disease) or sudden worsening of symptoms (such as might be explained by stroke).

Brain imaging is less commonly necessary in the evaluation of mood and behavior disturbance, particularly if such disturbance has been present for much of adulthood. Mood and behavior disturbance in association with focal neurological deficits or a history of neurological disease, on the other hand, should be investigated with neuroimaging. Stroke commonly causes depression and could be overlooked if its onset was silent. Seizure disorder and head injury often have psychiatric implications and may explain inappropriate behavior. Recently, for example, chronic traumatic encephalopathy in former athletes causing prominent depressive symptoms has gained new attention (McKee et al. 2009; Omalu et al. 2006). While psychiatric illnesses commonly impair cognition, further investigation with imaging is warranted when cognitive problems worsen in the face of improving mood or psychotic symptoms. This approach is particularly relevant with late-life-onset psychosis and when executive dysfunction is prominent. In such cases, the risk of frontotemporal dementia is high and the illness can be identified with structural and molecular imaging.

The diagnosis of Parkinson's disease (PD) does not require brain imaging (Gelb et al. 1999). However, imaging can play an important role in the evaluation of progressive motor disability when the onset of motor symptoms is ambiguous, there are complicating factors, additional neurological deficits are present, or there are nonmotor symptoms. When there is a history of stroke or head injury, these events may account for some or all of the symptoms depending on their localization, which can be determined with imaging. Rarely, familial parkinsonian disorders have a characteristic signature with imaging due to heavy metal deposition in the brain. In other cases, it may be difficult to distinguish the cause of tremor. PD, essential tremor, and tremor caused by cerebellar disease have differing imaging characteristics that may aid diagnosis. Finally, even after a diagnosis has been made, onset of cognitive deficits and rapid progression of motor disability over weeks (which could be caused by prion disease) warrant imaging.

Asking the Right Questions

The wide range of potential causes of neuropsychiatric symptoms requires that diagnostic questions be considered systematically. Diagnostic questions that imaging significantly aids in answering are listed in Table 7–2. Imaging modalities differ in their ability to address each question, and there is considerable clinical art in deciding on the selection and order of techniques. Because several disorders often contribute to an individual patient's symptoms, the clinician must address each diagnostic question in turn, even when investigations have identified a potential culprit. Depending on the clinical history and examination, all questions are not equally important, and that fact should be reflected in the types of imaging ordered and their priority. Fortunately, a single neuroimaging study usually addresses several clinical questions simultaneously. However, when the information provided by a single scanning modality is insufficient, additional imaging may be necessary. Neuroimaging is particularly valuable in difficult and atypical cases. Brain scanning may be the only way to conclusively disentangle multiple dementing disorders simultaneously contributing to a patient's intellectual decline.

TABLE 7–2. Diagnostic questions in neuropsychiatric evaluations most relevant to structural or molecular neuroimaging

Structural imaging
Is there a mass lesion?
Is there cerebrovascular disease?
Is there ventricular enlargement?
Is there generalized volume loss?
Is there focal volume loss?
Is there copper, iron, or manganese deposition?
Molecular imaging
What is the pattern of cerebral hypometabolism?
Is there loss of dopaminergic neurons?
Are there amyloid plaques?

Determining the Relevance of Findings

Achieving the full benefits of imaging requires integration of study results and their clinical context. Physicians ordering imaging studies are responsible for conveying to the radiologist or nuclear medicine specialist the diagnostic questions that need to be answered and indicating the clinical context. Even with this information, however, a radiologist alone cannot determine fully how findings relate to a patient's symptoms. A detailed understanding of the individual and his or her symptoms is needed to judge whether image abnormalities are clinically relevant. Unexpected abnormalities that are asymptomatic are common. For example, a population-based MRI study of 2,000 middle-aged and elderly subjects found asymptomatic brain infarcts in 7.2%, cerebral aneurysms in 1.8%, and benign primary tumors in 1.6% of the subjects (Vernooij et al. 2007). Consequently, the clinical context must be considered before deciding to act on any imaging abnormality. Imaging reports need not be taken at face value. Not all abnormalities are relevant or deserve further investigation. Exercising good clinical judgment and involving the radiologist, if necessary, can avoid needless, costly, and potentially risky additional testing, even when suggested in an imaging report.

A clinician often benefits from personally reviewing a scan to get a better sense of the extent and location of any abnormality. The size and number of lesions should correspond roughly with the severity of patient symptoms, and the type of findings should be consistent with the location of brain damage. Radiologists may be able to estimate the age of individual lesions and thus aid the comparison of imaging findings with a patient's clinical course. Whether or not the localization and timing of clinical symptoms and the imaging findings coincide is a reliable guide for deciding whether scan abnormalities are clinically important. Ideally, the care provider, radiologist, and nuclear medicine specialist work together to ensure that the best imaging techniques are used and that clinically meaningful information is appropriately incorporated into patient care.

TABLE 7–3. Potential errors and misuses of imaging

Utilization errors
Overuse—needlessly repeating studies or obtaining imaging studies using methods unlikely to contribute to a diagnosis, thus causing excessive costs without additional clinical benefit
Underuse—failure to utilize the imaging modality that could provide critical information for diagnosis
Omission—failure to incorporate significant imaging findings in diagnosis
Overdependence—using imaging results to decide whether there is dementia when clinical assessment alone is reliable, or using imaging results to make a diagnosis without utilizing other relevant clinical data
Interpretation errors
Overinterpretation—assigning a cause of dementia on the basis of clinically insignificant imaging findings
Misinterpretation—failing to recognize the presence of clinically significant lesions, causing errors in radiographic diagnosis
Inconsistent interpretation—variability between radiologists or from patient to patient in the description or clinical significance ascribed to identical imaging findings
Technical errors
Lack of reliability—inconsistent acquisition or processing of imaging data, causing misinterpretation
Artifact—failure to prevent or identify image acquisition or analysis errors that prevent the accurate interpretation of scans

Concerns About Use

Many concerns have been expressed about the appropriate use of neuroimaging in geriatric patients with neuropsychiatric illness (Table 7–3). Although these same concerns are relevant to the use of any diagnostic test, they seem to arise more often and are expressed more vigorously with evaluations of the elderly than with other populations.

Economic concerns have been particularly prominent in discussions about brain imaging in dementia. The high prevalence of cognitive problems, the increasing size of the aging population at high risk, and the expense of imaging studies all mean that costs of dementia evaluations are especially significant for insurers and society. Understandably, this expense causes diagnostic testing for dementia to be subjected to a higher degree of scrutiny. Furthermore, because current treatments for dementing disorders generally have only modest benefits, a robust link between imaging and treatment outcomes is difficult to document. On the other hand, the economic costs of failure to treat dementia and the expense of inappropriate care are also very high. Because an accurate diagnosis is the basis for rational management, imaging costs are easily justified if imaging is used appropriately and if it improves diagnostic accuracy. Evaluation costs are small when compared to the long-term costs of caring for patients with dementia over years. Unfortunately, cost-benefit analysis studies sometimes fail to consider the costs of inappropriate treatments, and the usual methods of cost containment tend to erect arbitrary barriers to access and can exacerbate some utilization errors and discourage definitive diagnosis. Insurance more readily reimburses test performance than the effort that would be needed to properly evaluate patients. As a result, physicians may order imaging repeatedly without reaching a specific diagnosis and may fail to use all the information relevant to dementia care that imaging provides. Improving providers' knowledge would be a more effective way to improve the cost-effectiveness of imaging in the long run. Overuse of and overdependence on imaging are most common when evaluations are incomplete or inadequate and when physicians lack confidence in their clinical skills. Lack of knowledge also causes errors of omission, which are exacerbated by barriers to obtaining timely testing.

Despite the potential value of unique information that neuroimaging can provide, many practitioners have considerable ambivalence about the use of neuroimaging in patients with suspected dementing illness. This ambivalence, which is uncommon with other brain disorders, deserves explanation because it contributes to misuse. In part, the ambivalence reflects a pervasive diagnostic and therapeutic nihilism that has not been fully overcome by the growing understanding of dementing diseases. Diagnostic efforts sometimes have been justified based solely on the potential for identifying reversible causes of dementia. With this approach, imaging often becomes a frustrating exercise because dementia is potentially reversible in only a small proportion of patients. It is now clear that accurate diagnosis is important regardless of whether symptoms can be reversed. Symptomatic and disease-specific treatments are available for most dementing diseases, and early diagnosis permits appropriate treatment to be initiated and can prevent complications. To achieve the goal of specific diagnosis, a "rule in" rather than "rule out" approach to neuroimaging is appropriate to identify characteristic findings of neurodegenerative disease and not simply mass lesions (Scheltens et al. 2002).

Interpretation errors also are critical. Although mass lesions can be identified and described, common and equally relevant neurodegenerative findings are not so clear-cut. Clinicians may find reports of imaging studies more confusing than helpful. For example, white matter changes are prevalent in dementing disorders, but factors critical to determining their clinical relevance (such as their location and extent) often are not included in radiologists' reports. Atrophy may be misjudged or focal atrophy overlooked.

Technical issues are especially relevant to imaging because of the complexity of performing studies. Attention to technical details is critical to ensure that neuroimaging results are reliable and is the primary responsibility of radiologists and nuclear medicine specialists. However, clinicians also can benefit from recognizing artifacts and being aware of methodological limitations. Until recently, imaging of patients with memory loss and dementia varied considerably from one institution to another. This is now changing due to the Alzheimer's Disease Neuroimaging Initiative (Mueller et al. 2005), a multisite, longitudinal study of normal cognitive aging, mild cognitive impairment, and early Alzheimer's disease (AD). This initiative has resulted in standardized image acquisition protocols for MRI and PET using a variety of scanner models and manufacturers, as well as the implementation of quality control methods with phantom studies and image processing methods that correct for geometric and signal variability. Data from the Alzheimer's Disease Neuroimaging Initiative are a public domain resource available to qualified investigators (https://www.loni.ucla.edu/ida/login.jsp). The Web site also provides technical details to encourage adoption of uniform imaging standards for dementia.

Molecular Neuroimaging

Molecular neuroimaging probes brain biochemistry by revealing the distribution of tracer quantities of radioactive-labeled drugs designed to participate in metabolism, interact with enzymes and transporters, occupy cellular receptors, or bind cellular and extracellular proteins. Molecular imaging can assess the characteristic biochemical signatures of dementing diseases as they evolve throughout the course of an illness. These methods are powerful but complex. Each tracer has unique properties described with a mathematical equation reflecting a "kinetic model" used to interpret counted emissions. Developing optimal synthesis methods, assessing the applicability of kinetic models, and performing necessary validation studies for clinical application often can take a decade or more to complete. As a consequence, only a few of the many potential molecular imaging strategies have reached clinical practice. Molecular imaging methods to measure cerebral blood flow and metabolism usually are equivalent in dementing illnesses and are the most established molecular imaging methods. Dopaminergic imaging and amyloid imaging also have great clinical promise for dementia care.

Choosing Between PET and SPECT

In recent years, the differences in the availability of PET and SPECT have changed dramatically. Previously, SPECT was much more accessible. Now, with the widespread use and reimbursement of PET in oncology, PET instruments have become common and PET radioisotopes are readily available. The choice between PET and SPECT primarily reflects the imaging agents that have been developed for each technology. The fundamental difference between PET and SPECT is the radioactive isotopes used in the two methods. Different instrumentation and acquisition algorithms are required to develop optimal images from positron-emitting and gamma-emitting tracers. Radiopharmaceuticals are valuable when they share the same properties as the substances labeled. The positron-emitting isotopes primarily used in PET (fluorine 18 and carbon 11) are much easier to insert into drugs and naturally occurring substances without altering biological activity than are the large, single photon–emitting isotopes commonly used in SPECT (technetium 99m and iodine 131). Therefore, interpreting and developing quantitative tracer kinetic models is much easier for PET than for SPECT. Furthermore, because positron annihilations produce two gamma rays oriented in opposite directions, PET inherently provides more accurate localization and better spatial resolution than does SPECT, which relies on single photon (gamma) emissions.

These theoretical differences have practical importance. The most commonly used SPECT tracers measure cerebral perfusion, whereas the most commonly used PET tracers measure glucose metabolism. Although glucose metabolism usually parallels cerebral perfusion, glucose uptake is more closely linked to neuronal activity. Consequently, the diagnostic accuracy of PET is superior to SPECT in differentiating AD from vascular dementia (Messa et al. 1994). In the past, SPECT has been more widely used than PET because of better reimbursement and broader availability. However, now that PET is becoming widely available and more frequently reimbursed by insurers, the technical advantages mean that PET likely will gradually replace SPECT in dementia evaluations. The subsequent discussion of molecular imaging, therefore, focuses primarily on PET.

Technical Considerations

Changes in the biological processes measured with molecular imaging occur at the cellular level and can be independent of structural change or reflect structural changes. Consequently, results from CT or MRI are critical for accurately interpreting molecular imaging scans. Many PET scanners now incorporate a CT scanner to help meld structural and molecular images. Unlike interpretation of findings in structural imaging studies, interpretation of PET and SPECT scans must consider many factors that can affect the activity and distribution of radioligands. For example, cerebral blood flow and metabolism are affected by patient medication, ambient room conditions, patient attributes such as open or closed eyes, and perhaps the patient's thoughts. Both current and recent medication use may affect the binding of neurotransmitter ligands. Thus, for molecular imaging, medication use and the conditions during scanning must be carefully recorded and controlled.

To decrease subject-to-subject variability, molecular imaging data are commonly "normalized," or adjusted by comparison to an average value in an image or a specified brain region. When this is done, the clinician cannot determine the absolute rate of biochemical reactions, only the value in one brain region relative to another. Nevertheless, the relative distribution of radiotracers has proven adequate for evaluating most disease changes. For glucose metabolism in dementia, there is no ideal region for normalization, but the pons seems to be best suited because pontine glucose metabolism is best preserved in AD (Minoshima et al. 1995).

Structural Neuroimaging

Dementing illnesses frequently alter brain structure. CT and MRI simplify diagnosis of tumors, stroke, and other focal destructive and mass lesions and are superior to radionuclide cisternography in identifying hydrocephalus. As a result, structural imaging was quickly adopted but not used routinely in dementia evaluations. Use of CT and MRI to recognize neurodegenerative diseases has been more challenging but has evolved sufficiently to show utility for this purpose also.

Choosing Between CT and MRI

As discussed in Chapter 6 ("Imaging the Structure of the Aging Human Brain"), CT and MRI provide similar but not identical information about brain structure (Figure 7–1). CT provides superlative anatomical information about bone and intracranial calcifications, ventricles, and sulci. Because X rays are linear, CT scans more accurately represent the location of brain lesions and are preferable in cases of head trauma and for surgical applications. In contrast, determining the size and relative position of brain structures with MRI depends on precise measurement of magnetic gradients and incorporating corrections to compensate for gradient variations that differ from scan to scan. Failure to apply these corrections accurately causes misleading spatial distortions. For most applications relevant to dementia, the advantages of CT usually are outweighed by its limitations. CT is subject to beam-hardening artifacts that appear adjacent to densely radiopaque objects, such as the temporal bone. This produces dense linear intensities, disrupting structural detail in the inferior temporal lobe and posterior fossa.

MRI has many advantages in dementia evaluations. It offers greater resolution and contrast, making it possible to precisely delineate gray matter and identify white matter hyperintensities in the aging brain. MRI possesses superior three-dimensional imaging capabilities, allowing high-resolution coronal and sagittal views of the brain to be obtained routinely and providing better visualization of small brain areas that are important in cognition (e.g., hippocampi and mammillary bodies). Altering acquisition parameters also allows MRI to emphasize specific properties of magnetic susceptibility and to provide more definitive and detailed information than is possible with CT. Furthermore, MRI can be performed repeatedly without the risks of radiation exposure associated with CT. Physicians have been largely unaware of the high cumulative levels of radiation to which many patients have been exposed from clinical studies, and this exposure is raising increasing concern (Brenner and Hall 2007). For these reasons, MRI is preferable to CT for neuropsychiatric evaluations, unless there is a contraindication. Most of the subsequent discussion of structural imaging therefore focuses on MRI, although often CT can provide similar results.

Technical Considerations

MRI produces images that maximize sensitivity to specific tissue characteristics by varying the timing and repetition of radiofrequency pulse sequences and signal acquisition parameters (see Figure 7–1). T_1-weighted images are most useful for defining anatomical structures. T_2-weighted and spin-echo images are best suited for detecting white matter lesions. Some protocols are especially valuable in dementia evaluations. Fluid-attenuated inversion recovery (FLAIR) images highlight white matter abnormalities seen in T_2-weighted images while suppressing signals in cerebrospinal fluid (CSF); this enhances visual contrast and helps distinguish widened capillary spaces from white matter pathology. Diffusion-weighted imaging is sensitive to subtle changes in brain water content and diffusivity and is used for diffusion tensor imaging and tractography. The degree of water content and diffusivity evolves after ischemic injury, so diffusion-weighted imaging can be used to estimate the age of vascular lesions. Diffusion-weighted imaging also is the most sensitive method for detecting spongiform pathology. Pulse sequences designed to highlight paramagnetic properties of hemoglobin are the basis for functional MRI and can identify microhemorrhages associated with amyloid angiopathy and normal aging. Gradient-echo imaging is the most widely used protocol for identifying hemorrhage. There is less experience with susceptibility-weighted imaging, but it appears to be even more sensitive (Haacke et al. 2007).

Ferromagnetic objects are a major obstacle and risk to the performance of MRI. Because high magnetic fields can propel objects containing iron into the scanner, imaging centers take extensive precautions to exclude inadvertent entry of metal objects. This can become a significant barrier, especially for acutely ill patients. For elderly patients, the most common contraindication is the presence of ferromagnetic implants or foreign bodies. Sometimes, unexpected small metal particles from trauma in the distant past are discovered and cause only minor interference with imaging. In other cases, when history is difficult to obtain, X-ray films must be obtained to scout for metal before proceeding with MRI. Although procedures have been developed so that patients with artificial joints generally can be scanned safely, MRI is hazardous with pacemakers, some mechanical valves, and metal-containing sutures and surgical devices. In general, these are serious contraindications to MRI, and careful queries are needed to avoid unknowingly scanning such patients. Many centers, however, have developed procedures for doing brain imaging in patients with pacemakers and defibrillators when the justification for the procedure is very high (Naehle et al. 2009; Nazarian et al. 2006; Sommer et al. 2006). A cardiology consultation is obtained to determine whether the patient is pacemaker dependent. If not, the pacemaker can be deactivated under the supervision of a cardiologist, who remains present throughout the MRI while the patient is closely monitored and then reprograms the device. Tattoos with metal-containing dyes can cause skin burns in high-field (>1.5T) scanners. Furthermore, dental work and foreign objects, including jewelry, can cause severe image distortions and artifacts and should be removed when possible. Another problem, especially for individuals with claustrophobia, is the confining space during MRI. Imaging is most effective when the gap between patient and magnet is minimized, so small-bore scanners are preferred. Some less confining "open" scanners, if available, can be appropriate in certain situations. MRI scanning requires more time than does CT; therefore, MRI may require sedation of certain patients, or CT may be preferred for patients who have claustrophobia or a movement disorder or for those who are less able to cooperate.

Choosing the Best Imaging Modality

Clinical neuroimaging can be divided broadly into structural and molecular methods. Structural methods produce images from absorption of X rays using CT or from measuring magnetic susceptibility of protons with MRI. Molecular methods count emissions from radioactive isotopes that produce either positrons in PET or gamma emission in SPECT. Structural and molecular methods provide different and complementary information about the brain. Although some MRI methods partially reflect brain function, these methods either are not generally available for clinical use or have uncertain clinical utility in dementia. Molecular imaging provides some information about brain structure, but this information can only be inferred after biochemical data are disentangled, and the result is much less detailed information about brain anatomy than CT or MRI provides. Consequently, structural and molecular imaging are best at addressing different clinical questions, and neither can replace the contributions of the other.

Framing the patient's problems as specific clinical questions can determine the imaging study most likely to be helpful (see Table 7–2). The American Academy of Neurology recommends that the initial evaluation of patients with dementia include structural neuroimaging with either noncontrast CT or MRI (Knopman et al. 2001). Focal neurological findings should raise suspicion of a structural lesion, but CT and MRI are justified by a reasonably high prevalence of abnormalities even when these are unsuspected after a careful medical history and examination (Chui and Zhang 1997). The role of molecular imaging in de-

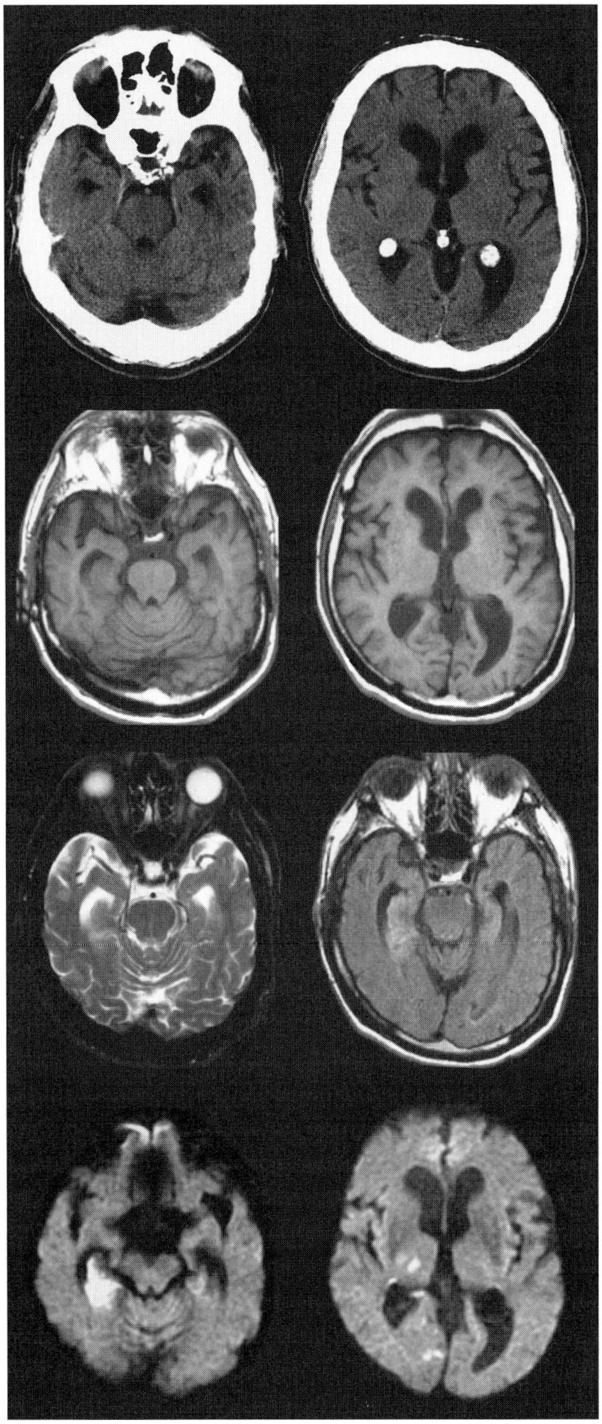

FIGURE 7–1. Computed tomography (CT) and magnetic resonance imaging (MRI) sequences identifying vascular lesions and volume loss.

Transaxial CT *(top row)* and MRI scans *(rows 2–4)* in an 82-year-old man referred for evaluation of profound memory loss. Although the family reported that the memory problems had begun abruptly over the previous few days, his physicians were doubtful. The CT scan shows widening of sulci and symmetrical enlargement of lateral ventricles. The skull and calcifications in the choroid plexus and pineal gland are bright and easily seen. No vascular or mass lesions are evident. On MRI, bone and calcified structures are not so readily visualized. Instead, fat in the scalp causes the high signal ring outside the brain seen in some images. T_1-weighted images *(row 2)* show sulci in greater detail than do CT scans, and gray and white matter can be distinguished. Ventricular size is similar, but brain boundaries are more sharply defined than with CT. A T_2-weighted image *(row 3, left)* provides less structural detail but highlights free water that causes high signal intensity in the orbits and cerebrospinal fluid (CSF). Slightly increased signal in the right hippocampus in the T_2 scan is even more apparent in the fluid-attenuated inversion recovery (FLAIR) image *(row 3, right)*, which suppresses signal in the CSF. This lesion becomes obvious on diffusion-weighted images *(row 4)*. On this sequence, recent strokes caused increased signal, and an acute stroke involving the right hippocampus and a small, punctate area in the right thalamus confirmed the family's report of recent, sudden memory loss.

mentia evaluations is not as firmly established. The biochemical changes revealed by PET and SPECT can often be inferred from the clinical history and examination or from the patient's response to medication. Nevertheless, when diagnostic uncertainty remains, molecular imaging can be useful in specific circumstances, as discussed in the section "Molecular Neuroimaging" earlier in this chapter.

Diagnostic Questions Most Relevant to Structural Neuroimaging

Is There a Mass Lesion?

The most obvious use of structural brain imaging is to identify a mass lesion. Focal neurological deficits indicative of brain injury, such as hemiparesis, visual field cut, or aphasia, warrant investigation with CT or MRI. Brain tumors, subdural hematomas, and brain abscesses are easily recognized. Most mass lesions in patients with dementia are identified when a brain scan is obtained to evaluate a focal neurological complaint rather than during a routine dementia evaluation. The most conspicuous exception is in elderly individuals for whom evaluations are delayed or incomplete. Imaging centers occasionally find unsuspected brain tumors and subdural hematomas when physicians inappropriately assumed that an elderly patient had AD without having considered other possibilities or incorrectly believed that a scan had been done previously. Fortunately, such diagnostic errors are becoming less common.

CT or MRI is needed when disruptive behavioral or personality changes occur de novo in middle or late adulthood. Frontal mass lesions often cause dementia and behavioral disturbance with few obvious focal neurological signs, so patients may not be scanned following early symptoms. Alternatively, behavioral symptoms in these patients initially may have been misinterpreted as purely psychiatric and brain imaging considered unnecessary.

Mass lesions are especially likely when dramatic dementia symptoms develop over a period of less than a year; this situation warrants a particularly diligent review of imaging results. Although it may seem obvious that a glioma, central nervous system lymphoma, or subdural hemorrhage can cause rapidly evolving cognitive problems, it is sometimes very difficult to obtain a consistent or accurate history about the timing of symptom onset.

Is There Cerebrovascular Disease?

Stroke and other cerebrovascular diseases are common causes of cognitive impairment and major reasons for obtaining structural neuroimaging in dementia evaluations. Although physicians traditionally seek a single cause of dementia, cerebrovascular disease frequently contributes to the severity of dementia when another dementing disease also is present. Mixed dementia involving both AD and vascular disease becomes increasingly common with age and is an increasing public health concern as the population becomes older (Langa et al. 2004). Indeed, more recent evidence suggests that mixed dementia is the most common cause of dementia in a community sample (Schneider et al. 2007).

Structural imaging, particularly MRI, is quite sensitive to cerebrovascular disease, so the major clinical challenge is to determine the significance of lesions that are found. Approximately 30% of elderly people have silent lacunar and cortical infarcts without clinical manifestations (Longstreth et al. 1998). Ideally, clinical relevance can be determined by correlating symptoms with the timing and location of the lesions. For example, in a demented patient with prominent language disturbance, vascular lesions would be expected to involve predominantly the left hemisphere. Careful review of all imaging data and a comparison of findings with different MRI sequences increase the sensitivity of identifying vascular lesions and estimating their age (see Figure 7–1). Nevertheless, relating imaging abnormalities with dementia can be difficult. History may be inadequate, and strokes are often asymptomatic (Price et al. 1997; Vermeer et al. 2002). Substantial motor and sensory recovery may obscure the signs of stroke by the time dementia is evaluated. Furthermore, the severity of dementia may preclude a detailed neurological examination, making it impossible to identify subtle deficits.

The extent of vascular lesions is critical to their clinical relevance and should be fully described as part of image interpretation. A larger number of strokes and more extensive white matter abnormalities increase the probability of dementia. Too often, clinical reports fail to distinguish minimal from extensive and confluent white matter abnormalities. The high sensitivity of MRI to changes in water content leads to overestimates of the clinical significance of deep white matter hyperintensities. White matter abnormalities are common in the elderly and should be evaluated critically because not all are pathological (Fazekas et al. 1993). Enlarged perivascular spaces cause increased signal on T_2-weighted images but can be distinguished by low signal with FLAIR imaging (Figure 7–2). Neurodegenerative disease can cause white matter abnormalities from wallerian degeneration and be indistinguishable from small vessel disease. Although the extent of white matter hyperintensity required for clinical significance is uncertain, one consensus group concluded that involvement of at least 25% of white matter was necessary for a clinical diagnosis of vascular dementia (Román et al. 1993).

Location of vascular lesions is also important. Even small thalamic infarcts can cause cognitive impairment (Mungas et al. 2001). Likewise, cognition may be negatively affected when white matter hyperintensities involve cholinergic projection pathways (Bocti et al. 2005; Selden et al. 1998). Cholinergic fibers originate in the nucleus basalis of Meynert and fan out as they ascend following a medial cingulate gyrus pathway and a lateral pathway that proceeds through the external capsule and claustrum into the centrum semiovale adjacent to the gray-white junction (Figure 7–3).

Evidence of cerebrovascular disease on neuroimaging is insufficient to exclude AD. AD pathology is often the primary factor for cognitive decline in older individuals with concurrent cerebrovascular injury (Fein et al. 2000), and approximately 30% of patients with AD at autopsy also have evidence of stroke (Gearing et al. 1995). When an individual has extensive vascular lesions, AD can be identified confidently when gradual cognitive decline occurs without change in vascular lesions. Gradient-echo MRI showing cortical microhemorrhages typical of cerebral amyloid angiopathy also provides indirect evidence of AD (Viswanathan and Chabriat 2006).

Although MRI is best for identifying vascular lesions, positron emission tomography with [^{18}F]fluorodeoxyglucose (FDG-PET) can help determine the cognitive consequences of these lesions. Stroke often causes metabolic abnormalities that are more extensive than structural lesions because of the loss of distant efferent nerve terminals. For example, a stroke damaging only the thalamus can cause ipsilateral cerebral cortical and contralateral cerebellar hypometabolism, reflecting the location of thalamic pathways (Pappata et al. 1990). These remote metabolic effects are clinically significant, and their localiza-

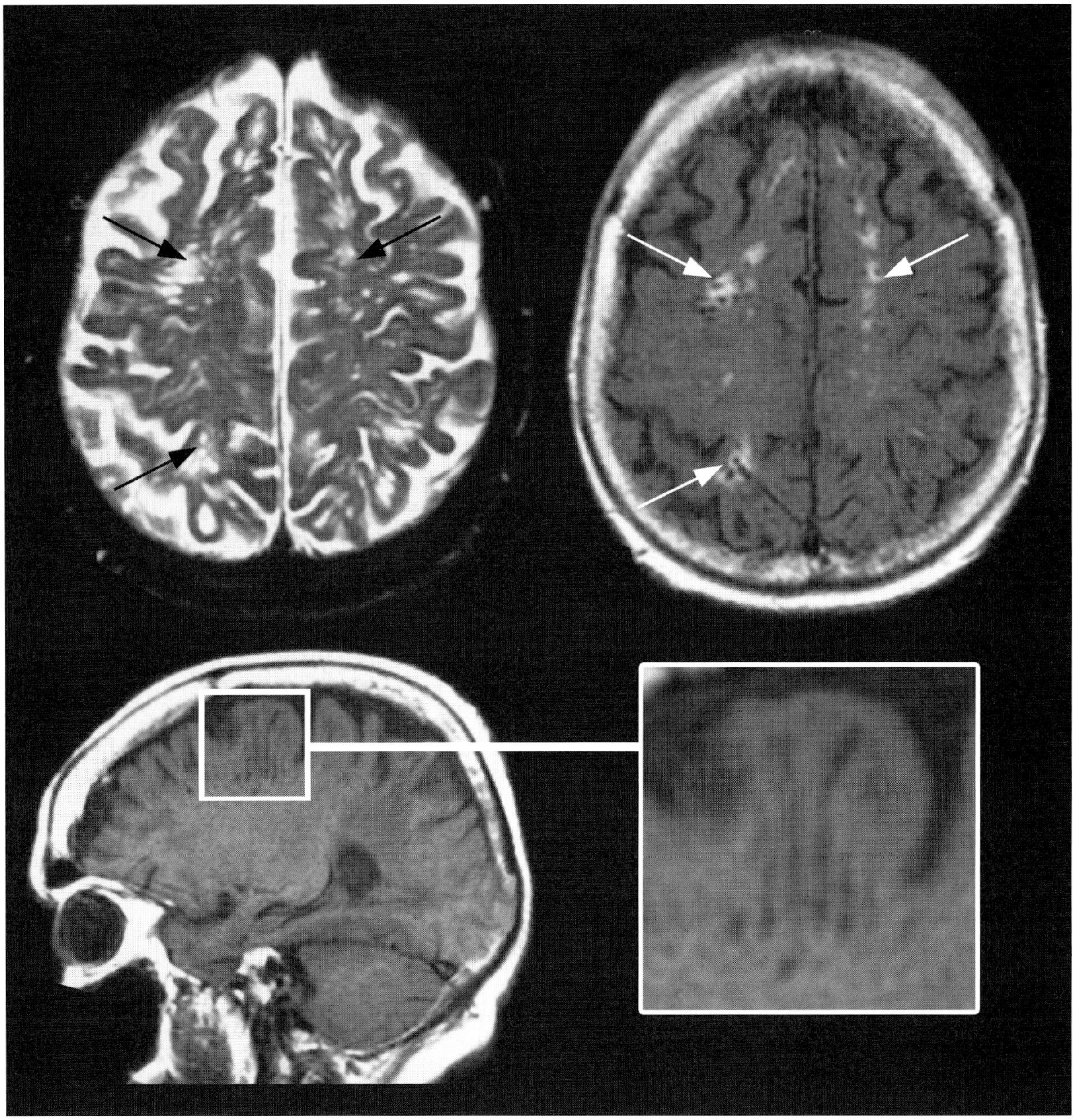

FIGURE 7–2. White matter hyperintensities due to enlarged perivascular spaces.

A T_2-weighted image *(top row, left)* shows multiple areas of increased signal in the white matter. Although similar to white matter changes seen in chronic small vessel disease, these have a linear pattern, and a fluid-attenuated inversion recovery (FLAIR) magnetic resonance image *(top row, right)* reveals that many of these hyperintensities have a central area of low signal due to suppression of cerebrospinal fluid in perivascular spaces *(arrows)*. Distinct features also are apparent in T_1-weighted sagittal images *(bottom row)*. Perivascular spaces are linear, running perpendicular to the brain surface following penetrating vessels *(inset on right)*. Areas of decreased signal in posterior periventricular areas have a patchy distribution characteristic of small vessel disease.

tion reflects the types of cognitive deficits observed. Cerebral cortical hypometabolism is the best predictor of whether subcortical lacunar stroke will cause dementia (Kwan et al. 1999).

Is There Ventricular Enlargement?

Ventricular enlargement can be an important indicator of a dementing disease, particularly if the disease is progressive. The presence of ventricular enlargement often is determined subjectively, but a simple alternative is to calculate the ratio of the maximal width of frontal horns to the maximal width of the inner skull, which normally is <0.30. Ventricular enlargement can be caused by abnormalities in CSF flow or loss of brain volume (hydrocephalus ex vacuo). Disorders of CSF dynamics are uncommon causes of dementia but are reliably

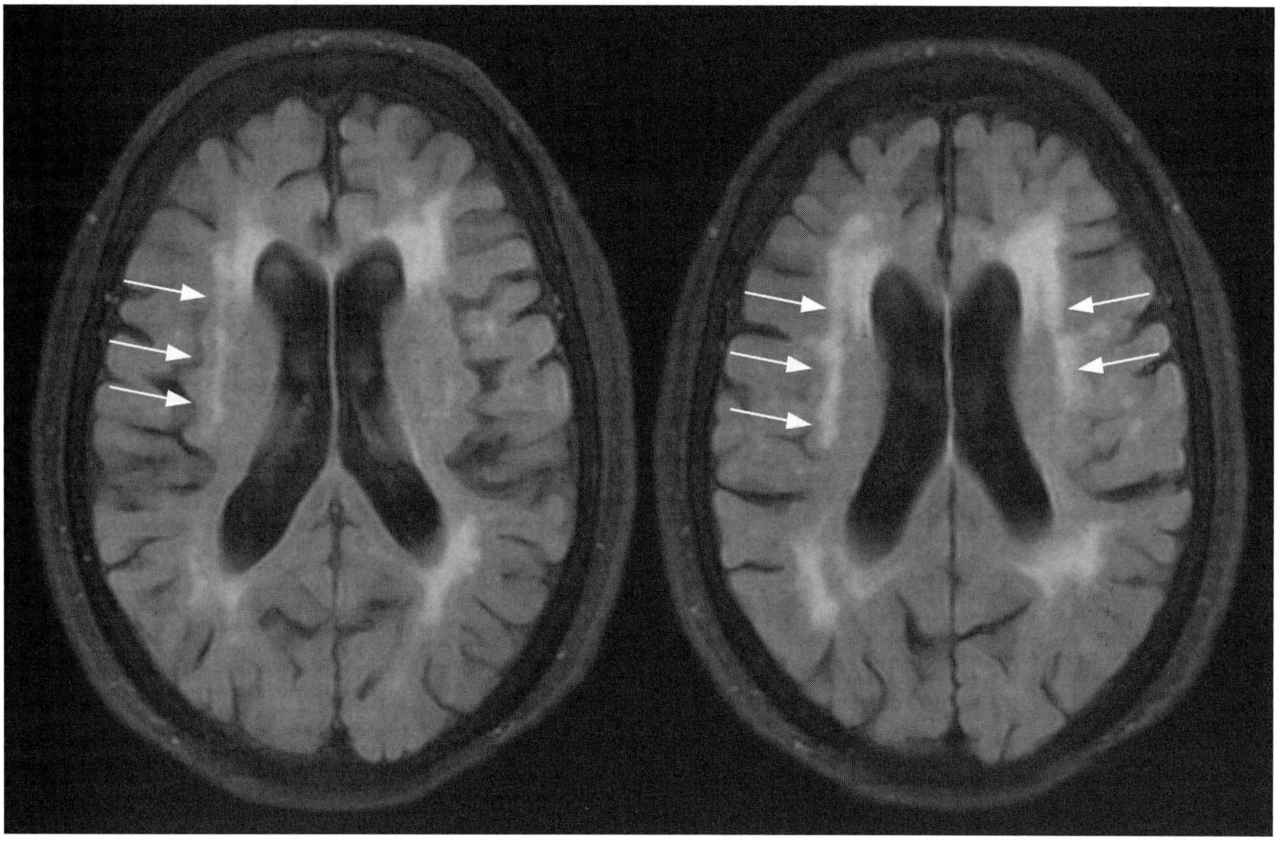

FIGURE 7–3. Critically located white matter hyperintensities.

The location of white matter abnormalities in this 75-year-old woman likely explains her mild memory deficits. Transaxial fluid-attenuated inversion recovery (FLAIR) scans show linear hyperintensities parallel to the margin of the gray-white junction coinciding with the distribution of ascending cholinergic fibers in the external capsule *(arrows)*. The scans also show "capping" of the frontal and posterior horns of the lateral ventricles, as often observed in cognitively normal individuals and of less clear clinical significance.

identified with CT and MRI. Both obstructive hydrocephalus and communicating hydrocephalus increase intracranial pressure, and patients present with headache and cognitive deficit. In obstructive hydrocephalus, the ventricular system balloons proximal to blockage of CSF flow. This obstruction commonly occurs at the cerebral aqueduct, causing disproportionate enlargement of third and lateral ventricles. Aqueductal flow of CSF can be measured precisely with MRI, allowing detection of even partial obstruction. MRI also can identify changes in periventricular brain water due to transependymal flow of CSF.

Structural imaging is essential in identifying normal pressure hydrocephalus, which causes the classic triad of mild dementia, gait apraxia, and urinary incontinence and which responds to ventricular shunting (Table 7–4). Ventricular CSF flow is unobstructed in normal pressure hydrocephalus, so all ventricles are similarly enlarged. Many imaging criteria have been proposed as possible predictors of response to ventricular shunting, but none has been found reliable (Relkin et al. 2005). The major challenge is to demonstrate that ventricular enlargement is not entirely attributable to cerebral atrophy. Consequently, ventricular enlargement should be disproportionately greater than sulcal enlargement. SPECT imaging is also supportive of the diagnosis of normal pressure hydrocephalus when radionuclide injected after lumbar puncture into the subarachnoid space fails to clear after 48–72 hours.

Ventricular enlargement due to hydrocephalus ex vacuo is a very common feature of AD and other neurodegenerative dementias. In these diseases, all ventricles expand roughly proportionate to enlargement of sulci. Unfortunately, relating the enlargement of ventricular volume to size of sulcal spaces remains a purely subjective determination. However, when sulci are prominent, loss of brain volume is the likely cause of ventricular enlargement and warrants further analysis to determine the pattern of volume loss.

Is There Generalized or Focal Volume Loss?

Loss of brain volume due to atrophy is seen at autopsy in AD and many other neurodegenerative diseases and is the most

TABLE 7–4. Structural imaging abnormalities in probable normal pressure hydrocephalus

Required findings

1. Ventricular enlargement not entirely attributable to cerebral atrophy or congenital enlargement (Evan's index >0.3 or comparable measure)
2. No macroscopic obstruction to cerebrospinal fluid flow
3. At least one of the following:
   a. Enlargement of the temporal horns of the lateral ventricles not entirely attributable to hippocampus atrophy
   b. Callosal angle of 40 degrees or more
   c. Evidence of altered brain water content, including periventricular signal changes on computed tomography and MRI not attributable to microvascular ischemic changes or demyelination
4. An aqueductal or fourth ventricular flow void on MRI

Other findings considered supportive

1. A brain imaging study performed before onset of symptoms showing smaller ventricular size or without evidence of hydrocephalus
2. Radionuclide cisternogram showing delayed clearance of radiotracer over the cerebral convexities after 48–72 hours
3. Cine MRI study or other technique showing increased ventricular flow rate
4. A SPECT-acetazolamide challenge showing decreased periventricular perfusion that is not altered by acetazolamide

Note. MRI=magnetic resonance imaging; SPECT=single-photon emission computed tomography.
Source. Adapted from Relkin et al. 2005.

consistently reported structural imaging abnormality in dementia. The development of CT offered an easy way to look for brain atrophy in living patients, but initial diagnostic studies were disappointing. It quickly became clear that the age of an individual was a significant determinant of brain volume and had to be considered. Brain atrophy on average was greater in AD patients than in cognitively normal elderly subjects of similar age, but significant overlap between individuals limited the diagnostic value of brain atrophy (Gado et al. 1982).

The decline in brain volume with age continues to be a major challenge (see Chapter 6, "Imaging the Structure of the Aging Human Brain"). Visual interpretation based on the subjective judgment of whether global brain volume is age appropriate varies considerably from one observer to another, is inconsistently applied, and is unreliable. When serial scans are available, diffuse progressive enlargement of CSF spaces over a year or two is easier to identify and suggests AD (Luxenberg et al. 1987). However, for diagnostic purposes, repeated scans add relatively little information to changes in cognition observed over the same time interval. Quantitative and focused approaches are more reliable. One method is to measure total brain volume using scans with uniform characteristics in all three dimensions. A second method is to consider the volume of specific brain regions commonly affected in neurodegenerative diseases.

Typical clinical MRI studies acquire images that have greater resolution in one plane than others to increase signal-to-noise ratio and often have gaps to speed imaging time. However, it is possible to acquire isovoxel images consisting of image elements that are contiguous and of equal size in all dimensions. Isovoxel images permit better delineation of boundaries between CSF, brain, and skull, and thus more accurate measurement of brain volume. Voxel-based morphometry, a computer-assisted approach, is able to distinguish groups of AD patients and nondemented individuals, and even patients with mild cognitive impairment (Chételat et al. 2002; Frisoni et al. 2002). However, the diagnostic sensitivity and specificity of this approach in individual patients have not yet been studied adequately to recommend its clinical adoption.

Changes in the volume of specific brain regions can be determined reliably with both subjective and quantitative methods. Pathology is so localized in some dementing diseases that focal atrophy often is easily recognized, especially when symptoms are severe. Caudate atrophy is characteristic of Huntington's disease and is most evident with coronal images. Progressive supranuclear palsy (PSP) causes midbrain and pontine atrophy, which is frequently apparent on sagittal MRI and can be used to distinguish it from other parkinsonian syndromes (Cosottini et al. 2007). If focal atrophy is evident, it can help confirm a suspected diagnosis, but sensitivity may not be high early in the course of the illness. Because brain size varies significantly with gender and age, these two factors need to be considered, particularly when evaluating the significance of quantitative volume measures.

The earliest pathological changes in AD occur in the entorhinal cortex, amygdala, and hippocampus (Braak and Braak 1991). Consequently, it is not surprising that AD causes medial temporal volume loss, which is apparent on MRI scans. Coronal views best visualize the hippocampus and should be obtained routinely in the evaluation of dementia (see Figure 7–2). The resolution of MRI also allows assessment of specific structures within the medial temporal lobe. Individual medial temporal structures can be outlined manually with good reliability, but this procedure is very tedious and time-consuming and has little clinical applicability. Several automated methods for assessing medial temporal volumes have been developed, but none has been widely adopted, and multicenter validation studies are still needed. Fortunately, hippocampal size is readily apparent on coronal MRI scans, and several studies have found that visual assessment has good sensitivity and specificity in distinguishing AD from normal aging (Scheltens et al. 2002). For example, one qualitative 0–4 scale using rating anchors based on the width of the choroid fissure, width of the temporal horn, and height of the hippocampus achieved specificity of 90%, although at this level sensitivity was only 41%. Medial temporal lobe atrophy also can help identify which patients with mild cognitive impairment will progress to dementia (Visser et al. 2002).

Frontotemporal dementia (FTD) also causes focal atrophy, particularly involving the superior frontal and anterior temporal cortex (Boccardi et al. 2003). Sometimes focal atrophy in these regions is evident on visual assessment. However, the sensitivity and specificity of this finding in individual patients have not been determined, and it is unclear how frequently focal atrophy is obvious at the time of initial assessment. Because the volume of brain regions varies considerably among individuals, focal abnormalities are more clearly pathological when they become more evident over time (Figure 7–4). Automated measurement of frontal and temporal volume and more recently available measurements of cortical thickness show distinctive abnormalities that correspond to clinical FTD syndromes (Du et al. 2007). In patients with progressive nonfluent aphasia, atrophy is asymmetric, primarily involving language regions (Gorno-Tempini et al. 2004). Quantitative measures of focal atrophy distinguish groups of FTD patients, AD patients, and cognitively normal individuals from each other. It is important to note that FTD also causes hippocampal and amygdalar atrophy (Boccardi et al. 2002, 2003). Consequently, medial temporal atrophy is probably an unreliable way to distinguish AD and FTD.

Is There Copper, Iron, or Manganese Deposition?

Heavy metals such as copper, iron, and manganese are paramagnetic and alter magnetic resonance (MR) signal. These metals accumulate in the brain in several neuropsychiatric diseases. Looking for evidence of metal deposition is particularly useful in evaluations of patients with familial or atypical movement disorders. On occasion, MR sequences that take advantage of the specific characteristics of heavy metals also are relevant to the evaluation of neurocognitive deficits.

Accumulation of copper is the basis for Wilson's disease, an autosomal recessive disease causing parkinsonism, dystonia, tremor, dementia, and often behavioral changes, including depression and psychosis. Although the clinical features of liver failure, pigmented corneal deposits, and progressive motor disability should lead to the diagnosis on clinical grounds, MRI abnormalities can aid early diagnosis and lead to a consideration of Wilson's disease that otherwise might have been overlooked. Wilson's disease causes midbrain, thalamic, basal ganglia, and brain stem hyperintensities on T_2-weighted images in a very high percentage of patients (Prashanth et al. 2010). This pattern of hyperintensities is nearly unique. The presence and extent of MRI abnormalities correlate with clinical severity; only genetic carriers who are asymptomatic lack MRI hyperintensities (Starosta-Rubinstein et al. 1987).

Iron is best visualized with gradient-echo and susceptibility-weighted imaging MRI sequences. Deposition of iron occurs in PD and other parkinsonian syndromes, and attempts have been made to exploit this to aid in differential diagnosis. Neurodegeneration with brain iron accumulation (also known as Hallervorden-Spatz disease) is an unusual autosomal dominant metabolic disorder characterized by relentless progression of gait impairment, rigidity, dystonic posturing, and mental deterioration, usually beginning in the second or third decades of life, but occasionally in midlife or even in the elderly. There is massive iron accumulation in the globus pallidus and substantia nigra, causing very prominent hypointense signal on MRI (Sethi et al. 1988).

Lesser degrees of iron deposition occur in PD and multiple system atrophy. Several reports demonstrate hypointensity in the substantia nigra in PD and hypointensity in the globus pallidus in multiple system atrophy (Kraft et al. 2002; Martin et al. 2008; von Lewinski et al. 2007). Although there have been efforts to exploit these differences to aid diagnosis, studies have been contradictory and lack postmortem confirmation of diagnosis. Manganese toxicity occasionally causes parkinsonism and is associated with increased signal in the striatum on T_1-weighted images and normal T_2-weighted scans (Racette et al. 2005).

Cortical microhemorrhages and superficial siderosis cause hemosiderin deposits in the cortex that can be visualized best. These abnormalities are asymptomatic and indicate the presence of congophilic angiopathy, which is very common in AD (Haacke et al. 2007; Linn et al. 2010). In some cases, detecting these abnormalities will provide important evidence supporting a diagnosis of AD. They may develop in the context of immunotherapy for AD (Boche et al. 2008). They also may indicate an increased risk of symptomatic cerebral hemorrhage in AD patients.

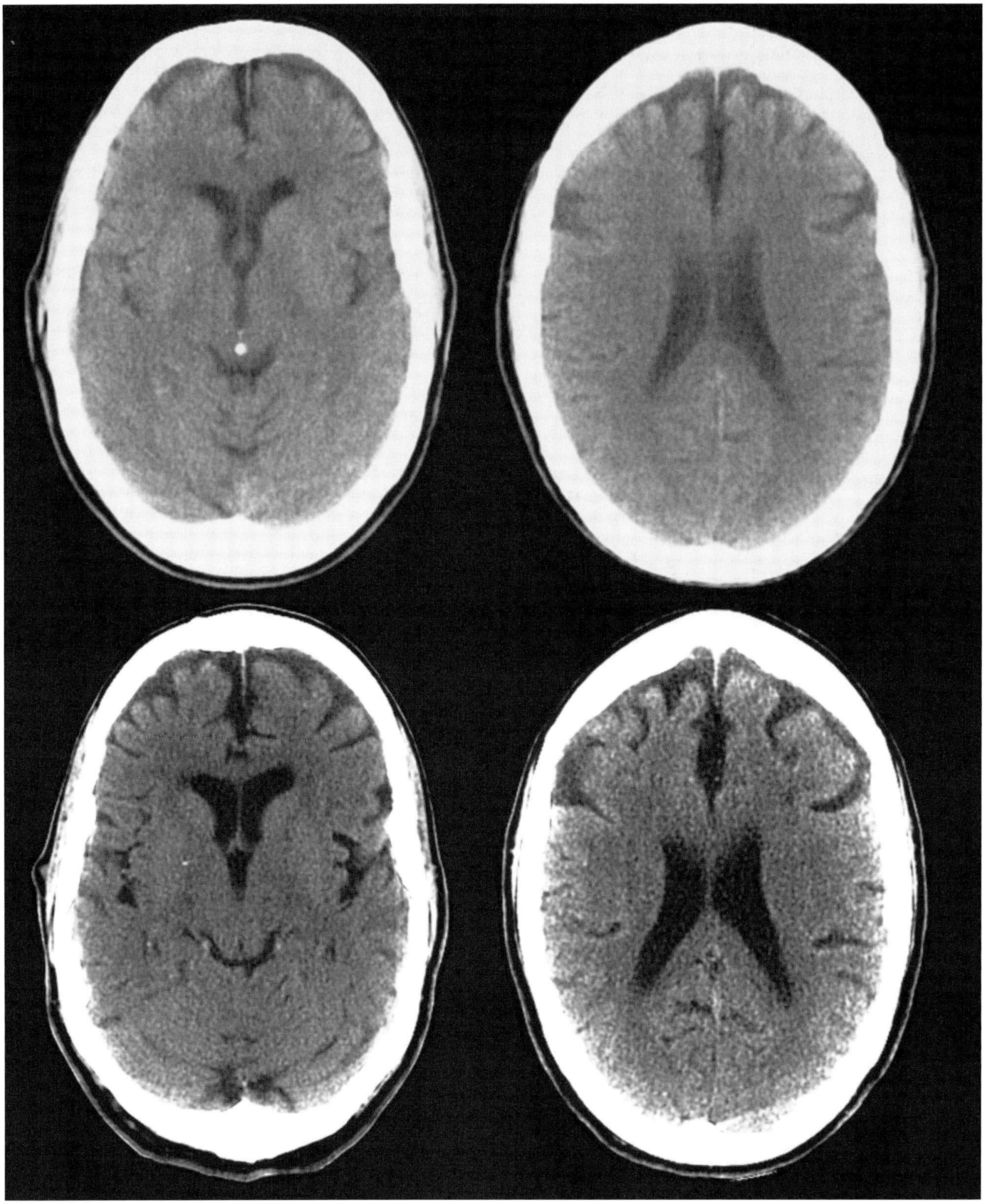

FIGURE 7–4. Progressive focal atrophy.

This woman had memory problems that were first noticed shortly after a minor automobile accident 2 years before her initial assessment at age 84 years. Sulci in the frontal cortex were somewhat more prominent in her initial scan *(top row)* but were considered to be of uncertain significance and perhaps due to her previous head injury. When her memory deficits remained mild and symptoms failed to progress as expected, another scan was obtained 6 years later *(bottom row)*. Atrophy was progressive and clearly predominant in frontal regions bilaterally. On reevaluation, it was evident that her major disability was due to a change in her personality and profound apathy rather than memory loss, symptoms that are consistent with frontotemporal dementia.

Diagnostic Questions Most Relevant to Molecular Neuroimaging

What Is the Pattern of Cerebral Hypometabolism?

Glucose is normally the brain's sole energy source, and glucose uptake primarily mirrors synaptic activity (Mata et al. 1980). FDG-PET images reflect brain activity over the 20–30 minutes following radioisotope injection. Therefore, these images can be used to examine a patient's responses to a task performed repeatedly over this uptake phase of the study. However, for clinical studies, individuals usually are asked to rest quietly in a darkened room. In cognitively normal individuals, cerebral metabolism is greatest in the basal ganglia, thalamus, cerebellum, and cerebral cortex; lower in the brain stem; and lowest in white matter (Figure 7–5). Glucose metabolic rates in the cerebral cortex are reasonably uniform. When eyes are left open, the visual cortex is activated and has higher glucose uptake.

FDG-PET is a sensitive indicator of the distribution of neuronal damage and synaptic failure. Images represent brain activity. Even though clinicians would profit from asking themselves what the pattern of hypometabolism is in every demented patient they encounter, FDG-PET is not always needed. The distribution of hypometabolism usually can be inferred accurately from the patient's history, examination, and relative cognitive deficits. Dementing diseases cause a global decline in glucose hypometabolism, with characteristic and distinctive patterns of regional predominance that evolve along with symptoms and reflect the selective vulnerability of different areas of the brain (Table 7–5).

Although the underlying disease determines the overall pattern of hypometabolism, individual differences in the regional intensity of the pattern are consistent with individual differences in clinical symptoms and follow classical principles of neurological localization. For example, patients with prominent language disturbance primarily have hypometabolism in the dominant hemisphere, patients with prominent visuospatial disturbance primarily have hypometabolism in the nondominant hemisphere, and patients with behavior disturbance have frontal hypometabolism. The observation that neuronal activity, as measured by cerebral metabolism, correlates with symptoms makes sense. What underlies brain function is the amount and effectiveness of neuronal activity, rather than simply the presence or loss of nerve cells. Although theoretically, inefficient brain activity caused by futile neuronal discharges or use of circuitous pathways could occur in dementia, these mechanisms would increase glucose metabolism and thus appear not to play a major role. Consequently, although the efficiency of neuronal activity is difficult to determine, decline in synaptic activity, rather than neuronal inefficiency, appears to account for symptoms of dementia and is more consistent with the hypometabolism observed with FDG-PET. Metabolic imaging may be even more reflective of patient symptoms than is pathological examination, which is unable to elucidate all of the physiological consequences of brain injury. Pathological hallmarks identified microscopically have uncertain effects on neuronal function, and the distribution of damage throughout the brain is difficult to delineate even at autopsy.

As with all imaging, FDG-PET is most helpful when used to answer specific questions after the differential diagnosis has first been narrowed with a careful history and examination. The most established clinical use of FDG-PET is to distinguish AD from FTD. Medicare and most insurance companies now reimburse for FDG-PET scans obtained for this indication when diagnosis remains unclear after completion of an otherwise comprehensive evaluation. AD and FTD are easily confused because they both lack distinctive neurological signs and have a similar progressive course. FTD typically causes predominant or disproportionate language deficits, with nonfluent progressive aphasia and semantic dementia (Adlam et al. 2006; Gorno-Tempini et al. 2004; Hodges and Patterson 2007). It also causes prominent behavior disturbance (Neary et al. 2005). Although these symptoms sometimes are distinctive enough to be diagnostic for FTD, these same kinds of symptoms also are frequently seen in AD. Indeed, patients with FTD often meet clinical criteria for AD (Varma et al. 1999).

FDG-PET is often very helpful in differentiating AD and FTD, despite their clinical similarities, because they have starkly contrasting patterns of hypometabolism. Foster et al. (2007) used FDG-PET scans from patients with pathologically confirmed disease to distinguish AD from FTD. In this study, visual interpretation of FDG-PET was based on the simple rule that FTD caused greater hypometabolism in anterior cingulate, anterior temporal, and frontal regions than in posterior cingulate and posterior temporoparietal cortex, whereas AD caused the opposite pattern to occur. After raters received brief training, diagnosis based on FDG-PET had greater interrater reliability (mean kappa=0.78) and diagnostic accuracy than clinical information alone. Furthermore, adding FDG-PET to clinical evaluation increased diagnostic accuracy, with a specificity of 97.6% and sensitivity of 86%, and with a positive likelihood ratio of 36.5 for FTD. FDG-PET was particularly helpful when raters were uncertain of their clinical diagnosis.

FDG-PET has not been as extensively studied in other situations involving considerable diagnostic uncertainty. Nevertheless, performing an FDG-PET scan and applying the current knowledge of how different dementing diseases affect the pattern of hypometabolism can be useful in specific circumstances. FDG-PET provides objective evidence of a neuro-

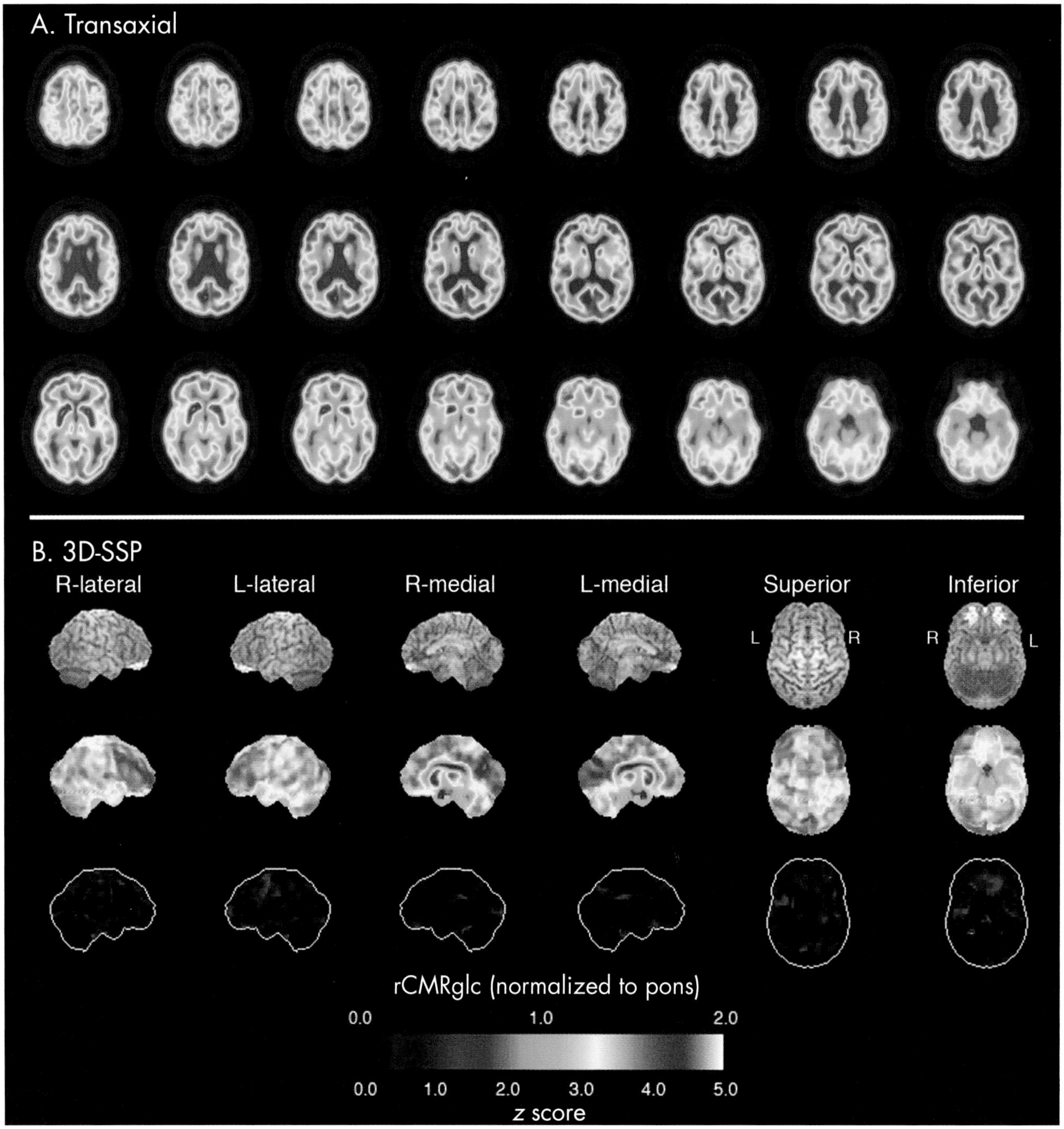

FIGURE 7–5. Fluorodeoxyglucose positron emission tomography (FDG-PET) image in a cognitively normal elderly individual.

FDG-PET scans produce up to 128 transaxial images, here truncated to the most relevant brain slices for easier display (**Panel A**). Rates of glucose metabolism (rCMRglc), in this case relative to pons, are displayed using a color scale shown below the images, with hotter colors representing higher rates of glucose metabolism. Analysis software programs allow scan data to be summarized and displayed in uniform space (**Panel B**), permitting direct comparison of scans from different individuals. One such program, three-dimensional stereotactic surface projection (3D-SSP), displays scan data from six perspectives, illustrated in a reference image of the brain surface *(Panel B, top row)*. Metabolism relative to pons *(Panel B, row 2)* is shown using the same color scale as in the transaxial images. A statistical map also can be constructed *(Panel B, row 3)*, showing the *z* score of surface pixels in this scan compared to 27 cognitively normal elderly people. Normal individuals have a relatively uniform and high metabolic rate throughout the cerebral cortex. In this case, there are no areas of the brain showing significant reductions in metabolic rate.

TABLE 7–5. Typical patterns of regional cerebral glucose metabolism in common dementing diseases

Disease	Pattern of glucose hypometabolism
Alzheimer's disease	Symmetric or asymmetric bilateral temporoparietal and posterior cingulate; lesser frontal association cortex; sparing of primary sensorimotor and visual cortex
Vascular dementia	Multifocal cortical and subcortical, correlating with structural imaging lesions
Parkinson's disease with dementia and dementia with Lewy bodies	Symmetric or asymmetric bilateral temporoparietal, posterior cingulate, and visual cortex; lesser frontal association cortex; sparing of primary sensorimotor cortex
Huntington's disease	Caudate nucleus and lesser frontal association cortex
Progressive supranuclear palsy	Caudate nucleus, putamen, thalamus, pons, primarily superior and anterior frontal cortex; sparing of cerebellum
Corticobasal degeneration	Asymmetric frontal, temporal, and parietal cortex and thalamus contralateral to limb apraxia

degenerative disease when medical history is ambiguous or informants are unavailable or unreliable. The pattern of hypometabolism may reveal important additional information when patients have an atypical clinical presentation or when diagnostic features are shared by two or more disorders. Because the patterns of hypometabolism in dementing diseases are complex, further detailed description is warranted.

Cerebral hypometabolism in AD is consistent in its typical sequence of regional involvement but varies in detail from patient to patient just as symptoms in individual patients can vary. Hypometabolism is first seen in the posterior cingulate gyrus (Minoshima et al. 1997). It then spreads to affect the association cortex in the parietal and posterior temporal lobes (Figure 7–6). Eventually, hypometabolism spreads to involve the prefrontal cortex and most of the brain. Although the relative decrease of metabolism in the posterior association cortex, compared with that in the anterior association cortex, remains throughout the course of AD, this discrepancy becomes harder to recognize as frontal regions become progressively more affected. As the surrounding frontal and parietal association cortex becomes more hypometabolic, the relative preservation of the primary sensorimotor cortex surrounding the central sulcus becomes increasingly evident. The occipital lobe, including the primary visual cortex, also is relatively spared. The caudate, putamen, and thalamus are spared relative to the cerebral cortex but are hypometabolic when compared to those of cognitively normal individuals of similar age (Foster et al. 1988). The cerebellum and brain stem are little affected in sporadic AD (Minoshima et al. 1995).

The initial involvement of the posterior cingulate gyrus in AD is perhaps unexpected because the hippocampus and medial temporal lobe appear to suffer the earliest damage on traditional neuropathological examination. Considerable evidence indicates that metabolic declines are greater in the posterior cingulate cortex and lateral temporal cortex because synaptic projections from the hippocampus and medial temporal cortex are damaged. Neurotoxic lesions in the entorhinal and perirhinal cortices in monkeys cause neocortical hypometabolism (Meguro et al. 1999). Anterior temporal lobectomy performed to treat epilepsy also causes posterior cingulate hypometabolism (Minoshima et al. 1999). Furthermore, hippocampal atrophy correlates with posterior cingulate hypometabolism in AD (Meguro et al. 2001).

Clinical criteria for AD have relatively poor specificity, and misdiagnoses occur in community practice and even at leading academic centers (Becker et al. 1994; Blacker et al. 1994; Mendez et al. 1992). FDG-PET is a promising method to improve AD diagnosis. Visual interpretation of FDG-PET scans has higher diagnostic accuracy than clinical evaluation alone when autopsy diagnosis is used as the gold standard. The diagnostic sensitivity (93%–94%) and specificity (73%–79%) of FDG-PET are better than those of clinical evaluation alone (sensitivities of 79%–85% and specificities of 50%–70%) (Hoffman et al. 2000; Lim et al. 1999; Silverman et al. 2001).

FTD causes glucose hypometabolism predominantly in anterior brain regions, including the frontal cortex, anterior cingulate cortex, and anterior temporal regions (Foster et al. 2005). As symptoms progress, deficits become more pervasive, but anterior regions remain predominantly affected, and primary motor-sensory and visual cortex and posterior association cortex are relatively spared. Several clinical phenotypes of FTD are recognized (see Chapter 16, "Alzheimer's Disease and the Frontotemporal Dementia Syndromes") and cause corresponding variations in this overall pattern of glucose hypometabolism (Miller et al. 1993). Patients with severe behavior disturbances tend to have predominant right hemisphere hypometabolism, whereas those with progressive aphasia exhibit more hypometabolism in the dominant hemisphere (Figure 7–7). Hypometabolism in some FTD patients is mostly in the anterior temporal cortex, but in others it is almost entirely limited to the frontal cortex. The reason for these individual variations is not yet understood (Foster et al. 2005).

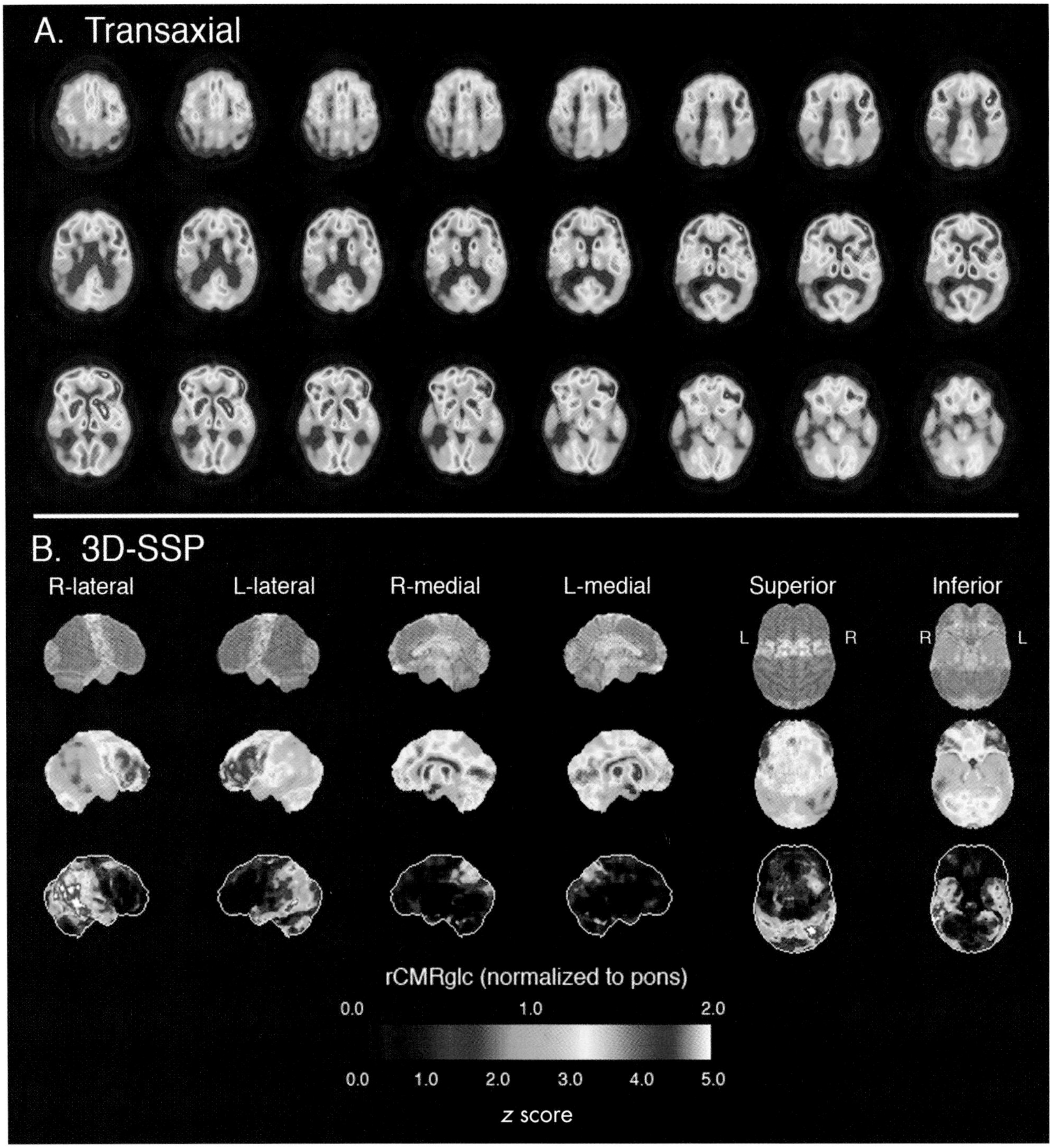

FIGURE 7–6. Fluorodeoxyglucose positron emission tomography (FDG-PET) in a patient with Alzheimer's disease (AD).

Transaxial (**Panel** A) and three-dimensional stereotactic surface projection (3D-SSP) displays (**Panel B**) of an FDG-PET scan from a patient with AD are shown. In this case, the reference image of the brain surface *(Panel B, top row)* has been colored to indicate areas typically most affected in AD (red=temporoparietal association cortex; orange=posterior cingulate cortex) and frontotemporal dementia (purple=frontal association cortex; blue=posterior cingulate cortex; green=anterior temporal cortex). AD causes glucose hypometabolism predominantly in posterior regions of the cerebral cortex *(Panel A; Panel B, row 2)*. The statistical map *(Panel B, row 3)* shows that some regions have hypometabolism 5 standard deviations (*z*=5) from that seen in 27 cognitively normal elderly individuals. Cerebral metabolism for glucose (rCMRglc) is shown relative to pons values.

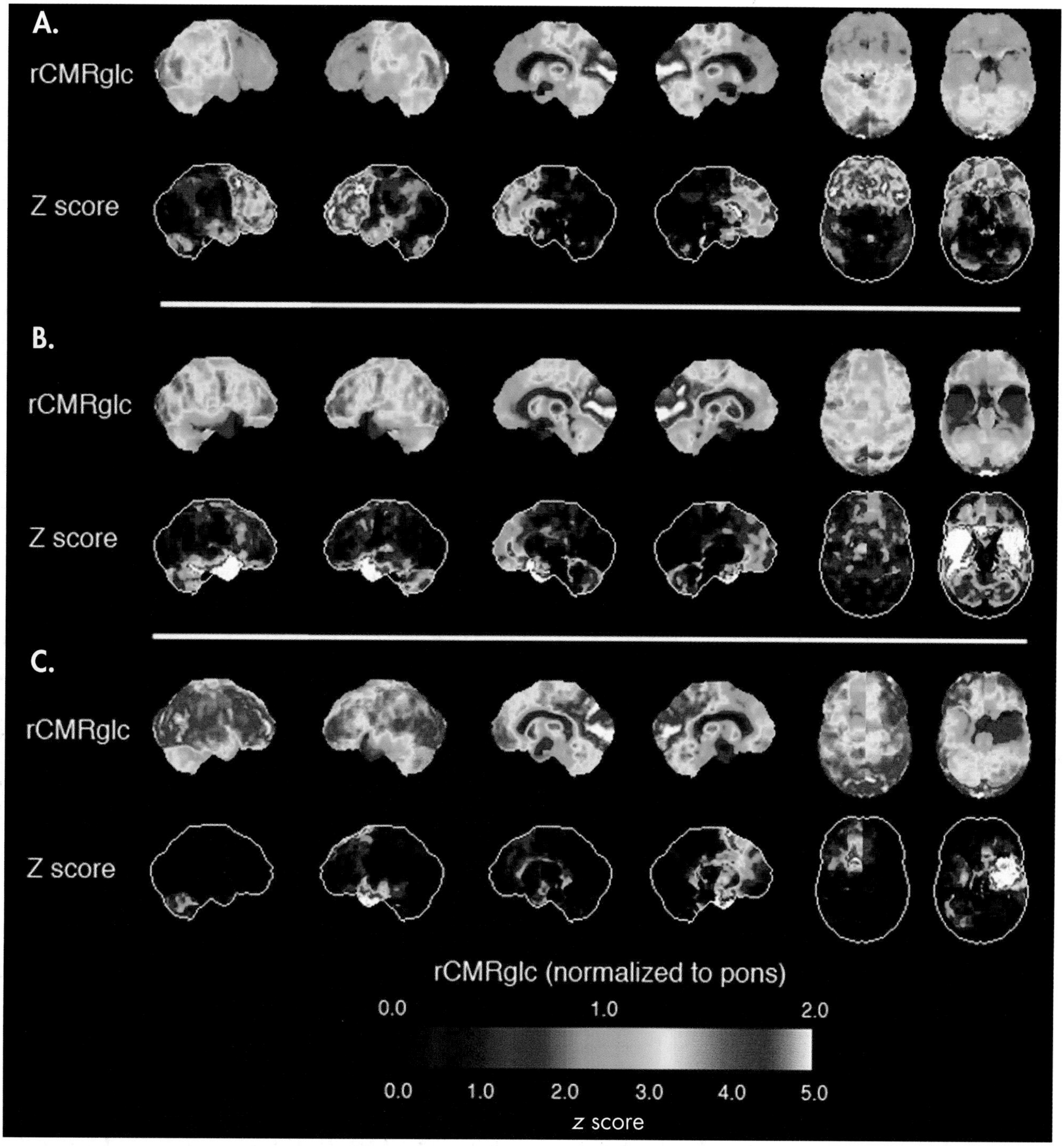

FIGURE 7–7. Fluorodeoxyglucose positron emission tomography (FDG-PET) in patients with frontotemporal dementia (FTD).

FDG-PET scans from three patients with FTD (**Panels A, B, and C**), displayed as three-dimensional stereotactic surface projection (3D-SSP) glucose metabolic (rCMRglc) and statistical (*z* score) maps as in Figures 7–5 and 7–6, illustrate the individual heterogeneity of this disorder. FTD causes glucose hypometabolism predominantly in frontal, anterior cingulate, and anterior temporal regions (see Figure 7–6), but its relative severity can vary considerably. Just as FTD causes several clinical syndromes, the pattern of glucose hypometabolism may differ from patient to patient. The cerebral hemispheres can have similar hypometabolism *(Panels A and B)* or significant metabolic asymmetry *(Panel C)*. Sometimes the frontal association cortex and anterior cingulate gyrus can be the primary sites of hypometabolism *(Panel A)*. In other cases, the anterior temporal lobes are predominantly affected *(Panels B and C)*, with variable involvement of other regions.

Dementia with Lewy bodies (DLB) and Parkinson's disease with dementia (PDD) both show a pattern of glucose hypometabolism similar to that in AD, with the added characteristic of occipital hypometabolism, whether or not there is also AD pathology (Ishii et al. 1998; Minoshima et al. 2001). The cause of occipital hypometabolism remains uncertain. The metabolic similarities of DLB and AD—that is, bilateral temporoparietal and lesser degrees of frontal hypometabolism—are not surprising given the frequent difficulty in clinically distinguishing these disorders. Current clinical criteria for DLB have good specificity but poor sensitivity, and patients with pathologically confirmed DLB often have been misdiagnosed as having AD (Weiner et al. 2003). Imaging with a dopaminergic marker may be particularly valuable in distinguishing AD from DLB (see "Is There Loss of Dopaminergic Neurons?" later in this chapter), but neuroimaging cannot distinguish DLB from PDD. Perhaps this is not surprising, because although clinical presentation and clinical criteria differ, the pathological findings in these two disorders are indistinguishable.

Distinctive patterns of glucose hypometabolism also have been identified in PSP and corticobasal degeneration. In most cases, the characteristic motor symptoms of PSP and corticobasal degeneration are sufficient for diagnosis, but the pattern of hypometabolism is occasionally helpful. FDG-PET findings differ between PSP and DLB and between PSP and PDD, even though there are similar abnormalities on dopaminergic imaging. Compared to cognitively normal subjects, patients with PSP have glucose hypometabolism in the caudate nucleus, putamen, thalamus, pons, and cerebral cortex (Foster et al. 1988). Declines of glucose metabolism are most prominent in the superior and anterior portions of the frontal cortex in a manner that is now better understood as causing a pattern typical of tauopathies (see Chapter 12, "Cognitive Impairment and Rehabilitation"). However, glucose metabolism in the cerebellar cortex is normal in PSP. This pattern can be helpful in distinguishing PSP from cerebellar degeneration, both of which have gait ataxia as an early symptom. Corticobasal degeneration is characterized by significant metabolic hemispheric asymmetry, just as the clinical symptoms are typically very asymmetric. Nearly the entire affected hemisphere, including frontal, temporal, and parietal regions, is involved. However, in addition to the asymmetry in the cerebral cortex, ipsilateral thalamic hypometabolism is evident, while the striatum seems relatively spared (Eidelberg et al. 1991). Although corticobasal degeneration, FTD, and PSP are now known to share tau pathology, they have remarkably different clinical symptoms and patterns of glucose hypometabolism.

Because FDG-PET is a measure of synaptic activity, it is reasonable to expect that synaptic activity is affected early in neurodegenerative diseases. Synaptic loss as an early sign of neurodegenerative disease has been best shown in AD, where synaptic failure precedes axonal loss and neuronal death (DeKosky and Scheff 1990; Selkoe 2002). When changes in metabolism first appear is unknown, but groups of individuals presumed to be at high risk for AD based on apolipoprotein ε4 genotype show metabolic changes long before symptoms are expected, particularly in the posterior cingulate gyrus, where hypometabolism begins in AD (Reiman et al. 1996; Small et al. 2000). Furthermore, several studies have shown that FDG-PET helps distinguish individuals with memory disturbance who later will develop AD. Many nondemented individuals with mild cognitive impairment show a pattern of cerebral glucose metabolism identical to that of patients with AD (see Figure 7–6). Moreover, patients with mild cognitive impairment are much more likely to develop AD over the subsequent few years if they exhibit AD patterns of glucose hypometabolism than if they do not (Anchisi et al. 2005; Berent et al. 1999; Chételat et al. 2003).

Is There Loss of Dopaminergic Neurons?

Dopaminergic function is affected in many neuropsychiatric diseases and dementing illnesses, including PD, DLB, PDD, and PSP. Furthermore, rigidity frequently develops in moderate and severe AD. The presence of parkinsonian features provides important clinical evidence of these disorders, but the sensitivity of clinical diagnosis is relatively low in most series. Molecular imaging provides a more objective and quantitative measure of dopaminergic function. Tracers are available to evaluate the integrity of dopaminergic neurons at several sites. Uptake of dopa, the dopamine precursor, can be measured with $[^{18}F]$fluorodopa. Radiotracers are available that bind to the vesicular monoamine transporter 2, which is responsible for storage of dopamine in synaptic vesicles, and to the dopamine transporter (DAT), which facilitates reuptake of dopamine into axons (Brooks et al. 2003). These tracers have been widely used in research studies, but none is currently available for clinical use in the United States or Canada. However, the SPECT DAT tracer $[^{123}I]\beta$-CIT (*N*-delta-[fluoropropyl]-2beta-carbomethoxy-3beta-[4-iodophenyl]tropane) is approved for clinical use in England and Europe to differentiate DLB from AD. These studies are relatively easy to interpret because after an initial uptake phase, remaining ligand is limited primarily to the striatum (site of dopaminergic projection axons from the substantia nigra). Both the amount and the morphological shape of binding can be helpful diagnostically, with normal distribution appearing in a comma shape, whereas with loss of dopamine neurons, posterior and caudal binding diminishes, causing a full-stop or circular pattern (Figure 7–8). In a prospective study of 288 demented patients with and without DLB who had acceptable $[^{123}I]\beta$-CIT scans, diagnostic accuracy, compared to consensus diagnosis based on the scan alone, was 85% for probable DLB, with a sensitivity of 77% and a specificity of 90% (McKeith et al. 2007). This compares fa-

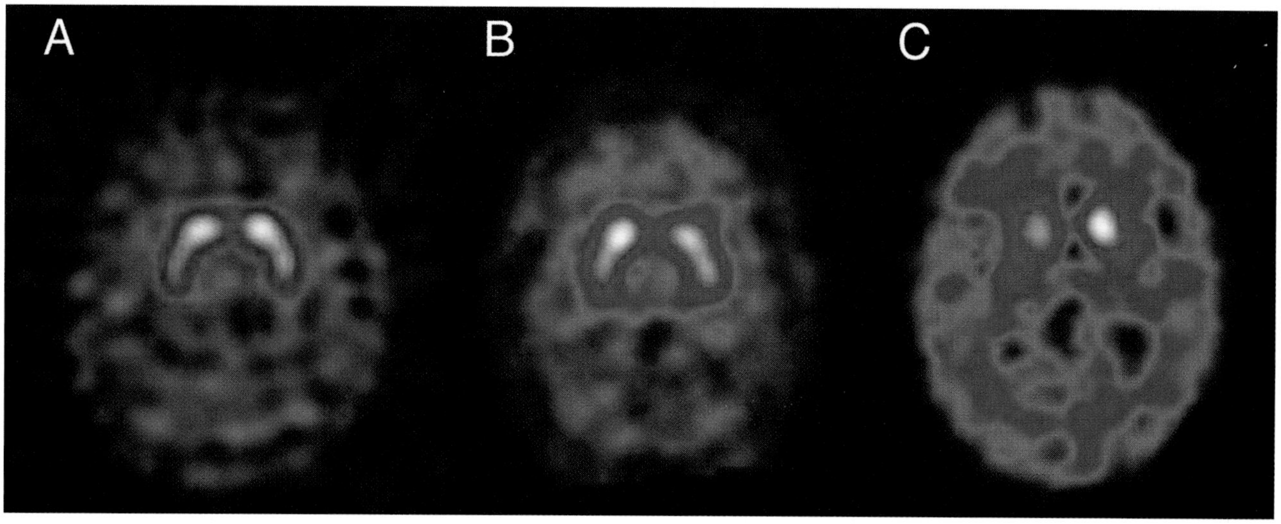

FIGURE 7–8. Dopamine imaging in patients with Alzheimer's disease (AD) and dementia with Lewy bodies (DLB).

β-CIT SPECT scans in a cognitively normal individual (**Panel A**), an 83-year-old patient with AD (**Panel B**), and an 81-year-old patient who has probable DLB (**Panel C**). Following an initial uptake phase that primarily reflects cerebral blood flow, static images shown here were obtained reflecting binding to dopamine uptake sites in the striatum. Binding is proportionate to the intensity of "hot" colors. Scans from the normal and AD subjects show a similar comma-like pattern. This is in contrast to the scan in the patient with DLB, which shows a more restricted full-stop pattern of uptake. In the DLB patient *(Panel C)*, the intensity of the striatum is asymmetric, with greater uptake in the left than in the right, a typical finding in both Parkinson's disease and DLB. Uptake in all images is displayed relative to cerebellum because absolute binding rates are not easily calculated in clinical studies.

β-CIT=*N*-delta-(fluoropropyl)-2beta-carbomethoxy-3beta-(4-iodophenyl)tropane; SPECT=single-photon emission computed tomography.

Source. Images are provided courtesy of GE Healthcare.

vorably to the average sensitivity of 49% for the clinical diagnosis of probable DLB when compared to autopsy diagnosis. Consequently, [^{123}I]β-CIT appears valuable for increasing the detection of DLB (specificity, but not sensitivity, of the clinical criteria for probable DLB is already high). Accuracy and specificity for possible DLB using both clinical and imaging criteria are considerably lower, and autopsy findings still are needed before clinicians can truly know whether imaging dopaminergic deficits in this situation are truly reliable.

As with other molecular imaging studies, a patient's use of drugs must be closely examined when interpreting scans of dopamine function. For example, bupropion and a number of other drugs affect [^{123}I]β-CIT scans. Because short-term use of levodopa or dopamine agonists and antagonists that act on postsynaptic dopamine receptors does not affect the scans, identifying DLB in patients receiving neuroleptic drugs should be possible without knowing for certain that parkinsonian symptoms are spontaneous. However, more study is needed to evaluate the effects of long-term treatment with dopaminergic agonists and antagonists on all ligands used in dopaminergic imaging (Ravina et al. 2005).

[^{123}I]β-CIT scans also can help differentiate PD from benign essential tremor (Catafau and Tolosa 2004; Marshall et al. 2006). PD has a decrease in striatal binding, whereas binding in essential tremor is normal. Usually, the clinical circumstances, including typical features and response to treatment, are sufficient for an accurate diagnosis. However, some patients may have both resting tremor, typical of PD, and an action tremor, typical of benign essential tremor. Traditionally, when both types of tremor are present, the most prominent determines the diagnosis. However, this judgment is very subjective, and this rule of thumb can be inaccurate. The onset of cognitive deficits in a patient with presumed essential tremor also raises doubts that can be resolved with dopamine imaging.

Although a positive scan may occasionally help confirm a diagnosis of PD or of PDD, it cannot distinguish PD from PDD or PD from either PSP or multiple system atrophy. One of the more intriguing opportunities is to improve diagnostic accuracy by assessing regional hypometabolism and dopaminergic function together. Use of a dopaminergic tracer provides an alternate and objective method of determining whether there is nigral pathology, which is always present in DLB. Simultaneous analysis of uptake and receptor binding phases of a dopaminergic tracer might substitute for a separate metabolic scan (Koeppe et al. 2005).

Are There Amyloid Plaques?

Undoubtedly, one of the most exciting developments in dementia imaging is the production of small-molecule radioactive probes for the in vivo assessment of AD pathology. These probes have generated intense interest, and remarkable progress has been made over a short time in the research necessary for modeling and validation. Both SPECT and PET agents have been proposed for amyloid imaging. Work is furthest along on the positron-emitting ^{11}C tracer Pittsburgh compound B (PIB), which is under active investigation at more than a dozen sites. This lipophilic tracer is a derivative of thioflavin-T and easily crosses the blood-brain barrier and appears to bind only fully formed plaques (Klunk et al. 2004; Mathis et al. 2002). A tracer kinetic model for PIB requires only venous access and uses a simple method for analysis (Price et al. 2005). PIB binding is much more evident in the cerebral cortex in patients with AD, whereas binding is similar in white matter and cerebral cortex in cognitively normal individuals (Figure 7–9). Amyloid imaging complements FDG-PET findings. Increased PIB binding can be seen when FDG-PET scans are normal. Preliminary studies indicate that binding of this tracer is not limited to patients with clinically diagnosed AD. Some elderly individuals who are not demented and some who have DLB also show increased PIB binding consistent with pathological studies (Rowe et al. 2007). The presence of increased PIB binding in nondemented elderly and in patients with mild cognitive impairment raises the question whether these findings will predict later development of AD (Forsberg et al. 2008). Furthermore, PIB binding is seen in some patients with clinically diagnosed FTD, suggesting that these individuals may actually have AD (Engler et al. 2008; Rabinovici et al. 2007). If further validation studies are successful, it may be possible to use amyloid imaging to study the evolution of neuritic plaques and their relationship to dementia symptoms and treatment response.

Other amyloid imaging agents are under active development. The tracer [^{11}C]SB-13, which is similar to [^{11}C]PIB, has been developed and partially validated (Verhoeff et al. 2004). PET amyloid tracers using ^{18}F, which has a longer half-life, also are under development. Another PET ligand, [^{18}F]FDDNP, has a different pattern of binding and appears to image both neurofibrillary tangles and neuritic plaques (Small et al. 2006). It is unclear whether this will have any advantages over imaging amyloid alone, but binding of [^{18}F]FDDNP does appear to increase as symptoms progress.

Special Situations

The causes of dementia that must be considered and the uses of neuroimaging are different when dementia progresses rapidly over a few weeks or months, when it begins before age 60 years, and when it appears to be inherited. Neuroimaging also can be particularly helpful in evaluating symptoms that evolve in the course of a progressive dementia.

Rapidly Progressive Dementia

Structural imaging is essential and MRI is clearly preferable to CT when evaluating a patient with rapidly progressive dementia. The superior sensitivity and flexibility of MRI are often extremely valuable in detecting multiple, small, disseminated lesions due to metastases or vasculitis, and vascular lesions from emboli due to endocarditis, cardiac thrombus, open-heart surgery, or a peripheral venous thrombus reaching the brain through a patent foramen ovale. Quickly identifying these conditions is critical because early treatment often can improve or stabilize the cognitive deficits.

Another advantage of MRI is its ability to detect prion diseases. Creutzfeldt-Jakob disease and other prion diseases very commonly cause focal increased signal on diffusion-weighted imaging, FLAIR, and proton-weighted MRI, and to a lesser extent on T_2-weighted imaging (Finkenstaedt et al. 1996; Na et al. 1999). Diffusion-weighted imaging appears most sensitive. It is important to recognize that CT scans and routine T_1-weighted MRI images may be normal in Creutzfeldt-Jakob disease. Therefore, the clinician may need to specifically request diffusion-weighted and FLAIR images and to focus the radiologist's attention to the suspected regions of interest, because the typical abnormalities of prion disease may not be recognized due to its low prevalence.

MRI diffusion changes are probably caused by gliosis and microscopic spongiform vacuolization. MRI abnormalities in typical, sporadic Creutzfeldt-Jakob disease are most often bilateral and symmetric, with increased signal in the putamen and caudate nuclei (Schroter et al. 2000). The cerebral cortex also can have focal abnormalities that have a distinctive ribbon appearance (Figure 7–10). By contrast, FLAIR images show diffuse abnormalities in stroke that involve both gray and white matter. The location of MRI changes in Creutzfeldt-Jakob disease can be either symmetric or asymmetric, reflects the distribution of prion pathology, and correlates with patient symptoms (Kropp et al. 1999; Mittal et al. 2002). In new variant Creutzfeldt-Jakob disease, acquired from exposure to bovine spongiform encephalopathy, increased signal typically occurs in the pulvinar of the thalamus (Zeidler et al. 2000). This so-called pulvinar sign has not been reported in sporadic or familial prion disease.

Young-Onset and Familial Dementia

Dementia occurring before the patient is age 60 years requires closer consideration of diseases that are uncommon later in life. Traumatic injury, brain tumors, and HIV and other sexu-

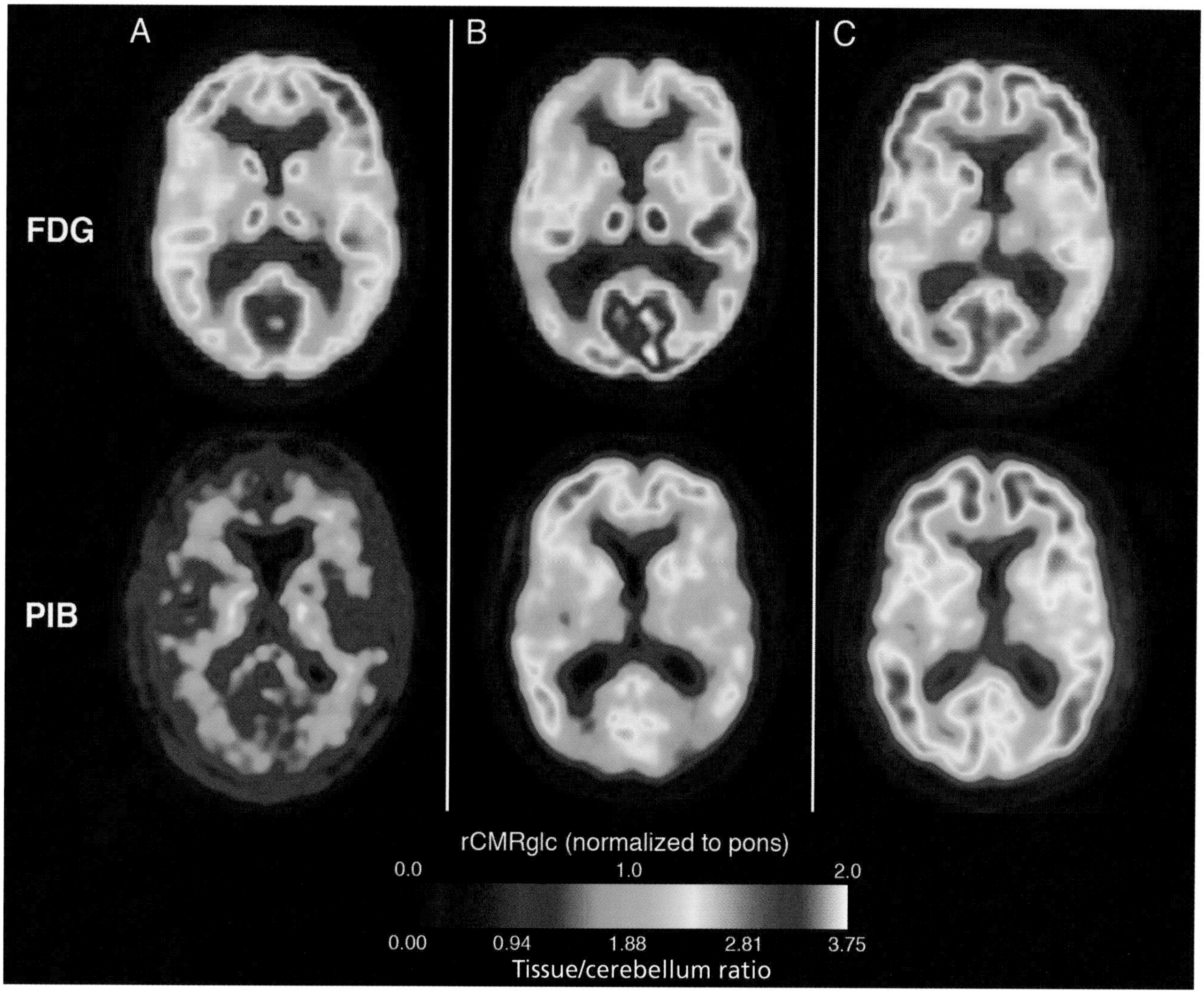

FIGURE 7–9. Amyloid positron emission tomography (PET) imaging.

Transaxial fluorodeoxyglucose positron emission tomography (FDG-PET) scans *(top row)* and amyloid PET scans with positron-emitting ^{11}C tracer Pittsburgh compound B (PIB) *(bottom row)* from a cognitively normal elderly individual and two patients with Alzheimer's disease (AD) are shown, using the color scale shown below the images. The normal subject (**Panel A**) has a normal distribution of FDG in the cerebral cortex, whereas both AD patients (**Panels B and C**) have predominant temporoparietal hypometabolism. Hypometabolism is greater in one AD patient *(Panel B)* than the other *(Panel C)* and also involves the right frontal cortex. Amyloid binding relative to the cerebellum is primarily evident in the white matter in the cognitively normal subject *(Panel A, bottom row)*. In the two AD patients, amyloid binding is much greater in the cerebral cortex, nearly obscuring the binding in the white matter. Amyloid binding is not closely correlated with the severity or distribution of glucose hypometabolism. The AD patient with the most pronounced cerebral hypometabolism *(Panel B)* has less ^{11}C-PIB binding than the other AD patient *(Panel C)*. Glucose metabolism is greatest in the visual cortex, where ^{11}C-PIB binding is not particularly high. Furthermore, there may be high amyloid binding in the frontal cortex *(Panel B)*, even if metabolism is little affected there *(Panel C)*.

ally transmitted infections are potential causes. FTD is nearly as common as AD in this age group. Young-onset dementia, which is often inherited, is another possibility. Some familial dementing disorders have distinctive imaging findings.

Cerebral autosomal dominant arteriopathy with subcortical infarcts and leukoencephalopathy (CADASIL) causes progressive dementia beginning in the third to sixth decades of life. This disease may go unrecognized for many years and be first identified only after the typical features are seen on brain scanning. Definitive diagnosis depends on identifying electron-dense inclusions in capillaries on biopsy or a causative *NOTCH3* mutation on chromosome 19. MRI shows lacunar infarcts and microhemorrhages that become more numerous over time. The most distinctive imaging feature of CADASIL

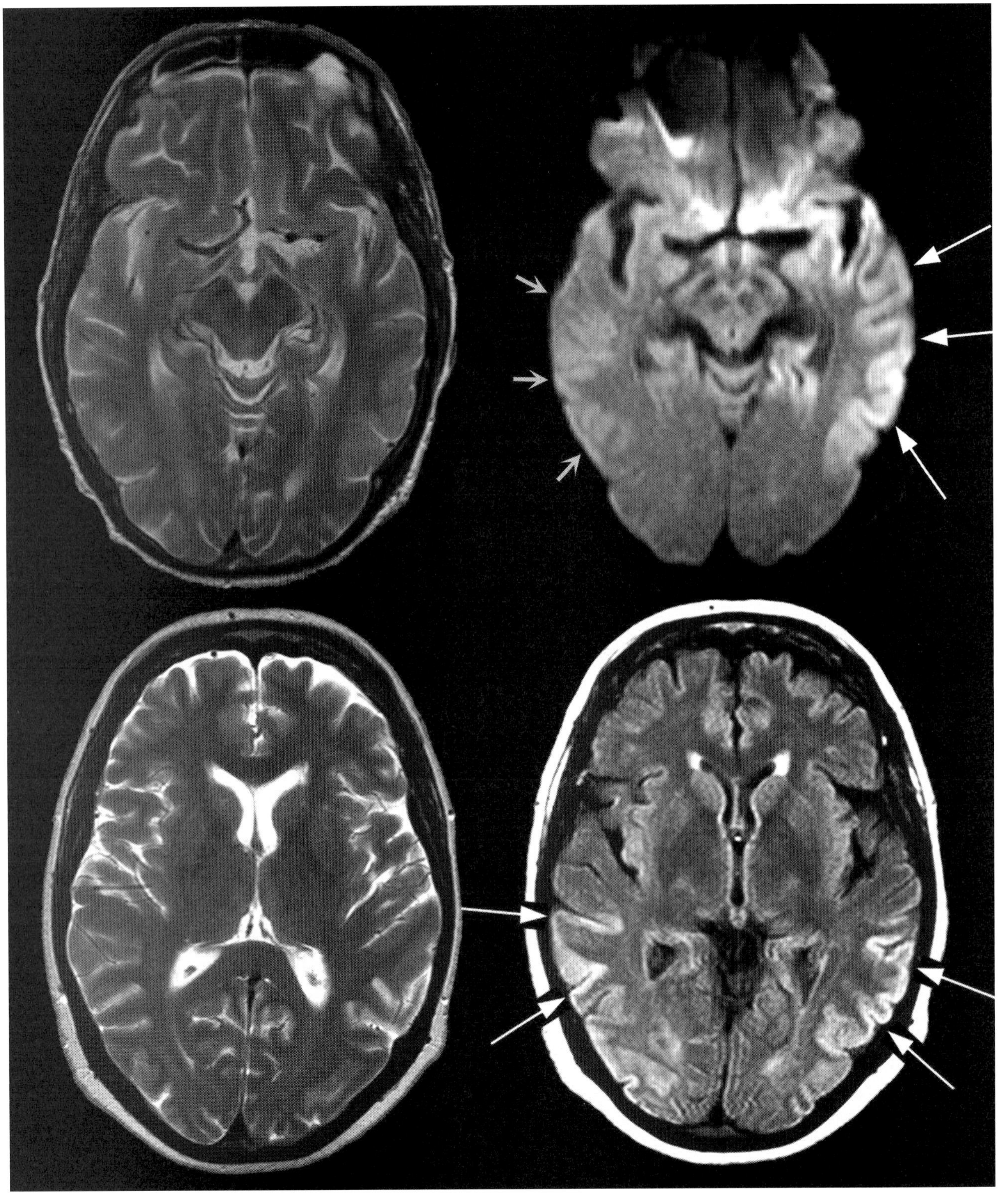

FIGURE 7–10. Magnetic resonance imaging in patients with Creutzfeldt-Jakob disease.

Magnetic resonance images show hyperintensities following the cortical ribbon in two patients with pathologically confirmed Creutzfeldt-Jakob disease. In one patient, a T_2-weighted image *(top row, left)* shows no abnormality, whereas the diffusion-weighted image *(top row, right)* shows increased signal in the left temporal lobe *(large arrows)* that is not seen on the right *(small arrows)*. The second patient also fails to show any abnormalities on a T_2-weighted image *(bottom row, left)*, although the fluid-attenuated inversion recovery (FLAIR) image shows increased signal in the temporoparietal cortical ribbon bilaterally *(large arrows)*.

is areas of hyperintensity in the anterior temporal lobes (Figure 7–11). In one study, a characteristic pattern of bilateral hyperintense white matter located directly below the cortical ribbon was found in all 40 patients with CADASIL, even in the youngest (van den Boom et al. 2003).

Familial AD also may have usual clinical and imaging findings. Some presenilin 1 mutations cause spastic paraparesis and can be associated with less dense cotton-wool plaques. In such cases, AD seems very aggressive and may involve areas that are usually spared, such as the primary motor cortex (Moretti et al. 2004). Likewise, some presenilin 1 mutations are associated with cerebellar amyloid plaques. Cerebellar glucose metabolism is usually normal in AD, but in these cases there may be cerebellar hypometabolism (Murrell et al. 2001).

Evolving Symptoms

When dementing diseases progress, imaging can help in understanding the cause of unexpected symptoms. In neurodegenerative diseases, symptoms are expected to evolve gradually and follow a typical course characteristic of each disorder. For example, worsening of memory loss or slow development of more severe language deficit in AD would not be surprising. Sometimes, however, the cause of dementia may be brought into question when the course of a patient's illness differs from that predicted by the clinical diagnosis (see Figure 7–4). In these cases, additional imaging studies are needed so appropriate treatment can be started.

It is impossible to consider all situations in which evolving symptoms warrant neuroimaging, but a few examples should be illustrative. Patients with AD are not expected to develop sudden hemiparesis or aphasia. If either occurs, an MRI is likely to show a cerebral infarct, subdural hematoma, or intracerebral hemorrhage. If apathy, inattention, perseveration, or loss of verbal fluency becomes more pronounced than memory loss in a patient thought to have AD, then FDG-PET is appropriate. In this case, the correct diagnosis may be FTD instead of AD. FDG-PET showing bilateral temporoparietal hypometabolism or abnormal amyloid imaging may help confirm AD when cognitive deficits worsen in a patient with vascular dementia, even though no new vascular lesions are seen with MRI.

Patients with dementia due to neurological disease almost uniformly have abnormal FDG-PET scans, whereas those with cognitive complaints for other reasons usually have normal scans. FDG-PET scans are abnormal even when symptoms of AD are mild. Thus, a normal pattern of glucose metabolism may provide additional assurance that the initial diagnosis was in error when a patient thought to have AD fails to get worse. FDG-PET also may be useful in differentiating neurodegenerative disease from cognitive impairment due to psychiatric illness, medication side effects, and malingering. Normal MRI and FDG-PET scans will help confirm that a patient is willfully unable to perform his or her daily care and does not have a dementing disease, even though he or she performs very poorly during the clinical examination and neuropsychological testing.

Emerging Neuroimaging Methods

With the rapid development of new technology, neuroimaging is providing important new insights about the mechanisms of neuropsychiatric illness and playing an increasing role in clinical care. Some promising methods can be incorporated into routine MRI scanning sessions and are already widely available. These include techniques to evaluate white matter integrity and connectivity with magnetic transfer imaging and diffusion tensor imaging, and magnetic resonance spectroscopy, which provides novel insight into brain energetics and biochemical pathways. Both have been discussed in Chapter 6 ("Imaging the Structure of the Aging Human Brain"). Despite the easy availability of these techniques, their role in neuropsychiatric practice is not yet established, and studies are needed to validate the interpretation of findings. Many other neuroimaging methods await further research and development. Those of greatest interest to neuropsychiatry are discussed below.

Advanced Image Analysis

Dramatic increases in computing power and significant advances in image processing algorithms and statistical methods will improve the accuracy of brain scan interpretation. Clinical studies still rely primarily on simple standard planar image displays and subjective interpretation of findings without reference to standardized data for comparison. However, much more can be done. Imaging data can be manipulated to show the brain in any angle of view or in four dimensions (by incorporating serial studies into processing algorithms). As scanner resolution has improved, the need to reduce this information to a more manageable form for interpretation has been compounded.

Advanced image analysis methods are widely used in research and can meet most practical challenges; however, regulatory and practical hurdles must be overcome before these methods are widely adopted in everyday medical practice. Nevertheless, these methods already have shown their clinical utility. Translating and warping images into a uniform stereotactic space permits individual and group comparisons (Herholz et al. 2002; Minoshima et al. 1995). New methods of image processing, such as three-dimensional stereotactic surface projection (3D-SSP) mapping, can reduce the number of images that have to be mentally manipulated for interpretation (see Figures 7–5 and 7–6). Peak pixel values for the lateral and

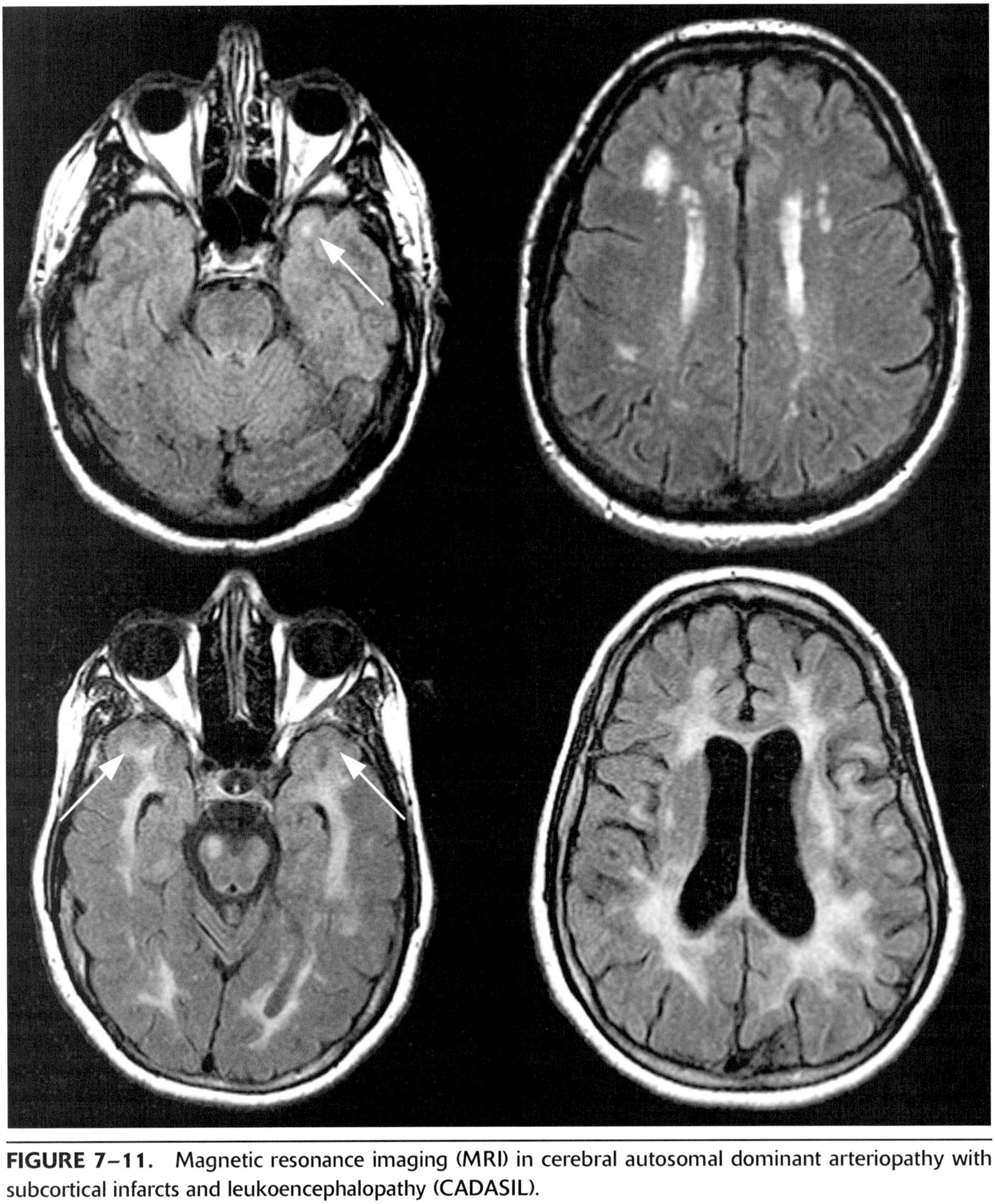

FIGURE 7–11. Magnetic resonance imaging (MRI) in cerebral autosomal dominant arteriopathy with subcortical infarcts and leukoencephalopathy (CADASIL).

The anterior temporal lobe is a notable site of predilection for hyperintensities in CADASIL. The MRI scan from a young patient who has a *NOTCH3* mutation but minimal clinical symptoms *(top row)* shows a few areas of white matter hyperintensity, including a characteristic lesion at the gray-white junction in the anterior temporal lobe *(arrow, left)*. A few hyperintensities are seen in the centrum semiovale. An older symptomatic and demented CADASIL patient *(bottom row)* has even more extensive and confluent white matter abnormalities in anterior temporal lobes bilaterally *(arrows, left)*. The image on the right shows confluent white matter hyperintensities involving most of the periventricular white matter. Similar hyperintensities occur in other forms of vascular dementia, so at this point, CADASIL usually can be recognized only when an autosomal dominant pattern of a similar illness in other family members is elicited.

medial brain surfaces are derived by 3D-SSP (Minoshima et al. 1995). The resulting summary images simplify scan displays and can be used to display statistical maps, making interpretation both quicker and more accurate (Burdette et al. 1996). Advanced imaging analysis methods also can improve the ability to recognize abnormalities in AD. The ability of 3D-SSP to display the medial surface of the brain makes it possible to demonstrate that the posterior cingulate gyrus is typically affected early in AD (Minoshima et al. 1994).

Accumulating databases of uniformly acquired images makes it possible to construct normative image atlases for statistical comparison with patient scans. These databases can be tailored to fit the profile of an individual patient. Statistical comparisons can help in deciding which changes recognized by the eye are truly significant and which are due to normal variation. The human brain recognizes asymmetries and contrasting patterns more easily than diffuse or gradual declines in image intensity. Using color scales to display images can be helpful but may also be deceptive. Brain scans provide an overwhelming mass of quantitative information; even a single image is composed of thousands of data points. New statistical methods have been developed to address the problem of simultaneously comparing thousands of nonindependent values. Approaches such as nonparametric permutation testing and false discovery ratio help ensure that statistical differences in imaging studies are dependable (Nichols and Hayasaka 2003; Nichols and Holmes 2002).

Neurotransmitter Imaging

Many molecular probes have been developed to examine neurotransmitter function. Cholinergic function is of particular interest in AD. AD damages cholinergic neurons, providing the basis for treatment of AD with cholinesterase inhibitors. With the development of appropriate radioactive ligands, molecular imaging can reveal the manner in which cholinergic deficits develop over time and their relationship to symptoms and patient characteristics. The radioactive-labeled vesamicol analogue IBVM binds to the presynaptic vesicular acetylcholine transporter and can serve as an in vivo marker of presynaptic cholinergic terminal density (Kuhl et al. 1996). Molecular imaging using the probe demonstrates that like glucose metabolism, there is a generally uniform distribution of cholinergic terminals throughout the neocortex in cognitively normal individuals. In AD, IBVM binding is decreased.

For technical reasons related to the efficacy of available radiotracers, accurately measuring cholinergic receptors is more challenging. However, significant alterations in muscarinic receptors do not appear to occur in AD (Zubieta et al. 2001). Perhaps most intriguing, observations have been made using a PET radioligand, such as 1-[^{11}C]methylpiperidin-4-yl propionate ([^{11}C]PMP), that binds to cholinesterase. Although cholinesterase is not a precise indicator of cholinergic neurons, both PET and postmortem studies find similar characteristic decreases of cholinesterase in AD (Kuhl et al. 1999). Peripheral red blood cell assays typically have been used to assess the potency of cholinesterase inhibitor drugs, even though it is inhibition in the central nervous system that is most relevant. PET studies with [^{11}C]PMP showed that a considerable discrepancy between central and peripheral cholinesterase inhibition may occur after acute treatment with donepezil. Although nearly complete acetylcholinesterase inhibition was expected from red blood cell assays, molecular imaging showed that an average of only 27% inhibition of cholinesterase occurred in the brain, indicating that more effective drugs could be developed (Kuhl et al. 2000).

Although these studies are informative and promising, the potential of cholinergic imaging to improve the diagnosis of dementing diseases or to guide choice of treatment has not yet been explored adequately.

Functional Magnetic Resonance Imaging

Functional MRI (fMRI) utilizes the principle of blood oxygen level–dependent (BOLD) contrast, or blood oxygenation level dependency of MR signals to assess local blood flow in response to a task or during the resting state. It exploits the paramagnetic properties of deoxyhemoglobin that alter the signal on MR images, and the observation that increased neuronal activity causes a transient increase in blood flow and temporarily decreases deoxyhemoglobin concentration. Under normal conditions, BOLD contrast in the brain reflects microvascular or venous blood.

Several acquisition protocols provide indirect measurement of blood flow based on BOLD contrast, including gradient-echo epiplanar imaging sequences and spin-echo protocols such as EPISTAR (echo-planar imaging and signal targeting with alternating radio frequency) (Edelman et al. 1994; Ogawa et al. 1990). No consensus has yet developed about which of these techniques is preferable. Spin-echo techniques appear more selective for capillary blood flow. Fast epiplanar data acquisition is more expensive but less influenced by blood flow and patient movement and may improve temporal resolution and signal-to-noise ratio.

Although fMRI has been used primarily to examine the anatomical correlates of cognitive function in cognitively normal individuals, an increasing number of studies have examined differences in nondemented elderly and those with mild memory impairment and dementia (Bookheimer et al. 2000; Dickerson et al. 2004; Lustig and Buckner 2004). A significant limitation of many fMRI paradigms is that impaired subjects have difficulty performing the cognitive tasks, making it impossible to study patients with more severe dementia. Comparison of subjects is difficult and requires either modification of task difficulty or adjustment for performance. Recent development of an alternative approach using fMRI signals between tasks permits assessment of "default mode activation" (Buckner et al. 2005). Rather than focusing on response to a cognitive stimulus, this strategy examines the coherence of responses between stimuli. This approach avoids problems of variable performance between subjects and within individual subjects during multiple trials and is a promising method for patients with dementia. Broad acceptance of a single cognitive paradigm and multicenter studies showing reliability and diagnostic accuracy are needed before fMRI is ready for clinical use in dementia evaluations.

Multimodal Imaging

Since different imaging methods reflect different pathological changes, it is not surprising that utilizing several molecular imaging techniques could improve diagnostic accuracy and uncover concurrent disorders. For example, dopamine and amyloid imaging would be needed to conclusively demonstrate DLB occurring with AD pathology. Timing of the appearance of imaging abnormalities in the course of illness also may be important in the selection of imaging methods. There is evidence that imaging abnormalities occur in a characteristic progressive order in AD (Jack et al. 2010). Amyloid PET appears to become abnormal first, often years before symptom onset, while FDG-PET abnormalities occur relatively early as synapses are lost and before hippocampal volume decreases. If this observation is correct, FDG-PET abnormalities in AD should occur only after amyloid binding is increased. Inconsistencies in the appearance of these abnormalities could have diagnostic and prognostic implications. Future longitudinal studies will help clinicians choose an imaging modality not only based on presumed diagnosis but also informed by symptom severity. Preclinical diagnosis of neuropsychiatric disorders now is a reasonable goal.

New Neuroimaging Applications

Monitoring Disease Progression and Drug Development

Neuroimaging could potentially be used to monitor disease progression and response to therapy. Cerebral atrophy and synaptic failure increase as dementia progresses in neurodegenerative disease, and these can be observed with MRI and FDG-PET. Imaging abnormalities also increase in vascular dementia as symptoms worsen. Several barriers, however, limit the clinical usefulness of imaging in monitoring disease progression. Precise measures of pathology often are not used in clinical studies. Accurately counting the number of small cerebral infarcts can even be difficult. Over time, test-retest variability of many imaging measures is uncertain. Scanner hardware and software are modified frequently. If the clinician is relying on visual interpretation, imaging changes need to be large and image acquisition and quality must be uniform to produce convincing evidence of disease progression. These requirements seldom are met in clinical practice. Furthermore, imaging is too expensive to replace cognitive measures for the care of individual patients.

These limitations are not as daunting when considering the use of imaging in clinical drug trials. Drug trials compare patient groups rather than making treatment decisions for individual patients. The economic realities also are different. The cost of developing a new drug is huge, and anything that would speed evaluation could save huge amounts of money. Imaging can assist new drug development at many levels. Drugs can be radiolabeled to study their distribution and pharmacokinetics. Imaging can be used to assess the effects of drugs on neurotransmitter function. The use of imaging to improve the accuracy of diagnosis in clinical trials could be expanded from MRI only to include FDG-PET and amyloid imaging. Imaging could help detect the earliest evidence of disease and identify subjects for earlier treatment. Despite the opportunities, the potential of imaging to speed drug development has not yet been fully realized.

Imaging biomarkers need to be validated as a surrogate measure of disease progression (Mueller et al. 2005). Imaging measures are more objective and likely to exhibit less variability than traditional clinical and neuropsychological outcome measures used in trials of drugs for dementia. MRI already has begun to be incorporated as an outcome measure of treatment response in clinical drug trials (Grundman et al. 2001). Only a few longitudinal studies of AD have used FDG-PET (Alexander et al. 2002), but others are under way. Clinical drug trials will benefit from using the best imaging measure of disease progression, allowing change to be detected over a period of a few months, rather than the much longer time now required. If this can be done, fewer patients will be needed to evaluate new treatments, more drugs can be tested, and studies will be less costly. This certainly is a worthwhile goal.

Personalized Medicine, Risk, and Prognosis

Dementing diseases affect individual patients in remarkably different ways. One patient with AD may be agitated, whereas another with the same dementia severity may be withdrawn. In personalized medicine, the clinician identifies the exact cause of disease early and selects the best treatment, taking into account the individual patient's unique physiology and response to the illness.

Imaging offers the opportunity to significantly advance the goals of this personalized approach to care. Preliminary studies suggest that FDG-PET and amyloid imaging might detect impending dementia in those at genetic risk and accurately predict dementia in those with memory impairment (Chételat et al. 2003; Drzezga et al. 2003; Reiman et al. 1996; Small et al. 2000). Molecular imaging can be used to identify individual variability in the distribution of pathology and to then tailor individualized therapies.

AD can cause focal and asymmetric clinical syndromes (Caselli 2000). Likewise, individuals with AD can have FDG-PET scans that appear remarkably different from each other but have recognizable variations on a distinctive pattern of hypometabolism. The cause of this metabolic variability is unknown but may affect prognosis and response to treatment. A significant barrier to understanding these phenomena has been the difficulty in recognizing when metabolic asymmetry is significant. Fortunately, new image analysis methods to tackle this problem are being developed and could mark a significant advance (Fletcher et al. 2007). As professionals learn more about dementing illnesses, it becomes clear that stereotypes are misleading. The full potential of therapeutics will not be realized until they can be tailored to address the variation of illness expression in individual patients.

Key Points

- Neuroimaging should be used to answer specific clinical questions.
- Unexpected imaging findings are frequent but may not be clinically relevant.
- Neuroimaging cannot be used to determine whether dementia is present.
- MRI is the preferred structural imaging method in dementia, unless contraindicated.
- MRI is sensitive in identifying vascular lesions, but clinical relevance must be considered.
- The pattern of cerebral hypometabolism reflects clinical symptoms.
- The pattern of cerebral hypometabolism can help distinguish AD from FTD.
- Amyloid plaques can be imaged with PET but may be asymptomatic; their prognostic implications are not yet clear.
- Emerging methods and new applications for neuroimaging in dementia promise an increasing role in dementia diagnosis and personalized care.

Recommended Readings

Herholz K, Herscovitch P, Heiss W-D: NeuroPET: PET in Neuroscience and Clinical Neurology. New York, Springer, 2004

McRobbie DW, Moore EA, Graves MJ, et al: MRI From Picture to Proton, 2nd Edition. New York, Cambridge University Press, 2007

Talairach J, Tournoux P: Co-Planar Stereotaxic Atlas of the Human Brain: 3-Dimensional Proportional System—An Approach to Cerebral Imaging. New York, Thieme Medical, 1988

References

Adlam AL, Patterson K, Rogers TT, et al: Semantic dementia and fluent primary progressive aphasia: two sides of the same coin? Brain 129:3066–3080, 2006

Alexander GE, Chen K, Pietrini P, et al: Longitudinal PET evaluation of cerebral metabolic decline in dementia: a potential outcome measure in Alzheimer's disease treatment studies. Am J Psychiatry 159:738–745, 2002

Anchisi D, Borroni B, Franceschi M, et al: Heterogeneity of brain glucose metabolism in mild cognitive impairment and clinical progression to Alzheimer disease. Arch Neurol 62:1728–1733, 2005

Becker JT, Boller F, Lopez OL, et al: The natural history of Alzheimer's disease. Description of study cohort and accuracy of diagnosis. Arch Neurol 51:585–594, 1994

Berent S, Giordani B, Foster N, et al: Neuropsychological function and cerebral glucose utilization in isolated memory impairment and Alzheimer's disease. J Psychiatr Res 33:7–16, 1999

Blacker D, Albert MS, Bassett SS, et al: Reliability and validity of NINCDS-ADRDA criteria for Alzheimer's disease. The National Institute of Mental Health Genetics Initiative. Arch Neurol 51: 1198–1204, 1994

Boccardi M, Pennanen C, Laakso MP, et al: Amygdaloid atrophy in frontotemporal dementia and Alzheimer's disease. Neurosci Lett 335:139–143, 2002

Boccardi M, Laakso MP, Bresciani L, et al: The MRI pattern of frontal and temporal brain atrophy in fronto-temporal dementia. Neurobiol Aging 24:95–103, 2003

Boche D, Zotova E, Weller RO, et al: Consequence of Abeta immunization on the vasculature of human Alzheimer's disease brain. Brain 131:3299–3310, 2008

Bocti C, Swartz RH, Gao F-Q, et al: A new visual rating scale to assess strategic white matter hyperintensities within cholinergic pathways in dementia. Stroke 36:2126–2131, 2005

Bookheimer SY, Strojwas MH, Cohen MS, et al: Patterns of brain activation in people at risk for Alzheimer's disease. N Engl J Med 343:450–456, 2000

Braak H, Braak E: Neuropathological staging of Alzheimer-related changes. Acta Neuropathol 82:239–259, 1991

Brenner DJ, Hall EJ: Computed tomography—an increasing source of radiation exposure. N Engl J Med 357:2277–2284, 2007

Brooks DJ, Frey KA, Marek KL, et al: Assessment of neuroimaging techniques as biomarkers of the progression of Parkinson's disease. Exp Neurol 184 (suppl 1):S68–S79, 2003

Buckner RL, Snyder AZ, Shannon BJ, et al: Molecular, structural, and functional characterization of Alzheimer's disease: evidence for a relationship between default activity, amyloid, and memory. J Neurosci 25:7709–7717, 2005

Burdette JH, Minoshima S, Vander Borght T, et al: Alzheimer's disease: improved visual interpretation of PET images by using three-dimensional stereotaxic surface projections. Radiology 198:837–843, 1996

Caselli RJ: Focal and asymmetric cortical degenerative syndromes. Adv Neurol 82:35–51, 2000

Catafau AM, Tolosa E: Impact of dopamine transporter SPECT using ^{123}I-ioflupane on diagnosis and management of patients with clinically uncertain parkinsonian syndromes. Mov Disord 19: 1175–1182, 2004

Chételat G, Desgranges B, De La Sayette V, et al: Mapping gray matter loss with voxel-based morphometry in mild cognitive impairment. Neuroreport 13:1939–1943, 2002

Chételat G, Desgranges B, de la Sayette V, et al: Mild cognitive impairment: can FDG-PET predict who is to rapidly convert to Alzheimer's disease? Neurology 60:1374–1377, 2003

Chui H, Zhang Q: Evaluation of dementia: a systematic study of the usefulness of the American Academy of Neurology's practice parameters. Neurology 49:925–935, 1997

Cosottini M, Ceravolo R, Faggioni L, et al: Assessment of midbrain atrophy in patients with progressive supranuclear palsy with routine magnetic resonance imaging. Acta Neurol Scand 116: 37–42, 2007

DeKosky ST, Scheff SW: Synapse loss in frontal cortex biopsies in Alzheimer's disease: correlation with cognitive severity. Ann Neurol 27:457–464, 1990

Dickerson BC, Salat DH, Bates JF, et al: Medial temporal lobe function and structure in mild cognitive impairment. Ann Neurol 56:27–35, 2004

Drzezga A, Lautenschlager N, Siebner H, et al: Cerebral metabolic changes accompanying conversion of mild cognitive impairment into Alzheimer's disease: a PET follow-up study. Eur J Nucl Med Mol Imaging 30:1104–1113, 2003

Du AT, Schuff N, Kramer JH, et al: Different regional patterns of cortical thinning in Alzheimer's disease and frontotemporal dementia. Brain 130:1159–1166, 2007

Edelman RR, Siewert B, Darby DG, et al: Qualitative mapping of cerebral blood flow and functional localization with echo-planar MR imaging and signal targeting with alternating radio frequency. Radiology 192:513–520, 1994

Eidelberg D, Dhawan V, Moeller JR, et al: The metabolic landscape of cortico-basal ganglionic degeneration: regional asymmetries studied with positron emission tomography. J Neurol Neurosurg Psychiatry 54:856–862, 1991

Engler H, Santillo AF, Wang SX, et al: In vivo amyloid imaging with PET in frontotemporal dementia. Eur J Nucl Med Mol Imaging 35:100–106, 2008

Fazekas F, Kleinert R, Offenbacher H, et al: Pathologic correlates of incidental MRI white matter signal hyperintensities. Neurology 43:1683–1689, 1993

Fein G, Di Sclafani V, Tanabe J, et al: Hippocampal and cortical atrophy predict dementia in subcortical ischemic vascular disease. Neurology 55:1626–1635, 2000

Fick DM, Cooper JW, Wade WE, et al: Updating the Beers criteria for potentially inappropriate medication use in older adults: results of a US consensus panel of experts. Arch Intern Med 163:2716–2724, 2003

Finkenstaedt M, Szudra A, Zerr I, et al: MR imaging of Creutzfeldt-Jakob disease. Radiology 199:793–798, 1996

Fletcher PT, Powell S, Foster NL, et al: Quantifying metabolic asymmetry modulo structure in Alzheimer's disease. Inf Process Med Imaging 20:446–457, 2007

Forsberg A, Engler H, Almkvist O, et al: PET imaging of amyloid deposition in patients with mild cognitive impairment. Neurobiol Aging 29:1456–1465, 2008

Foster NL, Gilman S, Berent S, et al: Cerebral hypometabolism in progressive supranuclear palsy studied with positron emission tomography. Ann Neurol 24:399–406, 1988

Foster NL, Koeppe RE, Giordani BJ, et al: Variations of the phenotype in frontotemporal dementias, in Genotype-Proteotype-Phenotype Relationships in Neurodegenerative Diseases. Edited by Cummings J, Hardy J, Poncet M, et al. Berlin, Springer-Verlag, 2005, pp 139–152

Foster NL, Heidebrink JL, Clark CM, et al: FDG-PET improves accuracy in distinguishing frontotemporal dementia and Alzheimer's disease. Brain 130:2616–2635, 2007

Frisoni GB, Testa C, Zorzan A, et al: Detection of grey matter loss in mild Alzheimer's disease with voxel based morphometry. J Neurol Neurosurg Psychiatry 73:657–664, 2002

Gado M, Hughes CP, Danziger W, et al: Volumetric measurements of the cerebrospinal fluid spaces in demented subjects and controls. Radiology 144:535–538, 1982

Gearing M, Mirra SS, Hedreen JC, et al: The Consortium to Establish a Registry for Alzheimer's Disease (CERAD), part X: neuropathology confirmation of the clinical diagnosis of Alzheimer's disease. Neurology 45:461–466, 1995

Gelb DJ, Oliver E, Gilman S: NINDS diagnostic criteria for Parkinson's disease. Arch Neurol 56:33–39, 1999

Gorno-Tempini ML, Dronkers NF, Rankin KP, et al: Cognition and anatomy in three variants of primary progressive aphasia. Ann Neurol 55:335–346, 2004

Grundman M, Sencakova D, Jack CR, et al: Use of brain MRI volumetric analysis in a mild cognitive impairment trial to delay the diagnosis of Alzheimer's disease, in Drug Discovery and Development for Alzheimer's Disease 2000. Edited by Fillet H, O'Connell A. New York, Springer, 2001, pp 24–32

Haacke EM, DelProposto ZS, Chaturvedi S, et al: Imaging cerebral amyloid angiopathy with susceptibility-weighted imaging. AJNR Am J Neuroradiol 28:316–317, 2007

Herholz K, Salmon E, Perani D, et al: Discrimination between Alzheimer dementia and controls by automated analysis of multicenter FDG PET. Neuroimage 17:302–316, 2002

Hodges JR, Patterson K: Semantic dementia: a unique clinicopathological syndrome. Lancet Neurol 6:1004–1014, 2007

Hoffman JM, Welsh-Bohmer KA, Hanson M, et al: FDG PET imaging in patients with pathologically verified dementia. J Nucl Med 41:1920–1928, 2000

Ishii K, Imamura T, Sasaki M, et al: Regional cerebral glucose metabolism in dementia with Lewy bodies and Alzheimer's disease. Neurology 51:125–130, 1998

Jack CR Jr, Knopman DS, Jagust WJ, et al: Hypothetical model of dynamic biomarkers of the Alzheimer's pathological cascade. Lancet Neurol 9:119–128, 2010

Klunk WE, Engler H, Nordberg A, et al: Imaging brain amyloid in Alzheimer's disease with Pittsburgh Compound-B. Ann Neurol 55:306–319, 2004

Knopman DS, DeKosky ST, Cummings JL, et al: Practice parameter: diagnosis of dementia (an evidence-based review). Report of the Quality Standards Subcommittee of the American Academy of Neurology. Neurology 56:1143–1153, 2001

Koeppe RA, Gilman S, Joshi A, et al: 11C-DTBZ and 18F-FDG PET measures in differentiating dementias. J Nucl Med 46:936–944, 2005

Kraft E, Trenkwalder C, Auer DP: T2*-weighted MRI differentiates multiple system atrophy from Parkinson's disease. Neurology 59:1265–1267, 2002

Kropp S, Schulz-Schaeffer WJ, Finkenstaedt M, et al: The Heidenhain variant of Creutzfeldt-Jakob disease. Arch Neurol 56:55–61, 1999

Kuhl DE, Minoshima S, Fessler JA, et al: In vivo mapping of cholinergic terminals in normal aging, Alzheimer's disease and Parkinson's disease. Ann Neurol 40:399–410, 1996

Kuhl DE, Koeppe RA, Minoshima S, et al: In vivo mapping of cerebral acetylcholinesterase activity in aging and Alzheimer's disease. Neurology 52:691–699, 1999

Kuhl DE, Minoshima S, Frey KA, et al: Limited donepezil inhibition of acetylcholinesterase measured with positron emission tomography in living Alzheimer cerebral cortex. Ann Neurol 48:391–395, 2000

Kwan LT, Reed BR, Eberling JL, et al: Effects of subcortical cerebral infarction on cortical glucose metabolism and cognitive function. Arch Neurol 56:809–814, 1999

Langa KM, Foster NL, Larson EB: Mixed dementia: emerging concepts and therapeutic implications. JAMA 292:2901–2908, 2004

Lim A, Tsuang D, Kukull W, et al: Clinico-neuropathological correlation of Alzheimer's disease in a community-based case series. J Am Geriatr Soc 47:564–569, 1999

Linn J, Halpin A, Demaerel P, et al: Prevalence of superficial siderosis in patients with cerebral amyloid angiopathy. Neurology 74:1346–1350, 2010

Longstreth WT, Bernick C, Manolio TA, et al: Lacunar infarcts defined by magnetic resonance imaging of 3660 elderly people: the Cardiovascular Health Study. Arch Neurol 55:1217–1225, 1998

Lustig C, Buckner RL: Preserved neural correlates of priming in old age and dementia. Neuron 42:865–875, 2004

Luxenberg JS, Haxby JV, Creasey H, et al: Rate of ventricular enlargement in dementia of the Alzheimer type correlates with rate of neuropsychological deterioration. Neurology 37:1135–1140, 1987

Marshall VL, Patterson J, Hadley DM, et al: Two-year follow-up in 150 consecutive cases with normal dopamine transporter imaging. Nucl Med Commun 27:933–937, 2006

Martin WR, Wieler M, Gee M: Midbrain iron content in early Parkinson disease: a potential biomarker of disease status. Neurology 70:1411–1417, 2008

Mata M, Fink DJ, Gainer H, et al: Activity-dependent energy metabolism in rat posterior pituitary primarily reflects sodium pump activity. J Neurochem 34:213–215, 1980

Mathis CA, Bacskai BJ, Kajdasz ST, et al: A lipophilic thioflavin-T derivative for positron emission tomography (PET) imaging of amyloid in brain. Bioorg Med Chem Lett 12:295–298, 2002

McKee AC, Cantu RC, Nowinski CJ, et al: Chronic traumatic encephalopathy in athletes: progressive tauopathy after repetitive head injury. J Neuropathol Exp Neurol 68:709–735, 2009

McKeith I, O'Brien J, Walker Z, et al: Sensitivity and specificity of dopamine transporter imaging with 123I-FP-CIT SPECT in dementia with Lewy bodies: a phase III, multicentre study. Lancet Neurol 6:305–313, 2007

Meguro K, Blaizot X, Kondoh Y, et al: Neocortical and hippocampal glucose hypometabolism following neurotoxic lesions of the entorhinal and perirhinal cortices in the non-human primate as shown by PET: implications for Alzheimer's disease. Brain 122:1519–1531, 1999

Meguro K, LeMestric C, Landeau B, et al: Relations between hypometabolism in the posterior association neocortex and hippocampal atrophy in Alzheimer's disease: a PET/MRI correlative study. J Neurol Neurosurg Psychiatry 71:315–321, 2001

Mendez MF, Mastri AR, Sung JH, et al: Clinically diagnosed Alzheimer disease: neuropathologic findings in 650 cases. Alzheimer Dis Assoc Disord 6:35–43, 1992

Messa C, Perani D, Lucignani G, et al: High-resolution technetium-99m-HMPAO SPECT in patients with probable Alzheimer's disease: comparison with fluorine-18-FDG PET. J Nucl Med 35:210–216, 1994

Miller BL, Chang L, Mena I, et al: Progressive right frontotemporal degeneration: clinical, neuropsychological and SPECT characteristics. Dementia 4:204–213, 1993

Minoshima S, Foster NL, Kuhl DE: Posterior cingulate cortex in Alzheimer's disease (letter). Lancet 344:895, 1994

Minoshima S, Frey KA, Foster NL, et al: Preserved pontine glucose metabolism in Alzheimer's disease: a reference region for functional brain analysis. J Comput Assist Tomogr 19:541–547, 1995

Minoshima S, Giordani BJ, Berent S, et al: Metabolic reduction in the posterior cingulate cortex in very early Alzheimer's disease. Ann Neurol 42:85–94, 1997

Minoshima S, Cross DJ, Foster NL, et al: Discordance between traditional pathologic and energy metabolic changes in very early Alzheimer's disease: pathophysiological implications. Ann N Y Acad Sci 893:350–352, 1999

Minoshima S, Foster NL, Sima AAF, et al: Alzheimer's disease versus dementia with Lewy bodies: cerebral metabolic distinction with autopsy confirmation. Ann Neurol 50:358–365, 2001

Mittal S, Farmer P, Kalina P, et al: Correlation of diffusion-weighted magnetic resonance imaging with neuropathology in Creutzfeldt-Jakob disease. Arch Neurol 59:128–134, 2002

Moretti P, Lieberman AP, Wilde EA, et al: Novel insertional presenilin 1 mutation causing Alzheimer disease with spastic paraparesis. Neurology 62:1865–1868, 2004

Mueller SG, Weiner MW, Thal LJ, et al: The Alzheimer's Disease Neuroimaging Initiative. Neuroimaging Clin N Am 15:869–877, 2005

Mungas D, Jagust WJ, Reed BR, et al: MRI predictors of cognition in subcortical ischemic vascular disease and Alzheimer's disease. Neurology 57:2229–2235, 2001

Murrell JR, Miravalle L, Foster NL, et al: Early-onset familial Alzheimer's disease (AD) from the first American report: a presenilin-1 (PS1) mutation found in descendants. J Neuropathol Exp Neurol 60:543, 2001

Na DL, Suh CK, Choi SH, et al: Diffusion-weighted magnetic resonance imaging in probable Creutzfeldt-Jakob disease: a clinical-anatomic correlation. Arch Neurol 56:951–957, 1999

Naehle CP, Strach K, Thomas D, et al: Magnetic resonance imaging at 1.5-T in patients with implantable cardioverter-defibrillators. J Am Coll Cardiol 54:549–555, 2009

Nazarian S, Roguin A, Zviman MM, et al: Clinical utility and safety of a protocol for noncardiac and cardiac magnetic resonance imaging of patients with permanent pacemakers and implantable-cardioverter defibrillators at 1.5 tesla. Circulation 114:1277–1284, 2006

Neary D, Snowden J, Mann D: Frontotemporal dementia. Lancet Neurol 4:771–780, 2005

Nichols T, Hayasaka S: Controlling the familywise error rate in functional neuroimaging: a comparative review. Stat Methods Med Res 12:419–446, 2003

Nichols TE, Holmes AP: Nonparametric permutation tests for functional neuroimaging: a primer with examples. Hum Brain Mapp 15:1–25, 2002

Ogawa S, Lee TM, Kay AR, et al: Brain magnetic resonance imaging with contrast dependent on blood oxygenation. Proc Natl Acad Sci U S A 87:9868–9872, 1990

Omalu BI, DeKosky ST, Hamilton RL, et al: Chronic traumatic encephalopathy in a National Football League player: part II. Neurosurgery 59:1086–1092, 2006

Pappata S, Mazoyer B, Tran DS, et al: Effects of capsular or thalamic stroke on metabolism in the cortex and cerebellum: a positron tomography study. Stroke 21:519–524, 1990

Prashanth LK, Sinha S, Taly AB, et al: Do MRI features distinguish Wilson's disease from other early onset extrapyramidal disorders? An analysis of 100 cases. Mov Disord 25:672–678, 2010

Price JC, Klunk WE, Lopresti BJ, et al: Kinetic modeling of amyloid binding in humans using PET imaging and Pittsburgh Compound-B. J Cereb Blood Flow Metab 25:1528–1547, 2005

Price TR, Manolio TA, Kronmal RA, et al: Silent brain infarction on magnetic resonance imaging and neurological abnormalities in community-dwelling older adults. The Cardiovascular Health Study. CHS Collaborative Research Group. Stroke 28:1158–1164, 1997

Rabinovici GD, Furst AJ, O'Neil JP, et al: 11C-PIB PET imaging in Alzheimer disease and frontotemporal lobar degeneration. Neurology 68:1205–1212, 2007

Racette BA, Antenor JA, McGee-Minnich L, et al: [^{18}F]FDOPA PET and clinical features in parkinsonism due to manganism. Mov Disord 20:492–496, 2005

Ravina B, Eidelberg D, Ahlskog JE, et al: The role of radiotracer imaging in Parkinson's disease. Neurology 64:208–215, 2005

Reiman EM, Caselli RJ, Yun LS, et al: Preclinical evidence of Alzheimer's disease in persons homozygous for the epsilon 4 allele for apolipoprotein E. N Engl J Med 334:752–758, 1996

Relkin N, Marmarou A, Klinge P, et al: Diagnosing idiopathic normal-pressure hydrocephalus. Neurosurgery 57(suppl):S4–S16, 2005

Román GC, Tatemichi TK, Erkinjuntti T, et al: Vascular dementia: diagnostic criteria for research studies: report of the NINDS-AIREN International Workshop. Neurology 43:250–260, 1993

Rowe CC, Ng S, Ackermann U, et al: Imaging beta-amyloid burden in aging and dementia. Neurology 68:1718–1725, 2007

Scheltens P, Fox N, Barkhof F, et al: Structural magnetic resonance imaging in the practical assessment of dementia: beyond exclusion. Lancet Neurol 1:13–21, 2002

Schneider JA, Arvanitakis Z, Bang W, et al: Mixed brain pathologies account for most dementia cases in community-dwelling older persons. Neurology 69:2197–2204, 2007

Schroter A, Zerr I, Henkel K, et al: Magnetic resonance imaging in the clinical diagnosis of Creutzfeldt-Jakob disease. Arch Neurol 57:1751–1757, 2000

Selden NR, Gitelman DR, Salamon-Murayama N, et al: Trajectories of cholinergic pathways within the cerebral hemispheres of the human brain. Brain 121:2249–2257, 1998

Selkoe DJ: Alzheimer's disease is a synaptic failure. Science 298:789–791, 2002

Sethi KD, Adams RJ, Loring DW, et al: Hallervorden-Spatz syndrome: clinical and magnetic resonance imaging correlations. Ann Neurol 24:692–694, 1988

Silverman DH, Small GW, Chang CY, et al: Positron emission tomography in evaluation of dementia: regional brain metabolism and long-term outcome. JAMA 286:2120–2127, 2001

Small GW, Ercoli LM, Silverman DH, et al: Cerebral metabolic and cognitive decline in persons at genetic risk for Alzheimer's disease. Proc Natl Acad Sci U S A 97:6037–6042, 2000

Small GW, Kepe V, Ercoli LM, et al: PET of brain amyloid and tau in mild cognitive impairment. N Engl J Med 355:2652–2663, 2006

Sommer T, Naehle CP, Yang A, et al: Strategy for safe performance of extrathoracic magnetic resonance imaging at 1.5 tesla in the presence of cardiac pacemakers in non-pacemaker-dependent patients: a prospective study with 115 examinations. Circulation 114:1285–1292, 2006

Starosta-Rubinstein S, Young AB, Kluin K, et al: Clinical assessment of 31 patients with Wilson's disease: correlations with structural changes on magnetic resonance imaging. Arch Neurol 44:365–370, 1987

van den Boom R, Lesnik Oberstein SA, Ferrari MD, et al: Cerebral autosomal dominant arteriopathy with subcortical infarcts and leukoencephalopathy: MR imaging findings at different ages—3rd–6th decades. Radiology 229:683–690, 2003

Varma AR, Snowden JS, Lloyd JJ, et al: Evaluation of the NINCDS-ADRDA criteria in the differentiation of Alzheimer's disease and frontotemporal dementia. J Neurol Neurosurg Psychiatry 66: 184–188, 1999

Verhoeff NP, Wilson AA, Takeshita S, et al: In-vivo imaging of Alzheimer disease beta-amyloid with [11C]SB-13 PET. Am J Geriatr Psychiatry 12:584–595, 2004

Vermeer SE, Koudstaal PJ, Oudkerk M, et al: Prevalence and risk factors of silent brain infarcts in the population-based Rotterdam Scan Study. Stroke 33:21–25, 2002

Vernooij MW, Ikram MA, Tanghe HL, et al: Incidental findings on brain MRI in the general population. N Engl J Med 357:1821–1828, 2007

Visser PJ, Verhey FR, Hofman PA, et al: Medial temporal lobe atrophy predicts Alzheimer's disease in patients with minor cognitive impairment. J Neurol Neurosurg Psychiatry 72:491–497, 2002

Viswanathan A, Chabriat H: Cerebral microhemorrhages. Stroke 37:550–555, 2006

von Lewinski F, Werner C, Jorn T, et al: T2*-weighted MRI in diagnosis of multiple system atrophy: a practical approach for clinicians. J Neurol 254:1184–1188, 2007

Weiner MF, Hynan LS, Parikh B, et al: Can Alzheimer's disease and dementias with Lewy bodies be distinguished clinically? J Geriatr Psychiatry Neurol 16:245–250, 2003

Zeidler M, Sellar RJ, Collie DA, et al: The pulvinar sign on magnetic resonance imaging in variant Creutzfeldt-Jakob disease. Lancet 355:1412–1418, 2000

Zhang Y, Baicker K, Newhouse JP: Geographic variation in the quality of prescribing. N Engl J Med 363:1985–1988, 2010

Zubieta JK, Koeppe RA, Frey KA, et al: Assessment of muscarinic receptor concentrations in aging and Alzheimer's disease with [11C]NMPB and PET. Synapse 39:275–287, 2001

PART III

Principles of Neuropsychiatric Treatment

8

Psychosocial Therapies

Glenise McKenzie, R.N., Ph.D.
Linda Teri, Ph.D.

Historically, it was believed that older adults were not good candidates for nonpharmacological psychotherapeutic interventions (Freud 1924). However, in the past several decades, awareness has been growing about the psychosocial issues confronting aging adults and about the value of psychotherapy as a tool for managing age-related change and maintaining quality of life. In this chapter, we focus on randomized controlled clinical trials that have investigated the efficacy of psychosocial approaches to enhancing psychosocial outcomes for older adults. The publications reviewed provide a clear starting point for neuropsychiatric practitioners to understand the current state of the science and apply this science to their ongoing care of older adults. To place this discussion in context, we examine recent studies focused on prevalent neuropsychiatric disturbances in this population, including depression, anxiety, and cognitive impairment. We also include studies addressing caregiver distress because of the primary role of caregivers in the treatment of older adults with cognitive impairment.

The empirical investigation of psychosocial treatments for older adults with neuropsychiatric disorders has evolved significantly over the past three decades. Numerous reviews (including both systematic reviews and meta-analyses) have evaluated the empirical literature on 1) the use of specific psychological interventions with older adults, such as cognitive-behavioral interventions (Satre et al. 2006), reminiscence and life review therapy (Bohlmeijer et al. 2007), and group psychotherapy (Payne and Marcus 2008); 2) psychosocial interventions for specific disorders, such as late-life depression (Pinquart et al. 2007; Wilson et al. 2008), late-life anxiety (Ayers et al. 2007; Thorp et al. 2009), neuropsychiatric symptoms of dementia (Livingston et al. 2005; Teri et al. 2005d), and insomnia (McCurry et al. 2007); and 3) psychosocial treatments for individuals with specific general medical illnesses, such as cancer (Maramaldi et al. 2008), cardiac disease (Peck and Ai 2008), diabetes (DeCoster 2008), and arthritis pain (Yoon and Doherty 2008).

This chapter provides an overview of the main psychosocial treatments that have been empirically evaluated with older adults. The literature reviewed in this chapter was identified through several electronic indexes (MEDLINE, Cumulative Index to Nursing and Allied Health Literature [CINAHL], PsychINFO), reference sections from identified articles, review articles, and consensus documents. Articles were included for review if they were 1) randomized controlled trials 2) of psychosocial treatments 3) with primary or secondary aims of improving emotional or psychological health 4) in samples of older adults (age 60 years and older) with or without cognitive impairment, and if they were 5) published in English 6) during the 10 years up to 2009. (For studies before 1999, see Teri and McCurry 1994, 2000.) Studies were excluded if they involved 1) other types of interventions (bright light therapy, electroconvulsive therapy, acupuncture, sensory therapies, pharmacology); 2) participants with specific general medical illnesses (i.e., individuals diagnosed with stroke, cancer, diabetes, Parkinson's disease); and 3) integrated care models that included general medical components. We identified more than 52 treatment outcome studies meeting our criteria. To facilitate this discussion, an overview of each study is shown in Tables 8–1 through 8–3, later in this chapter. Because some of the information in these articles was incomplete, information in the tables is presented as a guide for discussion, not a definitive statement of any study's intent. The exclusion of studies not meeting

Appreciation is extended to David La Fazia, Ph.D., for his assistance in the literature review for this chapter. Preparation of this chapter was supported in part by a grant from the National Institute on Aging (AG14777–06A2).

our criteria does not imply that the treatments they describe or their identified outcomes are unimportant or ineffective; rather, they are not included because an exhaustive review of the entire growing literature with geriatric patients would be beyond the scope of the present chapter.

Overview of Psychosocial Therapies

There is tremendous diversity in the nature of treatments included under the rubric "psychosocial." This diversity is evident in the articles we reviewed. For the purpose of organization and discussion, we provide in this section an overview of the three major psychosocial approaches represented in the studies reviewed here: 1) behavioral and cognitive-behavioral therapies, 2) psychodynamic psychotherapy, and 3) reminiscence and life review therapies.

Behavioral and Cognitive-Behavioral Therapies

Behavioral and cognitive-behavioral approaches have been widely used in the treatment of depression and anxiety in older adults. Behavioral therapy (BT) approaches derive from Lewinsohn's work (Lewinsohn et al. 1984) and were first applied to older adults by Teri and Logsdon (1990). The premise is that dementia-related behaviors can be altered by improvements in environmental stimuli and changes in caregiver responses to those behaviors. Cognitive-behavioral therapy (CBT) combines this behavioral view with cognitive theory (Beck et al. 1979): cognitive distortions are hypothesized to be the core disturbance maintaining psychological distress. Both BT and CBT seek to change the cognitive and/or behavioral context in which the disturbance occurs through use of a variety of specific techniques, such as providing new information, teaching problem-solving strategies, correcting skills deficits, modifying ineffective communication patterns, or changing the physical environment in which problems arise. Homework assignments are frequently given to supplement in-session interventions. Although specific treatment protocols vary, all BT and CBT approaches tend to be active and focused on solving specific, current day-to-day problems, rather than seeking global personality change in the client. It should be noted that in practice, the terms *psychoeducational therapy*, *problem-solving therapy*, and *cognitive-behavioral therapy* are often used interchangeably to refer to similar intervention strategies.

Evidence for the effectiveness of CBT with older adults has been well established over the past decade. For example, Payne and Marcus (2008) completed a meta-analysis of 44 studies, which included 17 CBT studies (delivered as group therapy), and found a moderate effect size for CBT (r=0.56; 95% confidence interval [CI]=0.44–0.65) in the treatment of a variety of psychological outcomes. Pinquart et al. (2007) focused on clinically depressed older adults and reported large effect sizes for cognitive and behavioral approaches overall (d=0.87) and for CBT specifically (d=1.12).

CBT has also been compared to pharmacotherapy for treating depression in the older adult population. One meta-analysis integrated data from 89 controlled studies of treatments for depressive conditions: 62 examined the effect of pharmacotherapy, and 32 examined the effect of psychotherapy (Pinquart et al. 2006). Overall effect sizes for the treatment of depression in older adults were moderate to large (d=–0.80), with no significant differences in effect sizes between psychotherapy (d=–1.09) and pharmacotherapy (d=–0.69). CBT, examined in 26 of the studies, yielded the largest effect (d=1.22) for improving depressive conditions in older adults.

Psychodynamic Psychotherapy

Psychodynamic approaches emphasize the importance of the therapeutic relationship as a mechanism of change, as well as the historical cause of current client behavior. The clients' psychological insight and ongoing emotional experience are considered critical for psychological progress, and the therapist is significantly less directive than CBT therapists. The evidence for effectiveness of psychodynamic approaches is limited. Pinquart et al. (2007) completed a meta-analysis of the effectiveness of psychosocial interventions and reported effect sizes for subcategories of treatment approaches. Of the 57 reviewed studies, 3 examined the effectiveness of psychodynamic therapies and reported an overall moderate effect size (d=0.76). Three additional studies were based on interpersonal therapy, with an overall small (nonsignificant) effect size (d=0.14).

Reminiscence and Life Review Therapies

In reminiscence therapy, older adults are encouraged to remember the past and to share their memories, either with a therapist or with peers, as a way of increasing self-esteem and social intimacy. This therapy is often highly directive and structured, with the therapist picking each session's reminiscence topic. In life review therapy, the therapist encourages the patient to recall past experiences, as well as to make an effort to reexperience old conflicts and rework them into a therapeutic resolution. In other words, life review is one form of reminiscence, designed to produce a better understanding and acceptance of past events (Butler 1963). In the clinical intervention literature, *reminiscence* and *life review* are often used as loosely interchangeable terms for any individual or group narrative therapy that encourages clients to remember and describe the past; however, there is some thought that reminiscence and life review activities are actually distinct psychological processes, and that these processes may significantly alter the effectiveness of reminiscence as a therapeutic technique (Watt and Wong 1991). Indeed, the conceptual differences between simple reminiscence and active life review have been considered by a number of authors (see Bohlmeijer et al. 2007).

The evidence for effectiveness of reminiscence therapy has grown in the past decade. For example, Pinquart et al.'s (2007) meta-analysis of effects of psychosocial interventions for older adults with clinical depression included eight outcome studies of reminiscence therapies and reported a large effect size (d=1.00; 95% CI=0.73–1.27). Bohlmeijer et al. (2007) conducted a meta-analysis of 15 outcome studies that included reminiscence or life review; the authors reported an overall medium effect size (d=0.54; 95% CI=0.33–0.75), with life review having a significantly greater effect on psychological outcomes than simple reminiscence.

Psychosocial Therapies Used With Older Adults and Caregivers

The studies included in this review involve three types of participants: 1) cognitively intact older adults, 2) cognitively impaired older adults, and 3) caregivers of older adults who are included in treatment to improve the status of the older adult.

Psychotherapy With Cognitively Intact Older Adults

Much of the psychotherapeutic research conducted with older adults has focused on the treatment of depression or anxiety. As discussed in Chapter 19, "Mood Disorders," and Chapter 20, "Anxiety Disorders," depression and anxiety are two of the most common neuropsychiatric disorders in older adults, yet they often go unrecognized and untreated (Administration on Aging 2001). In addition, depressed older adults have reported a preference for psychosocial treatments, yet only 8% of a sample of 1,801 depressed older adults received any psychosocial treatment for depression, and only 29% reported any effective treatment for depression in the past 3 months (Unutzer et al. 2003). Because older adults with chronic illnesses are at increased risk for developing depression or anxiety (Lenze et al. 2001) and because suicide rates for older adults are greater than for younger adults (Reynolds 1997), this lack of psychosocial treatment with older adults is a cause of concern. Fortunately, the literature has generally demonstrated that both acute and continuation psychosocial therapies can be effective. In this subsection, we review empirical studies of psychosocial interventions that were specifically designed to reduce depression or anxiety in cognitively intact older adults.

Cognitive-Behavioral Therapy

Nineteen of the articles meeting criteria for our review used CBT (Table 8–1). These studies all included depression or anxiety as a primary or secondary outcome and included criteria to exclude individuals with significant cognitive impairment. The studies included individual and group delivery of the therapy, and six studies examined the effectiveness of CBT combined with or compared with pharmacotherapy interventions.

Findings from these studies demonstrated that older adults respond positively to CBT aimed at treating late-life depression. For example, Floyd et al. (2004) compared individual cognitive therapy to cognitive bibliotherapy; both groups showed better outcomes than a delayed-treatment control group, there was no difference between the two intervention groups at follow-up, and posttreatment gains for both treatment groups were maintained at 2-year follow-up (Floyd et al. 2006). Haringsma et al. (2006) tested the effectiveness of a CBT-based psychoeducational course on coping with depression delivered to a group of self-referred older adults in a community-based mental health care system and reported significant improvement in depression and anxiety, with gains maintained at 14-month follow-up; however, 62% were still above the Center for Epidemiologic Studies Depression Scale cutoff for depression. Rokke et al. (1999) randomly assigned older adults to a waitlist control condition or to a cognitive or behavioral condition in which the treatment was either chosen or assigned. Both treatment conditions were effective in decreasing depression, and no differences were found between cognitive or behavioral groups or between having choice or not. However, participants who did choose the treatment were less likely to drop out of treatment.

Two studies focused on the effectiveness of cognitive-behavioral approaches in physically frail populations. Treatments were delivered to individuals in their homes. Gellis et al. (2007) compared the effectiveness of a brief problem-solving therapy (PST) intervention (six sessions) with usual care. The outcomes of interest were improving quality of life and depression symptoms in depressed older adults who were receiving acute home care services. The PST participants had a significant improvement in depression scores compared with those receiving usual care. In the second study, Scogin et al. (2007) tested the effectiveness of CBT (16–20 sessions) in treating Caucasian and African American medically ill older adults in rural areas. The CBT participants showed significant improvement in psychological symptoms (including depression and anxiety), and CBT was more beneficial for African Americans than for Caucasians on quality-of-life measures.

Outcome studies on late-life anxiety are consistent in demonstrating that older adults benefit from CBT. The majority of these studies targeted individuals with generalized anxiety disorder and provided evidence of significantly decreased levels of

TABLE 8–1. Psychotherapy with cognitively intact older adults

Study[a]	Sample population[b]	Intervention location and modality	Sample age (mean in years)	Treatment	Treatment duration and follow-up
Cognitive-behavioral therapy (CBT)					
Llewellyn-Jones et al. 1999	220 NH residents with depression 169 completed	Residential (self-care) in Australia	84	1. Collaborative model with consultation, training of practitioners in recognition of depression, and psychoeducation and health promotion of patients 2. Control: routine care	Not reported Follow-up at 9.5 months
Rokke et al. 1999	64 community residents with depression 40 completed 37% dropout; greatest in no-choice group (23% vs. 59%)	Outpatient clinic Individual	66 (range 60–86)	1. Choice (behavioral or cognitive) 2. No-choice (behavioral or cognitive) 3. Waitlist	Ten 1-hour weekly sessions Follow-up at 3 months
Barrowclough et al. 2001	55 referred from primary care and community with mix of anxiety disorders (GAD, panic) 43 completed	In-home Individual	72	1. CBT-RT 2. Supportive counseling	8–12 sessions Follow-up at 3, 6, and 12 months
Mohlman et al. 2003—Study 1	27 community residents with GAD 24 completed	Outpatient clinic Individual	66	1. CBT (standard version—Gorenstein protocol) 2. Waitlist	Thirteen 50-minute sessions followed by monthly booster sessions for 6 months Pre-post only
Mohlman et al. 2003—Study 2	15 community residents with GAD No dropouts	Outpatient clinic Individual	67	1. CBT—enhanced (with memory aides) 2. Waitlist	Thirteen 50-minute sessions followed by monthly booster sessions for 6 months Pre-post only
Stanley et al. 2003a	85 community residents with GAD (moderate to severe) 71 completed 16.5% dropout rate	Outpatient clinic Group	66	1. Group CBT (Stanley, Beck) 2. Minimal-contact control (phone contact)	15 group sessions Follow-up at 3, 6, and 12 months

TABLE 8–1. Psychotherapy with cognitively intact older adults *(continued)*

Study[a]	Sample population[b]	Intervention location and modality	Sample age (mean in years)	Treatment	Treatment duration and follow-up
Cognitive-behavioral therapy (CBT, *continued*)					
Stanley et al. 2003b	12 primary care clinic patients with GAD dx 9 completed 25% dropout	Outpatient clinic Individual	71	1. CBT—GAD/PC (education, relaxation, CBT, and sleep management skills) 2. Usual care	8 sessions Pre-post only
Wetherell et al. 2003	75 senior center and community residents with GAD 24% dropout	Outpatient clinic Group	67	1. Group CBT 2. Discussion group 3. Waitlist	12 sessions Follow-up at 6 months
Floyd et al. 2004 and Floyd et al. 2006 (2-year follow-up)	46 community residents with MDD or minor depression 31 completed	In-home Individual with phone call follow-up	68 (range 60–80)	1. Cognitive bibliotherapy (Feeling Good) 2. CBT (Beck-based manual) 3. Delayed-treatment control	1. Bibliotherapy: 4 telephone contacts over 1 month 2. CBT: 12–20 sessions for up to 16 weeks Follow-up at 3 months and 2 years
Arean et al. 2005	67 medical outpatients with MDD or dysthymia 50 completed	Outpatient clinic Group	65	1. Group CBT (based on Lewinsohn) 2. Clinical case management 3. Group CBT and case management	1. 18 sessions over 6 months 2. Weekly sessions over 6 months 3. Combo: Follow-up at 6 and 12 months
Haringsma et al. 2006	119 with depression dx, and 45% also with anxiety disorder Community mental health system in Netherlands 15% dropout	Outpatient clinic Group	—	1. Coping with depression course (BT—Lewinsohn) 2. Waitlist	10 weekly sessions, 2 hours each Follow-up at 2 and 14 months
Gellis et al. 2007	48 community residents receiving acute home health services 40 completed	In-home Individual	79 PST 80 usual care	1. PST 2. Usual care	6 sessions over 8 weeks Follow-up at 3 and 6 months
Scogin et al. 2007	134 rural older adults 57% African American 25% dropout	In-home Individual	75	1. CBT—manual (Thompson) 2. Minimal support	16–20 sessions with a 5.3-month average to completed treatment Follow-up at 3 and 6 months

TABLE 8–1. Psychotherapy with cognitively intact older adults *(continued)*

Study[a]	Sample population[b]	Intervention location and modality	Sample age (mean in years)	Treatment	Treatment duration and follow-up
CBT and/or pharmacotherapy					
Williams et al. 2000	415 primary care patients with minor depression 338 completed	PCP office Individual	71	1. Paroxetine 2. Placebo 3. PST	6 sessions in 11 weeks Follow-up at 11 weeks
Thompson et al. 2001	102 VA outpatients with MDD dx 30% dropout	Outpatient clinic (VA) Individual	66	1. Desipramine 2. CBT (manual based on Beck) 3. Desipramine and CBT	16–20 sessions in 3–4 months Pre-post only
Lynch et al. 2003	34 depression clinic patients with moderate to severe depression No dropouts	PCP office Group and individual phone calls	66 (range 60–80)	1. Medication and clinical management (Med) 2. Med+group DBT (with phone coaching)	DBT: 28 weeks of 2-hour sessions+30-minute weekly phone contact, followed by 6 months of phone calls Follow-up at 6 months
Gorenstein et al. 2005	42 volunteers with GAD wanting to decrease medication use 28 completed 33% dropout	Outpatient clinic Individual	68	1. CBT+MM (benzodiazepine taper) 2. MM (benzodiazepine taper)	8 sessions Follow-up at 6 months
Schuurmans et al. 2006	84 outpatients with anxiety disorder dx (GAD, panic, agoraphobia, social phobia) 52 completed 23% dropout	Outpatient clinic Group	70	1. Group CBT 2. Sertraline 3. Waitlist	CBT: Fifteen 1-hour sessions Meds: 8 (20-minute) clinic visits in 15 weeks Follow-up at 3 months
Wilkinson et al. 2009	45 outpatients with MDD; depressed in past 1 year and in remission for at least 2 months on antidepressant medication 36 completed	Outpatient office Group	73	1. Brief group CBT+antidepressant 2. Control: antidepressant treatment only	8 sessions Follow-up at 6 and 12 months

TABLE 8–1. Psychotherapy with cognitively intact older adults *(continued)*

Study[a]	Sample population[b]	Intervention location and modality	Sample age (mean in years)	Treatment	Treatment duration and follow-up
Psychodynamic therapy					
Reynolds et al. 1999	107 geropsychiatric clinic outpatients with unipolar recurrent MDD (currently in remission) 96 completed	Outpatient clinic Individual	67	Patients randomly assigned to one of four maintenance therapy conditions: 1. Nortriptyline 2. Nortriptyline and IPT 3. Placebo and IPT 4. Placebo	Monthly for 3 years or until recurrence of major depression episode
van Schaik et al. 2006	143 medical outpatients with MDD 120 completed	Outpatient clinic Individual	68	1. IPT 2. Care as usual	10 sessions in 5 months Follow-up at 6 months
Reminiscence or life review therapy					
Watt and Cappeliez 2000	42 older adults with moderate to severe depression 26 completed	Classroom Group	66	1. Group integrative reminiscence therapy 2. Group instrumental reminiscence therapy 3. Control: active socialization group	8 sessions in 3 months Control: 6 weekly sessions Follow-up at 3 months
Hanaoka and Okamura 2004	80 older adults 76 completed	NH or day care clients Group	82	1. Life review 2. Control: health discussion	Eight 1-hour sessions Follow-up at 3 months
Serrano et al. 2004	50 social services agency clients 43 completed	Research office Individual	77 (range 65–93)	1. Life review therapy group 2. Control: social assistance group	Six 1.5-hour sessions Pre-post only
Chao et al. 2006	24 older adults No dropouts	NH Group	78	1. Reminiscence group 2. Control	9 weekly sessions Pre-post only

Note. Completion and/or dropout rates and mean and/or range values are provided only when available in reference article.
BT=behavioral therapy; DBT= dialectical behavior therapy; dx=diagnosis; GAD=generalized anxiety disorder; GAD/PC=generalized anxiety disorder in primary care; IPT=interpersonal psychotherapy; MDD=major depressive disorder; med=medication; MM=medication management; NH=nursing home or long-term residential setting; PCP=primary care physician; PST=problem-solving therapy; RT=relaxation training; VA=Veterans Affairs.
[a]Studies cited together reported on subsamples of the same sample of the larger randomized clinical trial.
[b]Studies that identified subjects as diagnosed with MDD are specified; other studies may or may not have included subjects with MDD diagnosis.

anxiety, worry, and depression (Mohlman et al. 2003; Stanley et al. 2003a, 2003b; Wetherell et al. 2003). In individuals with a mix of anxiety disorders, significant improvements in self-reported anxiety and depression have also been reported (Barrowclough et al. 2001).

Two of the studies aimed at older adults with depression used multimodal approaches, combining case management strategies with a mix of components, including cognitive-behavioral strategies. For example, Llewellyn-Jones et al. (1999) found that a combined intervention (psychiatric consultation, psychoeducation, and health promotion activities) was superior to routine care in improving depression symptoms in nursing home residents. Arean et al. (2005) compared group CBT, case management, and their combination to treat depression in low-income older adults. Findings included a reduction in depression for case management and for combined case management plus CBT, but not for CBT alone.

CBT was either compared or combined with pharmacotherapy for treating depression in older adults in six of the reviewed studies. Williams et al. (2000) compared antidepressant treatment (paroxetine) with problem-solving treatment (based on CBT) in older adults with minor depression or dysthymia and found improvement for both treatment groups when compared with the control group; however, PST showed smaller benefits with slower onset when compared with medication treatment effects. Schuurmans et al. (2006) compared CBT to antidepressant treatment (sertraline) and reported improvements for both groups; however, there was a greater effect size for medication (d=0.94) than for group CBT (d=0.35). Three studies investigated the combination of pharmacotherapy and psychotherapy. Thompson et al. (2001) compared treatment with CBT alone and in combination with antidepressant medication (desipramine) in a sample of older adults with mild to moderate depression and found similar levels of improvement. Wilkinson et al. (2009) tested a brief group CBT for effectiveness in reducing recurrence of depression. The CBT plus antidepressant medication condition was compared with an antidepressant-only treatment condition. Individuals in the CBT plus antidepressant group had a 27.7% recurrence rate of depression, whereas those in the antidepressant-only group had a 44.4% recurrence rate (not significant). Lynch et al. (2003) compared antidepressant treatment alone with dialectical behavior therapy plus antidepressant therapy (selective serotonin reuptake inhibitor and/or tricyclic antidepressant medication) and found that the combination therapy significantly improved depressive symptoms. Additionally, the combined treatment group had a 71% remission rate, compared with a 47% rate in the medication-only group. In a novel study by Gorenstein et al. (2005), older adults who wanted to discontinue use of antianxiety medication (benzodiazepines) were randomly assigned either to receive CBT treatment while tapering medication or to taper medication without CBT. Both groups had equivalent decreases in their medication use. There were significant decreases in depression and anxiety levels in the participants who received CBT compared with levels in those who did not.

In summary, accumulating data support the effectiveness of CBT in treating depression in physically healthy and physically frail older adults without dementia. Evidence suggests that symptom improvements obtained with psychotherapy are equal to those found with pharmacotherapy and that psychotherapy may be associated with lower dropout rates during treatment than pharmacological interventions alone. A wide variety of CBT formats, including individual and group interventions, bibliotherapy, and variants of CBT (cognitive only, behavioral only, and CBT), have all produced reductions in depression or anxiety. In many studies, treatment gains have been maintained up to 1-year follow-up. Studies in this review that include multimodal approaches are limited in number and have mixed findings. The psychotherapy literature has focused primarily on community-residing volunteers diagnosed as having major depression; however, some studies have shown psychotherapy to be effective with milder or chronic depressive symptoms and with anxiety disorders as well.

Psychodynamic Psychotherapy

Our review identified only two controlled studies in the past decade that tested interpersonal psychotherapy (IPT) in older adults with depression or anxiety. Historically, however, some of the most extensive work examining the use of psychosocial interventions for treatment of late-life depression has compared IPT with nortriptyline. For example, Reynolds et al. (1999) followed a group of cognitively intact older adults who, after successful treatment for recurrent major depression with a combination of IPT and nortriptyline, were randomly assigned to maintenance treatment for 3 years with placebo, nortriptyline, or a combination of IPT plus placebo or IPT plus nortriptyline. Older patients benefited from active treatment (psychological or pharmacological treatment), and recurrence rates were most improved in the IPT plus nortriptyline group (Reynolds et al. 1999). In a study of medical outpatients with a diagnosis of major depressive disorder, van Schaik et al. (2006) compared IPT with usual care. IPT was more effective in decreasing symptoms of major depressive disorder when the two groups were compared at the end of treatment.

In summary, controlled studies of psychodynamic interventions with depressed or anxious older adults are limited. The use of IPT in combination with antidepressants has been shown to be most effective in decreasing recurrence rates of depression in older adults when compared with IPT alone. IPT by itself has also been effective in decreasing depression when compared with usual care; however, follow-up results have not been consistent.

Reminiscence and Life Review Therapies

Empirical trials have been conducted using reminiscence and life review therapies to reduce depression and anxiety in older adults. Although limited in number, these studies provide support for ongoing exploration of effectiveness and potential moderators. The four studies we reviewed include two that investigated reminiscence and two that explored life review therapy. Depression was a primary or secondary outcome measure, anxiety was not included as an outcome measure, and only two of the studies assessed for depressive conditions at baseline.

Watt and Cappeliez (2000) reported that integrative and instrumental reminiscence therapies produced significant improvement in depressive symptoms at completion of therapy and that the integrative reminiscence therapy group maintained gains at 3-month follow-up. Chao et al. (2006) tested a reminiscence group in older adults in a nursing home and reported positive but not significant improvement in depression scores compared with those of a waitlist control group. Serrano et al. (2004) attempted treating clinically significant depression in community-dwelling older adults with life review therapy and reported a significant decrease in depression scores compared with scores of adults in the social assistance control group. Hanaoka and Okamura (2004) investigated the effectiveness of a life review group for improving mood in individuals in nursing homes and day care settings. They reported significant improvement in depressive symptoms and hopelessness.

In summary, controlled trials investigating the effectiveness of reminiscence therapies in the treatment of depression or anxiety are limited. The four reviewed studies all considered and screened for cognitive impairment; however, the participants had diverse levels of depression at baseline. Nonsignificant findings were reported in one of the four studies. The approach to reminiscence or life review used for the treatment of geriatric depression has not been standardized, and many protocol variations have been used that could influence treatment outcome. Studies have shown that structured life review strategies may be more effective than simple narrative reminiscence.

Psychotherapy With Cognitively Impaired Older Adults

The previous section dealt with psychosocial interventions geared toward reducing depression or anxiety in cognitively intact older adults. However, there is growing interest in the psychosocial treatment of depression and anxiety in patients with cognitive impairment because both are commonly associated with dementia, and treatment can have a positive impact on the functional status of individuals with cognitive impairment (Teri and Wagner 1992; Teri et al. 2005c). In our review of the last decade of literature, we located nine randomized controlled clinical trials of psychosocial treatment of older adults with dementia in whom depression- and/or anxiety-related outcomes were reported (Table 8–2). Interestingly, although pharmacological treatment of depression in older adults remains a common approach to care, a review of randomized controlled trials on the use of antidepressant medication for the treatment of depression in dementia revealed only eight published placebo-controlled trials, and five of them failed to demonstrate efficacy (Olin et al. 2002). Thus, there is a clear need for more effective interventions for older adults with depression and dementia, and psychosocial approaches may offer alternatives to pharmacotherapy as well as ways to augment the latter's treatment effects. Therefore, we discuss the empirical studies that have been conducted specifically to reduce depression or anxiety in individuals with cognitive impairment.

Cognitive-Behavioral Therapy

Behavioral treatment approaches are focused on increasing pleasant interactions, decreasing unpleasant interactions, and developing skills necessary to alter the environment to obtain positive outcomes (Teri and Logsdon 1990). The person with dementia has limited ability to initiate pleasant interactions or to implement environmental changes. BT approaches for treating depression in persons with dementia are therefore often modified, in that the caregiver, as the person in greatest control of the environment, is targeted for training in the use of behavioral strategies (for more information about this framework, see Teri 1997). Five of the reviewed studies provided training to staff caregivers in long-term care settings, one to family caregivers, and two were delivered directly to the individuals with cognitive impairment.

The majority of the staff-focused BT interventions occurred in nursing homes. Proctor et al. (1999) evaluated the effectiveness of training long-term care staff to deliver BT-based depression interventions for residents with dementia. Staff training focused on establishing individualized, realistic goals for behavioral improvement, as well as on implementing behavioral strategies. The goals of treatment were to decrease behavioral disturbance and to decrease depression. The intervention also included ongoing supervision and support for behavioral plan development by members of a hospital outreach team. The intervention group showed significant change on depression at 6 months and significant differences on depression when compared with the control group.

Beck et al. (2002) also trained staff caregivers (hired for the study) to deliver two behavioral interventions to residents with dementia in a nursing home. There were three treatment groups (activities of daily living, psychosocial activity, and a combination). The goals of treatment were to reduce disruptive behaviors and improve mood. The analysis of videotaped interventions, using an observational measure of negative mood, showed a significant decrease in sad behaviors during treatment for the intervention groups but not for the control groups.

TABLE 8–2. Psychotherapy with cognitively impaired older adults

Study	Sample population	Intervention location and modality	Sample age (mean in years)	Treatment	Treatment duration and follow-up
Cognitive-behavioral therapy (CBT)					
Alexopoulos et al. 2003	25 older adults with MDD with executive dysfunction No dropouts	Home	74 (range 66–88)	1. Problem-solving therapy 2. Supportive therapy	Weekly for 12 weeks Pre-post only
Hyer et al. 2008–2009	25 depressed NH residents 24 completed	NH	79	1. CBT: group, individual, and staff support 2. Treatment as usual	2 individual coaching sessions, 13 group sessions, and staff support Pre-post only
Caregiver training and behavioral skill building (BT based)					
McCallion et al. 1999	120 NH residents with dementia 105 completed	NH	85	1. Communication skills training with CNAs 2. Waitlist control, normal facility in-services	5 group sessions and 4 individual sessions Duration not reported Follow-up at 6 months
Proctor et al. 1999	120 NH residents with dementia 105 completed	NH	83	1. Behavioral management training for staff 2. Usual care	Seven 1-hour training sessions and weekly follow-up support for 6 months Pre-post only
Beck et al. 2002	179 NH residents with dementia 127 completed	NH	84	1. Caregivers (hired for the study) conducted intervention containing behavioral strategies for ADLs, psychosocial activity, and both 2. Placebo: 1:1 with nurse daily 3. Usual care	Daily for 12 weeks Follow-up at 1 and 2 months
Lichtenberg et al. 2005	20 NH residents with dementia and depression No dropouts	NH	85	1. Behavioral therapy (aides trained to increase pleasant events for residents) 2. Usual care	3 sessions per week for 20–30 minutes each 3 months total Follow-up at 3 months

TABLE 8–2. Psychotherapy with cognitively impaired older adults *(continued)*

Study	Sample population	Intervention location and modality	Sample age (mean in years)	Treatment	Treatment duration and follow-up
Caregiver training and behavioral skill building (BT based, *continued*)					
Teri et al. 2005a	31 residents with dementia No dropouts	AL	86	1. Staff training on behavioral problem solving and increase in pleasant events for residents 2. Control	Two 4-hour workshops and 4 individual sessions for staff over 8 weeks Pre-post only
Reminiscence or life review therapy					
Lai and Kayser-Jones 2004	101 NH residents with dementia 86 completed	NH	85	1. Reminiscence (life story): individual 2. Social visits: individual 3. Control	Weekly for 6 weeks Follow-up at 6 weeks
Wang 2007	102 NH residents with dementia (mild, moderate, severe) 92 completed	NH	79	1. Reminiscence: group 2. Control	Weekly for 8 weeks Pre-post only

Note. Completion and/or dropout rates are provided only when available in reference article.
AD=Alzheimer's disease; ADLs=activities of daily living; AL=assisted living; BT=behavioral therapy; CNA=certified nursing assistant; MDD=major depressive disorder; NH=nursing home or long-term-care residential setting.

Improving effective verbal and nonverbal communication between nursing assistants and nursing home residents with dementia was tested in another BT-based training intervention (McCallion et al. 1999). Communication skills specific to the person's level of dementia, environmental modification, and approaches to problem behaviors were taught to and delivered to residents by nursing assistants. Depression scores were significantly decreased for the treatment group when compared with the waitlist control group. Additionally, withdrawal behaviors were significantly decreased in the treatment group when compared with the control group at baseline and 6-month follow-up.

Another project using behavioral strategies and designed to improve resident mood and decrease dementia-related behaviors took place in a newly opened dementia special care unit of a nursing home (Lichtenberg et al. 2005). Each week for 3 months, a trained nursing assistant provided three 20- to 30-minute behavioral sessions aimed at increasing pleasant events for residents. Although the treatment was appreciated by the residents, staff, and families, there were no differences in depressive symptoms when compared with usual care, and both groups had declines in behavioral disturbances.

In the only study thus far to investigate the efficacy of training staff in assisted-living residences, Teri et al. (2005a) trained direct care staff to use behavioral strategies (including problem solving, increasing pleasant events, and communication skills training) aimed at improving the affective and behavioral health of residents. Residents who were cared for by trained staff had a significant decrease in depression compared with the waitlist control group. Trained staff also showed improvement on outcome measures of their own depression and burden.

Two studies tested CBT interventions delivered directly to the individuals with cognitive impairment and depression. Alexopoulos et al. (2003) compared the efficacy of PST and supportive therapy in depressed older adults with cognitive dysfunction (in the absence of dementia syndrome, as evidenced by exclusion of individuals with Mini-Mental State Examination [MMSE] scores under 24). PST was more effective than supportive therapy in decreasing depressive symptoms. Participants improved skills in decision making, and their ability to generate alternatives was associated with improvements in depression. Hyer et al. (2008–2009) studied the effectiveness of a CBT intervention that included both individual and group modalities in a sample that included residents with some cognitive impairment, including mild dementia (mean MMSE score=23.6). Self-rated depression scores were significantly improved for the CBT group compared with the usual-care group. These studies provide further indication that depression in older adults with cognitive impairment may be treatable and that additional research exploring potential forms of treatment is warranted.

In summary, CBT and BT emphasize specific skill training and behavior change, and both have been shown to be effective in reducing depression in older adults with cognitive impairment and in those diagnosed with progressive dementing illnesses such as Alzheimer's disease. Evidence also suggests that treatment for depression in patients with dementia can improve caregivers' mood, even when treatment does not specifically focus on the caregiver. Although the empirical literature on the use of CBT and BT with patients who have dementia and their caregivers is still in its infancy, such positive early results warrant further investigation.

Reminiscence and Life Review Therapies

Reminiscence and life review techniques have also been used with depressed elderly patients with dementia in long-term-care settings. Reminiscence storytelling has been conducted in group (Wang 2007) and individual (Lai and Kayser-Jones 2004) formats. Specific topics or themes were suggested by staff, sometimes with the assistance of personal artifacts, newspapers, music, or other memorabilia used to stimulate residents' memories. Results of the two studies found that simple reminiscing led to reductions in depression and to improvements in social functioning for the confused participants. However, changes were not maintained over time.

Psychosocial Approaches for Family Caregivers of Persons With Dementia

The majority of assistance for community-dwelling older adults with dementia in the United States comes from family members, usually spouses or grown children who are themselves over age 50 years (Alzheimer's Association and National Alliance for Caregiving 2004). In the United States, an estimated 8.9 million people provide care for a relative over age 50 with dementia (Alzheimer's Association and National Alliance for Caregiving 2004), and the number of family caregivers is projected to increase 85%, to 37 million, by 2050 (Health and Human Services Assistant Secretary for Planning and Evaluation 2003). Providing care for an individual with dementia is often a difficult task that may negatively impact the caregiver's health, both emotionally (Covinsky et al. 2003) and physically (Lee et al. 2003; Schulz and Beach 1999). Thus, family caregivers are an important link in the care of older adults with dementia.

The last decade has seen a substantial increase in the number and quality of empirical studies investigating the effectiveness of various psychoeducational, psychotherapeutic, and self-help interventions used with family caregivers. Both systematic reviews (Belle et al. 2003; Gallagher-Thompson and Coon 2007; Pinquart and Sorensen 2006; Sorensen et al. 2006) and meta-analyses (Brodaty et al. 2003; Sorensen et al. 2002) have proliferated, attesting to the growth of this area. On the basis of a review identifying evidence-based psychological treatments for psychological distress in family caregivers providing care for older adults with cognitive impairments, Gallagher-Thompson and Coon (2007) reported that 14 of the 19 identified interventions were psychoeducational and yielded large effect sizes (0.81). In addition, three studies found CBT-based psychotherapy to be effective in improving depression and anxiety in family caregivers, with an average effect size of 1.20 (Gallagher-Thompson and Coon 2007). In this section, we discuss only those studies that include primary or secondary outcomes related to caregiver or care recipient depression or anxiety. In Table 8–3 and in the following text, these articles are grouped into two categories: those designed to teach family caregivers to manage emotional or behavioral issues of the care recipient's condition (care recipient focused) and those designed to enhance the caregiver's psychological functioning directly (caregiver focused).

The development and fruition of one multisite project may be viewed as addressing both of these domains. Resources for Enhancing Alzheimer's Caregiver Health (REACH) involved 1,222 caregivers across six sites in the United States (Schulz et al. 2003). Multicomponent interventions for ethnically and racially diverse family caregivers were investigated (Burgio et al. 2003; Burns et al. 2003; Eisdorfer et al. 2003; Gallagher-Thompson et al. 2003; Gitlin et al. 2003a, 2003b; Mahoney et al. 2003). In a meta-analysis of REACH interventions, active engagement in skills training significantly reduced depressive symptoms of caregivers compared with control conditions. Active treatment was more effective for Hispanics, nonspouses, and caregivers with lower education. The authors concluded that effective interventions need to include multiple components and be targeted to characteristics of the caregiver (Gitlin et al. 2003a).

Care Recipient–Focused Approaches

The term *care recipient* is used instead of *patient* or *client* to reflect that the person with a cognitive impairment who is receiving care may be residing independently, with family, or in a long-term-care setting—and thus may not consider himself or herself to be a patient or client. The general hypothesis of interventions focused on care recipients is that improving caregivers' skills for managing common dementia-related behaviors will aid both the care recipients (by decreasing the problems they experience) and the caregivers (by reducing their level of stress, burden, and/or depression). Interventions are aimed at building caregiver skills to enhance caregiver management of common emotional or behavioral issues related to a person with dementia.

Over the past decade, a variety of studies have taken place within the caregiver and care recipient's own home—delivered in person and/or by telephone—but findings across studies are inconsistent. For example, one study trained caregivers, in their homes for six sessions over 6 months, in behavioral and environmental management skills and found a significant improvement in caregiver mood, as well as a reduction in recipient behavioral occurrences, when compared with the control group (Gitlin et al. 2003b). The positive effects were still present at 12-month follow-up. In another study, caregivers received in-home training on behavioral and environmental management skills for 3–4 hours, followed by biweekly phone calls for 6 months, and they were compared with a minimal-contact control group (Buckwalter et al. 1999; Gerdner et al. 2002). Caregivers who received training had significant positive changes in depression and anxiety, which were maintained at 12-month follow-up. Burgio et al. (2003) also provided skills training in behavior management (17 sessions over 12 months) with phone call support in applying skills. Findings included decreased caregiver burden (reported levels of bother) but no change in levels of anxiety or depression in the treatment group compared with the minimal-support control group (phone calls only). Bourgeois et al. (2002) designed a combined format of a 3-hour group education session, followed by 11 in-home individual sessions (behavior management skills training), and compared the treatment group with a comparable-attention control group. They reported a significant improvement in patient depression symptoms postintervention; however, improvement was not maintained at 12-month follow-up. In another study, caregivers received problem-solving training on the telephone or in the home and were compared to a control group who received "friendly telephone" contact. No changes were reported in depression symptoms of the care recipients, but all three groups reported reduced burden for caregivers, with in-home training showing the greatest effect (Davis et al. 2004).

The most consistent findings in home settings have come from a series of studies by Teri and colleagues (2005b) in which a systematic and structured approach to caregiver training, incorporating skills training in communication, problem solving (ABCs of behavior management), and pleasant events (identifying and increasing pleasant activities and interactions), sought to enhance caregivers' skills with the goal of reducing care recipients' problems. This approach, called the Seattle Protocols, has been investigated via a series of randomized controlled clinical trials. The initial protocol was designed to reduce depression in care recipients with dementia (Teri et al. 1997). Seventy-two dyads of Alzheimer's disease patients and their caregivers were randomly assigned to two BT conditions and two control conditions. Study results indicated significant reductions in depression on standardized measures for care recipients in both behavioral conditions, but not for those in either control condition. Of care recipients in the BT conditions, 52% and 68% improved over the course of treatment, compared with 29% in the typical care and waitlist control conditions. Treatment effects were maintained at

TABLE 8–3. Psychosocial approaches for family caregivers of persons with dementia

Study	Sample population	Intervention location and modality	Sample age (mean in years)	Treatment	Treatment duration and follow-up
Care recipient–focused skill building in providing care (for the caregiver)					
Buckwalter et al. 1999	245 caregivers of persons with AD 174 completed	In-home Individual	64.6	1. Psychoeducational training in environmental and behavior management skills 2. Control: 2 in-home visits	3–4 hours of in-home training followed by biweekly phone calls for 6 months Follow-up at 12 months
Hepburn et al. 2001; Ostwald et al. 1999	117 families of persons with AD 94 completed	Classroom Group	65.6	1. Group workshop: psychoeducational and skill development for caregiving 2. Waitlist control	7 sessions (120 minutes) Follow-up at 5 months
Bourgeois et al. 2002	93 caregivers of patients with AD (majority spouses) 63 completed	Classroom and in-home Group and individual	73	1. Patient change: behavior management skills 2. Self change: caregiver-focused skills training 3. Control: comparable attention workshop	12 weeks: 1 week of 3-hour university training; 11 weeks of in-home visits with caregivers Follow-up at 3 and 6 months
Gerdner et al. 2002	237 caregivers of persons with dementia	In-home Individual	65	1. Progressively lowered stress threshold 2. Comparison: routine information and referrals for case management, community-based services, and support groups	4 hours of in-home intervention over 2 weeks Follow-up at 3, 6, 9, and 12 months
Burns et al. 2003	167 caregivers of persons with dementia At 2 years 76 remained (18% died; 28% lost to follow-up)	PCP office Individual	64	1. Behavior care management education 2. Enhanced: behavior management education+stress reduction training 1 and 2 in conjunction with care recipient PCP office visits	4 face-to-face sessions per year and follow-up phone calls at least monthly for 2 years (3 hours over 24 months) Pre-post (2-year intervention)
Burgio et al. 2003	140 dyads White and African American caregivers of persons with dementia 118 completed	In-home Individual	62	1. Skills training: behavior management, education, and phone calls 2. Minimal support (phone calls)	17 sessions over 12 months or telephone support Follow-up at 6 months

TABLE 8–3. Psychosocial approaches for family caregivers of persons with dementia *(continued)*

Study	Sample population	Intervention location and modality	Sample age (mean in years)	Treatment	Treatment duration and follow-up
Care recipient–focused skill building in providing care (for the caregiver, *continued*)					
Eisdorfer et al. 2003	225 family caregivers of persons with AD Cuban and white 147 completed (at 6 months)	In-home Individual and family	69	1. Family therapy: psychoeducation and restructuring of interactions between family members 2. Family therapy+computer telephone 3. Control: minimal support	14 in-home visits over 12 months Follow-up at 6, 12, and 18 months
Gitlin et al. 2003b; Gitlin 2005 (follow-up)	127 family caregivers of persons with dementia	In-home Individual	60	1. Home environmental and behavior management skill building 2. Control Individual in-home	6 sessions over 6 months Follow-up at 12 months
Mahoney et al. 2003	100 caregivers of persons with AD Dropouts not reported	In-home Telephone	61	1. Technology intervention: interactive voice response automated phone system; focused on helping caregivers manage problem behaviors; caregivers offered multiple components 2. Usual care	12 months Follow-up at 6, 12, and 18 months
Davis et al. 2004	71 family caregivers of persons with AD 61 completed	In-home Individual	65.1	1. Telephone problem-solving training 2. In-home problem-solving training 3. Friendly telephone contact (comparison group) Based on stress and coping model; taught behavioral problem-solving skills	Weekly sessions for 12 weeks Follow-up at 3 months
Mittelman et al. 2004	406 spousal caregivers of persons with AD Continuation of 1995 study	Home	71	1. Enhanced counseling and support (education and conflict resolution); also role-play to deal with problem behavior 2. Usual care	6 sessions of individual and family counseling; at 4 months, began attending weekly support group; received ad hoc counseling

TABLE 8–3. Psychosocial approaches for family caregivers of persons with dementia *(continued)*

Study	Sample population	Intervention location and modality	Sample age (mean in years)	Treatment	Treatment duration and follow-up
Care recipient–focused skill building in providing care (for the caregiver, *continued*)					
Mittelman et al. 2008	158 spouses of persons with AD 155 completed	Outpatient research clinics Individual and family	Range 60–89	1. Counseling/support and psychoeducation (AD person given donepezil) 2. Resource info and routine service (AD person given donepezil)	5 in-person sessions Follow-up at 3, 6, 9, 12, 18, and 24 months
Caregiver-focused approach					
Gallagher-Thompson et al. 2000	213 family caregivers of physically and/or cognitively impaired older adults (50% spouses) 177 completed	Classroom Group	60	1. Increased life satisfaction class (BT—Lewinsohn); increase in pleasant events 2. Problem-solving skills class 3. Waitlist/minimal-contact control	10 weekly 2-hour sessions Pre-post only
Marriott et al. 2000	42 family caregivers (with psychiatric morbidity) to person with dementia 41 completed	In-home Individual	63	1. CBT family intervention (education, stress management and coping skills training) 2. Control/in-depth family interview 3. Control/no interview	14 sessions with 2 weeks between each Follow-up at 3 and 6 months
Steffen 2000	33 caregivers to person with dementia 28 completed	In-home Individual and phone contact	64 (range 40–82)	1. Anger management: videotapes and phone call to home 2. Class on anger management 3. Waitlist control Videos and teaching based on CBT	In home: viewed 8- to 30-minute videos with 20-minute phone calls Class: Eight 90-minute sessions to watch video and discuss Pre-post only
Coon et al. 2003	169 women caregivers of person with dementia (60% wives, 40% daughters) 130 completed	Classroom Group	64	1 Anger management (CBT) 2. Depression management (BT) 3. Waitlist control	8 weekly 2-hour classes followed by 2 booster sessions (one per month) Follow-up at 3 months

TABLE 8–3. Psychosocial approaches for family caregivers of persons with dementia *(continued)*

Study	Sample population	Intervention location and modality	Sample age (mean in years)	Treatment	Treatment duration and follow-up
Caregiver-focused approach (*continued*)					
Gallagher-Thompson et al. 2003	213 women Latino and white Dropouts not reported	Classroom Group	57	1. Coping with caregiving (CBT); behavior and mood management (Beck and Lewinsohn) 2. Support group (Alzheimer's Association)	Ten 2-hour group sessions Follow-up at 3, 12, and 18 months
Teri et al. 2003	153 AD patients and family caregivers 140 completed	Home	Patient 78 Caregiver 70	1. Training in behavior management for family caregiver 2. Training in behavior management for caregiver and exercise for patient (30 minutes/day)	BT: 12 hour-long sessions; 2 per week for first 3 weeks and then 1 per week for next 4 weeks Follow-up at 6, 12, 18, and 24 months
Akkerman and Ostwald 2004	38 family caregivers (with anxiety) of persons with dementia 35 completed	Classroom Group	58 (range 34–85)	1. Group CBT focused on caregiver anxiety and management of anxiety 2. Waitlist control	9 weekly sessions Pre-post only
Belle et al. 2006	Racially diverse caregivers of a family member with dementia 212 Hispanic or Latino (188 completed) 219 white or Caucasian (204 completed) 211 black or African American (119 completed)	In-home Individual	79	1. Treatment group: targeted combination of enhancing mood management skills, stress management skills, self-care behaviors, social support, and management of care recipient problem behaviors 2. Control: 2 brief check-in calls during 6-month intervention	12 in-home and telephone sessions in 6 months Follow-up at 6 months
Gallagher-Thompson et al. 2007	55 Chinese women caring for person with dementia 45 completed	In-home	59	1. Telephone support 2. CBT program: aimed to decrease depression and stress in caregiver	6 sessions in 12 weeks Pre-post only

Note. Completion and/or dropout rates and mean and/or range values are provided only when available in reference article.
AD=Alzheimer's disease; BT=behavioral therapy; CBT=cognitive-behavioral therapy; NH=nursing home or long-term-care residential setting; PCP=primary care physician.

6-month follow-up, and baseline severity of depression was the only characteristic of care recipients that predicted treatment response (more depressed subjects were more likely to benefit from treatment). Interestingly, caregivers of individuals with dementia who were in the two BT conditions showed significant reductions in depression, but those on the waitlist did not. This latter finding was unexpected, because care recipients' depression was the only treatment target. Increased skill in behavior management, the availability of regular therapeutic support, and reduced depression in the family member with dementia were hypothesized to explain these added benefits.

In a more recent trial, which is included in this review, caregivers were taught a protocol that combined the Seattle Protocol with exercise to increase care recipients' physical activity and improve caregivers' physical and emotional health (Teri et al. 2003). A total of 153 dyads of caregivers and care recipients were enrolled. At posttest, active-treatment subjects improved significantly more than control subjects on primary outcomes of physical activity and depression, they exercised significantly more, and they had significantly fewer restricted-activity days. At 24 months, improvements in physical activity and mobility were maintained. For patients entering the study with higher levels of depression, significant improvements in depression were maintained at 24 months. There was also a trend for active-treatment patients to have less institutionalization due to behavioral disturbance throughout the 24-month follow-up period.

Two interventions were not delivered in-home. Hepburn et al. (2001) employed a group workshop (seven sessions of 120 minutes each) including the caregiver and other family members; it focused on education about dementia and practical skill development for caregiving. The caregiver group receiving treatment had a decrease in depressive symptoms when compared with the control group at 5-month follow-up. Another intervention was delivered to caregivers of individuals with dementia in conjunction with quarterly primary care office visits for the care recipient (Burns et al. 2003). Individual behavior management education was compared with enhanced care (individual stress reduction training in addition to behavior management education). The intervention included four face-to-face sessions a year and follow-up phone calls at least monthly for 2 years. Both groups of caregivers reported a decrease in depressive symptoms, with the enhanced-care participants having the greater decrease in symptoms.

Several studies combined psychoeducation with additional treatment components. For example, Mittelman et al. (2004) combined individual and family counseling, group support, and psychoeducation (conflict resolution and management of dementia-related behaviors). The intervention was aimed at improving the mood of caregivers and consisted of six individual and family counseling sessions for the first 2 months, followed by weekly support group meetings and ongoing counseling as needed for 1 year. Caregiver outcomes at 1 year included significant decreases in depressive symptoms for the active-treatment group compared with the usual-care control group and interestingly a decrease in nursing home placements for the care recipients. The improvements in depressive symptoms for the caregivers were sustained for 3.1 years. In a later study, Mittelman et al. (2008) added medication treatment (donepezil) for the care recipient as an additional treatment component. In this study, caregivers received five individual sessions of counseling/support and psychoeducation, and the care recipient received donepezil. Caregivers in the comparison group received usual care, and care recipients received donepezil. Depression scores decreased for caregivers in the combined condition, whereas they increased for caregivers who did not receive counseling. Effects were still present at 2-year follow-up.

Additional studies tested delivery of interventions compared with or enhanced by technological equipment. For example, Mahoney et al. (2003) designed an automated phone system with interactive voice response to provide on-demand education and support for caregivers related to managing dementia-related behaviors. The intervention was active for 12 months, and treatment outcomes were compared with those of a usual-care control group. Overall, there were no reductions in caregiver reports of depression or anxiety; however, intervention group caregivers with lower reported levels of mastery at baseline did report significant improvements in depression and anxiety symptoms when compared with those receiving usual care. In a multicomponent intervention, family therapy (structured ecosystems therapy) was compared with family therapy with the added component of a computer telephone (providing educational resources and online support group) (average of 19 hours). Findings included decreased depressive symptoms for family therapy with a computer telephone at 6- and 18-month follow-ups (Eisdorfer et al. 2003).

In summary, an array of interventions seeking to train caregivers to improve their own skills in order to reduce problems of care recipients has met with variable success. The most promising are those with clear skills training directly related to the outcomes of interest. More diffuse and generalized training appears less successful.

Caregiver-Focused Approaches

CBT is most commonly used in psychotherapeutic interventions for caregivers and focuses on assisting caregivers to identify and modify or cope with their own unhelpful thoughts and behaviors when providing care. The goal is to enhance caregivers' skills in managing their feelings of anger and depression and associated behaviors.

In a series of studies, Gallagher-Thompson and colleagues have investigated the effectiveness of CBT in combination with various strategies and in comparison with other approaches.

For example, one study found CBT more effective than either a problem-solving skills class or a control condition in improving caregiver depression (Gallagher-Thompson et al. 2000). Another study investigated the effectiveness of CBT-based anger management training compared with depression management training and a waitlist control in a group of ethnically diverse family caregivers. Caregivers in both treatment groups reported a significant increase in self-efficacy and a decrease in depressive symptoms (Coon et al. 2003). In another CBT-based intervention, group-delivered caregiver training, which focused on cognitive restructuring and behavior and mood management skills, was compared with a professionally led weekly support group condition. Overall, CBT was more effective in decreasing depression and improving self-efficacy (Gallagher-Thompson et al. 2003). Individual in-home CBT (six sessions in 6 weeks) was also compared with a telephone support program for Chinese women caring for a relative with dementia. The in-home CBT intervention was more effective in reducing depression (Gallagher-Thompson et al. 2007).

Additional studies have investigated the effectiveness of CBT and alternative delivery methods in treating anxiety and depression in family caregivers. In one study targeting anxiety, caregivers attended group sessions focused on developing cognitive and behavioral skills to reduce their own anxiety. Anxiety levels (self-reported and observed) significantly improved for the treatment group compared with the waitlist control group (Akkerman and Ostwald 2004). Marriott et al. (2000) tested CBT delivered individually (stress management techniques and cognitive coping skills) for family caregivers with symptoms of psychological distress. The comparison condition was participation in an in-depth semistructured interview and a no-contact control group. The treatment group reported a significant decrease in stress and depression at posttest and follow-up when compared with comparison and control groups. Steffen (2000) compared two delivery methods for CBT-based anger management training. One group watched eight videotapes at home with a telephone follow-up to reinforce learning and answer questions. The second treatment group attended eight class sessions to watch and discuss the videotapes. Both treatment groups reported reduced levels of anger and increased caregiver self-efficacy for managing disruptive behaviors when compared with the waitlist control group. However, only the caregivers viewing videotapes at home with follow-up phone calls had significant improvement in depressive symptoms.

As noted earlier in this section, the REACH investigators concluded that multiple-component and targeted interventions would be most effective in improving depression and burden in family caregivers. As a result, Belle et al. (2006) designed a study (REACH II) to test the effectiveness of a structured yet flexible multiple-component intervention, which included an aim of improving caregiver depression. Caregivers within each of the ethnic or racial groups were randomly assigned to treatment or control conditions. At 6-month follow-up, prevalence of clinical depression was lower in the treatment group than in the control group and remained significant after adjustment for race and ethnicity.

In summary, a variety of programs have focused on the caregivers themselves, with the goals of reducing burden and improving coping and well-being. The majority have shown improvements in caregivers' self-reports of depression and anxiety. Overall, treatment effects have been modest, and although follow-up reports are limited, eight studies reported that positive effects were maintained at follow-up. The past decade has broadened the scope of intervention location and delivery method. Interventions have been delivered individually, in groups, and remotely (telephones, online programs, and videos) to caregivers in their homes, in classrooms, and in primary care offices. The positive improvements related to cognitive and behavioral treatments across diverse delivery methods and locations lend support for broadening the use of these treatments.

Conclusion and Future Research Directions

Several conclusions can be drawn from the literature on the efficacy of psychosocial interventions with older adults. First, a variety of interventions have been studied in diverse populations of older adults. Behavioral and cognitive-behavioral strategies have generated the most empirical research, with moderate to large treatment effects. Overall, treatment has been found effective in decreasing depression or anxiety in cognitively intact older adults, and a few studies have shown effectiveness to be equal or superior to that of pharmacotherapeutic interventions. Some evidence indicates that improvements resulting from these treatments are better maintained at follow-up than those from the other treatment forms, but there are too few long-term outcome comparison studies to evaluate the strength of these findings.

Although research is less plentiful, there is also empirical evidence for the efficacy of BT and CBT and their variants in individuals with dementia, as well as for older adult caregivers. Together, these studies demonstrate the utility of working closely with caregivers—whether family or staff—to reduce depression in persons with dementia. When caregivers are not available, the situation is more problematic, and no studies have yet addressed this issue. In some cases, long-term improvements, such as delay in nursing home placement, were reported.

A variety of factors have been identified that may contribute to differential treatment effects across studies. These factors include patient variables, such as severity of symptoms at the onset of treatment, level of cognitive impairment, and patient preferences for type of treatment. Specific treatment variables have also been implicated in differential outcomes. For example, in therapy with patients in long-term-care settings and in outpatient therapy with caregivers, successful maintenance of therapeutic gains appears contingent upon ongoing, or at least periodic, therapy contact. Both group and individual therapy formats have been successful with older clients.

Although the empirical treatment literature has grown substantially in recent years, additional research is needed to examine the efficacy of psychosocial interventions with older adults. The controlled studies that have been conducted represent a mixture of behavioral, cognitive-behavioral, supportive, and educational techniques. Although increasing numbers of studies, particularly those focused on depression treatment, now have treatment manuals available, much of the research conducted with older adults is not well described, making replication or comparison across studies difficult. Little empirical research has been done on the impact of therapist or environmental variables on therapy outcome. The cultural, intrapersonal, familial, and health factors that are likely to impact treatment efficacy have yet to be systematically investigated. The intervention literature has tended to focus primarily on the management of pathological cognitive or emotional disorders. The challenges of normal aging deserve attention as well.

Additional research is needed to determine the duration of interventions necessary to maximize treatment impact and to establish strategies for generalization and maintenance once the active-treatment phase ends. In the studies reported in this chapter, therapy duration ranged from a single or few sessions to months or years; in some studies, subjects were exposed to different numbers of sessions over variable lengths of time. Clarifying the significance of this variable may be particularly important for older adults with chronic physical or social circumstances that have precipitated psychosocial intervention. Because therapy outcome is dependent on how psychosocial functioning is defined and measured, research is also needed to identify assessment instruments that are carefully validated, sensitive to expected changes, and appropriate for use with various elderly populations and in specialized contexts. The effectiveness of technological equipment in delivery of psychosocial interventions is a promising area for ongoing research. Among the studies reviewed for this chapter, there is tremendous variability in reported treatment outcomes, and the field would be well served by research that would help guide measurement selection in the future.

Given the growing number of older adults who are physically and cognitively impaired, it is surprising that there are so few controlled studies examining the psychosocial impact of physical disability and/or institutionalization on older adults. Additional "real-world" research examining treatment effectiveness in persons with multiple medical, psychiatric, and social disabilities is needed.

What is the take-home message for practicing clinicians? First, psychosocial treatments of depression and anxiety in older adults work. They should be implemented. Second, depression and anxiety in older adults do not remit over time. Overall, studies showed no change in waitlist or no-contact control groups. If older adults with depression or anxiety are not treated, they are unlikely to get better. Third, treatments should focus on helping older adults and older adult caregivers to understand and deal with depression and anxiety in a skill-oriented manner. Treatment providers should be flexible in their approach to addressing the dynamic nature of health and function and multifaceted in providing help with the diversity of problems besetting older adults and their caregivers.

Key Points

- Psychosocial treatments are effective in decreasing depression and anxiety in cognitively intact older adults and (in a limited number of studies) have been found equal or superior to pharmacotherapeutic intervention.
- Empirical evidence supports the efficacy of BT and cognitive-behavioral-based therapies in decreasing depression and anxiety in individuals with dementia, as well as in older adults who are caregivers for individuals with cognitive impairment.
- Current studies support the utility of training caregivers—whether family or staff—in CBT skills to successfully reduce depression and anxiety in persons with dementia.

Recommended Readings and Web Sites

Gallagher-Thompson D, Steffen AM, Thompson LW (eds): Handbook of Behavioral and Cognitive Therapies With Older Adults. New York, Springer, 2008

Knight BG: Psychotherapy With Older Adults, 3rd Edition. Thousand Oaks, CA, Sage, 2004

Alzheimer's Association: www.alz.org/index.asp. Web site provides information on the latest Alzheimer care strategies, research findings, and advocacy initiatives.

Family Caregiver Alliance: www.caregiver.org/caregiver/jsp/home.jsp. Community-based nonprofit organization addressing the needs of families and friends providing long-term care at home.

References

Administration on Aging: Older Adults and Mental Health: Issues and Opportunities. Rockville, MD, Department of Health and Human Services, 2001. Available at: http://www.globalaging.org/health/us/mental.pdf. Accessed September 2, 2010.

Akkerman RL, Ostwald SK: Reducing anxiety in Alzheimer's disease family caregivers: the effectiveness of a nine-week cognitive-behavioral intervention. Am J Alzheimers Dis Other Demen 19:117–123, 2004

Alexopoulos GS, Raue P, Areán P: Problem-solving therapy versus supportive therapy in geriatric major depression with executive dysfunction. Am J Geriatr Psychiatry 11:46–52, 2003

Alzheimer's Association and National Alliance for Caregiving: Families Care: Alzheimer's Caregiving in the United States 2004. Available at: http://www.alz.org/national/documents/report_familiescare.pdf. Accessed May 10, 2010.

Arean PA, Gum A, McCulloch CE, et al: Treatment of depression in low-income older adults. Psychol Aging 20:601–609, 2005

Ayers CR, Sorrell JT, Thorp SR, et al: Evidence-based psychological treatments for late-life anxiety. Psychol Aging 22:8–17, 2007

Barrowclough C, King P, Colville J, et al: A randomized trial of the effectiveness of cognitive-behavioral therapy and supportive counseling for anxiety symptoms in older adults. J Consult Clin Psychol 69:756–762, 2001

Beck AT, Rush AJ, Shaw BF, et al: Cognitive Therapy for Depression. New York, Guilford, 1979

Beck CK, Vogelpohl TS, Rasin JH, et al: Effects of behavioral interventions on disruptive behavior and affect in demented nursing home residents. Nurs Res 51:219–228, 2002

Belle SH, Czaja SJ, Schulz R, et al: Using a new taxonomy to combine the uncombinable: integrating results across diverse interventions. Psychol Aging 18:396–405, 2003

Belle SH, Burgio L, Burns R, et al: Enhancing the quality of life of dementia caregivers from different ethnic or racial groups: a randomized, controlled trial. Ann Intern Med 145:727–738, 2006

Bohlmeijer E, Roemer M, Cuijpers P, et al: The effects of reminiscence on psychological well-being in older adults: a meta-analysis. Aging Ment Health 11:291–300, 2007

Bourgeois MS, Schultz R, Burgio L, et al: Skills training for spouses of patients with Alzheimer's disease: outcomes of an intervention study. Journal of Clinical Geropsychology 8:53–73, 2002

Brodaty H, Green A, Koschera A: Meta-analysis of psychosocial interventions for caregivers of people with dementia. J Am Geriatr Soc 51:657–664, 2003

Buckwalter KC, Gerdner L, Kohout F, et al: A nursing intervention to decrease depression in family caregivers of persons with dementia. Arch Psychiatr Nurs 13:80–88, 1999

Burgio L, Stevens A, Guy D, et al: Impact of two psychosocial interventions on white and African American family caregivers of individuals with dementia. Gerontologist 43:568–579, 2003

Burns R, Nichols LO, Martindale-Adams J, et al: Primary care interventions for dementia caregivers: 2-year outcomes from the REACH study. Gerontologist 43:547–555, 2003

Butler RN: The life review: an interpretation of reminiscence in the aged. Psychiatry 26:65–76, 1963

Chao SY, Liu HY, Wu CY, et al: The effects of group reminiscence therapy on depression, self esteem, and life satisfaction of elderly nursing home residents. J Nurs Res 14:36–45, 2006

Coon DW, Thompson LW, Steffen A, et al: Anger and depression management: psychoeducational skill training intervention for women caregivers of a relative with dementia. Gerontologist 43:678–689, 2003

Covinsky KE, Newcomer R, Fox P, et al: Patient and caregiver characteristics associated with depression in caregivers of patients with dementia. J Gen Intern Med 18:1058–1059, 2003

Davis L, Burgio L, Buckwalter K, et al: A comparison of in-home and telephone-based skill training interventions with caregivers of persons with dementia. Journal of Mental Health and Aging 10:31–44, 2004

DeCoster VA: Diabetes treatments. J Gerontol Soc Work 50:105–129, 2008

Eisdorfer C, Czaja SJ, Loewenstein DA, et al: The effect of a family therapy and technology-based intervention on caregiver depression. Gerontologist 43:521–531, 2003

Floyd M, Scogin F, McKendree-Smith NL, et al: Cognitive therapy for depression: a comparison of individual psychotherapy and bibliotherapy for depressed older adults. Behav Modif 28:297–318, 2004

Floyd M, Rohen N, Shackelford JAM, et al: Two-year follow-up of bibliotherapy and individual cognitive therapy for depressed older adults. Behav Modif 30:281–294, 2006

Freud S: On Psychotherapy: Collected Papers, Vol 1. London, Hogarth Press, 1924

Gallagher-Thompson D, Coon DW: Evidence-based psychological treatments for distress in family caregivers of older adults. Psychol Aging 22:37–51, 2007

Gallagher-Thompson D, Lovett S, Rose J, et al: Impact of psychoeducational interventions on distressed family caregivers. Journal of Clinical Geropsychology 6:91–110, 2000

Gallagher-Thompson D, Coon DW, Solano N, et al: Change in indices of distress among Latino and Anglo female caregivers of elderly relatives with dementia: site-specific results from the REACH National Collaborative Study. Gerontologist 43:580–591, 2003

Gallagher-Thompson D, Gray HL, Tang PC, et al: Impact of in-home behavioral management versus telephone support to reduce depressive symptoms and perceived stress in Chinese caregivers: results of a pilot study. Am J Geriatr Psychiatry 15:425–434, 2007

Gellis ZD, McGinty J, Horowitz A, et al: Problem-solving therapy for late-life depression in home care: a randomized field trial. Am J Geriatr Psychiatry 15:968–979, 2007

Gerdner LA, Buckwalter KC, Reed D: Impact of a psychoeducational intervention on caregiver response to behavioral problems. Nurs Res 51:363–374, 2002

Gitlin LN, Belle SH, Burgio L, et al: Effect of multicomponent interventions on caregiver burden and depression: the REACH multisite initiative at 6-month follow-up. Psychol Aging 18:361–374, 2003a

Gitlin LN, Winter L, Corcoran M, et al: Effects of the home environmental skill-building program on the caregiver–care recipient dyad: 6-month outcomes from the Philadelphia REACH Initiative. Gerontologist 43:532–546, 2003b

Gitlin LN, Hauck WW, Dennis MP, et al: Maintenance of effects of the home environmental skill-building program for family caregivers and individuals with Alzheimer's disease and related disorders. J Gerontol A Biol Sci Med Sci. 60:368–374, 2005

Gorenstein EE, Kleber MS, Mohlman J, et al: Cognitive-behavioral therapy for management of anxiety and medication taper in older adults. Am J Geriatr Psychiatry 13:901–909, 2005

Hanaoka H, Okamura H: Study of effects of life review activities on the quality of life of the elderly: a randomized controlled trial. Psychother Psychosom 73:302–311, 2004

Haringsma R, Engels GI, Cuijpers P, et al: Effectiveness of the Coping With Depression (CWD) course for older adults provided by the community-based mental health care system in the Netherlands: a randomized controlled field trial. Int Psychogeriatr 18:307–325, 2006

Health and Human Services Assistant Secretary for Planning and Evaluation: The Future Supply of Long-Term Care Workers in Relation to the Aging Baby Boom Generation. Washington, DC, Department of Health and Human Services, 2003

Hepburn KW, Tornatore J, Center B, et al: Dementia family caregiver training: affecting beliefs about caregiving and caregiver outcomes. J Am Geriatr Soc 49:450–457, 2001

Hyer L, Yeager CA, Hilton N, et al: Group, individual and staff therapy: an efficient and effective cognitive behavioral therapy in long-term care. Am J Alzheimers Dis Other Dement 23:528–539, 2008–2009

Lai CK, Kayser-Jones J: A randomized controlled trial of a specific reminiscence approach to promote the well-being of nursing home residents with dementia. Int Psychogeriatr 15:33–49, 2004

Lee S, Colditz GA, Berkman L, et al: Caregiving and risks of coronary heart disease in U.S. women: a prospective study. Am J Prev Med 24:113–119, 2003

Lenze EJ, Rogers JC, Martire LM, et al: The association of late-life depression and anxiety with physical disability. Am J Geriatr Psychiatry 9:113–135, 2001

Lewinsohn PM, Antonuccio DO, Steinmetz J, et al: The Coping With Depression Course. Eugene, OR, Castalia, 1984

Lichtenberg PA, Kemp-Havican J, MacNeill SE, et al: Pilot study of behavioral treatment in dementia care units. Gerontologist 45: 406–410, 2005

Livingston G, Johnston K, Katona C, et al: Systematic review of psychological approaches to the management of neuropsychiatric symptoms of dementia. Am J Psychiatry 162:1996–2021, 2005

Llewellyn-Jones RH, Baikie KA, Smithers H, et al: Multifaceted shared care intervention for late life depression in residential care: randomised controlled trial. BMJ 319:676–682, 1999

Lynch TR, Morse JQ, Maendelson T, et al: Dialectical behavior therapy for depressed older adults: a randomized pilot study. Am J Geriatr Psychiatry 11:33–45, 2003

Mahoney DF, Tarlow BJ, Jones RN: Effects of an automated telephone support system on caregiver burden and anxiety: findings from the REACH for TLC intervention study. Gerontologist 43:556–567, 2003

Maramaldi P, Dungan S, Poorvu NL: Cancer treatments. J Gerontol Soc Work 50:45–77, 2008

Marriott A, Donaldson C, Tarrier N, et al: Effectiveness of cognitive-behavioural family intervention in reducing the burden of care in carers of patients with Alzheimer's disease. Br J Psychiatry 176:557–562, 2000

McCallion P, Toseland RW, Lacey D, et al: Educating nursing assistants to communicate more effectively with nursing home residents with dementia. Gerontologist 39:546–558, 1999

McCurry SM, Logsdon RG, Teri L, et al: Evidence-based psychological treatments for insomnia in older adults. Psychol Aging 22:18–27, 2007

Mittelman MS, Roth DL, Coon DW, et al: Sustained benefit of supportive intervention for depressive symptoms in caregivers of patients with Alzheimer's disease. Am J Psychiatry 161:850–856, 2004

Mittelman MS, Brodaty H, Wallen AS, et al: A three-country randomized controlled trial of a psychosocial intervention for caregivers combined with pharmacological treatment for patients with Alzheimer disease: effects on caregiver depression. Am J Geriatr Psychiatry 16:893–904, 2008

Mohlman J, Gorenstein EE, Kleber M, et al: Standard and enhanced cognitive-behavior therapy for late-life generalized anxiety disorder: two pilot investigations. Am J Geriatr Psychiatry 11:24–32, 2003

Olin JT, Katz IR, Meyers BS, et al: Provisional diagnostic criteria for depression of Alzheimer disease: rationale and background. Am J Geriatr Psychiatry 10:129–141, 2002

Ostwald SK, Hepburn KW, Caron W, et al: Reducing caregiver burden: a randomized psychoeducational intervention for caregivers of persons with dementia. Gerontologist 39:299-309, 1999

Payne KT, Marcus DK: The efficacy of group psychotherapy for older adult clients: a meta-analysis. Group Dyn 12:268–278, 2008

Peck MD, Ai AL: Cardiac conditions. J Gerontol Soc Work 50:13–44, 2008

Pinquart M, Sorensen S: Helping caregivers of persons with dementia: which interventions work and how large are their effects? Int Psychogeriatr 18:577–595, 2006

Pinquart M, Duberstein P, Lyness J: Treatments for later-life depressive conditions: a meta-analytic comparison of pharmacotherapy and psychotherapy. Am J Psychiatry 163:1493–1501, 2006

Pinquart M, Duberstein PR, Lyness JM: Effects of psychotherapy and other behavioral interventions on clinically depressed older adults: a meta-analysis. Aging Ment Health 11:645–657, 2007

Proctor R, Burns A, Stratton Powel H, et al: Behavioural management in nursing and residential homes: a randomised controlled trial. Lancet 35:26–29, 1999

Reynolds CF III: Treatment of major depression in later life: a life cycle perspective. Psychiatr Q 68:221–246, 1997

Reynolds CF III, Frank E, Perel JM, et al: Nortriptyline and interpersonal psychotherapy as maintenance therapies for recurrent major depression: a randomized controlled trial in patients older than 59 years. JAMA 281:39–45, 1999

Rokke PD, Tomhave JA, Jocic Z: The role of client choice and target selection in self-management therapy for depression in older adults. Psychol Aging 14:155–169, 1999

Satre DD, Knight BG, David S: Cognitive-behavioral interventions with older adults: integrating clinical and gerontological research. Prof Psychiatry Res Pr 37:489–498, 2006

Schulz R, Beach SR: Caregiving as a risk factor for mortality: the Caregiver Health Effects Study. JAMA 282:2215–2219, 1999

Schulz R, Burgio L, Burns R, et al: Resources for Enhancing Alzheimer's Caregiver Health (REACH): overview, site-specific outcomes, and future directions. Gerontologist 43:514–520, 2003

Schuurmans J, Comijs H, Emmelkamp PM, et al: A randomized, controlled trial of the effectiveness of cognitive-behavioral therapy and sertraline versus a waitlist control group for anxiety disorders in older adults. Am J Geriatr Psychiatry 14:255–263, 2006

Scogin F, Morthland M, Kaufman A, et al: Improving quality of life in diverse rural older adults: a randomized trial of a psychological treatment. Psychol Aging 22:657–665, 2007

Serrano JP, Latorre JM, Gatz M: Life review therapy using autobiographical retrieval practice for older adults with depressive symptomatology. Psychol Aging 19:272–277, 2004

Sorensen S, Pinquart M, Duberstein P: How effective are interventions with caregivers? An updated meta-analysis. Gerontologist 42:356–372, 2002

Sorensen S, Duberstein P, Gill D, et al: Dementia care: mental health effects, intervention strategies, and clinical implications. Lancet 5:961–973, 2006

Stanley MA, Beck JG, Novy DM, et al: Cognitive-behavioral treatment of late-life generalized anxiety disorder. J Consult Clin Psychol 71:309–319, 2003a

Stanley MA, Hopko DR, Diefenbach GJ, et al: Cognitive-behavior therapy for late life generalized anxiety disorder in primary care. Am J Geriatr Psychiatry 11:92–96, 2003b

Steffen A: Anger management for dementia caregivers: a preliminary study using video and telephone interventions. Behav Ther 31:281–299, 2000

Teri L: The relation between research on depression and a treatment program: one model, in Depression in Long Term and Residential Care: Advances in Research and Treatment. Edited by Rubinstein RL, Lawton MP. New York, Springer, 1997, pp 129–153

Teri L, Logsdon R: Assessment and management of behavioral disturbances in Alzheimer's disease. Compr Ther 16:36–42, 1990

Teri L, McCurry S: Psychosocial therapies, in The American Psychiatric Press Textbook of Geriatric Neuropsychiatry. Edited by Coffey C, Cummings J. Washington, DC, American Psychiatric Press, 1994, pp 662–682

Teri L, McCurry SM: Psychosocial therapies with older adults, in The American Psychiatric Press Textbook of Geriatric Neuropsychiatry, 2nd Edition. Edited by Coffey CE, Cummings J. Washington, DC, American Psychiatric Press, 2000, pp 861–890

Teri L, Wagner A: Alzheimer's disease and depression. J Consult Clin Psychol 3:379–391, 1992

Teri L, Logsdon RG, Uomoto J, et al: Behavioral treatment of depression in dementia patients: a controlled clinical trial. J Gerontol B Psychol Sci Soc Sci 52:159–166, 1997

Teri L, Gibbons LE, McCurry SM, et al: Exercise plus behavioral management in patients with Alzheimer disease: a randomized controlled trial. JAMA 290:2015–2022, 2003

Teri L, Huda P, Gibbons L, et al: STAR: a dementia-specific training program for staff in assisted living residences. Gerontologist 45:686–693, 2005a

Teri L, Logsdon RG, McCurry SM: The Seattle Protocols: advances in behavioral treatment of Alzheimer's disease, in Research and Practice in Alzheimer's Disease and Cognitive Decline. Edited by Vellas B, Grundman M, Feldman H, et al. New York, Springer, 2005b

Teri L, McCurry SM, Logsdon R, et al: Training community consultants to help family members improve dementia care: a randomized controlled trial. Gerontologist 45:802–811, 2005c

Teri L, McKenzie G, LaFazia D: Psychosocial treatment of depression in older adults with dementia. Clin Psychol 12:303–316, 2005d

Thompson LW, Coon DW, Gallagher-Thompson D, et al: Comparison of desipramine and cognitive behavioral therapy in the treatment of elderly outpatients with mild-to-moderate depression. Am J Geriatr Psychiatry 9:225–240, 2001

Thorp SR, Ayers CR, Nuevo R, et al: Meta-analysis comparing different behavioral treatments for late-life anxiety. Am J Geriatr Psychiatry 17:105–115, 2009

Unutzer J, Katon W, Callahan CM, et al: Depression treatment in a sample of 1,801 depressed older adults in primary care. J Am Geriatr Soc 51:505–514, 2003

van Schaik A, van Marwijk H, Ader H, et al: Interpersonal psychotherapy for elderly patients in primary care. Am J Geriatr Psychiatry 14:777–786, 2006

Wang JJ: Group reminiscence therapy for cognitive and affective function of demented elderly in Taiwan. Int J Geriatr Psychiatry 22:1235–1240, 2007

Watt LM, Cappeliez P: Integrative and instrumental reminiscence therapies for depression in older adults: intervention strategies and treatment effectiveness. Aging Ment Health 4:166–177, 2000

Watt LM, Wong PT: A taxonomy of reminiscence and therapeutic implications. J Gerontol Soc Work 16:37–57, 1991

Wetherell JL, Gatz M, Craske MG: Treatment of generalized anxiety disorder in older adults. J Consult Clin Psychol 71:31–40, 2003

Wilkinson P, Alder N, Juszczak E, et al: A pilot randomised controlled trial of a brief cognitive behavioural group intervention to reduce recurrence rates in late life depression. Int J Geriatr Psychiatry 24:68–75, 2009

Williams JW, Barrett J, Oxman T, et al: Treatment of dysthymia and minor depression in primary care: a randomized controlled trial in older adults. JAMA 284:1519–1526, 2000

Wilson KC, Mottram PG, Vassilas CA: Psychotherapeutic treatments for older depressed people. Cochrane Database of Systematic Reviews 2008, Issue 1. Art. No.: CD004853. DOI: 10.1002/14651858.CD004853.pub2

Yoon E, Doherty JB: Arthritis pain. J Gerontol Soc Work 50:79–103, 2008

to support the use of topiramate in any phase of bipolar disorder (Vasudev et al. 2006). The risk of cognitive impairment and mood destabilization with long-term treatment raises concerns about the use of topiramate to promote weight loss in patients taking mood stabilizers. Topiramate was effective for reexperiencing but not total symptom scores in PTSD in one study (Tucker et al. 2007), but in another study dropout rates due to adverse effects were so high that benefit as an adjunct for PTSD could not be demonstrated (Lindley et al. 2007).

Levetiracetam reduced mania scores in a 5-week open-label trial, although it did not produce additional benefit when combined with valproate (Kruger et al. 2008). Other open-label experience suggests that levetiracetam may not have any mood-stabilizing properties (Post et al. 2005). In a 6-month open-label study of zonisamide, obese remitted bipolar patients experienced significant weight loss, but almost three-fourths of the patients dropped out due to adverse effects on mood (Wang et al. 2008). The risk-benefit ratio for zonisamide to promote weight loss in patients with bipolar disorder therefore seems unacceptably high.

All antipsychotic drugs (see "Antipsychotic Drugs" later in this chapter) are effective for acute mania. As maintenance treatment, olanzapine appeared to reduce relapse over 18 months in patients with bipolar disorder (Tohen et al. 2006), although interpretation of this finding is limited by the use of sample enrichment and a single-symptom rating scale as the primary outcome measure. Quetiapine is approved as a treatment for bipolar depression based on two 8-week placebo-controlled trials; however, differences between placebo and quetiapine groups in these studies were not impressive, and there was no control for the effect of sedation and improved sleep (Thase et al. 2006). All studies of new anticonvulsants and atypical antipsychotic drugs in bipolar disorder have excluded patients with medical or neurological comorbidity as well as geriatric patients, making it impossible to extrapolate to these populations.

Verapamil has been found to have antimanic properties in most, but not all, controlled studies; negative studies have used lower dosages and shorter durations of treatment (Dubovsky 1995). Because it does not cause sedation or psychomotor impairment, verapamil is well tolerated by patients with dementia, although more frequent dosing may be difficult for these patients to remember. Nimodipine has been useful in a few studies of complex bipolar mood disorders (Post et al. 2000).

Uses in Neurological Disease

Lithium has been used to treat a number of recurrent disorders, including cluster headache and cyclical neutropenia. Induction of leukocytosis by lithium is used to treat leukopenia caused by chemotherapy for cancer and autoimmune disease. Lithium interferes with antidiuretic hormone (ADH; also known as vasopressin) signaling in the renal tubule, making it effective for counteracting the syndrome of inappropriate ADH secretion (SIADH). Lithium has occasionally been used to treat spasmodic torticollis and Huntington's disease.

Lithium has multiple neuroprotective effects that may provide mechanisms for amelioration of dementing disorders such as Alzheimer's disease (Yeh and Tsai 2008). A Danish database comparison of 16,238 people who purchased lithium and almost 1.5 million people who did not found that patients who continued to fill prescriptions for lithium had a decreased risk of all forms of dementia and for Alzheimer's disease in particular (Kessing et al. 2008). A magnetic resonance imaging study of 12 untreated bipolar patients, 17 lithium-treated bipolar patients, and 46 controls found that total gray matter volumes were significantly greater in lithium-treated patients than in the other groups (Sassi et al. 2002). The potential application of lithium as a neuroprotective agent is complicated by the frequent occurrence of cognitive impairment as an acute side effect of lithium.

Carbamazepine has been used to treat chronic pain. An antiexcitotoxic effect of lamotrigine could be helpful in degenerative disorders, although this has not been studied. Nimodipine is approved for the acute treatment of hemorrhagic stroke, although its effectiveness for this condition is not robust. Verapamil is a second-line treatment for migraine headache prophylaxis.

Dosing and Side Effects

A clear correlation between serum level and clinical response has been demonstrated for lithium in younger adults, with optimal levels said to be between 0.6 and 1.2 mM. No empirical support exists for the contention that lower dosages and lower serum levels are effective in elderly patients. Dosage increases should occur no more frequently than once a week because 90% of a steady state is reached in four half-lives. A single bedtime dose of lithium enhances adherence, decreases adverse effects, and has been found to be safe in elderly patients (Dubovsky 2005). If lower dosages are not effective and the patient is tolerating the medication, higher dosages are appropriate.

At least in the treatment of mania in younger neurologically healthy adults, a linear correlation appears to exist between serum level of divalproex and clinical response, with the optimal level being around 100 mg/dL (Allen et al. 2006). Therapeutic levels in older and neurologically ill patients and in maintenance therapy have not been studied. A correlation between serum level and clinical response has not been demonstrated for any of the other anticonvulsants used as alternatives to lithium. Typical dosages and levels of mood-stabilizing medications in geriatric neuropsychiatry are summarized in Table 9–16.

Lithium and anticonvulsants have neurological side effects (Table 9–17) and can aggravate cognitive impairment in

TABLE 9–16. Mood-stabilizing medications

Medication	Usual geriatric daily dosage, mg	Comments
Lithium	300–900	Therapeutic level usually 0.6–1.2 mM; some geriatric patients may respond to lower levels
Carbamazepine	300–1,200	Dosing thrice daily in younger adults, twice daily in older patients; no therapeutic level demonstrated
Valproate	125–1,000	Optimal level in mania ~100 mg/dL in younger patients; no therapeutic level demonstrated in older patients
Lamotrigine	25–100	Risk of severe rash with rapid dosage escalation
Verapamil	120–240	Usually given thrice daily to older patients.
Nimodipine	90–180	Requires frequent dosing; well tolerated by neurologically ill patients
Oxcarbazepine	600–1,500	Limited research in bipolar disorder; no research in bipolar disorder in elderly

dementia (Dubovsky 2005). Verapamil and nimodipine are better tolerated by patients with neurological illness, but fewer studies have been done of this class of medications in treating bipolar disorder. Interactions with neurological drugs are summarized in Table 9–18.

Antipsychotic Drugs

Antipsychotic drugs treat psychosis, regardless of its cause (see Chapter 21, "Psychosis"). These medications are not specific for any particular disorder, although they have been studied most extensively in schizophrenia, schizoaffective disorder, bipolar disorder, delusional disorder, psychotic depression, and Tourette's disorder, and to some extent in autism. First-generation antipsychotic drugs are called neuroleptics (from the Greek for "to clasp the neuron") because they treat psychosis and cause neurological side effects. The newer atypical antipsychotic drugs differ from the neuroleptics in that they produce less blockade of postsynaptic dopamine D_2 receptors and relatively more blockade of serotonin 5-HT_2 receptors. The combination of these effects, along with faster dissociation from D_2 receptors, reduces overall D_2 blockade, decreasing extrapyramidal and related side effects and presumably reducing the risk of tardive dyskinesia. However, experience with atypical antipsychotics has not been extensive enough to be certain that this is the case.

Major Classes

Several classes of neuroleptics (Table 9–19) are available and include the phenothiazines chlorpromazine, thioridazine, fluphenazine, perphenazine, and trifluoperazine; the butyrophenone haloperidol; the thioxanthene thiothixene; the diphenylbutylpiperidine pimozide; the dibenzazepine loxapine; and the dihydroindolone molindone. All classes of neuroleptics are broadly classified as high potency (i.e., smaller milligram doses are necessary to produce a given effect) or low potency. Low-potency neuroleptics such as chlorpromazine generally have longer elimination half-lives and active metabolites. Droperidol is a butyrophenone used as an anesthesia that can reduce agitation but does not treat psychosis. Atypical antipsychotic drugs (Table 9–20) include the dibenzodiazepine clozapine, the thiobenzodiazepine olanzapine, the dibenzothiazepines quetiapine and ziprasidone, the benzisoxazoles risperidone and paliperidone, and the quinolone aripiprazole.

Mechanisms of Action

Most drugs that have antipsychotic properties block postsynaptic dopamine D_2 receptors. D_2 occupancy of ~60% appears to be necessary for an antipsychotic effect, with greatest subjective well-being at this level of occupancy (de Haan et al. 2003). D_2 occupancy of 70% is associated with dysphoria and noncompliance; as D_2 occupancy approaches 78%, EPS are more prominent, usually without a greater antipsychotic effect. Clozapine and probably other atypical antipsychotics also antagonize dopamine D_1 and D_4 receptors.

Atypical antipsychotics have reduced D_2 occupancy and faster dissociation from the D_2 receptor, which permits less distortion of phasic dopamine signaling and less tolerance and upregulation of receptors. In addition, relatively greater blockade of serotonin 5-HT_2 receptors with atypical antipsychotic drugs reduces adverse effects of D_2 blockade and could confer additional antipsychotic and antidepressant effects. Aripiprazole differs from the other antipsychotic drugs in that it is a D_2 partial agonist. If synaptic dopamine availability is low, the partial agonist binds to the receptor and acts like dopamine, although not quite at potently as the actual neurotransmitter, and net

TABLE 9–17. Some neuropsychiatric side effects of mood stabilizers

Medication	System/Findings	Manifestations and comments
Lithium	Affective	Affective blunting
	Cognitive	Memory impairment, cognitive dulling, difficulty with word finding, confusion, dazed feeling; rule out hypothyroidism and hypercalcemia
	Extrapyramidal	Parkinsonism; antiparkinsonian drugs poorly tolerated
	Neuromuscular	Tremor, ataxia, dysarthria, incoordination, myoclonus; falls may result from ataxia, incoordination; tremor may improve with beta-blocker or single bedtime dose
	Intracranial	Pseudotumor cerebri; headache not always present; elevated CSF pressure may not remit after lithium discontinuation
	EEG	Generalized slowing, disorganization of background rhythm, REM sleep suppression, seizures
	Endocrine	Hyperparathyroidism common; hypercalcemia can cause confusion, depression, mania, weakness; hypothyroidism in 20% of adults; interference with insulin signaling may impair diabetes control
	Renal	Polyuria and polydipsia not more common in elderly patients; lithium does not cause or accelerate renal failure in elderly patients; nephrogenic diabetes insipidus may be reduced by amiloride, which reduces lithium transport into collecting duct; interstitial nephrosis and tubular and glomerular atrophy have been reported
Carbamazepine, oxcarbazepine	CNS	Ataxia, tremor, sedation, lethargy, diplopia, cognitive impairment, irritability, confusion, restlessness, seizures
	Neuroendocrine	SIADH; hyponatremia may cause confusion, delirium, myoclonus, or seizures
	Hypersensitivity	Rash in 10% that remits half the time; agranulocytosis risk is 2/525,000; routine CBCs do not predict bone marrow suppression; no bone marrow suppression with oxcarbazepine
Valproate	CNS	Sedation, ataxia, tremor, impaired memory
	Neuroendocrine	Weight gain, polycystic ovaries; polycystic ovarian syndrome in a minority with polycystic ovaries
	Hypersensitivity	Rash, hair loss; hepatotoxicity in 1/50,000 adults
Lamotrigine	CNS	Sedation, ataxia, memory impairment
	Hypersensitivity	Rash; severe rash in 1/5,000
Verapamil	CNS	Dizziness, headache, occasional extrapyramidal symptoms
Nimodipine	CNS	Dizziness, headache, nausea, flushed skin, nightmares

Note. CBC=complete blood count; CNS=central nervous system; CSF=cerebrospinal fluid; EEG=electroencephalogram; REM= rapid eye movement; SIADH=syndrome of inappropriate antidiuretic hormone secretion.

dopaminergic transmission increases. If synaptic dopamine concentrations are excessive, the partial agonist competes with dopamine for its receptor but has less of an effect on it, resulting in a net reduction of dopamine signaling. This dual action has been proposed to be useful for psychosis, which is thought to be related to increased dopamine signaling, and also for lack of motivation and withdrawal, which are thought to be related to reduced dopamine signaling in other regions. However, no actual evidence indicates that this hypothesis is correct, and aripiprazole has not been shown to be better for negative symptoms than any other antipsychotic drug.

Receptor effects probably explain only a portion of the action of antipsychotics. For example, clozapine and haloperidol modulate the expression of multiple genes involved in synaptic function and the regulation of intracellular calcium signaling (Kontkanen et al. 2002). Clozapine is also the only

TABLE 9–18. Some mood stabilizer interactions with neurological drugs

Medication	Interacts with	Result
Lithium	Antipsychotic drugs	Neurotoxicity; increased extrapyramidal side effects
	Clonazepam	Occasional neurotoxicity
	Tetracycline	Increased lithium toxicity
	ACE inhibitors	Increased lithium levels
	Calcium channel blockers	Additive cardiac slowing, neurotoxicity
	Carbamazepine	Neurotoxicity
	Ketamine	Lithium toxicity
	NSAIDs	Increased lithium level
	Valproate	Neurotoxicity
Carbamazepine	Valproate	Increased carbamazepine level; decreased valproate level
	Phenytoin, phenobarbital	Decreased levels of all medications
	Benzodiazepines	Decreased levels of alprazolam and clonazepam
	Corticosteroids	Decreased corticosteroid levels; false-positive dexamethasone suppression test
	Oral contraceptives	Decreased contraceptive efficacy
	Verapamil	Increased carbamazepine levels; neurotoxicity
Valproate	Benzodiazepines	Increased diazepam levels; absence seizures with clonazepam
	Ethosuximide, felbamate, phenobarbital, primidone, phenytoin	Increased anticonvulsant levels
	Salicylates	Increased unbound valproate; prolonged bleeding time, bruising
	Warfarin	Increased unbound warfarin
Lamotrigine	Carbamazepine, phenytoin, topiramate, phenobarbital, estrogen, lithium, fluoxetine	Decreased lamotrigine levels
	Valproate	Increased lamotrigine levels

Note. ACE=angiotensin-converting enzyme; NSAID=nonsteroidal anti-inflammatory drugs.

antipsychotic drug that has been shown to correct sensory gating abnormalities in schizophrenia, possibly through an action on an α-7 nicotinic receptor.

Indications

The best established use of antipsychotic drugs is in schizophrenia. Initial industry-supported research suggested that atypical antipsychotics were as effective as neuroleptics for positive symptoms (e.g., hallucinations, delusions, disorganization) and more effective for negative symptoms (e.g., social withdrawal, avolitional states). However, independently funded studies, such as the Clinical Antipsychotic Trial of Intervention Effectiveness (CATIE), found that the atypical antipsychotics are not substantially superior to neuroleptics for negative or positive symptoms and that the majority of patients treated in real-life settings discontinue medications of both classes at about the same rate (Lieberman et al. 2005). EPS in this study were no more likely with the neuroleptic perphenazine than with the atypical antipsychotics. Similarly, a British random-assignment study found no difference over 1 year in symptoms, quality of life, or functioning between atypical antipsychotics and neuroleptics (Jones et al. 2006).

TABLE 9–19. Neuroleptics

Medication	Usual geriatric daily dosage, mg	Comments
Phenothiazines		
Chlorpromazine	10–300	Low potency; long half-life and multiple active metabolites lead to accumulation in elderly; hypotensive and anticholinergic side effects are reasons to avoid parenteral use in elderly
Thioridazine	10–300	Low potency; dosages >800 mg in younger patients and possibly lower dosages in elderly cause pigmented retinopathy; significant QT prolongation associated with increased risk of sudden cardiac death; should usually be avoided in elderly
Fluphenazine	0.5–6 (oral) 0.07–3.5 (decanoate, enanthate depot/monthly)	High potency; fluphenazine decanoate used most frequently for nonadherence in schizophrenia
Perphenazine	2–20	Midpotency; most studied neuroleptic in psychotic depression
Trifluoperazine	10–75	Midpotency
Butyrophenone		
Haloperidol	0.25–8 (oral/iv) 5–250 (decanoate q 2–4 weeks)	High potency; therapeutic window in schizophrenia; intravenous haloperidol used for agitation in critical care unit, but torsades de pointes has been reported; decanoate used for nonadherence in schizophrenia; intramuscular formulations poorly tolerated by elderly
Thioxanthene		
Thiothixene	1–15	High potency; commonly studied in psychotic depression
Diphenylbutylpiperidine		
Pimozide	0.25–4	High potency; used for Tourette's disorder and monosymptomatic hypochondriasis; QT prolongation occurs but no reports of adverse cardiac events; should not be combined with other drugs with QT prolongation
Dibenzazepine		
Loxapine	10–100	Midpotency; metabolized to amoxapine, conferring antidepressant effects; effective as monotherapy for psychotic depression
Dihydroindolone		
Molindone	10–100	Midpotency; lowest risk of weight gain; recently withdrawn from market by manufacturer

Atypical antipsychotics were at one time thought to be particularly beneficial for improving cognition, but this effect seems to be related to reduced intrusive thinking and disorganization without as much interference with cognition by "cognitive parkinsonism" as occurs with the neuroleptics; no antipsychotic drug other than clozapine has been found to reduce the core cognitive dysfunction of schizophrenia, which involves deficient "gating" or filtering of irrelevant information. Clozapine is the only atypical antipsychotic that is clearly effective in refractory schizophrenia (as opposed to treatment failure caused only by being unable to tolerate antipsychotics). A meta-analysis of studies of atypical antipsychotics found that the effect size of clozapine compared with haloperidol (0.49) was almost as great as the effect size of haloperidol compared with placebo (0.60), whereas effect sizes compared with haloperidol of risperidone and olanzapine were 0.25 and 0.21, respectively. The other atypical antipsychotics were about as effective as haloperidol but with fewer adverse effects (Davis et al. 2003).

EPS are particularly problematic in the treatment of psychosis associated with Parkinson's disease. The initial ap-

TABLE 9–20. Atypical antipsychotic drugs

Medication	Usual geriatric daily dosage, mg	Comments
Dibenzodiazepine		
Clozapine	6.25–450[a]	Only atypical antipsychotic clearly effective in refractory schizophrenia; dose-dependent seizure risk; reversible agranulocytosis in 1%–2%; useful for psychosis in Parkinson's disease
Thiobenzodiazepine		
Olanzapine	2.5–15 po/1.25–10 im	Significant risk of weight gain and metabolic side effects
Dibenzothiazepines		
Quetiapine	25–200[a]	Sedation and short half-life useful as hypnotic in schizophrenia and bipolar disorder; some schizophrenia patients need higher-than-recommended dosages
Ziprasidone	5–80 po[a]/5–15 im	SSRI as well as atypical antipsychotic properties
Benzisoxazoles		
Risperidone	1–6 po/0.787–1.964 q 2–4 weeks depot	Greatest dopamine D_2 blockade of atypical antipsychotics
Paliperidone	1.5–6	Metabolite of risperidone in OROS sustained-release form; no clear advantage over risperidone
Quinolone		
Aripiprazole	2–15 po/2–6.25–15 im	Partial dopamine D_2 agonist; unpredictable extrapyramidal side effects

Note. SSRI = selective serotonin reuptake inhibitor.
[a]Given in two divided doses.

proach to this problem involves assessing whether anticholinergic delirium or excessive L-dopa administration is to blame, the latter being more likely if dyskinesias accompany psychosis. One way to diagnose this problem is to reduce the dosages of dopaminergic medications by 5%–10% at a time, being careful not to precipitate a bradykinetic crisis. Although low dosages of both quetiapine and olanzapine have been used successfully in patients with Parkinson's disease (Kurlan et al. 2007), exacerbation of the neurological disease is least likely with clozapine in a dosage of 6.25–25 mg/day, a dosage that can ameliorate psychosis in patients with Parkinson's disease.

All antipsychotic drugs are effective acutely for mania. Industry-sponsored studies have suggested that olanzapine (Tohen et al. 2006) and quetiapine (Vieta et al. 2008) may be useful adjuncts in the maintenance treatment of bipolar disorder. A couple of 8-week controlled trials sponsored by the manufacturer found reduction of depression rating scale scores in bipolar depression with quetiapine (Thase et al. 2006). However, because all industry-sponsored studies have used enriched samples and excluded patients with complex and comorbid conditions, the role of antipsychotic drugs in maintenance treatment, especially of nonpsychotic patients with bipolar disorder and any elderly and neurologically ill patients, remains to be demonstrated. Use of atypical antipsychotic drugs (e.g., quetiapine) to treat anxiety and insomnia requires a careful consideration of risks and benefits, especially in older patients.

Antipsychotic drugs are usually necessary adjuncts to antidepressants in the treatment of psychotic depression, which is not uncommon in older patients. Studies with neuroleptics suggested that high dosages of neuroleptics were needed for remission; it is not clear whether lower dosages of atypical antipsychotics are effective. Although no controlled studies have been reported to support this application, pimozide has been thought for many years to be particularly effective for monosymptomatic hypochondriasis, a form of late-onset delusional disorder possibly related to psychotic depression.

Dosing and Side Effects

Geriatric dosages of antipsychotic drugs are summarized in Tables 9–19 and 9–20. Most of these medications are administered once daily. However, twice-daily dosing is used for clozapine, quetiapine, and ziprasidone, with absorption of ziprasidone being increased by taking the medication with meals. In younger patients, peak concentrations usually occur within 2–4 hours (6–8 hours for pimozide) after oral dosing, 15–30 minutes after intramuscular administration, and immediately with intravenous haloperidol.

In the treatment of schizophrenia, serum levels of haloperidol exhibit a therapeutic window of ~5–15 ng/mL. Clozapine levels >400 ng/mL are more effective than lower levels. Correlations between serum levels and therapeutic effect have not been demonstrated for other antipsychotic drugs.

High-potency neuroleptics (i.e., neuroleptics that are used in lower dosages, such as haloperidol or fluphenazine) tend to have more neurological side effects but fewer anticholinergic and antihistaminic side effects and fewer active metabolites. Low-potency preparations, such as chlorpromazine and thioridazine, have a lower incidence of acute neurological side effects but more anticholinergic and sedative side effects, more weight gain, more hypotension, and more complex metabolism with more active metabolites and therefore more accumulation in elderly patients. Mid-potency neuroleptics, such as molindone and perphenazine, have somewhat more acute EPS than the low-potency drugs but fewer metabolic and sedative side effects.

Common acute EPS of all antipsychotic drugs include parkinsonism, dystonia, akathisia, and bradykinesia, which are most common with high-potency neuroleptics but can occur with any antipsychotic drug. In the treatment of schizophrenia, akathisia can be confused with agitation, leading to inappropriate increases in dosage, and bradykinesia can be misdiagnosed as negative symptoms. EPS are more common in male patients with brain disease and are more likely with higher dosages. Unless there is a history of significant EPS with antipsychotic drugs, pretreatment with anticholinergic medications is not recommended. Anticholinergic antiparkinsonian medications such as benztropine and trihexyphenidyl are usually used to treat parkinsonism, and intramuscular diphenydramine is used for acute dystonia. Benzodiazepines are more effective than anticholinergic drugs for akathisia. As all of these drugs are often poorly tolerated by older patients, the lowest possible antipsychotic dosage is recommended to reduce the risk that they will be needed.

Thanks to increased caution with antipsychotic drugs, greater awareness of adverse effects, and widespread use of atypical antipsychotics, the incidence of neuroleptic malignant syndrome (NMS) appears to have decreased to ~0.01%–0.02%, although the mortality rate is still ~10% when it does develop (Strawn et al. 2007). Features and treatment of NMS are summarized in Table 9–21. In 80% of cases, mental status changes precede systemic signs of NMS (Strawn et al. 2007), in which case they may be confused with the underlying psychiatric illness, resulting in dangerous increases in antipsychotic dosages. Although NMS may begin soon after starting an antipsychotic drug, onset may be delayed up to 30 days after the medication is begun. Autonomic signs and fever may be less obvious in older patients, and fever may be mistakenly attributed to comorbid urinary tract infections. Disastrous outcomes have occurred when agitation caused by NMS is attributed to the underlying illness and when elevated muscle enzyme levels are thought to be the result of multiple injections, leading to escalating dosages of the very drug that is causing the problem in the first place.

TABLE 9–21. Neuroleptic malignant syndrome

Signs	Fever Muscle rigidity Tachycardia Tachypnea Altered mental status Rhabdomyolysis
Laboratory findings	Leukocytosis Increased serum CK, aldolase, transaminases, LDH Metabolic acidosis Hypoxia Decreased serum iron concentration Normal CSF except decreased HVA
EEG	Generalized slowing
Neuroimaging	Normal
Differential diagnosis	CNS infections Heatstroke Serotonin syndrome Malignant catatonia Toxic delirium Nonconvulsive status epilepticus Thyrotoxicosis Pheochromocytoma
Complications	Renal failure Parkinsonism Catatonia
Treatment	Discontinue antipsychotic drug Support circulation Treat fever Parenteral lorazepam 0.5–2 mg Amantadine 100–200 mg/day Bromocriptine 1.25–45 mg/day Intravenous dantrolene 0.5–1.25 mg/kg initially, then 1 mg/kg every 6 hours ECT

Note. CK=creatine kinase; CNS=central nervous system; CSF=cerebrospinal fluid; ECT=electroconvulsive therapy; EEG=electroencephalogram; HVA=homovanillic acid; LDH=lactate dehydrogenase.

All of the atypical antipsychotic drugs have been associated with NMS, although at a lower rate than the neuroleptics. Other dopamine antagonists, such as metoclopramide, amoxapine, and prochlorperazine, can cause NMS, as can abrupt withdrawal of dopaminergic medications such as amantadine and L-dopa. The risk of recurrence of NMS with reintroduction of an antipsychotic drug is 30%, so these medications should be restarted cautiously at low initial dosages of medications that are less potent at D_2 receptor blockade.

Like NMS, catatonia is a form of extreme extrapyramidal reaction associated with antipsychotic drugs, especially the neuroleptics. Older patients with neurological impairments are particularly prone to develop antipsychotic drug–induced catatonia, which may then be mistaken for agitation. If the antipsychotic drug is continued, symptoms worsen, sometimes with life-threatening complications in older patients. In unclear situations, it is safer to withdraw antipsychotic drugs when agitation or behavioral slowing is worsening.

Extrapyramidal syndromes that may appear after chronic use of any antipsychotic drug include tardive dyskinesia, tardive dystonia, and tardive akathisia. The risk of tardive dyskinesia is ~5%–10%/year with the neuroleptics and ~0.5%/year with the atypical antipsychotics. Tardive dyskinesia often does not progress, especially if it is mild, and it remits about half the time with medication discontinuation, although it may take 3 years to resolve completely. Medications that have been used to treat tardive dyskinesia with mixed results include vitamin E, acetazolamide (combined with thiamine to reduce the risk of kidney stones), cholinergic agonists, and verapamil. Clozapine may also ameliorate tardive dyskinesia, although in rare cases it has been thought to cause tardive dyskinesia. Tardive dystonia, which is more disabling, has been treated with anticholinergic medications, benzodiazepines, clozapine, tetrabenazine, and botulinum toxin. Tardive akathisia is treated in the same manner as acute akathisia.

Weight gain occurs most frequently with the low-potency neuroleptics and with clozapine, olanzapine, risperidone, and quetiapine. A meta-analysis of published antipsychotic studies found that after 10 weeks of treatment, clozapine, olanzapine, thioridazine, chlorpromazine, quetiapine, and risperidone were associated with weight gain of roughly 10, 9.8, 7, 6, 5, and 4.8 pounds, respectively, whereas placebo, molindone, aripiprazole, and ziprasidone were weight neutral (Allison et al. 1999). Type 2 diabetes and hyperlipidemia have been reported most frequently with clozapine, olanzapine, and low-potency neuroleptics, but not always in association with weight gain (Gianfranesco et al. 2002). A consensus conference (American Diabetes Association et al. 2004) recommended regular monitoring for patients taking antipsychotic drugs chronically (Table 9–22). The recommendation is that unless nothing else has been effective, the medication be changed if weight increases by 5% or more or if glucose or lipid levels increase significantly.

Similar to some nonsedating antihistamines, erythromycin, and a number of other drugs, some antipsychotic drugs inhibit potassium efflux channels and prolong cardiac depolarization, resulting in lengthening of the QT interval. This effect can predispose patients to reentry arrhythmias, the most dangerous of which is torsades de pointes. This effect is marked with thioridazine, which has been associated with sudden cardiac death (Reilly et al. 2002). Ziprasidone is also associated with QTc prolongation. There are a few case reports of torsades associated with quetiapine, risperidone, and ziprasidone (Ray et al. 2009). Droperidol, a butyrophenone that does not have antipsychotic properties but is useful in the treatment of acute agitation, has a black box warning for QT prolongation (as do thioridazine and pimozide). The clinical implications of these effects are suggested by a review of Medicaid records of 44,218 patients taking neuroleptics, 46,089 patients taking atypical antipsychotic drugs, and 186,600 matched controls, in which Ray et al. (2009) reported that compared with controls, the incidence rate of sudden cardiac death was increased about twofold with both classes of medication, corrected for behavioral and cardiac risk factors. The risk was evident in patients taking antipsychotic drugs for less than 1 year, indicating that it was not explained by chronic metabolic effects of the medication.

In 2002, a joint letter from Health Canada and the manufacturer of risperidone indicated that in controlled trials, the risk of stroke in geriatric patients was twice as high with risperidone (4%) as with placebo (2%) (Passmore et al. 2008). In 2005, a black box warning was added to atypical antipsychotic drugs concerning an increased risk of cerebrovascular events and death in older patients taking these drugs. The FDA warning was based on a meta-analysis of 17 randomized controlled trials of olanzapine, risperidone, aripiprazole, and quetiapine for agitation in elderly patients with dementia that found a hazard risk of 1.6–1.7 with these drugs for cerebrovascular events (Friedman 2006). The warning was extended to ziprasidone and clozapine based on a presumed class effect, although not enough data were available on those medications (Passmore et al. 2008). Cohort studies of the neuroleptics have led to extension of the warning to neuroleptics as well as atypical antipsychotics (Passmore et al. 2008). In a sample of 10,615 Veterans Affairs patients over age 65 with a diagnosis of dementia, there was a significant difference between the overall 1-year mortality rate (18%) and the rates for patients taking neuroleptics (25.2%), atypical antipsychotics (22.6%), or both classes (29.1%), whereas the risk of death with other psychotropic medications was the same as that with no psychiatric medications (Kales et al. 2007). The conclusion from these studies is that although they are not contraindicated, there is

TABLE 9–22. Monitoring for metabolic side effects with chronic antipsychotic drug therapy

Factor	Baseline	4 weeks	8 weeks	12 weeks	Quarterly	Annually	Every 5 years
Personal/family history	X					X	
Body mass index	X	X	X	X	X		
Waist circumference	X					X	
Blood pressure	X			X		X	
Fasting blood sugar	X			X		X	
Fasting lipids	X			X			X

Source. American Diabetes Association 2004.

more evidence of potential harm than lack of harm when using the atypical antipsychotics in patients who are elderly and neurologically impaired (Passmore et al. 2008).

Antipsychotic drugs have been reported to accelerate cognitive decline in patients with cognitive impairment, even when other factors that affect cognition are controlled (Brooks and Hoblyn 2007). Atypical antipsychotics, especially olanzapine and risperidone, can also increase confusion, agitation, and delirium in patients with dementia (Brooks and Hoblyn 2007; Passmore et al. 2008).

Clozapine exhibits a dosage-dependent lowering of the seizure threshold, with a 5% incidence of seizures at dosages above 600 mg/day. Low-potency neuroleptics such as chlorpromazine lower the seizure threshold more than high-potency neuroleptics, and among the atypical antipsychotics olanzapine is more epileptogenic than risperidone (Brodtkorb and Mula 2006).

Interactions

Antipsychotic drugs can interact with a number of neurological medications. Some common examples are summarized in Table 9–23.

TABLE 9–23. Some interactions of antipsychotic and neurological medications

Medication	Interaction with	Result
Antipsychotic drugs	Opiates	Additive sedation
	SSRIs	Increased EPS
	Phenytoin	Increased free phenytoin levels due to displacement from binding protein; decreased antipsychotic level
	Valproate	Increased free antipsychotic levels
	Barbiturates	Decreased antipsychotic effect; increased barbiturate levels; additive sedation
Aripiprazole	Carbamazepine	Decreased antipsychotic level
Clozapine	Carbamazepine	Increased risk of agranulocytosis; combination contraindicated
	Benzodiazepines	Additive sedation; risk of respiratory arrest
Neuroleptics	Lithium	Increased risk of EPS
Neuroleptics, quetiapine, olanzapine, clozapine	Anticholinergic drugs	Additive anticholinergic effect; anticholinergic drug may impair absorption of antipsychotic drug and may increase risk of TD

Note. EPS=extrapyramidal side effects; SSRI=selective serotonin reuptake inhibitor; TD=tardive dyskinesia.
Source. Dubovsky 2005.

Treatment of Chronic Agitation in Neurological Disease

Agitation and psychosis are common in patients with dementia or brain damage, and antipsychotic drugs are among the most common treatments for these problems. However, despite industry-sponsored studies demonstrating superiority of atypical antipsychotics to placebo in the treatment of nonpsychotic agitation in patients with dementia, more recent research calls these results into question. For example, a meta-analysis of 15 randomized controlled trials in 5,110 agitated elderly patients with dementia, all but one study of which were industry sponsored, found that aripiprazole and risperidone, but not olanzapine, were superior to placebo in reducing agitation; insufficient data were available on quetiapine to draw any conclusion (Schneider et al. 2006a). The effective drugs were associated with only a 10% reduction in behavior and psychosis rating scale scores, which was statistically significant because of the large number of patients enrolled but not clinically important. The odds ratios of cerebrovascular adverse events were 2.13 for the atypical antipsychotics as a group and 3.43 for risperidone. In addition, all the antipsychotic drugs impaired cognition to the same degree that cholinesterase inhibitors would be expected to improve cognition.

In the Clinical Antipsychotic Trials of Intervention Effectiveness in Alzheimer's disease (CATIE-AD) study of 421 patients with Alzheimer's disease and agitation and/or psychosis who were randomly assigned for 36 weeks to atypical antipsychotic drugs or placebo, outpatients with dementia demonstrated no significant difference in discontinuation for any reason (the primary end point) for risperidone, olanzapine, quetiapine, and placebo; any apparent benefit because of a slightly but statistically significantly longer time to discontinuation for olanzapine was outweighed by time to discontinuation for adverse effects, which favored placebo over olanzapine (Schneider et al. 2006b). Olanzapine and risperidone produced significantly greater reduction of Neuropsychiatric Inventory (NPI) scores than placebo, but the total difference between these drugs and placebo was 3.5–7.6 points out of an average initial score of 37, suggesting that the difference may have been clinically trivial (Sultzer et al. 2008). Risperidone produced greater improvement on the psychosis subscale of the Brief Psychiatric Rating Scale (BPRS), and olanzapine and risperidone produced greater improvement on the hostile suspiciousness factor; because these were only retrospective secondary analyses and overall BPRS scores were no different between any active drug and placebo, these changes cannot be considered important. Aside from worsening of functioning with olanzapine, there were no differences between treatments in cognition, quality of life, care needs, or functioning.

A 1-year study of 933 Norwegian nursing home residents found clinically significant agitation, psychosis, anxiety, and depression as measured by the NPI in 84% of patients, and 75% of all patients were already taking antipsychotic drugs (Selbaek et al. 2008). No difference was found between patients who did and did not take psychotropic drugs of any kind in the prevalence or duration of these symptoms. The mean NPI score was higher in patients who received antipsychotic drugs, possibly because these drugs were more likely to be prescribed to more agitated patients, but NPI scores did not decrease more in patients who did than in those who did not take antipsychotic drugs. The severity of dementia increased over the year of follow-up, but NPI symptoms improved whether or not patients took psychotropic medications.

Considering all of these results, it would appear that atypical antipsychotics may be useful for short-term control of acute agitation in patients with dementia, especially if it is caused by psychosis, but that these medications are generally not preferable for chronic treatment (Passmore et al. 2008). Because the risk of acute neurological side effects such as EPS and NMS is increased in patients with neurological impairment, the high-potency neuroleptics such as haloperidol are generally not appropriate for the treatment of chronic agitation in older patients with dementia. Cardiovascular risks and anticholinergic side effects would make the low-potency neuroleptics, and thioridazine in particular, very poor choices for this population. There are, however, a number of other medication classes with varying levels of empirical support for treatment of agitation in patients with neurological impairment.

Cholinesterase inhibitors have been found to improve agitation in patients with Alzheimer's disease in some, but not all, studies (Lavretsky 2008), and improvement may evolve gradually over 3–6 months, although the effect is not robust (Passmore et al. 2008). These drugs have also been reported to improve agitation in patients with Parkinson's disease and Lewy body dementia (Passmore et al. 2008). Memantine produces statistically significant improvement of agitation in some dementias, but this is probably not clinically noticeable most of the time. Memantine has been reported to exacerbate agitation and hallucinations in patients with Lewy body dementia (Passmore et al. 2008).

A 12-week double-blind comparison of citalopram and risperidone found similar improvement of agitation and psychosis in patients with dementia, with significantly fewer adverse effects with citalopram (Pollock et al. 2007). Other SSRIs also appear to be effective, especially for unpredictable, unpremeditated aggression (Dubovsky and Thomas 1995). Trazodone, which is not particularly serotonergic but has 5-HT_2 antagonist properties that could be relevant, has been used for some time for agitation in dementia, but evidence is mixed

TABLE 9–24. Some side effects of herbal and complementary substances

Substance	System	Manifestations and comments
Ginkgo biloba	Allergic	Anaphylaxis, Stevens-Johnson syndrome
	CNS	Headache Rare intracranial hemorrhage Seizures
	Dermatological	Skin rash
	Gastrointestinal	Nausea, gastrointestinal distress, diarrhea
	Hematological	Increased bleeding time
St. John's wort	Cardiovascular	Cardiovascular collapse during anesthesia
	CNS	Confusion, dizziness, fatigue, headache, insomnia, restlessness, mania
	Dermatological	Exanthema, photosensitization, pruritis, skin rash
	Endocrine	Serotonin syndrome, sexual dysfunction
Valerian	Cardiovascular	Arrhythmias
	CNS	Headache, insomnia, psychomotor impairment, restlessness
Yohimbine	Cardiovascular	Hypertension, tachycardia
	CNS	Anxiety, insomnia, panic attacks, exacerbation of PTSD, tremor
	Dermatological	Exanthema
	Gastrointestinal	Nausea, vomiting, salivation

Note. CNS=central nervous system; PTSD=posttraumatic stress disorder.

(Passmore et al. 2008). Serotonergic properties of buspirone make it helpful in reducing unpredictable aggressive outbursts (Cantillon et al. 1996); however, like most effective treatments for episodic agitation, its onset of action may take a month or more, and dosages of 60 mg/day or more may be necessary (Passmore et al. 2008).

A large body of experience over the years has supported the efficacy of β-adrenergic-blocking agents, especially propranolol, for unpredictable, recurrent aggressive and violent outbursts in patients with dementia or brain damage (Brooke et al. 1992). Some patients respond to relatively low dosages, but others need 500 mg/day or more. Contrary to popular wisdom, propranolol rarely causes depression, but sedation, hypotension, and sexual dysfunction can be limiting side effects (Yudofsky 1992).

Valproate and carbamazepine have been reported to reduce agitation in patients with dementia, although controlled data are limited (Passmore et al. 2008). Interactions with other medications taken by older patients are not uncommon (see Table 19–18). Lithium has been reported to reduce agitation in patients with brain damage even when it is not associated with mania, often at levels lower than those used in bipolar disorder, but its use is complex. Impairment of cognition occurs in ~50% of people who take lithium, but as discussed earlier in "Mood-Stabilizing Medications," lithium has neuroprotective and antiapoptotic properties that could reduce the risk of further neuronal loss (Bearden et al. 2007).

Patients with dementia can have difficulty expressing depression and pain, especially in the presence of aprosodia. In this situation, either symptom is likely expressed as agitation. In the presence of a personal or family history of depression or depressive symptoms that are not clearly explained by the neurological illness, an empirical trial of an antidepressant may produce substantial improvement of agitation. Acetaminophen or low dosages of opioids may resolve agitation in patients who express chronic pain as agitation.

Reversal of the sleep-wake cycle is common in dementia. The patient may be awake but disoriented at night, resulting in nighttime wandering and agitation. During the day, the patient is out of bed but not physiologically awake, exacerbating confusion and agitation. Because the best cue to a disrupted sleep-wake cycle is bright light at the time of waking up, artificial bright light in the morning can normalize sleep and reduce agitation (Van Someren et al. 1997). Addition of melatonin at bedtime may further promote resynchronizing of the sleep-wake cycle with circadian cues (Passmore et al. 2008). Because plasma

TABLE 9–25. Some interactions of herbal remedies with other medications/substances

Herbal	Medication	Comments
Asian ginseng	Phenelzine	Mania with ginseng alone and in combination with phenelzine
Ginkgo biloba	ASA Rofecoxib Warfarin	Ginkgo has been associated with bleeding, both alone and in combination with ASA, rofecoxib, and warfarin, and with intracerebral hemorrhage when taken along with thrombolytic drugs
	Trazodone	Coma reported in one patient with Alzheimer's disease treated with ginkgo plus trazodone
Kava kava	Alprazolam	Delirium and coma
	Alcohol CNS depressants	Additive CNS depression
	Dopamine (e.g., L-dopa)	Interference with action of dopamine
Omega-3 fatty acids	Aspirin	Additive antiplatelet effect increases risk of bleeding
	Dong quai Evening primrose Feverfew *Ginkgo biloba* Ginseng Heparin Licorice NSAIDs	Additive anticoagulant effect increases risk of bleeding
	Oral hypoglycemics Insulin Metformin Sulfonylureas	Decreased efficacy of hypoglycemic agent; hyperglycemia
SAMe	MAOIs	Serotonin syndrome; hypertensive crisis
	SSRIs	Additive serotonergic effects
St. John's wort (SJW)	Amitriptyline	SJW decreases amitriptyline and nortriptyline AUC
	Cyclosporine	SJW induces CYP3A4 and lowers cyclosporine levels; may result in transplanted organ rejection
	Digoxin Midazolam	Reduced digoxin levels due to CYP3A4 induction Reduced midazolam levels due to CYP3A4 induction
	MAOIs	Serotonin syndrome
	Nefazodone, SSRIs, buspirone	Serotonin syndrome
	Narcotics	Prolonged CNS depression
	Oral contraceptives	Breakthrough bleeding
	Indinavir (protease inhibitor)	HIV treatment failure due to induction of CYP3A4 and 57% decrease in AUC
	Theophylline	Decreased theophylline levels
	Warfarin	Reduced anticoagulant effect
Valerian	Benzodiazepines	Additive CNS depression

TABLE 9–25. Some interactions of herbal remedies with other medications/substances *(continued)*

Herbal	Medication	Comments
Yohimbine	Antihypertensives	Antagonism of antihypertensive action
	Ephedrine	Increased risk of hypertension
	Morphine	Enhanced analgesic effect
	Naltrexone	Potentiation of effects of yohimbine; increased anxiety
	TCAs	Increased autonomic and central effects (anxiety) of yohimbine

Note. ASA= acetylsalicylic acid; AUC=area under curve; CNS=central nervous system; HIV=human immunodeficiency virus; MAOIs= monoamine oxidase inhibitors; NSAIDs=nonsteroidal anti-inflammatory drugs; SSRIs=selective serotonin reuptake inhibitors; TCAs= tricyclic antidepressants.

melatonin levels appear to decrease with age, adjunctive use of melatonin in older patients with dementia may be appropriate.

Alternative and Complementary Therapies

A 1999 survey found that 10% of adults in the United States used an herbal medicine in the previous year, spending $5.1 billion on these preparations; one in six patients taking prescription medications also took herbal remedies (de Smet 2002). Most of these products are considered dietary supplements by the FDA, so they can be marketed without demonstration of their efficacy or safety. The amount of active substance varies considerably in herbal preparations and may not correspond to what is written on the container.

Major Classes and Chemistry

Herbal and complementary therapies are produced in different ways and have diverse actions. *Ginkgo biloba* is an extract of the leaves of the maidenhair tree. *S*-adenosyl-L-methionine 1,4-butanedisulfonate (SAMe) is an amino acid derivative. Melatonin is produced in the pineal gland and at one time was produced commercially from animal brains. However, commercial melatonin is now synthetic. Pharmacological-grade melatonin is considered an investigational drug, whereas commercial preparations with various amounts of active melatonin are available commercially. St. John's wort (*Hypericum perforatum*; SJW) is made from dried above-ground parts of *Hypericum perforatum*. SJW has multiple constituents, including hypericin, pseudohypericin, phloroglucinols, phenylpropanes, flavonol derivatives, biflavones, proanthocyanidins, xanthones, and amino acids, making it difficult to know which is the active agent. Valerian root (*Valeriana officinalis*) contains iridoids, volatile oil, sesquiterpenes, pyridine alkaloids, caffeic acid derivatives, and glutamine. Commercial yohimbine is made from the dried bark of *Pausinystalia yohimbe*, which contains indole alkaloids and tannins. Lemon balm contains glycosides, caffeic acid derivatives, flavonoids, and triterpene acids. Omega-3 fatty acids contain eicosapentaenoic acid and docosahexaenoic acid. Omega-6 fatty acids contain dihomo-γ-linolenic acid and arachidonic acid.

Mechanisms of Action

The active components of ginkgo include flavonoids (benzodiazepine receptor agonists), proanthocyanidins, and other agents that act as platelet-activating factor inhibitors, antioxidants, inhibitors of nitric oxide production associated with tissue damage, free radical scavengers, and lipid peroxidation inhibitors (lipid peroxidation contributes to neuronal loss). In addition, flavonoids have anti-inflammatory and antibacterial effects. Components of SJW inhibit synaptic uptake of serotonin, dopamine, norepinephrine, GABA, L-glutamate, and melatonin. Valerian root inhibits GABA reuptake and increases GABA synthesis. One of the indole alkaloids (rauwolscine) in yohimbine is a selective α_2-adrenergic antagonist that increases norepinephrine release, resulting in a sympathomimetic effect. This effect can counteract adverse effects of excessive autonomic serotonergic neurotransmission on sexual function. Constituents of lemon balm have sedative, antioxidant, antiviral, antibacterial, and spasmolytic actions. SAMe is a methyl donor to biogenic amines, phospholipids, proteins, and nucleic acids.

Long-chain polyunsaturated fatty acids are needed for cell membrane functions, including receptor function, axon and dendrite growth, formation of new synapses, pruning of old synapses, actions of membrane-associated proteins, and cell signaling. Omega-3 fatty acids decrease the production of inflammatory cytokines and may improve membrane function by increasing production of membrane phospholipids in addition to antagonizing chronic inflammatory processes. Inhibition of protein kinase C by omega-3 fatty acids is thought to have the potential to be useful for mood disorders.

As noted earlier in the section "Medications for Anxiety and Insomnia" (under "Major Classes and Chemistry"), melatonin acts on melatonin M_1 and M_2 receptors in the suprachiasmatic nucleus to regulate a variety of circadian rhythms. Melatonin and melatonin receptor agonists can alter the timing but not the duration or quality of sleep (Montes et al. 2003). Such actions make melatonin agonists useful for disorders associated with desynchronization of these rhythms.

Indications

Melatonin is used to treat insomnia and jet lag, especially when combined with morning bright light, and has an NNT of only two (Herxheimer and Petrie 2002). Slow-release melatonin is not as effective, suggesting that a short-lived high peak level is important. Melatonin has also been used to improve the sleep disorder of dementia, although morning bright light may be more effective. The finding of abnormal melatonin release in recently abstinent alcoholics may predict that melatonin could be useful for insomnia associated with alcoholism.

SJW has been used to treat depression and anxiety. Although some placebo-controlled trials have demonstrated statistical superiority of SJW, its clinical efficacy has not been impressive. SJW may be comparable to low dosages of reference antidepressants in mild depression; however, it does not seem useful for more severe major depression (Hypericum Depression Trial Study Group 2002). The ability of SJW to inhibit growth of gram-positive bacteria has led to its use in treating wound infections, eczema, insect bites, and mild burns.

Two multicenter trials comparing SAMe to imipramine found that efficacy of SAMe was comparable to that of imipramine in major depression (Delle Chiaie et al. 2002), although the lack of a placebo control limits interpretation of the results.

A rationale for the use of omega-3 fatty acids for mood disorders emerged from studies suggesting an association of higher intake of seafood with lower rates of bipolar disorder and major depression. In a Cochrane Review, Montgomery and Richardson (2008) reported on one study of 75 patients with sufficient data to analyze that suggested a possible effect of omega-3 fatty acids on depression but not mania. Although insufficient data exist to warrant recommendation of routine use of omega-3 fatty acids in patients with mood disorders, these substances have been found useful for prevention of heart disease, and they may also be useful for arthritis, hyperlipidemia, Raynaud's syndrome, rheumatoid arthritis, and cyclosporine toxicity.

Ginkgo biloba is most frequently used to treat dementia, peripheral vascular disease, chronic headache, and tinnitus. Studies of cognitive improvement with ginkgo have been inconsistent, with better designed studies indicating less efficacy (Birks and Grimley Evans 2009).

Valerian is usually used to treat insomnia. It has been found to improve subjective assessments of sleep without daytime cognitive impairment (Vorbach et al. 1996), but no sleep laboratory studies have been performed. Valerian has also been used for anxiety, headache, restlessness, symptoms of menopause, and irritable bowel syndrome.

Lemon balm is sometimes used to treat anxiety and insomnia. In a single study, lemon balm was superior to placebo in reducing agitation and improving involvement in activities in 71 elderly nursing home residents with dementia (Ballard et al. 2002). Lemon balm is also used to treat palpitations and headache.

The primary use of yohimbine is to treat erectile dysfunction caused by antidepressants; it can also improve anorgasmia caused by antidepressants. Yohimbine is also used to increase salivary flow to treat medication-induced dry mouth, and it is occasionally used as an analgesic.

Dosing and Side Effects

Because they are classified as foods rather than drugs and their production is not regulated, the bioavailability of herbal preparations can vary substantially, and dosage recommendations are not precise. Following are average dosages of some over-the-counter preparations. Common side effects are summarized in Table 9–24.

Most studies find that pharmacological dosages of ~1 mg of melatonin are as effective as higher dosages at inducing sleep. However, bioavailability varies considerably in commercial preparations, the smallest available dose of which is 3 mg. With commercial preparations, dosages >5 mg are no more effective than 5 mg.

Usual dosages of SJW are 900–1,500 mg/day in divided doses. Lemon balm is administered as an oil (essential oil of *Melissa officinalis*) in a dose of 200 mg. Yohimbine is provided in a tablet containing 5.75 mg of active substance.

Interactions

Because drug-metabolizing enzymes evolved as a means of eliminating xenobiotics, herbal therapies are metabolized by the same enzymes that metabolize medications. Many medications are derived from plants, and they have similar targets. As a result, both pharmacokinetic and pharmacodynamic interactions between the two can occur. Some common interactions are noted in Table 9–25.

Key Points

- Major advances have been made in the psychopharmacological treatment of neuropsychiatric disorders. Despite greater ease of use of some newer treatments, all psychiatric medications have a significant risk of adverse effects and interactions with neurological drugs that requires careful consideration of therapy. Because mood, anxiety, and psychotic disorders are generally chronic or recurrent, maintenance treatment is often needed, with ongoing monitoring and adjustment of dosage.
- Many Axis I disorders in elderly patients are caused or aggravated by neurological dysfunction. Treating such syndromes is complicated by the sensitivity of the older nervous system to the toxic but probably not the therapeutic effects of psychotropic medications, as well as by interactions of psychotropic medications with the many neurological drugs taken by elderly patients. The sedating and anticholinergic tricyclic antidepressants and neuroleptics and the long-half-life benzodiazepines are especially problematic for older patients with neurological impairments. Short-half-life benzodiazepines may be appropriate choices for some patients with acute anxiety, but anxiety and insomnia in patients with overt brain disease often are better managed chronically with azapirones or antidepressants.
- Most mood-stabilizing medications are difficult to use in elderly neuropsychiatric patients. Lithium has clearly demonstrated neuroprotective properties, but impaired cognition is a common adverse effect. Calcium channel blockers are better tolerated by patients who are older and have neurological illness, but there is less empirical support for their use and frequent dosing is necessary. All antipsychotic drugs are being found to have significant risks in older patients, especially of adverse cerebrovascular and cardiovascular outcomes. The initial promise of the newer atypical antipsychotics that was demonstrated in industry-sponsored trials, especially for cognitive benefits, has been called into question by more recent government-sponsored research.
- Atypical antipsychotic drugs may be helpful acutely for agitation, but their common use for chronic behavioral control, especially of fluctuating nonpsychotic agitation, is not supported by available data, and their risks in elderly patients are significant. Beta-blocking agents, buspirone, selective serotonin reuptake inhibitors, lithium, and anticonvulsants appear safer, but they are not immediately effective. Morning artificial bright light can improve sleep phase reversals, which are thought to cause nighttime wandering and agitation and daytime confusion in patients with dementia, reducing the need for medications.
- Although as a general rule "less is more" for older patients with neurological impairments, slow increments of any psychotropic medications are appropriate. The approach to confusion and other neurological problems in geriatric pa-

tients should first involve withdrawing as many medications as possible. However, when psychotropic medications are necessary, some older patients need the same dosages and serum levels as younger adults. Most of the medications used in geriatric neuropsychiatry do not have as much empirical support as they do for younger patients, and therefore more care is required in their use.

- Herbal remedies are often thought to be benign because they are "natural." However, asbestos, radiation, and sunlight are also natural, yet they are not necessarily safe. Furthermore, anything that has positive effects can have negative actions, and as with medications, older patients may be more sensitive to adverse effects and interactions of naturopathic substances. In addition to over-the-counter medications, all patients should be asked about herbal and natural products that they may not consider drugs or medicines.

Recommended Readings and Web Sites

Astrand E, Astrand B, Antonov K, et al: Potential drug interactions during a three-decade study period: a cross-sectional study of a prescription register. Eur J Clin Pharmacol 63:851–859, 2007

Avorn J, Soumerai SB, Everitt DE, et al: A randomized trial of a program to reduce the use of psychoactive drugs in nursing homes. N Engl J Med 327:168–173, 1992

Brooks JO, Hoblyn JC: Neurocognitive costs and benefits of psychotropic medications in older adults. J Geriatr Psychiatry Neurol 20:199–214, 2007

Dubovsky SL: Clinical Guide to Psychotropic Medications. New York, WW Norton, 2005

Hilmer SN, Gnjidic D: The effects of polypharmacy in older adults. Clin Pharmacol Ther 85:86–93, 2009

Hilmer SN, McLachlan AJ, Le Couteur DG: Clinical pharmacology in the geriatric patient. Fundam Clin Pharmacol 21:217–230, 2007

Kales HC, Valenstein M, Kim HM, et al: Mortality risk in patients with dementia treated with antipsychotics versus other medications. Am J Psychiatry 164:1568–1576, 2007

Lavretsky H: Neuropsychiatric symptoms in Alzheimer's disease and related disorders: why do treatments work in clinical practice but not in the randomized trials? Am J Geriatr Psychiatry 16:523–527, 2008

Milton JC, Hill-Smith I, Jackson SH: Prescribing for older people. BMJ 336:606–609, 2008

Schwartz JB, Abernethy DR: Aging and medications: past, present, future. Clin Pharmacol Ther 85:3–10, 2009

Brown University Geriatric Psychopharmacology Update. Available at: http://www.accessmylibrary.com/coms2/browse_JJ_T106. Accessed May 13, 2010.

Skyscape. www.skyscape.com/estore/Physicians.aspx. Tool to access up to 600 medical resources through a single mobile app; also provides drug guides, medical alerts, journal summaries, and references from over 50 medical publishers.

References

Allen MH, Hirschfeld RM, Wozniak PJ, et al: Linear relationship of valproate serum concentration to response and optimal serum levels for acute mania. Am J Psychiatry 163:272–275, 2006

Allison DB, Mentore JL, Heo M: Antipsychotic-induced weight gain: a comprehensive research synthesis. Am J Psychiatry 156:1686–1696, 1999

American Diabetes Association, American Psychiatric Association, American Association of Clinical Endocrinologists, et al: Consensus development conference on antipsychotic drugs and obesity and diabetes. Diabetes Care 27:596–601, 2004

Astrand E, Astrand B, Antonov K: Potential drug interactions during a three-decade study period: a cross-sectional study of a prescription register. Eur J Clin Pharmacol 63:851–859, 2007

Ballard C, O'Brien J, Reichelt K, et al: Aromatherapy as a safe and effective treatment for the management of agitation in severe dementia: the results of a double-blind, placebo-controlled trial with Melissa. J Clin Psychiatry 63:553–558, 2002

Bauer M, Mitchner L: What is a "mood stabilizer"? An evidence-based response. Am J Psychiatry 161:3–18, 2004

Bearden CE, Thompson PM, Dalwani M, et al: Greater cortical gray matter density in lithium-treated patients with bipolar disorder. Biol Psychiatry 62:7–16, 2007

Birks J, Grimley Evans J: Ginkgo biloba for cognitive impairment and dementia. Cochrane Database of Systematic Reviews 2009, Issue 1. Art. No.: CD003120. DOI: 10.1002/14651858.CD003120.pub3

Brands B, Blake J, Marsh DC, et al: The impact of benzodiazepine use on methadone maintenance treatment outcomes. J Addict Dis 27:37–48, 2008

Brodtkorb E, Mula M: Optimizing therapy of seizures in adult patients with psychiatric comorbidity. Neurology 67 (suppl 4): S39–S44, 2006

Brooke MM, Patterson DR, Questad KA, et al: The treatment of agitation during initial hospitalization after traumatic brain injury. Arch Phys Med Rehabil 73:917–921, 1992

Brooks JO, Hoblyn JC: Neurocognitive costs and benefits of psychotropic medications in older adults. J Geriatr Psychiatry Neurol 20:199–214, 2007

Busto U, Sellers EM, Naranjo CA, et al: Withdrawal reaction after long-term therapeutic use of benzodiazepines. N Engl J Med 315:854–859, 1986

Calabrese JR, Bowden C, Sachs G, et al: A placebo-controlled 18-month trial of lamotrigine and lithium maintenance treatment in recently depressed patients with bipolar I disorder. J Clin Psychiatry 64:1013–1024, 2003

Cantillon M, Brunswick R, Molina D, et al: Buspirone vs. haloperidol: a double-blind trial for agitation in a nursing home population with Alzheimer's disease. Am J Geriatr Psychiatry 4:263–267, 1996

Conway CR, Chibnall JT, Nelson LA, et al: An open-label trial of adjunctive oxcarbazepine for bipolar disorder. J Clin Psychopharmacol 26:95–97, 2006

Davis JM, Chen N, Glick ID: A meta-analysis of the efficacy of second-generation antipsychotics. Arch Gen Psychiatry 60:553–564, 2003

de Haan L, van Bruggen M, Lavalaye J, et al: Subjective experience and D_2 receptor occupancy in patients with recent-onset schizophrenia treated with low-dose olanzapine or haloperidol: a randomized, double-blind study. Am J Psychiatry 160:303–309, 2003

Delle Chiaie R, Pancheri P, Scapicchio P: Efficacy and tolerability of oral and intramuscular S-adenosyl-L-methionine 1,4-butane-disulfonate (SAMe) in the treatment of major depression: comparison with imipramine in 2 multicenter studies. Am J Clin Nutr 76(suppl):1172S–1176S, 2002

de Smet PA: Herbal remedies. N Engl J Med 347:2046–2056, 2002

Dubovsky SL: Beyond the serotonin reuptake inhibitors: rationales for the development of new serotonergic agents. J Clin Psychiatry 55(suppl):34–44, 1994

Dubovsky SL: Calcium channel antagonists as novel agents for manic-depressive disorder, in American Psychiatric Press Textbook of Psychopharmacology. Edited by Schatzberg AF, Nemeroff CB. Washington, DC, American Psychiatric Press, 1995, pp 377–388

Dubovsky SL: Clinical Guide to Psychotropic Medications. New York, WW Norton, 2005

Dubovsky SL: Agents acting on the benzodiazepine receptor, in Comprehensive Textbook of Psychiatry, 9th Edition. Edited by Sadock B, Sadock V, Ruiz P. Baltimore, MD, Williams & Wilkins, 2009, pp 3044–3055

Dubovsky SL, Thomas M: Beyond specificity: effects of serotonin and serotonergic treatments on psychobiological dysfunction. J Psychosom Res 39:429–444, 1995

Dubovsky SL, Thomas M: Tardive dyskinesia associated with fluoxetine. Psychiatr Serv 47:991–993, 1996

Flint AJ: Recent developments in geriatric psychopharmacotherapy. Can J Psychiatry 39 (suppl 1):S9–S18, 1994

Friedman JH: Atypical antipsychotics in the elderly with Parkinson disease and the "black box" warning. Neurology 67:564–566, 2006

Furukawa TA, Streiner DL, Young LT, et al: Antidepressants and benzodiazepines for major depression. Cochrane Database of Systematic Reviews 2001, Issue 2. Art. No.: CD001026. DOI: 10.1002/14651858.CD001026

Gardner DM, Lynd LD: Sumatriptan contraindications and the serotonin syndrome. Ann Pharmacother 32:33–38, 1998

Georgotas A, McCue RE, Cooper TB: A placebo-controlled comparison of nortriptyline and phenelzine in maintenance therapy of elderly depressed patients. Arch Gen Psychiatry 46:783–786, 1989

Gerber PE, Lynd LD: Selective serotonin-reuptake inhibitor-induced movement disorders. Ann Pharmacother 32:692–698, 1998

Gianfranesco FD, Grogg AL, Mahmoud RA, et al: Differential effects of risperidone, olanzapine, clozapine and conventional antipsychotics on type 2 diabetes: findings from a large health plan database. J Clin Psychiatry 63:920–930, 2002

Hawes C, Morris JN, Phillips CD, et al: Development of the Nursing Home Resident Assessment Instrument in the USA. Age Ageing 26 (Suppl 2):19–25, 1997a

Hawes C, Mor V, Phillips CD, et al: The OBRA-87 nursing home regulations and implementation of the Resident Assessment Instrument: effects on process quality [see comments]. J Am Geriatr Soc 45:977–985, 1997b; comments 45:975–976, 1025–1028, 1997

Henderson S, Jorm AF, Scott LR, et al: Insomnia in the elderly: its prevalence and correlates in the general population. Med J Aust 162:22–24, 1995

Herxheimer A, Petrie KJ: Melatonin for the prevention and treatment of jet lag. Cochrane Database of Systematic Reviews 2002, Issue 2. Art. No.: CD001520. DOI: 10.1002/14651858.CD001520

Hilmer SN, Gnjidic D: The effects of polypharmacy in older adults. Clin Pharmacol Ther 85:86–93, 2009

Hilmer SN, Mager DE, Simosick EM, et al: A drug burden index to define the functional burden of medications in older people. Arch Intern Med 167:781–787, 2007

Hypericum Depression Trial Study Group: Effect of Hypericum perforatum (St John's wort) in major depressive disorder: a randomized controlled trial. JAMA 287:1807–1814, 2002

Jones PB, Barnes TR, Davies L, et al: Randomized controlled trial of the effect on quality of life of second- vs. first-generation antipsychotic drugs in schizophrenia: Cost Utility of the Latest Antipsychotic Drugs in Schizophrenia Study (CUtLASS 1). Arch Gen Psychiatry 63:1079–1087, 2006

Kales HC, Valenstein M, Kim HM, et al: Mortality risk in patients with dementia treated with antipsychotics versus other psychiatric medications. Am J Psychiatry 164:1568–1576, 2007

Katzung BG (ed): Basic and Clinical Pharmacology, 10th Edition. New York, McGraw-Hill, 2008

Kessing LR, Sondergard L, Forman JL, et al: Lithium treatment and risk of dementia. Arch Gen Psychiatry 65:1331–1335, 2008

Kontkanen O, Toronen P, Lakso M, et al: Antipsychotic drug treatment induces differential gene expression in the rat cortex. J Neurochem 83:1043–1053, 2002

Kruger S, Sarkar R, Pietsch R, et al: Levetiracetam as monotherapy or add-on to valproate in the treatment of acute mania: a randomized open-label study. Psychopharmacology 198:297–299, 2008

Krymchantowski AV, Silva MT, Barbosa JS, et al: Amitriptyline versus amitriptyline combined with fluoxetine in the preventative treatment of transformed migraine: a double-blind study. Headache 42:510–514, 2002

Kurlan R, Cummings J, Raman R, et al; Alzheimer's Disease Cooperative Study Group: Quetiapine for agitation or psychosis in patients with dementia and parkinsonism. Neurology 68:1356–1363, 2007

Laroche ML, Charmes JP, Bouthier G, et al: Inappropriate medications in the elderly. Clin Pharmacol Ther 85:94–97, 2009

Lavretsky H: Neuropsychiatric symptoms in Alzheimer disease and related disorders: why do treatments work in clinical practice but not in the randomized trials? Am J Geriatr Psychiatry 16:523–527, 2008

Lieberman JA, Stroup TS, McEvoy JP, et al: Effectiveness of antipsychotic drugs in patients with chronic schizophrenia. N Engl J Med 353:1209–1223, 2005

Lindley SE, Carlson EB, Hill K: A randomized, double-blind, placebo-controlled trial of augmentation topiramate for chronic combat-related posttraumatic stress disorder. J Clin Psychopharmacol 27:677–681, 2007

Loj J, Solomon GD: Migraine prophylaxis: who, why, and how. Cleve Clin J Med 73:793–816, 2006

McCleane G: Antidepressants as analgesics. CNS Drugs 22:139–156, 2008

McCue RE, Georgotas A, Nagachandran N, et al: Plasma levels of nortriptyline and 10-hydroxynortriptyline and treatment-related electrocardiographic changes in the elderly depressed. J Psychiatr Res 23:73–79, 1989

Milton JC, Hill-Smith I, Jackson SH: Prescribing for older people. BMJ 336:606–609, 2008

Mittmann N, Herrmann N, Shulman KI, et al: The effectiveness of antidepressants in elderly depressed outpatients: a prospective case series study. J Clin Psychiatry 60:690–697, 1999

Montes LG, Uribe MP, Sotres JC, et al: Treatment of primary insomnia with melatonin: a double-blind, placebo-controlled, crossover study. J Psychiatry Neurosci 28:191–196, 2003

Montgomery P, Richardson AJ: Omega-3 fatty acids for bipolar disorder. Cochrane Database of Systematic Reviews 2008, Issue 2. Art. No.: CD005169. DOI: 10.1002/14651858.CD005169.pub2

Pande AC, Feltner DE, Jefferson JW, et al: Efficacy of the novel anxiolytic pregabalin in social anxiety disorder: a placebo-controlled, multicenter study. J Clin Psychopharmacol 24:141–149, 2004

Pandi-Perumal SR, Srinivasan V, Spence DW, et al: Ramelteon: a review of its therapeutic potential in sleep disorders. Adv Ther 26:613–626, 2009

Panitch HS, Thisted RA, Smith RA: Randomized, controlled trial of dextromethorphan/quinidine for pseudobulbar affect in multiple sclerosis. Ann Neurol 59:780–787, 2006

Passmore M, Gardner DM, Polak Y, et al: Alternatives to atypical antipsychotics for the management of dementia-related agitation. Drugs Aging 25:381–398, 2008

Pollock BG, Mulsant BH, Sweet R: A double-blind comparison of citalopram and risperidone for the treatment of behavioral and psychotic symptoms associated with dementia. Am J Geriatr Psychiatry 15:942–952, 2007

Pollock BG, Forsyth CE, Bies RR: The critical role of clinical pharmacology in geriatric psychopharmacology. Clin Pharmacol Ther 85:89–93, 2009

Post RM, Pazzaglia PJ, Ketter TA, et al: Carbamazepine and nimodipine in refractory bipolar illness: efficacy and mechanisms, in Pharmacotherapy for Mood, Anxiety, and Cognitive Disorders. Edited by Halbreich U, Montgomery SA. Washington, DC, American Psychiatric Press, 2000, pp 77–110

Post RM, Altshuler LL, Frye MA, et al: Preliminary observations on the effectiveness of levetiracetam in the open adjunctive treatment of refractory bipolar disorder. J Clin Psychiatry 66:370–374, 2005

Rabkin JG, McElhiney MC, Rabkin R, et al: Modafinil treatment for fatigue in HIV+ patients: a pilot study. J Clin Psychiatry 65:1688–1695, 2004

Ray WA, Chung CP, Murry KT, et al: Atypical antipsychotic drugs and the risk of sudden cardiac death. N Engl J Med 360:225–235, 2009

Reilly J, Ayis SA, Ferrier IN, et al: Thioridazine and sudden unexplained death in psychiatric in-patients. Br J Psychiatry 180:515–522, 2002

Saarto T, Wiffen PJ: Antidepressants for neuropathic pain. Cochrane Database of Systematic Reviews 2007, Issue 4. Art. No.: CD005454. DOI: 10.1002/14651858.CD005454.pub2

Sassi R, Nicoletti M, Brambilla P, et al: Increased gray matter volume in lithium-treated bipolar disorder patients. Neurosci Lett 329: 243–245, 2002

Satel SL, Nelson JC: Stimulants in the treatment of depression: a critical overview. J Clin Psychiatry 50:241–249, 1989

Schneider LS, Dagerman KS, Insel PS: Efficacy and adverse effects of atypical antipsychotics for dementia: meta-analysis of randomized, placebo-controlled trials. Am J Geriatr Psychiatry 14:191–210, 2006a

Schneider LS, Tariot PN, Dagerman KS, et al: Effectiveness of atypical antipsychotic drugs in patients with Alzheimer's disease. N Engl J Med 355:1525–1538, 2006b

Schwartz JB, Abernethy DR: Aging and medications: past, present, future. Clin Pharmacol Ther 85:3–10, 2009

Selbaek G, Kirkevold O, Engedal K: The course of psychiatric and behavioral symptoms and the use of psychotropic medication in patients with dementia in Norwegian nursing homes: a 12-month follow-up study. Am J Geriatr Psychiatry 16:528–536, 2008

Shelton RC: Intracellular mechanisms of antidepressant drug action. Harv Rev Psychiatry 8:161–174, 2000

Shulman KI, Walker SE: Refining the MAOI diet: tyramine content of pizzas and soy products. J Clin Psychiatry 60:191–193, 1999

Shulman KI, Tohen M, Satlin A, et al: Mania compared with unipolar depression in old age. Am J Psychiatry 149:341–345, 1992

Smith D, Wesson DR: Benzodiazepines and other sedative-hypnotics, in American Psychiatric Press Textbook of Substance Abuse Treatment, 2nd Edition. Edited by Galanter M, Kleber HD. Washington, DC, American Psychiatric Press, 1999, pp 239–250

Strawn JR, Keck PE Jr, Caroff SN: Neuroleptic malignant syndrome. Am J Psychiatry 164:870–876, 2007

Sultzer DL, Davis SM, Tariot PN, et al: Clinical symptom response to atypical antipsychotic medications in Alzheimer's disease: phase 1 outcomes from the CATIE-AD effectiveness trial. Am J Psychiatry 165:844–854, 2008

Tardito D, Perez J, Tiraboschi E, et al: Signaling pathways regulating gene expression, neuroplasticity and neurotrophic mechanisms in the action of antidepressants: a critical review. Pharmacol Rev 58:115–134, 2006

Thase ME, Macfadden W, Weisler RH, et al: Efficacy of quetiapine monotherapy in bipolar I and II depression: a double-blind, placebo-controlled study (the BOLDER II study). J Clin Psychopharmacol 26:600–609, 2006

Tohen M, Calabrese JR, Sachs G, et al: Randomized, placebo-controlled trial of olanzapine as maintenance therapy in patients with bipolar I disorder responding to acute treatment with olanzapine. Am J Psychiatry 163:247–256, 2006

Tucker P, Trautman RP, Wyatt DB, et al: Efficacy and safety of topiramate monotherapy in civilian posttraumatic stress disorder: a randomized, double-blind, placebo-controlled study. J Clin Psychiatry 68:201–206, 2007

Vasudev K, Macritchie K, Geddes J, et al: Topiramate for acute affective episodes in bipolar disorder. Cochrane Database of Systematic Reviews 2006, Issue 1. Art. No.: CD003384. DOI: 10.1002/14651858.CD003384.pub2

Vieta E, Suppes T, Eggens I, et al: Efficacy and safety of quetiapine in combination with lithium or divalproex for maintenance of patients with bipolar I disorder. J Affect Disord 109:251–263, 2008

Vorbach EU, Gortelmeyer R, Bruning J: Therapy for insomniacs: effectiveness and tolerance of valerian preparations [in German]. Psychopharmakotherapie 3:109–115, 1996

Wagner GJ, Rabkin R: Effects of dextroamphetamine on depression and fatigue in men with HIV: a double-blind, placebo-controlled trial. J Clin Psychiatry 61:436–440, 2000

Wang PW, Yang YS, Chandler RA, et al: Adjunctive zonisamide for weight loss in euthymic bipolar disorder patients: a pilot study. J Psychiatr Res 42:451–457, 2008

Woolorton E: Triptan migraine treatments and antidepressants: risk of serotonin syndrome. CMAJ 175:874–875, 2006

Yeh HL, Tsai SJ: Lithium may be useful in the prevention of Alzheimer's disease in individuals at risk of presenile familial Alzheimer's disease. Med Hypotheses 71:948–951, 2008

Yudofsky SC: Beta-blockers and depression: the clinician's dilemma. JAMA 267:1826–1827, 1992

Zagnoni PG, Albano C: Psychostimulants and epilepsy. Epilepsia 43 (suppl 2):28–31, 2002

Zeeberg P, Olesen J, Jensen R: Medication overuse headache and chronic migraine in a specialized headache centre: field-testing proposed new appendix criteria. Cephalalgia 29:214–220, 2009

Ziere G, Dieleman JP, van der Cammen TJ, et al: Selective serotonin reuptake inhibiting antidepressants are associated with an increased risk of nonvertebral fractures. J Clin Psychopharmacol 28:411–417, 2008

10

Electroconvulsive Therapy and Related Treatments

C. Edward Coffey, M.D.
Charles H. Kellner, M.D.

Electroconvulsive therapy (ECT) is a sophisticated medical procedure that uses electrical stimulation applied to the scalp to induce a series of brief, controlled seizures in a patient who is under general anesthesia. ECT is a safe, rapidly acting, and highly effective treatment for certain severe neuropsychiatric disorders, most notably mood disorders (including those in patients with neurological disorders), some forms of schizophrenia, and syndromes such as delirium and catatonia (American Psychiatric Association 2001; U.K. ECT Review Group 2003).

In this chapter, we review the use of ECT as a treatment for neuropsychiatric disorders in elderly patients. We discuss the indications and efficacy, medical physiology, mechanisms of action, contemporary technique, and safety and adverse effects of this important procedure, as well as its unique role in patients with neurological disorders. In addition, we preview some experimental "brain stimulation" therapies that are related to ECT and that may hold promise for the future. These therapies include focal electrically administered seizure therapy (FEAST) and magnetic seizure therapy (MST). Other brain stimulation therapies are discussed in Chapter 11, "Brain Stimulation Therapies: Vagus Nerve Stimulation, Transcranial Magnetic Stimulation, Transcranial Direct Current Stimulation, and Deep Brain Stimulation."

ECT in Geriatric Neuropsychiatric Practice

Although precise data are not available, Hermann et al. (1995) estimated that ~4.9 patients per 10,000 population receive ECT annually in the United States. For years after its introduction in 1938, ECT was used primarily in younger adults because of concerns about its safety in older patients and in those with general medical comorbidity. Refinements in ECT technique (discussed in "Technique of ECT" later in this chapter) have largely obviated those initial concerns so that now a large proportion of patients receiving ECT are elderly, and this number will increase as the population continues to age. Kramer (1985) reviewed patterns of ECT use in California from 1977 to 1983 and found that the probability of receiving ECT increased with age of the patient. Patients ages 65 years and older were given ECT at a rate of 3.86/10,000 population, compared with 0.85/10,000 in those ages 25–44 years. In an analysis of the data on ECT use in California from 1984 to 1994, Kramer (1999) found similar patterns. Babigian and Guttmacher (1984) reviewed a massive data set from the Monroe County (New York) Psychiatric Case Register over three 5-year periods. They found that among patients hospitalized for the first time, those who received ECT were older than those who did not. Lambourn and Barrington (1986) surveyed the use of ECT from 1972 to 1983 in a British population of 3 million and found that ECT use was more common in patients (especially female patients) ages 60 years and older. In a study of 5,729 psychiatric admissions over 3 years, Malla (1988) found that patients who received ECT in general hospitals were significantly older than patients who did not receive ECT. Thompson et al. (1994) analyzed data from the National Institute of Mental Health Sample Survey program for 1980 and 1986, which included representative samples of psychiatric inpatients in the United States. They found that approximately one-third of ECT recipients were ages 65 years and older, a figure far out of proportion to the representation of that age group in the sample (8.2%). Rosenbach et al. (1997) studied a sample (~4,000 people) of Medicare Part B claims from 1987 to 1992 and found an ECT rate of 5.1/10,000 population. In an analysis of inpatient data from the 1993

Healthcare Cost and Utilization Project of the Agency for Healthcare Policy and Research, Olfson et al. (1998) found that ~10% of 22,761 patients admitted to a general hospital with a principal diagnosis of recurrent major depression received ECT that year. Increasing age was one of several patient variables associated with higher ECT use; persons ages 65 years and older were seven times more likely to receive ECT than were persons ages 18–34 years.

Several factors help to explain the frequent use of ECT in elderly patients. First, elderly individuals may be more sensitive to medication side effects, particularly the combination of antidepressants and antipsychotics typically required to treat psychotic depression. Second, evidence suggests that antidepressant pharmacotherapy may be less effective in elderly than in younger patients (Roose et al. 2004). In contrast, increasing age as a variable may be a positive predictor of ECT response (Black et al. 1993; Coryell and Zimmerman 1984; O'Connor et al. 2001; Tew et al. 1999). Third, elderly patients are more likely to have comorbid general medical or neurological disorders, which may complicate the use of psychotropic medications or limit their effectiveness (Mottram et al. 2006). For all these reasons, ECT is a critically important component of the neuropsychiatrist's tool kit used to treat mood disorders in elderly patients. Indeed, several studies have found that the use of ECT is one of the most important variables associated with a positive outcome in later-life depression (Bosworth et al. 2002; Philibert et al. 1995; Rubin et al. 1991; Zubenko et al. 1994). Finally, ECT appears to be at least as cost-effective as pharmacotherapy (Greenhalgh et al. 2005; McDonald 2006), and perhaps even more so in certain settings (Olfson et al. 1998).

Diagnostic Indications and Efficacy

ECT is indicated for the acute treatment of severe mood disorders (including depression or mania), certain forms of schizophrenia, and syndromes such as delirium and catatonia. ECT is also an effective form of continuation treatment for some of these conditions (discussed later in this chapter in "Technique of ECT"). The neurobiological effects of ECT may also prove salutary in other neuropsychiatric syndromes, such as Parkinson's disease (discussed later in this chapter in "ECT in Elderly Patients With Neurological Disorders").

Depression

The most common indication for ECT in all patients, including those who are elderly, remains the acute and maintenance treatment of depression, both major and bipolar. In elderly patients with depression, ECT is typically used as a second-line treatment, after patients have failed to respond to a trial of medication or have exhibited intolerance of the side effects of medication. ECT should be considered a first-line intervention in certain situations, however, such as when the presenting illness threatens the patient's life (e.g., severe suicide risk, severe melancholia with inanition and malnutrition, inability to comply with critical general medical care), when ECT is deemed safer than alternative treatments, or when the patient has a history of response to ECT or a preference for ECT (American Psychiatric Association 2001).

Six randomized controlled trials have found ECT superior to sham ECT in adults with depression (reviewed in Abrams 2002b). A reanalysis of one of these trials (the Nottingham trial; Gregory et al. 1985) found that the efficacy of ECT was also superior to sham ECT in elderly patients with depression (O'Leary et al. 1995). Although a Cochrane Review of the randomized evidence concluded that the data were too sparse to determine the efficacy of ECT in depressed elderly patients (Stek et al. 2003), subsequent reviews, which included the extensive nonrandomized literature, concluded that ECT is indeed effective in the acute treatment of depression in elderly patients (Dombrovski and Mulsant 2007; Flint and Gagnon 2002; Salzman et al. 2002; Van der Wurff et al. 2003).

The reported response rates to ECT among elderly patients with depression range from 63% to 98%, clearly demonstrating that increasing age, per se, does not have a negative impact on the effectiveness of ECT for depressive illness. In fact, evidence suggests that ECT may be even more effective in elderly patients than in younger age groups (O'Connor et al. 2001), and several reports have confirmed the efficacy and safety of ECT even in the "old-old" (the low end of which is variably defined as between ages 75 and 85) (Casey and Davis 1996; Cattan et al. 1990; Gormley et al. 1998; Manly et al. 2000).

ECT is reported to be 20%–45% more effective than pharmacotherapy for depression (see review by Abrams 2002b), as confirmed in two meta-analyses (Janicak et al. 1985; U.K. ECT Review Group 2003). This same therapeutic superiority of ECT over antidepressant pharmacotherapy has also been demonstrated in elderly patients (Folkerts et al. 1997; Salzman et al. 2002). No somatic therapy for depression has been shown to have efficacy superior to that of ECT (Sackeim 2005).

Certain clinical features may predict a particularly robust response to ECT among patients with depression. Data derived largely from mixed-age samples of adults suggest that a particularly good response to ECT is associated with the presence of psychosis, catatonia, pseudodementia, pathological guilt, anhedonia, agitation, and neurovegetative signs (Greenberg and Fink 1992; Hickie et al. 1996; Salzman 1982; Zorumski et al. 1988). These findings were confirmed in a prospective study involving 29 elderly patients (Fraser and Glass 1980), in which guilt, anhedonia, and agitation were identified as positive prognostic signs. In multiple studies, response to ECT has been particularly good in patients with delusional depression, compared with a nonpsychotic group (Hickie et al. 1996; Mulsant et al. 1991; Pande et al. 1990; Petrides et al. 2001; Wilkinson et al. 1993), although other studies have found no difference (O'Leary et al. 1995; Rich et al. 1984a, 1986; Sobin et al. 1996; Solan et al. 1988). Delusions are common in depressed elderly persons, and typically these patients respond poorly to pharmacotherapy. The use of ECT in agitated or psychotic elderly patients may spare them exposure to antipsychotic agents. This consideration is important, given the risks of antipsychotic drugs to induce motor (e.g., tardive dyskinesia), metabolic, and vascular complications in elderly patients (Jenike 1985; see also Chapter 9, "Geriatric Neuropsychopharmacology"). Suicide is a major concern for patients with depression, and the risk of this outcome is particularly high in elderly people (especially men). ECT is rapidly effective against suicidal ideation (Kellner et al. 2005), an advantage that is particularly important to elderly patients, who may respond more slowly to antidepressant medications than do younger patients (Mulsant et al. 2006).

A variety of biological markers for ECT response have been investigated in mixed-age samples, including the dexamethasone suppression test, the thyrotropin-releasing hormone test, and other neuroendocrine tests (Decina et al. 1987; Kamil and Joffe 1991; Kirkegaard et al. 1975; Krog-Meyer et al. 1984; Papakostas et al. 1981; Swartz 1993), as well as polysomnographic studies (Coffey et al. 1988; Grunhaus et al. 1996) and the apolipoprotein E polymorphism (Fisman et al. 2001). None of these laboratory studies appears to provide strong "state-specific" markers for major depressive illness, and data are inconsistent (Devanand et al. 1991) on whether they can be used serially to follow the course of ECT, predict outcome, or predict early relapse.

Several authors have attempted to identify predictors of nonresponse to ECT. In a retrospective study, Magni et al. (1988) compared elderly patients who responded to ECT and those who did not respond and found that physical illness during the index episode, fewer negative life events preceding the onset of the index episode, and prior depressive episodes of long duration were predictive of nonresponse to ECT. Other investigators have found that longer duration of the index episode predicts poorer outcome (Fraser and Glass 1980; Karlinsky and Shulman 1984). Previous courses of ECT and increased age at the time of first treatment with ECT have been linked with a slower response rate to ECT, with no effect on eventual positive outcome (Rich et al. 1984b; Salzman 1982; Shapira and Lerer 1999). There are conflicting data on whether pre-ECT medication resistance predicts nonresponse to ECT (Rasmussen et al. 2007a), with response rates ranging from 28% to 72% depending on the patient sample, definition of "medication resistance," and ECT treatment protocol (Dombrovski et al. 2005). The limited data, however, should not discourage the clinician from initiating a trial of ECT in patients with any of the aforementioned predictors of nonresponse. The fact that patients who receive ECT come from a selected population that is less responsive to antidepressant medication and generally is at greater risk for relapse underscores the value of this treatment for the most difficult-to-treat elderly patients.

Although few studies have directly compared residual depressive symptoms following ECT and following pharmacotherapy, full remission is likely to be more common following ECT (Hamilton 1982). Residual depressive symptoms have a serious impact on the quality of life and may result in chronicity of depression in elderly patients and increase the likelihood of relapse (Prien and Kupfer 1986). A number of studies have suggested that use of ECT is one of the most important variables in predicting a positive outcome of depression in elderly patients, with reduced chronicity, decreased morbidity, and possibly decreased mortality (Avery and Winokur 1976; Babigian and Guttmacher 1984; Philibert et al. 1995; Wesner and Winokur 1989; Zubenko et al. 1994).

Mania

Although extensive clinical experience indicates that ECT is effective for treating both manic and depressed phases of bipolar illness in elderly patients, formal data for this population are lacking. A small number of controlled studies involving relatively young mixed-age samples have found ECT to be superior to drug therapy (Mukherjee 1989; Mukherjee et al. 1988; Small et al. 1988, 1991). ECT appears to be particularly effective in mixed bipolar states and agitated mania, conditions that may become more prevalent as the illness becomes more chronic and refractory (Calabrese et al. 1993). ECT may be particularly suitable for elderly patients who have this more severe form of bipolar disorder. Also, morbidity from ECT is likely to be less risky than the general medical risks of a sustained period of mania in an older person.

Schizophrenia and Other Psychotic Disorders

No controlled data exist on the use of ECT in elderly patients with schizophrenia. ECT has been used in younger patients with this illness, and in these patients several features correlate with good outcome, including the presence of affective or catatonic features, an acute onset of illness with relatively brief duration of illness, and a history of response to ECT (American Psychiatric Association 2001; Braga and Petrides 2005; Tharyan and Adams 2005). ECT does not appear to be very effective for treating the chronic, residual phase of the illness with predominant negative features (Weiner and Coffey 1988). These "deficit" states become more common as the illness progresses (Kaplan and Sadock 2005) and thus may be highly represented in elderly patients with schizophrenia, although controlled data on this issue are lacking. To the best of our knowledge, there are no systematically collected data on the efficacy of ECT in patients with late-onset functional psychoses, such as late-onset schizophrenia.

Delirium and Catatonia

Although no controlled data have been reported on the use of ECT in patients with delirium (see Chapter 15, "Delirium"), numerous case and clinical series have documented its safety and effectiveness, irrespective of the underlying etiology of the delirium (see Krystal and Coffey 1997 for a review). Indeed, ECT has been used for the management of neuropsychiatric symptoms of delirium in Europe and Scandinavia for decades (Kramp and Bolwig 1981). The use of ECT in patients with delirium is generally reserved for those who have not responded to more standard general medical treatment (American Psychiatric Association 2001).

Catatonia is a potentially life-threatening syndrome whose symptoms overlap with those of delirium (see Chapter 15). A large clinical literature supports the effectiveness of ECT as a safe and rapidly effective treatment for catatonia and related conditions, such as neuroleptic malignant syndrome (Caroff et al. 2007; Fink and Taylor 2003).

Medical Physiology of ECT

The data on the physiology of ECT have been compiled largely from mixed-age adult samples, and to our knowledge, few data focus specifically on the physiology of ECT in elderly patients. Clearly, the myriad physiological changes that accompany an ECT seizure take on particular importance in elderly individuals, in whom general medical illnesses involving multiple organ systems are common. Of greatest importance are the physiological effects of ECT on the brain and the cardiovascular system. As described later in this chapter, modifications in ECT technique may be required in patients with brain or cardiovascular disease (see "Technique of ECT" and "ECT in Elderly Patients With Neurological Disorders").

Cerebral Physiology

With ECT, an electrical stimulus applied to the scalp is used to depolarize cerebral neurons and thereby produce a generalized cerebral seizure. The mechanism by which ECT seizures are propagated is not well understood. Bilateral ECT appears to lead to seizure generalization through direct stimulation of the diencephalon (a subcortical "pacemaker"), whereas seizures induced with unilateral stimulation may begin focally in the stimulated cortex and then generalize via corticothalamic pathways (Staton 1981).

During the initial phase of the induced seizure, electroencephalographic (EEG) activity is variable, consisting of patterns of low-voltage fast activity and polyspike rhythms. These patterns correlate with tonic or irregular clonic motor movements. With seizure progression, EEG activity evolves into a pattern of hypersynchronous polyspikes and waves that characterize the clonic motor phase. These regular patterns begin to slow and eventually disintegrate as the seizure ends, sometimes terminating abruptly in a flat electroencephalogram for several seconds (Weiner and Krystal 1993). The entire seizure typically lasts 30–60 seconds, and preseizure EEG rhythms are typically recovered within 20–30 minutes. It should be noted that although the scalp-recorded electroencephalogram implies that the ECT seizure is an all-or-none phenomenon, in fact the onset, duration, and EEG morphology of the seizure all vary according to the brain structures involved. The interictal (intertreatment) electroencephalogram typically shows mild slowing, particularly in frontal regions. These ictal and interictal EEG features vary with ECT technique (i.e., stimulus waveform, stimulus electrode placement, stimulus dosage, stimulus parameters, and treatment frequency and number), as well as with the patient's age. For example, increasing age is associated with shorter seizure duration; shorter slow-wave-phase duration; weaker overall strength and patterning; and lower early ictal, midictal, and postictal amplitudes (Krystal et al. 1995, 1998).

The ECT-induced seizure is also associated with a variety of transient and benign changes in cerebral physiology (reviewed in Abrams 2002b). In patients with depression, *cerebral blood flow* is typically reduced frontally at baseline, increased during the ECT seizure, and then either increased or decreased relative to baseline after ECT, depending in part on the timing and measurement technique employed. The increase in cerebral blood flow during the seizure produces a brief increase in intracranial pressure that is rarely of clinical consequence but is the reason for extreme caution when ECT is used in patients with space-occupying mass lesions. Studies of cerebral permeability generally confirm that the structural *integrity of the blood-brain barrier* is maintained during ECT, despite the rise in cerebral blood flow. A variety of changes in regional *cerebral glucose metabolism* (measured with positron emission tomography) are reported either during or after ECT (Nobler et al. 2001), but no consistent patterns have emerged. The effects of age on all these cerebral physiological changes have not been described systematically, although in animals, age is associated with increased blood-brain permeability changes after 10 electroconvulsive seizures (Oztas et al. 1990).

Cardiovascular Physiology

ECT results in a marked activation of the autonomic nervous system, and the relative balance of parasympathetic and sympathetic nervous system activity determines the observed cardiovascular effects (Applegate 1997). Vagal (parasympathetic) tone is increased during and immediately after administration of the electrical stimulus, and this may be manifested by bradycardia or even a brief period of asystole. With development of the seizure, activation of the sympathetic nervous system occurs, resulting in a marked increase in heart rate, blood pressure, and cardiac workload. Peripheral stigmata of sympathetic activation, including piloerection and gooseflesh, may also be observed. The tachycardia and hypertension continue through the ictus and generally end along with the seizure. Near or shortly after the end of the seizure, there may be a second period of increased vagal tone, which may be manifested by bradycardia and various dysrhythmias, including ectopic beats. As the patient awakens from anesthesia, there may be an additional period of increased heart rate and blood pressure as a result of arousal and further sympathetic outflow (Welch and Drop 1989).

The cardiovascular responses during ECT combine to produce an increase in myocardial oxygen demand and a decrease in coronary artery diastolic filling time. Transient electrocardiographic changes in the ST and T waves are seen in some patients during the procedure, but it is unclear whether these findings are related to myocardial ischemia (McCall 1997; Zvara et al. 1997). An alternative mechanism may be a direct effect of central nervous system stimulation on cardiac repolarization (Welch and Drop 1989). No corresponding increase in levels of cardiac enzymes has been found to accompany these electrocardiographic changes (Braasch and Demaso 1980). In a study of patients receiving ECT, Messina et al. (1992) obtained echocardiograms during and after ECT treatments and found transient regional wall motion abnormalities more often in patients with ST-T wave changes on electrocardiograms (ECGs), suggesting a period of demand myocardial ischemia. The clinical importance of these findings remains to be evaluated.

The effects of age on the cardiovascular response to ECT have been examined in only a few modern studies. Shettar et al. (1989) randomly assigned 19 patients (mean age 51 years; range 19–84 years) to ECT with pretreatment with glycopyrrolate or with placebo; the alternate pretreatment drug was used for the subsequent ECT treatment (i.e., each patient served as his or her own control). For both types of pretreatment, there was no correlation between age and length of poststimulus asystole. In two controlled studies of mixed-age samples that included elderly patients (Prudic et al. 1987; Webb et al. 1990), no relationship was found between age and ECT-induced changes in heart rate, blood pressure, or rate-pressure product. In a study of relatively younger patients (mean age 43 years; range 20–64 years), Huang et al. (1989) noted a significant inverse correlation between age and increases in blood pressure and rate-pressure product.

Although these results suggest that age, per se, is not associated with the extent of the cardiovascular response to ECT, these findings must be interpreted cautiously. Some of the subjects in these studies (especially those who were older) were also receiving antihypertensive drug therapy that may have attenuated their cardiovascular response to the treatments, and other clinical observations suggest that at least some elderly patients with cardiovascular disease may be at risk for marked increases in pulse and blood pressure during ECT (Applegate 1997; Zielinski et al. 1993; see also "Cardiovascular Side Effects" later in this chapter).

Mechanisms of Action of ECT

Despite considerable research into the neurobiology of ECT, its mechanism of action remains a mystery. ECT produces both acute and long-standing changes in brain chemistry, endocrinology, physiology, and neurogenesis and neuroplasticity (Holtzmann et al. 2007; Wahlund and von Rosen 2003). Current hypotheses of the mechanism of action of ECT focus on the *anticonvulsant effects* of the treatment (Sackeim 1999) or the extent and efficiency of *seizure generalization* throughout the brain and the resultant neurobiological effects in relevant brain regions (particularly prefrontal and diencephalic) (Abrams 2002b). It remains unclear, however, whether any of these neurobiological changes account for the clinical effects of ECT or whether they merely represent epiphenomena. Furthermore, the broad therapeutic spectrum of ECT (i.e., in addition to its antidepressant properties, ECT also exhibits antimanic, antipsychotic, anticonvulsant, and anticatatonic effects) would seem to make it unlikely that a single mechanism of action will explain all of these effects.

Technique of ECT

Pretreatment Evaluation

When a patient is referred for ECT, a formal pretreatment evaluation is carried out by a practitioner credentialed in ECT to 1) determine if ECT is indicated, 2) establish baseline measures of efficacy and cognitive side effects, 3) identify and treat any general medical conditions that may increase the risk of adverse effects (performed in conjunction with an anesthesia provider), 4) determine the setting (inpatient or outpatient) in which the treatments should be administered, 5) initiate the process of informed consent, and 6) prepare the patient and family or significant other for the procedure (American Psychiatric Association 2001; Coffey 1998).

The *indications for ECT* (discussed in "Diagnostic Indications and Efficacy" earlier in this chapter) are confirmed through a thorough neuropsychiatric history and examination (see Chapter 4, "Neuropsychiatric Assessment"). The patient's response to previous therapies, including ECT, should be thoroughly documented. Handedness should also be assessed because of its relevance to nondominant unilateral electrode placement (Kellner et al. 1997). Because the hand used for writing is a fallible indicator, patients should be asked which hand they use to throw a ball, cut with a knife, and so on (American Psychiatric Association 2001).

The neuropsychiatric history and examination also provide an opportunity to obtain *objective baseline data* essential for assessing the outcome of the course of ECT. A variety of measures of symptom severity are available for each diagnostic indication (e.g., the Montgomery-Åsberg Depression Rating Scale or the Hamilton Rating Scale for Depression for depression, the Brief Psychiatric Rating Scale for psychosis), and these can be used as markers of efficacy when administered regularly over the treatment course. Both clinician- and patient-rated instruments should be considered, given the potential dissociation between observer- and self-rated symptom severity. Measurement of baseline cognitive function (in particular, attention and memory) is essential to assess any cognitive side effects from the course of ECT. The ideal cognitive measure would be brief, inexpensive, simple to administer, and sensitive to change in both verbal and nonverbal spheres, and it would have multiple forms (to avoid practice effects). Although several instruments are available, none is ideal, and options range from a bedside mental status examination, to a brief instrument such as the Mini-Mental State Examination, to formal neuropsychological testing.

A general medical history and examination are also performed to identify any active *general medical problems*, with a focus on the brain, the cardiovascular system, the musculoskeletal system, the dentition, and the upper gastrointestinal tract. Any personal or family history of problems with anesthesia should also be noted. A limited laboratory evaluation (serum potassium, ECG) is sufficient for most patients, with other studies ordered only as clinically indicated. Consultation with anesthesia specialists is important because the provision of general anesthesia is associated with some, albeit small, medical risk. Indeed, an anesthesiologist experienced in ECT may also serve as the "general medical" consultant and can greatly facilitate the evaluation of patients with serious systemic illness. Although ECT has no "absolute" contraindications, serious disease of the brain (e.g., aneurysm, tumor), heart (ischemia or failure), or other systems (e.g., pheochromocytoma, retinal detachment) will require stabilization and optimal treatment and may necessitate additional consultation with other specialists, such as cardiologists, neurologists, or neurosurgeons.

Adjustments may also be required in some of the patient's *general medications*. Theophylline levels should be monitored closely or discontinued if possible, because high blood levels during ECT have been associated with status epilepticus (Fink and Sackeim 1998). Metrifonate and echothiophate are organophosphate medications that irreversibly inhibit cholinesterase and pseudocholinesterase, and may cause prolonged apnea when combined with succinylcholine and should not be given. In theory, the duration of succinylcholine muscle relaxation could be increased by cholinesterase inhibitors such as rivastigmine, donepezil, tacrine, and galantamine, which are used in patients with Alzheimer's disease (see Chapter 16, "Alzheimer's Disease and the Frontotemporal Dementia Syndromes"). However, case reports (Zink et al. 2002) and growing clinical experience suggest that acetylcholinesterase inhibitors may be continued safely during ECT. Otherwise, patients should take any required medications as scheduled.

Typically, *psychotropic medications* are stopped before ECT, with the exception of antipsychotics and possibly antidepressants (Farah et al. 1995). Lithium taken around the time of ECT has been linked to an increased occurrence of delirium and prolonged seizures (Weiner et al. 1980). For most patients, lithium can be discontinued or at least held for 1 day before ECT, with serum lithium levels kept as low as clinically feasible (Dolenc and Rasmussen 2005; Kellner et al. 1991a). Complete discontinuation of lithium may not be advisable for other patients with severe and recurrent mood disorder, particularly when ECT is used as a continuation/maintenance treatment. Thus, the decision to use lithium concurrent with ECT must be made on a case-by-case basis. Benzodiazepine use should be minimized or stopped, whenever possible, before ECT. Benzodiazepines may impair the induction or spread of the therapeutic seizure, thereby potentially decreasing treatment response (Kellner 1997b; Pettinati et al. 1986). The use of these agents by elderly patients may also theoretically increase their susceptibility to cognitive side effects from ECT. When necessary, the use of the lowest feasible doses of agents with relatively short half-lives and no active metabolites (e.g., lorazepam, oxazepam) has been recommended (American Psychiatric Association 2001). Similarly, anticonvulsant medications prescribed for psychiatric indications (e.g., mood stabilizers) should usually be tapered and discontinued before ECT, to avoid problems with seizure induction or effectiveness. Antidepressant medications are usually stopped to avoid cumulative cardiac and central nervous system side effects, although this practice is now being reconsidered, particularly with the newer agents (American Psychiatric Association 2001). Studies have reported conflicting findings on whether the addition of an antidepressant medication enhances the efficacy of ECT (Lauritzen et al. 1996; Mayur et al. 2000; Sackeim et al. 2009; Seager and Bird 1962).

Initiating the *informed consent process* is another essential element of the pre-ECT workup. Written informed consent for ECT is required from any patient with the capacity to give voluntary consent, and the consent form and process must be in compliance with all applicable laws, statutes, and standards. Patients who lack such a capacity may require the judicial appointment of a legal guardian to provide the consent. The American Psychiatric Association provides a pertinent sample of an informed consent document for ECT and discusses in detail the appropriate process for obtaining such consent (American Psychiatric Association 2001).

The complexities of voluntary consent for an elderly patient with a neuropsychiatric disorder are discussed in Chapter 14, "Ethical and Legal Issues." With the increased prevalence of cognitive impairment in elderly patients, competency to consent becomes a major issue, and the education of both patient and family becomes essential. This is also a time in the patient's life cycle when children are becoming increasingly responsible for their parents, and the patient's children should be involved in the consent process whenever possible. Of particular relevance to ECT, compared with younger patients, those over age 65 appear to be less aware that they can refuse ECT (Malcolm 1989).

Finally, the pre-ECT evaluation affords the clinician an opportunity to establish important interpersonal relationships with the patient and family. These relationships can be therapeutic and enhance patient satisfaction, as well as provide personal reward to the clinician.

ECT Procedure

In the United States, ECT is commonly given as a series of single treatments on alternate mornings, typically at a frequency of three times a week (on Monday, Wednesday, and Friday). Many patients receive the treatments on an outpatient basis, as long as certain precautions are taken (Fink et al. 1996). First, the patient's psychiatric illness must allow for safe management outside the hospital. Clearly, acute suicide risk or agitated psychosis often requires hospitalization. Second, the patient's general medical status should be stable enough for safe outpatient management. In addition, elderly persons are at risk for falling, and ECT may temporarily exacerbate this risk (Rao et al. 2008). Third, strong social support is required, because family members or others must transport the patient to and from the treatment facility, ensure that the patient takes nothing by mouth for at least 8 hours before a treatment session, and provide supervision between treatments (with particular attention paid to ensuring that the patient refrains from driving and making important financial or personal decisions while experiencing cognitive side effects) (Fink 1994). For some patients, it is helpful to administer the first (or several initial) ECT treatment(s) on an inpatient basis and then switch to outpatient treatments once it has been established that outpatient treatments can be administered safely and comfortably.

The treatment team consists of a psychiatrist, an anesthesiologist, and specially trained nursing personnel. ECT is typically given in either a special treatment suite or the recovery area of an operating room suite. Patients have been previously evaluated for treatment indications and coexisting general medical conditions by the ECT practitioner and anesthesia provider, appropriate treatment of these conditions has been implemented, and the consent process has been initiated. Patients should have nothing to eat or drink for at least 8 hours before treatment. The standard technique requires the establishment of a patent intravenous line. Electrodes for stimulation and for monitoring the seizure are applied according to appropriate technique (Kellner et al. 1997). Before anesthesia induction, a verbal "time-out" procedure should be conducted to confirm the patient's identity and details of the procedure (e.g., stimulus electrode placement, medication dosages). Administration of the anesthesia and maintenance of the patient's airway are under the direction of the anesthesia provider. The medication sequence includes anticholinergic premedication (glycopyrrolate or atropine) to prevent vagal-mediated cardiac slowing (if indicated), followed by an anesthetic (usually methohexital) and then succinylcholine for muscle relaxation. Throughout the procedure, the patient is ventilated with 100% oxygen by mask, and heart rate, ECG, blood pressure, and blood oxygen saturation are monitored.

Once the patient is asleep and thoroughly relaxed, a specially designed bite block is inserted into the patient's mouth, to protect the tongue and teeth from injury during jaw clenching as the electrical stimulus is applied (caused by direct electrical stimulation of the temporalis muscles). A predetermined electrical stimulus (see "Electrical Stimulus Mode, Waveform, and Dosing" later in this chapter) is delivered across electrodes placed on the patient's properly prepared scalp. Typically, a generalized seizure ensues and lasts from 30 to 60 seconds. The seizure is monitored by electroencephalography and by observation of the motor manifestations of the seizure, typically at the right ankle where a blood pressure cuff was inflated above systolic pressure immediately before administration of succinylcholine (the cuff is deflated once the seizure has ended). Ventilatory support is continued until the patient emerges from the anesthesia, and further recovery is provided in an environment with as little stimulation as possible. The entire procedure takes ~20 minutes, and patients are often able to have breakfast within 1 hour of the time of treatment. They are discharged shortly thereafter.

A typical acute course of ECT consists of 6 to 12 treatments, although occasionally patients may require fewer or more treatments to achieve full response. The treatment schedule is often modified in elderly patients to lessen cognitive side effects, with treatments given once or twice per week rather than three times per week (American Psychiatric Association 2001; Freeman 1995; Kellner et al. 1992; Lerer et al. 1995). ECT is stopped when maximal clinical improvement is thought to have been achieved or when further improvement is not noted between treatments. Special attention is then given to continuation/maintenance treatment with either medication or ECT.

Anesthesia Considerations

Brief, light general anesthesia is used during ECT to render the patient unconscious during (and thus amnesic for) the procedure. Methohexital is the agent of choice because it has a rapid onset and a brief duration of action, it induces minimal post-anesthesia confusion, and it is relatively inexpensive. Methohexital also appears to have a lesser anticonvulsant effect than thiopental or propofol (Bergsholm and Swartz 1996), which benefits seizure induction and spread. Still, because methohexital is an anticonvulsant and because the seizure threshold is often increased in elderly patients (see the following section), the lowest effective anesthetic dose is desirable. Because methohexital dosing is based on lean body mass, the required methohexital dosage in many elderly patients may be less than 1 mg/kg total body weight (Fragen and Avram 1990).

Etomidate is a reasonable alternative to methohexital, especially in cases of severe cardiovascular disease, but it is more expensive and is associated with pain on infusion, longer cognitive recovery time, and short-term adrenocortical suppression. Ketamine may be considered in patients with high seizure thresholds because of its proconvulsant properties, although it is somewhat slower acting and has a longer duration of action. Propofol, another alternative anesthetic agent, is well tolerated but has anticonvulsant properties and may be associated with shorter seizures (American Psychiatric Association 2001).

The preferred neuromuscular blocking agent for ECT is succinylcholine, primarily because it has rapid onset and a brief duration of action. The use of succinylcholine may require special consideration in elderly patients. Succinylcholine indirectly stimulates muscarinic cholinergic receptors in the sinus node, causing a prolonged depolarization followed by a depolarized state, which is resistant to further stimulation. The initial depolarization may contribute to bradycardia, especially if serial doses are required. This effect may be pronounced in patients receiving beta-blockers and in those with evidence of preexisting conduction delay, both frequently the case among elderly patients. Pretreatment with anticholinergics, such as atropine or glycopyrrolate, will block this bradycardic effect. Succinylcholine may also trigger life-threatening hyperkalemia in patients who have muscle wasting, a potential concern in some elderly patients who have severe inanition from melancholia or in those who have been relatively immobilized (e.g., from stroke or neuromuscular disorders). Use of a nondepolarizing muscle relaxant should be considered in these patients.

Intragastric pressure also increases with the use of succinylcholine, related to abdominal skeletal muscle fasciculation, and this may increase the risk of gastric reflux and aspiration. Certain groups of elderly patients (e.g., those with hiatal hernia, gastroparesis, or morbid obesity) are at risk for substantial gastroesophageal reflux during the procedure, with subsequent risk for aspiration pneumonitis (Zibrak et al. 1988). Smokers are particularly prone to morbidity from aspiration (Lichtor 1990). In these patients, additional strategies beyond withholding oral food and fluids before a session may be considered to decrease gastric acidity (e.g., premedication with histamine H_2 receptor antagonists or sodium citrate) and volume (e.g., premedication with metoclopramide) (Lichtor 1990).

Electrical Stimulus Mode, Waveform, and Dosing

The ECT stimulus should be delivered with a contemporary bidirectional, constant-current, brief-pulse device. A constant current provides for stable delivery of the ECT stimulus over a range of patient impedances. The brief-pulse waveform, with a pulse width of 0.5–2 milliseconds, is a more efficient and physiological stimulus for inducing seizures, relative to the sine wave current (phase period ~8.33 milliseconds) employed by early-model ECT devices, and therefore is associated with decidedly fewer cognitive side effects without loss of efficacy. The two major ECT devices currently produced in the United States—spECTrum by MECTA (Figure 10–1) and Thymatron System IV by Somatics (Figure 10–2)—are designed to deliver constant-current, brief-pulse stimulation, the use of which is strongly recommended by numerous professional organizations.

The *ECT stimulus intensity*, or stimulus dosage, should be sufficiently above the patient's seizure threshold to induce an effective seizure. Older patients require higher ECT stimulus intensities to elicit such seizures than do younger patients, because seizure threshold (the amount of electricity required to elicit a seizure) increases with age, as well as with gender (higher in males) and stimulus electrode placement (higher in bitemporal than in unilateral nondominant) (Coffey et al. 1995a; Sackeim et al. 1991). This age effect is believed to be the result of a decrease in the excitability of the brain but may also be partially due to increases in skull thickness (electrical resistance) with aging. It should be noted that the efficiency of seizure induction with the brief-pulse stimulus may vary as a function of the parameters (i.e., pulse width, frequency, duration, and current) of the stimulus set. For a given stimulus charge, those stimuli with shorter pulse widths and longer

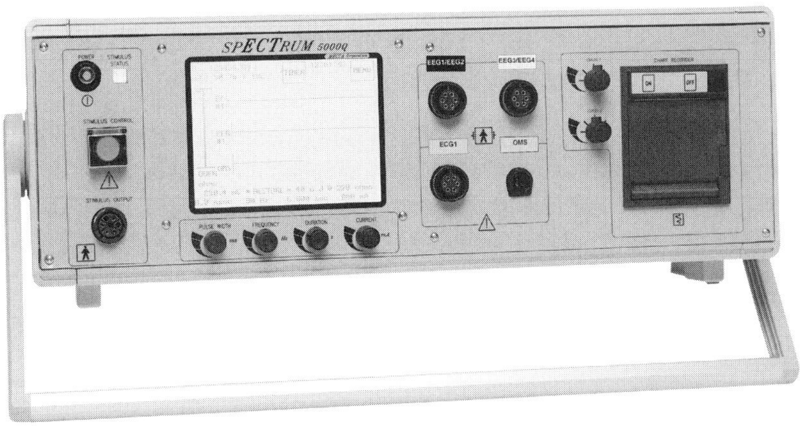

FIGURE 10–1. Frontal view of the spECTrum 5000Q ECT device by MECTA.

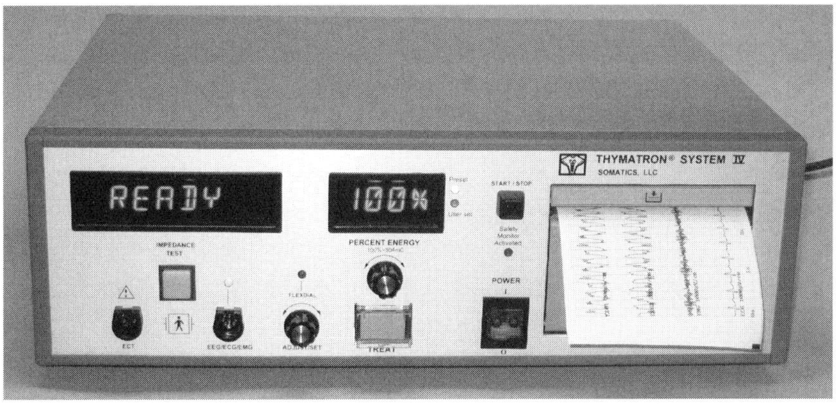

FIGURE 10–2. Frontal view of the Thymatron System IV ECT device by Somatics.

train durations are more efficient at seizure induction (i.e., are associated with a lower seizure threshold) than those with longer pulse widths. We recommend using parameter sets that employ pulse widths of 0.5–1 milliseconds. Research is under way to determine the clinical effects of even shorter pulse widths (so-called ultra-brief-pulse ECT) (Sackeim et al. 2008).

The precise stimulus dosage for optimal ECT has yet to be determined. Data in adult mixed-age samples suggest an interaction of stimulus dosage, stimulus parameters, electrode placement, and clinical efficacy. Bitemporal ECT is clinically effective at a stimulus dosage of 1.5–2.5 times seizure threshold (so-called moderate-dose ECT), but optimal unilateral nondominant ECT may require a stimulus dosage of ~4–6 times seizure threshold (so-called high-dose ECT) to match the efficacy of bitemporal ECT (McCall et al. 2000; Sackeim et al. 1993, 2000, 2008). In a study of 39 elderly inpatients with major depression, Stoppe et al. (2006) found similar rates of remission in those randomly assigned to high-dose unilateral nondominant ECT (88% remission) and in those who received moderate-dose bitemporal ECT (68% response rate). Thus, a critical factor in the efficacy of ECT appears to be the stimulus dosage relative to the patient's seizure threshold, adjusted for the effects of stimulus electrode placement.

The ECT specialist may use a number of options to determine the proper stimulus dosage for an individual patient (Coffey 2008). One approach is to employ a stimulus titration procedure at the first treatment to estimate initial seizure threshold and then adjust stimulus dosage upward accordingly at subsequent treatments (Coffey et al. 1995a). However, with this maneuver the first treatment can be assumed to be less than optimally effective if unilateral nondominant electrode placement is employed (because the seizure will be elicited by a "barely suprathreshold" stimulus dosage known to be subtherapeutic), and it carries a small risk of bradycardia and asystole associated with stimulation of the parasympathetic nervous system. These problems are obviated by an alternate "fixed-dose" method wherein the initial stimulus dose is set at 75%–100% of the maximum output (~576 mC) of contemporary U.S. ECT devices for right unilateral electrode placement or at approximately half the patient's age (in percentage of device output) for bilateral electrode placement (Petrides and Fink 1996). That dosage could then be titrated upward or downward at subsequent ECT treatments, using some established physiological "benchmark" of an "effective" seizure, such as peak heart rate or quantitative EEG metrics (e.g., percentage adequacy, postictal suppression index).

Seizure threshold increases during ECT (the well-known anticonvulsant effect), at times necessitating increases in stimulus dose during the course of therapy (Coffey et al. 1990, 1995b; Kellner et al. 1997). This effect does not appear to be more pronounced in elderly patients, but because this population has a higher initial seizure threshold, some older patients may eventually require stimulus intensities during their course of treatment that exceed the maximal dosage of the ECT device (Krystal et al. 2000; Lisanby et al. 1996). In this setting, successful seizure induction may be accomplished with the use of more efficient stimulus parameter sets (as discussed above) or by a switch to a proconvulsant anesthetic agent such as ketamine.

Stimulus Electrode Placement

ECT is generally administered through stimulus electrodes placed bitemporally, bifrontally, or in a unilateral nondominant position (the right side for most patients). The choice of stimulus electrode placement is complex. Studies in mixed-age samples of adults suggest that right unilateral ECT has fewer cognitive side effects, but as noted above, unless stimulus dosage and electrode application are carefully prescribed and certain medications restricted, treatment efficacy may be limited with this placement. Bilateral (bitemporal) electrode placement may be more reliably effective but may be associated with greater cognitive side effects (for a review, see Abrams 2002b).

Few studies have addressed the issue of electrode placement specifically in elderly patients. In a meta-analysis of the early literature, Pettinati et al. (1986) found a trend for improved efficacy in elderly patients receiving bilateral treatment. In one of the few controlled studies, Fraser and Glass (1980) assigned 29 elderly patients with depression to either unilateral or bilateral ECT two times a week. Stimulus-dosing strategies were unclear. No group differences were observed in terms of therapeutic response or memory performance after ECT, but those subjects randomly assigned to bilateral electrode placement required more time to become reoriented after the fifth ECT treatment. More recently, Stoppe et al. (2006) randomly assigned 39 elderly inpatients to unilateral or bitemporal high-dose ECT and found similar remission rates (88% and 68%, respectively) but fewer cognitive side effects with unilateral ECT. No studies have examined whether the effects of cerebral disease or age-related structural brain changes modify the therapeutic or adverse effects of unilateral versus bilateral ECT in elderly patients.

Thus, limited data exist to guide the choice of ECT electrode placement in elderly patients with neuropsychiatric illness. A reasonable approach in most elderly patients is to begin with unilateral nondominant ECT at a sufficiently high stimulus dosage; if minimal or no response is seen by the fifth or sixth treatment, then switch to bilateral ECT at moderate stimulus dosage. Because bilateral ECT may be associated with a statistically greater likelihood of response, it may be considered the treatment of choice in patients in urgent need of care. If intolerable cognitive side effects develop with bilateral ECT, the treatment may be changed to unilateral ECT once the affective disorder has begun to respond (other techniques for lessening cognitive side effects are discussed later in this chapter in "Adverse Effects of ECT and Their Management"). Finally, atypical electrode placements (e.g., left unilateral, right frontotemporal–left frontal, or bifrontal) may be clinically useful in some elderly patients (Bailine et al. 2000; Kellner 1997a, 2000; Little et al. 2004).

Seizure Monitoring

The ECT seizure should be monitored to confirm that a seizure has occurred and to determine when it has ended (Kellner et al. 1997; Weiner and Krystal 1993). The seizure may be monitored indirectly by observation of the motor response (convulsion) of a "cuffed" extremity, but additional monitoring with ictal electroencephalogram is now considered the standard of care. The ictal electroencephalogram has been studied using sophisticated computer analysis to determine whether seizure "potency" (and treatment efficacy) may be predicted by various indices such as amplitude, regularity, or coherence (Krystal et al. 1995, 1996; Weiner and Krystal 1993). Newer ECT devices now provide quantitative estimates of various ictal EEG indices, but their routine clinical utility is limited at present by their sensitivity to EEG artifacts, variation in EEG lead placement, and interindividual and intraindividual variation in the ictal electroencephalogram (Krystal et al. 1998).

Treatment Frequency and Number

A course of 6 to 12 treatments is usually required for treatment of an acute episode of major or bipolar depression, although fewer or more treatments are sometimes needed. Patients with schizophrenia may require a larger number of treatments. In the United States, the treatments are typically given thrice weekly, but in Europe a twice-weekly schedule is often employed.

The treatments are continued until the patient has reached a maximum level of response, at which point their frequency is tapered in preparation for continuation treatment. As discussed above, the ECT treatment technique should be modified (e.g., switch stimulus electrode placement, increase stimulus dosage) if no improvement is seen by the sixth treatment.

Alternative treatments should be considered if no response is observed by 8 to 10 treatments, although in some cases a longer series of treatments will be necessary.

Continuation/Maintenance Treatment

Because mood disorders are increasingly recognized as chronic, relapsing conditions, successful acute treatment should be followed by some form of continuation or maintenance treatment to prevent relapse or recurrence of the mood episode (see Chapter 19, "Mood Disorders"). Studies in mixed-age samples of adults with major depressive disorder have found 6-month relapse rates as high as 50% for patients initially responsive to antidepressants who were subsequently withdrawn from the medications (Prien and Kupfer 1986). Relapse rates following successful pharmacotherapy for major depression are substantially reduced by continuation of antidepressant medication at full dosage (Frank et al. 1990). Similarly high rates of relapse have been noted in adults with depression following ECT response when no form of continuation therapy was given (Jarvie 1954). The risk of relapse after successful acute ECT may be particularly high (especially in the first 4 months following ECT) in patients with major depression who were resistant to medication or who displayed psychotic symptoms during their index episode of illness (Grunhaus et al. 1995; Sackeim et al. 1993).

For continuation treatment in patients with *major depression* who are successfully treated with ECT acutely, there are two options: combination pharmacotherapy or continuation ECT. Controlled data suggest that continuation pharmacotherapy with nortriptyline and lithium (6-month relapse rate of 39%) is superior to nortriptyline alone (6-month relapse rate of 60%), which is in turn superior to placebo (6-month relapse rate of 84%), in preventing relapse of major depression in adults who have responded to an acute course of ECT (Sackeim et al. 2001). Continuation treatment with ECT is another option for continuation/maintenance treatment following successful acute ECT treatment, particularly in patients who have psychotic depression or those who were resistant to medication during the index episode (Fink 2007). Controlled data in a mixed-age sample of adults with major depression indicated that continuation ECT is comparable to continuation pharmacotherapy (nortriptyline and lithium) following a successful acute course of brief-pulse bitemporal ECT given at 1.5 times seizure threshold (6-month relapse rates of 37% and 32%, respectively) (Kellner et al. 2006). These data extend clinical reports of successful continuation ECT in elderly patients with major depression (Clark et al. 1989; Dubin et al. 1992; Loo et al. 1991; Monroe 1991; Thienhaus et al. 1990).

Continuation/maintenance ECT typically involves single treatments administered on an outpatient basis, initially at weekly intervals and then gradually reduced in frequency to every 4–8 weeks, as the patient's symptoms allow. The increased interval between treatments results in fewer cognitive side effects than during an acute course of ECT, and this has led to the suggestion that bilateral electrode placement may be preferred for continuation/maintenance ECT. The logistical factors in outpatient ECT are defined in the report by the Task Force on Ambulatory ECT of the Association for Convulsive Therapy (Fink et al. 1996).

No controlled data have been reported to inform the choice of whether to use pharmacotherapy or ECT for continuation treatment following successful ECT in patients with major depression. In clinical practice many clinicians use the rule "what got you well is what will keep you well," which would lead to a recommendation for ECT provided that it was reasonably well tolerated. For at least some patients, however, the logistical issues involved in months or years of continuation ECT are simply not manageable, and they prefer to take their chances with medication.

As noted earlier in this chapter, patients with *bipolar disorder* may be successfully treated with ECT for acute mania or bipolar depression. Following such acute treatment, we generally recommend at least 9–12 months of maintenance treatment with ECT, although there are no controlled data on this issue. During this maintenance ECT course, we continue to withhold mood-stabilizing agents (e.g., lithium, anticonvulsants) to avoid their potential complications (discussed in "Pretreatment Evaluation" earlier in this chapter). On the other hand, some clinicians are concerned that breakthrough mood syndromes may occur as the frequency of the maintenance ECT treatments is decreased, and thus they prefer to administer a mood stabilizer between treatments, holding the dose a few days before a scheduled ECT treatment to avoid potential complications. Most patients with bipolar disorder require lifetime maintenance treatment with at least a mood stabilizer (e.g., lithium, anticonvulsants). Some clinical literature and our own experience suggest that ECT may serve this role (alone or in combination with psychotropic medication variously prescribed) in some patients who tolerate the procedure and related logistical issues well.

Following successful treatment with an acute course of ECT, most patients with *schizophrenia* receive maintenance treatment with antipsychotic medication (occasionally in combination with other psychotropic medications). The potential role of maintenance ECT in such patients has not been studied.

Adverse Effects of ECT and Their Management

The safety of ECT compares favorably with that of any treatment requiring general anesthesia. The mortality is variously reported as approximating 1 death per 80,000 treatments (the same as for general anesthesia for minor surgery) and may actually be decreasing with improved management of underlying general medical illnesses. To put these data into perspective, Abrams (2002b) noted that ECT is 10 times safer than childbirth.

Kroessler and Fogel (1993) compared the mortality during long-term follow-up of 65 depressed patients ages 80 and older who had been treated with ECT or antidepressant medication. Although the 2-year survival rate was 54% in the group treated with ECT and 90% in the group treated with medication, this group difference was probably related to more severe depression and physical illness in the patients who received ECT. The course of ECT itself was remarkably well tolerated by these elderly patients, with a median interval between ECT and time of death of 20 months. The authors called for further attention to general medical comorbidity as a prognostic factor in future outcome studies of geriatric depression. Abrams (2002a) noted that the estimated mortality rate among community-dwelling elderly patients (~0.26% per each 3 weeks) was an order of magnitude higher than that observed after a 3-week course of eight ECT treatments in elderly patients (~0.016%). As noted earlier in "Medical Physiology of ECT," the major physiological impact of ECT is on the heart, vasculature, and brain.

Cardiovascular Side Effects

A proportion of elderly patients referred for ECT have serious preexisting cardiovascular disease. Common cardiac conditions, such as hypertension, ischemic heart disease, atrial and ventricular arrhythmia, aneurysm, and conduction system disease, require evaluation and optimized treatment before ECT to minimize any adverse effects from the hemodynamic events that occur during ECT (Priebe 2000).

Uncontrolled retrospective studies comparing the cardiovascular complication rate of ECT in older and younger patients have found an increase in transient and treatable complications in elderly patients. In a nonblinded retrospective chart review of 293 patients, Alexopoulos et al. (1984) found cardiovascular complications in 9% of the patients ages 65 and older, compared with 1% of the patients under age 65. Cardiac ischemia, arrhythmia, hypertension, and congestive heart failure were the most common complications, although the vast majority of complications were not clearly temporally related to ECT and did not prevent the completion of treatment. Burke et al. (1987) conducted a similar retrospective chart review of 136 subjects, 30% of whom were ages 60 and older. Sine wave bilateral ECT was used in 85% of cases. These investigators found a cardiorespiratory complication rate of 15% in patients ages 60 and older, compared with 3% in those under age 60. Complications were correlated with the number of cardiovascular medications the patient was receiving, with more medication presumably indicating those patients with more cardiovascular illness. These complications did not affect treatment response. In a chart review of 81 elderly patients, Cattan et al. (1990) found a 36% cardiovascular complication rate with ECT in patients over age 80, compared with 12% in younger geriatric patients. As would be expected, the older patients had more general medical diagnoses and were receiving more cardiovascular medication than were the younger patients.

Two controlled studies of ECT in a total of 66 high-risk patients with cardiovascular disease have demonstrated the safety of ECT in elderly individuals. Zielinsky et al. (1993) compared the rate of cardiac complications in a group of 40 depressed patients (mean age 68.9 years; range 54–84 years) with serious preexisting cardiac disease (left ventricular impairment, conduction delay, and ventricular arrhythmias) with the rate of such complications in a group of 40 depressed patients (mean age 68.3 years; range 55–83 years) without cardiac disease. Not surprisingly, the group with preexisting cardiac disease had more complications. Most of the complications were transient (e.g., brief arrhythmias or increases in ectopy), however, and 38 of the 40 patients with cardiac disease were able to complete their course of ECT. Of note, this group of depressed patients with cardiac disease had even more difficulty with adverse cardiac effects from prior trials of tricyclic antidepressants; 11 of the 21 patients previously treated with tricyclic antidepressants had been forced to stop tricyclic treatment because of cardiovascular complications. Rice et al. (1994) used a case-control design to compare two groups of patients over age 50 receiving ECT. One group consisted of 26 patients at increased risk for cardiac complications, and 27 patients at standard risk made up the other group. Compared with the patients at standard risk for cardiac complications, patients in the high-risk group were older, had received more medical consultations before ECT, and experienced more minor medical complications from ECT. However, the two groups did not differ in terms of frequency of major medical complications, and no patients died or experienced permanent cardiac morbidity from ECT.

The data just reviewed suggest that ECT is a low-risk procedure, even for elderly patients (Applegate 1997). It is rare for ECT to be associated with severe cardiovascular complications, such as acute myocardial infarction, stroke, cardiovascular collapse, ventricular arrhythmia, or ruptured cerebral or aortic aneurysm. Still, prospective studies, carefully controlled for pretreatment severity of cardiovascular and other medical disease, are needed to evaluate the effects of age on cardiovascular complications of ECT.

Increasingly sophisticated general medical management during ECT helps to decrease the cardiovascular risk of treatment in elderly patients (Applegate 1997). The primary areas of concern are bradycardia, tachycardia, hypertension, and ventricular arrhythmia. Anticholinergic premedications (atropine and glycopyrrolate) may be used to prevent *vagally induced bradycardia*, but in elderly patients the use of these medications may be more complicated by confusion, tachycardia, constipation, and urinary retention. The method of serial electrical stimulations to determine a patient's seizure threshold (described earlier) may involve administration of subconvulsive stimuli, which may produce a vagal surge unaccompanied by the sympathetic outflow associated with a seizure. The use of this method, as well as the presence of conduction delay on the ECG, suggests the need for premedication with an anticholinergic, particularly if the patient is also receiving a beta-blocker medication. Outside of these clinical scenarios, some practitioners reserve the use of anticholinergic premedication for patients who develop substantial bradyarrhythmias during ECT.

A related issue is the safety of ECT in a patient with a vagus nerve stimulator (see Chapter 11, "Brain Stimulation Therapies"), the effects of which might be thought to be problematic if they add to the vagal effects of ECT. Although experience is limited, the safe use of ECT in a patient with the vagus nerve stimulator has been reported (Husain et al. 2002).

Although *hypertension* and *tachycardia* (mediated by sympathetic activation) are common during ECT, they are well tolerated by most patients, including elderly individuals (Webb et al. 1990). Therefore, it is usually unnecessary to routinely blunt the cardiovascular response to ECT in elderly patients unless such changes are extreme or are clearly associated with evidence of cardiovascular compromise. These robust hemodynamic responses may be attenuated by short-acting intravenous beta-blockers, such as labetalol or esmolol, or by nitroglycerine preparations (Howie et al. 1990; Stoudemire et al. 1990). It should be kept in mind that beta-blockers have anticonvulsant effects, and their use during ECT may limit the intensity of the ECT seizure and, in turn, its therapeutic potency. In addition, the acute use of antihypertensive medication may lead to clinically significant hypotension in elderly patients during the recovery period. Finally, in patients receiving adrenergic blockers, anticholinergic premedication should be considered so as to prevent a disproportionate decrease of sympathetic tone below parasympathetic tone, with resultant bradycardia (Abrams 2002b).

Marked *posttreatment ventricular ectopy* (multifocal or several consecutive premature ventricular contractions) may be treated with lidocaine (1–1.5 m/kg body weight). Because of its anticonvulsant properties, lidocaine should be given after termination of the seizure (Drop and Welch 1989). Stoudemire et al. (1990) found that ventricular ectopy could also be reduced by pretreatment with labetalol. The presence of a properly functioning implanted cardiac pacemaker is not a concern with ECT, provided the usual electrical safety precautions are followed (Abrams 2002b).

Cerebral Side Effects

There is no evidence that ECT causes structural brain damage (Devanand et al. 1994; Weiner 1984). Carefully controlled prospective brain imaging studies in humans reveal no changes in brain structure for up to 6 months after a course of ECT (Coffey 1993; Coffey et al. 1991), and other studies using proton magnetic resonance spectroscopy find that ECT is not associated with a decrease in the *N*-acetylaspartate signal, a sign of cell atrophy (Ende et al. 2000; Pfleiderer et al. 2003). Neuropathological studies in elderly humans who received numerous lifetime ECT treatments reveal no evidence of ECT-related injury (Scalia et al. 2007). Neuropathological studies in animals, including cell counts in regions thought to be at risk, reveal no evidence of brain damage when the seizures are induced under conditions that approximate standard clinical practice (i.e., when the seizures are temporally spaced, relatively brief, and modified by oxygenation and muscle relaxation). Furthermore, studies of the pathophysiology of seizure-induced structural brain damage in animals indicate that the conditions necessary for injury do not apply to the modern practice of ECT (Weiner 1984). In this regard, a brain metabolic imaging study of elderly patients with depression found no evidence of brain perfusion abnormalities at 1 year following a successful course of ECT (Navarro et al. 2004).

The robust cardiovascular responses associated with the ECT seizure have raised a theoretical concern that they may precipitate cerebrovascular events. The incidence of *cerebrovascular complications* with ECT is exceedingly rare, however. We are aware of only one reported case of ischemic stroke after ECT that was confirmed by brain imaging (Bruce et al. 2006). ECT has been given successfully to patients with cerebral aneurysms, with close management of blood pressure elevation (Krystal and Coffey 1997). An intracerebral hemorrhage reported in a normotensive patient during ECT was probably related to cerebral amyloid angiopathy (Weisberg et al. 1991). We know of no other reported case of intracerebral hemorrhage with ECT.

Cognitive Side Effects

The cognitive side effects of ECT include acute postictal confusion, impaired retrograde and anterograde memory, and occasionally interictal delirium. The extent of these adverse effects is related to certain patient factors, such as increased age (see Gardner and O'Connor 2008 for a review), general medical disease burden, and preexisting cognitive impairment, and to ECT technique factors (sine wave stimulus waveform, bitemporal electrode placement, grossly suprathreshold stimulus dosage, increased number or frequency of treatments, poor oxygenation during the procedure, and certain concomitant medications, such as lithium and anticholinergics) (see *The Journal of ECT,* Volume 24, No. 1, Special Issue: Cognitive Effects of ECT, 2008).

Acute Postictal Disorientation

Most patients experience mild disorientation immediately upon awakening during the post-ECT recovery process, which typically resolves within an hour or so (Calev et al. 1993). In a study focusing on elderly patients, Fraser and Glass (1978) measured time to recovery of full orientation in nine elderly patients with depression who received ECT in which electrode placement alternated (e.g., unilateral placement in one treatment followed by bilateral placement in the next treatment). When comparing these reorientation times with those reported in the literature for younger patients, the investigators observed that recovery in elderly patients took five times longer for unilateral treatment and nine times longer for bilateral treatment. Recovery time after bilateral ECT increased cumulatively over the course of ECT and with closer spacing of treatments. No such relationship was found for unilateral ECT. In a subsequent study of 29 elderly patients with depression randomly assigned to courses of either unilateral (n=13) or bilateral (n=16) sine wave ECT, Fraser and Glass (1980) found significantly longer reorientation times after the fifth ECT session among patients receiving bilateral treatments (32.8 minutes) than among those receiving unilateral treatments (9.5 minutes). In contrast to the group undergoing bilateral ECT, patients receiving unilateral ECT had a significant reduction in recovery time from the first to the last treatment.

In a study of subjective side effects during ECT, Devanand et al. (1995) found that older patients actually reported fewer severe cognitive symptoms (i.e., confusion/disorientation and amnesia) than did younger patients.

Agitated Delirium on Emergence From Anesthesia

Approximately 10% of patients receiving ECT experience an acute agitated delirium on emergence from anesthesia, characterized by restlessness, disorientation, combativeness, and poor response to commands. Age does not appear to be a risk for this complication (Devanand et al. 1989). This complication is usually managed effectively with supportive care, although occasionally treatment with intravenous benzodiazepines (e.g., midazolam, diazepam) or other sedatives (e.g., methohexital, propofol) may be required.

Interictal Delirium

In a small proportion of patients, ECT is associated with more prolonged disorientation and even frank interictal delirium. Most studies evaluating interictal delirium in elderly patients have used disorientation as a measure rather than the full DSM criteria for delirium. In a retrospective study involving 136 patients receiving mainly bilateral sine wave ECT, Burke et al. (1987) found disorientation (confusion severe enough to alter the treatment plan) in 18% of patients older than age 60, compared with 13% of younger patients. This incidence increased to 25% for patients over age 75. In a retrospective study in which mostly bilateral (waveform not specified) ECT was administered, Alexopoulos et al. (1984) found a somewhat greater incidence of confusion (disorientation to time, place, and person) in elderly patients (12.6%) than in younger patients (9.6%). Cattan et al. (1990) conducted a study involving primarily bilateral or combination bilateral-unilateral sine wave ECT and found a nonsignificant trend for more frequent severe disorientation (defined functionally by interference in ward activities) in elderly patients over age 80 (59%, n=39), compared with those patients 65–80 years old (45%, n=42).

In the study by Alexopoulos et al. (1984), elderly patients with a history of underlying brain disease were found to have higher levels of severe post-ECT confusion than were the young patients, suggesting that baseline cerebral impairment may increase the risk of adverse cognitive effects of ECT.

In several studies, subcortical brain disease has been implicated in the development of interictal delirium with ECT. We have found subcortical gray and white matter lesions to be more extensive in elderly patients who developed a prolonged interictal delirium during a course of ECT (Figiel et al. 1990). Still, the majority of these patients were able to continue ECT, with no decline in expected treatment response. All patients were free of delirium 1 week after ECT (Coffey et al. 1989; Figiel et al. 1990). The specificity of subcortical disease in producing delirium after ECT was further suggested by Martin et al. (1992), who found that patients with ischemic lesions of the caudate nucleus had a 92% incidence of delirium during ECT. Patients with a previous stroke in other brain regions had the same incidence of delirium as did a group of elderly depressed nonstroke control subjects receiving ECT (Martin et al. 1992). In a prospective study of seven consecutive patients with Parkinson's disease, Figiel et al. (1991) found a 100% incidence of interictal delirium during a course of ECT. The delirium lasted 7–21 days, longer than is typical, but 86% of patients recovered from depression.

In summary, although the duration and severity of acute post-ECT disorientation may increase with age, the majority of elderly patients appear to recover their orientation within 60 minutes of the treatment. In the small percentage of elderly patients who develop more prolonged confusion or frank delirium, underlying cerebral impairment may be contributory, especially dysfunction of the basal ganglia. Clearly, more research is needed in a larger number of elderly patients to characterize post-ECT confusion and to identify its risk factors, including the effects of preexisting cerebral impairment.

Amnesia

The depressive syndrome (as well as many other psychiatric syndromes) causes impairment in new learning. An acute course of contemporary brief-pulse ECT may improve this deficit as it improves the depression, but the treatment also causes a new deficit in memory such that newly learned information is rapidly forgotten. Explicit (especially autobiographical) memories are affected (implicit memory is spared), and both anterograde and retrograde deficits are seen, particularly for events that occurred closest to the time of treatment. This memory deficit is typically relatively mild and is presumed to be secondary to transient disruption of medial temporal lobe function. The anterograde amnesia typically resolves within a few weeks of ECT, whereas the retrograde deficit may resolve more gradually. Persistent and severe retrograde amnesia has been reported rarely following ECT (Sackeim 2000), but the interpretation and significance of such reports remain controversial (Abrams 2002a).

Given the large body of data on the amnestic effects of ECT, it is surprising that there has been relatively little controlled research on age as a risk factor (Abrams 1997; Calev et al. 1993; Fink 1979). Some (Fromholt et al. 1973; Heshe et al. 1978) but not all (d'Elia and Raotma 1977; Strömgren et al. 1976) early studies found that ECT-induced amnesia is worse in older patients. Zervas et al. (1993) examined age effects on memory in a study comparing twice-weekly and three-times-weekly brief-pulse bilateral ECT administered using contemporary techniques (given at "moderately suprathreshold" stimulus intensity). The sample consisted of 42 inpatients with a mean age (±SD) of 53.5±16.1 years; no patient was older than 65 years, however. Correlations were found between age and decrements in retrograde memory 1–3 days after the end of ECT but not at 1 month or 6 months posttreatment. Age was also correlated with decrements in verbal anterograde memory acutely and 1 month after ECT (but not 6 months after ECT) and with changes in figural anterograde memory acutely and 6 months after ECT. McElhiney et al. (1995) examined autobiographical memory in a mixed-age sample (mean age [±SD] 54±13.9 years) of 75 patients with depression randomly assigned with regard to electrode placement and stimulus intensity. Age was found to be a predictor of lower recall of autobiographical memories after ECT. In a follow-up report on this sample, the pre-ECT modified Mini-Mental State Examination score was predictive of the extent of retrograde autobiographical amnesia both 1 week and 2 months after ECT (Sobin et al. 1995). This study provided evidence in support of the conventional clinical wisdom that preexisting cognitive deficit is a risk factor for more severe ECT-induced amnesia.

Memory performance has been reported to improve with successful ECT in elderly patients with the pseudodementia of depression (Reynolds et al. 1987; Stoudemire et al. 1995). In the study by Fraser and Glass (1980) described earlier, all elderly patients showed impairment of memory function before ECT; during treatment, however, memory improved and was normal in all patients by 3 weeks after completion of the ECT course. No group differences were found on the basis of electrode placement.

Relatively little research has been done regarding the effects of age on subjective memory complaints after ECT (Prudic et al. 2000). As noted previously, Devanand et al. (1995) found that older patients actually reported fewer severe cognitive symptoms (i.e., confusion/disorientation and amnesia) than did younger patients.

In summary, controlled data appear to support the clinical wisdom that elderly patients are at greater risk for the cognitive side effects of ECT. More work is needed in a larger number of elderly patients (especially very old patients) to characterize the extent and severity of ECT-induced amnesia and to identify relevant risk factors, including the effects of preexisting cerebral impairment.

Managing Cognitive Side Effects During ECT

Recommendations for lessening ECT amnesia in elderly patients focus on risk factors related to the patients, as well as on aspects of the treatment technique. Patients should have their general medical health optimized as much as possible before commencing ECT, and concomitant medications with potential adverse effects on memory should be discontinued when possible. The ECT technique should employ proper anesthetic technique, a contemporary constant-current brief-pulse device, and careful consideration of the relative merits of unilateral versus bilateral stimulus electrode placement. If intolerable cognitive side effects develop, the frequency of treatments could be reduced from thrice to twice weekly (e.g., Monday and Friday). A variety of "memory-enhancing" pharmacological agents (e.g., indomethacin, piracetam, naloxone, choline, donepezil, and herbals) have been explored in animal models of ECT as well as in humans, but the data are insufficient to support routine clinical use at this time (Prakash et al. 2006; Prudic et al. 1998; Rao et al. 2002; Tang et al. 2002).

Side Effects in Other Organ Systems

Other organ systems that may be impaired in elderly patients need to be evaluated before ECT and include the lungs, bones, eyes, and teeth. Pulmonary status should be optimized before ECT. Patients with severe chronic obstructive pulmonary disease and carbon dioxide retention may require special ventilatory strategies during the treatment (Abrams 2002b). Pneumonia secondary to aspiration of gastric contents may occur rarely during ECT (Alexopoulos et al. 1984; Karlinsky and Shulman 1984).

Patients with osteoporosis, spinal disk disease, or spondylosis may require increased muscular relaxation during ECT. Such patients may require succinylcholine doses of at least 1–

1.5 mg/kg body weight, and they require careful attention to clinical evidence of adequate relaxation (e.g., loss of reflexes or tone, and disappearance of fasciculations) before delivery of the stimulus. Kellner et al. (1991b) reported the safe treatment of a patient with osteoporosis and cervical spondylosis with multiple subluxations of the cervical spine using succinylcholine doses of 1.3 mg/kg weight.

Because ECT produces a transient increase in intraocular pressure, patients with chronic open-angle glaucoma should receive their eyedrops before ECT. As noted earlier in "Technique of ECT," treatment with echothiophate, an irreversible cholinesterase inhibitor, should be stopped several days before ECT. Patients with acute closed-angle glaucoma or retinal detachment should be stabilized before ECT and watched closely by an ophthalmologist during an ECT course.

When a patient's teeth are loose, decayed, or asymmetrical, the risk of dental injury during ECT may be increased. A major portion of malpractice litigation with ECT is related to dental issues (Slawson 1985). A specially designed bite block must be inserted before delivery of the ECT stimulus. The tongue, cheeks, and lips must be kept clear of the clenching teeth. The bite block should be used even in edentulous patients. Occasionally, upper or lower dentures may be kept in place during the treatment to facilitate airway management. In patients with only a few remaining, and possibly loose, teeth, dental consultation or alternative bite block strategies (with the aim of shifting bite pressure to the molars) may be helpful (Welch 1993).

ECT in Elderly Patients With Neurological Disorders

Although mood disturbances are common in patients with neurological disorders, there are relatively few controlled data to inform their treatment (see chapters in Part IV, "Neuropsychiatric Syndromes and Disorders"). There are no controlled data on the safety and efficacy of ECT in depressed elderly patients with concomitant neurological disorders (Coffey et al. 2007; Van der Wurff et al. 2003); however, a substantial clinical experience suggests that ECT may be an important therapeutic option for many of these patients (Coffey et al. 2007; Evans et al. 2005; Krystal and Coffey 1997), particularly when there is an urgent need for rapid clinical improvement or when pharmacotherapy has been either ineffective or poorly tolerated. The safety of ECT in these patients depends critically on optimizing the treatment of the underlying neurological (and all other general medical) conditions and on modifying the technique of ECT where indicated to mitigate the procedure's physiological effects (e.g., increased intracranial pressure, increased blood pressure) (Coffey et al. 2007). In all such cases, a careful risk-benefit analysis should be conducted during the pre-ECT evaluation. In the following sections, we discuss some of the more common conditions in which ECT may be considered as a treatment option for elderly patients with a neurological disorder.

Dementia

As discussed in Chapter 16, "Alzheimer's Disease and the Frontotemporal Dementia Syndromes," depression is common in patients with dementia, and it has a critical impact on patients' survival and functional recovery. Treatment with antidepressant medications may help some but not all of these patients (see Chapter 19, "Mood Disorders").

A small clinical literature suggests that ECT may also be safe and effective for treating depression in patients with degenerative dementia, including those with Alzheimer's disease, vascular dementia, Friedreich's ataxia, and probable Lewy body dementia. In a literature review of 56 patients with dementia who received ECT for depression, Price and McAllister (1989) found the rate of response of depression to be 73%. ECT effectively treated depression in several subtypes of dementia, including senile dementia of the Alzheimer's type, multi-infarct dementia, and normal-pressure hydrocephalus, as well as the dementias of Parkinson's disease and Huntington's disease. Location of the stimulus electrodes was not specified in the majority of the cases reviewed. Nearly one-third of patients with dementia also had an improvement in cognition after ECT. Delirium was a relatively infrequent complication of ECT in these patients (overall occurrence of 21%), clearing by the time of discharge in all but 1 patient. Nelson and Rosenberg (1991) found that the ECT outcomes were similar in their 21 elderly patients with dementia and major depression, compared with a reference group of 84 elderly depressed patients without dementia. Rao and Lyketsos (2000) described their experience with 31 consecutive patients with dementia treated with ECT over a 5-year period at their institution. Approximately 68% of the sample was "clearly improved," and the most common adverse event was a transient delirium (seen in 49%). Rasmussen et al. (2003) described 7 patients with presumed Lewy body dementia who responded to ECT and tolerated the treatment well. Although these data are reassuring, prospective studies are needed to determine the efficacy and side effects of ECT in depressed patients with dementia.

To minimize cognitive side effects of ECT in patients with dementia, the ECT practitioner needs to pay special attention to issues of concomitant medications (including cholinesterase inhibitors, which may prolong the effect of succinylcholine as well as lower seizure threshold), electrode placement, and frequency of treatments (discussed earlier in "Technique of ECT"). Particular attention must be paid to issues of informed consent (see Chapter 14, "Ethical and Legal Issues").

Cerebrovascular Disease and Cerebral Aneurysm

As discussed in Chapter 25, "Cerebrovascular Disease," depression is common following stroke, and it has a critical impact on the patient's survival and functional recovery. Treatment with antidepressant medications may help some but not all such patients (see Chapter 19, "Mood Disorders").

Case reports and case series suggest that ECT may also be safe and effective for treating poststroke depression. In a retrospective chart review of 14 patients with poststroke depression (mean age 66 years) treated with ECT at Massachusetts General Hospital, Murray et al. (1986) found that 86% had marked improvement in depression after ECT. Apparently, no patient exhibited any worsening of neurological deficit, and although formal measures of cognitive status were not reported, 5 of the 6 patients with "cognitive impairment" before ECT showed lessening of this deficit after ECT. Currier et al. (1992) published retrospective data on 20 geriatric patients with poststroke depression treated with ECT at the same hospital, with predominantly nondominant unilateral electrode placement being used. A "marked or moderate response" to ECT was observed in 95% of the patients. No patient experienced any exacerbation of preexisting neurological deficits, but 3 patients exhibited "minor encephalopathic complications" (prolonged postictal confusion and amnesia) and 2 patients developed "severe interictal delirium requiring neuroleptics." Of note, 7 of their patients (37%) relapsed within a mean of 4 months after stopping ECT, despite ongoing maintenance drug therapy.

Elderly patients with no clinical history of stroke often have subcortical white matter hyperintensities on magnetic resonance images, which are believed to be evidence of ischemic cerebrovascular disease (see Chapter 19). Coffey et al. (1989) found a high rate (82%) of response to ECT in depressed patients with these magnetic resonance imaging findings, many of whom had been refractory to antidepressant drug therapy. In addition, the majority of the patients tolerated the course of ECT without major systemic or cognitive side effects. This positive outcome with ECT is especially notable given other data suggesting that subcortical ischemic disease may be associated with depressive illness that is resistant to treatment with antidepressant medications (Baldwin et al. 2004; Iosifescu et al. 2006).

The safety of ECT in a patient with cerebrovascular disease requires a thorough diagnostic assessment and optimal pre-ECT treatment of the cerebrovascular disease and any other general medical conditions. A diagnostic evaluation must clarify the precise etiology of the cerebrovascular event (arterial ischemic stroke vs. cerebral venous sinus occlusion vs. hemorrhagic stroke), and the treatment for that condition must be optimized. The clinician must also assess the potential effect of the underlying vascular disease on other organs impacted by ECT, notably the heart, and institute treatment when indicated. Before commencing ECT, it is preferable to wait at least several weeks if possible after the cerebral infarct to allow time for fragile cerebral vessels and tissue to heal, thereby reducing the theoretical risk of rupture from the increased cerebral blood flow. Occasionally, the ECT practitioner may employ antihypertensive medications during the ECT procedure to lessen the hemodynamic effects of the electrical stimulus and seizure.

The authors of several case and small series studies have reported on the safe and effective use of ECT in patients with intracranial aneurysm (including coil embolization) or various malformations, including arteriovenous malformations, venous angiomas, and cavernous hemangiomas (Okamura et al. 2006; Rasmussen and Flemming 2006; Zahedi et al. 2006). We are not aware of a report of patients with untreated cerebral aneurysm or malformation who experienced an intracranial hemorrhage with ECT. Nevertheless, we advise surgical correction of such lesions when indicated, before commencing ECT. If such surgery is not indicated, pharmacological attenuation of the hemodynamic responses during ECT should be considered.

Parkinson's Disease

As discussed in Chapter 24, "Parkinson's Disease and Movement Disorders," depression is common in patients with Parkinson's disease, and it has a critical impact on patients' survival and functional recovery. Treatment with antidepressant medications may help some but not all such patients (see Chapter 19, "Mood Disorders").

A small clinical literature suggests that ECT may be safe and effective for both the mood disorder and the motor disturbance associated with Parkinson's disease (reviewed by Kellner and Bernstein 1993). Interestingly, some patients experience improvement in motor symptoms but not improvement in mood, or vice versa (Kellner and Bernstein 1993).

A group of Swedish investigators (Andersen et al. 1987) performed the most methodologically rigorous trial of ECT in Parkinson's disease. In this double-blind, controlled, crossover design comparison of real ECT and sham ECT, 9 (82%) of 11 nondepressed elderly patients with the on-off phenomenon experienced substantial improvement in parkinsonian symptoms with ECT, with the improvement lasting 2–6 weeks. Sham ECT was ineffective. Nine patients received bilateral ECT (eight responded, one did not), and two patients received right unilateral ECT (one responded, one did not). Five to six treatments were given during the active phase of the trial. The stimulus-dosing strategy was not fully detailed in the report.

In a prospective naturalistic study, Douyon et al. (1989) studied seven patients with both Parkinson's disease and major depression. Substantial improvement in motor function was noted after only two bilateral treatments. Following an average of seven bilateral ECT treatments, with "just above threshold" stimulus dosing, mean New York University Parkinson's Disease Rating Scale scores decreased from 65 to 32 (51% improvement). Patients remained well, without further ECT, for 4 weeks to 6 months. Although initial scores on the Hamilton Rating Scale for Depression were determined for all seven patients (all scores were greater than 20), follow-up scores were determined for only four patients (these scores decreased by a mean of 50%). In another prospective naturalistic study, Zervas and Fink (1991) described the ECT treatment of four nondepressed elderly patients with severe, refractory Parkinson's disease. Three of the four patients received bilateral ECT. Stimulus-dosing strategies were not specified. Improvement in parkinsonism rating scores of 20%–40% was observed. Two patients were successfully treated with ongoing maintenance ECT, but once it was discontinued, the parkinsonism returned in both patients within 4–6 weeks. Aarsland et al. (1997) reported on two additional patients whose Parkinson's disease was successfully treated with maintenance ECT, and others have reported its utility for this purpose as well (Krystal and Coffey 1997; Wengel et al. 1998). Finally, ECT has also been found to be effective for neuroleptic-induced parkinsonism (Hermesh et al. 1992).

Because patients with parkinsonism may be at an increased risk of interictal delirium with ECT, we recommend commencing treatment with unilateral nondominant electrode placement. ECT may also be associated with dopaminergic side effects (dyskinesia, psychosis), in which case the dose of levodopa or other antiparkinsonian agents may need to be reduced carefully during the course of treatments. We do not recommend altering the dose of levodopa prior to ECT, because doing so may precipitate severe bradykinesia. Finally, ECT may also be performed safely in patients with Parkinson's disease and a deep brain stimulator, because the brain electrodes do not become dislodged or heated (Bailine et al. 2008).

Brain Tumor or Mass

Intracranial mass lesions and increased intracranial pressure are among the most serious risk factors for ECT. Patients with these conditions are at risk for developing noncardiogenic pulmonary edema, cerebral edema, brain hemorrhage, and cerebral herniation (Krystal and Coffey 1997; Maltbie et al. 1980). ECT may be administered safely and effectively to patients with small or slow-growing intracranial tumors or arachnoid cysts that have no associated swelling or increased intracranial pressure (Abrams 2002b; Coffey et al. 1987). The risks to individuals with more substantial masses may be reduced by surgically removing or debulking the mass when possible, and by trying to diminish the surrounding edema (e.g., steroids, diuretics, or hyperventilation during the treatment) and the rise in intracranial pressure during the treatment (e.g., by pretreatment administration of antihypertensive agents) (Rasmussen et al. 2007b). There is no report of safely delivered ECT prospectively given to a patient with documented increased intracranial pressure (Abrams 2002b). Subdural hematomas may require evacuation before ECT (Abrams 2002b).

Patients with normal-pressure hydrocephalus, including those with a shunt, may be treated safely and effectively with ECT, provided the shunt is determined to be patent, although such patients may be at increased risk of cognitive side effects. These patients (as well as others with prior brain surgery or head injury) may have a skull defect, which may increase the risk of cognitive side effects or injury if the stimulus electrode is placed nearby (allowing greater current density to be administered to the brain). In such cases, repositioning of the stimulus electrode is indicated.

Psychosocial Issues

In addition to its myriad biological effects, ECT has important intrapsychic and interpersonal effects. A powerful treatment, during which the patient is put to sleep and has an electrical stimulus delivered to the head, may arouse predictable fears and fantasies in the patient. Issues of trust and autonomy over one's body while in a vulnerable position may predominate, especially in patients with a history of trauma. Patient education—in particular, educational videotapes—may reduce these fears. Patients who are vulnerable to idealized fantasies of a nurturing, all-caring, supportive other may overvalue the ECT procedure and practitioner. Conversely, these patients may excessively devalue the treatment when their distorted expectations are not realized. Such patients may be at increased risk for a bad psychological outcome from the treatment. The ECT practitioner should challenge overidealization of the treatment, and the informed consent process should be firmly grounded in factual information. We have also found that for some patients, the experience of ECT is markedly improved if a family member or significant other is present during the procedure.

Patient attitude surveys have found that although ECT is poorly understood, those undergoing ECT typically find the experience no more upsetting than a trip to the dentist (Fox 1993; Hughes et al. 1981; Malcolm 1989). These results are limited, however, by a variety of methodological issues (Rose et al. 2003). Only a few studies have systematically examined the effects of age on patients' perception and knowledge of ECT. Malcolm (1989) found that patients over age 65 had less knowledge of the procedure before treatment and were also less fearful of it. In addition, fewer elderly patients viewed the treatment as frightening after completing a course of ECT. Sienaert et al. (2005) found no relation between a patient's age and degree of satisfaction with ECT, which in general was quite high even in the presence of memory complaints.

Medicolegal issues surrounding the use of ECT with elderly patients include the informed consent process (discussed earlier in this chapter), do-not-resuscitate (DNR) orders, and consideration of driving after ECT (see Chapter 14, "Ethical and Legal Issues"). A patient with DNR status may still experience improved quality of life with aggressive treatment of his or her affective disorder and may still be considered for ECT (Sullivan et al. 1992). In such cases, strategies for the management of major complications that could occur during ECT should be discussed with the patient and the family before treatment. Patients should not drive after an ECT course until cognitive side effects have substantially resolved (Fink 1994). This issue may be an especially sensitive one for elderly patients who consider driving a means of maintaining their mobility and functional independence.

Financial concerns are of increasing importance in today's cost-conscious health care marketplace. A growing literature suggests that ECT has economic advantages over other forms of treatment for severe mood disorders. The cost-effectiveness of ECT has been demonstrated both for inpatient treatment of the index episode and for maintenance therapy on an ambulatory basis (Markowitz et al. 1987; McDonald et al. 1998; Olfson et al. 1998; Steffens et al. 1995). Despite these advantages, there remains much variation in ECT reimbursement patterns, and it is not uncommon to encounter payers who will reimburse only for ECT when given on an inpatient basis. In addition, reimbursement rates are very low and thus discourage the use of this safe and highly effective treatment.

Novel Techniques for Inducing Therapeutic Seizures

As discussed earlier in the section "Cognitive Side Effects," data suggest that the efficacy and cognitive side effects of ECT may be determined in part by the site of the seizure initiation and by the pattern of seizure generalization. The antidepressant effects of ECT may be correlated with functional changes in prefrontal (among other) brain regions, whereas the amnestic effects of ECT are associated with functional and synaptic changes in the medial temporal lobes. Thus, at least in theory, the goal of the "brain stimulation" specialist is to employ strategies that induce relatively focal seizures in regions that modulate mood (e.g., perhaps the prefrontal region) and that limit spread of the seizure to the medial temporal region.

The use of unilateral nondominant stimulus electrode placement is one such strategy to spatially target the stimulus. Although it produces differences in seizure initiation and spread, as well as substantial differences in cognitive side effects relative to bilateral stimulation, the resultant seizure is still bilaterally generalized. A recent strategy to spatially target even more precisely the electrical stimulus in ECT is known as focal electrically administered seizure therapy (FEAST). This experimental technique couples novel electrode geometry with unidirectional (anode-cathode) stimulation. In nonhuman primates, FEAST has been shown to be a safe and reliable means of inducing a variety of seizure types, from focal to generalized (Berman et al. 2005). Research is under way to determine the applicability of FEAST in humans.

Substantial challenges remain, however, in the use of electrical stimulation to induce focal brain seizures, as a result of the physics of brain stimulation. When electricity is applied directly to the scalp, its flow is impeded by the scalp and the skull, resulting in a "smearing" of the electrical stimulus and a relative broadening of the field of brain stimulation. These factors are likely confounded by individual differences in the anatomy of the scalp and skull, making standardization across patients difficult. Therefore, research has turned to the use of other stimuli to induce a relatively focal therapeutic brain seizure, and among the most promising is magnetic stimulation.

As discussed in Chapter 11, "Brain Stimulation Therapies," seizures may be a side effect of repetitive transcranial magnetic stimulation when administered at high stimulus intensity. This observation has led to the suggestion that repetitive transcranial magnetic stimulation might be used as a means of inducing therapeutic seizures, a technique termed *magnetic seizure therapy* (MST). Relative to ECT, MST would have a theoretical advantage of more precise targeting of the stimulus, because magnetic fields pass through tissue (including scalp and skull) without impedance (i.e., without smearing). In addition, MST typically delivers magnetic stimulation that is relatively superficial, penetrating only ~2–4 cm beneath the scalp. Thus, MST offers the theoretical advantage of relatively more precise targeting of the seizure to superficial cortical structures presumed to mediate mood (perhaps the prefrontal brain region) while at the same time sparing stimulation of deeper structures, such as the hippocampus, associated with amnestic side effects (Lisanby and Peterchev 2007).

Indeed, research in nonhuman primates has demonstrated that 1) relative to electrical stimulation, the current induced by MST is less intense and relatively more discrete; and 2) the resulting seizures are relatively more focal and are associated with less neuroendocrine, autonomic, and neuroplastic responses, as well as with more benign acute cognitive side effects (Spellman et al. 2008). Several dozen patients with depression have now received MST on an experimental basis, and in general they have tolerated the procedure without any major adverse or unanticipated effects (for a review, see Marcolin and Padberg 2007). Consistent with the studies in nonhuman primates, these patients had more focal and less physiologically "intense" seizures than with ECT, and patients experienced less disorientation and fewer short-term amnestic side effects, at least for some types of memory (i.e., those mediated by the temporal lobes). No differences were seen between ECT and MST seizures in those cognitive functions presumably mediated by prefrontal brain regions. Thus, MST appears feasible and safe, and the fact that it has relatively mild autonomic effects might be a decided advantage over ECT in elderly patients with cardiovascular risks. More research is needed, however, to determine the efficacy of MST and to clarify a host of technical issues (coil selection, parameters of stimulation, pulse characteristics, power requirements, optimal anesthesia, and so forth) that impact the neurobiological effects of this intriguing procedure.

Conclusion

More than 70 years after its introduction, ECT remains a cornerstone of the treatment of severe affective disorder and selected other neuropsychiatric illnesses in elderly patients. ECT also appears to be an effective treatment in patients with preexisting brain disease and in some cases may even have a beneficial effect on the underlying neurological disorder. Continued advances in ECT technique have improved the efficacy of the procedure and reduced the risk of severe side effects. However, few controlled studies have compared the efficacy and safety of ECT versus pharmacotherapy in elderly patients. Further study is needed to determine the impact of age-related changes in brain structure or function and of preexisting cerebral disease on the beneficial effects of ECT in elderly patients. The mechanism of action of this important treatment remains to be fully elucidated.

Key Points

- ECT is an important treatment option for elderly patients with certain neuropsychiatric illnesses. It is most commonly used for the treatment of severe medication-resistant depression. For urgently ill depressed patients, ECT may be used as first-line treatment. It is also used to treat mania, schizophrenia, and catatonia. It is effective in depression-complicating dementia, stroke, and Parkinson's disease. It has also been shown to have a beneficial effect on the motor symptoms of Parkinson's disease.
- The cardiovascular and cerebral physiological changes that occur during ECT are particularly relevant for elderly patients with complex medical illnesses. Modern anesthesia techniques (e.g., using ultra-brief-acting barbiturates, muscle relaxants, and intravenous beta-blockers to control cardiac rate and blood pressure) make the procedure remarkably safe. The cognitive effects of ECT, particularly recent memory loss, may be mitigated by careful attention to technical issues in the administration of the procedure, including the use of right unilateral electrode placement and optimal stimulus dosing.
- ECT is most commonly administered as a series of 6 to 12 treatments targeting acute depressive or psychotic symptoms. It can also be used as a continuation or maintenance treatment, given on an outpatient basis every 1–8 weeks, with the goal of preventing a subsequent episode of illness.
- Novel and still experimental brain stimulation techniques hold out the possibility of inducing more focal cerebral seizures or stimulation but are not yet available for widespread clinical use. Careful attention to patient and family education and the informed consent process are important aspects of making ECT acceptable and nonthreatening to patients.

Recommended Readings

Abrams R: Efficacy of electroconvulsive therapy, in Electroconvulsive Therapy, 4th Edition. New York, Oxford University Press, 2002, pp 17–42

American Psychiatric Association Committee on Electroconvulsive Therapy: The Practice of Electroconvulsive Therapy: Recommendations for Treatment, Training, and Privileging, 2nd Edition. Washington, DC, American Psychiatric Publishing, 2001

Lisanby SH: Electroconvulsive therapy for depression. N Engl J Med 357:1939–1945, 2007

References

Aarsland D, Larsen JP, Waage O, et al: Maintenance electroconvulsive therapy for Parkinson's disease. Convuls Ther 13:274–277, 1997

Abrams R: The mortality rate with ECT. Convuls Ther 13:125–127, 1997

Abrams R: Does brief-pulse ECT cause persistent or permanent memory impairment? J ECT 18:71–73, 2002a

Abrams R: Electroconvulsive Therapy, 4th Edition. New York, Oxford University Press, 2002b

Alexopoulos GS, Shamoian CJ, Lucas J, et al: Medical problems of geriatric psychiatric patients and younger controls during electroconvulsive therapy. J Am Geriatr Soc 32:651–654, 1984

American Psychiatric Association Committee on Electroconvulsive Therapy: The Practice of Electroconvulsive Therapy: Recommendations for Treatment, Training, and Privileging, 2nd Edition. Washington, DC, American Psychiatric Association, 2001

Andersen K, Balldin J, Gottfries CG, et al: A double-blind evaluation of electroconvulsive therapy in Parkinson's disease with "on-off" phenomena. Acta Neurol Scand 76:191–199, 1987

Applegate RJ: Diagnosis and management of ischemic heart disease in the patient scheduled to undergo electroconvulsive therapy. Convuls Ther 13:128–144, 1997

Avery E, Winokur G: Mortality in depressed patients treated with electroconvulsive therapy and antidepressants. Arch Gen Psychiatry 33:1029–1037, 1976

Babigian HM, Guttmacher LB: Epidemiologic considerations in electroconvulsive therapy. Arch Gen Psychiatry 41:246–253, 1984

Bailine SH, Rifkin A, Kayne E, et al: Comparison of bifrontal and bitemporal ECT for major depression. Am J Psychiatry 157:121–123, 2000

Bailine SH, Kremen N, Kohen I, et al: Bitemporal electroconvulsive therapy for depression in a Parkinson disease patient with a deep-brain stimulator. J ECT 24:171–172, 2008

Baldwin R, Jeffries S, Jackson A, et al: Treatment response in late-onset depression: relationship to neuropsychological, neuroradiological and vascular risk factors. Psychol Med 34:125–136, 2004

Bergsholm P, Swartz CM: Anesthesia in electroconvulsive therapy and alternatives to barbiturates. Psychiatr Ann 26:709–712, 1996

Berman RM, Sackeim HA, Truesdale MD, et al: Focal electrically administered seizure therapy (FEAST): nonhuman primate studies of a novel form of focal brain stimulation (abstract). J ECT 21:57, 2005

Black DW, Winokur G, Nasrallah A: A multivariate analysis of the experience of 423 depressed inpatients treated with electroconvulsive therapy. Convuls Ther 9:112–120, 1993

Bosworth HB, McQuoid DR, George LK, et al: Time-to-remission from geriatric depression: psychosocial and clinical factors. Am J Geriatr Psychiatry 10:551–559, 2002

Braasch ER, Demaso DR: Effect of electroconvulsive therapy on serum isoenzymes. Am J Psychiatry 137:625–626, 1980

Braga RJ, Petrides G: The combined use of electroconvulsive therapy and antipsychotics in patients with schizophrenia. J ECT 21:75–83, 2005

Bruce BB, Henry ME, Greer DM: Ischemic stroke after electroconvulsive therapy. J ECT 22:150–152, 2006

Burke WJ, Rubin EH, Zorumski CF, et al: The safety of ECT in geriatric psychiatry. J Am Geriatr Soc 35:516–521, 1987

Calabrese JR, Woyshville MJ, Kimmel SE, et al: Mixed states and bipolar rapid cycling and their treatment with divalproex sodium. Psychiatr Ann 23:70–78, 1993

Calev A, Pass HL, Shapira B, et al: ECT and memory, in The Clinical Science of Electroconvulsive Therapy. Edited by Coffey CE. Washington, DC, American Psychiatric Press, 1993, pp 125–142

Caroff SN, Ungvari GS, Bhati MT, et al: Catatonia and prediction of response to electroconvulsive therapy. Psychiatr Ann 37:57–64, 2007

Casey DA, Davis MH: Electroconvulsive therapy in the very old. Gen Hosp Psychiatry 18:436–439, 1996

Cattan RA, Barry PP, Mead G, et al: Electroconvulsive therapy in octogenarians. J Am Geriatr Soc 38:753–758, 1990

Clarke TB, Coffey CE, Hoffman GW, et al: Continuation therapy for depression using outpatient electroconvulsive therapy. Convuls Ther 5:330–337, 1989

Coffey CE: Structural brain imaging and electroconvulsive therapy, in The Clinical Science of Electroconvulsive Therapy. Edited by Coffey CE. Washington, DC, American Psychiatric Press, 1993, pp 73–92

Coffey CE: The pre ECT evaluation. Psychiatr Ann 28:506–508, 1998

Coffey CE: Some brief thoughts on brief and ultra-brief pulse ECT. Brain Stimulat 1:86–87, 2008

Coffey CE, Hoffman G, Weiner RD, et al: Electroconvulsive therapy in a depressed patient with a functioning ventriculoatrial shunt. Convuls Ther 3:302–306, 1987

Coffey CE, Figiel GS, Djang WT, et al: Leukoencephalopathy in elderly depressed patients referred for ECT. Biol Psychiatry 24: 143–161, 1988

Coffey CE, Figiel GS, Djang WT, et al: White matter hyperintensity on magnetic resonance imaging: clinical and neuroanatomic correlates in the depressed elderly. J Neuropsychiatry Clin Neurosci 1:135–144, 1989

Coffey CE, Figiel GS, Weiner RD, et al: Caffeine augmentation of ECT. Am J Psychiatry 147:579–585, 1990

Coffey CE, Weiner RD, Djang WT, et al: Brain anatomic effects of ECT: a prospective magnetic resonance imaging study. Arch Gen Psychiatry 48:1013–1021, 1991

Coffey CE, Lucke J, Weiner RD, et al: Seizure threshold in electroconvulsive therapy, I: initial seizure threshold. Biol Psychiatry 37: 713–720, 1995a

Coffey CE, Lucke J, Weiner RD, et al: Seizure threshold in electroconvulsive therapy, II: The anticonvulsant effect of ECT. Biol Psychiatry 37:777–788, 1995b

Coffey CE, McAllister TW, Silver JM (eds): Guide to Neuropsychiatric Therapeutics. Philadelphia, PA, Lippincott Williams & Wilkins, 2007

Coryell W, Zimmerman M: Outcome following ECT for primary unipolar depression: a test of newly proposed response predictors. Am J Psychiatry 141:862–867, 1984

Currier MB, Murray GB, Welch CC: Electroconvulsive therapy for post-stroke depressed geriatric patients. J Neuropsychiatry Clin Neurosci 4:140–144, 1992

Decina P, Sackeim HA, Kahn DA, et al: Effects of ECT on the TRH stimulation test. Psychoneuroendocrinology 12:29–34, 1987

d'Elia G, Raotma H: Memory impairment after convulsive therapy: influence of age and number of treatments. Arch Psychiatr Nervenkr 223:219–226, 1977

Devanand DP, Briscoe KM, Sackeim HA: Clinical features and predictors of postictal excitement. Convuls Ther 5:140–146, 1989

Devanand DP, Sackeim HA, Lo ES, et al: Serial dexamethasone suppression tests and plasma dexamethasone levels. Arch Gen Psychiatry 48:525–533, 1991

Devanand DP, Dwork AJ, Hutchinson MSE, et al: Does ECT alter brain structure? Am J Psychiatry 151:957–970, 1994

Devanand DP, Fitzsimons L, Prudic J, et al: Subjective side effects during electroconvulsive therapy. Convuls Ther 11:232–240, 1995

Dolenc TJ, Rasmussen KG: The safety of electroconvulsive therapy and lithium in combination: a case series and review of the literature. J ECT 21:165–170, 2005

Dombrovski AY, Mulsant BH: For debate: the evidence for electroconvulsive therapy (ECT) in the treatment of severe late-life depression. Int Psychogeriatr 19:9–35, 2007

Dombrovski AY, Mulsant BH, Haskett RF, et al: Predictors of remission after electroconvulsive therapy in unipolar major depression. J Clin Psychiatry 66:1043–1049, 2005

Douyon R, Serby M, Klutchko B, et al: ECT and Parkinson's disease revisited: a "naturalistic" study. Am J Psychiatry 146:1451–1455, 1989

Drop LJ, Welch CA: Anesthesia for electroconvulsive therapy in patients with major cardiovascular risk factors. Convuls Ther 5:88–101, 1989

Dubin WR, Jaffe R, Roemer R, et al: The efficacy and safety of maintenance ECT in geriatric patients. J Am Geriatr Soc 40:706–709, 1992

Ende G, Braus DF, Walter S, et al: The hippocampus in patients treated with electroconvulsive therapy: a proton magnetic resonance spectroscopic imaging study. Arch Gen Psychiatry 57:937–943, 2000

Evans DL, Charney DS, Lewis L, et al: Mood disorders in the medically ill: scientific review and recommendations. Biol Psychiatry 58:175–189, 2005

Farah A, Beale MD, Kellner CH: Risperidone and ECT combination therapy: a case series. Convuls Ther 11:280–282, 1995

Figiel GS, Coffey CE, Djang WT, et al: Brain magnetic resonance imaging findings in ECT-induced delirium. J Neuropsychiatry Clin Neurosci 2:53–58, 1990

Figiel GS, Hassen MA, Zorumski C, et al: ECT-induced delirium in depressed patients with Parkinson's disease. J Neuropsychiatry Clin Neurosci 3:405–411, 1991

Fink M: Convulsive Therapy: Theory and Practice. New York, Raven, 1979

Fink M: Convalescence and ECT. Convuls Ther 10:301–303, 1994

Fink M: What we learn about continuation treatments from the collaborative electroconvulsive therapy studies. J ECT 23:215–218, 2007

Fink M, Sackeim HA: Theophylline and ECT. J ECT 14:286–290, 1998

Fink M, Taylor MA: Catatonia: A Clinician's Guide to Diagnosis and Treatment. New York, Cambridge University Press, 2003

Fink M, Abrams R, Bailine S, et al: Ambulatory electroconvulsive therapy: report of a task force of the Association for Convulsive Therapy. J ECT 12:42–55, 1996

Fisman M, Rabheru K, Hegele RA, et al: Apolipoprotein E polymorphism and response to electroconvulsive therapy. J ECT 17:11–14, 2001

Flint AJ, Gagnon N: Effective use of electroconvulsive therapy in late-life depression. Can J Psychiatry 47:734–741, 2002

Folkerts HW, Michael N, Tolle R, et al: Electroconvulsive therapy vs. paroxetine in treatment-resistant depression: a randomized study. Acta Psychiatr Scand 96:334–342, 1997

Fox HA: Patients' fear of and objection to electroconvulsive therapy. Hosp Community Psychiatry 44:357–360, 1993

Fragen RJ, Avram MJ: Barbiturates, in Anesthesia, 3rd Edition, Vol 1. Edited by Miller RD. New York, Churchill Livingstone, 1990, pp 225–242

Frank E, Kupfer DJ, Perel JM, et al: Three year outcomes for maintenance therapies in recurrent depression. Arch Gen Psychiatry 47:1093–1099, 1990

Fraser RM, Glass IB: Recovery from ECT in elderly patients. Br J Psychiatry 133:524–528, 1978

Fraser RM, Glass IB: Unilateral and bilateral ECT in elderly patients: a comparative study. Acta Psychiatr Scand 62:13–31, 1980

Freeman CP (ed): The ECT Handbook: The Second Report of the Royal College of Psychiatrists' Special Committee on ECT. London, Royal College of Psychiatrists, 1995

Fromholt P, Christensen AL, Strömgren LS: The effects of unilateral and bilateral electroconvulsive therapy on memory. Acta Psychiatr Scand 49:466–478, 1973

Gardner BK, O'Connor DW: A review of the cognitive effects of electroconvulsive therapy in older adults. J ECT 24:68–80, 2008

Gormley N, Cullen C, Walters L, et al: The safety and efficacy of electroconvulsive therapy in patients over age 75. Int Geriatr Psychiatry 13:871–874, 1998

Greenberg L, Fink M: The use of electroconvulsive therapy in geriatric patients. Clin Geriatr Med 8:349–354, 1992

Greenhalgh J, Knight C, Hind D, et al: Clinical and cost-effectiveness of electroconvulsive therapy for depressive illness, schizophrenia, catatonia and mania: systematic reviews and economic modelling studies. Health Technol Assess 9:1–156, 2005

Gregory S, Shawcross CR, Gill D: The Nottingham ECT study: a double-blind comparison of bilateral, unilateral and simulated ECT in depressive illness. Br J Psychiatry 146:520–524, 1985

Grunhaus L, Dolberg O, Lustig M: Relapse and recurrence following a course of ECT: reasons for concern and strategies for further investigation. J Psychiatr Res 29:165–172, 1995

Grunhaus L, Shipley JE, Eiser A, et al: Polysomnographic studies in patients referred for ECT: pre-ECT studies. Convuls Ther 12:224–231, 1996

Hamilton M: The effect of treatment on the melancholia (depressions). Br J Psychiatry 140:223–230, 1982

Hermann RC, Dorwart RA, Hoover CW, et al: Variation in the use of ECT in the United States. Am J Psychiatry 152:869–875, 1995

Hermesh H, Aizenberg D, Friedberg G, et al: Electroconvulsive therapy for persistent neuroleptic-induced akathisia and parkinsonism: a case report. Biol Psychiatry 31:407–411, 1992

Heshe J, Röder E, Theilgaard A: Unilateral and bilateral ECT: a psychiatric and psychological study of therapeutic effect and side effects. Acta Psychiatr Scand Suppl 275:1–180, 1978

Hickie I, Mason C, Gordon P, et al: Prediction of ECT response: validation of a sign-based (CORE) system for defining melancholia. Br J Psychiatry 169:68–74, 1996

Holtzmann J, Polosan M, Baro P, et al: ECT: from neuronal plasticity to mechanisms underlying antidepressant medication effect (in French). Encephale 33:572–578, 2007

Howie MB, Black HA, Zvar AD, et al: Esmolol reduces autonomic hypersensitivity and length of seizures induced by electroconvulsive therapy. Anesth Analg 71:384–388, 1990

Huang KC, Lucas LF, Tsueda K, et al: Age-related changes in cardiovascular function associated with electroconvulsive therapy. Convuls Ther 5:17–25, 1989

Hughes J, Barraclough BM, Reeve W: Are patients shocked by ECT? J R Soc Med 74:283–285, 1981

Husain MM, Montgomery JH, Fernandes P, et al: Safety of vagus nerve stimulation with ECT. Am J Psychiatry 159:1243, 2002

Iosifescu DV, Renshaw PF, Lyoo IK, et al: Brain white-matter hyperintensities and treatment outcome in major depressive disorder. Br J Psychiatry 188:180–185, 2006

Janicak PG, Davis JM, Gibbons RD, et al: Efficacy of ECT: a meta-analysis. Am J Psychiatry 142:297–302, 1985

Jarvie H: Prognosis of depression treated by electric convulsive therapy. BMJ 1:132–134, 1954

Jenike MA: Handbook of Geriatric Psychopharmacology. Littleton, MA, PSG Publishing, 1985

Kamil R, Joffe RT: Neuroendocrine testing in electroconvulsive therapy. Psychiatr Clin North Am 14:961–970, 1991

Kaplan HI, Sadock BJ (eds): Synopsis of Psychiatry, 9th Edition. Baltimore, MD, Williams & Wilkins, 2005, pp 253–269

Karlinsky H, Shulman KI: The clinical use of electroconvulsive therapy in old age. J Am Geriatr Soc 32:183–186, 1984

Kellner CH: Left unilateral ECT: still a viable option? Convuls Ther 13:65–67, 1997a

Kellner CH: Seizure interference by medications: how big a problem (editorial)? Convuls Ther 13:1–3, 1997b

Kellner CH: High-dose right unilateral ECT. J ECT 16:209–210, 2000

Kellner CH, Bernstein HJ: ECT as a treatment for neurological illness, in The Clinical Science of Electroconvulsive Therapy. Edited by Coffey CE. Washington, DC, American Psychiatric Press, 1993, pp 183–210

Kellner CH, Nixon DW, Bernstein HJ: ECT-drug interactions: a review. Psychopharmacol Bull 27:595–609, 1991a

Kellner CH, Tollhurst JE, Burns CM: ECT in the presence of severe cervical spine disease. Convuls Ther 7:52–55, 1991b

Kellner CH, Monroe RR Jr, Pritchett J, et al: Weekly ECT in geriatric depression. Convuls Ther 8:245–252, 1992

Kellner CH, Coffey CE, Beale MD, et al: Handbook of ECT. Washington, DC, American Psychiatric Press, 1997

Kellner CH, Fink M, Knapp R, et al: Relief of expressed suicide intent by ECT: a consortium for research in ECT study. Am J Psychiatry 162:977–982, 2005

Kellner CH, Knapp RG, Petrides G, et al: Continuation ECT versus pharmacotherapy for relapse prevention in major depression: a multi-site study from CORE. Arch Gen Psychiatry 63:1337–1344, 2006

Kirkegaard C, Norlem N, Lauridsen UB, et al: Protirelin stimulation test and thyroid function during treatment of depression. Arch Gen Psychiatry 32:1115–1118, 1975

Kramer BA: Use of ECT in California, 1977–1983. Am J Psychiatry 142:1190–1192, 1985

Kramer BA: Use of ECT in California, revised: 1984–1994. J ECT 15:245–251, 1999

Kramp P, Bolwig T: Electroconvulsive therapy in acute delirious states. Compr Psychiatry 22:368–371, 1981

Kroessler D, Fogel B: Electroconvulsive therapy for major depression in the oldest old. Am J Geriatr Psychiatry 1:30–37, 1993

Krog-Meyer I, Kirkegaard C, Kijne B, et al: Prediction of relapse with the TRH test and prophylactic amitriptyline in 39 patients with endogenous depression. Am J Psychiatry 141:945–948, 1984

Krystal AD, Coffey CE: Neuropsychiatric considerations in the use of electroconvulsive therapy. J Neuropsychiatry Clin Neurosci 9: 283–292, 1997

Krystal AD, Weiner RD, Coffey CE: The ictal EEG as a marker of adequate stimulus intensity with unilateral ECT. J Neuropsychiatry Clin Neurosci 7:295–303, 1995

Krystal AD, Weiner RD, Gassert D, et al: The relative ability of 3 ictal EEG frequency bands to differentiate ECT seizures on the basis of electrode placement, stimulus intensity, and therapeutic response. Convuls Ther 12:13–24, 1996

Krystal AD, Coffey CE, Weiner RD, et al: Changes in seizure threshold over the course of electroconvulsive therapy affect therapeutic response and are detected by ictal EEG ratings. J Neuropsychiatry Clin Neurosci 10:178–186, 1998

Krystal AD, Dean MD, Weiner RD, et al: ECT stimulus intensity: are present ECT devices too limited? Am J Psychiatry 157:963–967, 2000

Lambourn J, Barrington PC: Electroconvulsive therapy in a sample British population in 1982. Convuls Ther 2:169–177, 1986

Lauritzen L, Odgaard K, Clemmesen L, et al: Relapse prevention by means of paroxetine in ECT-treated patients with major depression: a comparison with imipramine and placebo in medium term continuation therapy. Acta Psychiatr Scand 94:241–251, 1996

Lerer B, Shapira B, Calev A, et al: Antidepressant and cognitive effects of twice- versus three-times-weekly ECT. Am J Psychiatry 152: 564–570, 1995

Lichtor JL: Psychological preparation and preoperative medication, in Anesthesia, 3rd Edition, Vol 1. Edited by Miller RD. New York, Churchill Livingston, 1990, pp 895–928

Lisanby SH, Peterchev AV: Magnetic seizure therapy for the treatment of depression, in Advances in Biological Psychiatry, Vol 23: Transcranial Brain Stimulation for Treatment of Psychiatric Disorders. Edited by Marcolin MA, Padberg F. Basel, Switzerland, Karger, 2007, pp 155–171

Lisanby SH, Devanand DP, Nobler MS, et al: Exceptionally high seizure threshold: ECT device limitations. Convuls Ther 12:156–164, 1996

Little JD, Atkins MR, Munday J, et al: Bifrontal electroconvulsive therapy in the elderly: a 2-year retrospective. J ECT 20:139–141, 2004

Loo H, Galinowski A, DeCarvalho W, et al: Use of maintenance ECT for elderly depressed patients (letter). Am J Psychiatry 148:810, 1991

Magni G, Fisman M, Helmes E: Clinical correlates of ECT-resistant depression in the elderly. J Clin Psychiatry 49:405–407, 1988

Malcolm K: Patients' perceptions and knowledge of electroconvulsive therapy. Psychiatric Bulletin 13:161–165, 1989

Malla AK: Characteristics of patients who receive electroconvulsive therapy. Can J Psychiatry 33:696–701, 1988

Maltbie AA, Wingfield MS, Volow MR, et al: Electroconvulsive therapy in the presence of brain tumor. J Nerv Ment Dis 168:400–405, 1980

Manly DT, Oakley SP, Bloch RM: Electroconvulsive therapy in old-old patients. Am J Psychiatry 8:232–236, 2000

Marcolin MA, Padberg F (eds): Transcranial brain stimulation for treatment of psychiatric disorders, in Advances in Biological Psychiatry, Vol 23: Transcranial Brain Stimulation for Treatment of Psychiatric Disorders. Edited by Marcolin MA, Padberg F. Basel, Switzerland, Karger, 2007, pp i–x

Markowitz J, Brown R, Sweeney J, et al: Reduced length and cost of hospital stay for major depression in patients treated with ECT. Am J Psychiatry 144:1025–1029, 1987

Martin M, Figiel G, Mattingly G, et al: ECT-induced interictal delirium in patients with a history of CVA. J Geriatr Psychiatry Neurol 5:149–155, 1992

Mayur PM, Gangadhar BN, Subbakrishna DK, et al: Discontinuation of antidepressant drugs during electroconvulsive therapy: a controlled study. J Affect Disord 58:37–41, 2000

McCall WV: Cardiovascular risk during ECT: managing the managers (editorial). Convuls Ther 13:123–124, 1997

McCall WV, Reboussin DM, Weiner RD, et al: Titrated moderately suprathreshold vs. fixed, high-dose right unilateral electroconvulsive therapy: acute antidepressant and cognitive effects. Arch Gen Psychiatry 57:438–444, 2000

McDonald WM: Is ECT cost-effective? JECT 22:25–29, 2006

McDonald WM, Phillips VL, Figiel GS, et al: Cost-effective maintenance treatment of resistant geriatric depression. Psychiatr Ann 28:47–52, 1998

McElhiney MC, Moody BJ, Steif BL, et al: Autobiographical memory and mood: effects of electroconvulsive therapy. Neuropsychology 9:501–517, 1995

Messina AG, Paranicas M, Katz B, et al: Effect of electroconvulsive therapy on the electrocardiogram and echocardiogram. Anesth Analg 75:511–514, 1992

Monroe RR: Maintenance electroconvulsive therapy. Psychiatr Clin North Am 14:947–960, 1991

Mottram PG, Wilson K, Strobl JJ: Antidepressants for depressed elderly (review). Cochrane Database of Systematic Reviews 2006, Issue 1. Art. No.: CD003491. DOI: 10.1002/14651858. CD003491. pub2

Mukherjee S: Mechanisms of the antimanic effects of electroconvulsive therapy. Convuls Ther 5:227–243, 1989

Mukherjee S, Sackeim HA, Lee C: Unilateral ECT in the treatment of manic episodes. Convuls Ther 4:74–80, 1988

Mulsant BH, Rosen J, Thornton JE, et al: A prospective naturalistic study of electroconvulsive therapy in late-life depression. J Geriatr Psychiatry Neurol 4:3–13, 1991

Mulsant BH, Houck AP, Gildengers AG, et al: What is the optimal duration of a short-term antidepressant trial when treating geriatric depression? J Clin Psychopharmacol 26:113–120, 2006

Murray GB, Shea V, Conn DK: Electroconvulsive therapy for post-stroke depression. J Clin Psychiatry 47:258–260, 1986

Navarro V, Gasto C, Lomena F, et al: No brain perfusion impairment at long-term follow-up in elderly patients treated with electroconvulsive therapy for major depression. J ECT 20:89–93, 2004

Nelson JP, Rosenberg DR: ECT treatment of demented elderly patients with major depression: a retrospective study of safety and efficacy. Convuls Ther 7:157–165, 1991

Nobler MS, Oquendo MA, Kegeles LS, et al: Decreased regional brain metabolism after ECT. Am J Psychiatry 158:305–308, 2001

O'Connor MK, Knapp R, Husain M, et al: The influence of age on the response of major depression to electroconvulsive therapy: a CORE report. Am J Psychiatry 9:382–390, 2001

Okamura T, Kudo K, Sata N, et al: Electroconvulsive therapy after coil embolization of cerebral aneurysm. J ECT 22:148–149, 2006

O'Leary D, Gill D, Gregory S, et al: Which depressed patients respond to ECT? The Nottingham results. J Affect Disord 33:245–250, 1995

Olfson M, Marcus S, Sackeim HA, et al: Use of ECT for the inpatient treatment of recurrent major depression. Am J Psychiatry 155: 22–29, 1998

Oztas B, Kaya M, Camurcu S: Age-related changes in the effect of electroconvulsive shock on the blood-brain barrier permeability in rats. Mech Ageing Dev 51:149–155, 1990

Pande AC, Grunhaus LJ, Haskett RF, et al: Electroconvulsive therapy in delusional and non-delusional depressive disorder. J Affect Disord 19:215–219, 1990

Papakostas Y, Fink M, Lee J, et al: Neuroendocrine measures in psychiatric patients: course and outcome with ECT. Psychiatry Res 4:55–64, 1981

Petrides G, Fink M: The "half-age" stimulation strategy for ECT dosing. Convuls Ther 12:138–146, 1996

Petrides G, Fink M, Husain M, et al: ECT remission rates in psychotic versus nonpsychotic depressed patients: a report from CORE. J ECT 17:244–253, 2001

Pettinati HM, Mathisen KS, Rosenberg J, et al: Meta-analytical approach to reconciling discrepancies in efficacy between bilateral and unilateral electroconvulsive therapy. Convuls Ther 2:7–17, 1986

Pfleiderer B, Michael N, Erfurth A, et al: Effective electroconvulsive therapy reverses glutamate/glutamine deficit in the left anterior cingulum of unipolar depressed patients. Psychiatry Res 122: 185–192, 2003

Philibert RA, Richards L, Lynch CF, et al: Effect of ECT on mortality and clinical outcome in geriatric unipolar depression. J Clin Psychiatry 56:390–394, 1995

Prakash J, Kotwal A, Prabhu HRA: Therapeutic and prophylactic utility of the memory-enhancing drug donepezil hydrochloride on cognition of patients undergoing electroconvulsive therapy: a randomized controlled trial. J ECT 22:163–168, 2006

Price TRP, McAllister TW: Safety and efficacy of ECT in depressed patients with dementia: a review of clinical experience. Convuls Ther 5:61–74, 1989

Priebe HJ: The aged cardiovascular risk patient. Br J Anaesth 85:763–778, 2000

Prien R, Kupfer D: Continuation drug therapy for major depressive episodes: how long should it be maintained? Am J Psychiatry 143:18–23, 1986

Prudic J, Sackeim HA, Decina P, et al: Acute effects of ECT on cardiovascular functioning: relations to patient and treatment variables. Acta Psychiatr Scand 75:344–351, 1987

Prudic J, Sackeim HA, Spicknall K: Potential pharmacologic agents for the cognitive effects of electroconvulsive treatment. Psychiatr Ann 28:40–46, 1998

Prudic J, Peyser S, Sackeim HA: Subjective memory complaints: a review of patient self-assessment of memory after electroconvulsive therapy. J ECT 16:121–132, 2000

Rao V, Lyketsos CG: The benefits and risks of ECT for patients with primary dementia who also suffer from depression. Int J Geriatr Psychiatry 15:729–735, 2000

Rao SK, Andrade C, Reddy K, et al: Memory protective effect of indomethacin against electroconvulsive shock–induced retrograde amnesia in rats. Biol Psychiatry 51:770–773, 2002

Rao SS, Daly JW, Sewell DD: Falls associated with electroconvulsive therapy among the geriatric population: a case report. J ECT 24:173–175, 2008

Rasmussen KG, Flemming KD: Electroconvulsive therapy in patients with cavernous hemangiomas. J ECT 22:272–273, 2006

Rasmussen KG, Russell JC, Kung S, et al: Electroconvulsive therapy for patients with major depression and probable Lewy Body dementia. J ECT 19:103–109, 2003

Rasmussen KG, Mueller M, Knapp RG, et al: Antidepressant medication treatment failure does not predict lower remission with ECT for major depressive disorder: a report from the Consortium for Research in Electroconvulsive Therapy. J Clin Psychiatry 68: 1701–1706, 2007a

Rasmussen KG, Perry CL, Sutor B, et al: ECT in patients with intracranial masses. J Neuropsychiatry Clin Neurosci 19:191–193, 2007b

Reynolds CF, Perel JM, Kupfer DJ, et al: Open-trial response to antidepressant treatment in elderly patients with mixed depression and cognitive impairment. Psychiatry Res 21:111–122, 1987

Rice EH, Sombrotto LB, Markowitz JC, et al: Cardiovascular morbidity in high-risk patients during ECT. Am J Psychiatry 151:1637–1641, 1994

Rich CL, Spiker DG, Jewell SW, et al: DSM-III, RDC, and ECT: depressive subtypes and immediate response. J Clin Psychiatry 45:14–18, 1984a

Rich CL, Spiker DG, Jewell SW, et al: The efficacy of ECT, I: response rates in depressive episodes. Psychiatry Res 11:167–176, 1984b

Rich CL, Spiker DG, Jewell SW, et al: ECT response in psychotic versus nonpsychotic unipolar depressives. J Clin Psychiatry 47:123–125, 1986

Roose SP, Sackeim HA, Krishnan KRR, et al: Antidepressant pharmacotherapy in the treatment of depression in the very old: a randomized, placebo-controlled trial. Am J Psychiatry 161:2050–2059, 2004

Rose D, Wykes T, Leese M, et al: Patients' perspectives on electroconvulsive therapy: systematic review. BMJ 326:1–5, 2003

Rosenbach ML, Hermann RC, Dorwart RA: Use of electroconvulsive therapy in the Medicare population between 1987 and 1992. Psychiatr Serv 48:1537–1542, 1997

Rubin EH, Kinsoherf DA, Wehrman SA: Response to treatment of depression in the old and very old. J Geriatr Neurol 4:65–70, 1991

Sackeim HA: The anticonvulsant hypothesis of the mechanisms of action of ECT: current status. J ECT 15:5–26, 1999

Sackeim HA: Memory and ECT: from polarization to reconciliation. J ECT 16:87–96, 2000

Sackeim HA: Electroconvulsive therapy in late-life depression, in Clinical Geriatric Psychopharmacology. Edited by Salzman C. Philadelphia, PA, Lippincott Williams & Wilkins, 2005

Sackeim HA, Devanand DP, Prudic J: Stimulus intensity, seizure threshold, and seizure duration: impact on the efficacy and safety of electroconvulsive therapy. Psychiatr Clin North Am 14: 803–843, 1991

Sackeim HA, Prudic J, Devanand DP, et al: Effects of stimulus intensity and electrode placement on the efficacy and cognitive effects of electroconvulsive therapy. N Engl J Med 328:839–846, 1993

Sackeim HA, Prudic J, Devanand DP, et al: A prospective, randomized, double-blind comparison of bilateral and right unilateral ECT at different stimulus intensities. Arch Gen Psychiatry 57: 425–434, 2000

Sackeim HA, Haskett RF, Mulsant BH, et al: Continuation pharmacotherapy in the prevention of relapse following electroconvulsive therapy: a randomized controlled trial. JAMA 285:1299–1307, 2001

Sackeim HA, Prudic J, Nobler MS, et al: Effects of pulse width and electrode placement on the efficacy and cognitive effects of electroconvulsive therapy. Brain Stimulat 1:71–83, 2008

Sackeim HA, Dillingham EM, Prudic J, et al: Effect of concomitant pharmacotherapy on electroconvulsive therapy outcomes. Arch Gen Psychiatry 66:729–737, 2009

Salzman C: Electroconvulsive therapy in the elderly patient. Psychiatr Clin North Am 5:191–197, 1982

Salzman C, Wong E, Wright BC: Drug and ECT treatment of depression in the elderly, 1996–2001: a literature review. Biol Psychiatry 52:265–284, 2002

Scalia J, Lisanby SH, Dwork AJ, et al: Neuropathologic examination after 91 ECT treatments in a 92-year-old woman with late-onset depression. J ECT 23:96–98, 2007

Seager CP, Bird RL: Imipramine with electrical treatment in depression: a controlled trial. J Mental Sci 108:704–707, 1962

Shapira B, Lerer B: Speed of response to bilateral ECT: an examination of possible predictors in two controlled trials. J ECT 15:202–206, 1999

Shettar MS, Grunhaus L, Pande AC, et al: Protective effects of intramuscular glycopyrrolate on cardiac conduction during ECT. Convuls Ther 5:349–352, 1989

Sienaert P, De Becker T, Vansteelandt K, et al: Patient satisfaction after electroconvulsive therapy. J ECT 21:227–231, 2005

Slawson P: Psychiatric malpractice: the electroconvulsive therapy experience. Convuls Ther 1:195–203, 1985

Small JG, Klapper MH, Kellams JJ, et al: ECT compared with lithium in the management of manic states. Arch Gen Psychiatry 45:727–732, 1988

Small JG, Milstein V, Small IF: Electroconvulsive therapy for mania. Psychiatr Clin North Am 14:887–903, 1991

Sobin C, Sackeim HA, Prudic J, et al: Predictors of retrograde amnesia following ECT. Am J Psychiatry 152:995–1001, 1995

Sobin C, Prudic J, Devanand DP, et al: Who responds to electroconvulsive therapy? Br J Psychiatry 169:322–328, 1996

Solan WJ, Khan A, Avery DH, et al: Psychotic and nonpsychotic depression: comparison of response to ECT. J Clin Psychiatry 49:97–99, 1988

Spellman T, McClintock S, Terrace H, et al: Differential effects of high-dose magnetic seizure therapy and electroconvulsive shock on cognitive function. Biol Psychiatry 63:1163–1170, 2008

Staton RD: Electroencephalographic recording during bitemporal and unilateral non-dominant hemisphere (Lancaster position) electroconvulsive therapy. J Clin Psychiatry 42:264–269, 1981

Steffens DC, Krystal AD, Sibert TE, et al: Cost effectiveness of maintenance ECT (letter). Convuls Ther 11:283–284, 1995

Stek M, Wurff van der FFB, Hoogendijk W, et al: Electroconvulsive therapy for the depressed elderly. Cochrane Database of Systematic Reviews 2003, Issue 2. Art. No.: CD003593. DOI: 10.1002/14651858.CD003593

Stoppe A, Louza M, Rosa M, et al: Fixed high-dose electroconvulsive therapy in the elderly with depression: a double-blind, randomized comparison of efficacy and tolerability between unilateral and bilateral electrode placement. J ECT 22:92–99, 2006

Stoudemire A, Knos G, Gladson M, et al: Labetalol in the control of cardiovascular responses to electroconvulsive therapy in high-risk depressed medical patients. J Clin Psychiatry 51:508–512, 1990

Stoudemire A, Hill CD, Morris R, et al: Improvement in depression-related cognitive dysfunction following ECT. J Neuropsychiatry Clin Neurosci 7:31–34, 1995

Strömgren LS, Christensen AL, Fromholt P: The effects of unilateral brief-interval ECT on memory. Acta Psychiatr Scand 54:336–346, 1976

Sullivan MO, Ward NG, Laxton A: The woman who wanted electroconvulsive therapy and do-not-resuscitate status. Gen Hosp Psychiatry 14:204–209, 1992

Swartz CM: Clinical and laboratory predictors of ECT response, in The Clinical Science of Electroconvulsive Therapy. Edited by Coffey CE. Washington, DC, American Psychiatric Press, 1993, pp 53–71

Tang WK, Ungvari GS, Leung HCM: Effect of piracetam on ECT-induced cognitive disturbances: a randomized, placebo-controlled, double-blind study. J ECT 18:130–137, 2002

Tew JD, Mulsant BH, Haskett RF, et al: Acute efficacy of ECT in the treatment of major depression in the old-old. Am J Psychiatry 156:1865–1870, 1999

Tharyan P, Adams CE: Electroconvulsive therapy for schizophrenia. Cochrane Database of Systematic Reviews 2005, Issue 2. Art. No.: CD000076. DOI: 10.1002/14651858.CD000076.pub2

Thienhaus OJ, Margletta S, Bennett JA: A study of the clinical efficacy of maintenance ECT. J Clin Psychiatry 51:141–144, 1990

Thompson JW, Weiner RD, Myers CP: Use of ECT in the United States in 1975, 1980, and 1986. Am J Psychiatry 151:1657–1661, 1994

U.K. ECT Review Group: Efficacy and safety of electroconvulsive therapy in depressive disorders: a systematic review and meta-analysis. Lancet 361:799–808, 2003

van der Wurff FB, Stek ML, Hoogendijk WJG, et al: The efficacy and safety of ECT in depressed older adults, a literature review. Int J Geriatr Psychiatry 18:894–904, 2003b

Wahlund B, von Rosen D: ECT of major depressed patients in relation to biological and clinical variables: a brief overview. Neuropsychopharmacology 28:S21–S26, 2003

Webb MC, Coffey CE, Saunders WR, et al: Cardiovascular response to unilateral electroconvulsive therapy. Biol Psychiatry 28:758–766, 1990

Weiner RD: Does ECT cause brain damage? Behav Brain Sci 7:1–53, 1984

Weiner RD, Coffey CE: Indications for use of electroconvulsive therapy, in American Psychiatric Press Review of Psychiatry, Vol 7. Edited by Frances AJ, Hales RE. Washington, DC, American Psychiatric Press, 1988, pp 458–481

Weiner RD, Krystal AD: EEG monitoring of ECT seizures, in The Clinical Science of Electroconvulsive Therapy. Edited by Coffey CE. Washington, DC, American Psychiatric Press, 1993, pp 93–109

Weiner RD, Whanger AD, Erwin CW, et al: Prolonged confusional state and EEG seizure following concurrent ECT and lithium use. Am J Psychiatry 137:1452–1453, 1980

Weisberg LA, Elliott D, Mielke D: Intracerebral hemorrhage following electroconvulsive therapy. Neurology 41:1849, 1991

Welch CA: ECT in medically ill patients, in The Clinical Science of Electroconvulsive Therapy. Edited by Coffey CE. Washington, DC, American Psychiatric Press, 1993, pp 167–182

Welch CA, Drop LJ: Cardiovascular effects of ECT. Convuls Ther 5:35–43, 1989

Wengel SP, Burke WJ, Pfeiffer RF, et al: Maintenance electroconvulsive therapy for intractable Parkinson's disease. Am J Geriatr Psychiatr 6:263–269, 1998

Wesner RB, Winokur G: The influence of age on the natural history of unipolar depression when treated with electroconvulsive therapy. Eur Arch Psychiatry Neurol Sci 238:149–154, 1989

Wilkinson AM, Anderson DN, Peters S: Age and the effects of ECT. Int J Geriatr Psychiatry 8:401–406, 1993

Zahedi S, Yang C, O'Hanlon D, et al: Electroconvulsive therapy and venous angiomas. J ECT 22:228–230, 2006

Zervas IM, Fink M: ECT for refractory Parkinson's disease. Convuls Ther 7:222–223, 1991

Zervas IM, Calev A, Jandorf L, et al: Age-dependent effects of electroconvulsive therapy on memory. Convuls Ther 9:39–42, 1993

Zibrak JD, Jensen WA, Bloomingdale K: Aspiration pneumonitis following electroconvulsive therapy in patients with gastroparesis. Biol Psychiatry 24:812–814, 1988

Zielinski RJ, Roose SP, Devanand DP, et al: Cardiovascular complications of ECT in depressed patients with cardiac disease. Am J Psychiatry 150:904–909, 1993

Zink M, Sartorius A, Lederbogen F, et al: Electroconvulsive therapy in a patient receiving rivastigmine. J ECT 18:162–164, 2002

Zorumski CF, Rubin EH, Burke WJ: Electroconvulsive therapy for the elderly. Hosp Community Psychiatry 39:643–647, 1988

Zubenko GS, Mulsant BH, Rifai AH, et al: Impact of acute psychiatric inpatient treatment on major depression in late life and prediction of response. Am J Psychiatry 151:987–994, 1994

Zvara DA, Brooker RF, McCall WV, et al: The effects of esmolol on ST-segment depression and arrhythmias after electroconvulsive therapy. Convuls Ther 13:165–174, 1997

11

Brain Stimulation Therapies

Vagus Nerve Stimulation, Transcranial Magnetic Stimulation, Transcranial Direct Current Stimulation, and Deep Brain Stimulation

Mark S. George, M.D.
Edmund S. Higgins, M.D.
Ziad H. Nahas, M.D.

In contrast with Chapter 10, which covers electroconvulsive therapy (ECT) and two newer techniques designed to produce intentional therapeutic seizures (focal electrically administered seizure therapy and magnetic seizure therapy), in this chapter we describe the rapidly expanding field of nonseizure-producing techniques, in which the brain is focally stimulated using a range of methods, none of which intentionally causes a seizure. These methods essentially deliver a dose of electricity to the brain that ultimately improves behavior and emotions. We first describe and review the noninvasive methods of testing circuit-based theories and treating neuropsychiatric diseases that do not involve implanting electrodes into the brain or on its surface. These techniques are vagus nerve stimulation (VNS), transcranial magnetic stimulation (TMS), and transcranial direct current stimulation (tDCS). We conclude the chapter by discussing the most invasive method of nonconvulsive brain stimulation, called deep brain stimulation (DBS), or a superficial variant, called epidural cortical stimulation. This rapidly changing and fertile area is beginning to impact neuropsychiatric practice, with particular relevance for geriatric psychiatry because elderly patients are more susceptible to systemic medication side effects. Within the last 10 years, the U.S. Food and Drug Administration (FDA) has approved three of these approaches as therapies for different neuropsychiatric conditions, and several of the approvals, particularly in psychiatry, were within the past 5 years.

For each of these technologies, we briefly describe the technique and the major ideas concerning mechanisms of action and then touch on safety. We also overview the research and clinical uses. There are now entire journals devoted to the field of brain stimulation (Sackeim and George 2008) and entire books devoted to each of the individual techniques (e.g., George and Belmaker 2006) as well as in-depth overviews (e.g., Higgins and George 2009). The interested reader is referred to these. This chapter focuses on a quick and precise introduction to each technology from a neuropsychiatric perspective, with a focus on emerging clinical applications and research uses pertinent to the preceding chapters and theories.

One of the recurring themes regarding each of the techniques is finding the optimum dose of electricity needed for adequate treatment. Termed *use parameters,* these include the pulse width, current direction, intensity, frequency, duty cycle, and overall dose as well as dosing scheme. The future of the promising field of brain stimulation will undoubtedly involve better translating the knowledge gained about appropriate use parameters from preclinical cellular and nonhuman animal studies into clinical brain stimulation therapeutic uses.

Vagus Nerve Stimulation

The idea of stimulating the vagus nerve to modify central brain activity has been pursued for over 100 years. However, not until the mid-1980s did methods became available to efficiently stimulate the vagus nerve in man and animals. Although we may think that the vagus nerve primarily delivers signals from the brain to the periphery, in actuality the majority of information travels in the opposite direction: from the organs to the brain. Consequently, stimulating the vagus nerve can affect the brain.

Description of Method

Although the vagus nerve can be stimulated in several different ways, even transcutaneously, for all intents and purposes VNS in the modern literature refers to a technique in which a surgeon (for human studies) or researcher (for nonhuman animal uses) wraps a unidirectional wire around the vagus nerve in the neck. This wire is then connected to a battery-operated generator that is implanted subcutaneously in the left chest wall. The generator intermittently sends an electrical current through the wire and thus through the nerve, which then conveys a signal via neural impulses into the brain stem (George et al. 2000) (Figure 11–1).

In the United States, VNS implantation is usually an outpatient procedure performed by neurosurgeons. It can be done under local anesthesia if a patient is too frail for anesthesia induction. The battery in the device generates an intermittent electrical stimulation that is delivered to the vagus nerve. Clinicians following the patient control the frequency and intensity of the stimulation. Adjustments to the stimulation parameters are transmitted from a computer operated by the treating physician to the VNS device by a handheld infrared wand placed over the device.

The stimulating wire wrapped around the left nerve is directional, and this unidirectional feature likely helps minimize efferent side effects from stimulating vagal efferent (descending) fibers. However, some patients have had the leads accidentally reversed, without noticeable harm (Koo et al. 2001).

The vagus nerve is actually a large nerve bundle, composed of different-sized nerves (both unmyelinated and myelinated). The vagus nerve is thus a complex structure, and the current form of VNS is imprecise in activating discrete nerves within the bundle. Microsurgical techniques might theoretically allow for more focal VNS.

Indications and Clinical Uses

The first self-contained devices were implanted in humans in 1988 in patients with medically unresponsive epilepsy. Results were positive in two large acute double-blind, controlled studies of VNS in patients with treatment-resistant epilepsy (Ben-Menachem et al. 1994; Handforth et al. 1998). Low-dose stimulation (low intensity, low number of pulses per day) served as the control in comparison to high stimulation. In this difficult-to-treat population, seizure frequency decreased 28%–31% in the high-stimulation group compared to baseline while dropping only 11%–15% in the low-stimulation group.

Although few patients with VNS implants are able to stop their anticonvulsant medications, many are able to reduce the number of daily medications. This is clinically important in childhood epilepsy, because many children experience deleterious cognitive side effects from the anticonvulsants (Ferrie and Patel 2009; Shahwan et al. 2009).

Long-term follow-up studies have shown that the time course to respond to VNS is gradual, with continued improvement for up to 1 year and then stabilization of effect. There appear to be no problems regarding tolerance to VNS. The patient with the longest exposure to VNS has had the system operating for 17 years. VNS has assumed a small but significant role in epilepsy practice for those patients who have tried and failed two anticonvulsants.

VNS became available for use in Europe in 1994 and was given an FDA indication for epilepsy in the United States in 1997.

In 1997, one of the authors (M.S.G.), along with John Rush, Harold Sackeim, and later Lauren Marangell, began an initial pilot study of VNS for patients with treatment-resistant depression (Rush et al. 2000; Sackeim et al. 2001b). Several lines of evidence suggesting that VNS might be helpful for patients with depression included anecdotal reports of mood improvement in VNS-implanted epilepsy patients and functional imaging studies demonstrating that VNS increased activity in several regions of the brain thought to be involved with depression (Henry et al. 1998). This open-label study with 59 patients with treatment-resistant depression demonstrated good results—a 30% response rate and a 15% remission rate—at 10 weeks. Even more encouraging were the extended results (Marangell et al. 2002; Nahas et al. 2005); patients continued to improve long after the acute phase of the trial and were clinically better at 1 year than at 3 months. This pattern is unusual in the treatment of depression, especially in a difficult-to-treat cohort with prior tolerance to antidepressants (Rush et al. 2006a, 2006b). A more recent European trial found slightly better results, but with the same side effects and time course of response (Schlaepfer et al. 2008b).

A pivotal randomized, double-blinded multicenter trial of VNS was not as encouraging. In this underpowered trial, active VNS failed to statistically separate from sham treatment. The response rates for the acute treatment of treatment-resistant depression were 15% for active treatment and 10% for sham treatment (Rush et al. 2005a). The age range in this study was 18–65 years, and thus no controlled data are available for elderly patients.

A parallel but nonrandomized group was also studied and compared with those patients who received VNS in Rush et al.'s (2005a) pivotal trial. The two groups were followed for 12 months, during which time both groups received similar treatment (medications and ECT), but one of the two groups also received VNS (Rush et al. 2005b). At the end point the response rates were significantly different: 27% for the VNS

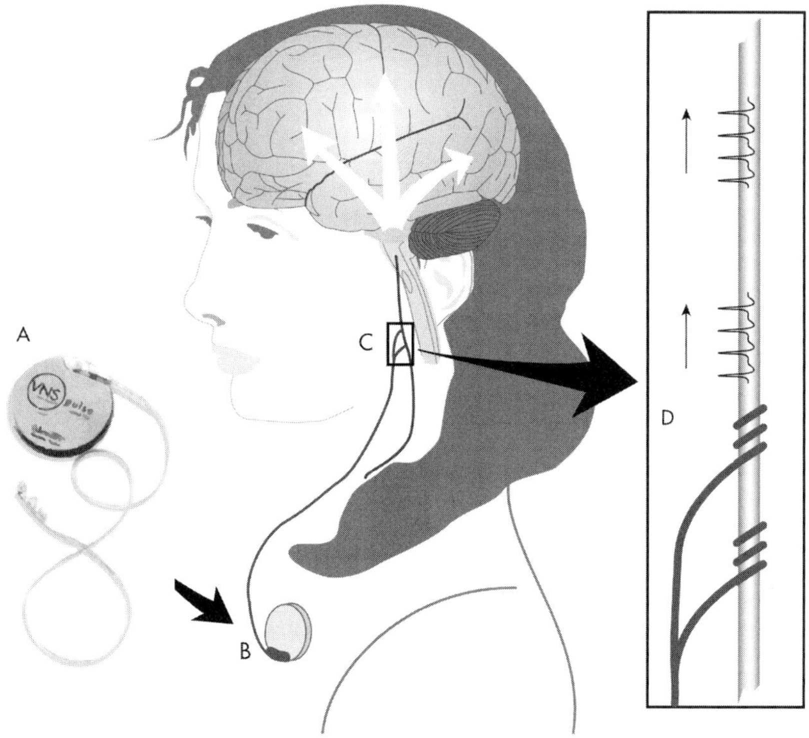

FIGURE 11–1. Clinical vagus nerve stimulation (VNS).

The VNS generator (A) contains a small battery that generates electrical impulses. A surgeon implants the generator subcutaneously over the chest (B) and attaches the electrodes to the left vagus nerve (C). Intermittent signals from the VNS device travel up the vagus nerve (D) and enter the medulla.

Source. Reprinted from Higgins ES, George MS: *Brain Stimulation Therapies for Clinicians.* Washington, DC, American Psychiatric Publishing, 2009, p. 81. Used with permission. Copyright © 2009 American Psychiatric Publishing.

group and 13% for the treatment as usual group (George et al. 2005).

The FDA considered all these studies when evaluating VNS for depression and was most impressed with the long-term enduring benefits for this difficult-to-treat population and the potential doubling of the chances of response (George et al. 2005). In 2005, the FDA approved VNS to treat patients with chronic or recurrent depression, either unipolar or bipolar, and with a history of failing to respond to at least four antidepressant trials. Because VNS is FDA approved for treatment-resistant depression in the absence of Class I evidence of efficacy, insurance companies have resisted reimbursing the implant. Thus, currently VNS is not making a large clinical impact for depression treatment, and the field awaits a much-needed adequately powered randomized controlled trial (RCT), which unfortunately has not been started due to financial concerns on the part of the manufacturer.

It is disappointing that the overall antidepressant response rate to VNS plus medications at 1 year is less than 50%, because VNS is costly and requires a surgical implantation. However, many studies are now showing that patients with treatment-resistant depression have poor outcomes to traditional medication treatment (Fekadu et al. 2009; Rhebergen et al. 2009; Rush et al. 2006a, 2006b; ten Doesschate et al. 2009; Trivedi et al. 2006; Yiend et al. 2009). Attempts to predict who is more likely to respond to VNS have not been successful.

Several other potential VNS clinical applications, reasoning from the known role of the vagus, include obesity (Roslin and Kurian 2001), craving (Bodenlos et al. 2007), pain (Borckardt et al. 2005, 2006a), traumatic brain injury (Colombo et al. 2008; Neese et al. 2007; Ottani et al. 2009), and anxiety (George et al. 2008). These trials, all with small sample sizes, suggest potential efficacy in these domains, but RCTs are needed.

With respect to geriatric neuropsychiatry, a Swedish group implanted VNS devices in 17 patients with Alzheimer's disease (Merrill et al. 2006; Sjögren et al. 2002). The researchers serially measured cognition and cerebrospinal fluid for up to 1 year and found improvement over expected natural declines in over half of the subjects. The small sample size and lack of a sham control group limit the interpretations that can be drawn from the trial, but VNS at least appears tolerable in a geriatric cohort with dementia.

Putative Mechanisms of Action

The vagus nerve (tenth cranial nerve) enters the brain at the medulla. It is the longest cranial nerve extending into the chest and abdominal cavity. *Vagus* comes from the Latin word for wandering, and this nerve is remarkably complex, both in its route through the body and in the variety of information it passes bidirectionally between the brain and the viscera. Traditionally, the vagus nerve has been conceptualized as modulating the parasympathetic tone of the internal organs (efferent functions). However, 80% of the signals traveling through the vagus nerve actually go from the organs back into the brain (afferent) (Foley and DuBois 1937).

In 1938, Bailey and Bremer stimulated the vagus nerve of cats and reported that this synchronized the electrical activity in the orbital cortex. In 1949, Paul MacLean and Karl Pribram carried out similar studies with anesthetized monkeys. Using an electroencephalogram (EEG) recording, they found that VNS generated slow waves over the lateral frontal cortex (Maclean 1990). The afferent fibers traveling in the vagus terminate largely in the nucleus tractus solitarius (NTS) in the medulla. The NTS, in turn, innervates the noradrenergic nucleus locus coeruleus (LC) both directly (Van Bockstaele et al. 1999a, 1999b) and indirectly via the rostral ventrolateral medulla (Van Bockstaele et al. 1989), which sends strong projections to LC neurons (Aston-Jones et al. 1986; Ennis and Aston-Jones 1988). LC neurons project extensively throughout the neuraxis, providing prominent noradrenergic innervation in the orbitofrontal cortex and the insula, including somatotopically defined regions that may represent emotional (limbic) information (Aston-Jones 2004). Thus, it is plausible that the NTS regulates norepinephrine release in the forebrain through its descending projections to LC afferents in the nucleus paragigantocellularis. In addition, these connections reveal that many vagus afferent fibers connect transsynaptically to areas of the limbic brain that regulate emotion. It is no surprise then that a person who grieves has the perception of having a "broken heart" or that a person who is nervous or anxious has the sensation of "butterflies in the stomach." This misplacement concerning the source of the sensory signal may reflect the fact that vagal cardiac fibers terminate in brain regions where the limbic system and gut sensations overlap.

Jake Zabara in the mid-1980s was perhaps the first person to demonstrate convincingly the therapeutic benefits of VNS, although many had been considering this avenue before Zabara (Groves and Brown 2005). Zabara discovered in a canine model of (strychnine-induced) epilepsy that repetitive electrical stimulation of the vagus nerve was able to acutely terminate a motor seizure. Importantly, he also found that the anticonvulsant benefits could outlast the period of stimulation by a factor of four (Zabara 1985a, 1985b, 1992). Constant stimulation was not required for enduring anticonvulsive effects.

Safety

No additional safety concerns are involved in using VNS with elderly patients, and VNS can be implanted under local anesthesia. Additionally, because VNS has no deleterious cognitive side effects and no interactions with other drugs, it has specific advantages for elderly patients. The adverse events associated with VNS fall into two categories: those associated with the complications of the surgery and those resulting from the side effects of stimulation.

The risks associated with surgery are minimal (O'Reardon et al. 2006). Wound infections are infrequent (<3%) and managed with antibiotics. Pain at the surgical site almost always resolves within 2 weeks. Although left vocal cord paresis persists rarely after surgery (<1 in 1,000), it usually resolves slowly over the ensuing weeks.

Temporary asystole during the initial testing of the device is a rare but serious surgical complication. In ~1 out of 1,000 cases, asystole has been reported in the operating room during initial lead testing. It may be a result of aberrant electrical stimulation resulting from poor hemostatic control; that is, blood in the surgical field causes arcing of the current, and the cardiac branch becomes depolarized. Fortunately, no deaths have been reported, and normal cardiac rhythm has always been restored. Postoperatively these patients have been able to safely use VNS. More importantly and surprisingly given the known efferent VNS effects, no cardiac events have been reported when the device is turned on for the first time after surgery.

The most common side effects associated with stimulation are hoarseness, dyspnea, and cough. They are dose dependent, correlate with stimulation intensity, and can be minimized with reductions in the stimulation parameters. Interestingly, most side effects decrease with time (Sackeim et al. 2001b). Hoarseness or voice alteration is the most persistent problem. Between 30% and 60% of patients continue to experience this side effect during times of stimulation; however, for reasons that are unclear, this problem also diminishes over months to years. As mentioned before, one would speculate that VNS might induce a parasympathetic response, but this has been aggressively monitored and has not been an issue.

VNS therapy also affects respiration during sleep and has been shown to worsen preexisting obstructive sleep apnea–hypopnea syndrome by increasing the number of apneas and hypopneas (Ebben et al. 2008; Holmes et al. 2003; Marzec et al. 2003; Papacostas et al. 2007). VNS should be used cautiously in patients with sleep apnea or be supplemented with continuous positive airway pressure.

Research Uses

Because of the cost and invasive nature of VNS, no human studies have been done in healthy adults. Some researchers have proposed transcutaneous VNS involving either stimulation in the neck through the skin or stimulation of a dermatome of skin in the ear that is vagally mediated (Huston et al. 2007; Kraus et al. 2007). Studies of VNS implantation in patients with epilepsy or depression have revealed that VNS causes discrete changes in limbic structures, including the cingulate gyrus, the hippocampus, and the insula (Chae et al. 2003; Henry 2002; Henry et al. 1999). The specific network activated depends on the choice of the use parameters (Mu et al. 2004), suggesting that with more extensive knowledge, the VNS signal could be "directed" within groups of patients or even individually (Lomarev et al. 2002). Human studies using functional magnetic resonance imaging (fMRI) and positron emission tomography (PET) techniques demonstrate that VNS induces neuronal activity changes within the amygdala, hippocampus, and thalamus, all targets of the LC (Henry et al. 1998, 1999; Lomarev et al. 2002; Mu et al. 2004). These regional changes evolve over time and vary with clinical response (Nahas et al. 2007). Additionally, VNS produces interesting improvements in cognition (Boon et al. 2006; Borghetti et al. 2007; Helmstaedter et al. 2001; Sackeim et al. 2001a; Smith et al. 2006), perhaps linked to its influence on the central LC–norepinephrine system. Improvements in verbal recognition memory (Clark et al. 1999) and enhanced working memory (Sackeim et al. 2001a) have also been reported. VNS also has effects on sleep and arousal states. VNS decreases daytime sleepiness in humans (Malow et al. 2001) and promotes increased attention and arousal in animals (Lockard et al. 1990). These findings suggest that VNS may be a potent modulator of cognition via influences on ascending arousal systems. Cerebrospinal fluid studies have found increases in serotonin and norepinephrine metabolites following VNS.

The VNS animal studies to date have been more extensive, although progress in this area was at one time slowed by the lack of small portable generators that fit in rats. Now that these are available for rats, VNS studies have shown the importance of the LC in the signal propagation (Krahl et al. 1998, 2001) and have also revealed long-term changes in raphe firing, unlike serotonin-acting medications (Biggio et al. 2009; Dorr and Debonnel 2006; Manta et al. 2009). These long-term changes in raphe firing may be somehow connected to the slow but durable anticonvulsant and antidepressant effects of VNS.

Studies in rodents have examined the functional relationship between the vagus nerve and the LC, in addition to the anatomical circuit connections summarized above. VNS induces expression of the immediate early gene c-fos in LC neurons (Naritoku et al. 1995). Several studies have linked the LC to the seizure-suppressant effects of vagal activity. Thus, lesions of the LC attenuate the antiepileptic effects of VNS in the rat (Krahl et al. 1998). Anatomical targets of LC projections also show electrophysiological and neurochemical changes following VNS. Amygdala, hippocampal, and insular cortex neurons all show enhanced neuronal activity after VNS (Radna and MacLean 1981a, 1981b). Microdialysis studies in animals demonstrate that VNS potentiates norepinephrine release in both the amygdala (Hassert et al. 2004) and the hippocampus (Miyashita and Williams 2003). VNS also induces c-fos expression in each of these structures, as well as in other LC targets including the thalamus (Naritoku et al. 1995). Thus, anatomical findings demonstrate that the vagus and LC are connected via well-specified relay nuclei, and functional studies show that these circuits contribute to forebrain activity. These findings demonstrate that chemical or electrical stimulation of the vagus nerve alters LC activity and that of its forebrain targets, suggesting that the therapeutic effects of VNS may involve the LC–noradrenergic system.

Researchers recently have been investigating the role that VNS might have on inflammation and the immune response (Ottani et al. 2009; Pavlov 2008; Van Der Zanden et al. 2009).

Transcranial Magnetic Stimulation

Description of Method

TMS involves inducing an electrical current within the brain using pulsating magnetic fields that are generated outside the brain near the scalp. The essential feature is using electricity to generate a rapidly changing magnetic field, which in turn produces electrical impulses in the brain. A typical TMS device produces a fairly powerful magnetic field (~1.5–3 teslas) but only very briefly (milliseconds). TMS is not simply the application of a static or constant magnetic field to the brain.

By 1820, scientists had discovered that passing an electrical current through a wire induces a magnetic field. In 1832, Michael Faraday demonstrated that the inverse was also true—passing a wire through a magnetic field generates an electrical current (Faraday 1965). Thus, a changing magnetic field can generate electrical current in nearby wires, nerves, or muscles. A static magnet will not generate a current. For most TMS applications, the electricity induced from the pulsating magnet, and not the magnetic field itself, likely produces neurobiological effects.

In 1959, Kolin et al. demonstrated that a fluctuating magnetic field could stimulate a peripheral frog muscle in preparation. However, the modern era of TMS did not start until 1985, when Anthony Barker in Sheffield, England, described the use of a noninvasive magnetic device resembling modern TMS instruments (Barker et al. 1985). The device was slow to recharge and quick to overheat, but it was able to stimulate spinal cord roots, as well as superficial human cortex.

TMS requires a unit to store and deliver a charge (called a capacitor) and an electromagnetic coil (typically round in the shape of a doughnut or two round side-by-side coils connected in a figure eight) (Figure 11–2). A system can be cumbersome (resembling a small refrigerator), although some systems are portable and weigh less than 20 lbs (Epstein 2008; Huang et al. 2009). The devices are regulated by the FDA for general safety, and most machines have FDA approval for sale in the United States. They are also regulated regarding a company's ability to advertise a product's therapeutic use for a particular disorder. In the United States, a device manufactured by Neuronetics (www.neuronetics.com) was approved by the FDA in 2008 for treating depression (O'Reardon et al. 2007).

Early TMS devices emitted only a single brief pulse. Modern devices can generate a rapid succession of pulses, called repetitive TMS (rTMS). These devices are used for behavioral research or clinical treatments and can discharge on and off for several minutes. For example, the typical treatment for depression is a 20- to 40-minute session, 5 days a week for 4–6 weeks. Because of the importance of keeping the patient still and correctly placing the device, the patient reclines in a chair, and the device is held securely against his or her head while the patient is awake and alert, without needing anesthesia.

The TMS coil generates a magnetic field impulse that can reach only the outer layers of the cortex (Davey et al. 2004). The main effect of the impulse penetrates only 2–3 cm below the device (Roth et al. 1994; Rothwell et al. 1999). However, a deep TMS device has been invented and is in early clinical trials for depression and several other indications (Roth et al. 2002, 2005).

When the TMS device produces a pulse over the motor cortex, descending fibers are activated and volleys of electrical impulses descend through connected fibers into the spinal cord and out to the peripheral nerve, where the TMS impulse being transmitted through these fibers can ultimately cause a muscle to twitch. The minimum amount of energy needed to produce contraction of the thumb (abductor pollicis brevis) is called the motor threshold (MT) (Fitzgerald et al. 2006; Fox et al. 2006; Sacco et al. 2009). Because MT is so easy to generate and varies widely across individuals, it is used as a measure of general cortical excitability, and most TMS studies (both research and clinical) report the TMS intensity as a function of individual MT rather than as an absolute physical value (Di Lazzaro et al. 2008). Although this convention has helped in making TMS safer, it is severely insufficient in that MT is referenced only to each machine and thus is not a universal number. Future work is focusing on more universal, constant measures of the magnetic field delivered.

In general with TMS, a stronger, more intense pulse results in more activation of the central nervous system (CNS) tissue, as well as a wider area of activation. The effect with changes in frequency is more complex. It is believed that frequencies of <1/second (<1 Hz) are inhibitory (Hoffman and Cavus 2002). This may be because low-frequency TMS more selectively stimulates the inhibitory γ-aminobutyric acid (GABA) neurons or because this frequency is long-term depression (LTD)-like. Conversely, higher-frequency stimulation is behaviorally excitatory (Ziemann et al. 2008). However, high-frequency TMS over some brain regions can temporarily block or knock out the function of that part of the brain (Epstein et al. 1996; Pascual-Leone et al. 1991).

A different kind of magnetic stimulator is being developed by Neuralieve (www.neuralieve.com) for home use by patients with migraine headaches. This handheld device delivers a single large pulse. When the patient experiences the aura phase of an impending headache, he or she holds the device to the back of the head and directs the pulse toward the occipital cortex (Ambrosini and Schoenen 2003; Clarke et al. 2006). Early results have been positive.

Putative Mechanisms of Action

TMS can produce different brain effects depending on the brain region being stimulated, the frequency of stimulation, and the use parameters (intensity, frequency, duty train), as well as whether the brain region is engaged or "resting." Thus, it is difficult to review a single "mechanism of action" for TMS. However, in general, a single pulse of TMS over a cortical region such as the motor cortex causes large neurons to depolarize; that is, the powerful transient magnetic field induces current to flow in neurons in superficial cortex (induced current). Both modeling and simple testing have shown that the fibers that are most likely to depolarize are those that are perpendicular to the coil and are bending within the gyrus (Amassian et al. 1990, 1992; Lisanby et al. 1998a, 1998b). Some lower TMS intensities do not cause large neuron depolarization but can still affect resting membrane potentials and thus alter brain activity and behavior. The most striking positive phenomena that TMS can produce are motor twitches (thumb, hand, arm, or leg movement) when applied over motor cortex or phosphenes when placed over the occiput. To date, TMS cannot reproduce old memories, thoughts, sensations, or percepts apart from the scalp sensation of the coil.

rTMS can produce measurable effects lasting for minutes to hours after the train. As mentioned earlier, in general, rTMS at frequencies of >1 Hz are excitatory, and those of <1 Hz are inhibitory. One particular TMS sequence builds directly from the neurobiological studies of long-term potentiation and long-term depression, and is called theta burst because it has short bursts of TMS at theta frequencies (Di Lazzaro et al. 2005; Stagg et al. 2009).

TMS over some cortical regions can produce a transient disruption of behavior. This is most striking when the coil is placed over Broca's area and the clinician can produce a transient expressive aphasia. Much interest involves whether TMS can produce short-term or even longer-term changes in plas-

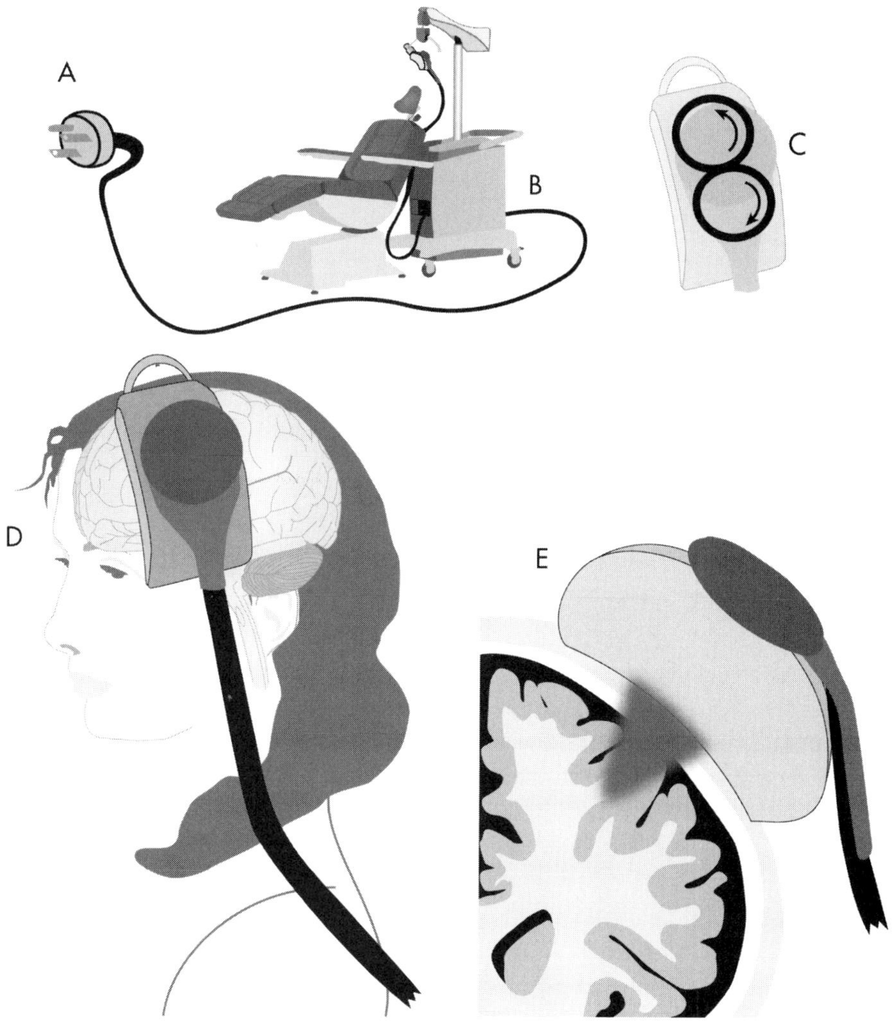

FIGURE 11–2. Transcranial magnetic stimulation (TMS).

Current from the wall (A) is used to charge a bank of large capacitors (B). These capacitors send a pulsing electrical current to the coils (C) resting on the scalp (D). The powerful but brief electrical current in the coil creates a transient magnetic field that passes unimpeded through the skin and skull and results in electrical impulses in neurons in superficial cortex under the coil (E). Depending on the type of cell that is engaged, this then results in secondary transsynaptic effects.

Source. Reprinted from Higgins ES, George MS: *Brain Stimulation Therapies for Clinicians.* Washington, DC, American Psychiatric Publishing, 2009, p. 106. Used with permission. Copyright © 2009 American Psychiatric Publishing.

ticity (Ziemann et al. 2008). Simple studies in motor and visual systems clearly indicate the potential for this approach (Miniussi et al. 2008), which is now being applied in studies of poststroke recovery and other forms of rehabilitation (Hummel et al. 2008; Pape et al. 2009).

Coupling TMS with electrophysiological measures allows the clinician to use TMS as a measure of motor cortex excitability and then to measure how behavior, medications, or other interventions might change excitability. Several groups are using this TMS excitability measurement technique to investigate new CNS-active compounds (Li et al. 2004, 2009; Paulus et al. 2008; Ziemann et al. 2008).

Coupling TMS with imaging (PET, single-photon emission computed tomography [SPECT], fMRI, or blood oxygenation level–dependent [BOLD] fMRI) allows the clinician to directly stimulate circuits and then image the resultant changes (George et al. 2007; Siebner et al. 2009). Regarding the neuropsychiatric uses of TMS for depression or pain, at a molecular level TMS is known to have similar effects as those seen with ECT, such as increased monoamine turnover, increased brain-derived neurotrophic factor (BDNF), and normalization of the hypothalamic-pituitary-adrenal (HPA) axis.

The initial use of daily prefrontal TMS to treat depression was based on the theory that clinical depression involves an imbalanced relationship between prefrontal cortex and limbic regions involved in mood regulation (insula, cingulate gyrus, amygdala, and hippocampus) (George et al. 1994). Only limited direct support indicates that this is occurring, although work by Maier and colleagues directly supports the causal role of medial prefrontal cortex in mitigating and reversing chronic learned helplessness. Stimulatory fibers from prefrontal cortex are critical in this model (Baratta et al. 2007; Christianson et al. 2008a, 2008b; Hutchinson et al. 2008).

Safety

In general, TMS is regarded as safe and without enduring side effects. No reported lasting neurological, cognitive, or cardiovascular sequelae have been reported. However, because TMS can alter brain function and is a relatively new technology, vigilance is required. The interested reader should refer to the results from an earlier international conference on TMS safety (Wassermann 1997). An update has been drafted following a more recent international consensus conference (Rossi et al. 2009).

Inducing a seizure is the primary safety concern with TMS, and advanced age is not a known risk factor. There have been fewer than 20 reported seizures induced with TMS, with a sample size of several thousand. The risk is less than 0.5%. Most of these patients were healthy volunteers without a history of epilepsy. Fortunately, there are no reports that the individuals affected experienced recurrence. Also, each of the seizures occurred during TMS administration when the patient was sitting down and near an investigator. Additionally, all of the seizures were self-limited without the patient needing medications or other interventions. Published safety tables concerning the proper intensity, frequency, and number of stimuli (Wassermann 1997) have helped minimize the number of seizures in the past 10 years. Of the reported cases, the majority were receiving TMS to the motor cortex—the most epileptogenic region of the cortex. Additionally, most (but not all) patients who experienced seizures were receiving trains of stimulation outside of suggested limits. These cases suggest that TMS-induced seizures will remain a small but significant adverse event even in patients without histories of seizures and even when TMS is used within suggested guidelines.

Studies in rabbits as well as some human studies suggest that TMS can cause hearing loss (Counter et al. 1990; Loo et al. 2001); therefore, subjects, patients, and operators should wear earplugs. Because of the increased vulnerability of elderly individuals to hearing loss, it is especially important to make sure that older patients receiving TMS wear good snug-fitting earplugs during treatments. After a patient reported a temporary hearing loss following TMS, an extensive study of auditory threshold was conducted before and after 4 weeks of TMS in over 300 patients. No changes were found. Nevertheless, patients should wear earplugs when receiving TMS.

Headaches are the most common complaint after TMS; however, O'Reardon et al. (2007) found no difference in headache frequency between sham and active conditions in a large trial. Repeated analyses of neurocognitive functioning of TMS patients have not found any enduring negative effects from the procedure (Avery et al. 2008; Little et al. 2000). After a session, patients or subjects are able to drive home and return to work. Research by Jorge et al. (2008) suggests that TMS is well tolerated by elderly patients, with no additional safety or cognitive concerns, even in those who have recently had a stroke.

Clinical Studies

Largely because of its noninvasiveness, TMS has been investigated as a potential treatment in almost all neuropsychiatric conditions. Until only recently, there has not been a TMS industry to promote or perform this work, and thus much of the clinical work has been performed at single sites without industry funding and with relatively small sample sizes.

Depression has been the condition most widely studied with TMS. Three initial studies from Europe used TMS over the vertex as a potential antidepressant (Grisaru et al. 1994; Hoflich et al. 1993; Kolbinger et al. 1995). In the United States, George et al. (1995, 1996, 1997b) performed initial safety studies in healthy controls, an open study, and then a double-blind controlled trial of TMS for 2 weeks. TMS research has now dramatically grown, but without much change in many of the initial treatment choices (coil location, frequency, dosing). There have now been several meta-analyses of the procedure (Ridding and Rothwell 2007). In one meta-analysis of rTMS for depression, Mitchell and Loo (2006) examined 25 published sham-controlled studies and concluded that left prefrontal TMS provided statistical superiority over sham treatment for patients with depression. However, they also concluded that the clinical benefits are marginal in the majority of reports and that considerable uncertainty remains concerning the optimal stimulation parameters. Two more positive meta-analyses suggest that the overall effect size with TMS in major depression is at least as good as that of standard pharmacotherapy (Lam et al. 2008; Schutter 2008). Those clinical features that appear to be associated with greater response include younger age, lack of refractoriness to antidepressants, and no psychotic features (Avery et al. 2008).

The largest multisite trial to date, which resulted in FDA approval, was by Neuronetics. The company sponsored a multisite double-blind study of 301 medication-free patients with major depression. Patients were randomly assigned to active TMS or sham treatment, which they received for 4–6 weeks (O'Reardon et al. 2007). There was some controversy about the results of the trial. Before conducting the experiment, the company chose a continuous variable, the change from baseline on the Montgomery-Åsberg Depression Rating Scale (MADRS), as the primary outcome measure (and did not tell investigators in the field) while using the Hamilton Rating Scale for Depression (Ham-D) as the entry criteria. At 6 weeks, however, the continuous measured MADRS change from baseline for the active treatment group was not quite statistically different from that for the control group (P=0.058). The Ham-D scores, considered secondary outcome measures, were indeed superior for those in the active treatment group. The company argued, successfully for the publication, for exclusion of six subjects with entry MADRS scores that were very low and could not reflect clinical improvement. Thus, the manuscript was published as a positive trial, but the FDA initially rejected the application and agreed to approval only after reviewing response data on subgroups. Because such a large effect was seen in those who were less treatment resistant, the FDA labeling is for the treatment of major depressive disorder in adult patients who have failed to achieve satisfactory improvement from one prior antidepressant treatment at or above the minimal effective dosage and duration in the current episode. In clinical practice, only about one in four treatment trials meets criteria for minimal dosage and duration, so the research treatment-resistance number in the trial translates in clinical practice to patients with a moderate level of treatment resistance (Dew et al. 2005; Joo et al. 2005; Oquendo et al. 2003).

These mixed results from this large pivotal trial reflect the current status of TMS for depression. Most investigators agree that daily left prefrontal TMS for several weeks has antidepressant effects and is safe and well tolerated. This treatment will likely be ideal for some patients. However, the efficacy data in trials to date are not as robust as some investigators would like, and many await the results of larger ongoing trials and better understanding of the mechanisms of action. For example, a large European trial failed to find a statistically significant difference, but the researchers likely used an active sham condition as well as examined TMS as an augmentation rather than stand-alone treatment (Herwig et al. 2007). The National Institutes of Health has funded a large multisite trial in depression (George et al. 2010), and the U.S. Department of Veterans Affairs has launched a large cooperative study of daily left prefrontal TMS in 300 veterans with depression.

With respect to geriatric neuropsychiatry, some investigators have questioned whether prefrontal TMS would work to treat geriatric depression. As outlined in Chapter 19, "Mood Disorders," geriatric depression differs from earlier-onset depression in that it is less responsive to treatment with medications, it responds better to ECT, and patients are more sensitive to medication side effects and drug-drug combinations. Some of the early TMS depression studies reported that prefrontal TMS did not work to treat geriatric depression (Figiel et al. 1998). In trying to understand these findings, we wondered whether the TMS signal was actually reaching the prefrontal cortex in elderly patients with increased prefrontal atrophy (Kozel et al. 2000). In a group of elderly patients with depression, we used magnetic resonance imaging (MRI) scans to measure prefrontal atrophy, calculated how much additional intensity would be needed to reach the patients' cortex, and then delivered this MRI-determined adequate dose in an open-label trial. We had good antidepressant responses and found that the average intensity needed to reach prefrontal cortex in this elderly sample was 117% of MT (Nahas et al. 2001, 2004). More recent work by Jorge et al. (2008) in Iowa has confirmed that TMS is likely an important therapeutic tool in treating vascular depression.

Another recent development in terms of TMS positioning has highlighted that better understanding of the TMS methods used will likely boost clinical antidepressant efficacy. The early National Institute of Mental Health studies used a rough measurement technique known as the 5-cm rule to place the TMS coil roughly over the prefrontal cortex (George et al. 1995, 1996, 1997b). Because the location of the motor strip varies across individuals, and skull size (hat size) also varies, this simple rule results in a large variation of actual location on scalp. Although this technique is obviously insufficient, it has nevertheless been used in most trials, including the one for FDA approval (Herwig et al. 2001). One study suggested that the 5-cm rule resulted in 30% of patients being treated over supplementary motor area rather than prefrontal cortex. Two retrospective analyses of clinical trials in which brain imaging was performed to document the coil location have independently confirmed that a coil position that is anterior and lateral is associated with a better clinical response with active but not sham TMS (Hasey 2008; Herbsman et al. 2009). An Australian group performed an RCT and found that a more anterior and lateral location indeed produced a superior antidepressant response compared with the 5-cm position (Fitzgerald et al. 2009). These findings suggest that the TMS effect is not nonspecific and that the location of the coil clearly matters, even within broad boundaries of a specific lobe. It is not clear whether individualized location will be needed or used or whether general algorithms will suffice for most patients.

Auditory hallucinations are part of the positive symptoms of schizophrenia. These types of hallucinations are believed to result from aberrant activation of the language perception area at the junction of the left temporal and parietal cortices (Higgins and George 2007). Low-frequency TMS has been used to potentially inhibit this area in patients with schizophrenia and provide relief from auditory hallucinations. In a meta-analysis, Aleman et al. (2007) examined the efficacy of low-frequency TMS as a treatment of resistant auditory hallucinations in schizophrenia. Ten sham-controlled studies have incorporated 212 patients. The review concluded that TMS was effective in reducing auditory hallucinations. Unfortunately, TMS had no effect on other positive symptoms or the cognitive deficits of schizophrenia. Larger studies are needed to definitely establish the efficacy, tolerability, and utility of TMS for schizophrenia.

There have been four RCTs of intermittent daily prefrontal TMS to treat negative symptoms in patients with schizophrenia. Only one of these studies was positive (Fitzgerald and Daskalakis 2008).

Tinnitus is a common, often disabling disorder, which has no adequate treatment. Up to 8% of adults over age 50 have tinnitus, a condition that can be quite distressing. Recent fMRI studies have identified increased activity in the auditory cortex in patients with tinnitus. Low-frequency TMS offers a possible mechanism to inhibit the overactive auditory cortex that may be producing tinnitus. Several small controlled trials from one research group in Germany have produced impressive results in treating patients with tinnitus (Langguth et al. 2008). Larger multicenter studies are needed to see if these positive effects can be replicated.

Numerous small controlled studies have evaluated the utility of TMS in patients with pain. Multiple brain sites have been tested, including prefrontal cortex, motor cortex, and parietal cortex (Andre-Obadia et al. 2006; Lefaucheur 2004; Lefaucheur et al. 2001a, 2001b; Pridmore and Oberoi 2000; Rollnik et al. 2003). In general, TMS provides effective pain relief in these different locations in diverse pain conditions. Unfortunately, the effect of TMS on pain only lasts for a short duration. Consequently, the utility of TMS as a practical treatment for chronic pain conditions has yet to be established.

Recent studies suggest that TMS may have some utility in managing acute pain (see also Chapter 23, "Pain"). In two different studies of patients recovering from gastric bypass surgery, each patient received 20 minutes of real or sham TMS administered to the prefrontal cortex. Then the patient's use of self-administered morphine was followed over the next 48 hours. Those receiving real TMS used 40% less morphine in the next 24 hours, with the majority of the reduction occurring in the first 8 hours after TMS (Borckardt et al. 2006b, 2008).

As mentioned earlier in "Description of Method," Neuralieve's handheld device is being studied as a treatment for migraine headaches. Preliminary results have been encouraging (Ambrosini and Schoenen 2003; Clarke et al. 2006). Larger studies are under way.

Following an ischemic event to the motor cortex, the brain attempts to reorganize the damaged networks. Indeed, the extent of reorganization correlates with the clinical recovery of motor function. TMS may accelerate the reorganization process and therefore enhance recovery (Hummel et al. 2008; Miniussi et al. 2008; Pape et al. 2009). It is unclear which types of TMS may be beneficial in stroke recovery. High-frequency TMS to the affected area may enhance reorganization. Alternatively, low-frequency TMS to the opposite intact hemisphere is believed to reduce the interference from the nonstroke side. Some believe that too much input from the unaffected side of the brain impedes recovery. Reducing excitability with low-frequency TMS may enhance recovery.

Ridding and Rothwell (2007) reviewed the studies of TMS in stroke recovery. Although the total number of patients in controlled trials was only 87, the results were encouraging. Clearly, larger studies are needed, but the results suggest that TMS might be able to improve the natural healing process after a stroke (Kew et al. 1994; McKay et al. 2002; Ridding and Rothwell 1995, 2007).

Theoretically, low-frequency TMS could be used to treat cortical epilepsy. Early studies showed that TMS could reduce EEG epileptiform abnormalities. Initial case studies were positive. In a controlled study of daily TMS over the cortical site of seizures for 1 week, Theodore et al. (2002) found a statistically significant reduction in seizures. However, the authors concluded that TMS treatment was not clinically significant. More recently, in another controlled trial, Cantello et al. (2007) concluded that "active" rTMS was no better than placebo for seizure reduction. Although the idea of using inhibitory doses of TMS to calm cortical targets is intriguing, the controlled trials to date have not been very successful.

Research Uses

Space does not permit a thorough overview of TMS research uses, other than to highlight the active research areas. TMS can be used as a measure of cortical excitability and has been used to investigate medication effects, emotional states, plasticity in learning and stroke recovery, sleep (Massimini et al. 2007; Tononi and Koch 2008), and a host of disease states. TMS can be combined with brain imaging to directly stimulate circuits and image the resultant changes (Figure 11–3). When precisely applied over critical brain regions, TMS can help causally determine whether a brain region is involved in a behavior and how information flows through the brain during a task (Figure 11–4). Despite the excitement over the possibilities, little hard evidence suggests at this time that TMS might be used to actually augment task performance, memory formation, or recovery from injury.

Transcranial Direct Current Stimulation

Description of Method

Perhaps one of the simplest ways of focally stimulating the brain is with tDCS. Similar techniques were practiced almost immediately after electricity was "discovered" in the late 1800s. Passing a direct current through muscle or the brain was in vogue in Europe. For example, one of Jean-Martin Charcot's

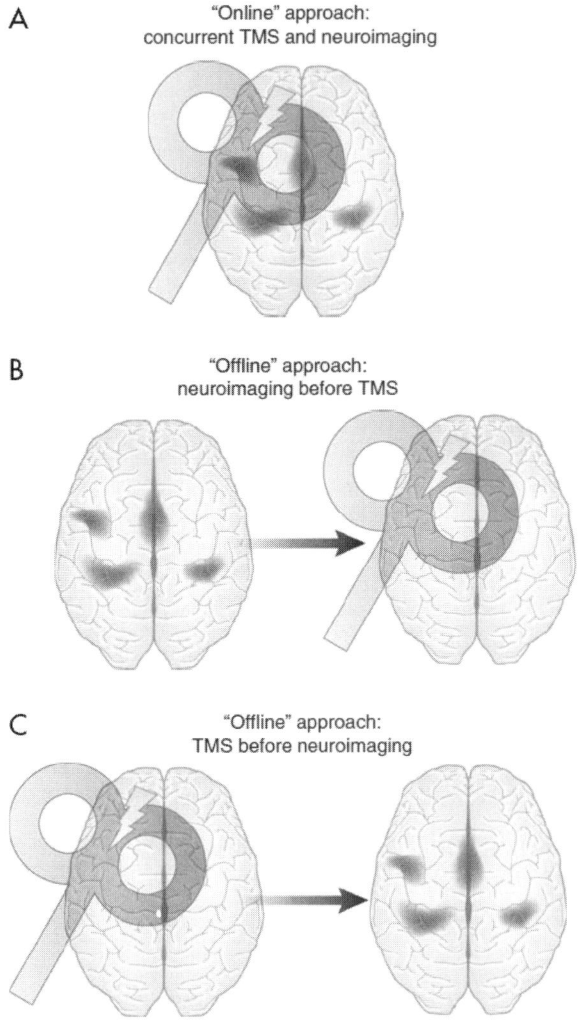

FIGURE 11–3. Brain stimulation and imaging.

The combination of brain imaging with brain stimulation allows for more direct examination of the role of circuit activity in brain-behavior relationships. Historically most brain imaging has been relatively passive, and changes in a circuit occur along with a behavior, but causality is not known. By combining actual stimulation with imaging, the clinician can move a step closer to causal statements, as well as prepare the stage for potential clinical translation and therapeutic uses of brain stimulation approaches. In general, the clinician can image simultaneously with stimulation (**Panel A**), or the clinician can use the brain imaging result (structural or functional or some combination) to guide the placement of the brain stimulation (in this case transcranial magnetic stimulation [TMS]) (**Panel B**). Finally, the clinician can stimulate a region with TMS or transcranial direct current stimulation, produce brain changes, and then use brain imaging to examine changes in circuit behavior (**Panel C**).

Source. Adapted from Siebner HR, Bergmann TO, Bestmann S, et al.: "Consensus Paper: Combining Transcranial Stimulation With Neuroimaging." *Brain Stimulation: Basic, Translational, and Clinical Research in Neuromodulation* 2:58–80, 2009.

residents, Georges Duchenne de Boulogne, traveled around Paris with a small battery and passed electricity through patients' muscles, examining the effects on numerous disorders and using it to better understand muscle-nerve innervations, particularly in the muscular dystrophies (George 1994). Others began applying direct current through the brain. Due to lack of patient benefits, this technique was largely dropped as a treatment in Europe and the United States.

For reasons that are not clear, tDCS has been an area of active research in Russia during the 1940s up until the present time. It was sometimes called "electrosleep therapy" because patients would sometimes nap or sleep during the 30-minute treatments (Gomez and Mikhail 1978). Most of the tDCS done in Russia was not delivered in clinical trials and was largely anecdotally used for the treatment of alcoholism, pain, depression, or a combination of these disorders (Feighner et al. 1973).

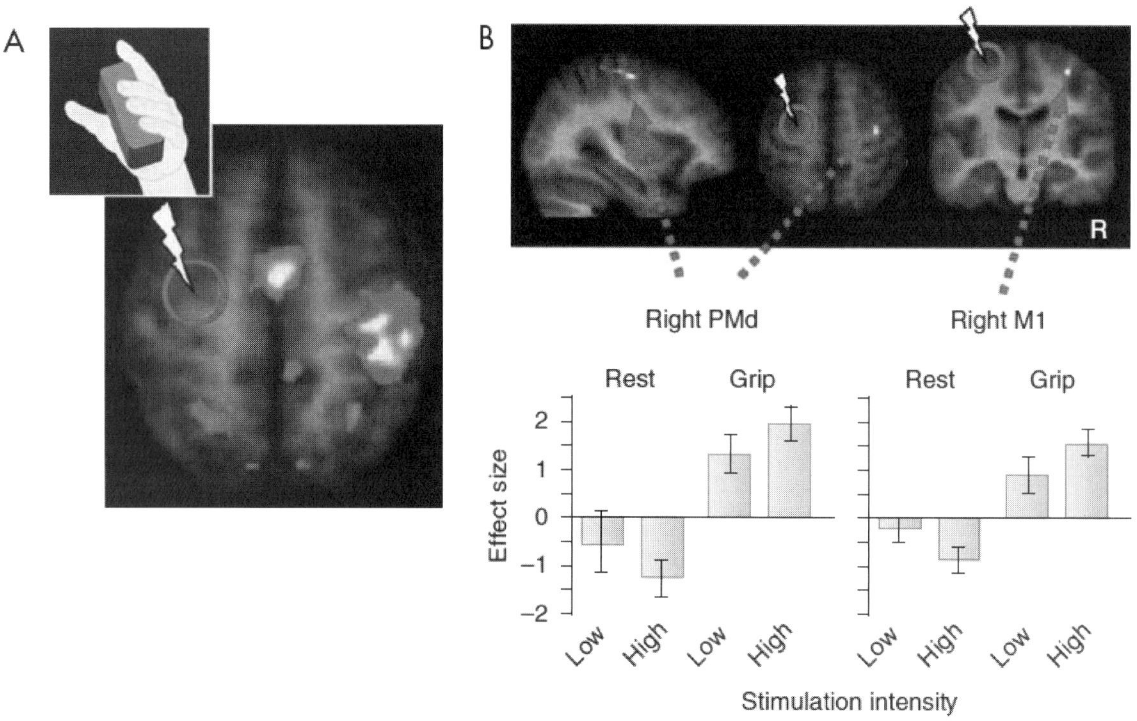

FIGURE 11–4. State-dependent interregional interactions evoked by transcranial magnetic stimulation (TMS) interleaved with functional magnetic resonance imaging.

Some groups can actually use TMS within a magnetic resonance imaging (MRI) scanner (Bohning et al. 1998). These images show the following: **Panel A:** The main effect of left-hand grip, irrespective of stimulation intensity. This illustrates how the clinician can obtain blood oxygenation level–dependent (BOLD) activation maps during concurrent application of TMS pulses (5 pulses, 11 Hz) inside an MRI scanner. **Panel B:** Task-state dependent effects of TMS on causal interactions in the human motor system. At rest, TMS applied to the left dorsal premotor cortex (PMd) increased activity in contralateral PMd and primary motor cortex (M1) at high stimulation intensity (110% of resting motor threshold), compared with stimulation at a lower control intensity (70% active motor threshold). By contrast, this effect was reversed during a simple motor task that activated right PMd and M1. Now high-intensity stimulation increased task-related activity, compared with lower-intensity stimulation. The results show that TMS can causally affect activity in contralateral regions and that these influences are dependent on the activation state of these regions.

Source. Adapted from Siebner HR, Bergmann TO, Bestmann S, et al.: "Consensus Paper: Combining Transcranial Stimulation With Neuroimaging." *Brain Stimulation: Basic, Translational, and Clinical Research in Neuromodulation* 2:58–80, 2009.

Walter Paulus and his group in Göttingen, Germany, have led a resurrection of this technology, and there is now active investigation of tDCS, with over 100 articles in the last 10 years in peer-reviewed journals (Paulus 2003). Clearly, tDCS has an effect on the brain—it can boost cortical excitability and improve memory in healthy people (Boggio et al. 2006, 2007). Whether these effects can be used therapeutically remains to be determined (George et al. 2009; Nitsche et al. 2008).

Quite simply, tDCS involves passing a weak (usually ≤1 mA) direct current through the brain between two electrodes. The current enters the brain from the anode, travels through the tissue, and exits out the cathode (Figure 11–5). Some researchers refer to the procedure as either cathodal tDCS or anodal tDCS depending on which electrode is placed over the region that is being modified.

The administration of tDCS is relatively easy. Many researchers simply use damp sponges as the electrodes. These can be placed anywhere on the scalp and are held in place with an elastic headband.

Putative Mechanisms of Action

Exactly what happens to the brain with tDCS remains unknown. However, experiments with animals and humans, and even direct recordings from individual neurons, provide a general idea. The cathode (which is negative) is where the electrical current exits the brain. A smaller exiting cathode can produce a more focal delivery of charge to a brain region, as more current lines up underneath the exit. Thus, the size of the brain region being affected can be shaped or influenced by changing the size of the cathodal electrode (smaller size is more focused)

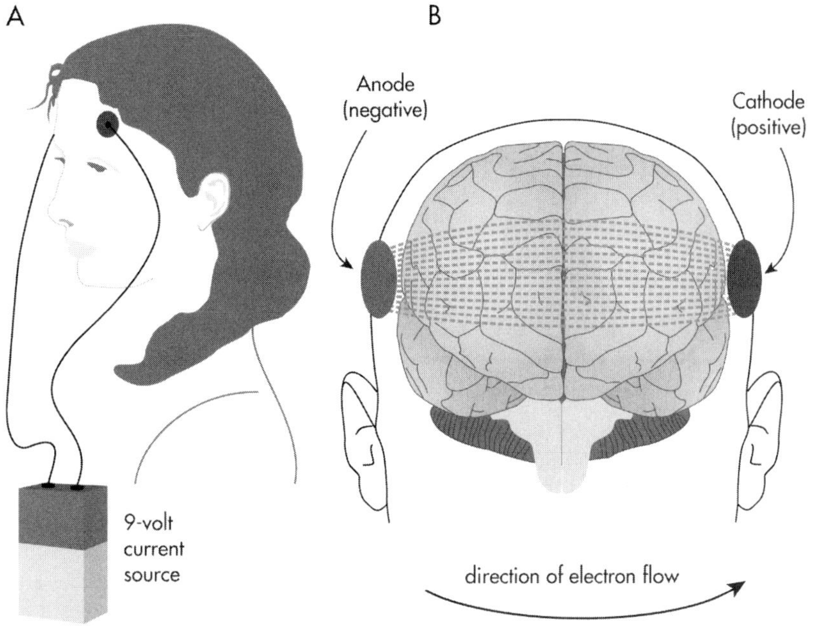

FIGURE 11–5. Transcranial direct current stimulation (tDCS).

Panel A: A tDCS device uses an anode and cathode connected to a direct current source much like a 9-volt battery. **Panel B:** The direct current passes through the intervening tissue, with some shunting through the skull, but much of it passes through the brain and changes resting electrical charge, particularly under the cathode.

Source. Reprinted from Higgins ES, George MS: *Brain Stimulation Therapies for Clinicians.* Washington, DC, American Psychiatric Publishing, 2009, p. 150. Used with permission. Copyright © 2009 American Psychiatric Publishing.

(Borckardt et al. 2009) or by changing the size and location of the anodal electrode (Datta et al. 2008; Nitsche et al. 2007).

The behavioral effects of what happens under the exiting cathode are not necessarily as simple as one would hope. In most studies, the area under the anode is more active (or excited), and the area under the cathode is more inhibited (Radman et al. 2008). It is likely that there are general shifts in cell membrane resting potentials and propensity for depolarization. Thus, tDCS is shifting the entire "set point" for overall excitability for a brain region, somewhat like a catalyst does in a chemical reaction. For example, stimulation of the motor regions produces such results, and this is being exploited as a possible treatment for stroke.

The brain is enormously complex, however, and in some studies the brain region under the anode has been behaviorally *inhibited*. For example, in one study examining the latency of a visual evoked response, 10 minutes of anodal tDCS reduced visual evoked potential amplitudes, whereas 10 minutes of cathodal tDCS increased amplitudes for several minutes following stimulation (Accornero et al. 2007). Thus, in this study, behavioral inhibition was observed under the anode and excitation under the cathode. Apparently, the different regions of the brain with varied morphology, layering, and cellular composition have different responses to direct current stimulation.

Because the human head is a poor conductor of electricity, tDCS and ECT are inefficient at stimulating the brain; at least 50% of the current is lost to the surrounding tissue. Thus, more electricity is needed than with direct invasive techniques, such as DBS, or with TMS (where the magnetic field passes through the skull).

Finally, as with all stimulation techniques, the ability to induce enduring effects, beyond the time of administration, is essential for practical clinical applications. With tDCS, the focal and behavioral changes appear to persist for at least some time after the electrodes are removed. In studies of tDCS on motor cortex, for example, tDCS-induced inhibition or excitation can last for several minutes to an hour or so (Fregni et al. 2006). Whether therapeutic changes can endure for weeks or months remains to be determined.

Safety

Side effects of tDCS depend on the type of electrode, the gel or contact agent used, the placement of the electrode, the choice of anodal or cathodal tDCS, the intensity of the stimulation, and the length of time the patient is treated (Poreisz et al. 2007). The older prefrontal treatment literature reported that skin burns could occur and that some patients felt uncomfortable or even had dizziness. Several case studies in the modern literature also report skin lesions or burns following tDCS (Palm et al. 2008).

Poreisz et al. (2007) reported results from 567 patients and subjects who had received tDCS in challenge studies over the motor, parietal, or occipital cortex. Remarkably, no patient requested that stimulation be terminated. About 70% of subjects noticed a mild tingling sensation under the electrode. One-third of subjects felt fatigue after treatment, and one-third also felt "itching" under the electrode. Less frequent complaints were headache (11%), nausea (3%), and insomnia (1%).

Research and Clinical Studies

Much of the most recent work with tDCS has dealt with its behavioral effects on healthy controls. Although it is beyond the scope of this chapter to review exhaustively these more basic behavioral studies, it is clear that tDCS can focally excite or inhibit the brain. This impressive and growing body of research strongly suggests that potential clinical uses of tDCS are yet to be discovered.

Numerous small studies with healthy volunteers have shown that tDCS can enhance motor function and control. The next logical step is to apply the technique to patients whose motor control has been damaged due to a stroke. The unique qualities of tDCS offer possibilities beyond just stimulating the damaged tissue. Some research suggests that constraining the unaffected, healthy side of the brain actually improves healing. This process is similar to constraining the good arm and forcing the patient to use the impaired arm to improve recovery following a stroke. Theoretically, tDCS could be used to excite the damaged side while inhibiting the healthy side. When the anode is placed over the brain injury, it should excite the neurons beneath it. Likewise, if the cathode is placed over the healthy side, it should provide some inhibition of those neurons. In summary, however, the work in stroke is still preliminary without large clear effects in well-conducted sham-controlled trials (Alonso-Alonso et al. 2007; Fregni and Pascual-Leone 2007; Hummel et al. 2008; Nitsche et al. 2008; Schlaug and Renga 2008; Schlaug et al. 2008).

As with all of the more recent stimulation techniques, research groups have been trying out the technology with many neuropsychiatric disorders. Single-site small sample studies with adult participants have suggested some positive effects of tDCS in treating pain, migraine, fibromyalgia, depression, and epilepsy. None of the studies were large or multisite, however, and the sample sizes have been small (George et al. 2009). Further work is needed to see if these early promising studies can be replicated.

In summary, tDCS is an exciting tool, but there are no clinically useful applications at the moment. Like many of the stimulation techniques, tDCS followed the interesting pattern of discovery, overuse, misuse, and then a reawakening with more modern approaches. This technique likely will be clinically useful in the near future for some conditions, especially when coupled with pharmacological and behavioral approaches to reshaping circuit behavior in health or disease.

Deep Brain Stimulation

Description of Method

The first implantable cardiac pacemaker was installed in 1958 in Sweden (Nicholls 2007). Although originally designed to increase the pace of a bradycardic heart, it has evolved into a device that can sense and respond to numerous inappropriate rhythms. In 1980, the first cardioverter-defibrillator was implanted. Such devices detect tachycardias and shock the heart back into a normal rhythm. Many of these are silent, except when they detect an abnormal electrocardiographic pattern. This concept is called *responsive stimulation*.

In the mid-1980s, Alim-Louis Benabid and his colleagues in France were using brain stimulation to map the best location to remove the ventral intermediate nucleus of the thalamus for Parkinson's disease (PD) and essential tremor (ET). Like Wilder Penfield before them, they used focal electrical brain stimulation to locate the most appropriate section to remove. They noted that acute stimulation of the ventral intermediate nucleus at frequencies >60 Hz immediately suppressed the tremors (Benabid et al. 1993). Furthermore, the effects were lost when the stimulation was stopped. In 1987, they began pilot studies of chronic stimulation for patients who had already been thalamotomized on one side. With positive results of stimulation at either the subthalamic nucleus (STN) or globus pallidus interna (GPi), they began bilateral stimulation with an implanted devise that is now FDA approved for PD patients resistant to L-dopa.

The FDA approved DBS in 1997 as a treatment for ET and has since expanded the approval to include PD and dystonia and most recently obsessive-compulsive disorder (OCD). The indications for dystonia and OCD are only for "compassionate use." DBS allows reversible neurosurgical interventions with fewer neurological complications than ablative resection. Theoretically, if the stimulation does not work, the surgeon can simply withdraw the thin wire, leaving the brain largely unchanged, unlike after resective surgery.

The DBS device, which looks much like a VNS device, comprises three components: the impulse generator, the extension, and the electrodes (Figure 11–6). The impulse generator is a battery-operated device placed subcutaneously, usually below the clavicle (although some generators are small enough to rest in a cavity in the skull). As with the VNS device, a clinician can externally calibrate the generator to optimize the benefits and minimize the side effects. The wire extension running subcutaneously through the neck transmits the electrical signal from the impulse generator to the electrodes in the brain. The probes are usually placed bilaterally in subcortical brain regions.

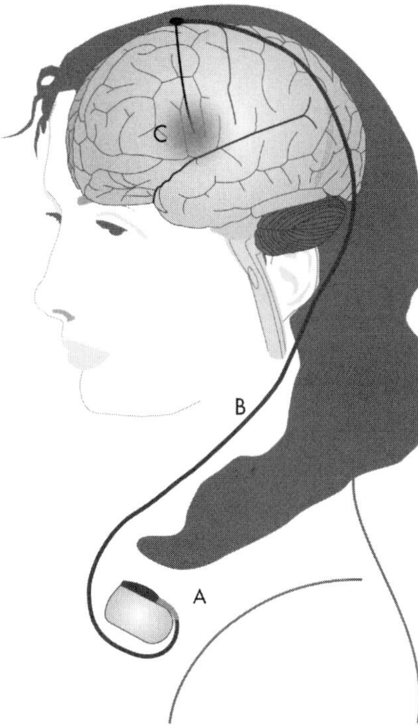

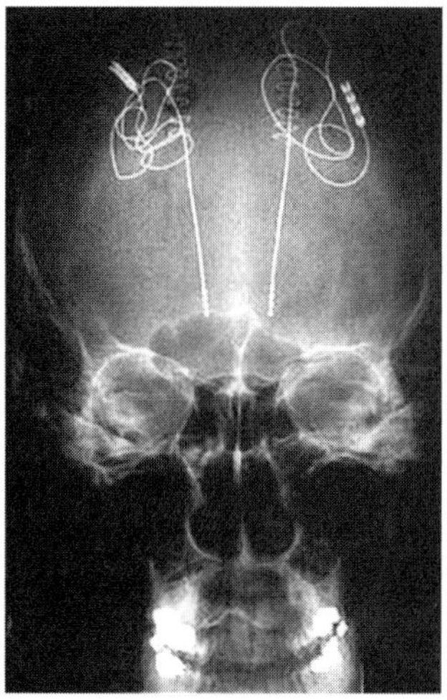

FIGURE 11–6. Deep brain stimulation.

The impulse generator (A), the extension (B), and the electrode implanted into subcortical regions of the brain (C).

Source. Reprinted from Higgins ES, George MS: *Brain Stimulation Therapies for Clinicians.* Washington, DC, American Psychiatric Publishing, 2009, p. 106. Used with permission. Copyright © 2009 American Psychiatric Publishing. X-ray image on right provided with permission by Helen Mayberg.

Typically, but not always, the neurosurgery to implant the device is performed under a combination of general and local anesthesia. Local anesthesia is used for a portion of the implant procedure to allow the patient to participate in the proper placement of the electrode. For example, with ET the neurosurgeon wants to find the location that maximally quiets the tremors. However, with dystonia, which can take months to show benefits, the placement is done under general anesthesia. The electrode is simply placed in the best possible location using image guidance.

The active portion of the probe usually contains four electrodes that can emit electrical signals. The four sites on the lead of the probe can be controlled to optimize the effect on the target site. By adjusting which electrodes emit a signal, clinicians can mold the DBS effect (Butson and McIntyre 2008; Miocinovic et al. 2009). Activation of different electrodes in the probe changes the electrical signal, which in turn modifies the parts of the brain stimulated and ultimately determines the effect of DBS on the patient (Grill and McIntyre 2001).

As with the other brain stimulation treatments, many use parameters can be adjusted with DBS, not only which electrode emits a current. Voltage, pulse width, frequency, and duty cycle (constantly on vs. intermittent) are other variables that can be adjusted with DBS. For example, a possible setting for PD might be 3.5 volts, pulse width of 60, and frequency of 130 Hz. Changing these variables can alter the effects of the stimulation.

As with cardiac pacemakers, integrating and coordinating the stimulation based on feedback from the brain has become possible with a system called *responsive neural stimulation* (Morrell 2006; Skarpaas and Morrell 2009; Sun et al. 2008). Responsive neural stimulation entails the addition of a microprocessor designed to sense the brain's electrical signals (through electroencephalography, or more accurately, electrocorticography) and deliver pulses when abnormal activity is detected. A large multisite clinical trial is under way in epilepsy, designed for potential FDA approval.

Another promising invasive nonconvulsive brain stimulation technique is cortical brain stimulation, or extradural cortical stimulation. In this case, the electrodes are placed directly on the surface of the cortex below the skull but on top of the dura mater. This procedure may be useful for problems that arise from disorders in the cortical gray matter, such as when a seizure focus is in the cortex.

Putative Mechanisms of Action

The mechanisms of action of DBS are incompletely understood (Kern and Kumar 2007). However, the frequency of the stimulation is important. For certain indications such as tremor, frequencies of >100 Hz seem to be most effective, whereas frequencies of <50 Hz are of no benefit. The stimulation remains localized (~2–3 mm) because the intensity of the current is small. The pulse width may determine the parts of the neuron that are affected. Longer pulse widths influence the cell body, whereas shorter pulse widths have more effect on the axons. These parameters (frequency, intensity, pulse width, etc.) can be modified to influence effects and side effects (Butson and McIntyre 2008).

The ultimate effect of constant high-frequency DBS is reversible inhibition of the stimulated site, and the results of focal stimulation like this are similar to those seen with ablative surgery to the same region. Exactly how high-frequency stimulation "shuts down" the target site remains a mystery. Theories include "neuronal jamming" such that signals emitting from the site are incomprehensible and ineffective downstream. Other researchers have speculated that constant high-frequency DBS activates inhibitory GABA neurons. Still others speculate that DBS stimulates reciprocal inhibitory neurons or neurons passing through the region and acting elsewhere (Gradinaru et al. 2009). DBS and the other focal stimulation methods will continue to improve as researchers understand more about how to intermittently stimulate neurons to produce different long-term changes in circuit behavior. Current use parameters will eventually appear quite crude.

Perhaps the best understanding of DBS effects is in its use for PD (see Chapter 24, "Parkinson's Disease and Movement Disorders"). The pathology of PD is centered on the basal ganglia, and the disease process starts with gradual destruction of the substantia nigra, which in turn has devastating effects on the other nuclei of the basal ganglia (Bear et al. 2006). This process occurs subclinically without external symptoms, because the system has some reserve and is able to compensate for mild losses.

The downstream effect of a diminished signal coming out of the substantia nigra is to enhance signals coming out of other nuclei. This action has the effect of "putting the brakes on movement"; that is, increased signals from the STN and GPi result in increased inhibition of the ventrolateral nucleus of the thalamus (Purves et al. 2004). The goal of DBS as currently used for PD is to inhibit the enhanced inhibiting signals. In other words, high-frequency DBS (or ablative surgery) "releases the brakes," thus allowing movement to occur more normally. The two best locations for DBS for PD are the STN and the GPi. By inhibiting these nuclei with a DBS electrode, the brakes are removed and movement flows.

Clinical and Research Uses

Parkinson's Disease

The pivotal trials testing for DBS with PD patients who were no longer responding to medications were conducted at 18 centers in the late 1990s (Deep-Brain Stimulation for Parkinson's Disease Study Group 2001). Although no patients received a sham implantation, double-blind assessments were conducted at 6 months by assessing motor function with the stimulator turned on and again when turned off. Many of these patients were elderly.

The two neuroanatomical sites for implantation used in the original studies were the STN and the GPi. Although no head-to-head trial has been conducted, the STN has become the preferred site for most surgeons. Since the publication of the pivotal studies, further research continues to support benefits from DBS for the movement disorders associated with PD. A 5-year follow-up of the first 49 patients to receive bilateral stimulation of the STN found continued improvement in motor function (Krack et al. 2003). A meta-analysis of 45 studies concluded that motor function improved by 54% in patients with STN stimulation and by 40% in patients with GPi stimulation (Weaver et al. 2005).

More recently, a randomized study compared DBS with medical management in patients with PD (Deuschl et al. 2006). The authors reported superior motor function as well as improved quality of life for the patients receiving stimulation and medication compared with those receiving medication only. This study also provided a better assessment of adverse events. Although the patients receiving medication alone experienced greater overall frequency of side effects (64% vs. 50%), the patients with DBS had a greater incidence of serious adverse events (13% vs. 4%), including one death from intracerebral hemorrhage.

Finally, it is important to remember that DBS for PD only improves motor function. The natural progression of akinesia, postural instability, and cognitive function is unaffected by DBS.

Essential Tremor

The treatment of tremors was actually the first use of DBS and continues to be a major application of the device (Wichmann and DeLong 2006). ET is the most common cause of tremor, but several other kinds of tremors respond to DBS, including brain stem (Holmes) tremor as well as tremors associated with PD or multiple sclerosis. The ventral intermediate nucleus of the thalamus is the usual site for placement of the DBS electrodes. The stimulation of this location appears to be effective for most forms of tremor regardless of the etiology.

The pivotal trials of DBS for parkinsonian tremor or ET were conducted in Europe at 13 neurosurgical centers (Limousin et al. 1999), in which 110 patients were implanted. The results were reported at 12-month follow-up. Patients' upper and lower limb tremors were significantly reduced in 85% of the patients. Postural tremors were reduced in 89%.

Numerous subsequent studies have continued to demonstrate beneficial effects of DBS for ET (Wichmann and DeLong 2006). Specifically, the procedure has an enduring and positive effect on quality of life.

Dystonia

Early work involving ablation of either the GPi or the STN led others to try DBS for dystonia (Wichmann and DeLong 2006), with the GPi the most common site of stimulation. Pivotal trials were never conducted because of the belief that the eventual market demand in dystonia was insufficient to justify industry funding of such a study. However, remarkable individual responses with DBS led the FDA to grant approval on a "compassionate use" basis or humanitarian device exemption (Horgan 2005).

In a randomized, double-blind, sham-controlled European study of 40 patients with primary segmental or generalized dystonia (Kupsch et al. 2006), half the patients received stimulation immediately, and the other half were delayed by 3 months. After 3 months, patients were blindly rated on the basis of video exams and in comparison to baseline. Patients who received stimulation had significant improvements in movement scores (39%) and disability (38%). Patients in the sham group had small nonsignificant improvements.

Chronic Pain

DBS for chronic pain has been studied sporadically for over 50 years, although only in the past 20 years has the technology existed for continued stimulation (Kringelbach et al. 2007). Numerous small studies have followed the effects of stimulation of various regions for various different forms of pain. In general, it is believed that stimulation of the periventricular-periaqueductal gray matter is best for nociceptive pain, whereas stimulation of the sensory thalamic nuclei is best for neuropathic pain (Kern and Kumar 2007). The reports look encouraging. However, as with the ablation studies, results are not so straightforward.

In the 1990s, Medtronic (the manufacturer of the DBS device; http://professional.medtronic.com) conducted two multicenter trials of DBS for chronic pain while also conducting studies for PD and ET (Coffey 2001). The results of the pain studies were disappointing (high dropout rate and poor efficacy), and the manufacturer abandoned the studies and did not apply for FDA approval. A definitive large randomized multicenter trial establishing sufficient efficacy has not yet been conducted.

Cortical stimulation. Another option for chronic pain entails stimulation of the motor cortex. In this procedure, the electrodes are placed directly on the dura mater over the motor cortex where the pain is located. Although this use is not FDA approved, it is relatively common (Birknes et al. 2006). At our institution (Medical University of South Carolina), the neurosurgeon asks for a TMS mapping evaluation of the motor cortex before surgery to have a better understanding of the location of the desired section of the motor cortex, representing an example of how the different stimulation technologies cross-fertilize.

Depression

Subgenual cingulate. The use of DBS in patients with treatment-resistant depression recently has been widely reported in the lay press. Although DBS is an exciting new option for depressed patients who fail all other therapies, the enthusiasm is perhaps premature. To date, very few patients have been treated (<50 in the world), and properly blinded studies have not been conducted. To make matters even more confusing, the different research groups are using different technologies and stimulating varying sites in the brain.

The most widely cited work is that by Helen Mayberg and her group originally in Toronto, Ontario, and now at Emory University in Atlanta, Georgia (Mayberg et al. 2005). It had previously been noted that compared with controls, patients with depression showed greater activity in the subgenual cingulate cortex, or what is also called Brodmann area 25 (George et al. 1997a; Wu et al. 1992). Research by a different group replicated and extended these insights (Greicius et al. 2007); in this study, the resting activity in the subgenual cingulate correlates with the duration of the episode of depression. Other research had shown that those patients with depression who respond to treatment show a decrease in activity in the subgenual cingulate (Wu et al. 1992). Finally, earlier neurosurgical cingulate ablation studies also reported ~70% partial or full response at 2- to 3-year follow-up (Laitinen 1979, 2004; Laitinen and Vilkki 1972; Vilkki 1977).

With this background, the Toronto group implanted bilateral electrodes in six patients with treatment-resistant depression in an open-label fashion as an adjunctive treatment to continuing medications. The electrodes were actually placed in the white matter fiber tracts next to the subgenual cingulate because that location of the cingulate is hard to reach. At 6 months, 4 of the 6 patients were responders (Mayberg et al. 2005). In a more recent publication by this group on 14 more patients, Lozano et al. (2008) reported that at 6 months, there was a 60% response rate and 35% remission rate, with similar findings at 1-year follow-up.

Nucleus accumbens. Thomas Schlaepfer and his group in Germany have experimented with stimulating the nucleus accumbens (Schlaepfer et al. 2008a). They postulated that activity in the nucleus accumbens is insufficient in depressed patients, which may explain the anhedonia and lack of motivation these patients experience. Schlaepfer's group implanted DBS electrodes in three patients with extremely resistant forms of depression. They reported that clinical ratings improved for all three patients when the stimulator was on and worsened when the stimulator was turned off (Schlaepfer et al. 2008a).

Although the study was small and of short duration, it is of particular interest because of its similarities to the work Robert Heath was conducting in the 1950s and 1960s. Heath also implanted stimulating devices to enhance pleasure in patients with depression (Heath 1964; Heath and Guerrero-Figueroa 1968; Heath and Mickle 1960). Ultimately, he found that the benefits dissipated with time. It will be important to establish whether modern DBS has enduring efficacy.

A different multisite group is implanting the electrodes in a manner that interrupts the white matter tracts connecting the cingulate to the orbitofrontal cortex. The tip of these electrodes abuts on the nucleus accumbens. The FDA calls this approach ALICNA (anterior limb of the internal capsule, nucleus accumbens), and some refer to it as ventral caudate, ventral striatum (VC/VS). In a study of 15 treatment-resistant patients, this group added DBS to stable background medication and found that about half of the patients responded at 6 and 12 months, with less than one-third achieving remission (Dougherty et al. 2007). Although the patients had some worsening of suicidal thoughts, they made no suicide attempts. A more recent report of these 15 patients found a 40% remission rate at 1-year follow-up (Greenberg et al. 2008; Malone et al. 2009).

Obsessive-Compulsive Disorder

For patients with severe, unremitting OCD, ablative neurosurgery has been an option. Small lesions of the anterior capsule or anterior cingulate have been effective in about one-third of the patients. DBS offers the option of interrupting the obsessive circuitry without destroying tissue. However, only sequential case studies have been reported, and no large comprehensive study has been conducted. Greenberg et al. (2006) published the best report. They followed eight patients, all under age 65, for 36 months after implantation. They reported that four patients had improvements of >35% on the OCD scale, while an additional two had improvements of >25%. Based on these data and others, in 2009 the FDA granted a humanitarian device exemption for DBS in OCD.

Summary of Clinical Uses

DBS is FDA approved and is effective for treatment-resistant PD, and it is also FDA approved through a device exemption for dystonia, ET, and most recently OCD. Cortical stimulation over motor cortex has been used for many years by neurosurgeons for intractable pain. There are other exciting case series of DBS for depression, but large RCTs are needed. It is important to know if the effects seen are DBS related or are caused by the insertion effect of the microtrauma of passing the wire. Given the history of the overrapid adoption of frontal lobotomies, it is important to proceed cautiously with DBS for other conditions, because of potential morbidity and even mortality (Freeman and Watts 1950).

Safety

The most serious potential risk associated with DBS is from the neurosurgical procedure, particularly bleeding and stroke (Kern and Kumar 2007). This risk generally ranges from 1% to 3%. If a stroke occurs, it usually occurs during or within a few hours of surgery. Another risk is infection, which occurs in ~4%–5% of patients. If an infection occurs, it is usually not life threatening but may require immediate removal of the entire DBS system. It is important to realize that DBS, almost alone among the brain stimulation treatments, has a small but nevertheless real risk of death (<1% depending on the location and type of electrodes). Of note, because it requires anesthesia, ECT also has a theoretical risk of death, but it is only ~1 in 50,000 inductions.

DBS may lead to neuropsychiatric problems (Wichmann and DeLong 2006). Some patients have developed paresthesias or involuntary movements. Other patients have developed cognitive side effects or mood changes that range from disinhibition, gambling, or even worse, suicide. Most of these problems can be eliminated with adjustments to the stimulating parameters, but they are important to recognize. The dopaminergic medications used to treat PD have been reported to increase impulsive behavior, such as pathological gambling (Dodd et al. 2005). A group at the University of Arizona recently demonstrated with a computer game that STN DBS for PD may also increase impulsiveness (Frank et al. 2007). The DBS patients were quicker to rush their choices when their stimulators were on.

Postmortem analyses of brains from patients with long-term DBS have revealed some subtle findings. Mild gliosis (proliferation of inflammatory cells of the brain) has been found around the electrode. Moderate cell loss proximal to the electrode tip has also been found. Thus, it is not entirely accurate to say that DBS is totally reversible, because in most cases the passing of the stimulating electrode does produce local changes that are not reversible.

Other Techniques

The field of brain stimulation is rapidly growing and transforming. For example, in a 2009 issue of *Science*, two reports suggested that more invasive DBS might be replaced with simpler surface-based approaches to stimulation (Fuentes et al. 2009; Gradinaru et al. 2009). Thus, even spinal cord stimulators, electroacupuncture, or simple transcutaneous electrical nerve stimulation units might become more widely used as the field learns more about the underlying neurobiology of circuits and ways to interact with them. The field is evolving rapidly (George and Sackeim 2008; Higgins and George 2009; Sackeim and George 2008). We have listed the current known

TABLE 11–1. Major brain stimulation techniques and their indications as approved by the U.S. Food and Drug Administration (FDA)

Device	Disease	Current FDA status
Vagus nerve stimulation	Epilepsy	General approval
	Treatment-resistant depression	General approval
Transcranial magnetic stimulation	Treatment-resistant depression, unipolar depression	General approval
	Migraine prophylaxis	Clinical trials under way
Transcranial direct current stimulation		No FDA-approved indication
Deep brain stimulation	Parkinson's disease	General approval
	Dystonia	Humanitarian device exemption approval
	Obsessive-compulsive disorder	Humanitarian device exemption approval
	Epilepsy	Clinical trials under way
	Treatment-resistant depression	Clinical trials under way

techniques discussed in this chapter in Table 11–1 and have indicated those with FDA approval.

Future Directions and Clinical Implications

Dale's principle (one neuron, one transmitter) is clearly outdated. An analogy to this outdated approach—one transmitter and one disease (e.g., dopamine and schizophrenia)—is also likely outdated. The data reviewed in this chapter and this volume clearly suggest that the near future of brain stimulation therapies involves understanding focal pharmacology and the ways in which several neurotransmitters interact in discrete brain regions and circuits to drive behaviors and create disease.

This revolution in basic mechanisms of understanding at a circuit level is occurring simultaneously with an explosion of new technologies for interacting with the brain through direct and indirect stimulation. These approaches vary drastically from traditional neuropsychopharmacology, with profound differences in dosing, tolerance, and compliance. The field is just beginning to understand some of the more basic underlying principles in brain stimulation therapies.

The future is bright for brain stimulation therapies because of this simultaneous growth in the knowledge of the neurobiology of circuits and the technology of brain stimulation methods. Over the past decade, brain stimulation methods have already transformed or at least significantly impacted the treatment of PD, epilepsy, dystonia, OCD, and depression. Hopefully, this rapid pace will continue, and 10 years from now, the field will be using none of the current methods but rather another generation of brain stimulation methods honed on the knowledge flowing from basic science and imaging.

Key Points

- Several recent brain stimulation methods do not involve producing a seizure.
- The most widely studied are transcranial magnetic stimulation (TMS), vagus nerve stimulation (VNS), and deep brain stimulation (DBS).
- Both TMS and VNS have recently been FDA approved for treatment of depression. VNS is also approved to treat epilepsy.

- TMS appears to have special promise in treating geriatric depression because it is nonsystemic, has no cognitive side effects, and does not require repeated general anesthesia.
- DBS is widely used for treating tremor and Parkinson's disease, especially in elderly patients. It is approved through a humanitarian device exemption for treating obsessive-compulsive disorder. It is still experimental for treating depression and other neuropsychiatric applications.

Recommended Reading

Higgins ES, George MS: Brain Stimulation Therapies for Clinicians. Washington, DC, American Psychiatric Publishing, 2009

References

Accornero N, Li Voti P, La Riccia M, et al: Visual evoked potentials during direct current cortical polarization. Exp Brain Res 178: 261–266, 2007

Aleman A, Sommer IE, Kahn RS: Efficacy of slow repetitive transcranial magnetic stimulation in the treatment of resistant auditory hallucinations in schizophrenia: a meta-analysis. J Clin Psychiatry 68:416–421, 2007

Alonso-Alonso M, Fregni F, Pascual-Leone A: Brain stimulation in poststroke rehabilitation. Cerebrovasc Dis 24 (suppl 1):157–166, 2007

Amassian VE, Quirk GJ, Stewart M: A comparison of corticospinal activation by magnetic coil and electrical stimulation of monkey motor cortex. Electroencephalogr Clin Neurophysiol 77:390–401, 1990

Amassian VE, Eberle L, Maccabee PJ, et al: Modelling magnetic coil excitation of human cerebral cortex with a peripheral nerve immersed in a brain-shaped volume conductor: the significance of fiber bending in excitation. Electroencephalogr Clin Neurophysiol 85:291–301, 1992

Ambrosini A, Schoenen J: The electrophysiology of migraine. Curr Opin Neurol 16:327–331, 2003

Andre-Obadia N, Peyron R, Mertens P, et al: Transcranial magnetic stimulation for pain control: double-blind study of different frequencies against placebo, and correlation with motor cortex stimulation efficacy. Clin Neurophysiol 117:1536–1544, 2006

Aston-Jones G: Locus coeruleus, A5 and A7 noradrenergic cell groups, in The Rat Nervous System. Edited by Paxinos G. San Diego, CA, Elsevier/Academic Press, 2004, pp 259–294

Aston-Jones G, Ennis M, Pieribone VA, et al: The brain nucleus locus coeruleus: restricted afferent control of a broad efferent network. Science 234:734–737, 1986

Avery DH, Isenberg KE, Sampson SM, et al: Transcranial magnetic stimulation in the acute treatment of major depressive disorder: clinical response in an open-label extension trial. J Clin Psychiatry 69:441–451, 2008

Bailey P, Bremer F: A sensory cortical representation of the vagus nerve. J Neurophysiol 1:405–412, 1938

Baratta MV, Christianson JP, Gomez DM, et al: Controllable versus uncontrollable stressors bi-directionally modulate conditioned but not innate fear. Neuroscience 146:1495–1503, 2007

Barker AT, Jalinous R, Freeston IL: Non-invasive magnetic stimulation of human motor cortex. Lancet 1:1106–1107, 1985

Bear MF, Connors BW, Paradiso MA (eds): Neuroscience: Exploring the Brain. Baltimore, MD, Lippincott Williams & Wilkins, 2006

Benabid AL, Pollak P, Seigneuret E, et al: Chronic VIM thalamic stimulation in Parkinson's disease, essential tremor and extrapyramidal dyskinesias. Acta Neurochir Suppl 58:39–44, 1993

Ben-Menachem E, Mañon-Espaillat R, Ristanovic R, et al: Vagus nerve stimulation for treatment of partial seizures, I: a controlled study of effect on seizures. First International Vagus Nerve Stimulation Study Group. Epilepsia 35:616–626, 1994

Biggio F, Gorini G, Utzeri C, et al: Chronic vagus nerve stimulation induces neuronal plasticity in the rat hippocampus. Int J Neuropsychopharmacol 12:1209–1221, 2009

Birknes JK, Sharan A, Rezai AR: Treatment of chronic pain with neurostimulation. Prog Neurol Surg 19:197–207, 2006

Bodenlos JS, Kose S, Borckardt JJ, et al: Vagus Nerve Stimulation Acutely Alters Food Craving in Adults With Depression. Appetite 48:145–153, 2007

Boggio PS, Ferrucci R, Rigonatti SP, et al: Effects of transcranial direct current stimulation on working memory in patients with Parkinson's disease. J Neurol Sci 249:31–38, 2006

Boggio PS, Bermpohl F, Vergara AO, et al: Go-no-go task performance improvement after anodal transcranial DC stimulation of the left dorsolateral prefrontal cortex in major depression. J Affect Disord 101:91–98, 2007

Bohning DE, Shastri A, Nahas Z, et al: Echoplanar BOLD fMRI of brain activation induced by concurrent transcranial magnetic stimulation. Invest Radiol 33:336–340, 1998

Boon P, Moors I, De Herdt V, et al: Vagus nerve stimulation and cognition. Seizure 15:259–263, 2006

Borckardt JJ, Kozel FA, Anderson B, et al: Vagus nerve stimulation affects pain perception in depressed adults. Pain Res Manag 10:9–14, 2005

Borckardt JJ, Anderson B, Kozel FA, et al: Acute and long-term VNS effects on pain perception in a case of treatment-resistant depression. Neurocase 12:216–220, 2006a

Borckardt JJ, Weinstein M, Reeves ST, et al: Postoperative left prefrontal repetitive transcranial magnetic stimulation reduces patient-controlled analgesia use. Anesthesiology 105:557–562, 2006b

Borckardt JJ, Reeves ST, Weinstein M, et al: Significant analgesic effects of one session of postoperative left prefrontal cortex repetitive transcranial magnetic stimulation: a replication study. Brain Stimul 1:122–127, 2008

Borckardt JJ, Linder KJ, Ricci R, et al: Focal electrically administered therapy: device parameter effects on stimulus perception in humans. J ECT 25:91–98, 2009

Borghetti D, Pizzanelli C, Maritato P, et al: Mismatch negativity analysis in drug-resistant epileptic patients implanted with vagus nerve stimulator. Brain Res Bull 73:81–85, 2007

Butson CR, McIntyre CC: Current steering to control the volume of tissue activated during deep brain stimulation. Brain Stimul 1:7–15, 2008

Cantello R, Rossi S, Varrasi C, et al: Slow repetitive TMS for drug-resistant epilepsy: clinical and EEG findings of a placebo-controlled trial. Epilepsia 48:366–374, 2007

Chae JH, Nahas Z, Lomarev M, et al: A review of functional neuroimaging studies of vagus nerve stimulation (VNS). J Psychiatr Res 37:443–455, 2003

Christianson JP, Benison AM, Jennings J, et al: The sensory insular cortex mediates the stress-buffering effects of safety signals but not behavioral control. J Neurosci 28:13703–13711, 2008a

Christianson JP, Paul ED, Irani M, et al: The role of prior stressor controllability and the dorsal raphe nucleus in sucrose preference and social exploration. Behav Brain Res 193:87–93, 2008b

Clark KB, Naritoku DK, Smith DC, et al: Enhanced recognition memory following vagus nerve stimulation in human subjects. Nat Neurosci 2:94–98, 1999

Clarke BM, Upton AR, Kamath MV, et al: Transcranial magnetic stimulation for migraine: clinical effects. J Headache Pain 7:341–346, 2006

Coffey RJ: Deep brain stimulation for chronic pain: results of two multicenter trials and a structured review. Pain Med 2:183–192, 2001

Colombo J, Shoemaker WC, Belzberg H, et al: Noninvasive monitoring of the autonomic nervous system and hemodynamics of patients with blunt and penetrating trauma. J Trauma 65:1364–1373, 2008

Counter SA, Borg E, Lofqvist L, et al: Hearing loss from the acoustic artifact of the coil used in extracranial magnetic stimulation. Neurology 40:1159–1162, 1990

Datta A, Elwassif M, Bansal V, et al: A system and device for focal transcranial direct current stimulation using concentric ring electrode configurations. Brain Stimul 1:318, 2008

Davey KR, Epstein CM, George MS, et al: Modeling the effects of electrical conductivity of the head on the induced electrical field in the brain during magnetic stimulation. Clin Neurophysiol 114:2204–2209, 2004

Deep-Brain Stimulation for Parkinson's Disease Study Group: Deep-brain stimulation of the subthalamic nucleus or pars interna of the globus pallidus in Parkinson's disease. N Engl J Med 345: 956–963, 2001

Deuschl G, Schade-Brittinger C, Krack P, et al: A randomized trial of deep-brain stimulation for Parkinson's disease. N Engl J Med 355:896–908, 2006

Dew RE, Kramer SI, McCall WV: Adequacy of antidepressant treatment by psychiatric residents: the Antidepressant Treatment History Form as a possible assessment tool. Acad Psychiatry 29:283–288, 2005

Di Lazzaro V, Pilato F, Saturno E, et al: Theta-burst repetitive transcranial magnetic stimulation suppresses specific excitatory circuits in the human motor cortex. J Physiol 565:945–950, 2005

Di Lazzaro V, Ziemann U, Lemon RN: State of the art: physiology of transcranial motor cortex stimulation. Brain Stimul 1:345–362, 2008

Dodd ML, Klos KJ, Bower JH, et al: Pathological gambling caused by drugs used to treat Parkinson disease. Arch Neurol 62:1377–1381, 2005

Dorr AE, Debonnel G: Effect of vagus nerve stimulation on serotonergic and noradrenergic transmission. J Pharmacol Exp Ther 318:890–898, 2006

Dougherty DD, Malone D, Carpenter L, et al (eds): Long-Term Outcomes of Ventral Capsule/Ventral Striatum DBS for Highly Treatment-Resistant Depression. Boca Raton, FL, American College of Psychopharmacology, 2007

Ebben MR, Sethi NK, Conte M, et al: Vagus nerve stimulation, sleep apnea, and CPAP titration. J Clin Sleep Med 4:471–473, 2008

Ennis M, Aston-Jones G: Activation of locus coeruleus from nucleus paragigantocellularis: a new excitatory amino acid pathway in brain. J Neurosci 8:3644–3657, 1988

Epstein CM: A six-pound battery-powered portable transcranial magnetic stimulator. Brain Stimul 1:128–130, 2008

Epstein CM, Lah JJ, Meador K, et al: Optimum stimulus parameters for lateralized suppression of speech with magnetic brain stimulation. Neurology 47:1590–1593, 1996

Faraday M: Effects on the production of electricity from magnetism (1831), in Michael Faraday. Edited by Williams LP. New York, Basic Books, 1965, p 531

Feighner JP, Brown SL, Olivier JE: Electrosleep therapy: a controlled double blind study. J Nerv Ment Dis 157:121–128, 1973

Fekadu A, Wooderson SC, Markopoulo K, et al: What happens to patients with treatment-resistant depression? A systematic review of medium to long term outcome studies. J Affect Disord 116:4–11, 2009

Ferrie CD, Patel A: Treatment of Lennox-Gastaut syndrome (LGS). Eur J Paediatr Neurol 13:493–504, 2009

Figiel GS, Epstein C, McDonald WM, et al: The use of rapid rate transcranial magnetic stimulation (rTMS) in refractory depressed patients. J Neuropsychiatry Clin Neurosci 10:20–25, 1998

Fitzgerald PB, Daskalakis ZJ: A review of repetitive transcranial magnetic stimulation use in the treatment of schizophrenia. Can J Psychiatry 53:567–576, 2008

Fitzgerald PB, Fountain S, Daskalakis ZJ: A comprehensive review of the effects of rTMS on motor cortical excitability and inhibition. Clin Neurophysiol 117:2584–2596, 2006

Fitzgerald PB, Hoy K, McQueen S, et al: A randomized trial of rTMS targeted with MRI based neuro-navigation in treatment-resistant depression. Neuropsychopharmacology 34:1255–1262, 2009

Foley JO, DuBois F: Quantitative studies of the vagus nerve in the cat: the ratio of sensory and motor studies. J Comp Neurol 67:49–67, 1937

Fox PT, Narayana S, Tandon N, et al: Intensity modulation of TMS-induced cortical excitation: primary motor cortex. Hum Brain Mapp 27:478–487, 2006

Frank MJ, Samanta J, Moustafa AA, et al: Hold your horses: impulsivity, deep brain stimulation, and medication in parkinsonism. Science 318:1309–1312, 2007

Freeman W, Watts JW: Psychosurgery in the Treatment of Mental Disorder and Intractable Pain, 2nd Edition. Springfield, IL, Charles C Thomas, 1950

Fregni F, Boggio PS, Santos MC, et al: Noninvasive cortical stimulation with transcranial direct current stimulation in Parkinson's disease. Mov Disord 21:1693–1702, 2006

Fregni F, Pascual-Leone A: Technology insight: noninvasive brain stimulation in neurology: perspectives on the therapeutic potential of rTMS and tDCS. Nat Clin Pract Neurol 3:383–393, 2007

Fuentes R, Petersson P, Siesser WB, et al: Spinal cord stimulation restores locomotion in animal models of Parkinson's disease. Science 323:1578–1582, 2009

George MS: Reanimating the face: early writings by Duchenne and Darwin on the neurology of facial emotion expression. J Hist Neurosci 3:21–33, 1994

George MS, Belmaker RH: TMS in Clinical Psychiatry. Washington, DC, American Psychiatric Publishing, 2006

George MS, Sackeim HA: Brain stimulation, revolutions, and the shifting time domain of depression. Biol Psychiatry 64:447–448, 2008

George MS, Ketter TA, Post RM: Prefrontal cortex dysfunction in clinical depression. Depression 2:59–72, 1994

George MS, Wassermann EM, Williams WA, et al: Daily repetitive transcranial magnetic stimulation (rTMS) improves mood in depression. Neuroreport 6:1853–1856, 1995

George MS, Wassermann EM, Williams WA, et al: Changes in mood and hormone levels after rapid-rate transcranial magnetic stimulation (rTMS) of the prefrontal cortex. J Neuropsychiatry Clin Neurosci 8:172–180, 1996

George MS, Ketter TA, Parekh PI, et al: Blunted left cingulate activation in mood disorder subjects during a response interference task (the Stroop). J Neuropsychiatry Clin Neurosci 9:55–63, 1997a

George MS, Wassermann EM, Kimbrell TA, et al: Mood improvement following daily left prefrontal repetitive transcranial magnetic stimulation in patients with depression: a placebo-controlled crossover trial. Am J Psychiatry 154:1752–1756, 1997b

George MS, Sackeim HA, Rush AJ, et al: Vagus nerve stimulation: a new tool for brain research and therapy. Biol Psychiatry 47:287–295, 2000

George MS, Rush AJ, Marangell LB, et al: A one-year comparison of vagus nerve stimulation with treatment as usual for treatment-resistant depression. Biol Psychiatry 58:364–373, 2005

George MS, Bohning DE, Li X, et al: Neuroimaging of rTMS effects on the brain, in Transcranial Brain Stimulation in Mental Disorders. Edited by Marcolin M, Padberg F. Berlin, Germany, Karger, 2007, pp 35–52

George MS, Ward HE, Ninan PT, et al: A pilot study of vagus nerve stimulation (VNS) for treatment-resistant anxiety disorders. Brain Stimul 1:112–121, 2008

George MS, Padberg F, Schlaepfer TE, et al: Controversy: repetitive transcranial magnetic stimulation or transcranial direct current stimulation shows efficacy in treating psychiatric diseases (depression, mania, schizophrenia, obsessive-compulsive disorder, panic, posttraumatic stress disorder). Brain Stimul 2:14–21, 2009

George MS, Lisanby SH, Avery D, et al: Daily left prefrontal transcranial magnetic stimulation therapy for major depressive disorder: a sham-controlled randomized trial. Arch Gen Psychiatry 67:507–516, 2010

Gomez E, Mikhail AR: Treatment of methadone withdrawal with cerebral electrotherapy. Br J Psychiatry 134:111–113, 1978

Gradinaru V, Mogri M, Thompson KR, et al: Optical deconstruction of parkinsonian neural circuitry. Science 324:354–359, 2009

Greenberg BD, Malone DA, Friehs GM, et al: Three-year outcomes in deep brain stimulation for highly resistant obsessive-compulsive disorder. Neuropsychopharmacology 31:2384–2393, 2006

Greenberg BD, Gabriels LA, Malone DA Jr, et al: Deep brain stimulation of the ventral internal capsule/ventral striatum for obsessive-compulsive disorder: worldwide experience. Mol Psychiatry 15:64–79, 2008

Greicius MD, Flores BH, Menon V, et al: Resting-state functional connectivity in major depression: abnormally increased contributions from subgenual cingulate cortex and thalamus. Biol Psychiatry 62:429–437, 2007

Grill WM, McIntyre CC: Extracellular excitation of central neurons: implications for the mechanisms of deep brain stimulation. Thalamus Relat Syst 1:269–277, 2001

Grisaru N, Yarovslavsky U, Abarbanel J, et al: Transcranial magnetic stimulation in depression and schizophrenia. Eur Neuropsychopharmacol 4:287–288, 1994

Groves DA, Brown VJ: Vagal nerve stimulation: a review of its applications and potential mechanisms that mediate its clinical effects. Neurosci Biobehav Rev 29:493–500, 2005

Handforth A, DeGiorgio CM, Schachter SC, et al: Vagus nerve stimulation therapy for partial-onset seizures: a randomized active-control trial. Neurology 51:48–55, 1998

Hassert DL, Miyashita T, Williams CL: The effects of peripheral vagal nerve stimulation at a memory-modulating intensity on norepinephrine output in the basolateral amygdala. Behav Neurosci 118:79–88, 2004

Heath RG: Pleasure response of human subjects to direct stimulation of the brain: physiologic and psychodynamic considerations, in The Role of Pleasure in Behavior. Edited by Heath RG. New York, Hoeber, 1964, pp 219–243

Heath RG, Guerrero-Figueroa R: Stimulation of the human brain: spontaneous and evoked electroencephalographic responses. Acta Neurol Latinoam 14:116–124, 1968

Heath RG, Mickle WA: Evaluation of seven years experience with depth electrode studies in human patients, in Electrical Studies of the Unanesthetized Brain. Edited by Ramey ER, O'Doherty D. New York, Hoeber, 1960, pp 214–247

Helmstaedter C, Hoppe C, Elger CE: Memory alterations during acute high-intensity vagus nerve stimulation. Epilepsy Res 47: 37–42, 2001

Henry TR: Therapeutic mechanisms of vagus nerve stimulation. Neurology 59 (suppl 4):S15–S20, 2002

Henry TR, Bakay RA, Votaw JR, et al: Brain blood flow alterations induced by therapeutic vagus nerve stimulation in partial epilepsy, I: acute effects at high and low levels of stimulation. Epilepsia 39:983–990, 1998

Henry TR, Votaw JR, Pennell PB, et al: Acute blood flow changes and efficacy of vagus nerve stimulation in partial epilepsy. Neurology 52:1166–1173, 1999

Herbsman T, Avery D, Ramsey D, et al: More lateral and anterior prefrontal coil location is associated with better repetitive transcranial magnetic stimulation antidepressant response. Biol Psychiatry 66:509–515, 2009

Herwig U, Padberg F, Unger J, et al: Transcranial magnetic stimulation in therapy studies: examination of the reliability of "standard" coil positioning by neuronavigation. Biol Psychiatry 50: 58–61, 2001

Herwig U, Fallgatter AJ, Hoppner J, et al: Antidepressant effects of augmentative transcranial magnetic stimulation: randomised multicentre trial. Br J Psychiatry 191:441–448, 2007

Higgins ES, George MS: The Neuroscience of Clinical Psychiatry: The Pathophysiology of Behavior and Mental Illness. Baltimore, MD, Lippincott Williams & Wilkins, 2007

Higgins ES, George MS: Brain Stimulation Therapies for Clinicians. Washington, DC, American Psychiatric Publishing, 2009

Hoffman RE, Cavus I: Slow transcranial magnetic stimulation, long-term depotentiation, and brain hyperexcitability disorders. Am J Psychiatry 159:1093–1102, 2002

Hoflich G, Kasper S, Hufnagel A, et al: Application of transcranial magnetic stimulation in the treatment of drug-resistant major depression. Hum Psychopharmacol 8:361–365, 1993

Holmes MD, Chang M, Kapur V: Sleep apnea and excessive daytime somnolence induced by vagal nerve stimulation. Neurology 61:1126–1129, 2003

Horgan J: The forgotten era of brain chips. Sci Am 293:66–73, 2005

Huang Y, Sommer M, Thickbroom GW, et al: Consensus: new methodologies for brain stimulation. Brain Stimul 2:2–13, 2009

Hummel FC, Celnik P, Pascual-Leone A, et al: Controversy: noninvasive and invasive cortical stimulation show efficacy in treating stroke patients. Brain Stimul 1:370–382, 2008

Huston JM, Gallowitsch-Puerta M, Ochani M, et al: Transcutaneous vagus nerve stimulation reduces serum high mobility group box 1 levels and improves survival in murine sepsis. Crit Care Med 35:2762–2768, 2007

Hutchinson MR, Coats BD, Lewis SS, et al: Proinflammatory cytokines oppose opioid-induced acute and chronic analgesia. Brain Behav Immun 22:1178–1189, 2008

Joo JH, Solano FX, Mulsant BH, et al: Predictors of adequacy of depression management in the primary care setting. Psychiatr Serv 56:1524–1528, 2005

Jorge RE, Moser DJ, Action L, et al: Treatment of vascular depression using repetitive transcranial magnetic stimulation. Arch Gen Psychiatry 65:268–276, 2008

Kern DS, Kumar R: Deep brain stimulation. Neurologist 13:237–252, 2007

Kew JJ, Ridding MC, Rothwell JC, et al: Reorganization of cortical blood flow and transcranial magnetic stimulation maps in human subjects after upper limb amputation. J Neurophysiol 72: 2517–2524, 1994

Kolbinger HM, Hoflich G, Hufnagel A, et al: Transcranial magnetic stimulation (TMS) in the treatment of major depression: a pilot study. Hum Psychopharmacol 10:305–310, 1995

Kolin A, Brill NQ, Broberg PJ: Stimulation of irritable tissues by means of an alternating magnetic field. Proc Soc Exp Biol Med 102:251–253, 1959

Koo B, Ham SD, Sood S, et al: Human vagus nerve electrophysiology: a guide to vagus nerve stimulation parameters. J Clin Neurophysiol 18:429–433, 2001

Kozel FA, Nahas Z, deBrux C, et al: How coil-cortex distance relates to age, motor threshold, and antidepressant response to repetitive transcranial magnetic stimulation. J Neuropsychiatry Clin Neurosci 12:376–384, 2000

Krack P, Batir A, Van Blercon N, et al: Five-year follow-up of bilateral stimulation of the subthalamic nucleus in advanced Parkinson's disease. N Engl J Med 349:1925–1934, 2003

Krahl SE, Clark KB, Smith DC, et al: Locus coeruleus lesions suppress the seizure-attenuating effects of vagus nerve stimulation. Epilepsia 39:709–714, 1998

Krahl SE, Senanayake SS, Handforth A: Destruction of peripheral C-fibers does not alter subsequent vagus nerve stimulation-induced seizure suppression. Epilepsia 42:586–589, 2001

Kraus T, Hösl K, Kiess O, et al: BOLD fMRI deactivation of limbic and temporal brain structures and mood enhancing effect by transcutaneous vagus nerve stimulation. J Neural Transm 114: 1485–1493, 2007

Kringelbach ML, Jenkinson N, Owen SLF, et al: Translational principles of deep brain stimulation. Nat Rev Neurosci 8:623–635, 2007

Kupsch A, Benecke R, Muller J, et al: Pallidal deep brain stimulation in primary generalized or segmental dystonia. N Engl J Med 355: 1978–1990, 2006

Laitinen LV: Emotional responses to subcortical electrical stimulation in psychiatric patients. Clin Neurol Neurosurg 81:148–157, 1979

Laitinen LV: Personal memories of the history of stereotactic neurosurgery. Neurosurgery 55:1420–1428; discussion 1428–1429, 2004

Laitinen LV, Vilkki J: Stereotactic ventral anterior cingulotomy in some psychological disorders, in Psychosurgery. Edited by Hitchcock E, Laitinen L, Kjeld V. Springfield, IL, Charles C Thomas, 1972, pp 242–252

Lam RW, Chan P, Wilkins-Ho M, et al: Repetitive transcranial magnetic stimulation for treatment-resistant depression: a systematic review and metaanalysis. Can J Psychiatry 53:621–631, 2008

Langguth B, de Ridder D, Dornhoffer JL, et al: Controversy: does repetitive transcranial magnetic stimulation/transcranial direct current stimulation show efficacy in treating tinnitus patients? Brain Stimul 1:192–205, 2008

Lefaucheur JP: Transcranial magnetic stimulation in the management of pain. Suppl Clin Neurophysiol 57:737–748, 2004

Lefaucheur JP, Drouot X, Keravel Y, et al: Pain relief induced by repetitive transcranial magnetic stimulation of precentral cortex. Neuroreport 12:2963–2965, 2001a

Lefaucheur JP, Drouot X, Nguyen JP: Interventional neurophysiology for pain control: duration of pain relief following repetitive transcranial magnetic stimulation of the motor cortex. Neurophysiol Clin 31:247–252, 2001b

Li X, Teneback CC, Nahas Z, et al: Interleaved transcranial magnetic stimulation/functional MRI confirms that lamotrigine inhibits cortical excitability in healthy young men. Neuropsychopharmacology 29:1395–1407, 2004

Li X, Ricci R, Large CH, et al: Lamotrigine and valproic acid have different effects on motorcortical neuronal excitability. J Neural Transm 116:423–429, 2009

Limousin P, Speelman JD, Gielen F, et al: Multicentre European study of thalamic stimulation in parkinsonian and essential tremor. J Neurol Neurosurg Psychiatry 66:289–296, 1999

Lisanby SH, Luber B, Schroeder C, et al: Intracerebral measurement of rTMS and ECS induced voltage in vivo. Biol Psychiatry 43 (suppl):100S, 1998a

Lisanby S, Luber B, Schroeder C, et al: rTMS in primates: intracerebral measurement of rTMS and ECS induced voltage in vivo. Electroencephalogr Clin Neurophysiol 107:79, 1998b

Little JT, Kimbrell TA, Wassermann EM, et al: Cognitive effects of 1- and 20-hertz repetitive transcranial magnetic stimulation in depression: preliminary report. Neuropsychiatry Neuropsychol Behav Neurol 13:119–124, 2000

Lockard JS, Congdon WC, DuCharme LL: Feasibility and safety of vagal stimulation in monkey model. Epilepsia 31 (suppl 2):S20–S26, 1990

Lomarev M, Denslow S, Nahas Z, et al: Vagus nerve stimulation (VNS) synchronized BOLD fMRI suggests that VNS in depressed adults has frequency/dose dependent effects. J Psychiatr Res 36:219–227, 2002

Loo C, Sachdev P, Elsayed H, et al: Effects of a 2- to 4-week course of repetitive transcranial magnetic stimulation on neuropsychological functioning, electroencephalogram, and auditory threshold in depressed patients. Biol Psychiatry 49:615–623, 2001

Lozano AM, Mayberg HS, Giacobbe P, et al: Subcallosal cingulate gyrus deep brain stimulation for treatment-resistant depression. Biol Psychiatry 64:461–467, 2008

Maclean PD: The Triune Brain in Evolution: Role in Paleocerebral Functions. New York, Plenum, 1990

Malone DA Jr, Dougherty DD, Rezai AR, et al: Deep brain stimulation of the ventral capsule/ventral striatum for treatment-resistant depression. Biol Psychiatry 65:267–275, 2009

Malow BA, Edwards J, Marzec M, et al: Vagus nerve stimulation reduces daytime sleepiness in epilepsy patients. Neurology 57:879–884, 2001

Manta S, Dong J, Debonnel G, et al: Optimization of vagus nerve stimulation parameters using the firing activity of serotonin neurons in the rat dorsal raphe. Eur Neuropsychopharmacol 19:250–255, 2009

Marangell LB, Rush AJ, George MS, et al: Vagus nerve stimulation (VNS) for major depressive episodes: one year outcomes. Biol Psychiatry 51:280–287, 2002

Marzec M, Edwards J, Sagher O, et al: Effects of vagus nerve stimulation on sleep-related breathing in epilepsy patients. Epilepsia 44:930–935, 2003

Massimini M, Ferrarelli F, Esser SK, et al: Triggering sleep slow waves by transcranial magnetic stimulation. Proc Natl Acad Sci U S A 104:8496–8501, 2007

Mayberg HS, Lozano AM, Voon V, et al: Deep brain stimulation for treatment-resistant depression. Neuron 45:651–660, 2005

McKay DR, Ridding MC, Thompson PD, et al: Induction of persistent changes in the organisation of the human motor cortex. Exp Brain Res 143:342–349, 2002

Merrill CA, Jonsson MA, Minthon L, et al: Vagus nerve stimulation in patients with Alzheimer's disease: additional follow-up results of a pilot study through 1 year. J Clin Psychiatry 67:1171–1178, 2006

Miniussi C, Cappa SF, Cohen LG, et al: Efficacy of repetitive transcranial magnetic stimulation/transcranial direct current stimulation in cognitive neurorehabilitation. Brain Stimul 1:326–336, 2008

Miocinovic S, Lempka SF, Russo GS, et al: Experimental and theoretical characterization of the voltage distribution generated by deep brain stimulation. Exp Neurol 216:166–176, 2009

Mitchell PB, Loo CK: Transcranial magnetic stimulation for depression. Aust N Z J Psychiatry 40:406–413, 2006

Miyashita T, Williams CL: Enhancement of noradrenergic neurotransmission in the nucleus of the solitary tract modulates memory storage processes. Brain Res 987:164–175, 2003

Morrell M: Brain stimulation for epilepsy: can scheduled or responsive neurostimulation stop seizures? Curr Opin Neurol 19:164–168, 2006

Mu Q, Bohning DE, Nahas Z, et al: Acute vagus nerve stimulation using different pulse widths produces varying brain effects. Biol Psychiatry 55:816–825, 2004

Nahas Z, Teneback CC, Kozel A, et al: Brain effects of TMS delivered over prefrontal cortex in depressed adults: role of stimulation frequency and coil-cortex distance. J Neuropsychiatry Clin Neurosci 13:459–470, 2001

Nahas Z, Li X, Kozel FA, et al: Safety and benefits of distance-adjusted prefrontal transcranial magnetic stimulation in depressed patients 55–75 years of age: a pilot study. Depress Anxiety 19:249–256, 2004

Nahas Z, Marangell LB, Husain MM, et al: Two-year outcome of vagus nerve stimulation (VNS) for treatment of major depressive episodes. J Clin Psychiatry 66:1097–1104, 2005

Nahas Z, Teneback C, Chae JH, et al: Serial vagus nerve stimulation functional MRI in treatment-resistant depression. Neuropsychopharmacology 32:1649–1660, 2007

Naritoku DK, Terry WJ, Helfert RH: Regional induction of Fos immunoreactivity in the brain by anticonvulsant stimulation of the vagus nerve. Epilepsy Res 22:53–62, 1995

Neese SL, Sherill LK, Tan AA, et al: Vagus nerve stimulation may protect GABAergic neurons following traumatic brain injury in rats: an immunocytochemical study. Brain Res 1128:157–163, 2007

Nicholls M: Pioneers of cardiology: Rune Elmqvist, MD. Circulation 115:f109–f111, 2007

Nitsche MA, Doemkes S, Karakose T, et al: Shaping the effects of transcranial direct current stimulation of the human motor cortex. J Neurophysiol 97:3109–3117, 2007

Nitsche MA, Cohen LG, Wassermann EM, et al: Transcranial direct current stimulation: state of the art 2008. Brain Stimul 1:206–223, 2008

Oquendo MA, Baca-Garcia E, Kartachov A, et al: A computer algorithm for calculating the adequacy of antidepressant treatment in unipolar and bipolar depression. J Clin Psychiatry 64:825–833, 2003

O'Reardon JP, Cristancho P, Peshek AD: Vagus nerve stimulation (VNS) and treatment of depression: to the brainstem and beyond. Psychiatry 3:54–63, 2006

O'Reardon JP, Solvason HB, Janicak PG, et al: Efficacy and safety of transcranial magnetic stimulation in the acute treatment of major depression: a multisite randomized controlled trial. Biol Psychiatry 62:1208–1216, 2007

Ottani A, Giuliani D, Mioni C, et al: Vagus nerve mediates the protective effects of melanocortins against cerebral and systemic damage after ischemic stroke. J Cereb Blood Flow Metab 29:512–523, 2009

Palm U, Keeser D, Schiller C, et al: Skin lesions after treatment with transcranial direct current stimulation (tDCS). Brain Stimul 1:386–387, 2008

Papacostas SS, Myrianthopoulou P, Dietis A, et al: Induction of central-type sleep apnea by vagus nerve stimulation. Electromyogr Clin Neurophysiol 47:61–63, 2007

Pape TL, Rosenow J, Lewis G, et al: Repetitive transcranial magnetic stimulation-associated neurobehavioral gains during coma recovery. Brain Stimul 2:22–35, 2009

Pascual-Leone A, Gates JR, Dhuna A: Induction of speech arrest and counting errors with rapid-rate transcranial magnetic stimulation. Neurology 41:697–702, 1991

Paulus W: Transcranial direct current stimulation (tDCS). Suppl Clin Neurophysiol 56:249–254, 2003

Paulus W, Classen J, Cohen LG, et al: State of the art: pharmacologic effects on cortical excitability measures tested by transcranial magnetic stimulation. Brain Stimul 1:151–163, 2008

Pavlov VA: Cholinergic modulation of inflammation. Int J Clin Exp Med 1:203–212, 2008

Poreisz C, Boros K, Antal A, et al: Safety aspects of transcranial direct current stimulation concerning healthy subjects and patients. Brain Res Bull 72:208–214, 2007

Pridmore S, Oberoi G: Transcranial magnetic stimulation applications and potential use in chronic pain: studies in waiting. J Neurol Sci 182:1–4, 2000

Purves D, Augustine GJ, Fitzpatrick D, et al: Neuroscience, 3rd Edition. Sunderland, MA, Sinauer, 2004

Radman T, Ramos R, Brumberg JC, et al: Role of cortical cell type and neuronal morphology in electric field stimulation. Brain Stimul 1:247–248, 2008

Radna RJ, MacLean PD: Vagal elicitation of respiratory-type and other unit responses in basal limbic structures of squirrel monkeys. Brain Res 213:45–61, 1981a

Radna RJ, MacLean PD: Vagal elicitation of respiratory-type and other unit responses in striopallidum of squirrel monkeys. Brain Res 213:29–44, 1981b

Rhebergen D, Beekman AT, Graaf R, et al: The three-year naturalistic course of major depressive disorder, dysthymic disorder and double depression. J Affect Disord 115:450–459, 2009

Ridding MC, Rothwell JC: Reorganisation in human motor cortex. Can J Physiol Pharmacol 73:218–222, 1995

Ridding MC, Rothwell JC: Is there a future for therapeutic use of transcranial magnetic stimulation? Nat Rev Neurosci 8:559–567, 2007

Rollnik JD, Däuper J, Wüstefeld S, et al: Repetitive magnetic stimulation for the treatment of chronic pain conditions. Suppl Clin Neurophysiol 56:390–393, 2003

Roslin M, Kurian M: The use of electrical stimulation of the vagus nerve to treat morbid obesity. Epilepsy Behav 2:S11–S16, 2001

Rossi S, Hallett M, Rossini PM, et al: Safety, ethical considerations, and application guidelines for the use of transcranial magnetic stimulation in clinical practice and research. Clin Neurophysiol 120:2008–2039, 2009

Roth BJ, Momen S, Turner R: Algorithm for the design of magnetic stimulation coils. Med Biol Eng Comput 32:214–216, 1994

Roth Y, Zangen A, Hallett M: A coil design for transcranial magnetic stimulation of deep brain regions. J Clin Neurophysiol 19:361–370, 2002

Roth Y, Zangen A, Voller B, et al: Transcranial magnetic stimulation of deep brain regions: evidence for efficacy of the H-coil. Clin Neurophysiol 116:775–779, 2005

Rothwell JC, Hallett M, Berardelli A, et al: Magnetic stimulation: motor evoked potentials. The International Federation of Clinical Neurophysiology. Electroencephalogr Clin Neurophysiol Suppl 52:97–103, 1999

Rush AJ, George MS, Sackeim HA, et al: Vagus nerve stimulation (VNS) for treatment-resistant depressions: a multicenter study. Biol Psychiatry 47:276–286, 2000

Rush AJ, Marangell LB, Sackeim HA, et al: Vagus nerve stimulation for treatment-resistant depression: a randomized, controlled acute phase trial. Biol Psychiatry 58:347–354, 2005a

Rush AJ, Sackeim HA, Marangell LB, et al: Effects of 12 months of vagus nerve stimulation in treatment-resistant depression: a naturalistic study. Biol Psychiatry 58:355–363, 2005b

Rush AJ, Kraemer HC, Sackeim HA, et al: Report by the ACNP Task Force on response and remission in major depressive disorder. Neuropsychopharmacology 31:1841–1853, 2006a

Rush AJ, Trivedi MH, Wisniewski SR, et al: Bupropion-SR, sertraline, or venlafaxine-XR after failure of SSRIs for depression. N Engl J Med 354:1231–1242, 2006b

Sacco P, Turner D, Rothwell JC, et al: Corticomotor responses to triple-pulse transcranial magnetic stimulation: effects of interstimulus interval and stimulus intensity. Brain Stimul 2:36–40, 2009

Sackeim HA, George MS: Brain stimulation—basic, translational and clinical research in neuromodulation: why a new journal? Brain Stimul 1:4–6, 2008

Sackeim HA, Keilp JG, Rush AJ, et al: The effects of vagus nerve stimulation on cognitive performance in patients with treatment-resistant depression. Neuropsychiatry Neuropsychol Behav Neurol 14:53–62, 2001a

Sackeim HA, Rush AJ, George MS, et al: Vagus nerve stimulation (VNS) for treatment-resistant depression: efficacy, side effects, and predictors of outcome. Neuropsychopharmacology 25:713–728, 2001b

Schlaepfer TE, Cohen MX, Frick C, et al: Deep brain stimulation to reward circuitry alleviates anhedonia in refractory major depression. Neuropsychopharmacology 33:368–377, 2008a

Schlaepfer TE, Frick C, Zobel A, et al: Vagus nerve stimulation for depression: efficacy and safety in a European study. Psychol Med 38:651–661, 2008b

Schlaug G, Renga V: Transcranial direct current stimulation: a noninvasive tool to facilitate stroke recovery. Expert Rev Med Devices 5:759–768, 2008

Schlaug G, Renga V, Nair D: Transcranial direct current stimulation in stroke recovery. Arch Neurol 65:1571–1576, 2008

Schutter DJ: Antidepressant efficacy of high-frequency transcranial magnetic stimulation over the left dorsolateral prefrontal cortex in double-blind sham-controlled designs: a meta-analysis. Psychol Med 39:65–75, 2008

Shahwan A, Bailey C, Maxiner W, et al: Vagus nerve stimulation for refractory epilepsy in children: more to VNS than seizure frequency reduction. Epilepsia 50:1220–1228, 2009

Siebner HR, Bergmann TO, Bestmann S, et al: Consensus paper: combining transcranial stimulation with neuroimaging. Brain Stimul 2:58–80, 2009

Sjögren MJ, Hellström PT, Jonsson MA, et al: Cognition-enhancing effect of vagus nerve stimulation in patients with Alzheimer's disease: a pilot study. J Clin Psychiatry 63:972–980, 2002

Skarpaas TL, Morrell MJ: Intracranial stimulation therapy for epilepsy. Neurotherapeutics 6:238–243, 2009

Smith DC, Tan AA, Duke A, et al: Recovery of function after vagus nerve stimulation initiated 24 hours after fluid percussion brain injury. J Neurotrauma 23:1549–1560, 2006

Stagg CJ, Wylezinska M, Matthews PM, et al: The neurochemical effects of theta burst stimulation as assessed by magnetic resonance spectroscopy. J Neurophysiol 101:2872–2877, 2009

Sun FT, Morrell MJ, Wharen RE Jr: Responsive cortical stimulation for the treatment of epilepsy. Neurotherapeutics 5:68–74, 2008

ten Doesschate MC, Koeter MW, Bockting CL, et al: Health related quality of life in recurrent depression: a comparison with a general population sample. J Affect Disord 120:126–132, 2009

Theodore WH, Hunter K, Chen R, et al: Transcranial magnetic stimulation for the treatment of seizures: a controlled study. Neurology 59:560–562, 2002

Tononi G, Koch C: The neural correlates of consciousness: an update. Ann N Y Acad Sci 1124:239–261, 2008

Trivedi MH, Rush AJ, Wisniewski SR, et al: Evaluation of outcomes with citalopram for depression using measurement-based care in STAR*D: implications for clinical practice (see comments). Am J Psychiatry 163:28–40, 2006

Van Bockstaele EJ, Pieribone VA, Aston-Jones G: Diverse afferents converge on the nucleus paragigantocellularis in the rat ventrolateral medulla: retrograde and anterograde tracing studies. J Comp Neurol 290:561–584, 1989

Van Bockstaele EJ, Peoples J, Telegan P: Efferent projections of the nucleus of the solitary tract to peri-locus coeruleus dendrites in rat brain: evidence for a monosynaptic pathway. J Comp Neurol 412:410–428, 1999a

Van Bockstaele EJ, Peoples J, Valentino RJ: Anatomic basis for differential regulation of the rostrolateral per-locus coeruleus region by limbic afferents. Biol Psychiatry 46:1352–1363, 1999b

Van Der Zanden EP, Boeckxstaens GE, de Jonge WJ: The vagus nerve as a modulator of intestinal inflammation. Neurogastroenterol Motil 21:6–17, 2009

Vilkki J: Late psychological and clinical effects of subrostral cingulotomy and anterior mesoloviotomy in psychiatric illness, in Neurosurgical Treatment in Psychiatry, Pain, and Epilepsy. Edited by Sweet WS, Obrador S, Martin-Rodriguez JG. Baltimore, MD, University Park Press, 1977, pp 253–259

Wassermann EM: Report on risk and safety of repetitive transcranial magnetic stimulation (rTMS): suggested guidelines from the International Workshop on Risk and Safety of rTMS (June 1996). Electroencephalogr Clin Neurophysiol 108:1–16, 1997

Weaver F, Follett K, Hur K, et al: Deep brain stimulation in Parkinson disease: a meta-analysis of patient outcomes. J Neurosurg 103: 956–967, 2005

Wichmann T, DeLong MR: Deep brain stimulation for neurologic and neuropsychiatric disorders. Neuron 52:197–204, 2006

Wu JC, Gillin JC, Buchsbaum MS, et al: Effect of sleep deprivation on brain metabolism of depressed patients. Am J Psychiatry 149: 538–543, 1992

Yiend J, Paykel E, Merritt R, et al: Long term outcome of primary care depression. J Affect Disord 118:79–86, 2009

Zabara J: Peripheral control of hypersynchronous discharge in epilepsy. Electroencephalogr Clin Neurophysiol 61(suppl):S162, 1985a

Zabara J: Time course of seizure control to brief, repetitive stimuli. Epilepsia 26:518, 1985b

Zabara J: Inhibition of experimental seizures in canines by repetitive vagal stimulation. Epilepsia 33:1005–1012, 1992

Ziemann U, Paulus W, Nitsche MA, et al: Consensus: motor cortex plasticity protocols. Brain Stimul 1:164–182, 2008

12

Cognitive Impairment and Rehabilitation

Hal S. Wortzel, M.D.
David B. Arciniegas, M.D., F.A.N.P.A., C.B.I.S.T.

To address the neurorehabilitative needs of older persons with cognitive impairments, one needs a thorough understanding of each patient's cognitive and functional strengths and limitations. Unfortunately, diagnostic assessments anchored to the conditions described in the *Diagnostic and Statistical Manual of Mental Disorders*, 4th Edition, Text Revision (DSM-IV-TR; American Psychiatric Association 2000), frequently afford too limited a view of the cognitive problems experienced by many older patients. Despite general agreement that the DSM-IV-TR approach to delirium, Alzheimer's disease, and some of the amnestic disorders (e.g., alcohol-induced persisting amnestic disorder, also known as Korsakoff's syndrome) is clinically useful, less agreement exists on the usefulness of this approach to the diagnosis and treatment of non-Alzheimer's dementias (e.g., frontotemporal dementia, dementia due to traumatic brain injury [TBI], vascular dementia, dementia due to Huntington's disease) and of memory disorders with presentations that are not predominated by defective new learning/encoding. Additionally, many older individuals with stroke, TBI, or other neuropsychiatric conditions may develop focal neurobehavioral syndromes—one of the aphasias, apraxias, agnosias, or a dysexecutive syndrome—rather than delirium, an amnestic disorder, or overt dementia. These focal cognitive impairments are subsumed collectively under the DSM-IV-TR category cognitive disorder not otherwise specified, but they are potentially disabling problems that require domain-specific assessment and domain-specific interventions.

To be helpful in developing a useful clinical diagnosis and treatment plan for the older adult with cognitive impairment, an evaluation must be sensitive to these considerations. We recommend beginning this type of evaluation with a dimensional (rather than categorical diagnostic) approach that includes assessment of cognitive, emotional, behavioral, and sensorimotor abilities, the four principal domains of neuropsychiatric function. As discussed in Chapter 15, "Delirium," and Chapter 16, "Alzheimer's Disease and the Frontotemporal Dementia Syndromes," assessment across all of these neuropsychiatric domains is necessary to characterize accurately the strengths and weaknesses of each patient for both diagnostic and treatment planning purposes. While acknowledging the necessity of broad-based neuropsychiatric assessment, we focus more narrowly on the evaluation and rehabilitation of impaired cognition (not due to delirium and not manifesting as frank dementia) in the older adult. We begin by describing a general framework for understanding and evaluating cognitive impairments, and then we review general principles of the evaluation and treatment of cognitive impairments in older adults. Thereafter, we discuss cognitive domain–specific diagnostic and therapeutic issues.

Cognitive Domains

It is useful to consider cognition as a neuropsychiatric dimension that is organized into a relative hierarchy of increasing complexity (Arciniegas and Beresford 2001). This hierarchy parallels the neuroanatomy on which cognition is predicated. Arousal occupies the lower end of the hierarchy and is supported by "lower" brain areas (reticular formation, reticulothalamic connections, diencephalic structures). Conversely, executive function occupies the upper end of the cognitive hierarchy and is supported by "higher" frontal cortical structures and cortical-subcortical circuits. This hierarchy complements the framework presented in Chapter 3, "Neurobiological Basis of Behavior."

Between the base and the top of this cognitive hierarchy are the other major discrete but functionally interactive cognitive domains: arousal and hyperarousal, attention and processing speed, recognition, memory, language, praxis, visuospatial function, and executive function. Each of these cognitive domains is predicated on a set of increasingly complex neural structures organized in a similar hierarchical manner. Primary sensory cortex (and information-filtering pathways leading and connected to it) supports selective attention, and connections to inferolateral frontal and related corticothalamocortical circuits support sustained attention and working memory. Secondary sensory association cortices support recognition (gnosis), and limbic (amygdalar)–sensory connections and secondary motor-subcortical circuits support implicit (procedural) memory. Systems of increasing complexity support the higher and more complex cognitive functions. Many of these complex systems rely on, or incorporate, the neuroanatomy supporting these lower cognitive functions, as well as tertiary sensory association cortices, medial temporal areas (e.g., entorhinal-hippocampal complex, among others), quaternary (frontal) association areas, the subcortical structures to which they are connected, and the white matter making those connections.

This hierarchical framework for cognition may be used to inform the clinical approach to the evaluation of cognitive function, as well as to understand the clinical presentation and neuroanatomical basis of the cognitive disorders. When structural or functional disruptions occur at the base of this hierarchy, disorders of arousal result (e.g., coma, vegetative and minimally conscious states, and delirium, in decreasing order of severity). Given this low-level foundational disruption, the capacity for cognition at levels above arousal is also disrupted. These problems are examples of "bottom-up" disturbances of cognition. Conversely, impairments at the upper end of the hierarchy—that is, with executive function—produce not only problems in the intrinsic executive functions, such as abstraction, judgment, and problem solving (see "Executive Function" later in this chapter), but also difficulties with executive control of the so-called lower cognitive functions, such as attention, memory, and language. When multiple areas of cognition not including arousal are impaired—that is, memory and one other in the DSM-IV-TR framework or three or more in the approach advocated by Cummings and Benson (1992)—a dementia is diagnosed and its anatomy is understood as multifocal. Through this hierarchical approach to understanding cognition and its neuroanatomical basis, the evaluation and treatment of the older patient with cognitive impairments is facilitated.

General Principles of Cognitive Evaluation and Treatment

Cognitive complaints are common among older persons with neuropsychiatric disorders. In some cases, cognitive impairments are the defining features of the clinical presentation. In other circumstances (e.g., TBI, stroke, Parkinson's disease), cognitive impairments are but one aspect of a multidimensional set of neuropsychiatric disturbances. In either context, the severity and functional consequences of cognitive problems vary with a host of premorbid (e.g., age, education), condition-specific (e.g., degenerative, traumatic, demyelinating), and associated psychiatric, medical, and psychosocial factors. Regardless of the context in which they develop, however, cognitive impairments are a potential source of disability for affected persons and of distress for patients and their families.

Interview and Examination

The evaluation of cognitive impairments in the older adult requires a thorough neuropsychiatric history focused on not only the reported cognitive problem but also the identification of underlying medical, neurological, and psychiatric (including substance use) disorders, as well as contributing medication and psychosocial factors. Regarding the cognitive problem, it is important first to determine whether it is a subjective one (cognitive complaint), an objective one (cognitive impairment), or both. The types of cognitive problems experienced and the course of the problem (i.e., acute vs. insidious onset; intermittent vs. persistent impairment; static vs. progressive decline) are important to identify next.

Although many patients present for evaluation of "memory" problems, frequently the problem experienced by the patient reflects impairment in another cognitive domain instead of or in addition to memory. Listening to the complaint with these other domains of cognition in mind will shed light not only on the specific problem requiring treatment but also on the differential diagnosis for that problem. This process requires a careful history, "bedside" cognitive testing, and often additional assessments.

This information then needs to be put into context by ascertaining the patient's premorbid cognitive and functional status. Obtaining collateral history from reliable informants (e.g., observers, data describing prior function) is essential, for the purpose of both corroborating (or not) the patient's reports and identifying other important historical information about which the patient with cognitive impairment may be unaware or unable to report. During the interview of a reliable informant, the interviewer needs to clarify whether the patient's current cognitive abilities represent a functionally important decline from his or her baseline; whether they are manifestations of a known medical, neurological, psychiatric (e.g., depression, anxiety), or substance use problem; and what, if any, interventions or strategies to compensate for these problems have been attempted by the patient or others. Identifying and interpreting cognitive complaints with respect to each of these issues are necessary for developing a refined differential diagnosis and formulating appropriate treatment goals and strategies.

Neuropsychiatric assessment was discussed in detail in Chapter 4. Examination of the adult with cognitive impairment begins with a detailed general physical and neurological examination. In addition to screening for focal, lateralizing, or other abnormal findings on the neurological examination, examination for subtle neurological signs (i.e., primitive reflexes or frontal release signs) may also be diagnostically informative (Hogan and Ebly 1995; Molloy et al. 1991). The general mental status examination is performed next and then supplemented with standardized assessments of cognitive function. A variety of such assessments are available, some of which are the Mini-Mental State Examination (MMSE; Folstein et al. 1975); various versions of the Clock Drawing Test; the Frontal Assessment Battery (Dubois et al. 2000); the EXIT25, a measure of executive function (Royall et al. 1992); and the Behavioral Dyscontrol Scale (Kaye et al. 1990). A combination of these measures, usually the MMSE and one or two others (e.g., Clock Drawing Test and the Frontal Assessment Battery), affords a relatively brief but broad assessment of cognitive function. Because performance on these measures is strongly influenced by both age and education, interpreting performance by comparison against normative data (which are available for each of these commonly used measures) rather than by simple cutoff scores is essential. Through comparison to age- and education-adjusted performance expectations, these screening assessments of cognition provide information that clarifies whether the patient's presentation includes cognitive complaints, cognitive impairments, or both.

When screening assessments fail to identify impairments in the cognitive domains that are suggested by patient complaints or history, or when the pattern of impairment on these assessments is inconsistent with the diagnosis otherwise suggested by the history and examination, formal neuropsychological assessment may be helpful (see Chapter 5, "Neuropsychological Assessment"). This testing is most useful when it includes not only an assessment of cognition but also evaluation of psychiatric and psychological processes (particularly anxiety and depression) that are known to adversely affect performance on cognitive assessment measures.

The selection of additional diagnostic assessments varies with the clinical context. Serum laboratory assessments for common reversible causes of cognitive impairment (e.g., those related to vitamin B_{12} and thyroid-stimulating hormone) are recommended (Knopman et al. 2001); when justified by the clinical history, other assessments of serum (e.g., human immunodeficiency virus, rapid plasma reagin, antinuclear antibody, liver function, electrolytes, complete blood count) and urine (e.g., urinalysis, urine toxicology) may be appropriate. When epilepsy or delirium is suspected, electroencephalography may inform the diagnostic assessment. Consistent with the Report of the Quality Standards Subcommittee of the American Academy of Neurology (Knopman et al. 2001), structural brain imaging (preferably magnetic resonance imaging [MRI]) is strongly recommended in the evaluation of all patients with cognitive impairment, as well as those with suspected dementia (see Chapter 6, "Imaging the Structure of the Aging Human Brain").

Treatment

The foundation of neuropsychiatric treatment of older patients with cognitive impairment, as with all patients, is a strong therapeutic alliance and promotion of treatment adherence. This foundation is sometimes challenging to build because many patients with cognitive impairments have limited awareness of the nature, severity, or functional consequences of their deficits and, therefore, of the need for either a relationship with the physician or the recommended treatments. In this context, a patient's apparent resistance to diagnosis and treatment may reflect psychological denial (not wanting to be labeled as "brain damaged" or "demented"), but more often the resistance is a manifestation of deficits in self-monitoring and awareness of illness (i.e., anosognosia). Despite the ongoing challenge to the treatment relationship and the patient's adherence to treatment presented by unawareness of illness, developing and maintaining a therapeutic alliance with such a patient, as well as with the patient's family and caregivers, is essential.

As a general rule, the treatment of cognitive impairments in the older adult is guided usefully by understanding the anticipated course of those impairments. When cognitive impairments occur in association with, or as a result of, a condition that might reasonably be expected to produce or exacerbate cognitive complaints and/or impairments (e.g., depression, anxiety, substance use disorders, sleep disturbances, endocrine problems, metabolic perturbations, nutritional deficits, adverse effects of medication), initial treatment is directed at the amelioration of that condition. Among patients with delirium or a dementing disorder that is potentially reversible (e.g., dementia due to depression, endocrine or nutritional disorders, infectious encephalopathies), treatment of the underlying cause and, in some cases, symptomatic management of the cognitive impairments are appropriate. Among patients with progressive neurodegenerative or neurological disorders (e.g., Alzheimer's disease, Parkinson's disease), augmenting current cognitive functions to the greatest extent possible, delaying progression of symptoms when possible, and improving quality of life despite persistence and/or progression of symptoms are appropriate treatment goals, particularly in the absence of disease-modifying (or curative) therapies. For patients experiencing cognitive impairments as a result of an injury or other condition that can be reasonably expected to produce static cognitive dysfunction and functional limitations (e.g., individuals with TBI, focal vascular events, radiation- or chemotherapy-induced brain injury, neurodevelopmental disorders), symptomatic treatment using nonpharmacological (usually rehabilitative) and pharmacological interventions is reasonable. Among such patients, the prognosis for cognitive and functional recovery typically varies as a function of the patient's age at onset of such problems, as well as the nature, severity, and chronicity (i.e., time since onset) of the disorder causing the cognitive and functional impairments.

As a treatment plan is developed, integrating neuropsychiatric treatment with treatment provided by other clinicians is necessary. Older patients with cognitive impairments frequently receive concurrent treatments from multiple clinicians; the likelihood that such treatments are working at cross-purposes is reduced by regular and effective communication among clinicians.

Nonpharmacological interventions, including some types of cognitive rehabilitation, are effective for the treatment of some cognitive impairments, particularly among persons with static brain disorders (e.g., TBI, stroke, hypoxic-ischemic brain injury, and possibly schizophrenia). Domain-specific nonpharmacological, and particularly rehabilitative, treatments of cognitive impairment are described in the following sections of this chapter. In general, these interventions seek to remediate or compensate for cognitive impairment through the use of performance monitoring, feedback, and skills or strategy training. Such interventions may be regarded as successful to the extent that they generalize beyond the context of treatment (i.e., improve the patient's function in settings besides the clinician's office).

Even in the absence of referral to an occupational therapist, speech-language therapist, or neuropsychologist for formal cognitive rehabilitation, the geriatric neuropsychiatrist can assist the patient and caregivers to develop several strategies that may limit the adverse effects of cognitive impairment on functional performance. For example, identifying and modifying environmental antecedents to cognitive failures and the affective/behavioral problems they produce may facilitate improvements in functional cognition, reduce disability, and alleviate patient and caregiver distress. Outlining daily events and challenges and scheduling them to coincide with periods when the individual is well rested and refreshed may limit the adverse effects of physical and/or cognitive fatigue on the patient's function. Performance on everyday tasks and interpersonal interactions may also be improved substantially simply by adjusting patient and family expectations (e.g., by teaching others to wait longer for verbal responses, to not respond or perform immediately for the individual, to allow longer intervals to accomplish tasks). Encouraging the use of so-called cognitive prosthetics, such as memory notebooks, timers with alarms and messages, task lists, and verbal or nonverbal cues from others (or by signage posted in the patient's environment), is often quite helpful for impairments in attention, working memory, declarative memory, and executive function. Use of cognitive prosthetics may also reduce performance failure- or frustration-related affective responses (e.g., anxiety, crying, anger, agitation). Similarly, assistive technologies such as communication devices, smartphones, and global positioning devices also may help to compensate for impairments in language, topographical orientation, and executive function. Even informal consultation with speech and occupational therapists experienced in the selection and use of such technologies may help the geriatric neuropsychiatrist identify interventions of these sorts to use in the context of patient treatment.

Pharmacotherapy of cognitive impairments in older adults is best regarded as an adjunct to nonpharmacological therapies. Common clinical experience suggests that the tendency among most physicians, including many neuropsychiatrists, is to prescribe medications as the first-line intervention for cognitive impairments. The individual response to pharmacotherapy is highly variable, with respect to both specific agents and dosages. Although some medications used for these purposes may be useful, in our experience patients and families report more benefit from the nonpharmacological interventions noted above than from most "cognition-enhancing" medications. This is not to suggest that the use of such agents be avoided but instead that they should not be regarded (or employed) as substitutes for the types of rehabilitative interventions and compensatory strategies described above. Indeed, their use may enhance the effectiveness of nonpharmacological interventions (Huber et al. 1997).

A "start-low, go-slow" approach is prudent when prescribing neuroactive agents to persons with neuropsychiatric disorders, although standard dosages of such agents are often required. Because no medications have been approved by the U.S. Food and Drug Administration (FDA) for the treatment of the cognitive impairments described in this chapter, individual treatment remains a matter of clinical judgment and empirical trial. With this in mind, assessing and documenting treatments' effects (whether beneficial, adverse, or absent) is very important. Serial assessment of the target domain(s) of cognition for which treatments are prescribed entails administration of standardized (bedside or formal neuropsychological) assessments, as well as evaluation of the effects of treatment on a patient's function in everyday life. Accurate recording of the response to treatment, whether nonpharmacological or pharmacological, and sharing those results with the patient and his or her caregivers may facilitate engagement in and adherence to prescribed treatments, when such are effective, and decreases the likelihood of maintaining or repeating unsuccessful treatments.

Cognitive Domain–Specific Diagnostic and Therapeutic Issues

In the sections that follow, we proceed through the hierarchy of cognition and address cognitive impairments and their rehabilitation. In each section, we describe a domain of cognition and briefly review the characteristic impairments and neuroanatomical bases of cognitive impairments in that domain. We also discuss the pharmacological and neurorehabilitative interventions that may improve impairments in each of these cognitive domains.

Arousal and Hypoarousal

Arousal denotes a state of wakefulness that is a prerequisite to the ability to respond to internal or external stimuli. Arousal exists on a continuum, with pathological extremes at either end. Coma represents an extreme state of *hypoarousal,* whereas manic excitement, severe anxiety (including the hypervigilance and heightened reactivity of posttraumatic stress disorder), and agitated delirium represent examples of conditions in which extreme hyperarousal features prominently. These latter conditions and their treatments are discussed in Chapter 15, "Delirium," and Chapter 20, "Anxiety Disorders." Here, we focus on the evaluation and treatment of disorders of hypoarousal.

States of diminished arousal are consequences of many conditions, including TBI, hypoxic-ischemic brain injury, cerebrovascular events, metabolic disturbances, medication or substance intoxication, cerebral neoplasms, advanced neurodegenerative conditions, and congenital or developmental disorders, among others. Hypoarousal reflects structural and/or functional impairment of one or more elements of the selective distributed reticulothalamic, thalamocortical, and reticulocortical networks that serve this cognitive function.

Cholinergic projections arising from the pendunculopontine and laterodorsal tegmental nuclei constitute the reticulothalamic portion of this system. These projections terminate in the body and also the reticular nucleus of the thalamus, the balance of activity between which modulates thalamic activity and, therefore, arousal. Glutamatergic projections from the thalamus to the cortex (i.e., thalamocortical projections) activate cortex and prepare it for information processing; that processing is modulated further by reticulocortical dopaminergic, noradrenergic, serotonergic, and cholinergic projections. The balance of activity within and between reticulothalamic, thalamocortical, and reticulocortical systems influences level of arousal. Injury to or dysfunction of these components of the arousal system will impair this cognitive function. Impairments of arousal, also known as disorders of consciousness, include coma, vegetative states (whether transient or persistent), minimally conscious state (MCS), and delirium. Because the last of these is addressed in detail in Chapter 15, "Delirium," it will not be discussed further here.

Coma represents a complete failure of the arousal system, and therefore it is the most extreme form of hypoarousal. The comatose patient is unconscious, demonstrates neither spontaneous eye opening nor sleep-wake cycles, and fails to arouse with even the most vigorous or noxious sensory stimulation.

Vegetative state is a condition wherein simple arousal ("core" consciousness) is relatively preserved, but self-awareness and environmental awareness ("higher" consciousness) are absent. Despite these impairments, patients in vegetative states may retain the capacity for spontaneous and/or stimulus-induced arousal and may demonstrate sleep-wake cycles. Although a vegetative state is often temporary, experienced as a person transitions from coma to more normal states of arousal, in some cases it may last for longer periods. When this condition persists for more than a few weeks, the term *persistent vegetative state (PVS)* is used to describe it.

MCS describes a condition in which a person demonstrates inconsistent but clearly discernible behavioral evidence of both core consciousness and higher consciousness. The latter includes the ability to follow simple commands, offer gestural or verbal "yes" or "no" responses (regardless of their accuracy), make intelligible verbalizations, and/or perform purposeful (even if rudimentary) behaviors. In this context, purposeful behaviors include movements or affective responses that occur as meaningful and contextually relevant responses to environmental stimuli and that do not simply reflect reflexive behavior.

Although significant hypoarousal is often identified easily by a simple observational examination, distinguishing among coma, vegetative states, and MCS can be challenging. Anchoring the diagnosis to the descriptions above is essential, because the severity of the condition and its duration carry prognostic information (Clark et al. 2007; Dolce et al. 2008; Schnakers et al. 2008). Useful steps to include in the evaluation of a patient who is hypoaroused are offered by Giacino et al. (2002). These include 1) maximizing arousal by ensuring that adequate stimulation is provided; 2) reducing or eliminating factors that may impair arousal—for example, ensuring adequate treatment of seizures and other medical problems and avoiding sedating medications; 3) avoiding the use of verbal or physical stimuli that are likely to evoke reflexive, rather than purposeful, responses; 4) employing command-follow tasks that are appropriate to the patient's motor abilities; 5) assessing behavioral responses broadly through the use of a wide array of eliciting stimuli; 6) minimizing potentially distracting environmental stimuli; 7) performing serial assessments systematically through both observation and use of reliable measurements; and 8) observing interactions between the patient and others as a means of collecting clinical data and identifying types of interactions (or individuals) that garner the best responses from the patient.

Essential elements of the diagnostic evaluation include laboratory assessments directed at the identification of metabolic, endocrine, toxic, and other potential medical etiologies. Additionally, structural neuroimaging (computed tomography [CT] or MRI) is also recommended because it provides both diagnostic and prognostic information. Electroencephalography and evoked potentials, particularly somatosensory evoked potentials, can also be useful as methods of identifying causes of or contributors to hypoarousal (e.g., seizures) and for making prognostic determinations (Brenner 2005; Carter and Butt 2005).

A noteworthy confound to the identification of disorders of impaired arousal is the locked-in syndrome. Patients with this condition do not have a disorder of arousal but instead are unable to move or communicate due to paralysis of almost all voluntary motor function (except eye movement) resulting from damage to the ventral pons. Although a thorough neurological examination combined with the behavioral observations described above is generally sufficient to distinguish this syndrome from disorders of impaired arousal, there are rare cases in which voluntary eye movements are impaired and thereby result in a pseudocoma or pseudovegetative presentation. Owen and Coleman (2008) described such a case and demonstrated that functional MRI [fMRI] may reveal preserved cognitive function in patients who otherwise appear to be vegetative. Although the application of the imaging paradigm they described requires further clinical validation, their example suggests that functional neuroimaging may come to play an important role in the evaluation of patients presenting with possible impairments of arousal.

When causative or contributory medical conditions are present, treatment directed at such conditions is a prerequisite to any other intervention for patients with impaired arousal. Concurrently, supportive care and active prevention of additional medical complications are essential. The patient's environment should be managed such that facilitating cues promoting adaptive engagement are maximized while distractions and potential sources of overstimulation (including pain and unnecessary procedures) are minimized. Lighting and meals should be coordinated to facilitate entrainment of circadian rhythms, and particularly sleep-wake cycles. Coma stimulation protocols may be useful; these involve the delivery of structured sensory stimulation, theoretically augmenting the recovery of sensory awareness and return from coma. In light of the favorable safety profile of such interventions, a time-limited trial of coma stimulation is a reasonable treatment option for coma, PVS, and MCS, despite the limited evidence supporting this practice (Lombardi et al. 2002).

Although no pharmacological options have been approved by the FDA for the treatment of coma, PVS, or MCS, the neurochemistry of arousal systems suggests catecholaminergic, glutamatergic, and/or cholinergic targets. Amantadine is supported by evidence from two separate double-blind, placebo-controlled investigations (Meythaler et al. 2002; Whyte et al. 2005) and thus is recommended as first-line treatment for disorders of consciousness. Other agents for which benefits have been reported for persons with these disorders include bromocriptine (Passler and Riggs 2001), levodopa (Patrick et al. 2003), pramipexole (Patrick et al. 2003), methylphenidate (Hornyak et al. 1997; Plenger et al. 1996; Worzniak and Fetters 1997), lamotrigine (Pachet et al. 2003; Showalter and Kimmel 2000), modafinil (Rivera 2005), and zolpidem (Clauss et al. 2000; Cohen and Duong 2008), among others. The evidence supporting the use of these other agents is limited, and neither the consistency of benefits nor the risks attendant to their use in this context have been fully described. Nonetheless, among patients in whom amantadine is ineffective or tolerated poorly, these medications may be considered second-line treatments for disorders of consciousness. As with all medications discussed in this chapter, clinicians are advised to familiarize themselves with prescribing information for these agents—and particularly side effects, drug interactions, and contraindications—before administering them to older adults with impaired arousal.

Attention and Processing Speed

Attention refers to the ability to direct, select, and maintain focus on a stimulus. Subsumed under attention are the component processes of selective attention (filtering information to identify an attentional target), sustained attention (maintaining attention on a selected target), and divided attention (focusing on two or more stimuli at the same time). *Processing speed* refers to the rate at which an individual processes and reacts to stimuli or information and is manifested clinically as reaction time or response latency. Disorders of attention and processing speed commonly complicate many neuropsychiatric conditions, and we consider these disorders together in this section.

Attentional processes are supported by several large-scale neural networks involving cortical, subcortical, brain stem, and white matter elements. Disturbances in the structure or function of any of these networks may produce attentional impairments (Mesulam 2000). Given the wide distribution of these networks, such impairments are common consequences of many neuropsychiatric conditions, including TBI, stroke, hypoxic-ischemic brain injuries, multiple sclerosis, Lewy body disease, toxic or infectious encephalitides, neurotoxic injuries, metabolic conditions, endocrine disorders, and many major psychiatric disorders, among others.

Electrophysiological and functional imaging studies indicate that the component domains of selective, sustained, and divided attention are each supported by distinct but interconnected neural substrates. These include the systems involved in arousal, described in the previous section, as well as primary and secondary sensory cortices, heteromodal parietal cortical areas, medial temporal (i.e., hippocampal and entorhinal) areas, the striatum and pallidum, several prefrontal (i.e., cingulate, inferolateral, and dorsolateral) cortices, and the axonal connections between them (Arciniegas and Topkoff 2004; Bledowski et al. 2004; Mesulam 2000). Spatial attention is generally regarded as a specialized attentional function that is lateralized to the nondominant (usually the right) hemisphere (Mesulam 2000). Reduction in processing speed, though often comorbid with attentional impairment, is most often related to disturbances involving the structure and/or function of cerebral white matter (Aukema et al. 2009). The anatomy of attention is modulated by multiple neurochemical systems, including dopamine, norepinephrine, serotonin, acetylcholine, glutamate, and γ-aminobutyric acid (GABA) (Arciniegas and Silver 2006; Arciniegas and Topkoff 2004; Bledowski et al. 2004).

Although severe impairments in attention or processing speed are often immediately apparent on observational examination, more subtle manifestations may be missed by commonly used bedside cognitive screening tools, such as the MMSE, which includes no timed tasks of attention. Augmenting the clinical assessment with vigilance (Lewis and Rennick 1979) or cancellation tasks (Mesulam 1985), continuous performance tasks (Conners 2000), or batteries specifically designed for the detailed assessment of this cognitive domain (e.g., the Trail Making Test [Reitan 1958] or the Test of Everyday Attention [Robertson et al. 1994, 1996]) is useful for diagnosing, clarifying, and monitoring recovery from impairments of attention and processing speed (see also Chapter 5, "Neuropsychological Assessment").

Nonpharmacological interventions are the first-line treatment for impairments of attention and processing speed. Environmental and/or lifestyle adjustments, particularly those that eliminate or minimize distractions and that reduce the potential for internal or environmental overstimulation, should be implemented. Engaging patients and caregivers in realistic appraisal of the time required to complete tasks successfully, including direct observation and timing of their performance, may help them allot adequate time for such tasks and thereby decrease the adverse consequences of unrealistic time demands (including anxiety) on task performance. Such appraisals may also help the patient and caregivers develop reasonable expectations about such matters and about the patient's anticipated level of productivity (or, conversely, need for functional support) at home and/or at work. In addition to allotting an appropriate amount of time and support for daily tasks, building defined periods of rest and recovery into the patient's schedule may further enhance function.

Cognitive rehabilitation may be useful, particularly if focused specifically on remediation of attentional impairments and/or compensatory strategy development. Although some authors have reported marginal benefit from such exercises (Lincoln et al. 2000; Riccio and French 2004), attention training appears to be useful when provided to highly motivated patients with relatively mild impairments in the late (not the acute) period following TBI or stroke (Cicerone et al. 2000, 2005; Rohling 2009). Attention training is most useful when it is functionally oriented (i.e., designed to address actual tasks the patient performs in daily life rather than simply office-based exercises).

Pharmacological treatment of impaired attention and/or processing speed is often a useful adjunct to nonpharmacological treatment (Michel and Mateer 2006). The most common pharmacological strategies for these purposes include catecholaminergic and cholinergic augmentation. The former approach is the one more widely used, and methylphenidate, dextroamphetamine, and mixed amphetamine salts are the agents used most often for these purposes. Although the use of these agents for impaired attention among persons with neurological disorders is driven by their use among persons with attention-deficit/hyperactivity disorder (ADHD) (Biederman et al. 2004; Jadad et al. 1999), the effects among persons with neurological disorders are often more pronounced on processing speed than on attention per se (Whyte et al. 2002). Despite such differences, however, these agents—and methylphenidate more specifically—are generally regarded as the first-line pharmacological treatments of attention and processing speed impairments that are due to neurological injuries.

Despite commonly expressed concerns regarding the cardiovascular safety of methylphenidate, carefully conducted studies of this agent among persons with TBI (Alban et al. 2004), other acquired brain injuries (Burke et al. 2003), or adult ADHD demonstrate modest increases in heart rate and/or systolic blood pressure that are usually not clinically significant. Similarly, these agents do not typically affect seizure frequency adversely (Feldman et al. 1989; Wroblewski et al. 1992). Accordingly, the literature does not support a priori prohibitions of the use of these agents in this population. Nonetheless, it remains prudent to establish baseline cardiovascular and/or seizure characteristics before initiating treatment and to monitor for changes when prescribing methylphenidate or other stimulant medications to older persons with attention and/or processing speed impairments.

When methylphenidate or other stimulants are ineffective or tolerated poorly, alternative medications may be considered. These agents, reviewed in detail by Arciniegas and Silver (2006) and Silver et al. (2009b), include levodopa, amantadine, bupropion (sustained-release formulation), modafinil, and the cholinesterase inhibitors. Among the cholinesterase inhibitors, donepezil's relative ease of use, favorable side-effect profile, and limited drug-drug interactions make it a reasonable first-choice agent from this medication class for use in the older adult with attention and processing speed impairments. Galantamine, particularly in its extended-release formulation, and transdermal rivastigmine are acceptable agents as well, although published reports of their use for the treatment of conditions other than dementia (or mild cognitive impairment) are few (Silver et al. 2006, 2009a).

For patients who are partial responders to stimulant medications, augmentation of stimulants with another agent is reasonable. Given that the principal beneficial effects of most of the nonstimulant medications are attributable (directly or indirectly) to the augmentation of cerebral catecholaminergic function, rational pharmacotherapy suggests that augmentation of a stimulant be undertaken using an agent with a complementary (rather than redundant) mechanism of action (e.g., a cholinesterase inhibitor). When an agent of this type is added to a stimulant with beneficial results, it is prudent to taper the dosage of the stimulant to arrive at the minimally necessary dosage of both agents required to effect optimal cognitive improvement.

Recognition

Agnosia describes a sensory domain–specific inability to recognize objects resulting from impaired integration of sensory information at a cortical level (cortically based perception), impaired attachment of meaning to those percepts (association), or both. Patients with agnosia typically present with this problem in a single sensory domain (i.e., visual, auditory, tactile, or, at least theoretically, olfactory or gustatory). The sensory domain–specific presentation allows for distinguishing these patients clinically from those with impaired naming (anomia): patients with agnosia are unable to recognize a stimulus presented in the affected domain (e.g., visual) but remain able to recognize (and name) it when it is presented in an unaffected domain (e.g., auditory or tactile).

The most common type of agnosia is visual, which is frequently subdivided into apperceptive and associative types. Visual apperceptive agnosias refer to the inability to recognize, discriminate between, and copy visual stimuli despite intact primary cortical sensory processing. Visual apperceptive agnosia is therefore distinguished from cortical blindness, a condition in which a patient has a cortically based failure to perceive visual stimuli. In visual associative agnosias, the ability to perceive the constituent elements of a visual stimulus is preserved, but the stimulus is nonetheless not recognized; in contrast, in visual apperceptive agnosia, the ability to copy the stimulus remains intact.

The following are common types of visual agnosias:

- *Object agnosia:* inability to identify objects; this usually affects recognition of some, but not all, object categories
- *Form agnosia:* inability to recognize the whole object due to impaired recognition of one or more of its parts
- *Shape agnosia:* inability to recognize the shape of the object despite recognition of its other features (color, size, etc.)
- *Finger agnosia:* inability to recognize fingers on the hand; this is a feature of Gerstmann's syndrome, in which agraphia (inability to write), acalculia (inability to calculate), and left-right disorientation co-occur
- *Mirror agnosia:* inability to recognize objects or activity in either the left or right field of view
- "*Pure word blindness,*" also known as alexia without agraphia: inability to read despite preserved perception of letters, words, and/or sentences (evidenced by the patient's ability to copy the text that he or she cannot "read"); preserved ability to write; and otherwise normal language
- *Color agnosia:* inability to recognize colors despite the ability to distinguish between colors (distinguished from central achromatopsia, a cortically based impairment of color perception)
- *Simultanagnosia:* inability to synthesize multiple elements in a simultaneously displayed visual presentation into a cohesive whole despite recognition of the constituent elements of the viewed scene
- *Prosopagnosia:* inability to recognize familiar faces (sometimes including the patient's own face)

Visual agnosia is a prominent feature of Balint's syndrome, an acquired disturbance in the ability to perceive the visual field as a whole resulting from the combination of simultanagnosia, optic ataxia (an impairment of visually guided reaching), and oculomotor apraxia (an impairment of saccadic initiation). Deficits in face recognition, although not frank prosopagnosia, also may contribute to Capgras syndrome; this is a delusional misidentification syndrome in which the patient believes that a familiar person has been replaced by an impostor or exact double despite recognition of the familiarity of that person's appearance and behavior. Deficits in face recognition also contribute to impaired social development among patients with Asperger's disorder.

The auditory agnosias are conditions in which the ability to recognize auditory stimuli is impaired despite intact primary auditory sensory processing. Auditory agnosia is therefore distinguished from cortical deafness, a condition in which there is a cortically based failure to perceive auditory stimuli. Auditory agnosia, as a specific condition, denotes an inability to recognize environmental sounds (e.g., a dog's bark, a car engine). Auditory/verbal information agnosia, also known as "pure word deafness," denotes an inability to recognize verbal stimuli in the absence of impaired language comprehension. Receptive amusia refers to an inability to recognize music.

Tactile agnosia is the inability to recognize somatosensory stimuli. Common forms of tactile agnosia include astereognosia, an inability to recognize objects by touch, and agraphesthesia, an inability to recognize a number or letter written on the skin (usually the palm or first finger).

Other forms of agnosia include olfactory agnosia, the inability to recognize stimuli by smell, and gustatory agnosia, the inability to identify stimuli by taste. Anosognosia refers to an inability to recognize disease in oneself. Although sometimes used to describe impaired ability to recognize nondominant (usually left) hemiplegia, this term is used more commonly to refer to an unawareness of motor and cognitive deficits as well as a lack of awareness of illness.

Because intact primary sensory function is a required element of the agnosias, the evaluation for agnosia begins with a thorough elementary neurological examination. Additionally, because agnosia must be distinguished from anomia (alone or as part of another aphasia), a detailed language examination is required. Formal neuropsychological testing may be helpful when questions regarding the presence, type, and severity of a suspected agnosia remain despite a careful bedside examination. In addition to identifying impairments, identifying preserved recognition in other sensory modalities is vital to the design of compensatory strategies for agnosia.

Unfortunately, little evidence is available to support the effectiveness of formal rehabilitative interventions for the treatment of the agnosias (Behrmann et al. 2005; Burns 2004). Additionally, there is no evidence supporting pharmacotherapy for these conditions. Assisting the patient and family in the adaptation to disability is essential, and creative development of compensatory strategies that capitalize on preserved recognition functions and other cognitive strengths is required of the geriatric neuropsychiatrist. Consultation with a speech-language and/or occupational therapist experienced in the care of persons with disorders of recognition may be useful toward these ends.

Memory

Memory refers to the ability to learn, store, and retrieve information. Memory is not a unitary cognitive domain but instead denotes several different neurocognitive functions that are predicated on multiple neuroanatomical networks. Given the frequency with which the geriatric neuropsychiatrist will encounter memory impairments, evaluating and describing memory dysfunction adeptly and accurately are essential skills. At a minimum, clinicians in this discipline should be able to distinguish between declarative memory and procedural memory and to differentiate between the processes of memory encoding and memory retrieval.

Declarative memory, the ability to learn, store, and retrieve factual information, requires first an intact sensory-cortical pathway through which to acquire (learn) new information. From primary and secondary association cortices, highly processed multimodal sensory information is transmitted from parietal heteromodal association cortices to the entorhinal-hippocampal complex. When that incoming multimodal sensory information produces a sufficiently robust signal in the hippocampus (a process that, at least in part, necessitates amygdala-hippocampal interactions that attach a motivational-emotional, or "survival-related," valence to that information), the process of long-term potentiation within the network processing that information is initiated. By forming stable synapses within that network, long-term potentiation—a glutamatergically mediated and cholinergically dependent process—serves as the neural basis for encoding (Giovannini 2006; Kullmann and Lamsa 2007). Because the hippocampus is necessary for encoding declarative information, the process of new learning of declarative information is described as hippocampally dependent. The processing stream into which the hippocampus projects via the hippocampal-forniceal-mammillothalamic pathway engages frontal areas (particularly the dorsolateral prefrontal cortex) in the process of consolidating new memories.

After consolidation, volitional retrieval of declarative information requires prefrontal structures to activate the selective distributed networks in which that information was originally encoded. In contrast to new learning, volitional retrieval of previously learned (consolidated) information is not hippocampally dependent but instead is frontally dependent. Declarative memory is also highly associative, as evidenced by nonvolitional (or automatic) retrieval: reactivation of nearly any part of the neural networks (including their sensory elements) involved in the original encoding of that information results in retrieval of that information.

Procedural memory refers to the ability to learn, store, and retrieve how to do things and overlaps considerably with praxis. It is predicated on the development and fine-tuning of the sensorimotor-frontal-subcortical-cerebellar networks that are necessary for learning and efficiently retrieving complex sensorimotor routines. Procedural memory therefore is not hippocampally dependent, and its function and dysfunction are dissociable from declarative memory.

Working memory involves the process of holding information in mind, or "online," for a brief period immediately after a stimulus leaves the sensory field. Everyday examples of working memory include a person's maintaining in mind a phone number just heard or read until the person writes it down or dials it and a patient's ability to hold in mind a three-word set presented to him or her before repeating those words back to the examiner (as on the registration portion of the MMSE). Working memory therefore overlaps with and extends the process of sustained attention. When working memory is impaired, patients typically experience difficulties with new learning (and, by extension, memory retrieval), as well as with executive operations on information in working memory (e.g., information reversal tasks such as digit span backwards, serial subtractions, paced auditory serial addition tasks, n-back tasks).

Amnesia denotes an impairment of memory. Although often used only to describe impairments in declarative memory (particularly new learning), the term applies broadly to impairments of declarative or procedural memory, encoding or new learning, and recall or retrieval of previously learned information. Amnesia can be anterograde (inability to form new memories subsequent to the event that produced the amnesia), retrograde (inability to recall information acquired before the event that produced the amnesia), or both (global). Because the term *amnesia* may be used to refer to any of the types of memory impairment, when using this term, one should clarify its referent by providing specific descriptions of type and severity of the memory functions that are impaired. When such clarity is lacking, erroneous inferences and conclusions regarding diagnosis and the relationship between amnesia and other concurrently experienced neuropsychiatric symptoms are inevitable.

The neuroanatomy of memory offers a foundation for interpreting the putative neurobiological bases for amnesia in its various forms. Impaired declarative new learning is generally associated with dysfunction of the hippocampal-forniceal-mammillothalamic pathway, whereas impaired volitional retrieval of declarative information is associated with dysfunction of the frontal-subcortical systems necessary for reactivation of the neural network in which such information is represented. Impaired procedural memory is generally associated with subcortical dysfunction (e.g., as in Parkinson's and Huntington's diseases) and manifests as difficulty learning new (generally motor or behavioral) routines.

When declarative memory impairments develop, anterograde amnesia is the rule. Although rare cases of pure retrograde amnesia due to mechanical trauma or vascular injury have been reported, the occurrence of retrograde amnesia is usually concurrent to anterograde amnesia of greater severity. With regard to the content of the retrograde amnesia, information acquired proximate to the time of onset of memory dysfunction is more severely affected than information acquired more remotely (Ribot's law). In other words, events immediately preceding the acquisition of the condition producing the memory impairment (e.g., TBI or hypoxic-ischemic brain injury) may be lost, but previously learned semantic and autobiographical information is relatively preserved.

Patients and their families or caregivers frequently use the term *memory problems* as the chief complaint in initial clinical encounters. Although it is sometimes the most correct term to describe a patient's cognitive difficulties, it is not uncommon to find that the patient's problems are more directly referable to difficulties in other cognitive domains, such as attention, language, recognition, or executive function. Careful history and examination are therefore necessary to confirm that the patient's problem in fact involves memory rather than another cognitive function. The history obtained should capture information surrounding the onset of the memory impairment, its course, and any possible contributing etiologies. The use of bedside assessments is very helpful in the assessment of memory. Particularly helpful in neuropsychiatric practice is the MMSE, which contains several items that assess memory: a three-item registration task (assessing working memory), a three-item recall task (assessing new learning/encoding and retrieval of the three items presented in the registration task), and two five-item assessments of temporal and geographic orientation (requiring attention, new learning, and retrieval). Although these constitute only a cursory evaluation when compared to formal neuropsychological testing of memory, they can provide valuable information regarding the presence and type of memory problem experienced by a patient. In particular, the three-item recall task—when augmented with semantic and recognition cues in the case of failed spontaneous recall—may be used to distinguish between impairments in new learning/encoding and retrieval. Patients unable to recall the items even with the aid of semantic and/or recognition cues are likely to have a defect in memory encoding, whereas those who succeed with such cues have intact encoding but problems with memory retrieval. Although patients are scored only on their spontaneous recall, developing a differential diagnosis for those with impaired performance on this task is facilitated by this simple addition to the MMSE.

Assessment of semantic and autobiographical information may be accomplished by asking the patient about his or her personal, family, and medical history, as well as about general knowledge, knowledge of topics relevant to the patient's schooling or work, and historical facts with which persons of the patient's age and culture are expected to be familiar. Obtaining answers to questions about personal, family, medical, or other issues from a family member or person familiar with the patient is needed to assess the facts' accuracy (or their indication of memory impairment).

Although procedural memory is not generally assessed by neuropsychiatric clinicians, it is an important function about which to obtain information, particularly in patients with impaired declarative memory. Because declarative memory and procedural memory are psychologically and anatomically dissociable, patients with impairments in one function may retain preserved abilities in the other. This pattern has been consistently observed in patients with Alzheimer's disease (van Halteren-van Tilborg et al. 2007), among other conditions.

Capitalizing on intact procedural memory may sustain or enhance the functional independence of such patients despite their declarative memory impairments.

Environmental and lifestyle adjustments may be useful in addressing persisting memory difficulties. Sources of overstimulation and distraction should be eliminated to the greatest extent possible. Rehearsal of new information may assist with encoding, and written or verbal environmental cues may facilitate retrieval of information such that the functional consequences of memory problems are substantially minimized. Patients with impairments of working memory may allocate an excessive amount of processing resources to sustain near-normal cognitive performance, resulting in early fatigue (McAllister et al. 2004). Allowing time for rest and recovery after periods of cognitive exertion may help optimize functional ability. Memory prosthetics, such as memory books and various technologies, enhance cued memory retrieval and are an important component of treatment and rehabilitation (Cicerone et al. 2000, 2005). These interventions appear to be most effective when provided to patients with memory impairments secondary to TBI or stroke, particularly among those with mild impairments and motivation to improve.

No agents have been specifically approved by the FDA for the treatment of memory impairment alone. However, the neurochemistry of memory suggests that strategies augmenting cholinergic systems, stabilizing glutamatergic systems, and augmenting catecholaminergic function may be useful. Evidence from case reports, open-label trials, and small-scale double-blind, placebo-controlled studies indicates that cholinesterase inhibitors are helpful for impairments in new learning and memory retrieval across many etiologies (Devi and Silver 2000). For impairments of working memory, catecholaminergic augmentation, typically with methylphenidate, may be of benefit (Barch 2004; McAllister et al. 2004). We generally employ donepezil as first-line treatment of declarative memory impairments due to neurological disorders, although sustained-release galantamine and transdermal rivastigmine are also reasonable choices for these purposes. Memantine may prove useful alone or in combination with a cholinesterase inhibitor for patients who fail to respond to such first-line treatments. Memantine is an uncompetitive *N*-methyl-D-aspartate (NMDA) receptor antagonist and may augment dopaminergic function in frontal-subcortical circuits. For patients who are unwilling to try these medication options or for those who appreciate no benefit from them, cytidine 5′-diphosphocholine (CDP-choline) may be helpful (Fioravanti and Yanagi 2005). However, lack of FDA regulation and the incomplete safety profile of this agent preclude our formally recommending use of this agent presently.

Language

The various types of aphasia involve impairments in one or more of the four principal components of language: fluency, repetition, comprehension, and/or naming (Table 12–1). Aphasias are the result of damage to neural networks of the dominant (usually left) hemisphere, which support the syntactic and semantic aspects of language. *Fluency* is defined as the ability to produce phrases of six or more words with normal syntax and without undue word-finding pauses; impairments in this language function define the nonfluent aphasias (Broca's, transcortical motor), also sometimes described as the anterior aphasias given their involvement of frontal structures. *Comprehension* refers to the ability to recognize written or spoken symbols across multiple sensory modalities and to attach linguistic meaning to them. Impairments in this domain are the defining feature of Wernicke's and transcortical sensory aphasias, also referred to as the posterior aphasias given their involvement of temporoparietal areas. *Repetition* involves the reproduction of phrases without error; isolated impairment in this component of language (with relative preservation of others) defines conduction aphasia. *Naming* refers to the ability to linguistically identify actions and objects across multiple sensory domains; impairments of naming are observed in all of the aphasias, and this type of impairment is the defining (isolated) feature of anomic aphasia. Impairments in all of these language components constitute global aphasia.

Injury to the homologous neuroanatomical networks of the nondominant (usually right) hemisphere results in aprosodia, an impairment of the melodic, affective, and kinesic components of language that add meaning to and enhance linguistic communication. As with the language functions of the dominant hemisphere, fluency, comprehension, and repetition are core elements of prosody. Nonfluent (anterior) aprosodia manifests as flat and monotonous speech that is absent of the normal inflections that communicate relevant affect or that allow modulation of intonation to change the meaning of language (e.g., "He's a great guy" spoken literally vs. sarcastically). Comprehension aprosodia represents as an inability to understand the intonations, kinesics, and affective import of the language of others. The inability to repeat prosody constitutes conduction aprosodia.

Disorders of language (aphasias) must be differentiated from impairments in the motor aspects of speech (dysarthria) and voice (dysphonia). Aphasias must also be differentiated from agnosia, an impairment in sensory domain–specific recognition. Unlike anomia, in which object naming is impaired regardless of the sensory modality in which the object-to-be-named is presented, agnosia represents a sensory domain–specific impairment in recognition (e.g., the patient with visual agnosia may not be able to name an object presented visually but can do so when the same object is presented via tactile or

TABLE 12–1. Classification of the aphasias

Aphasia	Fluency	Repetition	Comprehension	Naming
Global	–	–	–	–
Broca's	–	–	+	–
Transcortical motor	–	+	+	–
Conduction	+	–	+	–
Wernicke's	+	–	–	–
Transcortical sensory	+	+	–	–
Mixed transcortical	–	+	–	–
Anomic	+	+	+	–

Note. + indicates that the function is relatively intact; – indicates that the function is impaired, although the degree of impairment may vary from mild (as in the transcortical and anomic aphasias) to severe (as in Broca's and Wernicke's aphasias).

auditory means). A specific example of the importance of distinguishing between aphasia and agnosia is alexia without agraphia (pure word blindness), in which the patient has an acquired impairment of reading with preservation of writing and also all other language functions. This classic disconnection syndrome reflects inability to communicate visual input from the visual cortices (typically as a result of a lesion of the posterior dominant hemisphere affecting visual cortex and also the callosal fibers carrying visual information from the nondominant hemisphere) to dominant hemisphere language cortex.

Impairments in functional communication, whether aphasia, aprosodia, both, or more subtle disturbances of language, are common features of many neuropsychiatric conditions (e.g., the primary progressive aphasia and semantic dementia variants of frontotemporal dementia, stroke, TBI, Alzheimer's disease, dementia with Lewy bodies, infectious or neoplastic conditions, schizophrenia) and are particularly common sequelae of stroke (Bakheit 2004; Berthier 2005). The evaluation for aphasia requires careful examination of each of the major language domains. Verbal and written tests are administered to establish fluency, comprehension, repetition, and naming abilities. Assessment of fluency involves evaluation of verbal and written phrase length, word-finding ability, and syntactic (grammatical) structure. Comprehension is assessed during the interview, as well as by direct assessment of the patient's responses to yes/no, true/false, and short-story questions; note that the three-step comprehension task on the MMSE is actually a test of ideational praxis, and impaired performance on it requires dissection of the patient's performance into its language- and praxis-related components. Repetition is assessed by asking the patient to repeat simple, complex, or agrammatical statements (e.g., "no ifs, ands, or buts"), and naming assessment involves evaluating the patient's ability to name objects (e.g., pen, watch) and their parts (e.g., pen cap, ballpoint, watch band, stem of watch). Consultation with a speech-language pathologist and/or neuropsychologist may be required to characterize language deficits and to formulate a language rehabilitation plan. When such consultations cannot be obtained for logistical or financial reasons, the geriatric neuropsychiatrist may consider using the Mississippi Aphasia Screening Test for these purposes (Nakase-Thompson et al. 2005).

Aphasias, aprosodias, and nonaphasic functional communication impairments are amenable to cognitive rehabilitation (Cicerone et al. 2000, 2005; Rohling 2009); referral to a speech-language therapist experienced in addressing these impairments is recommended for patients with such problems. Treatment of the patient with aphasia balances the provision of opportunities for the patient to communicate independently with the provision of compensatory and supported communication strategies. "Constraint-induced" aphasia therapy (i.e., emphasizing independent communication) appears to facilitate improvement in language abilities and reduces patients' feelings of frustration and/or inadequacy (Pulvermuller et al. 2001). If the patient is unable to be engaged in formal aphasia therapy for logistic or financial reasons, compensatory and supported communication strategies based on the principles of such therapy can be facilitated by the geriatric neuropsychiatrist. These strategies include emphasis on direct, simple, and concrete statements (by and to the patient) and use of communication boards with objects and/or pictures to which that patient and others may refer when communicating. Among patients with aprosodias, encouraging communication of affect directly (i.e., verbalizing feelings such as sadness, happiness, anger) rather than by inference from the manner in which the patient communicates (or interprets the communication of others) is essential.

FDA-approved medication treatment options for aphasias are lacking, and the pharmacological literature is essentially limited to small-scale open-label studies involving dopaminergic or cholinergic augmentation (Berthier 2005). Notable exceptions to this statement are several single-site randomized, placebo-controlled studies of speech therapy augmented with piracetam (Greener et al. 2001), donepezil (Berthier et al. 2006), or bromocriptine (Ashtary et al. 2006; Bragoni et al. 2000), demonstrating that these treatments afford greater improvement in aphasia than do speech therapy and placebo. Given methylphenidate's potential benefits for motor recovery and mood following stroke (Grade et al. 1998), it may be a useful pharmacological augmentation strategy for patients with poststroke aphasia as well.

Praxis

Praxis refers to the ability to perform skilled purposeful movement on demand, and *apraxia* denotes impairment of this ability that cannot be attributed to sensory, motor, or language disturbances. Apraxia may involve axial, limb, and/or whole body movements, and three major subtypes of apraxia are generally agreed upon. *Limb-kinetic apraxia* refers to the inability to execute precise individual finger movements on demand. Because impaired performance of such tasks is frequently attributable to elementary motor impairment, limb-kinetic apraxia is not universally accepted as a true apraxia. *Ideomotor apraxia* denotes the inability to perform gestural (pantomime) movements to verbal command despite preservation of the same movement in a naturalistic setting. This apraxia may affect not only pantomime on command but also spontaneous, environmentally relevant movements. Ideomotor apraxia frequently involves both axial and limb movements. *Ideational apraxia* refers to the inability to carry out a complex sequence of movements despite preserved ability to correctly execute the individual components of that sequence.

Ideational apraxia occurs most often in the setting of acute confusional states, dementias, and other disorders affecting frontal-subcortical function, and it overlaps conceptually and clinically with impairments of executive function and/or attention (Weintraub 2000). Approximately 13%–28% of stroke survivors experience some degree of apraxia, with left-sided lesions being twice as likely to produce this impairment (Donkervoort et al. 2000; Pedersen et al. 2001; Zwinkels et al. 2004). Apraxia is also a relatively common feature of various neurodegenerative disorders, including corticobasal degeneration, Alzheimer's disease, dementia with Lewy bodies, Parkinson's disease, frontotemporal dementia, and progressive supranuclear palsy, among others. Apraxia may also adversely affect the patient's ability to make use of other cognitive functions, whether intact or impaired, and also diminish the patient's functional status (Saeki et al. 1995).

Praxis is a function of the dominant hemisphere, and its anatomy is in close proximity with that supporting language. Areas supporting praxis include the left inferior parietal lobule, premotor cortex, supplementary motor area, and other aspects of the left frontal convexity, as well as the corpus callosum. It has been suggested that the core deficits in ideomotor apraxia reflect defects in movement representations that are coded in premotor association areas of the dominant hemisphere, thereby explaining the frequent co-occurrence of ideomotor apraxia and nonfluent aphasia (Leiguarda 2001).

Establishing that the patient possesses the sensory, motor, and language comprehension functions necessary to perform a skilled, purposeful movement on demand is a prerequisite to the evaluation for apraxia. Limb-kinetic apraxia is typically tested with instructions to pantomime finely graded finger movements, such as buttoning a shirt or performing pincer or tapping movements. Ideomotor apraxia is assessed by asking the patient to pantomime various axial, limb, and whole body movements (e.g., brushing teeth, dealing cards, using scissors, blowing out a match). Ideational praxis is assessed by observing requested performance of multistep tasks, such as the three-step command on the MMSE. Several bedside assessments of praxis are available and may be a useful guide to such evaluations (Almeida et al. 2002; Zwinkels et al. 2004). Additionally, consultation with a speech-language pathologist, occupational therapist, and/or neuropsychologist may be diagnostically useful and assist with treatment planning.

Some evidence, chiefly derived from small-scale uncontrolled treatment trials, supports compensatory strategy training in the rehabilitation of apraxia from stroke and TBI (Cappa et al. 2005; Cicerone et al. 2000, 2005). However, the treatment of apraxia in other contexts, in particular neurodegenerative disease, is often challenging. Simple interventions such as reduction of task complexity, where possible, as well as setting up the required task elements (e.g., objects, their locations, their order), may facilitate performance despite apraxia. When such interventions are not successful, direct supervision, assistance of varying degrees, or complete elimination of some tasks (e.g., stovetop cooking) may be required, or in some cases, patients may need to be placed in assisted living or another setting in which tasks are performed for patients.

The literature regarding pharmacotherapy of apraxia is underdeveloped. Case reports suggest that some forms of apraxia may respond to levodopa (Yamada et al. 2004), amantadine (Yasuoka et al. 2001), or donepezil (Kim et al. 2005). However, the number of reports is too limited to warrant recommendation of these agents for the treatment of apraxia; further study of the pharmacological treatment of apraxia is needed.

Visuospatial Function

Visuospatial function refers to a constellation of complex visual processing abilities, including spatial awareness and attention, awareness of self-other and of self-object spatial relationships, visuospatial memory, and interpretation and navigation of extrapersonal space. The prototypical impairment of visuospatial function is unilateral hemispace neglect, an inability to attend to sensory events in one hemispace (usually, but not always, the left) in the absence of elementary sensorimotor deficits that better account for this impairment. Although unilateral visual neglect is often the most salient form of impaired spatial attention, impairment is frequently multimodal, involving hemi-inattention to auditory and somatosensory stimuli as well as reduced motor exploration of the affected hemispace (Mesulam 2000). In its more subtle form, unilateral hemi-inattention, impairments may become apparent only by direct examination.

Another relatively common form of visuospatial dysfunction is topographic disorientation, which denotes an acquired inability to learn and/or retrieve information related to spatial orientation between places. This impairment may make navigating one's environment difficult or impossible. Patients with this problem may complain of or be brought to clinical attention as a result of "getting lost" in new or even previously familiar places.

Impaired constructional ability (i.e., difficulty with figure copying) is frequently but incorrectly described as "constructional apraxia." Construction tasks require normal visual acuity, recognition, visuospatial function (including spatial attention), executive function, and the motor abilities to carry out the task. When visual function and motor ability are normal, impaired constructional ability is a manifestation of spatial inattention (including unilateral neglect), executive dysfunction, or both and is not an apraxia. Similarly, "dressing apraxia" is a misnomer. Dressing involves aligning the axis of the body and/or limb with the garment to be donned and requires normal visual acuity, recognition, visuospatial function (including spatial attention), executive function, and the motor abilities to carry out the task. Again, when visual function and motor ability are normal, impaired dressing ability is best understood as a manifestation of spatial inattention (including unilateral neglect), executive dysfunction, or both and is not an apraxia.

Disorders of visuospatial function are a common feature of many neurological disorders, particularly those affecting the structure and/or function of the nondominant (typically right) hemisphere through a lesion (e.g., stroke, tumor) or neurodegenerative disorder (e.g., Alzheimer's disease, dementia with Lewy bodies, corticobasal degeneration, posterior cortical atrophy). Despite the high frequency of visuospatial dysfunction across many dementing conditions, impairment of this function is not included in the DSM-IV-TR criteria for dementia.

Visuospatial function is supported by a distributed neural network involving the reticular system, thalamus, superior colliculus, striatum, parietal cortex, and frontal eye fields. There is marked nondominant hemispheric specialization for this cognitive domain, with the nondominant parietal cortex playing a particularly vital role within the extended network supporting spatial attention. Visuospatial memory is in large part supported by the parahippocampal place area, a portion of the parahippocampal gyrus (Epstein and Kanwisher 1998). Cholinergic and dopaminergic deficits have been implicated in the development of impaired visuospatial function.

The evaluation for visuospatial dysfunction requires careful assessment of sensory and motor function, as well as memory, language, recognition, praxis, and executive function; deficits in any of these may lead secondarily to visuospatial impairments. Bedside assessment tools, such as line bisection, target cancellation tasks, and reading tasks, are often useful. Construction tasks (e.g., figure copy or clock drawing tasks) may reveal hemispace neglect. Among patients with hemi-inattention, testing for extinction to bilateral simultaneous stimulation may reveal this impairment. Visuospatial memory may be assessed by asking the patient to locate a particular building in a city or to map out the route from one location to another. Identification of impaired dressing ability requires observation of the patient performing such tasks.

Environmental modifications, while always an important component of cognitive rehabilitation, are particularly essential for patients with visuospatial dysfunction. Tasks should be modified such that key items are set up within the patients' unaffected hemispace—particularly for patients with true neglect syndromes, which involve not only impairment of visuospatial processing in the affected hemispace but also persistent and dense unawareness of the presence of that hemispace. Among patients with incomplete neglect syndromes (i.e., hemispatial inattention), cues to draw attention to the affected hemispace may be useful; nonetheless, taking steps to remove or reduce hazards within the neglected hemispace is crucial to maintaining patient safety. The patient's room may be set up to maximize observation and engagement; for instance, the bed might be placed such that the door lies to the patient's unaffected side. Cognitive rehabilitation of visuospatial dysfunction may be useful, with compensatory training being the first-line intervention (Cappa et al. 2005; Cicerone et al. 2000, 2005; Rohling 2009).

Clinical reports and expert opinions suggest that cholinesterase inhibitors, uncompetitive NMDA receptor antagonists, or catecholamine augmentation may be of benefit for visuospatial impairment. However, no medication options have been approved by the FDA, and the state of evidence does not permit recommendation of pharmacotherapy targeting isolated deficits in this cognitive domain.

Executive Function

Executive function refers to a collection of higher cognitive functions, including categorization and abstraction; problem solving; self-direction; planning and organization of cognition and behavior; independence from external environmental contingencies; maintenance of and facile shifting between information or behavior sets; and executive control of more "basic" cognitive functions such as attention, working memory, systematic memory searching and information retrieval, language (lexical fluency and functional communication), praxis, and visuospatial function. Judgment and insight are also generally considered executive functions, although the concept of self-awareness (which overlaps conceptually and clinically with insight) extends beyond executive function alone. Such impairments are increasingly recognized as a component of many primary psychiatric disorders and as a major contributor to both functional disability and caregiver burden (Fogel 1994; Royall et al. 1998).

Executive dysfunction is a common feature of many neuropsychiatric conditions, particularly those affecting the structure or function of one or more elements of the frontal-subcortical circuits (see Chapter 3, "Neurobiological Basis of Behavior"). Executive dysfunction may arise as a result of injury to or dysfunction of either the closed-loop or open-loop elements of the dorsolateral prefrontal-subcortical circuit. The closed-loop elements include the dorsolateral surface of the frontal lobes, dorsolateral head of the caudate nucleus, lateral aspect of the globus pallidus interna, and rostrolateral substantia nigra (elements of the "direct" circuit); the dorsal globus pallidus externa and lateral subthalamic nucleus (elements of the "indirect" circuit); the parvocellular portions of the ventral anterior and mediodorsal thalamus; and the white matter connections between these structures. The open-loop elements of this circuit include the other cortical areas that project to and from it, as well as the white matter connections between these other cortical areas and the dorsolateral prefrontal-subcortical circuit. These open-loop elements permit the dorsolateral prefrontal-subcortical circuit to serve as a controller of the processing within and interaction between more "basic" cognitive functions.

The anterior cingulate- and the lateral orbitofrontal-subcortical circuits serve motivation and comportment, respectively. The structures and functions of these circuits are distinct from but reciprocally interactive with the dorsolateral prefrontal-subcortical circuit and may thereby modify (for better or worse) executive function. The function of the prefrontal-subcortical circuits is also modulated by multiple neurotransmitters, including glutamate (the primary excitatory neurotransmitter), acetylcholine, dopamine, norepinephrine, serotonin, and GABA (the primary inhibitory neurotransmitter), among others. Executive dysfunction therefore may arise as a result not only of structural problems but also of disruption of normal neurochemical modulation.

Patients with mild executive dysfunction (and preserved insight) may present independently for evaluation and treatment of this problem. In many cases, however, executive dysfunction is accompanied by (and contributes to) impaired insight, leading others (e.g., relatives, friends, employers) to bring the patient for evaluation and treatment. In either case, the evaluation of the patient will require a careful description of the others' concern(s). As noted earlier, many patients and their families use terms such as "memory problems," "forgetfulness," or "trouble concentrating" to describe problems that in fact reflect executive dysfunction. The history therefore should seek to clarify the manifesting problem following the principles of general evaluation described earlier in this chapter. Obtaining reliable historical information from collateral sources, particularly from individuals familiar with the patient's premorbid and current daily functioning, is especially important in the evaluation for executive dysfunction.

The MMSE, despite being a useful bedside tool for other cognitive domains (attention, language, and memory), does not adequately assess executive function and is not appropriate to use as a stand-alone screening assessment for executive dysfunction. The Frontal Assessment Battery (Dubois et al. 2000) and the EXIT25 (Royall et al. 1992) are particularly useful screening measures for executive dysfunction, and normative data with which to interpret performance are available for both (Appollonio et al. 2005; Royall et al. 2004); when executive dysfunction is suspected, addition of one of these measures to the bedside cognitive examination is recommended. Strict adherence to the administration and scoring procedures for these measures is essential; flexibility in their administration and/or charity in their scoring may falsely elevate the patient's score and inadvertently mask subtle but diagnostically and functionally important performance problems. When there are concerns about the fidelity of the bedside examination, or when the examination and history are discordant, formal neuropsychological testing and also performance-based evaluations (usually performed by occupational therapists) may be required to identify executive dysfunction.

Compensatory strategy training is generally recommended in the treatment of executive dysfunction resulting from TBI, stroke, and other neurological conditions, particularly among highly motivated patients with relatively mild impairments and preserved insight (Cicerone et al. 2000, 2005). Cognitive rehabilitation of executive dysfunction also may be useful for persons with schizophrenia and other forms of severe persistent mental illness (Kurtz 2003). For patients with more severe impairments, particularly those whose lack of insight and judgment can sap investment in treatment, therapy is most usefully directed toward caregiver training, particularly the development of caregiver skills needed to provide "executive" structure, optimize safety, and maximize the patient's function at home and elsewhere. The provision of cognitive rehabilitation for executive dysfunction is best provided by collaborative intervention between the geriatric neuropsychiatrist and a speech-language therapist, occupational therapist, and/or neuropsychologist experienced in this field.

When multimodal neurorehabilitative treatment is not available or feasible, the geriatric neuropsychiatrist may still offer relatively simple but effective interventions that are informed by cognitive rehabilitation approaches. Because the patient with a dysexecutive syndrome is often stimulus bound, highly distractible, and relatively easily overwhelmed, minimizing commotion and undue environmental influences is an important initial step in management. Simple and concrete written, verbal, and manual cues may serve to maximize functional independence. Electronic and/or written organizers or day planners may serve as auxiliary frontal lobes, helping patients to remain on task and successfully navigate activities of daily living. Additionally, engaging family and caregivers in the development, implementation, and maintenance of such strategies is an essential element of successful nonpharmacological treatment of executive dysfunction.

Despite the frequency with which executive dysfunction is encountered in clinical neuropsychiatric populations, no treatments have been approved by the FDA for this problem. Nonetheless, the literature offers insight into pharmacotherapies that may be useful for this purpose. When executive deficits coexist with impairments of arousal, attention, or processing speed, methylphenidate is recommended as first-line treatment. Subjective reports of improvement should be judged against objective data, because psychostimulants are also often effective in the treatment of depression, motivation, and fatigue. When executive dysfunction presents along with deficits in memory (either encoding or retrieval), cholinesterase inhibitors are recommended as first-line pharmacological treatment. Treatment of executive deficits is largely a matter of empirical trial; some patients will respond to methylphenidate or cholinesterase inhibitors alone, some will respond to the combination of both, and some will not respond at all. If other agents, such as memantine or amantadine, are used for this purpose, care should be taken to follow the general principles of pharmacotherapy presented earlier in this chapter. Similarly, selection of agents for the treatment of comorbid affective or behavioral symptoms, such as psychosis, should be informed by their effects on executive function and implemented so as to limit adverse effects on executive function and/or to improve executive function through rational pharmacotherapy (Cuesta et al. 2001).

Emerging Therapies for Cognitive Impairments

The approach to cognitive impairment and rehabilitation described in this chapter may be very useful in clinical situations involving conditions that defy current diagnostic schemes and well-established treatment strategies and those conditions whose neurobiology remains incompletely characterized. However, enormous progress has been made in the study of the phenomenology and neurobiology of many neuropsychiatric conditions that result in cognitive impairments. Such progress may soon afford opportunities to provide etiological, rather than purely symptomatic, interventions. For the geriatric neuropsychiatrist, advances in the genetics and proteomics of neurodegenerative dementias, including Alzheimer's disease, frontotemporal dementia, Huntington's disease, and prion diseases, among others, suggest the possibility of treatments that may improve a broad range of neuropsychiatric problems arising from these conditions by treating their underlying cause. While the current state of the science often makes dimensional approaches to diagnosis and management most fruitful, the deft geriatric neuropsychiatrist will remain abreast of developments and incorporate these definitive diagnostic and therapeutic measures as they emerge.

For example, elucidation of the role of the frontal-subcortical circuits and of nigral degeneration in Parkinson's disease has led to anatomically targeted treatment of this condition in the form of deep brain stimulation (DBS). This neurosurgical intervention targets either the subthalamic nucleus or the pallidum internum, ameliorates hyperactivity in these structures, and improves movement abnormalities resulting from dysfunction of the motor circuits in which these structures participate (Deuschl 2009). Such improvements also enhance quality of life for patients with Parkinson's disease (Deuschl 2009; Deuschl et al. 2006; Weaver et al. 2009). Although DBS does not correct the underlying pathology in Parkinson's disease, it provides symptomatic improvement that is predicated upon precise knowledge of the neuroanatomical bases of this condition. In this regard, DBS represents an etiologically and neuroanatomically based neuropsychiatric intervention that may provide a model for the development of similar interventions for the treatment of cognitive impairments.

Another promising line of research for a treatment of neuropsychiatric illness involves the use of embryonic and adult human stem cells. Recognizing the complex ethical issues and diverse sentiments evoked by this kind of work, the American Academy of Neurology and American Neurological Association (2005) acknowledge sufficient potential for "breakthrough therapies" and therefore offer their support for ongoing stem cell research. It is possible that the introduction of such cells into a brain that has been injured (e.g., TBI, stroke, hypoxic-ischemic brain injury) or that is degenerating (e.g., Alzheimer's disease, Parkinson's disease, Huntington's disease) might be anatomically and functionally restorative (Harting et al. 2008; Maegele and Schaefer 2008). The mechanisms by which grafted or injected stems cells integrate into neurobehaviorally important brain areas remain uncertain. Animal studies and preclinical trials suggest that stem cells may be able to differentiate into and replace lost neural tissue, potentially yielding functional recovery. Additionally, grafted cells may provide trophic support to injured brain areas, promoting vasculogenesis, as well as encouraging survival, migration, and differentiation of endogenous precursor cells. At present, the precise neurochemical environment that enables stem cells to migrate to injured brain regions and to survive, differentiate into neurons, and incorporate into existing neural circuitry requires further elucidation. Successful use of such cells requires the development of techniques that facilitate cell replacement, provide trophic support, ensure protection from oxidative stress, and adequately control growth-inhibitory mechanisms (Chang et al. 2007). Nonetheless, the potential for this emerging therapy to definitively treat neuropsychiatric conditions resulting in cognitive impairment is sufficient to impel further research along these lines.

Although the prospect of genetic therapies for neuropsychiatric conditions, including cognitive impairment, is enticing, many challenges must be surmounted before such therapies can be safely and effectively undertaken. Chief among these challenges is the effective delivery of genetic vectors to brain tissue. The blood-brain barrier prevents many gene expression vectors from reaching target neurons. Local injection of vector via craniotomy avoids this obstacle, but this mode of delivery is far too localized to provide adequate treatment for many, frequently multifocal, neuropsychiatric conditions. Further complicating delivery of genetic treatments are the risks associated with viral vectors, which may cause insertional mutations and potentially produce cancers. The risk of brain inflammation is also substantial, particularly when viral vectors are used. The advent of molecular "Trojan horses," capitalizing on the blood-brain barrier's receptor-mediated transport mechanisms to ferry gene vectors across, may provide one solution to some of these challenges. Additionally, episomal gene expression systems may avoid the risks of random insertion into the genome, but such vectors are highly susceptible to nuclear degradation enzymes and would thus require frequent readministration. Once a therapeutic gene is successfully introduced, however, methods by which to ensure that the appropriate level of expression occurs will be required (Schlachetzki et al. 2004).

As with stimulator and stem cell therapies, genetic treatments of neuropsychiatric conditions, particularly of cognitive impairments, remain promising but distant prospects. Nonetheless, progress toward the development of these treatments is being made, portending a future wherein definitive disease-specific treatments feature prominently in the geriatric neuropsychiatrist's therapeutic armamentarium. Concurrent with providing the types of evaluations and treatments described in this chapter and elsewhere in this volume, we encourage geriatric neuropsychiatrists to keep abreast of the development of these and other emerging technologies and their potential applications to the care of older adults with cognitive impairments.

Key Points

- Although focal cognitive impairments are subsumed collectively under the DSM-IV-TR category cognitive disorder not otherwise specified, they represent potentially disabling problems that require domain-specific assessment and interventions.
- A hierarchical framework for cognition may be used to inform the clinical approach to the evaluation of cognition and also to understand the clinical presentation and neuroanatomical bases of cognitive impairments.
- Older patients with cognitive impairments frequently receive concurrent treatments from multiple clinicians; the likelihood that such treatments are working at cross-purposes is reduced by regular and effective communication among clinicians.
- Domain-specific nonpharmacological treatments of cognitive impairment seek to remediate or compensate for cognitive impairment through the use of performance monitoring, feedback, and skills or strategy training. Such interventions may be regarded as successful to the extent that they generalize

beyond the context of treatment (i.e., improve the patient's function in settings beyond the clinician's office).

- Pharmacotherapy of cognitive impairment in the older adult is best regarded as an adjunct to nonpharmacological therapies. A "start-low, go-slow" approach is prudent when prescribing neuroactive agents to persons with neuropsychiatric disorders, although standard dosages of such agents are often required. Accurate recording of the response to treatment and sharing of those results with the patient and caregivers may facilitate engagement in and adherence to prescribed treatment and decrease the likelihood of maintaining or repeating unsuccessful treatments.
- Although neurosurgical, regenerative, and genetic therapies for cognitive impairments are not available presently, the deft geriatric neuropsychiatrist will remain abreast of neuroscientific developments and incorporate definitive diagnostic and therapeutic measures as they emerge.

Recommended Readings

Arciniegas DB, Silver JM: Pharmacotherapy of posttraumatic cognitive impairments. Behav Neurol 17:25–42, 2006

Cappa SF, Benke T, Clarke S, et al: EFNS guidelines on cognitive rehabilitation: report of an EFNS task force. Eur J Neurol 12:665–680, 2005

Cicerone KD, Dahlberg C, Kalmar K, et al: Evidence-based cognitive rehabilitation: recommendations for clinical practice. Arch Phys Med Rehabil 81:1596–1615, 2000

Cicerone KD, Dahlberg C, Malec JF, et al: Evidence-based cognitive rehabilitation: updated review of the literature from 1998 through 2002. Arch Phys Med Rehabil 86:1681–1692, 2005

Liepert J: Pharmacotherapy in restorative neurology. Curr Opin Neurol 21:639–643, 2008

Mesulam M-M: Principles of Behavioral and Cognitive Neurology. Oxford, UK, Oxford University Press, 2000

References

Alban JP, Hopson MM, Ly V, et al: Effect of methylphenidate on vital signs and adverse effects in adults with traumatic brain injury. Am J Phys Med Rehabil 83:131–137; quiz 138–141, 167, 2004

Almeida QJ, Black SE, Roy EA: Screening for apraxia: a short assessment for stroke patients. Brain Cogn 48:253–258, 2002

American Academy of Neurology and American Neurological Association: Position statement regarding the use of embryonic and adult human stem cells in biomedical research. Neurology 64: 1679–1680, 2005

American Psychiatric Association: Diagnostic and Statistical Manual of Mental Disorders, 4th Edition, Text Revision. Washington, DC, American Psychiatric Association, 2000

Appollonio I, Leone M, Isella V, et al: The Frontal Assessment Battery (FAB): normative values in an Italian population sample. Neurol Sci 26:108–116, 2005

Arciniegas DB, Beresford TP: Neuropsychiatry: An Introductory Approach. Cambridge, UK, Cambridge University Press, 2001

Arciniegas DB, Silver JM: Pharmacotherapy of posttraumatic cognitive impairments. Behav Neurol 17:25–42, 2006

Arciniegas DB, Topkoff JL: Applications of the P50 evoked response to the evaluation of cognitive impairments after traumatic brain injury. Phys Med Rehabil Clin N Am 15:177–203, viii, 2004

Ashtary F, Janghorbani M, Chitsaz A, et al: A randomized, double-blind trial of bromocriptine efficacy in nonfluent aphasia after stroke. Neurology 66:914–916, 2006

Aukema EJ, Caan MW, Oudhuis N, et al: White matter fractional anisotropy correlates with speed of processing and motor speed in young childhood cancer survivors. Int J Radiat Oncol Biol Phys 74:837–843, 2009

Bakheit AM: Drug treatment of poststroke aphasia. Expert Rev Neurother 4:211–217, 2004

Barch DM: Pharmacological manipulation of human working memory. Psychopharmacology (Berl) 174:126–135, 2004

Behrmann M, Marotta J, Gauthier I, et al: Behavioral change and its neural correlates in visual agnosia after expertise training. J Cogn Neurosci 17:554–568, 2005

Berthier ML: Poststroke aphasia: epidemiology, pathophysiology and treatment. Drugs Aging 22:163–182, 2005

Berthier ML, Green C, Higueras C, et al: A randomized, placebo-controlled study of donepezil in poststroke aphasia. Neurology 67:1687–1689, 2006

Biederman J, Spencer T, Wilens T: Evidence-based pharmacotherapy for attention-deficit hyperactivity disorder. Int J Neuropsychopharmacol 7:77–97, 2004

Bledowski C, Prvulovic D, Goebel R, et al: Attentional systems in target and distractor processing: a combined ERP and fMRI study. Neuroimage 22:530–540, 2004

Bragoni M, Altieri M, Di Piero V, et al: Bromocriptine and speech therapy in non-fluent chronic aphasia after stroke. Neurol Sci 21:19–22, 2000

Brenner RP: The interpretation of the EEG in stupor and coma. Neurologist 11:271–284, 2005

Burke DT, Glenn MB, Vesali F, et al: Effects of methylphenidate on heart rate and blood pressure among inpatients with acquired brain injury. Am J Phys Med Rehabil 82:493–497, 2003

Burns MS: Clinical management of agnosia. Top Stroke Rehabil 11:1–9, 2004

Cappa SF, Benke T, Clarke S, et al: EFNS guidelines on cognitive rehabilitation: report of an EFNS task force. Eur J Neurol 12:665–680, 2005

Carter BG, Butt W: Are somatosensory evoked potentials the best predictor of outcome after severe brain injury? A systematic review. Intensive Care Med 31:765–775, 2005

Chang YC, Shyu WC, Lin SZ, et al: Regenerative therapy for stroke. Cell Transplant 16:171–181, 2007

Cicerone KD, Dahlberg C, Kalmar K, et al: Evidence-based cognitive rehabilitation: recommendations for clinical practice. Arch Phys Med Rehabil 81:1596–1615, 2000

Cicerone KD, Dahlberg C, Malec JF, et al: Evidence-based cognitive rehabilitation: updated review of the literature from 1998 through 2002. Arch Phys Med Rehabil 86:1681–1692, 2005

Clark DE, Lucas FL, Ryan LM: Predicting hospital mortality, length of stay, and transfer to long-term care for injured patients. J Trauma 62:592–600, 2007

Clauss RP, Guldenpfennig WM, Nel HW, et al: Extraordinary arousal from semi-comatose state on zolpidem: a case report. S Afr Med J 90:68–72, 2000

Cohen SI, Duong TT: Increased arousal in a patient with anoxic brain injury after administration of zolpidem. Am J Phys Med Rehabil 87:229–231, 2008

Conners CK: Conners' Continuous Performance Test II: Computer Program for Windows Technical Guide and Software Manual. North Towanda, NY, Multi-Health Systems, 2000

Cuesta MJ, Peralta V, Zarzuela A: Effects of olanzapine and other antipsychotics on cognitive function in chronic schizophrenia: a longitudinal study. Schizophr Res 48:17–28, 2001

Cummings JL, Benson DF: Dementia: A Clinical Approach. Boston, MA, Butterworth-Heineman, 1992

Deuschl G: Neurostimulation for Parkinson disease. JAMA 301:104–105, 2009

Deuschl G, Schade-Brittinger C, Krack P, et al: A randomized trial of deep-brain stimulation for Parkinson's disease. N Engl J Med 255:896–908, 2006

Devi G, Silver J: Approaches to memory loss in neuropsychiatric disorders. Semin Clin Neuropsychiatry 5:259–265, 2000

Dolce G, Quintieri M, Serra S, et al: Clinical signs and early prognosis in vegetative state: a decisional tree, data-mining study. Brain Inj 22:617–623, 2008

Donkervoort M, Dekker J, van den Ende E, et al: Prevalence of apraxia among patients with a first left hemisphere stroke in rehabilitation centres and nursing homes. Clin Rehabil 14:130–136, 2000

Dubois B, Slachevsky A, Litvan I, et al: The FAB: a Frontal Assessment Battery at bedside. Neurology 55:1621–1626, 2000

Epstein R, Kanwisher N: A cortical representation of the local visual environment. Nature 392:598–601, 1998

Feldman H, Crumrine P, Handen BL, et al: Methylphenidate in children with seizures and attention-deficit disorder. Am J Dis Child 143:1081–1086, 1989

Fioravanti M, Yanagi M: Cytidinediphosphocholine (CDP-choline) for cognitive and behavioural disturbances associated with chronic cerebral disorders in the elderly. Cochrane Database of Systematic Reviews 2005, Issue 2. Art. No.: CD000269. DOI: 10.1002/14651858.CD000269.pub3

Fogel BS: The significance of frontal system disorders for medical practice and health policy. J Neuropsychiatry Clin Neurosci 6: 343–347, 1994

Folstein MF, Folstein SE, McHugh PR: "Mini-mental state": a practical method for grading the cognitive state of patients for the clinician. J Psychiatr Res 12:189–198, 1975

Giacino JT, Ashwal S, Childs N, et al: The minimally conscious state: definition and diagnostic criteria. Neurology 58:349–353, 2002

Giovannini MG: The role of the extracellular signal-regulated kinase pathway in memory encoding. Rev Neurosci 17:619–634, 2006

Grade C, Redford B, Chrostowski J, et al: Methylphenidate in early poststroke recovery: a double-blind, placebo-controlled study. Arch Phys Med Rehabil 79:1047–1050, 1998

Greener J, Enderby P, Whurr R: Pharmacological treatment for aphasia following stroke. Cochrane Database of Systematic Reviews 2001, Issue 4. Art. No.: CD000424. DOI: 10.1002/14651858.CD000424

Harting MT, Sloan LE, Jimenez F, et al: Subacute neural stem cell therapy for traumatic brain injury. J Surg Res 153:188–194, 2008

Hogan DB, Ebly EM: Primitive reflexes and dementia: results from the Canadian Study of Health and Aging. Age Ageing 24:375–381, 1995

Hornyak JE, Nelson VS, Hurvitz EA: The use of methylphenidate in paediatric traumatic brain injury. Pediatr Rehabil 1:15–17, 1997

Huber W, Willmes K, Poeck K, et al: Piracetam as an adjuvant to language therapy for aphasia: a randomized double-blind placebo-controlled pilot study. Arch Phys Med Rehabil 78:245–250, 1997

Jadad AR, Boyle M, Cunningham C, et al: Treatment of attention-deficit/hyperactivity disorder. Evid Rep Technol Assess (Summ) i–viii, 1–341, 1999

Kaye K, Grigsby J, Robbins LJ, et al: Prediction of independent functioning and behavior problems in geriatric patients. J Am Geriatr Soc 38:1304–1310, 1990

Kim E, Lee Y, Lee J, et al: A case with cholinesterase inhibitor responsive asymmetric posterior cortical atrophy. Clin Neurol Neurosurg 108:97–101, 2005

Knopman DS, DeKosky ST, Cummings JL, et al: Practice parameter: diagnosis of dementia (an evidence-based review). Report of the Quality Standards Subcommittee of the American Academy of Neurology. Neurology 56:1143–1153, 2001

Kullmann DM, Lamsa KP: Long-term synaptic plasticity in hippocampal interneurons. Nat Rev Neurosci 8:687–699, 2007

Kurtz MM: Neurocognitive rehabilitation for schizophrenia. Curr Psychiatry Rep 5:303–310, 2003

Leiguarda R: Limb apraxia: cortical or subcortical. Neuroimage 14:S137–S141, 2001

Lewis RF, Rennick PM: Manual for the Repeatable Cognitive-Perceptual-Motor Battery. Grosse Point Park, MI, Axon, 1979

Lincoln NB, Majid MJ, Weyman N: Cognitive rehabilitation for attention deficits following stroke. Cochrane Database of Systematic Reviews 2000, Issue 4. Art. No.: CD002842. DOI: 10.1002/14651858.CD002842

Lombardi FFL, Taricco M, De Tanti A, et al: Sensory stimulation for brain injured individuals in coma or vegetative state. Cochrane Database of Systematic Reviews 2002, Issue 2. Art. No.: CD001427. DOI: 10.1002/14651858.CD001427

Maegele M, Schaefer U: Stem cell-based cellular replacement strategies following traumatic brain injury. Minim Invasive Ther Allied Technol 17:119–131, 2008

Manly T, Robertson IH, Anderson V, et al: The Test of Everyday Attention for Children (TEA-CH). Bury St. Edmonds, UK, Thames Valley Test Company, 1999

McAllister TW, Flashman LA, Sparling MB, et al: Working memory deficits after traumatic brain injury: catecholaminergic mechanisms and prospects for treatment—a review. Brain Inj 18:331–350, 2004

Mesulam MM: Principles of Behavioural Neurology. Philadelphia, PA, FA Davis, 1985

Mesulam MM: Attentional networks, confusional states, and neglect syndromes, in Principles of Behavioral and Cognitive Neurology. Edited by Mesulam MM. New York, Oxford University Press, 2000, pp 174–256

Meythaler JM, Brunner RC, Johnson A, et al: Amantadine to improve neurorecovery in traumatic brain injury–associated diffuse axonal injury: a pilot double-blind randomized trial. J Head Trauma Rehabil 17:300–313, 2002

Michel JA, Mateer CA: Attention rehabilitation following stroke and traumatic brain injury: a review. Eura Medicophys 42:59–67, 2006

Molloy DW, Clarnette RM, McIlroy WE, et al: Clinical significance of primitive reflexes in Alzheimer's disease. J Am Geriatr Soc 39: 1160–1163, 1991

Nakase-Thompson R, Manning E, Sherer M, et al: Brief assessment of severe language impairments: initial validation of the Mississippi Aphasia Screening Test. Brain Inj 19:685–691, 2005

Owen AM, Coleman MR: Detecting awareness in the vegetative state. Ann N Y Acad Sci 1129:130–138, 2008

Pachet A, Friesen S, Winkelaar D, et al: Beneficial behavioural effects of lamotrigine in traumatic brain injury. Brain Inj 17:715–722, 2003

Passler MA, Riggs RV: Positive outcomes in traumatic brain injury–vegetative state: patients treated with bromocriptine. Arch Phys Med Rehabil 82:311–315, 2001

Patrick PD, Buck ML, Conaway MR, et al: The use of dopamine enhancing medications with children in low response states following brain injury. Brain Inj 17:497–506, 2003

Pedersen PM, Jorgensen HS, Kammersgaard LP, et al: Manual and oral apraxia in acute stroke, frequency and influence on functional outcome: the Copenhagen Stroke Study. Am J Phys Med Rehabil 80:685–692, 2001

Plenger PM, Dixon CE, Castillo RM, et al: Subacute methylphenidate treatment for moderate to moderately severe traumatic brain injury: a preliminary double-blind placebo-controlled study. Arch Phys Med Rehabil 77:536–540, 1996

Pulvermuller F, Neininger B, Elbert T, et al: Constraint-induced therapy of chronic aphasia after stroke. Stroke 32:1621–1626, 2001

Reitan RM: Validity of the Trail Making Test as an indicator of organic brain damage. Percept Mot Skills 8:271–276, 1958

Riccio CA, French CL: The status of empirical support for treatments of attention deficits. Clin Neuropsychol 18:528–558, 2004

Rivera VM: Modafinil for the treatment of diminished responsiveness in a patient recovering from brain surgery. Brain Inj 19:725–727, 2005

Robertson IH, Ward T, Ridgeway V, et al: The Test of Everyday Attention. Bury St. Edmunds, UK, Thames Valley Test Company, 1994

Robertson IH, Ward T, Ridgeway V, et al: The structure of normal human attention: The Test of Everyday Attention. J Int Neuropsychol Soc 2:525–534, 1996

Rohling M: Effectiveness of cognitive rehabilitation following acquired brain injury: a meta-analytic re-examination of Cicerone et al.'s (2000, 2005) systematic reviews. Neuropsychology 23:20–39, 2009

Royall DR, Mahurin RK, Gray KF: Bedside assessment of executive cognitive impairment: the executive interview. J Am Geriatr Soc 40:1221–1226, 1992

Royall DR, Cabello M, Polk MJ: Executive dyscontrol: an important factor affecting the level of care received by older retirees. J Am Geriatr Soc 46:1519–1524, 1998

Royall DR, Palmer R, Chiodo LK, et al: Declining executive control in normal aging predicts change in functional status: the Freedom House Study. J Am Geriatr Soc 52:346–352, 2004

Saeki S, Ogata H, Okubo T, et al: Return to work after stroke: a follow-up study. Stroke 26:399–401, 1995

Schlachetzki F, Zhang Y, Boado RJ, et al: Gene therapy of the brain. Neurology 62:1275–1281, 2004

Schnakers C, Ledoux D, Majerus S, et al: Diagnostic and prognostic use of bispectral index in coma, vegetative state and related disorders. Brain Inj 22:926–931, 2008

Showalter PE, Kimmel DN: Stimulating consciousness and cognition following severe brain injury: a new potential clinical use for lamotrigine. Brain Inj 14:997–1001, 2000

Silver JM, Koumaras B, Chen M, et al: Effects of rivastigmine on cognitive function in patients with traumatic brain injury. Neurology 67:748–755, 2006

Silver JM, Koumaras B, Meng X, et al: Long-term effects of rivastigmine capsules in patients with traumatic brain injury. Brain Inj 23:123–132, 2009a

Silver JM, McAllister TW, Arciniegas BD: Depression and cognitive complaints following mild traumatic brain injury. Am J Psychiatry 166:653–661, 2009b van Halteren-van Tilborg IA, Scherder EJ, Hulstijn W: Motor-skill learning in Alzheimer's disease: a review with an eye to the clinical practice. Neuropsychol Rev 17:203–212, 2007

Weaver F, Follett F, Stern M, et al: Bilateral deep brain stimulation vs best medical therapy for patients with advanced Parkinson disease: a randomized controlled trial. JAMA 301:63–73, 2009

Weintraub S: Neuropsychological assessment of mental state, in Principles of Behavioral and Cognitive Neurology. Edited by Mesulam MM. New York, Oxford University Press, 2000, pp 121–173

Whyte J, Vaccaro M, Grieb-Neff P, et al: Psychostimulant use in the rehabilitation of individuals with traumatic brain injury. J Head Trauma Rehabil 17:284–299, 2002

Whyte J, Katz D, Long D, et al: Predictors of outcome in prolonged posttraumatic disorders of consciousness and assessment of medication effects: a multicenter study. Arch Phys Med Rehabil 86:453–462, 2005

Worzniak M, Fetters MD, Comfort M: Methylphenidate in the treatment of coma. J Fam Pract 44:495–498, 1997

Wroblewski BA, Leary JM, Phelan AM, et al: Methylphenidate and seizure frequency in brain injured patients with seizure disorders. J Clin Psychiatry 53:86–89, 1992

Yamada S, Matsuo K, Hirayama M, et al: The effects of levodopa on apraxia of lid opening: a case report. Neurology 62:830–831, 2004

Yasuoka T, Ikeda M, Maki N, et al: A case of corticobasal degeneration of which movemental disturbances were improved by administration of amantadine (in Japanese). No To Shinkei 53: 781–785, 2001

Zwinkels A, Geusgens C, van de Sande P, et al: Assessment of apraxia: inter-rater reliability of a new apraxia test, association between apraxia and other cognitive deficits and prevalence of apraxia in a rehabilitation setting. Clin Rehabil 18:819–827, 2004

13

Neuropsychiatry in the Long-Term-Care Setting

Adam Rosenblatt, M.D.
Quincy M. Samus, Ph.D.

A great deal has changed in the field of long-term care (LTC) since the last edition of this textbook was published in 2000. Notable changes include the reinvention of the LTC continuum, the rise of assisted living (AL) as an alternative to nursing homes for elderly people unable to live independently, greater oversight and regulation of restraint and sedation practices in the LTC settings, and the emergence of a pharmacopeia for Alzheimer's disease (AD) and potentially other forms of dementia. These changes have sparked a sometimes acrimonious series of conversations about caring for this population, with topics including differences between psychiatric treatment versus management of behavior, ways to measure and maximize quality of life for persons with dementia, and whether treatment is cost-effective.

Continuum of Long-Term Care

The continuum-of-care concept is founded on the principle that a range of supports should be available to older adults with chronic conditions depending on their needs and that these supports should be offered in the least restrictive environment while promoting independence and personal control (Moody 2006). Because health and social needs tend to fluctuate in older adults, the care continuum should offer options of care that take account of and respond to the changing needs of the individuals (Brickner et al. 1987).

The rapid growth of the older population (Federal Interagency Forum on Aging Related Statistics 2006), the devolution of decision making on health policy and funding from the federal government to states (Caro and Morris 2002), the rising costs of health care (Goodall and Ginsberg 2008), and a societal shift toward consumer-directed health care have all contributed to a reinvention of the way that health and social services are conceptualized, incorporated, and delivered in the care continuum (Maddox and Bolda 2009). Nursing homes and hospitals remain staples in the system; however, recent momentum generated by these various influences has led to innovative alternatives to high-cost, high-intensity services. Notably, AL, an intermediary form of residential LTC, and community-based end-of-life care, such as hospices, are examples of innovations that have come into increasing demand over the past several decades. Other examples of health and social support systems in the continuum of care include adult day care, senior centers, homemaker or housekeeping services, companion/friendly visitor services, personal care, home health care, and outpatient medical and mental health care (Moody 2006).

It is widely hoped that the trend toward increased emphasis on in-community and home-based alternatives in the care continuum may reduce use of acute care such as emergency room visits and inpatient hospitalizations as well as delay entry into nursing homes, thus achieving some potential cost savings and increasing quality of life. The effect of this trend is arguable, however. Although recent projections by the Congressional Budget Office suggest that the proposed Affordable Choices Act, a program that would increase access to community- and home-based alternatives for people with chronic conditions, may reduce the federal budget deficit in the short term by about $58 billion during the 2010–2019 period (Elmendorf 2009), this shift toward care in community-based alternatives may already be contributing to an increase in the overall levels of disability and neuropsychiatric morbidity found among elders who do utilize residential care settings, namely AL facilities. Thus, recognition has been increasing regarding the importance of psychiatry and the mental health profession in these residential care settings.

The topic of LTC is of central importance in the field of geriatric neuropsychiatry, as well in the current discussions of health reform. This chapter is devoted to discussion of the epidemiology, management, and impact of mental health conditions and changes in these elements that have occurred with recent developments in evidence-based medicine, pharmacological advances, and increased regulatory oversight of LTC settings.

Nursing Homes

Modern nursing homes are descended from the almshouses and mental institutions of the nineteenth century. Like those mental institutions, which once contained dairies and vegetable gardens for the residents to grow food, nursing homes have become "medicalized" over the years, to the extent that they now resemble hospital wards, with nurses' stations, uniformed staff, drug carts, and medical charts. The policies and procedures of most nursing homes are in fact based on the so-called medical model (Coleman 1995). Nursing homes, defined by the Social Security Act, are institutions that primarily provide skilled nursing care, rehabilitation care, or regular health care to individuals who require such care as a result of a health condition but whose primary condition is not a mental health condition (Social Security Administration 2009). However, as discussed later in this chapter (see "Epidemiology"), mental disorders are often comorbid with other medical conditions. The need for "skilled" as opposed to "custodial" care is the dividing line that once crossed, permits possible eligibility for federal funds, such as Medicare reimbursement, to cover some or all of the costs of care. This distinction between skilled and custodial care may be an artificial one, a distinction prejudicial to those whose disability stems, for example, from the behavioral consequences of dementia rather than from osteoarthritis, and has several possible unintended consequences.

The majority of nursing homes are certified by Medicaid or Medicare (or both), whereas the remainder are not certified but are licensed by individual states. Most nursing homes (about 92%) offer skilled nursing care (Jones et al. 2009) and are referred to as skilled nursing facilities (SNFs), a distinction that relates to the availability of higher intensity services and treatments, and the type of reimbursement for such services that may be received (i.e., Medicare). (Hereafter, we refer to nursing homes as a generality of this setting and SNF if the study or data being discussed was specifically from this type of nursing home.) Because of rapid hospital discharges and shorter lengths of stay, trends have shown that SNFs are now serving patients with greater postacute medical needs and those with the most severe disabilities (Bishop 1999). For example, about 70% of the primary diagnoses at admission to nursing homes are medical disorders or acute illnesses such as heart disease, acute and chronic respiratory diseases, or endocrine disorders (Jones et al. 2009). Registered nurses are on staff, and physician visits are conducted on-site. Medications are almost always administered to residents by the staff, and a host of other medical interventions and procedures are available within the facility, such as physical therapy, tube feeding, wound care and dressing changes, and respiratory treatments.

SNFs, like hospitals, are a very costly form of care. In 2007, the average base cost per year for SNF care in the United States was $69,715–$77,380 per resident (MetLife 2008), which contributed to a total cost of $131.3 billion, an increase of 4.8% from the year before (Centers for Medicare and Medicaid Services 2009). Projections suggest that total nursing care costs could actually increase 1.7-fold, to an estimated $226 billion, over the next decade (Centers for Medicare and Medicaid Services 2009) due to the increasing number of people who will be at risk for needing these services. Medicaid is the primary payer for nursing home services, funding about 66% of all national nursing home expenditures, with 33% of the total Medicaid budget spent on LTC services (Mollica et al. 2005).

Given the high cost of nursing home care and the hospital-like setting of many SNFs (Hawes 2001), AL has been the most rapidly growing form of LTC since the early 1990s (American Association of Retired Persons 2002; National Center for Assisted Living 2001), whereas SNFs are increasingly serving subacute patients and those with the highest medical needs (Spillman and Black 2006). At present, more than 1 million people are probably living in assisted living facilities (ALFs) in the United States (Hawes 2001; Mollica 2002), and according to the report given by the Commission on Affordable Housing and Health Facility Needs for Seniors in the 21st Century (2002), the number of ALF units occupied by individuals ages 65 and older may increase by almost 50% from 1999 to 2020. In contrast to the implicit medical model of SNFs, the AL movement is based on an explicitly social model of care, which focuses on provision of a more desirable homelike environment (Morgan et al. 2001) and on maximization of independence, quality of life, and the ability to "age in place" without having to move to another setting (Assisted Living Quality Coalition 1998; National Center for Assisted Living 2001). However, the underrecognition of dementia and other mental health conditions that has plagued nursing homes, combined with a failure to appreciate the conditions' progressive nature, has cast doubt on the practicality of "aging in place" as a goal. AL is now widely viewed as an integral intermediary component of the LTC continuum that fills the gap between home-delivered care and institutional-style care for many elders who cannot live independently in the community (National Center for Assisted Living 2001).

ALFs, which are much less expensive than SNFs, are funded almost entirely by private dollars, from the savings and pensions of their residents and whatever family members can supply. To contain nursing home costs, most states use Medicaid funds to help keep older adults with disabilities in the community setting. As of 2004, 44 states provided some sort of funding for AL, mostly through Medicaid waiver programs (Mollica et al. 2005). Typically, eligibility for Medicaid waivers requires that individuals meet criteria for a nursing home level of care, in effect diverting those who would have otherwise gone to SNFs into AL or transitioning individuals out of SNFs. This eligibility requirement can make finding the right environment for otherwise healthy elders with dementia and limited assets extremely challenging.

Case Vignette 1

An 81-year-old African American widower with dementia, a retired factory worker, is admitted to an inpatient psychiatric unit for insomnia and paranoia after repeated temper outbursts with his granddaughter. He has no psychiatric history, and his only medical problem is moderate hypercholesterolemia. His family has been trying to care for him at home, but it has been very difficult because he is not sleeping at night and his behavior has been getting worse. His score on the Mini-Mental State Examination (MMSE; Folstein et al. 1975) is 13/30. In the hospital he responds very well to the therapeutic environment and a small dose of neuroleptic medication, but his sleep-wake cycle remains disturbed. The treatment team recommends that he have 24-hour supervision. The family is unable to provide this level of support at home and cannot afford a home health aide. The unit social worker attempts to place him in an SNF but is unable to demonstrate his need for "skilled" care. He has no financial assets to pay for AL and receives only a small Social Security pension. His state's waiver program has a 3-year waiting list. He is discharged back to the care of his family. Two weeks later, he falls at home and fractures a hip. He is admitted to a medical unit, and his documented need for skilled nursing care now facilitates his admission to an SNF.

Epidemiology

Rates of both dementia (see Chapter 16, "Alzheimer's Disease and the Frontotemporal Dementia Syndromes") and associated behavioral problems in nursing homes are quite high and appear to be increasing, probably as a consequence of changing populations and greater detection. The 1977 National Nursing Home Survey reported a 57% rate of "chronic brain syndrome" or "senility" (National Center for Health Statistics 1979) among residents living in nursing homes. This rate was 63% in 1985 (National Center for Health Statistics 1987) and perhaps as high as 70%–80% in 1996 (Krauss et al. 1997). However, a review of the National Nursing Home Survey from 1999 found that only 42% of nursing home residents ages 65 and older had an ICD-9-CM (World Health Organization 1978) code of AD, senile dementia, or arteriosclerotic dementia recorded in their medical charts (Bernstein and Remsburg 2007). It remains to be seen whether rates of dementia in nursing homes will remain that high or will decline as more persons with dementia move into ALFs.

In a literature review of studies designed to assess the prevalence of behavioral problems among nursing home residents with cognitive impairments, Zuidema et al. (2007) reported that more than 80% of residents sampled had behavioral problems. Although the prevalence of specific behavioral problems ranged considerably among studies, the most frequent problems appeared to be delusions (3%–54%), depressed mood (8%–74%), anxiety (7%–69%), apathy (17%–84%), aggression or agitation (48%–82%), and physical aggression (11%–44%). The collection of studies reviewed suggested that these behavioral problems were positively associated with male gender, more severe dementia, certain types of psychotropic medications, and use of physical restraints (Zuidema et al. 2007).

In a study of 454 residents newly admitted to eight SNFs, the overall rate of psychiatric disorders was 80.2%, which could be divided into dementia complicated by depression, delusions, or delirium (27.1% of the entire sample; 40.2% of all patients with dementia); uncomplicated dementia (40.3% of the entire sample); and other psychiatric disorders such as affective disorders and schizophrenia (12.8%) (Rovner et al. 1990). Dementia was by far the most common specific diagnosis (67.4%) and could be broken down into AD (37.9% of the entire sample), vascular dementia (17.8% of the entire sample), and other dementia syndromes or causes of dementia. Of the 32.6% of patients without dementia, more than one-third (or 12.8% of the entire sample) had psychiatric disorders such as affective disorder (31.8% of those without dementia) or schizophrenia (7.4% of those without dementia).

Another study involved 187 consecutive patients admitted to a model nursing home program for patients with dementia (Tariot et al. 1993). Among new residents, 60% had AD, 16% had vascular dementia, and the remainder had other forms of dementia. The average MMSE score was 9. Patients had high rates of noncognitive psychiatric problems, including delusions (40%), major depression (21%), sleep disorders (36%), and hallucinations (15%). Of the patients, 40% had been physically aggressive and 49% had wandered in the 2 weeks before admission. Ninety-two percent had at least one behavioral disturbance.

One might expect prevalence rates of cognitive impairment and dementia to be lower in AL facilities than in SNFs, but the rates are in fact highly similar. Depending on the criteria and method of assessment, indirect estimates range from 20% to 50% (Hawes et al. 1999; Lair and Lefkowitz 1990), but these data may be affected by underreporting. Studies using direct estimates of cognitive impairment generate generally higher estimates, from 40% to 63% (Hawes et al. 1999; Magsi and Malloy 2005; Morgan et al. 2001; Quinn et al. 1999). The

Maryland Assisted Living (MD-AL) Study (Rosenblatt et al. 2004) is the only study to have employed a comprehensive in-person assessment (including a psychiatric examination and a detailed cognitive battery) and to apply DSM-IV criteria (American Psychiatric Association 1994). Of 198 randomly selected participants from 22 facilities, 134 (68%) met DSM-IV criteria for dementia, whereas 7% of residents who did not meet criteria for dementia were diagnosed with another clinically significant cognitive disorder, for a 74% rate of cognitive disorder. AD was the most common type of dementia (69%), followed by mixed dementia or dementia not otherwise specified (28%), vascular dementia (13%), and Lewy body disease (<1%). Although most AL residents with dementia were in the mild to moderate ranges, over a quarter had MMSE scores of <10 (Rosenblatt et al. 2004).

Behavioral disturbances, most of them related to dementia, are also quite common in AL, with cross-sectional prevalence rates from the Collaborative Studies of Long-Term Care (CS-LTC) ranging from 36% to 49% among AL residents (Morgan et al. 2001). About 34% of all AL residents had weekly problematic episodes (Gruber-Baldini et al. 2004), and between 42% and 56% of residents with dementia had a behavioral disturbance in the previous 2 weeks (Boustani et al. 2005). In the MD-AL Study, in the previous month, 83% of residents with dementia had at least one neuropsychiatric symptom, such as agitation, irritability, pacing, anxiety, or delusions, and 70% had clinically significant symptoms (Leroi et al. 2007). The presence of depression, dementia, worse overall cognitive impairment, or functional impairment was strongly associated with behavioral symptoms of all types in the CS-LTC (Gruber-Baldini et al. 2004).

In the AL setting, dementia is correlated with disability (Burdick et al. 2005), use of resources such as staff time (Arling and Williams 2003; Rosenblatt et al. 2004), and caregiver stress (Bruce et al. 2005). Behavioral symptoms of dementia, such as agitation, aggression, apathy, and irritability, also explained about 30% of the variance in quality of life for AL residents with dementia in the MD-AL Study (Samus et al. 2005), and residents with dementia exited the ALF (in almost all instances due to death or discharge to a higher level of care) an average of 209 days sooner than those without dementia (Lyketsos et al. 2007).

Of the specific psychiatric conditions found in AL residents, depression is the most common (see Chapter 19, "Mood Disorders"). In some studies, depressive symptoms are rated on a scale such as the Cornell Scale for Depression in Dementia (Alexopoulos et al. 1988), and a cutoff is used to determine clinically significant symptoms, generating prevalence rates from 13% to 24%. Rates of depressive symptoms in the subset of residents with dementia are often considerably higher (Samus and Rosenblatt 2008). The MD-AL Study was the only study to use DSM-IV standards, demonstrating a prevalence of mood disorders of 18% (Rosenblatt et al. 2004). Depression and other psychiatric disorders have been shown to correlate with discharge from AL to higher levels of care (Dobbs et al. 2006; Watson et al. 2003). Depression is also related to both subjective and proxy-rated quality of life (Samus et al. 2005).

In the MD-AL Study, residents with depression showed greater medical comorbidity and greater dependence in performing activities of daily living, spent a greater number of days in bed per month, and were less likely to participate in organized activities. Forty-three percent of depressed residents and only 40% of severely depressed residents were receiving antidepressants. Sixty percent of depressed residents had no regular source of psychiatric care (Watson et al. 2006).

Anxiety disorders (see Chapter 20, "Anxiety Disorders") and primary psychotic disorders, such as schizophrenia (see Chapter 21, "Psychosis"), are also significant problems. Anxiety is often comorbid with depression and dementia, conditions that are very common in AL residents. Schizophrenia is fairly uncommon in older adults in community settings, but it may be more common in residential care settings such as AL because of the supportive environment.

A number of other neuropsychiatric and neurodegenerative conditions are prevalent in the LTC setting, may be comorbid with other forms of dementia, and present challenges to care and treatment. Parkinsonism may be present in approximately 7% of nursing home residents (Tse et al. 2008). Associated challenges include fall risk, cognitive impairment, communication difficulties, and a host of neuropsychiatric symptoms (see Chapter 24, "Parkinson's Disease and Movement Disorders"). Common psychiatric syndromes in LTC residents with Parkinson's disease include depression, apathy, anxiety, disinhibition, sleep disturbance, and psychosis (Marsh 2000). Psychosis in Parkinson's disease is sometimes related to the use of dopaminergic medications for the movement disorder or may relate to on-off fluctuations and can include striking visual hallucinosis. Little therapeutic research has been done on this topic. Antidepressant treatment for persons with Parkinson's disease tends to be governed by an appreciation of side effects, and management of psychosis may include nonpharmacological management, adjustment of antiparkinsonian medications, and judicious use of neuroleptics (Marsh 2000). In some cases, the progressive nature of the movement disorder may necessitate transition to a higher level of care sooner than cognitive or behavioral symptoms would suggest.

It is difficult to estimate the proportion of nursing home residents with poststroke conditions (see Chapter 25, "Cerebrovascular Disease") because many are transient residents, relying on the facility for rehabilitation, whereas others may have strokes after admission. The 2004 National Nursing Home Survey (U.S. Department of Health and Human Services 2004) gave a prevalence of 24% among long-term nursing home residents. The 2006 Overview of Assisted Living (National Center for Assisted Living 2006) gave a rate of approximately 14% for AL residents. A review of the MD-AL Study data indicated that hemiparesis was observed in approximately 7% of randomly selected AL residents given a neurological examination.

In AL and nursing home residents, numerous poststroke conditions may be a focus of concern and include depression, anxiety, catastrophic reactions, pathological affect, and psychosis (see Chapter 25). Depression and anxiety may also limit recovery in stroke patients who are primarily seeking rehabilitation in the nursing home setting. A number of trials have demonstrated response to antidepressants in poststroke patients with depression and pathological affect, but the misperception that depression is an "understandable" psychological reaction to having a stroke contributes to undertreatment (Chemerinski and Robinson 2000). Communication difficulties caused by aphasia and dysarthria may make psychiatric syndromes in LTC residents with stroke more difficult to assess and diagnose, and physical impairments such as hemiparesis or visual field cuts may necessitate a higher level of care than would have been expected based on the residents' other functional abilities.

Treatment

The treatment of dementia and its associated behavioral manifestations must begin with detection, if not a formal diagnosis (see Chapter 16, "Alzheimer's Disease and the Frontotemporal Dementia Syndromes"). Even when clinicians understand its high prevalence in nursing home and AL settings, dementia remains underdiagnosed, particularly in the AL setting. In a study using MMSE cutoff scores, 61% of AL residents identified as having cognitive impairment did not have a dementia diagnosis (Magsi and Malloy 2005). In the MD-AL Study, 20% of dementia cases went unrecognized by family members and 22% by professional caregivers as compared to an expert "gold standard" evaluation (Rosenblatt et al. 2004). Factors associated with nonrecognition were higher MMSE, better functional abilities, and fewer behavioral problems (Maust et al. 2006). Nonetheless, the average MMSE score in individuals with unrecognized dementia was only 18. In addition to precluding coordinated treatment, failure to recognize dementia prevents patients and family members from receiving an accurate prognosis. Even when a case of dementia is identified, effort is rarely made to subtype it as AD, vascular dementia, or another form. When such attributions are made, they are frequently wrong and not based on established diagnostic criteria. For example, a resident may be given a diagnosis of vascular dementia solely on the basis of cardiac risk factors. Adverse consequences can result when caregivers do not appreciate the special vulnerabilities of residents with dementia and the usually progressive nature of the illness.

Case Vignette 2

A 79-year-old widowed white male retired music professor with a doctoral degree has moved to AL. When asked about his memory, he describes an insidious onset and 3- to 4-year history of forgetfulness and difficulty with complex tasks. Both of his parents had dementia in late life. His daughter reports that he asks repetitive questions. He recently gave up driving after he went to the parking lot to get his car to pick up his daughter at a restaurant and was gone for 40 minutes. Both he and his daughter agree that the problem has been slowly getting worse. The patient brings with him a magnetic resonance imaging scan of the brain, ordered by his primary care doctor. The written interpretation is "mild to moderate cortical atrophy, as is often seen in people of this age." He is articulate but displays occasional word-finding difficulty. His primary care doctor has documented a normal neurological examination and a score of 27/30 on the MMSE. The doctor wrote in his notes that he suspects "a component of vascular disease and a component of depression" and prescribed an antidepressant for the patient.

Once in AL, he tends to keep to himself, rarely socializing with others or going to activities, and remains in his room with the door shut, sleeping, watching television, or playing on the electronic keyboard he brought with him. His room is cluttered with memorabilia, books, and sheet music. When spoken to, he is always congenial. Sometimes he comes out of his room in the middle of the night, fully dressed in a suit and tie, but is cooperative when asked to return to bed. A few months after admission, a second sedating antidepressant is added to his medication regimen for insomnia. He gets up at 3 A.M. one night, trips over a pile of books, and breaks a hip, causing him to be transferred to a nursing facility.

Given the vulnerability of elderly persons with dementia (see Chapter 9, "Geriatric Neuropsychopharmacology"), nonpharmacological interventions are a vital part of the management of dementia in LTC. These techniques include environmental modifications, creation of a routine daily schedule, prevention of accidents and falls, adequate nutrition and hydration, support for activities of daily living, good sleeping habits, access to primary care, and use of specific interpersonal approaches by caregivers (Rabins et al. 2006). A number of clinical researchers have attempted to combine these elements into a more formal multicomponent disease management regimen in both ambulatory and LTC settings.

The Staff Training in Assisted Living Residences (STAR) program (Teri et al. 2005) included a small randomized trial of a dementia-specific staff training intervention involving 31 residents and 25 staff at four ALs (see Chapter 8, "Psychosocial Therapies"). The trial, which did not include pharmacotherapy, demonstrated statistically significant differences on residents' behavioral disturbance, depression, and anxiety, as well as on measures of the impact on staff.

The PREVENT study (Callahan et al. 2006), conducted in a community-dwelling population, included pharmacotherapy for AD, enacted by the subjects' primary care physicians, and a guided behavioral intervention, carried out by their family caregivers. This regimen was based on a series of protocols aimed at common behavioral symptoms of dementia, such as asking repetitive questions or wandering, and essentially encapsulated the advice that an experienced clinician would give during an office visit. The authors found that the treatment group had significantly fewer behavioral and psychological symptoms of dementia, as measured by the Neuropsychiatric Inventory, than did the usual-care group. Caregivers of this group also experienced significant improvements both in distress related to behavioral symptoms and in depression.

Restraint

The Omnibus Budget Reconciliation Act of 1987, which contains regulations concerning the use of physical restraint and psychotropic medicines in nursing homes, has been generally credited with reducing the use of mechanical restraints and the nontherapeutic use of psychoactive drugs such as antipsychotics (so-called chemical restraint) in this setting. Nevertheless, physical restraints such as Posey vests and geri-chairs remain fairly common in nursing homes (Snowden and Roy-Byrne 1998) and in some instances have actually been associated with an increase in serious falls (Capezuti et al. 1996). Use of restraints in nursing homes may be justifiable in emergencies, when a resident presents a risk to self or others; for a resident while waiting for a more definitive intervention, such as during the assessment of delirium; or in some cases of extreme fall risk. The clinician should document the reason for the restraint, describe what alternatives have been considered or tried, and frequently reassess the need for ongoing use. Educational programs for staff members on other ways to deal with combative behavior, environmental changes to reduce the risk of falls, and careful consideration of treatable causes of agitation may help to reduce their use (American Psychiatric Association 2006).

Pharmacotherapy

Five drugs have been approved by the U.S. Food and Drug Administration for the treatment of AD, and four are commonly prescribed: the acetylcholinesterase inhibitors (ACIs) donepezil, rivastigmine, and galantamine, and the *N*-methyl-D-aspartate receptor antagonist memantine. All are symptom-treating rather than disease-modifying therapies. These agents have been shown in controlled studies to modestly improve scores on measures of cognitive function, such as the MMSE or the Cognitive subscale of the Alzheimer's Disease Assessment Scale; measures of functional abilities; and measures of behavioral disturbance, such as the Neuropsychiatric Inventory.

The effects of the ACIs and memantine can be subtle and must be observed against a background of expected cognitive decline. A reasonably sensitive quantitative instrument such as the MMSE is important for detecting initial improvement, demonstrating treatment effects to the patient and caregivers, and following the patient longitudinally. Patients and families should be helped to understand that improvements will usually be mild and that the patients' condition will continue to deteriorate but perhaps not as severely. Families, caregivers, and even some clinicians tend to lose heart when the patient who showed a response to an anti-AD drug crosses the initial baseline, and they sometimes conclude that the drug has stopped working. Unnecessary discontinuation at this point sometimes leads to a sharp decline in function. In other cases, AD medication may be discontinued inadvertently; for example, one physician might stop the medication in the context of an acute medical problem or episode of delirium, and another physician may not restart it when the problem is over. Even in the hospice setting, continued AD pharmacotherapy may play a role in maintaining quality of life.

Case Vignette 3

An 86-year-old widowed woman has been living in an ALF for 3 years. She has been diagnosed with AD, has a usual MMSE of 12/30, and has been taking donepezil plus memantine. Her son and daughter-in-law visit at least twice a week, and she enjoys the company, although she does not always remember her daughter-in-law's name. They no longer take her out for lunch because she has become incontinent. Recently, she has been losing weight and was diagnosed with a metastatic carcinoma, with a life expectancy of several months. The decision was made for her to move to the nursing home section of her facility and enter a hospice program there. As part of the discontinuation of medications not necessary for "comfort," her doctor has discontinued both of her cognitive enhancers. She has difficulty adapting to the new setting and is often awake at night. Three weeks after moving, she no longer recognizes her son and has to be fed at mealtimes. She looks fearful and repeatedly calls out "Help me!" even when nothing appears to be wrong.

The decision of how long to continue use of ACIs and memantine is currently a matter of individual clinical judgment, but an AD drug need not be discontinued at some arbitrary point if the patient tolerates it well and clearly showed an initial response. Whether the ACIs produce long-term benefits, such as an improvement in mortality or institutionalization rates, is not clear. Some observational studies seem to demonstrate lower institutionalization rates for community-dwelling AD patients who continue to take ACIs (Geldmacher et al. 2003), whereas other studies do not (AD2000 Collaborative Group 2004). It may be easier to show an effect in persons who already live in an institutional setting. The MD-AL Study, an observational study, demonstrated 30% longer survival in AL for those residents with dementia who were rated by an expert panel as receiving adequate treatment of any type (Lyketsos et al. 2007), as well as 228 days longer survival for AL residents with AD who were taking an ACI (Rosenblatt et al. 2008). Issues of cost and long-term outcomes are still unresolved but should not prevent clinicians from attempting to provide symptom relief. Even small gains in function can be very important to patients and their families when the baseline is already quite impaired.

Another important strategy in the management of LTC residents includes control of vascular risk factors that might worsen dementia; these include hypertension, hyperglycemia, and hyperlipidemia (Papademetriou 2005). This approach is consistent with the American Association for Geriatric Psychiatry's position statement on dementia care (Lyketsos et al. 2006), but it may run counter to some physicians' ideas of not wanting to be too "aggressive" in LTC settings. The important distinction is that the aim is not necessarily to prolong the patient's life but rather to maintain quality of life and prevent an escalation in the cost of caring for the resident.

Consensus seems to exist on the need for aggressive treatment of depression in the LTC population, because depression is common, underrecognized, undertreated, and associated with significant morbidity (Samus et al. 2005; Watson et al. 2006). Obstacles to identifying depression in elderly patients can include comorbidity with dementia, associated communication difficulties, and presence of common physical conditions, such as pain or fatigue, which may mimic or obscure common somatic manifestations of depression (Ayalon 2008). Like treatment of behavioral symptoms of dementia, treatment of depression is an underresearched topic, with some evidence supporting the efficacy of psychotherapy in those patients who are able to participate (Bharucha et al. 2006). Although the efficacy of antidepressants in elderly people is not really in dispute (Mukai and Tampi 2009), results in studies specifically in the nursing home setting or in patients with comorbid dementia have been equivocal (Magai et al. 2000). The same principles apply as to pharmacotherapy for behavioral problems in dementia—namely, the clinician should perform a thorough assessment, consider nonpharmacological means, assess the response and continued need for treatment, and employ a collaborative care approach (Ayalon 2008).

Perhaps because most psychoactive medications are not prescribed to LTC residents by psychiatrists, overtreatment of conditions such as depression, anxiety, and insomnia may be just as large a problem as undertreatment. In our experience, many LTC residents are placed on agents such as antidepressants, benzodiazepines, hypnotics (including antidepressants and neuroleptics used as hypnotics), and so-called mood stabilizers for unclear reasons, often soon after admission to the facility. These are often residents without dementia who display behavioral problems or who verbalize complaints about mood, anxiety, or sleep during the settling-in process. The response to treatment and the ongoing need for these medications may be inadequately assessed. Although these medications may play a useful role in individual cases, all have potentially serious side effects and some, such as neuroleptics, have scant evidence for general efficacy (Sink et al. 2005). We often encounter residents without dementia who have no idea that they are taking a medication for depression. In some cases, neither the family, nor the professional caregiver, nor the current physician can explain the original indication for the drug. A Swedish randomized nursing home study found no ill effects from discontinuation of selective serotonin reuptake inhibitors in such cases (Ulfvarson et al. 2003). Finally, the avoidance of unnecessarily anticholinergic or deliriogenic medicines in this population (Fick et al. 2003) is just as much a part of "treatment" as the use of cognitive-enhancing agents (see Chapter 15, "Delirium," and Chapter 29, "Neuropsychiatric Disorders Associated With General Medical Therapies").

Conclusion

Problems in the psychiatric treatment of LTC residents have much to do with perceptions. On the one hand, those who care and advocate for residents of these facilities, out of a desire to maintain residents' autonomy, may fail to appreciate how frequently dementia and other psychiatric problems occur in this setting. This lack of recognition may lead to the delivery of programs that are appropriate for only a minority of the facility's population. On the other hand, some clinicians, especially those who do not work regularly in LTC settings, tend to view being institutionalized as having "lost the battle" and to view continued intervention as overaggressive or, worse, futile. The work of advocacy organizations and ongoing longitudinal and interventional research by dedicated professionals are helping to portray these settings as the living, changing communities that they are. Given current demographic trends, it is now more important than ever to understand the unique circumstances, assets, and vulnerabilities of LTC residents, most particularly in the area of psychiatric treatment.

Key Points

- The LTC continuum for older persons with mental health conditions has shifted focus to community-based care, with the goals of incorporating consumer decision-making and preferences and of obtaining high-quality care in the least restrictive environment possible.

- AL has risen as an alternative residential LTC setting due to the reinvention of the LTC continuum.
- Neuropsychiatric conditions, especially cognitive disorders such as dementia, are extremely common in LTC residents and may continue to be underrecognized and undertreated.
- Use of evidence-based medicine and new pharmacological treatments aimed at symptom amelioration and enhanced quality of life for residents with mental disorders in residential LTC is a priority for consumers, regulators, and health care providers. Given the current demographic trends, further work needs to be done to ensure that residents receive high-quality psychiatric care.

Recommended Readings and Web Sites

Commission on Affordable Housing and Health Facility Needs for Seniors in the 21st Century: Part III: Key Demographic Findings and Projections. Final report delivered to Congress on June 28, 2002. Available at: http://govinfo.library.unt.edu/seniorscommission/pages/final_report/keydemo.html. Accessed June 24, 2010.

Rabins PV, Lyketsos CG, Steele CD: Practical Dementia Care, 2nd Edition. New York, Oxford University Press, 2006

Reichman WE, Katz PR: Psychiatry in Long-Term Care, 2nd Edition. New York, Oxford University Press, 2009

Zimmerman S, Sloane PD, Eckert JK (eds): Assisted Living: Needs, Practices, and Policies in Residential Care for the Elderly. Baltimore, MD, Johns Hopkins University Press, 2001

Zuidema SU, Derksen E, Verhey FR, et al: Prevalence of neuropsychiatric symptoms in a large sample of Dutch nursing home patients with dementia. Int J Geriatr Psychiatry 22:632–638, 2007

Administration on Aging: http://www.aoa.gov

U.S. Department of Health and Human Services National Clearinghouse for Long-Term Care Information: Understanding LTC: Definitions and Risks. October 2008. Available at: http://www.longtermcare.gov/LTC/Main_Site/Understanding_Long_Term_Care/Basics/Basics.aspx. Accessed June 24, 2010.

References

AD2000 Collaborative Group: Long-term donepezil treatment in 565 patients with Alzheimer's disease (AD2000): randomized double-blind trial. Lancet 363:2105–2115, 2004

Alexopoulos GS, Abrams RC, Young RC, et al: Cornell Scale for Depression in Dementia. Biol Psychiatry 23:271–284, 1988

American Association for Retired Persons: In Brief: Before the Boom: Trends in Long-Term Supportive Services for Older Americans With Disabilities. Washington, DC, American Association for Retired Persons, 2002

American Psychiatric Association: Diagnostic and Statistical Manual of Mental Disorders, 4th Edition. Washington, DC, American Psychiatric Association, 1994

American Psychiatric Association: American Psychiatric Association Practice Guidelines for the Treatment of Psychiatric Disorders: Compendium 2006. Washington, DC, American Psychiatric Publishing, 2006

Arling G, Williams A: Cognitive impairment and resource use of nursing home residents: a structural equation model. Med Care 41:802–812, 2003

Assisted Living Quality Coalition: Assisted Living Quality Initiative: Building a Structure That Promotes Quality. Washington, DC, Assisted Living Quality Coalition, 1998

Ayalon L: Depression recognition and treatment in long-term care: future directions. Expert Rev Neurother 8:1005–1007, 2008

Berstein AB, Remsburg RE: Estimated prevalence of people with cognitive impairment: results from nationally representative community and institutional surveys. Gerontologist 47:350–354, 2007

Bharucha AJ, Dew MA, Miller MD, et al: Psychotherapy in long-term care: a review. J Am Med Dir Assoc 7:568–580, 2006

Bishop CE: Where are the missing elders? The decline in nursing home use, 1985 and 1995. Health Aff 18:146–155, 1999

Boustani M, Zimmerman S, Williams CS, et al: Characteristics associated with behavioral symptoms related to dementia in long-term care residents. Gerontologist 45(suppl):56–61, 2005

Brickner PW, Lechich AJ, Lipsman R, et al: Long-Term Health Care: Providing a Spectrum of Services to the Aged. New York, Basic Books, 1987

Bruce DG, Paley GA, Nichols P, et al: Physical disability contributes to caregiver stress in dementia caregivers. J Gerontol A Biol Sci Med Sci 60:345–349, 2005

Burdick DJ, Rosenblatt A, Samus QM, et al: Predictors of functional impairment in residents of assisted-living facilities: The Maryland Assisted Living Study. J Gerontol A Biol Sci Med Sci 60:258–264, 2005

Callahan C, Boustani M, Unverzagt F, et al: Effectiveness of collaborative care for older adults with Alzheimer disease in primary care: a randomized controlled trial. JAMA 295:2148–2157, 2006

Capezuti E, Evans L, Strumpf N, et al: Physical restraint use and falls in nursing home residents. J Am Geriatr Soc 44:627–633, 1996

Caro F, Morris R: Devolution and Aging Policy. New York, Haywood Press, 2002

Centers for Medicare and Medicaid Services: Table 2: national health expenditure amounts, and annual percent change by type of expenditure: calendar years 2003–2018, in National Health Care Expenditure Projections 2008–2018. 2009. Available at: http://www.cms.hhs.gov/NationalHealthExpendData/downloads/proj2008.pdf. Accessed June 24, 2010.

Chemerinski E, Robinson RG: The neuropsychiatry of stroke. Psychosomatics 41:5–14, 2000

Coleman BJ: European models of long-term care in the home and community. Int J Health Serv 25:255–274, 1995

Commission on Affordable Housing and Health Facility Needs for Seniors in the 21st Century: Part III: Key Demographic Findings and Projections. Final report delivered to Congress on June 28, 2002. Available at: http://govinfo.library.unt.edu/seniorscommission/pages/final_report/keydemo.html. Accessed June 24, 2010.

Dobbs D, Hayes J, Chapin R, et al: The relationship between psychiatric disorders and the ability to age in place in assisted living. Am J Geriatr Psychiatry 14:613–620, 2006

Elmendorf DW: Letter to Senator Kay Hagan on July 6, 2009. Available at: http://www.cbo.gov/ftpdocs/104xx/doc10436/07–06-CLASSAct.pdf. Accessed June 24, 2010.

Federal Interagency Forum on Aging Related Statistics: Older Americans Update 2006: Key Indicators of Well-Being, 2006. Available at: http://www.aoa.gov/agingstatsdotnet/Main_Site/Data/2006_Documents/OA_2006.pdf. Accessed June 24, 2010.

Fick D, Cooper J, Wade W, et al: Updating the Beers criteria for potentially inappropriate medication use in older adults: results of a U.S. consensus panel of experts. Arch Intern Med 163:2716–2724, 2003

Folstein M, Folstein S, McHugh P: "Mini-Mental State": a practical method for grading the cognitive state of patients for the clinician. J Psychiatr Res 12:189–198, 1975

Geldmacher DS, Provenzano G, McRae T, et al: Donepezil is associated with delayed nursing home placement in patients with Alzheimer's disease. J Am Geriatr Soc 51:937–944, 2003

Goodall S, Ginsberg PB: High and Rising Health Care Costs: Demystifying U.S. Health Care Spending. Robert Wood Johnson Foundation Policy Brief 16. 2008. Available at: http://www.rwjf.org/files/research/101508.policysynthesis.costdrivers.brief.pdf. Accessed June 24, 2010.

Gruber-Baldini AL, Boustani M, Sloane PD, et al: Behavioral symptoms in residential care/assisted living facilities: prevalence, risk factors, and medication management. J Am Geriatr Soc 52:1610–1617, 2004

Hawes C: Introduction, in Assisted Living: Needs, Practices, and Policies in Residential Care for the Elderly. Edited by Zimmerman S, Sloane PD, Eckert JK. Baltimore, MD, Johns Hopkins University Press, 2001, pp 1–6

Hawes C, Rose M, Phillips C: A National Study of Assisted Living for the Frail Elderly: Results from a National Survey of Facilities. Beachwood, OH, Myers Research Institute, 1999

Johnson CL, Grant LA: The Nursing Home in American Society. Baltimore, MD, Johns Hopkins University Press, 1985

Jones AL, Dwyer LL, Bercovitz AR, et al: The National Nursing Home Survey: 2004 overview. Vital Health Stat 13 (167):1–155, 2009

Krauss NA, Freiman NP, Rhoades JA, et al: Medical Expenditure Panel Survey, Nursing Home Update, 1996 (AHCPR Publ No 97-0036). Washington, DC, U.S. Government Printing Office, 1997

Lair TJ, Lefkowitz DC: Mental Health and Functional Status of Residents of Nursing and Personal Care Homes: National Medical Expenditure Survey Research Findings (DHHS Publ No PHS 90-3470). Rockville, MD, Agency for Health Care Policy and Research, 1990

Leroi I, Samus QM, Rosenblatt A, et al: A comparison of small and large assisted living facilities for the diagnosis and care of dementia: the Maryland Assisted Living Study. Int J Geriatr Psychiatry 22:224–232, 2007

Lyketsos C, Colenda C, Beck C, et al: Position statement of the American Association for Geriatric Psychiatry regarding principles of care for patients with dementia resulting from Alzheimer disease. Am J Geriatr Psychiatry 14:561–572, 2006

Lyketsos CG, Samus QM, Baker A, et al: Effect of dementia and treatment of dementia on time to discharge from assisted living facilities: The Maryland Assisted Living Study. J Am Geriatr Soc 55:1031–1037, 2007

Maddox GL, Bolda EJ: The continuum of caring in the long term: movement toward the community, in Textbook of Geriatric Psychiatry, 4th Edition. Edited by Blazer DG, Steffens DC. Washington, DC, American Psychiatric Publishing, 2009, pp 587–599

Magai C, Kennedy G, Cohen CI, et al: A controlled clinical trial of sertraline in the treatment of depression in nursing home patients with late-stage Alzheimer's disease. Am J Geriatr Psychiatry 8:66–74, 2000

Magsi H, Malloy T: Underrecognition of cognitive impairment in assisted living facilities. J Am Geriatr Soc 53:295–298, 2005

Marsh L: Neuropsychiatric aspects of Parkinson's disease. Psychosomatics 41:15–23, 2000

Maust DT, Onyike CU, Sheppard JME, et al: Predictors of caregiver unawareness and nontreatment of dementia among residents of assisted living facilities: the Maryland Assisted Living Study. Am J Geriatr Psychiatry 14:668–675, 2006

MetLife Mature Market Institute: The MetLife Market Survey of Nursing Home and Assisted Living Costs, October 2008. Available at: http://www.metlife.com/assets/cao/mmi/publications/studies/mmi-2008-nursing-home-%20assisted-living-cost%20-survey.pdf. Accessed June 24, 2010.

Mollica R: State Assisted Living Policy: 2002, Vol. 2007. Washington, DC, National Academy for State Health Policy, 2002

Mollica R, Johnson-Lamarche H, O'Keeffe J: State Residential Care and Assisted Living Policy: 2004. Washington, DC, U.S. Department of Health and Human Services, 2005

Moody HR: Aging: Concepts and Controversies, 5th Edition. Thousand Oaks, CA, Pine Forge Press, 2006

Morgan LA, Gruber-Baldini A, Magaziner J: Resident characteristics, in Assisted Living: Needs, Practices, and Policies in Residential Care for the Elderly. Edited by Zimmerman S, Sloane PD, Eckert JK. Baltimore, MD, Johns Hopkins University Press, 2001, pp 144–172

Mukai Y, Tampi RR: Treatment of depression in the elderly: a review of the recent literature on the efficacy of single- versus dual-action antidepressants. Clin Ther 31:945–961, 2009

National Center for Assisted Living: Facts and Trends: The Assisted Living Sourcebook. Washington, DC, National Center for Assisted Living, 2001

National Center for Assisted Living: 2006 Overview of Assisted Living. Washington, DC, National Center for Assisted Living, 2006

National Center for Health Statistics: 1977 Summary for the U.S.: Vital and Health Statistics, Series B, No 43 (DHHS Publ No PMS 79-1794). Washington, DC, U.S. Government Printing Office, 1979

National Center for Health Statistics: Preliminary Data From the 1985 National Nursing Home Survey: Advance Data From Vital and Health Statistics, No 142 (DHHS Publ No PMS 87-1250). Hyattsville, MD, U.S. Public Health Service, 1987

Papademetriou V: Hypertension and cognitive function: blood pressure regulation and cognitive function: a review of the literature. Geriatrics 60:20–22, 24, 2005

Quinn ME, Johnson MA, Andress EL, et al. Health characteristics of elderly personal care home residents. J Adv Nurs 30:410–417, 1999

Rabins P, Lyketsos C, Steele C. Practical Dementia Care, 2nd Edition. New York, Oxford University Press, 2006

Rosenblatt A, Samus QM, Steele CD, et al: The Maryland Assisted Living Study: prevalence, recognition, and treatment of dementia and other psychiatric disorders in the assisted living population of central Maryland. J Am Geriatr Soc 52:1618–1625, 2004

Rosenblatt A, Samus QM, Onyike CU, et al: Acetylcholinesterase inhibitor use in assisted living: patterns of use and association with retention. Int J Geriatr Psychiatry 23:178–184, 2008

Rovner BW, German PS, Broadhead J, et al: The prevalence and management of dementia and other psychiatric disorders in nursing homes. Int Psychogeriatr 2:13–24, 1990

Samus QM, Rosenblatt A: The epidemiology and care of mental health conditions in assisted living: current practices and emerging knowledge, in Psychiatry in Long-Term Care. Edited by Reichmann W, Katz PR. New York, Oxford University Press, 2008, pp 484–516

Samus QM, Rosenblatt A, Steele C, et al: The association of neuropsychiatric symptoms and environment with quality of life in assisted living residents with dementia. Gerontologist 45(suppl): 19–26, 2005

Sink KM, Holden KF, Yaffe K: Pharmacological treatment of neuropsychiatric symptoms of dementia: a review of the evidence. JAMA 293:596–608, 2005

Snowden M, Roy-Byrne P: Mental illness and nursing home reform: OBRA-87 ten years later. Psychiatr Serv 49:229–233, 1998

Social Security Administration: Compilation of the Social Security Laws, Including the Social Security Act, As Amended and Related Enactments Through January 1, 2009, Vol 1. Social Security Act § 1919. 2009. Available at: http://www.ssa.gov/OP_Home/ssact/ssact.htm. Accessed June 24, 2010.

Spillman BC, Black KJ: The Size and Characteristics of the Residential Care Population: Evidence from Three National Surveys. Washington, DC, U.S. Department of Health and Human Services, 2006

Tariot PN, Podgorski CA, Blazina L, et al: Mental disorders in the nursing home: another perspective. Am J Psychiatry 150:1063–1069, 1993

Teri L, Huda P, Gibbons L, et al: STAR: a dementia-specific training program for staff in assisted living residences. Gerontologist 45:686–693, 2005

Tse W, Libow LS, Neufeld R, et al: Prevalence of movement disorders in an elderly nursing home population. Arch Gerontol Geriatr 46:359–366, 2008

Ulfvarson J, Adami J, Wredling R, et al: Controlled withdrawal of selective serotonin reuptake inhibitor drugs in elderly patients in nursing homes with no indication of depression. Eur J Clin Pharmacol 59:735–740, 2003

U.S. Department of Health and Human Services, National Center for Health Statistics: National Nursing Home Survey. Washington, DC, U.S. Department of Health and Human Services, 2004

Watson LC, Garrett JM, Sloane PD, et al: Depression in assisted living: results from a four-state study. Am J Geriatr Psychiatry 11: 534–542, 2003

Watson LC, Lehmann S, Mayer L, et al: Depression in assisted living is common and related to physical burden. Am J Geriatr Psychiatry 14:876–883, 2006

World Health Organization: International Classification of Diseases, 9th Revision, Clinical Modification. Ann Arbor, MI, Commission on Professional and Hospital Activities, 1978

Zuidema SU, Derksen E, Verhey FR, et al: Prevalence of neuropsychiatric symptoms in a large sample of Dutch nursing home patients with dementia. Int J Geriatr Psychiatry 22:632–638, 2007

14

Ethical and Legal Issues

Daniel C. Marson, J.D., Ph.D.
Andrea C. Solomon, Ph.D.

Clinicians and scientists working with older adults with cognitive or psychiatric disorders face varied and complex ethical and legal issues. These issues include impairment of decision-making capacity and associated issues of informed consent and legal competency, declining independence and autonomy, end-of-life issues such as quality of life and right to die, conflicts of interest, and issues related to geriatric health care policy and regulation. In this chapter, we consider such issues within the context of geriatric neuropsychiatry, setting forth guiding principles and describing practical implications for physicians, mental health professionals, and researchers working with older adults. Although the concepts discussed in this chapter are relevant to a range of geriatric patients, particular emphasis is placed on patients with neurodegenerative diseases such as Alzheimer's disease (AD), Parkinson's disease (PD), and Huntington's disease (HD), given the intrinsic salience of ethical and legal issues in these populations (see Chapter 16, "Alzheimer's Disease and the Frontotemporal Dementia Syndromes," and Chapter 24, "Parkinson's Disease and Movement Disorders").

Several aspects of neurodegenerative disease make ethical and legal issues of aging especially germane to this population (Marson et al. 2000a). First, neurodegenerative disease involves *progressive cognitive impairment and ultimately the loss of all decision-making capacities* (Melnick and Dubler 1984). In that the basis of ethics in the Western world is predicated on engaging a rational autonomous self, dementia inherently raises ethical issues by undermining the rationality and autonomy of patients (Whitehouse 2000). As abilities for memory, judgment, reasoning, and planning erode, patients with progressive dementia eventually lose decisional capacity in every sphere of life. Specific capacities that are lost include the capacity to drive, to manage finances, to make medical decisions, and to manage all personal affairs. It is this stark reality of neurodegenerative disease—progressive impairment and eventual loss of autonomous decision-making—that sets the context for understanding ethical and legal issues in geriatric neuropsychiatry (Marson et al. 2000a).

Second, neurodegenerative dementing disorders are *distinctly human disease processes* (Melnick and Dubler 1984). Because AD, PD, HD, and related diseases are disorders of higher cortical and subcortical function, research progress depends on the use of human subjects with dementia and their blood and tissue samples. This is not to say that progress in this field is dependent solely on human studies. On the contrary, extensive and elegant translational neuroscience studies have yielded well-characterized animal models of neurodegenerative diseases, and this work is clinically and scientifically critical. Nevertheless, many questions necessitate the use of human subjects with neurodegenerative disease and the use of human blood or tissue. Such research raises ethical and legal challenges associated with obtaining informed consent from persons with potentially compromised decisional capacity.

Third, neurodegenerative diseases primarily affect older adults in the *later stages of life*. As noted by Whitehouse (2000), these stages of life are associated with biological and functional decline and with concerns about quality of life, end of life, and quality of death. Many hard decisions involving competing values confront patients and families, as well as clinicians and researchers working with these patients, at this time of life.

Finally, the *protracted course* (Marson et al. 2000a) of neurodegenerative diseases contributes to the ethical and legal dilemmas faced by clinicians, scientists, and policy makers. For

Supported by grants from the National Institute on Aging (1P50 AG16582 [Alzheimer's Disease Research Center] and R01 AG21927), the National Institute of Mental Health (R01 MH55427), and the National Institute of Child Health and Human Development (R01 HD053074).

instance, individuals with AD live ~3.5–8 years after diagnosis (Brookmeyer et al. 2002), and the average life span following symptom onset in HD is ~15–20 years (Ho et al. 2001). As a neurodegenerative disease progresses, the patient typically experiences gradual cognitive, emotional, and functional declines, with eventual loss of competency, development of various disabilities, emergence of other health problems, and a need for increasing levels of care. As a result, clinicians and scientists working in the field of geriatric neuropsychiatry face an ever-evolving and often intensifying set of ethical and legal issues.

In this chapter, we provide a general overview of key ethical and legal issues in geriatric neuropsychiatry. We begin by presenting key *principles in bioethics*—foundational precepts that have historically guided how human beings care for one another. We then address the doctrine of *informed consent* and its significance to both the treatment and the study of patients, particularly those with dementia. The doctrine of informed consent, in turn, provides a segue to the key topic of *competency*—that minimal level of decisional capacity required by society and the legal system for individuals to act autonomously. We discuss competencies encountered in clinical settings, such as treatment consent capacity, research consent capacity, and driving, and also touch on competencies encountered more commonly in legal settings, such as financial capacity and testamentary capacity. *Surrogate decision-making* and *advance directives* are addressed next in the chapter. In addition to discussing traditional instructional and proxy directives for health care (e.g., living wills and durable powers of attorney), we address the use of advance directives for scientific research. Next, we turn to challenging clinical and ethical issues regarding *end-of-life treatment* that clinicians encounter in working with older adults, in particular those patients with neurodegenerative dementias. In this section, we consider quality of life, end-of-life decision-making, limiting of medical treatment, and assisted suicide/euthanasia. Finally, we address *geriatric mental health policy issues*, specifically the clinical and fiscal crisis in geriatric mental health care, as well as the use of evidence-based practices (EBPs) in geriatric mental health.

Principles in Bioethics

Professional ethics may be considered from a variety of philosophical and theoretical frameworks. For instance, Sadler et al. (2003) noted that ethical problems in modern medicine are often considered within the context of either dilemma-based (i.e., conflict-based) ethics or virtue (i.e., agent-based) ethics. However, regardless of the overarching framework, there are commonly recognized foundational principles for ethical behavior in the health care professions and in research involving human subjects. Much of modern bioethics reflects awareness of and adherence to four specific ethical principles: *beneficence, nonmaleficence, respect for the individual and autonomy*, and *justice*. As noted previously by others (Tidswell et al. 2008), these principles are virtually ubiquitous in medical bioethics and are found historically in ethical guidelines ranging from the Hippocratic Oath to the Belmont Report (National Commission for the Protection of Human Subjects of Biomedical and Behavioral Research 1979).

Beneficence and Nonmaleficence

The principles of *beneficence* and *nonmaleficence* hold that clinicians and scientists should "promote good" and "do no harm" to persons (National Commission for the Protection of Human Subjects of Biomedical and Behavioral Research 1979), and together they reflect a foundational tenet of the Hippocratic Oath. The precept here is that the health care professional or researcher should strive to act in the best interests of the patient or subject. This principle extends beyond simply protecting the individual from harm and includes taking active steps to secure the well-being of the patient or subject (American Psychological Association 2002; National Commission for the Protection of Human Subjects of Biomedical and Behavioral Research 1979). Ultimately, the guiding principles of beneficence and nonmaleficence direct the clinician and scientist to maximize benefits and minimize risks to the patient or research subject.

Autonomy

The principle promoting *respect for persons and individual autonomy* refers to the idea that persons are viewed as autonomous agents with the right to deliberate, make decisions, and engage in self-directed actions (National Commission for the Protection of Human Subjects of Biomedical and Behavioral Research 1979; Tidswell et al. 2008). The American Psychiatric Association's (2009) ethics code reflects this principle: "The psychiatrist should diligently guard against exploiting information furnished by the patient and should not use the unique position of power afforded him/her by the psychotherapeutic situation to influence the patient in any way not directly relevant to the treatment goals" (p. 7). Included in the principle of respect for autonomy is the notion that persons must be provided with information regarding the risks and benefits of an action so they can engage in autonomous decision-making regarding the action (Tidswell et al. 2008). Moreover, this principle holds that persons with diminished capacity for autonomy should be protected (American Psychological Association 2002; National Commission for the Protection of Human Subjects of Biomedical and Behavioral Research 1979). The American Psychological Association's (2002) Ethical Principles of Psychologists and Code of Conduct states that "special safeguards may be necessary to protect the rights and welfare of persons or communities whose vulnerabilities impair autonomous decision-making" (p. 1063). In the case of neurodegenerative disease, patients who lose the ability to engage in autonomous decision-making due to dementia would thus be entitled to protection according to this principle.

Justice

The principle of *justice* holds that clinicians and scientists should strive to achieve fairness in distribution of risks and benefits. As stated in the Belmont Report, "An injustice occurs when some benefit to which a person is entitled is denied without good reason or when some burden is imposed unduly" (National Commission for the Protection of Human Subjects of Biomedical and Behavioral Research 1979, p. 6). For the clinician, this principle has to do with fairness in resource allocation (Tidswell et al. 2008). For instance, the American Psychological Association's (2002) interpretation of this principle states that "fairness and justice entitle all persons to access to and benefit from the contributions of psychology and to equal quality in the processes, procedures, and services being conducted by psychologists" (p. 1062). For the scientist, this principle holds that the benefits and risks of research should be distributed equally among equally deserving persons (National Commission for the Protection of Human Subjects of Biomedical and Behavioral Research 1979). An oft-cited example of injustice in this context is the Tuskegee syphilis study, in which a group of African American men were denied available treatments for syphilis in a study of the untreated course of the disease. The risks of this study were unfairly limited to African American men, despite the fact that the disease did not solely affect that particular racial group or gender.

In addition to the four foundational principles outlined above, specific disciplines routinely recognize other guiding ethical standards. For instance, the ethics code for psychologists emphasizes as well the principles of *fidelity*, *responsibility*, *integrity*, and *respect for personal dignity and individual differences* (American Psychological Association 2002). Physicians, mental health professionals, and scientists also commonly ascribe to standards of *confidentiality*, *compassion*, and *mitigation of pain* (Tidswell et al. 2008).

Although by no means intended as an exhaustive list, this overview highlights some of the ethical principles that are relevant for clinicians and scientists working with older adults and provides a conceptual framework in which to consider the specific ethical and legal issues that are explored in the following sections. One final important point to consider is that ethical guidelines are necessarily somewhat fluid, reflecting the ever-evolving nature of ethical and legal issues. As noted by the American Psychiatric Association (2009), these guidelines "are not designed as absolutes and will be revised from time to time so as to be applicable to current practices and problems" (p. 4). For instance, two new ethical principles were recently adopted by the American Medical Association: "A physician shall, while caring for a patient, regard responsibility to the patient as paramount" and "A physician shall support access to medical care for all people" (American Psychiatric Association 2009, p. 5).

Informed Consent

The medicolegal doctrine of informed consent is the cornerstone for the protection of the rights of medical patients and human participants in research (Marson et al. 2000a; Sachs 1994). The informed consent doctrine specifies that to be legally valid, a consent to medical treatment or research participation must be informed, voluntary, and competent (Kapp 1992). At the heart of this doctrine is the ethical responsibility to respect an individual's personal autonomy and inherent right of self-determination (Kapp 1992; Marson et al. 2000a). The informed consent doctrine applies to all diagnostic and therapeutic medical interventions performed by health care professionals and to all human subjects research protocols and procedures. In the absence of valid treatment consent, any action (even one as seemingly harmless as merely touching a patient) on the part of the health care professional is technically considered a battery, even if benign and intended to benefit (Marson et al. 2000a). From a legal perspective, informed consent is considered as essential to the practice of medicine as are patient care and technical skill on the part of the physician (Marson et al. 2000a; Mazur 1986).

The loss of capacity to give informed consent is a common consequence of many neurological and psychiatric disorders and is an inevitable consequence of most neurodegenerative diseases that cause dementia. Thus, treatment and research with these patients raise special concerns regarding consent capacity, the appropriate procedures for obtaining informed consent, and the need in some cases for proxy consent. In the following sections, we briefly discuss the origins of the informed consent doctrine and identify the legal elements of informed consent and their ethical implications (Marson et al. 2000a).

Origins

Although it is now ubiquitous throughout medicine and human subjects research, the doctrine of informed consent evolved from the field of surgery. The earliest documented case of an alleged lack of patient consent for a surgical procedure occurred in 1767 (*Slater v. Baker and Stapleton* 1767) and was followed by increasing numbers of such cases by the turn of the twentieth century (Mazur 1986). It was in one such case that Justice Cardozo uttered the famous dictum that "every human being of adult years and sound mind has a right to determine what shall be done with his own body" (*Schloendorff v. Society of New York Hospital* 1914). This principle of self-determination remains a fundamental aspect of the contemporary informed consent doctrine (Marson et al. 2000a; Mazur 1986).

The modern doctrine of informed consent was established several decades ago, in the landmark cases of *Canterbury v. Spence* (1972) and *Cobbs v. Grant* (1972). These cases established the physician's responsibility to provide the patient with sufficient medical treatment information that a "reasonable man" would need to make an informed decision about his treatment. The modern doctrine promotes patient participation in medical decision-making, supports self-determination and rational decision-making in medical treatment settings, and encourages collaborative decision-making between patient and physician as well as between researcher and study participant. This notion of collaborative decision-making is dependent 1) on the clinician or scientist providing technical information and contributing professional judgment and advice to the patient or research participant and 2) on the patient or research participant making a final decision based on his or her personal values, beliefs, and preferences (Munetz et al. 1985). The informed consent doctrine reflects and enforces the U.S. constitutional concern with the individual's right to be free from the conduct of others that affronts bodily integrity, privacy, and autonomy (Meisel et al. 1977). This doctrine is embedded firmly in American jurisprudence and forms a recognized basis for physician liability in the 50 states and the District of Columbia (Marson et al. 2000a).

Elements of Informed Consent

Informed consent is generally conceptualized as comprising three fundamental elements: the informed element, the voluntary element, and the competency element (Kapp 1992; Meisel et al. 1977; Tepper and Elwork 1984). Each of these fundamental aspects of informed consent is uniquely relevant in geriatric neuropsychiatry, particularly for those clinicians and scientists working with patients with a dementia. Health care professionals and researchers in geriatric neuropsychiatry have an ethical responsibility to ensure that the consent decisions of individuals with cognitive impairment are adequately informed, voluntary, and competent (Marson et al. 2000a).

The Informed Element

The informed element specifies that a patient or research participant must be provided with sufficient information to afford a knowledgeable or intelligent decision to consent to or refuse the treatment or research study (Kapp 1992). For instance, a physician must communicate specific information to the patient, including the clinical diagnosis, the nature and purpose of the proposed intervention, the associated risks and benefits of the procedure, the available treatment alternatives and their associated risks and benefits, and any other information that is relevant to the treatment decision (Capron 1974; Waltz and Scheuneman 1970). Similarly, a scientific investigator must furnish sufficient information regarding the research study's purpose, procedures, risks, and benefits, as well as the rights of the research participant, so as to allow the potential participant to make an informed decision about research participation (High 1992).

In the case of the individual with cognitive impairment or dementia, impairments in comprehension, encoding, and processing of consent information create challenges for adequate disclosure of this information (Marson and Harrell 1999; Marson et al. 1995b, 1996). Individuals with dementia may have limited abilities to assimilate consent information via standard approaches of oral dialogue and a written consent form, necessitating adaptations in the method of presentation. For instance, complex consent information can be presented in simple language and syntax (Marson et al. 1995b; Taub et al. 1981) (e.g., a consent form can be written at a sixth-grade reading level), in manageable segments or chunks (Grisso and Appelbaum 1991), and on multiple occasions to facilitate rehearsal (Taub et al. 1981). In addition, alternative methods of presentation, such as pictures, videotapes, and DVDs, have been used successfully as nonverbal adjuncts or independent approaches (Jeste et al. 2009). Accommodations such as these may improve the quantity and quality of information disclosure and transfer, thereby enhancing the consent process for individuals with cognitive impairment (Marson et al. 2000a).

The Voluntary Element

The voluntary element requires that in making his or her decision, the patient or research participant must be free from coercion, unfair persuasion, and inducement (Capron 1974). It is the ethical responsibility of the physician and investigator to ensure that indirect or covert influences on the patient's decision be kept to a minimum. The individual must be allowed to freely accept or refuse a medical intervention and to freely participate or refuse to participate in a research study (Grisso 1986; Tepper and Elwork 1984). An agreement that is obtained under duress to accept treatment or to participate in a research study or an agreement that is induced by fraud or misrepresentation is legally invalid.

It must be acknowledged that some element of indirect coercion may be unavoidable in any health care encounter (Kapp 1992) and that older adults are generally more vulnerable to such influences (Kapp 1992). This issue is of particular importance for clinicians and scientists working with older patients with neuropsychiatric conditions. Patients with neurodegenerative disease, for instance, are extremely vulnerable, due in part to their progressive cognitive impairments and loss of insight (American College of Physicians 1989; Caralis 1994; Melnick and Dubler 1984). In addition, older adults with neurological or psychiatric disorders may be overly willing to suspend their own available judgment and unreservedly accept the advice or recommendations of professionals. In a qualitative study of treatment consent capacity, we found that patients with AD were very prone to inappropriately delegate decision-making authority to others, particularly physicians (Marson et al. 1999).

Accordingly, clinicians and scientists must actively seek to ensure that their own values and interests do not bias the consent decisions of their patients or potential research participants. Relevant medical or research information must be presented clearly and in a neutral manner. The clinician or scientist has an implicit ethical obligation to inform patients of their right to make their own decisions (Meisel et al. 1977). The goal of the clinician or scientist working with a cognitively compromised patient should always be to obtain a consent that is as voluntary as possible.

The Competency Element

The third fundamental element of the informed consent doctrine requires that the patient or research participant be competent to consent. Competency has generally been defined as the "minimal threshold imposed by society under which individuals retain the power to make decisions for themselves" (Appelbaum and Gutheil 1991, p. 218). With respect to informed consent, competency refers to the individual's cognitive and emotional capacity to consent to a treatment or research study, to refuse treatment or research participation, and to select among treatment alternatives (Grisso 1986; Tepper and Elwork 1984). The competency element of the informed consent doctrine is aimed specifically at promoting a minimal level of decision-making ability, as well as supporting patient autonomy (voluntariness) and informed decision- making (Marson et al. 2000a).

Competency is perhaps the most problematic element of informed consent within the context of geriatric neuropsychiatry. Although under the law an adult (including an individual with dementia) is presumed to be competent until proven otherwise (Kapp 1992), patients with dementia are at high risk for impairment or loss of competency. Nevertheless, as society ages, clinicians and scientists have an increasing imperative to treat individuals with neurodegenerative disease and dementia and to foster their participation in research. Individuals with AD, for example, are increasingly asked to consent to certain medical and research procedures, such as functional neuroimaging, antidepressant and other psychopharmacological medications, placebo-controlled drug trials involving experimental agents, and lumbar puncture (Marson et al. 2001), each of which requires a valid informed consent. In these and similar instances, the clinician or scientist is charged with carefully assessing the individual's level of consent capacity. In situations where competency has been lost, proxy consent from a legally authorized representative must be obtained (High 1992; Marson et al. 2000a). In the subsequent competency section, we address consent capacity in more detail.

In summary, the informed consent doctrine is a cornerstone of ethical clinical practice and scientific research. Both clinicians and scientists must take appropriate steps to obtain informed, voluntary, and competent consent from patients and potential research participants. In situations where competency is diminished or lost, surrogate decision-making measures will need to be implemented.

Competency

As noted in the previous section, competency can be conceptualized as a legally defined and enforced "minimal threshold" under which persons have authority to make decisions for themselves (Appelbaum and Gutheil 1991). More broadly, competency refers to an individual's legal capacity or ability to make autonomous decisions, to engage in reasoning and deliberation, to understand and communicate information, and to possess goals and values (Appelbaum and Gutheil 1991; President's Commission for the Study of Ethical Problems in Medicine and Biomedical and Behavioral Research 1982). As discussed above, patients with neuropsychiatric disorders are at risk for decisional impairments that can threaten legal competency. For instance, patients with dementia may be unable to make rational decisions regarding medical treatments or participation in research, may no longer be able to understand or conduct financial matters, or may have lost knowledge—of both personal assets and potential heirs—needed to make a new will. Thus diminished competency poses important ethical and legal challenges for clinicians and scientists working with older adults. In the sections below, we consider key principles regarding competency in geriatric neuropsychiatry and then briefly examine the specific competencies of treatment consent capacity, driving capacity, financial capacity, and testamentary capacity.[1] We conclude this section by describing steps that can be taken to minimize the complications associated with anticipated future loss of competency.

[1]The topic of competency in geriatric neuropsychiatry has become too broad for comprehensive coverage here. The interested reader is directed to a series of capacity assessment handbooks for attorneys, judges, and psychologists published jointly by the American Bar Association Commission on Law and Aging and the American Psychological Association (2005, 2008; American Bar Association Commission on Law and Aging et al. 2006).

Key Principles

Capacity Versus Competency

The terms *capacity* and *competency*, although often used interchangeably (Marson 2001a), have historically referred to somewhat distinct concepts (Kapp 1992). The term *capacity* generally refers to a clinical judgment made by a health care professional, whereas determinations of *competency* are made by a judge or other legal professional. In arriving at a clinical judgment regarding capacity, a clinician must consider a patient's history, behavioral presentation, and cognitive and functional abilities. Importantly, a clinical judgment of incapacity does not itself permit the formal transfer of decisional authority to another person (except in the case of a "springing" durable power of attorney, which may be explicitly designed to go into effect upon such a clinical judgment). Nevertheless, patients and families often accept and behave in accordance with the physician's or other health care professional's judgment regarding the patient's capacity, which confers a certain quasi-adjudicative status on the clinical judgment.

In contrast, a legal determination of incompetency by a judge formally alters an individual's legal status and necessitates appointment of a surrogate decision-maker (e.g., a guardian). This change in legal status may be limited to specific transactions (e.g., making a will) or may impact the individual's autonomy more globally (e.g., through appointment of a guardian or conservator). In considering the distinction between capacity and competency, it is helpful to note that a *clinical* judgment regarding capacity is but one of many pieces of evidence that may bear upon a *legal* judgment of competency. That is, a judge may consider clinical capacity assessments as part of his or her determination regarding competency but will evaluate other sources of information as well, including lay testimony, statutes, case law precedent, and principles of equity and justice.

Despite the clear conceptual distinction between capacity and competency, practical usage of these terms has become increasingly intertwined. A recent trend in the legal sphere (in particular within the area of guardianship law) has been to invoke the term capacity as a replacement for the older term competency, the latter term having fallen into disfavor (American Bar Association Commission on Law and Aging and American Psychological Association 2008). In addition, clinicians often use the term *competency evaluation* synonymously with *capacity assessment*. Ultimately, it is important to be mindful of the conceptual distinction between capacity and competency, although the terms are increasingly used synonymously in practice (Marson 2001a). Clinicians are likely to encounter situations in which they need to educate the patient, family, and in some instances, the attorney regarding the clinician's role in capacity assessment and the distinction between clinical and legal judgments regarding competency and capacity. In the interest of clarity, it may be helpful to employ language that clearly differentiates judgments of *clinical* competency and capacity from those of *legal* competency and capacity to avoid confusion. In this chapter, the terms capacity and competency are generally used in reference to a clinical context, unless otherwise indicated.

Multiple Competencies

Competency is not a unitary construct. The law recognizes numerous distinct competencies that draw on a range of functional skills and abilities. Specific competencies that are commonly considered within geriatric neuropsychiatry include the capacity to drive, to consent to medical treatment, to make a will, to manage financial affairs, and ultimately to manage all of one's personal affairs. These competencies involve distinct functional abilities and skills that distinguish them from one another (Grisso 1986). For instance, the cognitive and physical skills requisite for driving are arguably quite distinct from those involved in making a will (Marson 2001a). In addition, issues regarding a specific competency typically unfold within a specific and somewhat individualized context (Grisso 1986). For example, questions related to an individual's clinical capacity to consent to treatment almost invariably arise in a medical setting. From a practical clinical standpoint, the concept of multiple competencies suggests that rather than asking, "Is the individual competent?" the clinician should ask, "Does the individual have the capacity to do X in Y context?" (Marson et al. 1994).

Presumption of Competency

In the United States, the legal system presumes that an adult is competent until proven otherwise (Spar 2000). The burden of proof in a legal proceeding lies with the party alleging that a person is incompetent. Thus, despite diagnosis and dementia severity, a patient with advanced AD is presumed to be competent until shown otherwise.

Limited Competency

Competency evaluation has historically been viewed as a dichotomous determination with an outcome of being either competent or incompetent (American Bar Association Commission on Law and Aging and American Psychological Association 2008; Appelbaum and Gutheil 1991). The concept of limited competency reflects a more sophisticated view of the dimensional aspects of the construct. An individual with cognitive impairment may be able to perform certain activities within a general functional domain, but be unable to perform other activities within that domain. For instance, an older adult with mild dementia may be able to use a checkbook and manage small sums of money but be incapable of making complex investment and financial decisions. In this example, the individual might be said to have limited competency to manage his or her financial affairs.

Limited competency is recognized by the legal system through the judicial appointment of limited guardianships and conservatorships. Limited competency in the context of geriatric neuropsychiatry, and in particular neurodegenerative dementia, places additional challenges on judges and other legal personnel, because they must continue to monitor the individual and his or her declining residual capacities over time. However, limited competency also affords an important opportunity for the "judge as craftsman" to develop a limited order recognizing the deficits as well as the specific preserved abilities of the individual (American Bar Association Commission on Law and Aging et al. 2006, p. 13).

Intermittent Competency and Legal Restoration of Competency

Clinicians working with older adults need to recognize that a patient's competency or incompetency is not necessarily a static condition (Marson 2001a). For example, a patient with a long-standing history of a major illness such as schizophrenia or bipolar disorder experiences symptom fluctuations that may periodically compromise his or her ability to engage in medical decision-making, whereas the individual may be fully competent to make such decisions during periods of relative health. Also, an older adult with dementia may initially have limited competency for managing his or her financial affairs, but the individual may eventually progress to the point that he or she is not capable of carrying out any financial activity. These examples illustrate the importance of periodic reevaluations in cases where competency may be expected to change over time. In fact, in some cases, a neuropsychiatric condition may resolve with treatment or time, leaving a formerly incompetent individual capable of once again engaging in autonomous decision-making. The legal system allows for restoration of competency in such cases through a formal court hearing and judicial decision (American Bar Association Commission on Law and Aging et al. 2006).

Neuropsychiatric Diagnosis: Not Equivalent With Incompetence

A diagnosis of dementia or other neuropsychiatric disorder does not correspond to incompetence (Marson 2001a). In fact, individuals with dementia or psychiatric illness may be competent to engage in a variety of autonomous acts, including consenting to medical treatment or research, driving, or balancing a checkbook. Clinical diagnostic information, although highly relevant, is not sufficient for making determinations of competency. The critical component in any evaluation of competency is an analysis of the individual's functional abilities relative to performing a specific act in its context (American Bar Association Commission on Law and Aging and American Psychological Association 2008).

Cognitive Impairment: Not Equivalent With Incompetence

A related but distinct point is that cognitive or mental status test findings cannot, in isolation, determine questions of competency (Marson 2001a). Cognitive and neuropsychological evaluations are important for diagnosing dementia and assessing severity of cognitive impairment, and they certainly are relevant to issues of competency. Nonetheless, a cognitive assessment by itself does not resolve the competency question (Grisso 1986; High 1992). Clinical observations and evidence, such as that obtained via neuropsychological evaluation, must be linked to the specific capacities in question (Grisso 1986). For instance, documenting that a patient has deficits in attention, language comprehension, and reasoning abilities is relevant to a competency determination only when these deficits are meaningfully linked with competency-specific functional impairments, such as the impaired ability to express a treatment preference, to understand the nature and purpose of a will, or to operate a motor vehicle (American Bar Association Commission on Law and Aging and American Psychological Association 2008; Marson et al. 1995a, 1996, 1997a).

Values and Competency

The importance of considering an individual's personal goals and values has been increasingly emphasized in the competency assessment literature (American Bar Association Commission on Law and Aging and American Psychological Association 2008). That is, an individual's medical (or other) decision-making process will typically be motivated by factors that are significant to the individual and that signify quality of life in his or her mind. Such factors include, but are not limited to, religious beliefs or values, a desire to preserve life, a need or desire for autonomy and independence, and a concern about becoming a burden on one's family or caretakers. Clinicians and other professionals charged with making determinations of competency should consider whether an individual's decision process is consistent with his or her known long-standing values and goals. At the same time, it is also true that an individual's values can change over time, and "fluctuating statements of values do not necessarily indicate incapacity" (American Bar Association Commission on Law and Aging and American Psychological Association 2008, p. 54). Nevertheless, the consistency of an individual's current choices with his or her established belief system and preferences is one important aspect to consider in evaluating competency.

Medical Decision-Making Capacity

Medical decision-making capacity, or treatment consent capacity, refers to a patient's "ability to understand the significant benefits, risks, and alternatives to proposed health care and to make and communicate a health-care decision" (Uniform Health-Care Decisions Act of 1993, § 1[3]). Medical decision-making capacity is a fundamental aspect of individual autonomy, because it concerns intimate decisions about the care of a person's body and mind (Marson 2001a). It is distinctive in that it is a "generic" instrumental activity of daily life common to all independent community-dwelling older adults. Independently functioning adults are generally presumed to possess medical decision-making capacity and are expected to exercise this capacity in encounters and treatment decisions with physicians and other health care providers (Marson and Dreer 2006; Marson and Harrell 1999). Accordingly, the law presumes, until proven otherwise, that adults have the capacity to make medical decisions for themselves.

Clinicians routinely encounter older patients with a variety of organic or psychiatric illnesses that result in impairment or loss of medical decision-making capacity. For instance, individuals with neurodegenerative diseases such as AD and PD experience progressive declines in memory, judgment, reasoning, and planning that interfere with their abilities to comprehend, encode, and process treatment information; to reach a decision about treatment or research; and to communicate this decision to their physician or to the study investigator. In addition, due to the heightened incidence and prevalence of medical illnesses that come with aging, older adults must make a disproportionately higher number of personal medical decisions compared with other age groups (Marson and Harrell 1999). In this regard, patients with dementia are increasingly called on to make medical treatment decisions as new therapeutics are introduced (Morris 2002). Consent capacity is also an ethical issue in the research sphere, because patients with dementia increasingly must choose whether to participate in clinical research (Kim et al. 2001).

Medical decision-making capacity is unique from other forms of capacity in that it occurs most often within a medical rather than a legal setting, and its determination primarily relies on physicians, psychologists, and other health care professionals, as opposed to legal professionals. These determinations do not adjudicate competency in a formal legal sense, but they often result in a similar loss of decision-making power for the patient (Marson and Hebert 2008a). Although clinical determinations of treatment consent capacity are rarely subject to judicial review, several distinct thresholds or standards of competency, drawn from case law and the psychiatric literature (Roth et al. 1977), inform and guide clinical judgment in this area:

- S1: capacity to *evidence* a treatment choice
- [S2]: capacity to *make the reasonable choice*
- S3: capacity to *appreciate* the consequences of a treatment choice
- S4: capacity to *reason about treatment/provide rational reasons for a treatment choice*
- S5: capacity to *understand* the treatment situation and treatment choices

These standards represent different thresholds for evaluating capacity to consent (Marson et al. 1994). For instance, S1 (evidencing a choice) requires only that an individual be able to communicate a treatment choice. In contrast, S3 (appreciating consequences) is of moderate difficulty and requires that the individual appreciate the way in which a treatment choice will personally affect him or her. The fourth standard, S4 (providing rational reasons), references an individual's ability to supply rational reasons for his or her treatment choice. Finally, S5 (understanding) is a comprehension standard and requires that the individual demonstrate conceptual and factual knowledge regarding the medical condition, symptoms, and treatment choices and their respective risks and benefits. As a side note, these four standards are relevant also to other competencies to consent, such as capacity to consent to research, as well as to decisional capacity in general.

In addition to the four standards described above, a fifth consent standard is described as the ability to make the "reasonable" treatment choice in cases in which the alternative choice is manifestly unreasonable (Roth et al. 1977). This standard, which we reference as [S2], is somewhat distinct insofar as it emphasizes outcome rather than the decision-making process itself. Under this standard, an individual who fails to make a decision that is roughly congruent with the decision that a "reasonable" person in like circumstances would make is considered incompetent. Due to the subjectivity inherent in determining what constitutes a *reasonable* choice (Tepper and Elwork 1984), [S2] is not an accepted legal standard for judging consent capacity. Consequently, we reference [S2] in brackets to distinguish it from the other established legal standards. Nevertheless, [S2] is a useful threshold for understanding treatment preferences of patients with neurodegenerative disorders (Dymek et al. 2001).

Assessment of Medical Decision-Making Capacity

A clinical judgment of impaired medical decision-making capacity can have significant ramifications for patients and families, as well as for clinicians. Diminished or lost decisional capacity impacts patients' autonomy and psychological well-being and creates substantial patient disability and caregiving burdens for families (Marson and Dreer 2006; Moye and Marson 2007). Sound clinical assessment of medical decision-making capacity is thus an important issue in geriatric neuropsychiatry (Marson et al. 1997b). Historically, clinical assessment of decisional capacity has been confined to subjective clinical interview. Practice has been limited by a lack of objective assessment tools and, more important, limited competency assessment knowledge and training among physicians, psychologists, and other health care professionals (American Bar Association Commission on

Law and Aging and American Psychological Association 2008; Sadler et al. 2003). However, significant progress has been made in recent years toward the development of reliable and valid methods for assessing medical decision-making capacity (American Bar Association Commission on Law and Aging and American Psychological Association 2008).

Psychometric Tools for Assessing Medical Decision-Making Capacity

Over the past 20 years, a number of instruments have been developed for assessing medical decision-making capacity in various clinical populations (Dunn et al. 2006; Grisso and Appelbaum 1991; Marson et al. 1995b, 1997b, 2000b; Vellinga et al. 2004). These measures bring objectivity and psychometric rigor to the assessment of decisional capacity via standardized content and administration procedures, quantitative scoring, and use of normative data for interpretation. These tools represent an important advance in the field of competency research, which historically has relied heavily on subjective clinical interviews as the norm for assessment.

Our own laboratory has developed an instrument for use in assessing the capacity of patients with dementia to consent to medical treatment. The Capacity to Consent to Treatment Instrument (CCTI; Marson et al. 1995b) includes two clinical vignettes (i.e., neoplasm vignette and cardiac vignette), which were designed to test competency within the context of defined legal standards of consent capacity. The vignettes present hypothetical medical problems and symptoms, and the examinee is presented with two alternative treatment choices with associated risks and benefits. The vignettes are presented to the examinee both orally and in written form in an uninterrupted disclosure format (Grisso and Appelbaum 1991). The examinee then answers questions aimed at assessing consent capacity according to the five specific standards, S1–S5, described above.

Using the CCTI, we have investigated medical decision-making capacity in geriatric neuropsychiatric populations, such as patients with AD (Griffith et al. 2005; Marson et al. 1995b, 1996), amnestic mild cognitive impairment (MCI) (Okonkwo et al. 2008), and PD and cognitive impairment/dementia (Marson and Dymek 2004; Martin et al. 2008b). Overall, our findings indicate that consent capacity shows early impairment in patients with MCI and PD patients with cognitive impairment without dementia, and more substantial impairment in patients with AD and PD with dementia. Other researchers such as Karlawish (2008) and Kim et al. (2001) have arrived at similar findings.

Together, these empirical findings underscore the importance of careful assessment of consent capacity in older adults with cognitive impairment. Ideally, a comprehensive assessment approach would be used, which might incorporate some or all of the following: clinical interview, cognitive assessment, psychodiagnostic assessment, and psychometric assessment of medical decision-making capacity, as well as assessment of the individual's values (American Bar Association Commission on Law and Aging and American Psychological Association 2008).

Driving Capacity

Another competency frequently encountered in geriatric neuropsychiatry is the capacity to operate an automobile. Driving is a fundamental aspect of mobility and a central aspect of U.S. culture (American Bar Association Commission on Law and Aging and American Psychological Association 2008). As clinicians who work with older adults will attest, the threat of loss of driving privileges represents a direct challenge to many older individuals' sense of autonomy and independence. At the same time, there are serious societal consequences associated with allowing an impaired older individual to continue driving. The core tension in bioethics between individual autonomy on the one hand and protection of the individual and society on the other is epitomized by the issue of whether to allow a cognitively impaired older adult to continue to drive.

Clinicians are increasingly asked to make judgments regarding an individual's competency to drive and are expected (and in some states required) to report a patient's medical condition to authorities if the condition is thought to pose a driving-related safety risk to the patient or others (Bacon et al. 2007a). However, some parties have argued that requiring physicians to report patients to authorities may negatively impact the physician-patient relationship (Bacon et al. 2007a). In addition, it is not clear that mandated reporting will promote safety, because patients and families may simply withhold information that would suggest impaired driving capacity (Bacon et al. 2007a). Further complicating matters for the clinician is that accurate assessment of driving capacity is often not feasible for the health care provider. In contrast to other capacities discussed here, clinicians working with older adults are often not well positioned to make determinations of driving capacity, because such judgments are best made using on-the-road testing or driving simulators (Kay et al. 2008). Consequently, some parties have suggested that the appropriate role of the physician in this context is to make appropriate assessment referrals and to facilitate the family's decision-making process regarding the individual's capacity to drive (Sadler et al. 2003).

As part of the normal aging process, and particularly in cases of neurological or psychiatric illness, driving ability will gradually decline over the years (Bacon et al. 2007a; Spar 2000). This fact highlights the importance of regular reassessment, which can be accomplished via standardized road tests administered by the appropriate government agency. To the extent possible, the older individual should be actively involved in the ongoing dialogue concerning his or her driving abilities (Bacon et al. 2007a; Sadler et al. 2003). In many cases of early dementia, a graduated approach to limiting driving may be taken while an individual's judgment and insight may still be relatively intact. For instance, the individual may elect to drive only during the day and/or only in familiar, low-traffic areas. Often, voluntary adaptations such as these are prompted by an episode of getting lost or by involvement in an accident (Sadler et al. 2003).

As an older individual's cognitive and/or physical health deteriorates, the clinician and family increasingly face concerns for both the patient's safety and the safety of the public at large. When an individual with cognitive or physical limitations poses a risk to self or the public and is unwilling to refrain from driving, it may be necessary for the family to take action such as confiscating the individual's car keys or impounding the vehicle. As noted by a number of commentators (Bacon et al. 2007a; Sadler et al. 2003; Spar 2000), such actions are ethically justifiable, given the imminent safety risks involved.

The American Academy of Neurology has published guidelines for physicians working with patients whose medical conditions may impact driving capacity (Bacon et al. 2007a). The group supports *optional* physician reporting to authorities concerning patients whose medical conditions may impact driving safety, "especially in cases where public safety has already been compromised, or it is clear that the person no longer has the skills needed to drive safely" (p. 1176). In addition, the organization emphasizes the need for development of tools and instruments for assessing driver safety, "both in terms of helping physicians recognize when a driver should be referred for evaluation, and assisting state officials in conducting such an evaluation" (p. 1177).

Financial Capacity

The financial capacity of older adults is also a growing clinical issue for physicians and other health care professionals (Marson et al. 2009). Families increasingly look to health care providers to address issues of their loved ones' declining financial skills and decision-making. Among higher-order abilities, financial capacity has particular significance to independent functioning of older adults (Marson et al. 2000c). Financial capacity comprises a broad range of conceptual, pragmatic, and judgment abilities that range from basic skills such as counting coins and currency to more complex skills such as paying bills, managing a checkbook, and exercising financial judgment (Marson 2001b). Similar to driving and mobility, it is a core aspect of individual autonomy in our society and represents a cognitively complex set of knowledge and skills vulnerable to cognitive aging and dementia (Marson 2001b; Marson et al. 2000c).

Impairment and loss of financial capacity have a number of important consequences for individuals and families, as well as important implications for health care and legal professionals (Marson 2001b; Marson and Zebley 2001; Marson et al. 2000c). Diminished or lost financial capacity has important economic consequences. For instance, individuals with neurodegenerative disease or dementia often have difficulties paying their bills and carrying out basic financial tasks (Marson et al. 2000c). These individuals are also at increased risk for making decisions that endanger assets needed for their own long-term care or that are intended for distribution to family members through a will.

Important psychological consequences are also associated with diminished or lost financial capacity. Loss of control over one's own finances involves loss of a core aspect of personal independence and can lead to depression and other psychological problems (Moye 1996).

Diminished or lost financial capacity also places older individuals at increased risk for financial exploitation, victimization, and vulnerability to elder abuse, a finding of particular ethical and legal importance (Marson et al. 2000a; Nerenberg 1996). There are daily media accounts of older adults victimized in consumer fraud and other scams (Walton 2002). Older adults are also the victims of undue influence exercised by family members, professionals, and third parties (Marson et al. 2000c; Spar and Garb 1992).

Finally, compromised financial capacity can trigger important legal issues of guardianship and conservatorship (Grisso 1986; Marson et al. 2000a). Disproportionately high numbers of older adults are involved in conservatorship proceedings, often due to dementia and other mental and medical illnesses affecting financial competency in this age group (Grisso 1986).

As with medical decision-making capacity and driving, sound assessment practices need to be employed in making judgments of patients' financial capacity. Financial capacity has received increased empirical attention in recent years, and researchers have developed psychometric assessment tools for evaluating financial capacity (Marson 2001b; Marson et al. 2000c). Our own laboratory has produced the Financial Capacity Instrument (FCI; Griffith et al. 2003; Marson et al. 2000c), which affords direct, objective, quantitative assessment of an individual's ability to engage in various financial tasks. The FCI assesses general domains of financial capacity (e.g., basic monetary skills, financial judgment), as well as performance on specific financial tasks; the tasks reflect more basic financial skills that comprise domain-level capacities (e.g., the domain of financial judgment encompasses skills such as making investment decisions). The measure has good reliability and validity (Griffith et al. 2003; Marson and Hebert 2008b) and has demonstrated sensitivity to declines in financial abilities associated with various neurological conditions (Griffith et al. 2003; Marson et al. 2000c, 2006; Martin et al. 2008a; Sherod et al. 2009).

Studies with the FCI have demonstrated significant impairment of financial abilities in patients with both mild and moderate AD (Marson and Hebert 2008b; Marson et al. 2000c). At the domain level, patients with mild AD have been shown to perform significantly below healthy older adult controls on all domains of financial activity, with the exception of basic monetary skills. Our data indicate that patients with moderate AD perform significantly below controls and patients with mild AD on all financial domains. At the task level, patients with mild AD have been shown to perform equivalently with older controls on simple tasks such as naming and counting coins and currency, understanding parts of a checkbook, and detecting risk of mail fraud. However, patients with mild AD have difficulty performing more complex financial tasks, such as applying financial concepts (e.g., choosing the best interest rate), obtaining exact change for vending machine use, understanding and using a bank statement, and making an investment decision. Our findings also demonstrate that patients with moderate AD are substantially impaired on all financial tasks, relative to both normal older adults and persons with mild AD. At the global level, patients with mild AD exhibit substantial impairment in financial capacity relative to older controls, and patients with moderate AD are impaired relative to both controls and patients with mild AD (Marson and Hebert 2008b; Marson et al. 2000c).

Based on these initial findings, Marson et al. (2000c) proposed preliminary clinical guidelines for assessment of the financial capacity of patients with mild and moderate AD:

> 1) Patients with mild AD are at significant risk for impairment in most financial activities, in particular complex activities like checkbook and bank statement management. Areas of preserved autonomous financial activity should be carefully evaluated and monitored.
> 2) Patients with moderate AD are at great risk for loss of all financial activities. Although each AD patient must be considered individually, it is likely that most patients with moderate AD will be unable to manage their financial affairs. (p. 883)

Declines in financial capacity have also been observed in persons with MCI (Griffith et al. 2003; Sherod et al. 2009). Relative to cognitively normal older adults, individuals with MCI demonstrate mild impairments on domains of financial conceptual knowledge, checkbook and bank statements, financial judgment, and bill payment. More specifically, persons with MCI have relative difficulty with tasks requiring practical application of financial concepts, understanding and using a bank statement, and prioritizing and preparing bills for mailing. However, persons with MCI perform significantly better than persons with mild AD on most domain-level financial activities and task-specific abilities. Importantly, our data indicate that not all patients with MCI demonstrate these impairments, suggesting heterogeneity in financial performance in this prodromal dementia group. Nonetheless, these results suggest that significant, albeit mild, decline in financial abilities is an aspect of functional change associated with MCI and may play a role in the eventual conversion of patients from MCI to AD. Accordingly, clinicians should monitor over time the financial capacity of individuals with MCI (Marson et al. 2009). Such monitoring entails inquiring about changes in a patient's capacity as part of routine clinic visits, keeping in mind important aspects of financial capacity, such as financial management and judgment. As needed, a formal assessment of financial capacity may be pursued, which would incorporate a variety of available and relevant information sources, including a clinical interview, cognitive assessment, psychodiagnostic assessment, psychometric assessment of financial capacity, and values assessment (American Bar Association Commission on Law and Aging and American Psychological Association 2008).

Testamentary Capacity

From time to time, professionals in the area of geriatric neuropsychiatry may encounter referral questions concerning testamentary capacity. *Testamentary capacity* refers to an individual's ability to make a will and is a competency related to but also distinct from financial capacity (American Bar Association Commission on Law and Aging and American Psychological Association 2008). The freedom to choose how one's property and other possessions will be disposed of following death is a fundamental right under Anglo-American law (Marson et al. 2004). However, the law of testation specifies that a testator (person making the will) must have *testamentary capacity* or *competency* (Black 1968). If testamentary capacity is lacking at the time of execution of the will, the will is invalid and void in effect (Perr 1991).

Conceptually, testamentary capacity falls within the broader concept of financial capacity, but for reasons of legal history and tradition, it is treated by legal professionals as a distinct capacity (Marson and Hebert 2008c). Each state jurisdiction, through its statutes and case law, sets forth legal elements or criteria for testamentary capacity. Although requirements vary across states, four general criteria have been identified: a testator must 1) know what a will is, 2) have knowledge of his or her potential heirs, 3) have knowledge of the nature and extent of his or her assets, and 4) have a general plan of distribution of assets to heirs. The absence of one or more of these elements of testamentary capacity can serve as grounds for a court to invalidate a will. A will can also fail if the testator has an insane delusion that specifically affects the testator's creation or amendment of a will (Marson and Hebert 2008c).

As with medical decision-making, driving, and financial capacities, sound assessment of testamentary capacity in older adults is very important. Although the field of testamentary capacity assessment is comparatively young, there is increasing conceptual and clinical interest in this area (American Bar Association Commission on Law and Aging and American Psychological Association 2008; Marson et al. 2004; Spar and Garb 1992). In addition, efforts are under way to empirically assess testamentary capacity and develop tools designed to assess the cognitive and functional abilities involved in testamentary capacity. Our research group has developed and is field-testing the Testamentary Capacity Instrument (K.R. Hebert, F.R. Scogin, D.C. Marson, Birmingham, Alabama, February 2009), a psychometric instrument for empirically assessing testamentary capacity.

Undue influence is a separate issue that clinicians can encounter in legal cases of testamentary capacity. Although the testator may possess testamentary capacity, the law requires that a testator be free from undue influence by another individual who may profit from a new will or a codicil (i.e., a legal amendment of an existing will) (Spar et al. 1995). As such, a validly executed will may be separately voided by the court if the volition of the testator is judged to have been supplanted by an individual exercising undue influence over him or her.

Neurocognitive and psychiatric disorders in general, and dementia in particular, increase the susceptibility of older adults to undue influence (Haldipur and Ward 1996). Indicators of undue influence include the active participation of the coercing party in attaining a will and/or controlling the testamentary act, the role of the coercing party as an adviser or confidant to the testator and the coercing party's use of this relationship to influence the way in which the testator disposes of his or her assets, and provisions within the will that are inconsistent with prior and/or subsequent expressions of the testator's intent in executing a will (Marson et al. 2004).

Legal Steps in Response to Possible or Anticipated Future Loss of Competency

All adults, whether cognitively intact or not, should consider and plan for the possibility of future loss of competency. Sometimes, an individual and family receive a clear warning of impending future incapacity (e.g., positive genetic testing for HD, or diagnosis of amnestic MCI or early AD). In most situations, some simple, practical steps can be taken to minimize the complications associated with anticipated future loss of competency (Sadler et al. 2003).

One common action is to *draft and execute a will and estate plan*. We recommend that individuals and families consult with appropriate professionals to ensure that the will and estate plan are prepared appropriately. Such professionals might include an attorney, financial planner, trust officer, accountant, and insurance agent, to name a few. Individuals and families may also find it helpful to *prepare an inventory of assets and liabilities*. This inventory might include a list of important documents (e.g., property deeds, insurance policies, financial statements) and their location (Sadler et al. 2003).

An increasingly common practice is to *establish durable powers of attorney* (see subsequent section on surrogate decision-making and advance directives) (Sadler et al. 2003). A durable power of attorney identifies a proxy decision-maker for the management of one's health care and/or property. In the event of an incapacitating injury or illness, a durable power of attorney for financial affairs allows for the management of the individual's property in accordance with his or her previously expressed wishes. As discussed above, a medical power of attorney identifies a proxy for medical decision-making. Because the legal definitions and limitations of powers of attorney vary across jurisdictions, local statues should be consulted. Finally, the use of a durable power of attorney is efficient and cost-effective compared with the expense, delay, and potential travail of guardianship/conservatorship proceedings through the probate courts (Marson et al. 2000a). However, in some situations, such as those involving intractable family conflict, a court-appointed guardianship/conservatorship with ongoing judicial oversight provides the best resolution to an individual's loss of competency.

Surrogate Decision-Making and Advance Directives

When an older individual loses decisional capacity, surrogate forms of decision-making for health care and other issues become necessary (American College of Physicians 1989; Marson et al. 2000a). Forms of surrogate decision-making include instructional directives such as living wills, proxy directives such as durable powers of attorney for health care and finances, and court-appointed guardians and/or conservators. In addition, most states statutorily prescribe a hierarchy of family members allowed to provide consent for medical procedures, even if no prior proxy or other appointment had been arranged (American Bar Association Commission on Law and Aging and American Psychological Association 2008).

When an advance directive is not in place, surrogate decision-making raises a host of ethical and practical considerations (Marson et al. 2000a). These include deciding who should make medical care and research decisions for the incompetent individual, as well as determining on what basis such surrogate decisions should be made. From an ethical standpoint, such decisions should be similar to ones the individual might make if still competent (i.e., substituted judgment) and should reflect that individual's premorbid values and wishes. If those values are not ascertainable, the decision should be made in the "best interests" of the individual (Cox and Sachs 1994). These ethical goals are complicated by the practical difficulties inherent in reliably determining an incompetent patient's best interests and prior wishes about medical care and research involvement (Marson et al. 2000a).

Accordingly, although mechanisms exist for surrogate decision-making in the absence of evidence of a patient's wishes, it is preferable to have an advance directive in place. An *advance directive* is a written or oral statement made by a competent individual that identifies a proxy who will be responsible for making health care decisions when the individual is no longer capable of making his or her own decisions (proxy directive), or that specifies the medical procedures and types of care that the individual would accept or refuse under certain medical circumstances (instructional directive) (Doukas and Reichel 1993). Advance directives, therefore, afford families, physicians and other health care professionals, and legal professionals valuable information about an individual's preferences, values, and decisions while he or she was still mentally competent, which can guide the surrogate decision-making process. An American Academy of Neurology position paper on laws and regulations concerning life-sustaining treatment states that "decisions regarding the treatment of patients should be anchored in terms of each patient's own values, preferences, and goals of care, as best understood, which determine what is best for each patient" (Bacon et al. 2007b, p. 1097).

Proxy Directives

As noted in the previous paragraph, advance directives can be either proxy or instructional. A *proxy directive* is a form of advance directive in which a competent person appoints a specific individual to make or enforce future health care, financial, and other decisions on behalf of the person should the person be deemed incompetent (Doukas and Reichel 1993). Most scholars in the field of competency as well as most health care professionals favor the use of a proxy directive "because it empowers a living, breathing human advocate who can speak for the patient at the critical juncture and with whom the health care team can communicate and interact in the patient's stead" (Kapp 1992, pp. 215–216). This issue is particularly relevant in geriatric neuropsychiatry, where patients with neurodegenerative dementias may experience a protracted disease course and associated period of incompetence and for whom a series of complex decisions may need to be made.

Perhaps the most common form of proxy directive is the *durable power of attorney,* which designates an individual to act or make decisions for a patient at which time he or she becomes incompetent. A durable power of attorney differs from a regular power of attorney by virtue of its *durability*, which means that it remains in effect (or takes effect, in the case of the springing durable power of attorney) upon the incapacity of its executor (Doukas and Reichel 1993). For example, a durable power of attorney for health care (i.e., a medical power of attorney) permits a competent individual to appoint in advance a known, trusted person to make future health care decisions according to a set of values, preferences, and guidelines articulated by the individual.

There are different views regarding the way in which a proxy decision-maker should proceed (Sadler et al. 2003). According to the *substituted judgment* standard, the proxy is charged with deciding not on the basis of his or her own beliefs but on the basis of the patient's views of what is right and good. In accordance with this standard, the proxy should have intimate awareness of and respect for the individual's personal values, beliefs, and preferences regarding health care decisions. Alternatively, the *best interests* standard holds that the proxy should act in the best interests of the patient. Neither standard is without flaws (Sadler et al. 2003), but the best interests standard may afford the patient less protection insofar as its ambiguity allows the proxy more flexibility to insert his or her own personal preferences into the decision-making process.

Although proxy decision-makers should ideally be free from conflicts of interest, this can be difficult to avoid in practice. Often the proxy is a spouse or child of the patient, and this proxy may have personal motivations for proceeding in contradiction to the patient's personal values or best interests. For instance, a grieving adult child of a terminal patient with advanced dementia may be unwilling to adhere to the patient's previously expressed wishes that he or she not receive life-sustaining medical treatment, such as artificial nutrition or hydration. In this case, the proxy may be acting in his or her own interests rather than the patient's, due to grief (e.g., "I'm not ready for Mom to go"), denial (e.g., "Maybe she will get better"), or guilt (e.g., "I can't be the one to pull the plug"). Unfortunately, proxies may also have financial motivations that can impede the ability to act in accordance with the patient's wishes or best interests, such as the spouse or family member who stands to inherit a large sum of money upon the patient's death. These examples highlight the importance of early planning and written clarification of the patient's wishes while he or she remains competent.

Instructional Directives

An *instructional directive* is an advance directive that outlines an individual's medical treatment preferences without designating a specific agent or proxy. Instructional directives are typically broad in scope and articulate an individual's values and desires regarding the withholding or withdrawal of life-sustaining medical treatment (Cox and Sachs 1994). One such instructional directive is the *values history*, which is a document specifying and prioritizing an individual's beliefs, values, and preferences with the goal of guiding future clinical decision-making (Crane et al. 2005). Perhaps the most widely recognized instructional directive is the *living will*, a document that outlines instructions regarding life-sustaining medical treatments that are to be withheld or withdrawn if the individual is terminally ill.

Although instructional directives are often quite broad and general, they can be designed, with forethought and careful drafting, to provide explicit treatment instructions and preferences in a range of situations. Nonetheless, by virtue of their static written form, they often may fail to address unanticipated potential medical circumstances. This issue may be particularly true in the context of geriatric neuropsychiatry, given the often extended course of neurodegenerative and other diseases and the emergence of unforeseen general medical problems or events. Specific instructional directives have also been criticized on the basis that they can overlook the patient's general beliefs and values (Brett 1991).

Advance Directives for Research Participation

The applicability of advance directives for participation in scientific research has also been a topic of increasing interest in the field of geriatric neuropsychiatry (American College of Physicians 1989; Dresser 2001; Sachs et al. 1994). The purpose of an advance directive for research participation is to obtain consent from a still competent individual that will support the individual's continued research participation after he or she becomes incompetent to give such consent. According to the American College of Physicians (1989), the advance directive should also designate a proxy to supervise the individual's subsequent participation in the research protocol after he or she loses competency. The concept here is that the proxy should serve as an advocate for the individual's interests during the consent process at the time of future research participation and should have no conflict of interest (High 1992). However, the involvement of a proxy decision-maker for research consent should not overshadow the importance of obtaining assent of the potential research participant (Sachs et al. 1994).

Advance directives for research participation are generally more problematic than health care and financial advance directives. In contrast to medical treatment, research participation typically affords minimal benefit to the individual other than possible altruistic reward. In addition, individuals and families generally have little motivation for outlining their wishes for future participation in scientific research (Sachs et al. 1994). There is also a relative lack of family communication about individuals' preferences regarding research participation, compared with communication regarding health care preferences. This lack of communication makes it difficult to ascertain and act in accordance with the individual's wishes at the time of future research participation (Sachs et al. 1994).

End-of-Life Issues

Clinicians working with older adults with neuropsychiatric disorders commonly encounter complex ethical and legal issues surrounding the end of life (Marson et al. 2000a). For example, virtually all patients with neurodegenerative dementias have unremitting disease courses that inevitably lead to death. Because most of these patients will be incompetent in the terminal phase of their illness, decisions about end-of-life treatment have to be made by legal representatives, family members, and/or physicians (Marson et al. 2000a). Situations inevitably arise in which nothing more can be done for the patient clinically and in which continued treatment may be more cruel than kind. Thus, prospective planning is important for addressing end-of-life issues in these patients. Sadler et al. (2003) noted the importance of ongoing discussions between patients, families, and clinicians concerning end of life and emphasized in particular the need for repeated conversations over time. Such discussions afford families and clinicians the opportunity to evaluate over time an individual's preferences under different circumstances, as well as the pattern and relative stability of the patient's expressed wishes. These considerations can inform surrogate decision-making later if necessary. As discussed in the following subsections, topics relevant to end of life include quality of life, end-of-life decision-making, limiting medical treatment, and physician-assisted suicide and euthanasia.

Quality of Life

Quality of life is an increasingly important metric of care for clinicians, family members, and other caregivers (Logsdon et al. 2007). Whitehouse and Rabins (1992) contended that quality of life is "not an isolated concept to be included as one of many measurements of the benefits of our care, but rather…it is the central goal of our professional activity, driving the organization of both our clinical and research efforts" (p. 136). Physicians and other health care professionals need to recognize the importance of developing interventions that not only impact cognitive, functional, and behavioral symptoms but also improve quality of life (Whitehouse and Rabins 1992).

Quality of life appears to be a multidimensional construct that embraces subjective values of the patient; a range of physical, psychological, and social variables; and situational context (Marson et al. 2000a). The empirical literature on quality of life in patients with dementia has converged on several common factors that appear particularly important, including the patient's involvement in pleasurable activities and personally meaningful activities and the patient's ability to perform activities of daily living (Logsdon et al. 2007). These factors highlight the importance of maintaining an appropriate balance between the patient's independence and his or her safety (as well as the safety of others)—a recurrent theme for clinicians working with older adults who have cognitive impairment. To the extent possible, fostering continued (limited) independence (while not compromising safety) can help maintain the patient's sense of personal worth and quality of life.

The quality of life of older adult patients with neuropsychiatric impairment may be difficult at times to ascertain. This is particularly true in more severe dementias in which expressive and receptive language deficits are significant and the ability to communicate has been lost. However, some evidence suggests that patients in the early to middle stages of dementing diseases, such as dementia of the Alzheimer's type, are still able to reliably articulate their own perceptions of their quality of life (Logsdon et al. 2007; Thorgrimsen et al. 2003). Caregiver reports are often essential to consider when evaluating the quality of life of older individuals with cognitive and/or psychiatric disorders (Kurz et al. 2008).

It is important that physicians consider quality-of-life issues in end-of-life treatment of patients with neuropsychiatric diseases (Caralis 1994; Marson et al. 2000a). Responsible medical care in these situations involves a proper balancing of the interests in preserving life with those of providing comfort and a compassionate death. Objectivity and attention to the patient's own life values are of critical importance here. On the one hand, the life of an individual with even the most severe dementia should not be undervalued. For instance, family members and others may incorrectly assume that a patient is miserable without fully considering his or her behavior, attitude, affect, and mood (Sadler et al. 2003); studies have shown that individuals with dementia frequently rate their overall quality of life as good or excellent, despite experiencing losses that appear devastating (Logsdon et al. 2007). On the other hand, the unreflective use of life-sustaining medical treatments or cardiopulmonary resuscitation on a terminally ill patient with dementia may be viewed as cruel, insofar as it ignores the inevitability and naturalness of death (Wanzer et al. 1984).

In summary, a sea change is occurring in physicians' views and approach to end-of-life care. The historical medical imperative to emphasize quantity of life rather than quality of life is receiving increased scrutiny and criticism (Whitehouse 2000). Quality-of-life considerations, based on patient directives, family member accounts, and the physician's own professional and personal experience, are informing decisions about appropriate care of patients with dementia (Caralis 1994). As properly noted by Sidler et al. (2008), end-of-life care is shifting "from the focus on curative and often aggressive, potentially harmful approaches, to an acknowledgement of palliative care, enabling issues of quality of life and care to take precedence over an undue and irrational insistence on the idea of the sanctity of life" (p. 284).

End-of-Life Decision-Making

The primary task faced by clinicians in most end-of-life situations is one of weighing the anticipated burdens and benefits of a proposed medical intervention (Kapp 1992; Marson et al. 2000a). If a proposed intervention has a good chance of temporarily improving the patient's condition (e.g., reducing pain or discomfort), poses little risk, and leaves the patient with a reasonable quality of life, the intervention would likely be in the best interest of the patient. However, many interventions at end of life are accompanied by at least some degree of uncertainty regarding outcome. In addition, as noted in the previous subsection, it may be difficult to ascertain a patient's actual quality of life, particularly during the end stages of a terminal disease. Therefore, some ambiguity inherently attends end-of-life decisions. In many situations, the burdens associated with treatment may outweigh the benefits of medical intervention, calling into question what (if any) treatment lies in the patient's best interests (Marson et al. 2000a).

Because end-of-life decisions are inherently private and medical in nature, most courts have historically maintained that they are best resolved without judicial involvement (Kapp 1992). However, this area has seen a marked increase in legislative activity and media attention in recent years, as exemplified by the popularized case of Theresa Schiavo (Bacon et al. 2007b). In fact, since Ms. Schiavo's death in 2005, legislators have proposed bills in several states that would severely limit physicians' ability to withdraw or withhold life-sustaining medical treatments such as artificial nutrition and hydration. These bills would also give elected officials unprecedented rights to challenge both the administration and the withdrawal of life-sustaining medical treatment (Bacon et al. 2007b).

It is generally agreed that decisions about end-of-life issues are best made through a process of discussion and negotiation involving the patient (when competent), family and/or significant others, health care personnel, and possibly an institutional ethics committee (Kapp 1992; Marson et al. 2000a; Sidler et al. 2008). It is critical that all parties involved attend to the patient's personal values, beliefs, and preferences. Optimally, wherever possible, discussions should occur outside of a medical crisis atmosphere.

Limiting Medical Treatment

The ethical and legal principle of self-determination holds that a competent adult has the right to make personal medical treatment decisions, including the right to refuse life-sustaining medical treatments (Truog et al. 2008). *Life-sustaining medical treatment* refers to any intervention intended to prolong life, such as artificial nutrition and hydration, and cardiopulmonary life support. "Do not" orders, which are written documents requesting that particular types of life-sustaining medical treatments be withheld under certain future circumstances, are common means by which patients (and families) communicate a refusal to receive treatment. The most prevalent type of "do not" order is the order not to initiate cardiopulmonary resuscitation, commonly referred to as a do-not-resuscitate order, or a no-code order.

As with all medical treatment decisions, a patient's decision to refuse life-sustaining measures must be voluntary, informed, and competent. In situations of diminished or lost decisional capacity, such decisions are made by a surrogate decision-maker. As discussed earlier in "Surrogate Decision-Making and Advance Directives," formal procedures exist for appointing surrogate decision-makers (e.g., health care power of attorney) and/or providing instructions under certain medical circumstances (e.g., living will). Surrogate decision-making also often proceeds in an informal manner according to the principle of family-centered care, which views patients within the context of multiple relationships and an overall social structure (Truog et al. 2008). The influence of this principle in modern palliative care is reflected in the accepted notion of collaborative decision-making among the patient (when possible), family, and health care providers (Sidler et al. 2008). However, in some instances, the physician may encounter a patient who does not have an advance directive, such as a living will or medical power of attorney, and whose wishes are unknown to either the family members or the health care provider. In these cases, it is advisable to consult the health care institution's ethics committee, the existence of which is required of all health care organizations, according to The Joint Commission (McCarrick 1992).

When a patient or family refuses treatment at the end of life, the primary goal of the health care provider is that of maintaining the integrity and comfort of the patient and providing him or her relief from suffering (Sidler et al. 2008). Remediation of physical discomfort can be provided through medical, psychological, and social means (Kapp 1992; Truog et al. 2008). In some situations, the patient may be unable to self-report pain and other symptoms, and evidence suggests that pain and suffering may be undertreated in end-of-life care due to difficulties in assessing behavioral indicators of these symptoms (Truog et al. 2008; see Chapter 23, "Pain"). The use of behavioral rating scales (Payen et al. 2001) designed to aid the physician in identifying behavioral and physiological variables that indicate pain has been recommended in this context. In addition to attending to the palliative needs of the patient, the physician's role in end-of-life care is increasingly seen as one involving education, communication, and collaboration with the patient's family. Accordingly, physicians should be mindful of the patient's and family's cultural and religious perspectives and should be prepared to deliver information in an accessible manner (Truog et al. 2008). Physicians are encouraged to "take seriously their responsibility to make recommendations and guide families in ways that accord with their decision-making preferences. Merely providing treatment alternatives and asking patients and families to choose among them may make the patients and families feel solely responsible for the decision to forgo life-sustaining treatment, and this practice contrasts with the preferred practice of shared decision-making" (Truog et al. 2008, p. 954).

Decisions to withhold or withdraw life-sustaining measures are difficult not only for patients and families but also for health care providers. As noted by Reynolds et al. (2007), "it is difficult to determine when it is appropriate to accept that a patient is dying, cease further aggressive treatment, and strengthen palliative support" (p. 920). The challenging nature of these decisions reflects a number of factors, including perceived moral distinction between withholding and withdrawing treatment; spiritual, religious, and cultural beliefs and practices; technological imperative; prognostic ambiguity; variability among practitioners; and caregiver discomfort with death (Reynolds et al. 2007; Truog et al. 2008).

Legal issues can also complicate issues of limiting medical care. Health care providers are frequently anxious about incurring potential criminal or civil liability as a result of withholding treatment (Kapp 1992; Lee 2005; Reynolds et al. 2007). However, these fears appear to be somewhat exaggerated (Lee 2005), and greater legal liability may exist in ignoring or overriding requests to withhold life-sustaining medical treatment than in limiting it in accordance with the patient's requests (Schermer 1990). In addition to legal ramifications, the escalating costs of health care add to the importance of limiting medical treatment on request. A legal precedent has been set that the provider will bear full financial responsibility for delivery of a treatment to which the patient or family objected (Kapp 1992).

Despite the complexity inherent in decisions regarding the limitation of medical treatments at end of life, a general ethical and legal consensus supporting this practice has emerged in the United States (Lee 2005; Truog et al. 2008). This consensus is based on legal decisions that 1) equate the acts of withholding care and of withdrawing life support, 2) distinguish between killing a patient and allowing a patient to die, and 3) allow the provision of medications for pain and other symptom relief "even when this may have the foreseen (but not intended) consequence of hastening death" (Truog et al. 2008, p. 955).

Physician-Assisted Suicide and Euthanasia

Looming behind the ethical issue of limiting medical treatment at end of life are the controversial topics of physician-assisted suicide and euthanasia. Although these terms are sometimes used interchangeably, they refer to distinct concepts. The European Association for Palliative Care (EAPC) Ethics Task Force defines *euthanasia* as "a doctor intentionally killing a person by the administration of drugs, at that person's voluntary and competent request" (Materstvedt et al. 2003, p. 98). Importantly, the EAPC Task Force specifies that neither the withholding or withdrawal of treatments nor terminal sedation (i.e., the use of sedatives to alleviate suffering during the last days of life) should be considered forms of euthanasia. *Physician-assisted suicide* is defined as "a doctor intentionally helping a person to commit suicide by providing drugs for self-administration, at that person's voluntary and competent request" (Materstvedt et al. 2003, p. 98).

Although currently permitted in only a handful of countries and jurisdictions, physician-assisted suicide and euthanasia are increasingly relevant topics for clinicians working with older adults. Both were legalized in the Netherlands in 2002 by the Dutch Euthanasia Act, also called the Termination of Life on Request and Assisted Suicide (Review Procedures) Act (Buiting et al. 2008). Euthanasia is permitted in Belgium, and Switzerland allows assisted suicide (Pereira et al. 2008). In 1997, the state of Oregon passed the Oregon Death With Dignity Act, which legalized physician-assisted suicide for Oregonians (Steinbrook 2008). The state of Washington recently followed suit, passing the Washington Death With Dignity Act in November 2008, which took effect on March 5, 2009 (Steinbrook 2008). Although physician-assisted suicide remains a hotly debated topic, similar legislation will likely be proposed in additional states in the United States. Some data suggest that approximately 25% of physicians and nurses have been approached by a patient or family with a request for assisted suicide or euthanasia (Reynolds et al. 2007). Perhaps even more surprising are the results of one study: of the 17% of 1,600 nurses surveyed who were approached with such requests, 16% obliged (Asch 1996). These data illustrate the importance of this issue and signal a trend toward increasing discussion, if not increasing acceptance, of an ethical and legal basis for assisted suicide and euthanasia.

As the U.S. population ages and the prevalence of incapacitating neurodegenerative diseases increases (Alzheimer's Association 2008; Jeste et al. 1999; Wan et al. 2005), physicians can expect to encounter an increasing number of cases in which requests of these kinds may arise. Such circumstances pose numerous challenges for physicians and other health care professionals, such as reconciling clinical practice standards, policy, and legislation with their own personal beliefs; managing conflict and resolving disputes among members of the treatment team; and participating in collaborative decision-making with the patient and family (Pereira et al. 2008; Reynolds et al. 2007). In addition, not only are physicians charged with judging the patient's competence (note that the specific requirement of competency is explicitly included in the definitions of physician-assisted suicide and euthanasia outlined above), but they also must consider potentially complicating factors such as the presence of depression (Aungst 2008). As noted by Whitehouse (2000), the requirement of competency in the current definitions of physician-assisted suicide and euthanasia suggests that future ethical issues will likely arise concerning the appropriateness of advance directives for euthanasia in patients with neurological and psychiatric disorders.

Geriatric Mental Health Policy Issues

Clinical and Fiscal Crisis of Geriatric Mental Health Care

Over a decade ago, Jeste et al. (1999) highlighted the emerging crisis of geriatric mental health care in the United States, noting that "the current research infrastructure, health care financing, pool of mental health care personnel with appropriate geriatric training, and mental health care delivery systems are extremely inadequate to meet the challenges posed by the expected increase in the number of elderly persons with mental illnesses" (p. 848). Indeed, as the first baby boomers approach retirement age, the prevalence of dementia and other geriatric neuropsychiatric conditions in the United States is expected to rise dramatically (Alzheimer's Association 2008; Jeste et al. 1999). Some estimates project that by 2030, there will be approximately 72 million adults over age 65 in the United States, representing an increase from 12% (in 2003) to 20% of the U.S. population (Wan et al. 2005). Moreover, the oldest-old population (persons ages 85 and older) is expected to reach 9.6 million by 2030 and 20.9 million by 2050 (Wan et al. 2005). Advancing age is a major risk factor for cognitive impairment, and the prevalence of AD in persons ages 65 and older is anticipated to reach 7.7 million by 2030 and 11–16 million by 2050 (Alzheimer's Association 2008). In addition, the number of persons in the United States ages 65 and older with psychiatric conditions is projected to increase from approximately 4 million (in 1970) to 15 million by 2030 (Jeste et al. 1999). In the context of these figures, the need for policy directives and increased funding support in geriatric mental health care is alarmingly apparent.

There is an increasing comorbidity of general medical and neuropsychiatric illnesses in the geriatric population (Friedman and Steinhagen 2007). Neuropsychiatric symptoms are common in dementia, with prevalence estimates ranging from 50% to 80% (Weintraub and Katz 2005). With comorbid general medical and mental illnesses comes increased disability, with associated greater health care demands and an increased need for patient supervision and assistance with activities of daily living (Friedman and Steinhagen 2007). Unfortunately, some data suggest that the specialized mental health care needs of these older patients are not being met. Older adults with mental disorders are more likely to seek psychiatric treatment from a general practitioner than a mental health specialist (Friedman and Steinhagen 2007; Jeste et al. 1999), and many of these patients receive no mental health services (Bartels and Drake 2005). Moreover, older adults with mental disorders are more likely to receive inadequate mental health care than are both younger patients with mental disorders and older patients without mental health problems (Bartels and Drake 2005).

These disturbing patterns reflect a variety of factors, including organizational and policy barriers to treatment access for older patients, underfunding of geriatric mental health care, shortage of professionals with appropriate training in geriatric mental health, ageism among providers, and lack of coordinated care (Bartels et al. 2002; Bruce et al. 2005; Jeste et al. 1999). Inadequate access to mental health care for older adults has substantial costs for individual patients (i.e., patient outcomes) as well as society at large (i.e., health care expenditures). In older adults, mental health problems are associated with increased risk for suicide, poorer cognitive status and overall physical health, greater disability, higher rates of health care service utilization, longer hospital stays, higher probability of nursing home placement, self-neglect, loss of independence, and overall reduced quality of life (Bruce et al. 2005; Friedman and Steinhagen 2007). From an economic perspective, these data translate to more health care dollars spent (Bruce et al. 2005). In the United States alone, the costs of depression in older patients have been estimated at $9 billion annually (Langa et al. 2004), and one report estimated that the worldwide cost of dementia in 2005 was over $315 billion (Wimo et al. 2007). As the world population ages, the clinical and economic burden of cognitive and psychiatric disorders in older adults is expected to increase markedly. Byock et al. (2009) noted that "nearly one quarter of Medicare and Medicaid expenditures occur during the last year of life, with no relationship between dollars spent and quality received" (p. 1).

Policy Implications of the Clinical and Fiscal Crisis

As the number of older adults with dementia and neuropsychiatric conditions continues to rise, nursing homes and other long-term-care facilities are expected to play an increasing role in the care of these patients (Bharani and Snowden 2005). In addition, primary care physicians can expect to encounter a growing number of older patients presenting with neurocognitive and neuropsychiatric symptoms (Jeste et al. 1999). In a health care system that is already failing (Bartels and Drake 2005), these realities suggest a clear imperative for policy directives aimed at improving the quality of mental health care for older adults.

Key issues related to improving the quality of geriatric mental health care include staffing, housing, access to palliative and hospice care, caregiver support, and access to health care in rural communities. In a survey of 463 citizens in New Hampshire, 94% of respondents favored the establishment and enforcement of minimum staffing requirements in nursing homes and assisted living facilities, and over 95% endorsed a need for expanding assisted housing options for older adults who are not fully independent but are not in need of skilled nursing care (Byock et al. 2009). Moreover, respondents overwhelmingly endorsed models of long-term care that include higher levels of staffing and attention to residents' quality of life. The results of the survey also indicate a clear preference among respondents for mandated insurance coverage of hospice and palliative care, increased access to palliative care in long-term-care settings, and increased access to hospice care. Regarding hospice care, over 80% of respondents favored removal of the current qualifying requirements of a 6-month life expectancy and the need to discontinue treatments aimed at treating the disease and prolonging life. Respondents also overwhelmingly endorsed the need for policy directives that provide support for caregivers of elderly patients (Byock et al. 2009) and that address the unique challenges of older adults in rural communities.

These data suggest that substantial changes are needed in the U.S. health care system to address the needs of patients and families coping with geriatric mental health issues. The critical need for a system-wide overhaul has been recognized by policy makers as well; the President's New Freedom Commission on Mental Health (established in 2002 under President George W. Bush) concluded that mental health services in this country are "fragmented, disconnected and often inadequate.... Instead of ready access to quality care, the system presents barriers that all too often add to the burden of mental illnesses for individuals, their families, and our communities" (President's New Freedom Commission on Mental Health 2003, p. 1). The commission's report sets forth several goals for improving mental health care, with specific recommendations for improving access to mental health services, improving mental health treatment in primary care settings, focusing on preventive medicine, and adopting EBPs.

Evidence-Based Practice in Geriatric Neuropsychiatric Health

In response to the growing crisis in geriatric mental health care, researchers have increasingly focused on identifying treatment protocols and health care policies that are both efficacious and cost-effective. The EBP movement, which emphasizes the importance of incorporating the current best scientific evidence into clinical practice (Sackett et al. 1997), has informed much of the progress in this area. Although EBP is often thought of as a guiding framework for the treatment of individual patients, the principles of EBP are also relevant for health care policy at a macro level. For instance, "Our limited health care resources should be applied to providing interventions that have proven effectiveness based on well-designed evaluation trials, with emphasis on randomized controlled trials" (Bartels et al. 2002, p. 1420).

Recognizing the need for increased scientific and clinical attention to geriatric mental health care, the Subcommittee on Older Adults (established as part of the President's New Freedom Commission on Mental Health) identified the widespread implementation of EBPs as a vital initiative for improving care quality for older adults with mental health conditions (Bartels and Drake 2005). In the December 2005 issue of *Psychiatric Clinics of North America*, which is devoted solely to EBP in geriatric psychiatry, evidence-based treatments for geriatric depression, bipolar disorder, anxiety disorders, substance abuse, and schizophrenia are reviewed (Bartels 2005). Of particular relevance are two articles addressing evidence-based interventions for psychosis, agitation, and other behavioral symptoms in neurodegenerative disease and dementia (Bharani and Snowden 2005; Weintraub and Katz 2005). These articles highlight the limitations of the current knowledge base regarding treatment of neuropsychiatric symptoms in patients with dementia and emphasize the need for further research in this area. Weintraub and Katz (2005) noted that "clinicians working with patients who have psychosis and agitation associated with dementia have a difficult task: applying scientific evidence and general principles to estimate the benefits versus the risks of alternative treatments for an individual patient even in the face of critical gaps in the information that is available to them" (p. 977).

Nonetheless, there is reason to be cautiously hopeful. With the new administration in Washington, D.C., and with the renewed focus on overhauling and reforming the current health care system—including the mental health system—there is likely to be additional funding available to support new research. This research can provide the information base critical to developing new evidence-based interventions and programs of care in geriatric neuropsychiatry.

Key Points

- Autonomy and self-determination, beneficence and nonmaleficence, and justice are core ethical principles that inform and guide clinical practice and research in geriatric neuropsychiatry.
- The medicolegal doctrine of informed consent is a cornerstone for the protection of the rights of medical patients and human research participants.
- Competency can be defined as a minimal threshold imposed by society under which individuals retain the power to make decisions for themselves.
- Neither neuropsychiatric diagnosis nor cognitive impairment is sufficient by itself to support a competency judgment. Rather, the critical component of a competency assessment is the analysis of an individual's functional abilities relative to performing a specific act in its context.
- Specific competencies commonly assessed within geriatric neuropsychiatry include the capacity to consent to medical treatment; to drive; to manage financial affairs; to make a will; and to manage one's personal affairs and live independently.
- A durable power of attorney is an efficient and cost-effective means of transferring decisional authority, in contrast to the expense and delay of guardianship/conservatorship proceedings in the probate courts.
- End-of-life issues in geriatric neuropsychiatry include quality of life, end-of-life decision-making, limiting medical treatment, and assisted suicide and euthanasia.
- A clinical and fiscal crisis currently exists in geriatric mental health care. The United States possesses inadequate research infrastructure, health care financ-

ing, mental health care personnel with appropriate geriatric training, and mental health care delivery systems in relation to the challenges posed by the rapidly aging society.

Recommended Readings

American Bar Association Commission on Law and Aging and American Psychological Association: Assessment of Older Adults With Diminished Capacity: A Handbook for Lawyers. Washington, DC, American Bar Association and American Psychological Association, 2005. Available at: http://www.apa.org/pi/aging/resources/guides/diminished-capacity.pdf. Accessed September 7, 2010.

American Bar Association Commission on Law and Aging and American Psychological Association: Assessment of Older Adults With Diminished Capacity: A Handbook for Psychologists. Washington, DC, American Bar Association and American Psychological Association, 2008. Available at: http://www.apa.org/pi/aging/programs/assessment/capacity-psychologist-handbook.pdf. Accessed September 7, 2010.

American Bar Association Commission on Law and Aging, American Psychological Association, National College of Probate Judges: Judicial Determination of Capacity of Older Adults in Guardianship Proceedings: A Handbook for Judges. Washington, DC, American Bar Association and American Psychological Association, 2006. Available at: http://www.apa.org/pi/aging/resources/guides/judges-diminished.pdf. Accessed September 7, 2010.

Bacon D, Williams MA, Gordon J: Position statement on laws and regulations concerning life-sustaining treatment, including artificial nutrition and hydration, for patients lacking decision-making capacity. Neurology 68:1097–1100, 2007

Bartels SJ (ed): Evidence-based geriatric psychiatry. Psychiatr Clin North Am 28:xiii–xv, 2005

Kapp M: Geriatrics and the Law: Patient Rights and Professional Responsibilities. New York, Springer, 1992

Marson DC, Ingram KK, Cody HA, et al: Assessing the competency of patients with Alzheimer's disease under different legal standards: a prototype instrument. Arch Neurol 52:949–954, 1995

Marson DC, Sawrie SM, Snyder S, et al: Assessing financial capacity in patients with Alzheimer disease: a conceptual model and prototype instrument. Arch Neurol 57:877–884, 2000

Moye J, Marson DC: Assessment of decision-making capacity in older adults: an emerging area of practice and research. J Gerontol B Psychol Sci Soc Sci 62:3–11, 2007

Reynolds S, Cooper AB, McKneally M: Withdrawing life-sustaining treatment: ethical considerations. Surg Clin North Am 87:919–936, viii, 2007

Truog RD, Campbell ML, Curtis JR, et al: Recommendations for end-of-life care in the intensive care unit: a consensus statement by the American College [corrected] of Critical Care Medicine. Crit Care Med 36:953–963, 2008

References

Alzheimer's Association: Alzheimer's Disease Facts and Figures: Ten Million U.S. Baby Boomers Will Develop Alzheimer's Disease. March 18, 2008. Available at: http://www.alz.org/national/documents/release_031808_2008_facts_and_figures.pdf. Accessed June 25, 2010.

American Bar Association Commission on Law and Aging and American Psychological Association: Assessment of Older Adults With Diminished Capacity: A Handbook for Lawyers. Washington, DC, American Bar Association and American Psychological Association, 2005. Available at: http://www.apa.org/pi/aging/resources/guides/diminished-capacity.pdf. Accessed September 7, 2010.

American Bar Association Commission on Law and Aging and American Psychological Association: Assessment of Older Adults With Diminished Capacity: A Handbook for Psychologists. Washington, DC, American Bar Association and American Psychological Association, 2008. Available at: http://www.apa.org/pi/aging/programs/assessment/capacity-psychologist-handbook.pdf. Accessed September 7, 2010.

American Bar Association Commission on Law and Aging, American Psychological Association, National College of Probate Judges: Judicial Determination of Capacity of Older Adults in Guardianship Proceedings: A Handbook for Judges. Washington, DC, American Bar Association and American Psychological Association, 2006. Available at: http://www.apa.org/pi/aging/resources/guides/judges-diminished.pdf. Accessed September 7, 2010.

American College of Physicians: Cognitively impaired subjects. Ann Intern Med 111:843–848, 1989

American Psychiatric Association: The Principles of Medical Ethics with Annotations Especially Applicable to Psychiatry, 2009 Edition Revised. Arlington, VA, American Psychiatric Association, 2009. Available at: http://www.psych.org/MainMenu/PsychiatricPractice/Ethics/ResourcesStandards/PrinciplesofMedicalEthics.aspx. Accessed June 25, 2010.

American Psychological Association: Ethical Principles of Psychologists and Code of Conduct. Am Psychol 57:1060–1073, 2002

Appelbaum P, Gutheil T: Clinical Handbook of Psychiatry and the Law, 2nd Edition. Baltimore, MD, Williams & Wilkins, 1991

Asch DA: The role of critical care nurses in euthanasia and assisted suicide. N Engl J Med 334:1374–1379, 1996

Aungst H: Death with dignity. Geriatrics 63:20–22, 2008

Bacon D, Fisher RS, Morris JC, et al: American Academy of Neurology position statement on physician reporting of medical conditions that may affect driving competence. Neurology 68:1174–1177, 2007a

Bacon D, Williams MA, Gordon J: Position statement on laws and regulations concerning life-sustaining treatment, including artificial nutrition and hydration, for patients lacking decision-making capacity. Neurology 68:1097–1100, 2007b

Bartels SJ (ed): Evidence-based geriatric psychiatry. Psychiatr Clin North Am 28:xiii–xv, 2005

Bartels SJ, Drake RE: Evidence-based geriatric psychiatry: an overview. Psychiatr Clin North Am 28:763–784, 2005

Bartels SJ, Dums AR, Oxman TE, et al: Evidence-based practices in geriatric mental health care. Psychiatr Serv 53:1419–1431, 2002

Bharani N, Snowden M: Evidence-based interventions for nursing home residents with dementia-related behavioral symptoms. Psychiatr Clin North Am 28:985–1005, 2005

Black H: Black's Law Dictionary, 4th Edition. St. Paul, MN, West Publishing, 1968

Brett AS: Limitations of listing specific medical interventions in advance directives. JAMA 266:825–828, 1991

Brookmeyer R, Corrada MM, Curriero FC, et al: Survival following a diagnosis of Alzheimer disease. Arch Neurol 59:1764–1767, 2002

Bruce ML, Van Citters AD, Bartels SJ: Evidence-based mental health services for home and community. Psychiatr Clin North Am 28:1039–1060, 2005

Buiting HM, Gevers JK, Rietjens JA, et al: Dutch criteria of due care for physician-assisted dying in medical practice: a physician perspective. J Med Ethics 34:e12, 2008

Byock IR, Corbeil YJ, Goodrich ME: Beyond polarization, public preferences suggest policy opportunities to address aging, dying, and family caregiving. Am J Hosp Palliat Care 26:200–208, 2009

Canterbury v Spence, 464 F2d 772, 787 (DC Cir), cert denied, 409 US 1064 (1972)

Capron A: Informed consent in catastrophic disease research and treatment. Univ PA Law Rev 123:340–438, 1974

Caralis P: Ethical and legal issues in the care of Alzheimer's patients. Med Clin North Am 78:877–893, 1994

Cobbs v Grant, 8 Cal 3d 229, 502 P2d 1, Cal Rptr 505 (1972)

Cox DM, Sachs GA: Advance directives and the patient self-determination act. Clin Geriatr Med 10:431–443, 1994

Crane MK, Wittink M, Doukas DJ: Respecting end-of-life treatment preferences. Am Fam Physician 72:1263–1268, 2005

Doukas D, Reichel W: Planning for Uncertainty: A Guide to Living Wills and Other Advance Directives for Health Care. Baltimore, MD, Johns Hopkins University Press, 1993

Dresser R: Advance directives in dementia research: promoting autonomy and protecting subjects. IRB 23:1–6, 2001

Dunn LB, Nowrangi MA, Palmer BW, et al: Assessing decisional capacity for clinical research or treatment: a review of instruments. Am J Psychiatry 163:1323–1334, 2006

Dymek MP, Atchison P, Harrell L, et al: Competency to consent to medical treatment in cognitively impaired patients with Parkinson's disease. Neurology 56:17–24, 2001

Friedman MB, Steinhagen KA: Geriatric Mental Health Policy for the 21st Century. September 2007. Available at: http://www.mhaofnyc.org/yusyin/toolkit/04GMHBriefingBook.ppt. Accessed June 25, 2010.

Griffith HR, Belue K, Sicola A, et al: Impaired financial abilities in mild cognitive impairment: a direct assessment approach. Neurology 60:449–457, 2003

Griffith HR, Dymek MP, Atchison P, et al: Medical decision-making in neurodegenerative disease: mild AD and PD with cognitive impairment. Neurology 65:483–485, 2005

Grisso T: Evaluating Competencies: Forensic Assessments and Instruments. New York, Plenum, 1986

Grisso T, Appelbaum P: Mentally ill and non-mentally ill patients' abilities to understand informed consent disclosure for medication. Law Hum Behav 15:377–388, 1991

Haldipur C, Ward M: Competence and other legal issues, in Psychological Treatment of Older Adults: An Introductory Text. Edited by Hersen M, Van Hasslet V. New York, Plenum, 1996, pp 103–125

High D: Research with Alzheimer's disease subjects: informed consent and proxy decision-making. J Am Geriatr Soc 40:950–957, 1992

Ho LW, Carmichael J, Swartz J, et al: The molecular biology of Huntington's disease. Psychol Med 31:3–14, 2001

Jeste DV, Alexopoulos GS, Bartels SJ, et al: Consensus statement on the upcoming crisis in geriatric mental health: research agenda for the next 2 decades. Arch Gen Psychiatry 56:848–853, 1999

Jeste DV, Palmer BW, Golshan S, et al: Multimedia consent for research in people with schizophrenia and normal subjects: a randomized controlled trial. Schizophr Bull 35:719–729, 2009

Kapp M: Geriatrics and the Law: Patient Rights and Professional Responsibilities. New York, Springer, 1992

Karlawish J: Measuring decision-making capacity in cognitively impaired individuals. Neurosignals 16:91–98, 2008

Kay L, Bundy A, Clemson L, et al: Validity and reliability of the on-road driving assessment with senior drivers. Accid Anal Prev 40:751–759, 2008

Kim S, Caine E, Currier G, et al: Assessing the competence of persons with Alzheimer's disease in providing informed consent for participation in research. Am J Psychiatry 158:712–717, 2001

Kurz A, Schulz M, Reed P, et al: Personal perspectives of persons with Alzheimer's disease and their carers: a global survey. Alzheimers Dement 4:345–352, 2008

Langa KM, Valenstein MA, Fendrick AM, et al: Extent and cost of informal caregiving for older Americans with symptoms of depression. Am J Psychiatry 161:857–863, 2004

Lee KF: Palliative care: good legal defense. Surg Clin North Am 85:287–302, 2005

Logsdon RG, McCurry SM, Teri L: Evidence-based interventions to improve quality of life for individuals with dementia. Alzheimers care today 8:309–318, 2007

Marson D: Loss of competency in Alzheimer's disease: conceptual and psychometric approaches. Int J Law Psychiatry 24:267–283, 2001a

Marson D: Loss of financial capacity in dementia: conceptual and empirical approaches. Neuropsychol Dev Cogn B Aging Neuropsychol Cogn 8:164–181, 2001b

Marson D, Dreer L: Assessing competency in patients with Alzheimer's disease, in Clinical Diagnosis and Management of Alzheimer's Disease. Edited by Gauthier S. London, Martin Dunitz, 2006, pp 325–340

Marson D, Dymek M: Competency in Parkinson's disease with dementia. J Ethics Law Aging 10:63–82, 2004

Marson D, Harrell LE: Neurocognitive models that predict physician judgments of capacity to consent in patients with mild Alzheimer's disease, in Medical Information Processing and Aging. Edited by Park D, Morrell R, Shifrin K. New York, Erlbaum, 1999, pp 109–126

Marson D, Hebert K: Capacity to consent to treatment, in Encyclopedia of Psychology and the Law, Vol 1. Edited by Cutler BL. Thousand Oaks, CA, Sage, 2008a, pp 51–54

Marson D, Hebert K: Financial capacity, in Encyclopedia of Psychology and the Law, Vol 1. Edited by Cutler BL. Thousand Oaks, CA, Sage, 2008b, pp 313–316

Marson D, Hebert K: Testamentary capacity, in Encyclopedia of Psychology and the Law, Vol 2. Edited by Cutler BL. Thousand Oaks, CA, Sage, 2008c, pp 798–801

Marson D, Zebley L: The other side of the retirement years: cognitive decline, dementia, and loss of financial capacity. Journal of Retirement Planning 4:30–39, 2001

Marson D, Schmitt FA, Ingram KK, et al: Determining the competency of Alzheimer patients to consent to treatment and research. Alzheimer Dis Assoc Disord 8(suppl):5–18, 1994

Marson D, Cody HA, Ingram KK, et al: Neuropsychologic predictors of competency in Alzheimer's disease using a rational reasons legal standard. Arch Neurol 52:955–959, 1995a

Marson D, Ingram KK, Cody HA, et al: Assessing the competency of patients with Alzheimer's disease under different legal standards: a prototype instrument. Arch Neurol 52:949–954, 1995b

Marson D, Chatterjee A, Ingram KK, et al: Toward a neurologic model of competency: cognitive predictors of capacity to consent in Alzheimer's disease using three different legal standards. Neurology 46:666–672, 1996

Marson D, Hawkins L, McInturff B, et al: Cognitive models that predict physician judgments of capacity to consent in mild Alzheimer's disease. J Am Geriatr Soc 45:458–464, 1997a

Marson D, McInturff B, Hawkins L, et al: Consistency of physician judgments of capacity to consent in mild Alzheimer's disease. J Am Geriatr Soc 45:453–457, 1997b

Marson D, Annis S, McInturff B, et al: Error behaviors associated with loss of competency in Alzheimer's disease. Neurology 53: 1983–1992, 1999

Marson D, Dymek M, Geyer J: Ethical and legal issues of clinical care and research, in Neurodegenerative Dementias. Edited by Trojanowski J, Clark C. New York, McGraw-Hill, 2000a, pp 425–435

Marson D, Earnst K, Jamil F, et al: Consistency of physicians' legal standard and personal judgments of competency in patients with Alzheimer's disease. J Am Geriatr Soc 48:911–918, 2000b

Marson D, Sawrie SM, Snyder S, et al: Assessing financial capacity in patients with Alzheimer disease: a conceptual model and prototype instrument. Arch Neurol 57:877–884, 2000c

Marson D, Dymek M, Geyer J: Informed consent, competency, and the neurologist. Neurology 7:317–326, 2001

Marson D, Huthwaite J, Hebert K: Testamentary capacity and undue influence in the elderly: a jurisprudent therapy perspective. Law Psychol Rev 28:71–96, 2004

Marson D, Savage R, Phillips J: Financial capacity in persons with schizophrenia and serious mental illness: clinical and research ethics aspects. Schizophr Bull 32:81–91, 2006

Marson D, Martin RC, Wadley V, et al: Clinical interview assessment of financial capacity in older adults with mild cognitive impairment and Alzheimer's disease. J Am Geriatr Soc 57:806–814, 2009

Martin R, Griffith HR, Belue K, et al: Declining financial capacity in patients with mild Alzheimer disease: a one-year longitudinal study. Am J Geriatr Psychiatry 16:209–219, 2008a

Martin RC, Okonkwo OC, Hill J, et al: Medical decision-making capacity in cognitively impaired Parkinson's disease patients without dementia. Mov Disord 23:1867–1874, 2008b

Materstvedt LJ, Clark D, Ellershaw J, et al: Euthanasia and physician-assisted suicide: a view from an EAPC Ethics Task Force. Palliat Med 17:97–101; discussion 102–179, 2003

Mazur D: What should patients be told prior to a medical procedure? Ethical and legal perspectives on medical informed consent. Am J Med 81:1051–1054, 1986

McCarrick PM: Ethics committees in hospitals. Kennedy Inst Ethics J 2:285–306, 1992

Meisel A, Roth L, Lidz C: Toward a model of the legal doctrine of informed consent. Am J Psychiatry 134:285–289, 1977

Melnick V, Dubler N: Clinical research in senile dementia of the Alzheimer type: suggested guidelines addressing the ethical and legal issues. J Am Geriatr Soc 32:531–536, 1984

Morris J: Challenging assumptions about Alzheimer's disease: mild cognitive impairment and the cholinergic hypothesis. Ann Neurol 51:143–144, 2002

Moye J: Theoretical frameworks for competency in cognitively impaired elderly adults. J Aging Stud 10:27–42, 1996

Moye J, Marson DC: Assessment of decision-making capacity in older adults: an emerging area of practice and research. J Gerontol B Psychol Sci Soc Sci 62:P3–P11, 2007

Munetz M, Lidz C, Meisel A: Informed consent and incompetent patients. J Fam Pract 20:273–279, 1985

National Commission for the Protection of Human Subjects of Biomedical and Behavioral Research: Belmont Report: Ethical Principles and Guidelines for the Protection of Human Subjects of Research. Washington, DC, U.S. Government Printing Office, 1979

Nerenberg L: Financial Abuse of the Elderly. Washington, DC, National Center on Elder Abuse, 1996

Okonkwo O, Griffith HR, Copeland JN, et al: Medical decision-making capacity in mild cognitive impairment: a three-year longitudinal study. Neurology 71:1474–1480, 2008

Payen JF, Bru O, Bosson JL, et al: Assessing pain in critically ill sedated patients by using a behavioral pain scale. Crit Care Med 29:2258–2263, 2001

Pereira J, Anwar D, Pralong G, et al: Assisted suicide and euthanasia should not be practiced in palliative care units. J Palliat Med 11: 1074–1076, 2008

Perr IN: Alleged brain damage, diminished capacity, mens rea, and misuse of medical concepts. J Forensic Sci 36:722–727, 1991

President's Commission for the Study of Ethical Problems in Medicine and Biomedical and Behavioral Research: Making Health Care Decisions, Vol 1. A Report on the Ethical and Legal Implications of Informed Consent in the Patient-Practitioner Relationship. Washington, DC, U.S. Government Printing Office, 1982

President's New Freedom Commission on Mental Health: Achieving the Promise: Transforming Mental Health Care in America. Rockville, MD, The President's New Freedom Commission on Mental Health, July 22, 2003. Available at: http://store.samhsa.gov/shin/content//SMA03-3831/SMA03-3831.pdf. Accessed January 4, 2011.

Reynolds S, Cooper AB, McKneally M: Withdrawing life-sustaining treatment: ethical considerations. Surg Clin North Am 87:919–936, viii, 2007

Roth L, Meisel A, Lidz C: Tests of competency to consent to treatment. Am J Psychiatry 134:279–284, 1977

Sachs G: Advance consent for dementia research. Alzheimer Dis Assoc Disord 8:19–27, 1994

Sachs GA, Stocking CB, Stern R, et al: Ethical aspects of dementia research: informed consent and proxy consent. Clin Res 42:403–412, 1994

Sackett DL, Richardson WS, Rosenberg WMC, et al: Evidence-Based Medicine: How to Practice and Teach EBM. Edinburgh, Scotland, Churchill Livingstone, 1997

Sadler JZ, Bernstein BE, Marson DC: Legal and ethical issues, in The Dementias: Diagnosis, Treatment, and Research. Edited by Weiner MF, Lipton AM. Washington, DC, American Psychiatric Publishing, 2003, pp 341–369

Schermer B: A practical guide for hospital counsel in decisions to withhold or withdraw medical treatment. J Health Hosp Law 23:264–266, 286, 1990

Schloendorff v Society of New York Hospital, 211 NY 125, 129 (1914)

Sherod MG, Griffith HR, Copeland J, et al: Neurocognitive predictors of financial capacity across the dementia spectrum: normal aging, mild cognitive impairment, and Alzheimer's disease. J Int Neuropsychol Soc 15:258–267, 2009

Sidler D, Arndt HR, van Niekerk AA: Medical futility and end-of-life care. S Afr Med J 98:284–286, 2008

Slater v Baker and Stapleton, 2 Wils. K.B. 359, 95 Eng. Rep. 860 (1767)

Spar J: Competency and related forensic issues, in The American Psychiatric Press Textbook of Geriatric Neuropsychiatry, 2nd Edition. Edited by Coffey CE, Cummings JL. Washington, DC, American Psychiatric Press, 2000, pp 945–963

Spar J, Garb A: Assessing competency to make a will. Am J Psychiatry 149:169–174, 1992

Spar J, Hankin M, Stodden A: Assessing mental capacity and susceptibility to undue influence. Behav Sci Law 13:391–403, 1995

Steinbrook R: Physician-assisted death: from Oregon to Washington State. N Engl J Med 359:2513–2515, 2008

Taub H, Kline G, Baker M: The elderly and informed consent: effects of vocabulary level and corrected feedback. Exp Aging Res 7: 137–146, 1981

Tepper A, Elwork A: Competency to consent to treatment as a psychological construct. Law Hum Behav 8:205–223, 1984

Thorgrimsen L, Selwood A, Spector A, et al: Whose quality of life is it anyway? The validity and reliability of the Quality of Life-Alzheimer's Disease (QoL-AD) scale. Alzheimer Dis Assoc Disord 17:201–208, 2003

Tidswell M, Jodka PG, Steingrub JS: Medical ethics and end-of-life care, in Irwin and Rippe's Intensive Care Medicine. Edited by Irwin RS, Rippe JM. Philadelphia, PA, Lippincott Williams & Wilkins, 2008, pp 2339–2349

Truog RD, Campbell ML, Curtis JR, et al: Recommendations for end-of-life care in the intensive care unit: a consensus statement by the American College [corrected] of Critical Care Medicine. Crit Care Med 36:953–963, 2008

Uniform Health-Care Decisions Act of 1993, § 1(3). Available at: http://www.law.upenn.edu/bll/archives/ulc/fnact99/1990s/uhcda93.htm. Accessed June 25, 2010.

Vellinga A, Smit JH, van Leeuwen E, et al: Instruments to assess decision-making capacity: an overview. Int Psychogeriatr 16:397–419, 2004

Walton V: Con man sentenced to 20 years. Birmingham News, February 2, 2002, p 11-A

Waltz J, Scheuneman T: Informed consent to therapy. Northwest University Law Review 64:628–650, 1970

Wan H, Sengupta M, Velkoff VA, et al: 65+ in the United States: 2005. Current Population Reports, Special Studies. Washington, DC, U.S. Census Bureau, 2005. Available at: http://www.census.gov/prod/2006pubs/p23–209.pdf. Accessed June 25, 2010.

Wanzer SH, Adelstein SJ, Cranford RE, et al: The physician's responsibility toward hopelessly ill patients. N Engl J Med 310:955–959, 1984

Weintraub D, Katz IR: Pharmacologic interventions for psychosis and agitation in neurodegenerative diseases: evidence about efficacy and safety. Psychiatr Clin North Am 28:941–983, 2005

Whitehouse P: Ethical issues, in The American Psychiatric Press Textbook of Geriatric Neuropsychiatry, 2nd Edition. Edited by Coffey CE, Cummings JL. Washington, DC, American Psychiatric Press, 2000, pp 935–944

Whitehouse P, Rabins PV: Quality of life and dementia. Alzheimer Dis Assoc Disord 6:135–137, 1992

Wimo A, Winblad B, Jonsson L: An estimate of the total worldwide societal costs of dementia in 2005. Alzheimers Dement 3:81–91, 2007

PART IV

Neuropsychiatric Syndromes and Disorders

15

Delirium

Larry E. Tune, M.D., M.A.S.
Marie A. DeWitt, M.D.

The term *delirium* originated from the Latin *delirare,* meaning "to deviate from a straight line" and from the Greek word *leros,* meaning "nonsense" (Adamis et al. 2007b; Lipowski 1990). Ancient Greeks and Romans recognized delirium as a distinct condition. The Greek physician Aretaeus differentiated acute conditions from chronic diseases and defined phrenitis and lethargus as the principal acute mental conditions. *Phrenitis* was defined as a syndrome characterized by restlessness, insomnia, and hallucinations. These symptoms contrasted with the undue quietness, dulling of the senses, and sleepiness characteristic of *lethargus.* Hippocrates wrote about the tendency of lethargus to cross over to phrenitis and vice versa. He attributed a poor prognosis to both of these conditions. The Persian physician Rhazes recognized not only the contrasting manifestations of agitated and lethargus deliriums but also their similarities—and he advocated for the use of one term, *sirsen,* to refer to both phrenitis and lethargus. Delirium was identified as a syndrome rather than a disease in the seventeenth century in Thomas Willis's treatise on mental disorders.

Numerous terms have been used to classify delirium. This alone complicates the dialogue on this topic across specialties. "Confusion" is widely used as a synonym for delirium. Outdated synonyms such as "altered mental status," "intensive care unit psychosis," "organic mental syndrome," "organic psychosis," "subacute befuddlement," and "acute confusional state" are used interchangeably with delirium. The *Diagnostic and Statistical Manual of Mental Disorders,* Third Edition (DSM–III; American Psychiatric Association 1980), provided operational diagnostic criteria for delirium, but it was classified as an "organic brain syndrome."

Current diagnostic requirements for delirium are set forth in DSM-IV-TR (American Psychiatric Association 2000). The essential feature of delirium is *inattention:* a disturbance of consciousness resulting in reduced clarity of awareness of the environment and reduced ability to focus, sustain, or shift attention. Additionally, a change in cognition or the development of a perceptual disturbance is required. Delirium reflects a change from previous level of functioning, develops over a relatively short period of time, and is usually attributed to single or multiple medical conditions, substance intoxication, or substance withdrawal.

Epidemiology

The prevalence of delirium varies widely according to the clinical setting and study population. Delirium in community-dwelling individuals is uncommon, with a point prevalence of 0.4% among those ages 18–64, 1% among those age 55 and older, and 14% among those age 85 years and older (Folstein et al. 1991). The prevalence of delirium was less than 1% in community-dwelling individuals without dementia age 75 and older (Andrew et al. 2006). In nursing homes and post–acute care settings, nearly 60% of the residents age 75 and older are delirious compared with 35% in personal care homes and 35% living independently with the assistance of home health services (Kiely et al. 2004; Roche 2003; Sandberg et al. 1998). Approximately 10% of individuals age 65 and older presenting to an emergency department have delirium (Elie et al. 2000; Murphy 2000). There is a 15%–25% prevalence of delirium at time of hospital admission (all age groups); in individuals age 65 and older, 30% are delirious on the day of hospital admission (Edlund et al. 2006; Inouye 2006). Another 10%–30% of the general hospital population develops delirium during their hospitalization (Inouye 2006). Delirium has been found to be

- More common in individuals with preexisting brain pathology. One study of acute stroke found a 13% prevalence of delirium in patients under age 85 years. Overall, delirium occurs in up to 50% of all patients after an acute stroke (Caeiro et al. 2004a; Ferro et al. 2002; McManus et al. 2007; Oldenbeuving et al. 2007). Of the patients with traumatic brain injury admitted to an inpatient neurological rehabilitation unit, 70% were delirious on admission, and delirium persisted at time of discharge in 30% of the patients (Nakase-Thompson et al. 2004). Dementia plus coexisting delirium is common. Nearly 15% of community-dwelling individuals and 50%–75% of hospitalized patients with dementia had superimposed delirium (Fick et al. 2002, 2005).

- Most prevalent in intensive care units (ICUs). Approximately 60% of patients younger than 65 and 70% of those age 65 and older have delirium during their hospitalization. Rates higher than 80% have been reported (Ely et al. 2001a, 2001c; Peterson et al. 2006). Nearly 75% of the patients in the surgical ICU and 67% of the patients in the trauma ICU (mean ages=55 and 41, respectively) were delirious during their ICU hospitalization (Pandharipande et al. 2007). Prevalence of delirium is higher in patients receiving mechanical ventilation (80%) compared with patients who did not require mechanical ventilation (50%) (Ely et al. 2001c).
- Common in postoperative patients. Rates vary drastically depending on the procedure performed. Fewer than 5% of patients undergoing cataract surgery, 40% of patients undergoing vascular surgery, and 60% of elderly traumatic orthopedic patients experience postoperative delirium (Amador and Goodwin 2005; Chang et al. 2008). The literature on postoperative delirium is complicated because preoperative delirium is rarely considered.
- Very common in hospitalized patients who are terminally ill or immunocompromised. The incidence of delirium in patients the first 30 days after bone marrow transplantation is between 50% and 75% (Fann 2000; Fann et al. 2002). Approximately 30%–40% of patients hospitalized with AIDS are delirious at the time of admission (Breitbart et al. 1996). Twenty-five percent of patients hospitalized with cancer and up to 40% of patients with cancer experience delirium (Fann 2000). Delirium near the end of life, sometimes referred to as *terminal delirium,* is quite common: 85% of individuals with a terminal illness develop delirium in the last weeks of life (Breitbart and Alici 2008; Lawlor et al. 2000b).

Outcomes

Delirium is associated with adverse outcomes. Mortality is substantially increased in delirious patients. In-hospital mortality may be as high as 30%, with an additional 25% mortality at 6 months posthospitalization, contributing to the total 60% mortality a year after hospitalization (Adamis et al. 2007a; Inouye et al. 1999b; Leslie et al. 2005). There is a positive correlation between delirium severity and mortality (Leslie et al. 2005; McAvay et al. 2006; McCusker et al. 2002).

In the elderly, delirium rarely resolves immediately or completely on resolution of the precipitating medical condition (Adamis et al. 2007a; Engel and Romano 2004; Inouye et al. 1998; Jackson et al. 2004; Katz et al. 2001; Marcantonio et al. 2003; McCusker et al. 2001, 2003; Sylvestre et al. 2006; Wacker et al. 2006). Inattention, disorientation, and impaired memory are the most common symptoms to persist (McCusker et al. 2003). Between 15% and 40% of patients who were delirious during hospitalization remained delirious at the time of hospital discharge (Inouye et al. 2007; McAvay et al. 2006). Delirium persisted for 45%, 33%, 25%, and 21% of patients at discharge, 1, 3, and 6 months, respectively (Cole et al. 2009). Poor outcomes (e.g., institutionalization, death) were strongly associated with persistent delirium. Delirious patients are twice as likely to have cognitive impairment at a 2-year follow-up compared with nondelirious matched control subjects (Dolan et al. 2000). Approximately 40%–55% of individuals had dementia by the end of 2-year follow-up, although as many as half of patients likely had undetected dementia before the delirious episode (Francis and Kapoor 1990; McCusker et al. 2001; Meagher 2001; Rahkonen et al. 2000, 2001). In cases of preexisting dementia, delirium accelerates the rate of cognitive decline of the underlying dementia (Fick et al. 2002).

Delirium is associated with a multitude of other negative outcomes. Delirious patients are at an increased risk for complications during their hospitalization, including falls, pressure ulcers, infections, and use of restraints. Length of hospitalization is increased by an average of 5–10 days, which is likely the result of behavioral manifestations of delirium complicating care and the need for placement into a facility on discharge (Adamis et al. 2006; Saravay et al. 2004). Nursing home placement is increased two- to threefold in delirious elderly hospitalized patients (Inouye et al. 1998; McAvay et al. 2006). In the ICU, delirium is associated with an increased risk of reintubation and is the strongest predictor of hospital length of stay (Ely et al. 2001a; Pun and Ely 2007). In postoperative patients, delirium is associated with increased risk of complications, longer recovery periods, longer hospitalizations, and increased long-term disability (Fann 2000).

Costs associated with delirium are estimated to be near $150 billion annually (compared with $92 and $258 billion spent for diabetes mellitus and cardiovascular disease, respectively; Inouye and Ferrucci 2006; Leslie et al. 2008). Medicare expenditures for hospitalization attributable to delirium are in excess of $7 billion annually (Inouye and Ferrucci 2006). Delirium is estimated to increase health care costs by more than $60,000 per delirious patient for the year following a delirious episode, with most of the cost burden attributed to nursing home care and inpatient expenses (Leslie et al. 2008).

Clinical Features and Presentation

The core symptom of delirium is *inattention,* which includes difficulty establishing, maintaining, or shifting attention (Burns et al. 2004). Impairment in attention may manifest as disorientation, impaired comprehension, distractibility, hypervigilance, disorganized thought process, poor concentration, and memory impairment. This inattention, which often go unnoticed, is usually present for at least 1–2 days before the onset of associated frank behavioral symptoms (Saravay et al. 2004). Disturbance of consciousness includes not only impairment in attention but also a reduced clarity of awareness. Both disorientation and memory impairment—specifically, working memory—are present in as many as 90% of patients (Gupta et al. 2008). Disorganized thought process as evidenced by the presence of tangentiality, loose associations, or circumstantiality occurs in up to 80% of delirious episodes (Gupta et al. 2008).

Behavioral symptoms are common in delirium. Psychotic symptoms, including hallucinations and delusions, occur in at least 50% of patients (Gupta et al. 2008; Webster and Holroyd 2000). Hallucinations are usually visual; however, less frequently auditory, tactile, olfactory, and gustatory hallucinations have been documented. Delusions often have an oneiroid (dreamlike or nightmarelike) quality and incorporate themes of impending danger, misidentification, or bizarre occurrences in the environment. Alterations or lability of mood and affect are found in 75% of cases (Gupta et al. 2008). Speech and language disturbances, including dysnomias, paraphasias, and incoherency, occur in more than half of delirious episodes (Gupta et al. 2008). Neurological symptoms, including dysgraphia, constructional apraxia, tremor, asterixis, myoclonus, and changes in reflex and tone, also may be present.

Disturbances in circadian rhythm manifesting as alterations in sleep patterns or as diurnal variation of symptoms are common. Nearly 60% of patients experience diurnal variation of symptoms, half have evening or nighttime delirium, and slightly fewer having fluctuating delirium throughout the day and night (Edlund et al. 2006). Disturbances in the normal wake-sleep cycle are found in as many as 95% of delirious patients. In many delirious individuals, the distinction between sleep and wakefulness is less obvious because wakeful periods may be experienced as dreamlike states, leaving a question as to whether delirium is better classified as a disorder of circadian rhythm or wakefulness (Gupta et al. 2008; Lipowski 1990).

Subtypes

Delirium is usually subclassified as hyperactive, hypoactive, and mixed (with features of both hyperactive and hypoactive) subtypes (Camus et al. 2000a; Liptzin and Levkoff 1992; Meagher et al. 2008b; Trzepacz and Dew 1995). The clinical significance of these subtypes is unclear. Few consistent data support the theory that the etiology, treatment, and outcome vary according to subtype. However, the lack of a universally accepted method for subtyping has made comparisons across studies difficult (Meagher et al. 2008a).

Agitation, combativeness, restlessness, and insomnia are generally suggestive of the hyperactive subtype, whereas somnolence, psychomotor retardation, and withdrawn affect are indicative of the hypoactive subtype—similar to Aretaeus's ancient distinction between phrenitis and lethargus, respectively. Table 15–1 shows examples of hypoactive and hyperactive symptoms. The active and disruptive symptoms of hyperactive delirium result in a higher rate of recognition of this subtype, whereas up to 80% of cases of hypoactive delirium are undetected (O'Keefe and Lavan 1999).

The frequencies of delirium subtypes differ according to study population and classification system used. Estimates for hyperactive, hypoactive, and mixed subtypes of delirious states range from 20% to 45%, 25% to 30%, and 40% to 50%, respectively, although many studies cite significantly higher rates of hypoactive delirium (Camus et al. 2000b; O'Keefe and Lavan 1999). Three-quarters of all delirious states are mixed or hypoactive (Stagno et al. 2004). In delirious ICU patients, nearly 40% have hypoactive, 55% have mixed, and as few as 2% have hyperactive subtypes (Peterson et al. 2006). In the trauma ICU and surgical ICU, the prevalence of hypoactive, mixed, and hyperactive subtypes of delirium was 60%–65%, 6%–9%, and 0%–1%, respectively (Pandharipande et al. 2007). Near the end of life, 80% of patients experience hypoactive delirium (Casarett et al. 2001).

Prodromal Phase

Delirium is usually defined as having an acute onset, with symptoms developing over a matter of hours to days. A prodromal phase has been recognized (Cole 2004; Duppils and Wikblad 2004; Gupta et al. 2008; Sirois 1988; Tune 2008), which may be as short as a few hours to as long as several weeks. Tune (2008) found that delirious symptoms in acutely hospitalized patients with dementia and delirium were often emerging up to 1 month before hospitalization. During this period, an individual may experience disorientation, memory difficulties, disorganized thought process, day-night confusion, and impaired concentration (de Jonghe et al. 2007; Tune 2008). Mood symptoms including anxiety, depression, and irritability may complicate recognition of the underlying subclinical delirium. Fatigue, sleep disturbance, vivid dreams, psychomotor restlessness, hypersensitivity to light or sound, headaches, and a sense of general uneasiness are also characteristics of this prodromal phase.

The prodromal phase of delirium may be understood as subsyndromal delirium, which is defined as the presence of

TABLE 15–1. Liptzin and Levkoff's (1992) examples of hypoactive and hyperactive symptoms on the Delirium Symptom Interview

Hyperactive symptoms	Hypoactive symptoms
Hypervigilance	Unawareness
Restlessness	Decreased alertness
Fast or loud speech	Sparse or slow speech
Irritability	Lethargy
Combativeness	Slowed movements
Impatience	Staring
Swearing	Apathy
Singing	
Laughing	
Uncooperativeness	
Euphoria	
Anger	
Wandering	
Easy startling	
Fast motor responses	
Distractibility	
Tangentiality	
Nightmares	
Persistent thoughts	

Source. Reprinted from Liptzin B, Levkoff SE: "An Empirical Study of Delirium Subtypes." *British Journal of Psychiatry* 161:843–845, 1992. Used with permission.

many of the core delirium features without satisfying the full diagnostic criteria for delirium (Levkoff et al. 1996). An estimated 30%–50% of patients in the ICU and postacute nursing home facilities have subsyndromal delirium (Marcantonio et al. 2005; Ouimet et al. 2007). Length of hospitalization, morbidity, and mortality for individuals with subsyndromal delirium are intermediate between those with and without delirium, supporting the theory that delirium exists along a continuum (Ouimet et al. 2007).

Neurobiology

Most neurobiological studies of delirium focus on disturbances in the circuitry or neurochemistry associated with consciousness, attentiveness, and cognition. It has been suggested that precipitants of delirium can usefully be divided into two distinct categories: direct brain insults and aberrant stress responses (MacLullich et al. 2008). Several biomarkers for delirium have been identified; however, the pathophysiology of delirium remains elusive. It is hypothesized that delirium may be an outcome after activation of either or both of two stress responses: inflammatory processes or activation of the limbic-hypothalamic-pituitary-adrenal axis (MacLullich et al. 2008).

Cholinergic Transmission

Acetylcholine is a central neurotransmitter involved in consciousness, memory, and attention (Flacker and Lipsitz 1999a; Hshieh et al. 2008; Lipowski 1987; Tune 2001). Cholinergic disruption may be the "final common pathway" of delirium. Several distinct animal models of delirium support this common pathway through the reduction of cerebral cholinergic neurotransmission (Flacker and Lipsitz 1999b; Trzepacz 1994; Tune 2001; Tune and Egeli 1999). Exposure to anticholinergic load as a result of the cumulative effects of multiple medications with anticholinergic properties is an accepted cause of delirium (Han et al. 2001; Mach et al. 1995; Tune and Bylsma 1991). This observed relation has led to the theory that anticholinergic burden or anticholinergic load is a frequent cause of delirium, especially in older adults (Tune 2000). In addition to individual differences in pharmacokinetics, innate anticholinergic activity, and lack of awareness of anticholinergic effects of drug metabolites, several medications commonly prescribed to elderly patients have unappreciated anticholinergic effects, which makes estimating anticholinergic burden from a list of medications inaccurate (Tune et al. 1992). Studies that use an anticholinergic radioreceptor assay to measure total serum anticholinergic activity have consistently found correlations between anticholinergic levels and the presence and the severity of delirium and performance on the Mini-Mental State Examination, whereas a decline in serum anticholinergic activity has been correlated with resolution of delirium (Caeiro et al. 2004b; Flacker and Lipsitz 1999b; Mulsant et al. 2003; Mussi et al. 1999; Tune and Egeli 1999; Tune et al. 1981, 1993). One study of four plasma esterase levels, including acetylcholinesterase, found lower plasma esterase levels among individuals who already had or were developing delirium when compared with individuals without delirium (White et al. 2005). Physostigmine, an acetylcholinesterase inhibitor, has been effective in reversing delirium associated with anticholinergic medications (Tune 2001).

Cholinergic deficiency can result from several different mechanisms, including impaired synthesis of acetylcholine, impaired cholinergic synaptic mechanisms, global stressors, and neurotransmitter imbalance (Hshieh et al. 2008). Associated with low albumin (a known risk factor for delirium), poor nutrition impairs acetyl coenzyme A production, thereby limiting acetylcholine synthesis. Postsynaptic muscarinic receptors such as the M_1 receptor subtype—which is involved in perception, attention, and cognitive functioning and found widely throughout the brain—have been implicated in delirium when they are competitively antagonized by anticholinergic compounds (Blass and Gibson 1999). Cerebral ischemia is associated with a stress response and a precipitous rise in levels of glutamate and acetylcholine, thereby disrupting acetylcholine synthesis and creating a state of cholinergic deficit (Hshieh et al. 2008). In general, the stress response can be activated by a variety of environmental and medical stressors, triggering cytokine release (Eikelenboom and Hoogendijk 1999). Cytokines may promote a cholinergic deficit state either directly by reducing choline acetyltransferase, which is necessary for the synthesis of acetylcholine, or indirectly by increasing permeability of the blood-brain barrier and altering the equilibrium of neurotransmitter systems (Broadhurst and Wilson 2001).

The cholinergic system is closely linked with monoamine activity. Dopamine, serotonin, or norepinephrine system perturbations may also alter cholinergic functioning. Age-related decreases in dopamine may contribute to the increased prevalence of delirium in older patients (Stagno et al. 2004). Dopamine excess is linked to decreases in acetylcholine and hyperactive delirium, offering a possible neurobiological explanation for the different presentations of delirium (Trzepacz 1999). The effectiveness of dopamine antagonists—most notably, antipsychotics—in the management of delirium may be the result of decreasing dopamine levels, which reciprocally increase acetylcholine.

Brain Pathology

It has been suggested that dementia and delirium are points along the same continuum of cognitive disorders because of the substantial overlap in their pathophysiology (Hshieh et al. 2008). Both delirium and dementia appear to share several pathophysiological features, including deficits in cholinergic transmission, decreased cerebral metabolism, and an inflammatory response (Eikelenboom and Hoogendijk 1999; Minger et al. 2000). A genetic study found an association among dementia, delirium, and apolipoprotein E-ε4 allele, which is associated with longer duration of delirium (Ely et al. 2007). Finally, conditions such as dementia of Alzheimer's type, which is associated with a state of cholinergic deficiency, increase vulnerability to delirium.

Cerebral lesions in delirious patients are more commonly localized to the right hemisphere. Follow-up neurological assessment in subjects who previously experienced an episode of delirium revealed impairments in right hemisphere tasks (Mach et al. 1996). Localized neuroanatomical lesions may be associated with particular symptom presentations during a delirious episode. Marked inattention may be due to disturbances in the nondominant posterior parietal cortex, whereas injury to the middle temporal gyrus and frontostriatal injury may lead to hyperactivity and hypoactivity subtypes, respectively (Mori and Yamadori 1987). Cortical atrophy, ventricular enlargement, and white matter lesions also have been associated with delirium; however, it is unclear if these findings could represent premorbid disease causing increased vulnerability in the development of delirium (Alsop et al. 2006; Soiza et al. 2008).

Cerebrovascular Flow and Cortical Activity

Neuroimaging studies of delirium are understandably limited. Changes in cerebrovascular flow have been observed in the midst of delirious episodes. During a delirious episode, global cerebral blood flow is reduced up to 40% (Alsop et al. 2006). In addition to a global reduction in cerebral blood flow, regional blood flow may be reduced (Yokota et al. 2003). Single-photon emission computed tomography (SPECT) scans suggest that regional reductions in blood flow may occur in the frontal or parietal lobes during a delirious episode. These changes in blood flow usually resolve on resolution of the delirium (Fong et al. 2006).

Electroencephalographic (EEG) monitoring during delirious episodes usually demonstrates increased slowing of cortical activity, as manifested by increased delta and theta waves, isolated to the anterior cingulate cortex and the right frontoparietal region (Jacobson and Jerrier 2000; Reischies et al. 2005). Delirium associated with withdrawal from alcohol and other sedatives usually yields electroencephalograms with fast, low-voltage activity (Engel and Romano 2004). Quantitative EEG studies in patients with delirium have reported significant reductions of relative power in alpha, increased theta and delta activity, and slowing of the peak and mean frequencies (Koponen et al. 1989).

Risk Factors

Several risk factors have been identified for delirium (Burns et al. 2004; Elie et al. 1998; Inouye 1994; Inouye and Charpentier 1996; Inouye et al. 1993; Laurila et al. 2008; Pisani et al. 2007). These variables may be classified as either predisposing or precipitating risk factors (Inouye 1999; Inouye and Charpentier 1996; Inouye et al. 1993; Laurila et al. 2008). The risk of developing delirium can be conceptualized as an inverse relation between 1) patient vulnerability, based on predisposing risk factors and protective factors; and 2) the severity of insult, caused by precipitating factors (Figure 15–1; Inouye and Charpentier 1996). Some of these risk factors are modifiable and provide a potential point of intervention to prevent or limit the course of delirium (see section "Management" later in this chapter).

Certain demographic and environmental factors are highly associated with risk of developing delirium. Age is consistently associated with an increased risk of delirium (Schuurmans et al. 2001). Education level is inversely associated with delirium risk, supporting the role of cognitive reserve as an attenuating

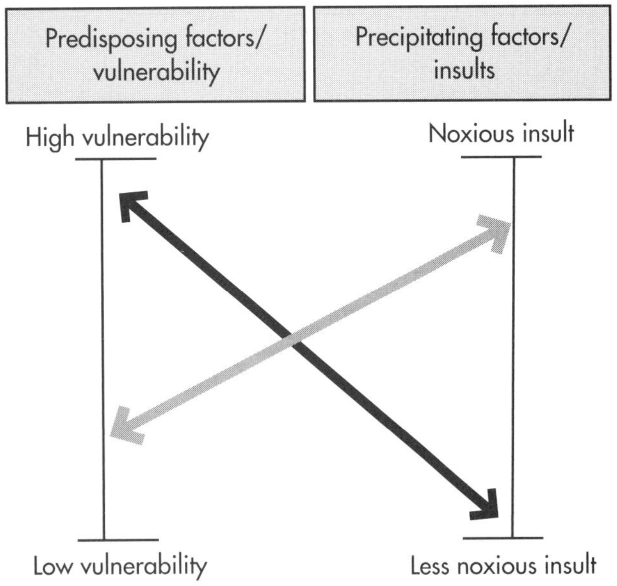

FIGURE 15–1. Risk of developing delirium.

There is an inverse relation between patient vulnerability (based on predisposing risk factors and protective factors) and the severity of insult (caused by precipitating factors).

Source. Reprinted from Inouye SK, Charpentier PA: "Precipitating Factors for Delirium in Hospitalized Elderly Persons: Predictive Model and Interrelationship With Baseline Vulnerability." *Journal of the American Medical Association* 275:852–857, 1996. Used with permission. Copyright© 1996 American Medical Association. All rights reserved.

factor of delirium vulnerability (Jones et al. 2006). Environmental factors such as unfamiliar surroundings, sensory deprivation, and sleep deprivation are risk factors for development of delirium. Clinically, this translates into an increased risk of delirium associated with room and staff changes, lack of hearing and visual aids, frequent nighttime awakenings, and limited cues indicating day or night. Placement in the ICU, the use of physical restraints, and the presence of an indwelling urinary catheter also have been associated with the development of delirium (Schuurmans et al. 2001).

Premorbid central nervous system pathology increases vulnerability to delirium. Preexisting cognitive impairment is a consistent risk factor across medical, surgical, and psychiatric patient populations. It is speculated that more than 50% of delirious patients have underlying mild cognitive impairment or dementia, and some studies suggest a much higher percentage. Direct insults to the brain such as recent stroke or traumatic brain injury significantly increase the risk of developing delirium. In the acute stroke population, the use of anticholinergic medications before the stroke, use of nonneuroleptic anticholinergic medications during hospitalization, medical complications, and intracranial hemorrhage were all independent predictors of development of delirium (Caeiro et al. 2004a, 2004b).

Presence and severity of comorbid medical conditions are well-established risk factors for delirium. Generally, conditions that trigger stress responses or cause direct brain insults are associated with increased vulnerability to delirium (MacLullich et al. 2008). Common specific risk factors include dehydration, malnutrition, electrolyte or metabolic abnormalities, hypoglycemia, hypoxia, infection, hepatic impairment, renal impairment, cardiac ischemia, and alcohol abuse. Surgery, the number of procedures performed during hospitalization, starting more than three newly prescribed medications during hospitalization, and the use of neuroleptics or narcotics were associated with an increased risk of delirium (Schuurmans et al. 2001).

Surgery conveys a greater risk of delirium for several potential reasons. These include the type of surgery, volume and electrolyte shifts, perioperative medication changes, reactive inflammatory response associated with surgery, and exposure to general anesthesia. Most general anesthetics are associated with development of postoperative delirium. Isoflurane is strongly associated with postoperative delirium and dementia (Xie et al. 2006). Additional specific risk factors vary according to the type of surgery (Fricchione et al. 2008). For all patients undergoing cardiac surgery, stroke was the most significant predictor of delirium, and need for urgent operation, intraoperative hemofiltration, operative time of greater than 3 hours, and high perioperative transfusion requirement were independent perioperative predictors of delirium (Bucerius et al. 2004). In older cardiac surgery patients, preoperative cardiogenic shock, cerebral or peripheral vascular disease, atrial fibrillation, diabetes mellitus, or a cardiac ejection fraction less than 30% increased the risk of developing postoperative delirium (Bucerius et al. 2004). In patients undergoing elective noncardiac surgery, greater preoperative risk was conferred with older age, alcohol abuse, impaired cognition, poor functional status, and markedly abnormal electrolytes, whereas perioperative factors that increased risk included prolonged waiting time for surgery, low intraoperative hemoglobin level, intraoperative blood loss, postoperative transfusions, and lower postoperative hematocrit level (Schuurmans et al. 2001). Patients may have delirium preoperatively. Nearly a third of elderly patients undergoing surgical correction of femoral neck fractures were found to have delirium *before* surgery (Edlund et al. 2001). Risk factors for the presence of preoperative delirium in this population included premorbid dementia, use of medications with anticholinergic properties, previous delirious episodes, and a history of indoor falls (Edlund et al. 2001). Both postoperative pain and the medications used to treat postoperative pain have been associated with delirium.

Medications deserve particular attention. Numerous classes of medication have been associated with development of delirium (see Chapter 9, "Geriatric Neuropsychopharmacology," for further discussion). It is estimated that medications may be the sole cause of delirium in up to 40% of delirious episodes in the elderly (Ancelin et al. 2006). Theoretically, nearly any substance that crosses the blood-brain barrier has the potential to cause delirium; however, some medications appear to be more deliriogenic than others. Psychoactive medications have been shown to be causally linked in at least 15% of delirium cases. Anesthetics, antibiotics, anticholinergics, β-blockers, calcium channel blockers, chemotherapeutics, corticosteroids, diuretics, histamine blockers, nonsteroidal anti-inflammatory agents, and opioids, among others, all have been associated with the development of delirium (Ancelin et al. 2006; Gaudreau et al, 2005). In this view, it is important to realize that many of these categories of medications have more than one effect. For example, anesthetics and most opiates have anticholinergic effects. Polypharmacy confers a markedly increased risk of development of delirium. As stated in the "Neurobiology" section earlier in this chapter, the cumulative anticholinergic load of most medications and their metabolites is not appreciated. The cumulative anticholinergic load of multiple medications, even at relatively low doses, in combination with the documented impairment in enzyme activity during a delirious episode, often initiates or prolongs delirious episodes.

Detection and Recognition

Delirium may be the manifesting feature of an undetected medical illness. Poor awareness of the symptoms of delirium, lack of implementation of standard screening instruments, and unfamiliarity with bedside evaluation for delirium result in most cases of delirium going unrecognized (Table 15–2).

Outside of psychiatric units, it is estimated that at least 50% of delirium cases are unrecognized by physicians. In one study, the overall rate of recorded diagnosis of delirium or a related diagnosis in hospitalized elderly veterans was only 4% (Kales et al. 2003). Emergency department physicians detect 35% of cases of delirium in older adults and use the term *delirium* in only 60% of these cases (Elie et al. 2000). Among patients given the diagnosis of delirium by a psychiatric consultation team, referring clinicians fail to establish the diagnosis of delirium or a confusional state in nearly 50% of cases. Referring clinicians were more likely to attribute symptoms to something other than delirium if the patient was oriented or had a history of major mental illness (Swigart et al. 2008). When elements of delirium are recognized, such as disorientation, they are frequently listed as a symptom without further consideration of delirium as a possible diagnosis (Engel and Romano 2004).

Nurses are in an excellent position to monitor for symptoms of delirium. They have the most extensive direct patient contact, and they are more likely to obtain collateral information from spouses, family, or caregivers (Schuurmans et al. 2001). However, the ability of nurses to accurately diagnose delirium is limited by their education and training (Inouye et al. 2001). More thorough clinical evaluation and a higher index of suspicion are appropriate when evaluating individuals who have preexisting dementia, vision impairment, and hypoactive symptoms or who are age 80 and older; nurses are less likely to recognize symptoms of delirium in these individuals (Inouye et al. 2001). A collaborative approach between nurses, who are able to document and monitor for symptoms over a period of hours, and physicians, who are trained at diagnosis, might decrease the number of unrecognized delirious episodes.

Delirium is usually undiagnosed in the ICU, which may be the result of its relatively common occurrence and subsequent view that the symptoms of delirium are "normal" or "expected" in this setting (Chevrolet and Jolliet 2007; Pandharipande et al. 2005). International and national governing professional bodies recommend that patients in the ICU be monitored daily for the development of delirium. Despite these recommendations, only 5%–40% of ICU professionals screen for delirium, with only 15%–50% of these professionals using a formal assessment tool (Ely et al. 2004; Thomason et al. 2005; Van Eijk et al. 2008).

Validated delirium screening scales include the Confusion Assessment Method (CAM), Delirium Symptom Interview, NEECHAM Confusion Scale, Cognitive Test for Delirium (CTD), and Delirium Observation Screening Scale. The CAM is likely the most recognized of the screening instruments and was developed on the basis of DSM-III-R criteria for delirium (American Psychiatric Association 1987). It has now been validated against DSM-IV criteria (American Psychiatric Association 1994; Inouye et al. 1990; Laurila et al. 2002). A version of the CAM for use in the ICU (CAM-ICU), specifically with mechanically ventilated patients, also has been validated (Ely et al. 2001b). Most screening instruments may be biased toward the recognition of the hyperactive subtype of delirium (Gupta et al. 2008; Meagher et al. 2008a). Additional instruments are available for assessing symptom severity. The Memorial Delirium Assessment Scale, Delirium Rating Scale—Revised-98 (DRS-R-98), Confusional State Evaluation, Delirium Severity Scale, Delirium Index, and Delirium-O-Meter were all developed to quantify severity of delirious symptoms.

TABLE 15–2. Clinical features of delirium and bedside clinical examination[a]

Disturbance of consciousness, arousal, awareness	**Disorganized thinking**
Ask the patient to describe surroundings with eyes closed and ask, "What color is the wall?" Ask the patient, "Are you feeling 100% awake?" and if not, "How awake do you feel?"	Ask patient an open-ended question (e.g., "Describe your medical condition."). Listen for rambling, incoherent speech or tangential and circumstantial thought process.
Attention disturbances	**Delusions**
Is the patient easily distracted by outside stimuli or overabsorbed in a task, such as picking at the bed sheet? Test digit span, starting with 3, 4, then 5 digits forward, followed by 3, 4, then 5 digits backward.	Ask patient, "Are you feeling unsafe here?" Find out from family or staff whether patient is acting in a paranoid, suspicious, hypervigilant, fearful, or hostile fashion.
Disorientation	**Psychomotor disturbances**
Check for orientation to time, place, and person. Test the limits of orientation (e.g., year, month, date, day, and time). Do not assume full orientation because patients know the year and the month.	Observe whether the patient is restless and agitated or slow and hypoactive. Use observations of family, staff, or both to assess psychomotor activity over previous 24 hours.
	Sleep-wakefulness cycle disturbances
Cognitive disturbances including memory impairment, executive dysfunction, aphasia, paraphasia, dysnomia, apraxia, agnosia	Determine from family, staff, or both whether the patient has been "awake most of the night, and asleep most of the day."
Test registration and immediate recall (use different words for successive evaluations). Test speech fluency, naming, reading, repetition, writing, comprehension. Perform Clock Drawing Test.[b]	**Acute onset, fluctuating course** Staff and family are often the best informants. The clinical presentation can be abrupt in onset (e.g., hours to days), and each of the symptoms of delirium can fluctuate over the course of a 24-hour period.
Perceptual disturbances (illusions, hallucinations)	**Neurological signs consistent with delirium (e.g., asterixis, frontal release signs, myoclonus)**
Ask specifically about hallucinations (e.g., "Are you seeing or hearing strange things?"). Use nursing or family member reports to determine incidents of perceptual disturbances.	These findings are supportive of delirium. An electroencephalogram can also be supportive of a delirium diagnosis (diffuse slowing) or can reveal seizure activity.

[a]Based on clinical experience assessing the *Diagnostic and Statistical Manual of Mental Disorders,* 4th Edition, Text Revision (DSM-IV-TR), components of delirium.

[b]Clock Drawing Test primarily assesses the severity of cognitive impairment. Despite its frequent use in the clinical setting, it has low utility in differentiating delirium from dementia when used alone.

Source. Reprinted from Breitbart W, Alici Y: "Agitation and Delirium at the End of Life: We Couldn't Manage Him." *Journal of the American Medical Association* 300:2898–2910, 2008. Used with permission.

Differential Diagnosis

Discriminating delirium from primary mood, psychotic, or cognitive disorders may be difficult because of the overlap of symptoms. Hypoactive delirium can mimic symptoms of depression (see Chapter 19, "Mood Disorders"), whereas hyperactive delirium may resemble a mixed, manic, or hypomanic mood state or an agitated depression (Leonard et al. 2008). Affective lability that waxes and wanes throughout the day is more common in delirium (Leonard et al. 2008). Hallucinations and delusions in delirium raise the possibility of a primary psychotic disorder such as schizophrenia (see Chapter 21, "Psychosis"). Simple, bizarre, or paranoid delusions and visual hallucinations usually occur during a delirious episode, whereas auditory hallucinations and complex or systematized delusions are more characteristic of schizophrenia. The disturbance of consciousness, fluctuations in symptoms, and acute to subacute onset associated with delirium contrast with the typically intact level of consciousness, consistency of symptoms, and chronic course of schizophrenia.

Distinguishing delirium from dementia (discussed in Chapter 16, "Alzheimer's Disease and the Frontotemporal Dementia Syndromes") can be challenging, especially when an individual's premorbid cognitive status is unknown. Most uncomplicated dementias lack the relatively acute onset, fluctuation in symptoms throughout the day and over the course of days, disturbed consciousness, and inattention that are characteristic of delirium. Neuropsychiatric symptoms are common in the course of the dementing process (Aalten et al. 2005). Distinguishing features of dementia with Lewy bodies (DLB)—with hallmark symptoms including disturbed attention, visual hallucinations, and fluctuation in symptoms—make it particularly difficult to differentiate from delirium; however, the presence of parkinsonian symptoms, autonomic dysfunction, or sensitivity to neuroleptics should raise suspicion for DLB. Several screening instruments, including the CAM, DRS-R-98, and CTD, have been validated in their ability to distinguish delirium from dementia, further supporting the role of validated screening instruments in evaluating for the presence of delirium.

Delirium superimposed on dementia is common and complicates the diagnosis of delirium. As many as 90% of hospitalized and 13% of community-dwelling individuals with dementia have comorbid delirium (Fick et al. 2002, 2005). Indeed, some investigators have speculated that dementia with psychosis or dementia with behavioral disturbance is a variant of dementia with superimposed delirium (Meagher and Trzepacz 2007; Minger et al. 2000). Delirium in individuals with dementia is phenomenologically similar to the delirium in individuals without dementia. However, patients with comorbid dementia tend to have an increased number of delirious symptoms, such as more psychomotor agitation, disorganized thinking, and disorientation (Cole et al. 2002).

Clinical Evaluation

Usually, multiple etiologies are identified for a single delirious episode. This leads to an unclear specific etiology in 50%–75% of cases (Camus et al. 2000b; Stagno et al. 2004). Fewer than 20% of patients have a single etiology of delirium, and approximately 90% have up to four possible etiologies (Camus et al. 2000b). Specific populations often have their particular vulnerabilities and precipitants (e.g., dehydration is one of the common causes of delirium among terminally ill cancer patients) (Lawlor et al. 2000a).

Delirium requires an immediate, comprehensive assessment. A complete general medical examination that includes vital signs with oxygen saturation, neurological examination, and mental status examination should be performed. A broad review of the patient's medical history that includes talking to informants (e.g., family, caregivers, and nursing staff) is important to elucidate important historical information, including accurate medication history and recent changes that may be associated with the onset of delirium. A comprehensive review of the patient's medication list and discontinuation of any unnecessary medications is appropriate. Basic laboratory tests include a complete blood count and blood chemistries with a complete set of electrolytes, glucose level, serum urea nitrogen level, creatinine level, and liver enzymes; in addition, urinalysis, electrocardiogram, and chest radiograph should be obtained. Additional tests and studies, including a urine drug screen, measurement of serum levels of medications, lumbar puncture, and neuroimaging, can be ordered as clinically indicated.

Management

The most effective delirium management intervention is prevention. Once delirium is present, a thorough search for underlying causes is indicated because frequently the etiology is multifactorial (see section "Clinical Evaluation" earlier in this chapter). The reversibility of delirium on prompt treatment of underlying causes should not be underestimated. Management involves the implementation or continuation of several nonpharmacological strategies and the use of pharmacological interventions if indicated. The goals of management are to

- Alleviate anxiety and fear
- Control behavior with the least restrictive means necessary
- Promote a healthy wake-sleep cycle with appropriate levels of alertness and arousal.

A critical component of delirium management is nonpharmacological intervention. Although a Cochrane Database review concluded that there was a lack of robust information supporting nonpharmacological prevention of delirium, several successful interventions have been published (Cole 2004; Flaherty et al. 2003; Inouye 2000, 2004; Siddiqi et al. 2007; Weber et al.. 2004). The Delirium Prevention Trial used the Hospital Elder Life Program (HELP) to target modifiable risk factors—such as cognitive impairment, sleep deprivation, immobility, visual and hearing impairments, and dehydration—and to implement standardized interventions. The intervention resulted in a substantial decrease in the incidence of delirium, number of delirious episodes, and total delirium days (Inouye et al. 1999a). Several other interventions that target population-specific risk factors have been used with inconsistent results (Bergmann et al. 2005; Bo et al. 2009; Inouye 2000; Marcantonio et al. 2001; Michaud et al. 2007; Milisen et al. 2005; Naughton et al. 2005; Pitkälä et al. 2006, 2008; Vollmer et al. 2007; Young et al. 2008).

Pharmacological Intervention

Medications to manage delirium should be restricted to situations in which the symptoms cause severe behavioral or emotional disturbance (e.g., severe agitation or anxiety) that places the patient or others at risk of harm or interferes with essential treatment and cannot be managed with nonpharmacological methods. Antipsychotics remain the medication class of choice in the pharmacological management of delirium (American Psychiatric Association 1999; Cook 2004). Antipsychotics have been associated with significant improvement in or complete alleviation of both cognitive and noncognitive delirious symptoms (Bourne et al. 2008). A Cochrane Database review concluded that randomized controlled trials provide evidence for the effectiveness of antipsychotics for the treatment of delirium (Lonergan et al. 2007).

Although no consensus has been reached on a preferred first-line antipsychotic agent, haloperidol is often advocated because of its few active metabolites; minimal sedating side effects; negligible anticholinergic side effects; and availability in oral, intramuscular, and intravenous formulations (Attard et al. 2008). A hallmark study evaluating the treatment of delirium in hospitalized patients with AIDS found that low doses of chlorpromazine or haloperidol resulted in significant improvement in symptoms with a very low prevalence of extrapyramidal side effects (Breitbart et al. 1996). The efficacy of various second-generation antipsychotics—risperidone, olanzapine, and quetiapine—has been supported in various studies, and case reports have indicated the effective use of ziprasidone and aripiprazole (Greco et al. 2005; Schwartz and Masand 2002; Tune 2002). Low-dose haloperidol (<3 mg/day), risperidone, and olanzapine were equally effective in treating delirium without significant differences in adverse effects (Lonergan et al. 2007). These data indicate that second-generation antipsychotics and haloperidol show equal efficacy in the management of delirium in acutely ill patients (Rea et al. 2007). The American Psychiatric Association guidelines support the use of haloperidol, olanzapine, risperidone, quetiapine, and ziprasidone (American Psychiatric Association 1999; Cook 2004). The Society for Critical Care Medicine recommends treating delirium in critically ill patients with haloperidol while monitoring for electrocardiogram changes—notably, QTc prolongation (Siegal 2003). Depending on the patterns and severity of the targeted behavior, antipsychotic medication can be made available on as-needed basis or, if necessary, scheduled. The antipsychotics can be tapered off over several days 1–2 weeks after resolution of the targeted delirium symptom and overall improvement in delirium symptoms.

Lorazepam has been used as a first-line treatment for delirium as either monotherapy or in combination with an antipsychotic agent. It has been associated with excessive sedation, disinhibition, increased confusion, and prolongation and worsening of delirium symptoms (Pisani et al. 2009). A review article concluded that treatment of non–alcohol withdrawal delirium with lorazepam alone was ineffective and often associated with treatment-limiting adverse effects (Bourne et al. 2008; Jackson and Lipman 2004). Benzodiazepines are no longer recommended for management of uncomplicated non–alcohol withdrawal–related delirium (Lonergan et al. 2009).

Nontraditional pharmacotherapy has been considered in unique populations and when standard interventions have failed. In patients with continued behavioral symptoms despite adequate use of haloperidol or the atypical antipsychotics, trials of methotrimeprazine or chlorpromazine, two phenothiazine neuroleptics, or augmentation with lorazepam has been studied (Breitbart and Strout 2000; Stagno et al. 2004). In delirious patients with Parkinson's disease, management should be focused on decreasing (where clinically possible) deliriogenic Parkinson's disease medications. If necessary, quetiapine or lorazepam may be used for symptom control as these agents are less likely to exacerbate Parkinson's disease (see Chapter 24, "Parkinson's Disease and Movement Disorders"). Approximately 25% of delirious terminally ill patients require sedation, often with propofol or lorazepam, to provide comfort and symptom control (Casarett et al. 2001; Namba et al. 2007). Benzodiazepines are a first-line pharmacological treatment for delirium secondary to benzodiazepine, barbiturate, or alcohol withdrawal, as well as for delirium related to seizures, neuroleptic malignant syndrome, and Parkinson's disease (American Psychiatric Association 1999; Cook 2004; Inouye 2006).

Prophylactic antipsychotics have been used in patients undergoing surgical interventions. Prophylactic haloperidol was evaluated in an older population undergoing elective hip surgery. Although it was not effective at preventing delirium, prophylactic haloperidol reduced the severity and duration of delirious episodes (Kalisvaart et al. 2005). Prophylactic risperidone reduced the incidence of delirium by nearly two-thirds among patients who underwent elective cardiac surgery (Prakanrattana and Prapaitrakool 2007). Prophylactic olanzapine decreased the incidence of postoperative delirium in an orthopedic population (Bourne et al. 2008).

A small body of evidence supports the therapeutic role of cholinesterase inhibitors in treating drug-induced delirium and delirium superimposed on dementia (Bourne et al. 2008; Moretti et al. 2004). Randomized double-blind, placebo-controlled trials of donepezil in the prevention of postoperative delirium found no statistically significant difference, although a trend was observed when compared with placebo (Liptzin et al. 2005; Sampson et al. 2007). One recent double blind, placebo controlled trial of adjunctive therapy with rivastigmine was terminated because of increased mortality associated with rivastigmine (van Eijk et al. 2010). In this study, a sample size of 440 subjects was originally planned. However, the trial was abruptly stopped after 104 subjects because of increased mortality in the rivastigmine group (22%; 12 of 54 subjects) compared with the placebo group (8%; 4 of 50 subjects). A Cochrane Database review concluded that no conclusive evidence supported the use of cholinesterase inhibitors in the management of delirium (Overshott et al. 2008).

The Patient's Experience

Personal accounts of individuals who recovered from delirium articulate the extreme confusion and fear experienced during a delirious episode (Breitbart et al. 2002; Laitinen 1996; Minnick et al. 2001; Schofield 1997). Delusions in delirium are often due to the patient's misinterpretation of the surrounding environment. For some individuals, the experience is so harrowing and persistent that posttraumatic stress disorder (PTSD) becomes a long-lasting complication (DiMartini et al. 2007). Development of PTSD among patients who were hospitalized in the ICU was more likely if they recalled delusional memories, which were often paranoid; experienced prolonged sedation; or were placed in physical restraints without sedation (Jones et al. 2007). The presence of short-term memory impairment, increased severity of delirium, and perceptual disturbances predicted less common recall of the delirious episode (Breitbart et al. 2002). Hypoactive delirium was as distressing as hyperactive delirium (Breitbart et al. 2002).

Delirious patients routinely experience fear, anxiety, and feelings of being threatened, leading to a sense of hopelessness, loneliness, and depression (O'Malley et al. 2008). Visual hallucinations were recalled as common experiences and frequently served as sources of anxiety and fright (O'Malley et al. 2008). Patients felt distressed and humiliated when they were unable to understand their environment or communicate with others. The delirious state was described as "a borderland between external reality and imagination…conscious and unconscious…past and present" (Andersson et al. 2002). These self-accounts underscore the importance of addressing fear and anxiety in patients with delirium 1) by instituting (at least) simple practice interventions such as providing a calming atmosphere, verbal and written explanations of current circumstances, frequent reorientation, and copious reassurance; and 2) by encouraging the presence of trusted individuals such as close family members.

Key Points

- Delirium is a disorder of inattention that is often accompanied by confusion, disorganized thinking, disorientation, perceptual disturbances, wake-sleep cycle disturbances, memory impairment, and changes in psychomotor activity and may be further classified into hyperactive and hypoactive subtypes based on level of arousal and psychomotor activity.
- Delirium is often the result of reduced brain cholinergic activity effectively creating a cholinergic-deficient state.
- The risk of developing delirium can be conceptualized as an inverse relation between vulnerability and burden of cumulative insults.
- Although often unrecognized, delirium is associated with poor outcomes, including worsening cognitive functioning, deteriorating physical status, and increased mortality.
- The primary management of delirium includes implementing preventive interventions, identifying and treating all possible underlying etiologies, liberally implementing nonpharmacological interventions, and judiciously administering low-dose antipsychotics when severe agitation or anxiety is present.
- Approximately half of the patients who recovered from a delirious episode recalled their experience and often remembered it as distressing.

Recommended Readings

Cole MG, Ciampi A, Belzile E, et al: Persistent delirium in older hospital patients: a systematic review of frequency and prognosis. Age Ageing 38:19–26, 2009

Cook IA: Guideline Watch: Practice Guideline for the Treatment of Patients With Delirium. Arlington, VA, American Psychiatric Association, 2004

Fick DM, Agostini JV, Inouye SK: Delirium superimposed on dementia: a systematic review. J Am Geriatr Soc 50:1723–1732, 2002

Fricchione GL, Nejad SH, Esses JA, et al: Postoperative delirium. Am J Psychiatry 165:803–812, 2008

Inouye SK: Delirium in older persons. N Engl J Med 354:1157–1165, 2006

Inouye SK, Bogardua ST Jr, Charpentier PA, et al: A multicomponent intervention to prevent delirium in hospitalized older patients. N Engl J Med 340:669–676, 1999

Tune L: The role of antipsychotics in treating delirium. Curr Psychiatry Rep 4:209–212, 2002

Tune LE, Egeli S: Acetylcholine and delirium. Dement Geriatr Cogn Disord 10:342–344, 1999

ICU Delirium and Cognitive Impairment Study Group: www.icudelirium.org

The Hospital Elder Life Program: http://hospitalelderlifeprogram.org

References

Aalten P, de Vugt ME, Jaspers N, et al: The course of neuropsychiatric symptoms in dementia, part I: findings from the two-year longitudinal Maasbed study. Int J Geriatr Psychiatry 20:523–530, 2005

Adamis D, Treloar A, Martin FC, et al: Recovery and outcome of delirium in elderly medical inpatients. Arch Gerontol Geriatr 43: 289–298, 2006

Adamis D, Treloar A, Darwiche FZ, et al: Associations of delirium with in-hospital and in 6-months mortality in elderly medical inpatients. Age Ageing 36:644–649, 2007a

Adamis D, Treloar A, Martin FC, et al: A brief review of the history of delirium as a mental disorder. Hist Psychiatry 18(72 pt 4):459–469, 2007b

Alsop DC, Fearing MA, Johnson K, et al: The role of neuroimaging in elucidating delirium pathophysiology. J Gerontol A Biol Sci Med Sci 61:1287–1293, 2006

Amador LF, Goodwin JS: Postoperative delirium in the older patient. J Am Coll Surg 200:767–773, 2005

American Psychiatric Association: Diagnostic and Statistical Manual of Mental Disorders, 3rd Edition. Washington, DC, American Psychiatric Association, 1980

American Psychiatric Association: Diagnostic and Statistical Manual of Mental Disorders, 3rd Edition, Revised. Washington, DC, American Psychiatric Association, 1987

American Psychiatric Association: Diagnostic and Statistical Manual of Mental Disorders, 4th Edition. Washington, DC, American Psychiatric Association, 1994

American Psychiatric Association: Practice guideline for the treatment of patients with delirium. Am J Psychiatry 156(5 Suppl):1–20, 1999

American Psychiatric Association: Diagnostic and Statistical Manual of Mental Disorders, 4th Edition, Text Revision. Washington, DC, American Psychiatric Association, 2000

Ancelin ML, Artero S, Portet F, et al: Non-degenerative mild cognitive impairment in elderly people and use of anticholinergic drugs: longitudinal cohort study. BMJ 332(7539):455–459, 2006

Andersson EM, Hallberg IR, Norberg A, et al: The meaning of acute confusional state from the perspective of elderly patients. Int J Geriatr Psychiatry 17:652–663, 2002

Andrew MK, Freter SH, Rockwood K: Prevalence and outcomes of delirium in community and non-acute care settings in people without dementia: a report from the Canadian Study of Health and Aging. BMC Med 4:15, 2006

Attard A, Ranjith G, Taylor D: Delirium and its treatment. CNS Drugs 22:631–644, 2008

Bergmann MA, Murphy KM, Kiely DK, et al: A model for management of delirious postacute care patients. J Am Geriatr Soc 53: 1817–1825, 2005

Blass JP, Gibson GE: Cerebrometabolic aspects of delirium in relationship to dementia. Dement Geriatr Cogn Disord 10:335–338, 1999

Bo M, Martini B, Ruatta C, et al: Geriatric ward hospitalization reduced incidence delirium among older medical inpatients. Am J Geriatr Psychiatry 17:760–768, 2009

Bourne RS, Tahir TA, Borthwick M, et al: Drug treatment of delirium: past, present and future. J Psychosom Res 65:273–282, 2008

Breitbart W, Alici Y: Agitation and delirium at the end of life: We couldn't manage him." JAMA 300:2898–2910, 2008

Breitbart W, Strout D: Delirium in the terminally ill. Clin Geriatr Med 16:357–372, 2000

Breitbart W, Marotta R, Platt MM, et al: A double-blind trial of haloperidol, chlorpromazine, and lorazepam in the treatment of delirium in hospitalized AIDS patients. Am J Psychiatry 153: 231–237, 1996

Breitbart W, Gibson C, Tremblay A: The delirium experience: delirium recall and delirium-related distress in hospitalized patients with cancer, their spouses/caregivers, and their nurses. Psychosomatics 43:183–194, 2002

Broadhurst C, Wilson K: Immunology of delirium: new opportunities for treatment and research. Br J Psychiatry 179:288–289, 2001

Bucerius J, Gummert JF, Borger MA, et al: Predictors of delirium after cardiac surgery delirium: effect of beating-heart (off-pump) surgery. J Thorac Cardiovasc Surg 127:57–64, 2004

Burns A, Gallagley A, Byrne J: Delirium. J Neurol Neurosurg Psychiatry 75:362–367, 2004

Caeiro L, Ferro JM, Albuquerque R, et al: Delirium in the first days of acute stroke. J Neurol 251:171–178, 2004a

Caeiro L, Ferro JM, Claro MI, et al: Delirium in acute stroke: a preliminary study of the role of anticholinergic medications. Eur J Neurol 11:699–704, 2004b

Camus V, Burtin B, Simeone I, et al: Factor analysis supports the evidence of existing hyperactive and hypoactive subtypes of delirium. Int J Geriatr Psychiatry 15:313–316, 2000a

Camus V, Gonthier R, Dubos G, et al: Etiologic and outcome profiles in hypoactive and hyperactive subtypes of delirium. J Geriatr Psychiatry Neurol 13:38–42, 2000b

Casarett DJ, Inouye SK, American College of Physicians-American Society of Internal Medicine End-of-Life Care Consensus Panel: Diagnosis and management of delirium near the end of life. Ann Intern Med 135:32–40, 2001

Chang YL, Tsai YF, Lin PJ, et al: Prevalence and risk factors for postoperative delirium in a cardiovascular intensive care unit. Am J Crit Care 17:567–575, 2008

Chevrolet JC, Jolliet P: Clinical review: agitation and delirium in the critically ill—significance and management. Crit Care 11:214, 2007

Cole MG: Delirium in elderly patients. Am J Geriatr Psychiatry 12:7–21, 2004

Cole MG, McCusker J, Dendukuri N, et al: Symptoms of delirium among elderly medical inpatients with or without dementia. J Neuropsychiatry Clin Neurosci 14:167–175, 2002

Cole MG, Ciampi A, Belzile E, et al: Persistent delirium in older hospital patients: a systematic review of frequency and prognosis. Age Ageing 38:19–26, 2009

Cook IA: Guideline Watch: Practice Guideline for the Treatment of Patients With Delirium. Arlington, VA, American Psychiatric Association, 2004. Available at: http://www.psychiatryonline.com/content.aspx?aid=147844. Accessed January 27, 2011.

de Jonghe JF, Kalisvaart KJ, Dijkstra M, et al: Early symptoms in the prodromal phase of delirium: a prospective cohort study in elderly patients undergoing hip surgery. Am J Geriatr Psychiatry 15:112–121, 2007

DiMartini A, Dew MA, Kormos R, et al: Posttraumatic stress disorder caused by hallucinations and delusions experienced in delirium. Psychosomatics 48:436–439, 2007

Dolan MM, Hawkes WG, Zimmerman SI, et al: Delirium on hospital admission in aged hip fracture patients: prediction of mortality and 2-year functional outcomes. J Gerontol A Biol Sci Med Sci 55:M527–M534, 2000

Duppils GS, Wikblad K: Delirium: behavioural changes before and during the prodromal phase. J Clin Nurs 13:609–616, 2004

Edlund A, Lundström M, Brännström B, et al: Delirium before and after operation for femoral neck fracture. J Am Geriatr Soc 49: 1335–1340, 2001

Edlund A, Lundström M, Karlsson S, et al: Delirium in older patients admitted to general internal medicine. J Geriatr Psychiatry Neurol 19:83–90, 2006

Eikelenboom P, Hoogendijk WJG: Do delirium and Alzheimer's dementia share specific pathogenetic mechanisms? Dement Geriatr Cogn Disord 10:319–324, 1999

Elie M, Cole MG, Primeau FJ, et al: Delirium risk factors in elderly hospitalized patients. J Gen Intern Med 13:204–212, 1998

Elie M, Rousseau F, Cole M, et al: Prevalence and detection of delirium in elderly emergency department patients. CMAJ 163:977–981, 2000

Ely EW, Gautam S, Margolin R, et al: The impact of delirium in the intensive care unit on hospital length of stay. Intensive Care Med 27:1892–1900, 2001a

Ely EW, Margolin R, Francis J, et al: Evaluation of delirium in critically ill patients: validation of the Confusion Assessment Method for the Intensive Care Unit (CAM-ICU). Crit Care Med 29:1370–1379, 2001b

Ely EW, Siegel MD, Inouye SK: Delirium in the intensive care unit: an under-recognized syndrome of organ dysfunction. Semin Respir Crit Care Med 22:115–126, 2001c

Ely EW, Shintani A, Truman B, et al: Delirium as a predictor of mortality in mechanically ventilated patients in the intensive care unit. JAMA 291:1753–1762, 2004

Ely EW, Girard TD, Shintani AK, et al: Apolipoprotein E4 polymorphism as a genetic predisposition to delirium in critically ill patients. Crit Care Med 35:112–117, 2007

Engel GL, Romano J: Delirium: a syndrome of cerebral insufficiency. J Neuropsychiatry Clin Neurosci 16:526–538, 2004

Fann JR: The epidemiology of delirium: a review of studies and methodological issues. Semin Clin Neuropsychiatry 5:64–74, 2000

Fann JR, Roth-Roemer S, Burington BE, et al: Delirium in patients undergoing hematopoietic stem cell transplantation: incidence and risk factors. Cancer 95:1971–1981, 2002

Ferro JM, Caeiro L, Verdelho A: Delirium in acute stroke. Curr Opin Neurol 15:51–55, 2002

Fick DM, Agostini JV, Inouye SK: Delirium superimposed on dementia: a systematic review. J Am Geriatr Soc 50:1723–1732, 2002

Fick DM, Kolanowski AM, Waller JL, et al: Delirium superimposed on dementia in a community-dwelling managed care population: a 3-year retrospective study of occurrence, costs, and utilization. J Gerontol A Biol Sci Med Sci 60:748–753, 2005

Flacker JM, Lipsitz LA: Neural mechanisms of delirium: current hypotheses and evolving concepts [published erratum appears in J Gerontol A Biol Sci Med Sci 54:B275, 1999]. J Gerontol A Biol Sci Med Sci 54:B239–B246, 1999a

Flacker JM, Lipsitz LA: Serum anticholinergic activity changes with acute illness in elderly medical patients. J Gerontol A Biol Sci Med Sci 54:M12–M16, 1999b

Flaherty JH, Tariq SH, Raghavan S, et al: A model for managing delirious older inpatients. J Am Geriatr Soc 51:1031–1035, 2003

Folstein MF, Bassett SS, Romanoski AJ, et al: The epidemiology of delirium in the community: the Eastern Baltimore Mental Health Survey. Int Psychogeriatr 3:169–176, 1991

Fong TG, Bogardus ST Jr, Daftary A, et al: Cerebral perfusion changes in older delirious patients using 99mTc HMPAO SPECT. J Gerontol A Biol Sci Med Sci 61:1294–1299, 2006

Francis J, Kapoor WN: Delirium in hospitalized elderly. J Gen Intern Med 5:65–79, 1990

Fricchione GL, Nejad SH, Esses JA, et al: Postoperative delirium. Am J Psychiatry 165:803–812, 2008

Gaudreau JD, Gagnon P, Roy MA, et al: Association between psychoactive medications and delirium in hospitalized patients: a critical review. Psychosomatics 46:302–316, 2005

Greco KE, Tune LE, Brown FW, et al: A retrospective study of the safety of intramuscular ziprasidone in agitated elderly patients. J Clin Psychiatry 66:928–929, 2005

Gupta N, de Jonghe J, Schieveld J, et al: Delirium phenomenology: what can we learn from the symptoms of delirium? J Psychosom Res 65:215–222, 2008

Han L, McCusker J, Cole M, et al: Use of medications with anticholinergic effect predicts clinical severity of delirium symptoms in older medical inpatients. Arch Intern Med 161:1099–1105, 2001

Hshieh TT, Fong TG, Marcantonio ER, et al: Cholinergic deficiency hypothesis in delirium: a synthesis of current evidence. J Gerontol A Biol Sci Med Sci 63:764–772, 2008

Inouye SK: The dilemma of delirium: clinical and research controversies regarding diagnosis and evaluation of delirium in hospitalized elderly medical patients. Am J Med 97:278–288, 1994

Inouye SK: Predisposing and precipitating factors for delirium in hospitalized older patients. Dement Geriatr Cogn Disord 10: 393–400, 1999

Inouye SK: Prevention of delirium in hospitalized older patients: risk factors and targeted intervention strategies. Ann Med 32:257–263, 2000

Inouye SK: A practical program for preventing delirium in hospitalized elderly patients. Cleve Clin J Med 71:890–896, 2004

Inouye SK: Delirium in older persons. N Engl J Med 354:1157–1165, 2006

Inouye SK, Charpentier PA: Precipitating factors for delirium in hospitalized elderly persons: predictive model and interrelationship with baseline vulnerability. JAMA 275:852–857, 1996

Inouye SK, Ferrucci L: Elucidating the pathophysiology of delirium and the interrelationship of delirium and dementia. J Gerontol A Biol Sci Med Sci 61:1277–1280, 2006

Inouye SK, van Dyck CH, Alessi CA, et al: Clarifying confusion: the Confusion Assessment Method: a new method for detection of delirium. Ann Intern Med 113:941–948, 1990

Inouye SK, Viscoli CM, Horwitz RI, et al: A predictive model for delirium in hospitalized elderly medical patients based on admission characteristics. Ann Intern Med 119:474–481, 1993

Inouye SK, Rushing JT, Foreman MD, et al: Does delirium contribute to poor hospital outcomes? A three-site epidemiologic study. J Gen Intern Med 13:234–242, 1998

Inouye SK, Bogardus ST Jr, Charpentier PA, et al: A multicomponent intervention to prevent delirium in hospitalized older patients. N Engl J Med 340:669–676, 1999a

Inouye SK, Schlesinger MJ, Lydon TJ: Delirium: a symptom of how hospital care is failing older persons and a window to improve quality of hospital care. Am J Med 106:565–573, 1999b

Inouye SK, Foreman MD, Mion LC, et al: Nurses' recognition of delirium and its symptoms: comparison of nurse and researcher ratings. Arch Intern Med 161:2467–2473, 2001

Inouye SK, Zhang Y, Jones RN, et al: Risk factors for delirium at discharge: development and validation of a predictive model. Arch Intern Med 167:1406–1413, 2007

Jackson JC, Gordon SM, Hart RP, et al: The association between delirium and cognitive decline: a review of the empirical literature. Neuropsychol Rev 14:87–98, 2004

Jackson KC, Lipman AG: Drug therapy for delirium in terminally ill adult patients. Cochrane Database of Systematic Reviews 2004, Issue 2. Art. No.: CD004770. DOI: 10.1002/14651858.CD004770

Jacobson S, Jerrier H: EEG in delirium. Semin Clin Neuropsychiatry 5:86–92, 2000

Jones C, Bäckman C, Capuzzo M, et al: Precipitants of post-traumatic stress disorder following intensive care: a hypothesis generating study of diversity in care. Intensive Care Med 33:978–985, 2007

Jones RN, Yang FM, Zhang Y, et al: Does educational attainment contribute to risk for delirium? A potential role for cognitive reserve. J Gerontol A Biol Sci Med Sci 61:1307–1311, 2006

Kales HC, Kamholz BA, Visnic SG, et al: Recorded delirium in a national sample of elderly inpatients: potential implications for recognition. J Geriatr Psychiatry Neurol 16:32–38, 2003

Kalisvaart KJ, de Jonghe JF, Bogaards MJ, et al: Haloperidol prophylaxis for elderly hip-surgery patients at risk for delirium: a randomized placebo-controlled study. J Am Geriatr Soc 53:1658–1666, 2005

Katz IR, Curyto KJ, TenHave T, et al: Validating the diagnosis of delirium and evaluating its association with deterioration over a one-year period. Am J Geriatr Psychiatry 9:148–159, 2001

Kiely DK, Bergmann MA, Jones RN, et al: Characteristics associated with delirium persistence among newly admitted post-acute facility patients. J Gerontol A Biol Sci Med Sci 59:M344–349, 2004

Koponen H, Partanen J, Pääkkönen A, et al: EEG spectral analysis in delirium. J Neurol Neurosurg Psychiatry 52:980–985, 1989

Laitinen H: Patients' experience of confusion in the intensive care unit following cardiac surgery. Intensive Crit Care Nurs 12:79–83, 1996

Laurila JV, Pitkala KH, Strandberg TE, et al: Confusion assessment method in the diagnostics of delirium among aged hospital patients: would it serve better in screening than as a diagnostic instrument? Int J Geriatr Psychiatry 17:1112–1119, 2002

Laurila JV, Laakkonen ML, Tilvis RS, et al: Predisposing and precipitating factors for delirium in a frail geriatric population [published erratum appears in J Psychosom Res 65:507, 2008]. J Psychosom Res 65:249–254, 2008

Lawlor PG, Fainsinger RL, Bruera ED: Delirium at the end of life: critical issues in clinical practice and research. JAMA 284:2427–2429, 2000a

Lawlor PG, Gagnon B, Mancini IL, et al: Occurrence, causes, and outcome of delirium in patients with advanced cancer: a prospective study. Arch Intern Med 160:786–794, 2000b

Leonard M, Agar M, Mason C, et al: Delirium issues in palliative care settings. J Psychosom Res 65:289–298, 2008

Leslie DL, Zhang Y, Holford TR, et al: Premature death associated with delirium at 1-year follow-up. Arch Intern Med 165:1657–1662, 2005

Leslie DL, Marcantonio ER, Zhang Y, et al: One-year health care costs associated with delirium in the elderly population. Arch Intern Med 168:27–32, 2008

Levkoff SE, Liptzin B, Cleary P, et al: Subsyndromal delirium. Am J Geriatr Psychiatry 4:320–329, 1996

Lipowski ZJ: Delirium (acute confusional states). JAMA 258:1789–1792, 1987

Lipowski ZJ: Clinical features, course, and outcome, in Delirium: Acute Confusional States. New York, Oxford University Press, 1990, pp 54–70

Liptzin B, Levkoff SE: An empirical study of delirium subtypes. Br J Psychiatry 161:843–845, 1992

Liptzin B, Laki A, Garb JL, et al: Donepezil in the prevention and treatment of post-surgical delirium. Am J Geriatr Psychiatry 13:1100–1106, 2005

Lonergan E, Britton AM, Luxenberg J: Antipsychotics for delirium. Cochrane Database of Systematic Reviews 2007, Issue 2. Art. No.: CD005594. DOI: 10.1002/14651858.CD005594.pub2

Lonergan E, Luxenberg J, Areosa Sastre A: Benzodiazepines for delirium. Cochrane Database of Systematic Reviews 2009, Issue 4. Art. No.: CD006379. DOI: 10.1002/14651858.CD006379.pub3

Mach JR Jr, Dysken MW, Kuskowski M, et al: Serum anticholinergic activity in hospitalized older persons with delirium: a preliminary study. J Am Geriatr Soc 43:491–495, 1995

Mach JR Jr, Kabat V, Olson D, et al: Delirium and right-hemisphere dysfunction in cognitively impaired older persons. Int Psychogeriatr 8:373–382, 1996

MacLullich AM, Ferguson KJ, Miller T, et al: Unravelling the pathophysiology of delirium: a focus on the role of aberrant stress responses. J Psychosom Res 65:229–238, 2008

Marcantonio ER, Flacker JM, Wright RJ, et al: Reducing delirium after hip fracture: a randomized trial. J Am Geriatr Soc 49:516–522, 2001

Marcantonio ER, Simon SE, Bergmann MA, et al: Delirium symptoms in post-acute care: prevalent, persistent, and associated with poor functional recovery. J Am Geriatr Soc 51:4–9, 2003

Marcantonio ER, Kiely DK, Simon SE, et al: Outcomes of older people admitted to postacute facilities with delirium. J Am Geriatr Soc 53:963–969, 2005

McAvay GJ, Van Ness PH, Bogardus ST Jr, et al: Older adults discharged from the hospital with delirium: 1-year outcomes. J Am Geriatr Soc 54:1245–1250, 2006

McCusker J, Cole M, Dendukuri N, et al: Delirium in older medical inpatients and subsequent cognitive and functional status: a prospective study. CMAJ 165:575–583, 2001

McCusker J, Cole M, Abrahamowicz M, et al: Delirium predicts 12-month mortality. Arch Intern Med 162:457–463, 2002

McCusker J, Cole M, Dendukuri N, et al: The course of delirium in older medical inpatients: a prospective study. J Gen Intern Med 18:696–704, 2003

McManus J, Pathansali R, Stewart R, et al: Delirium post-stroke. Age Ageing 36:613–618, 2007

Meagher D: Delirium episode as a sign of undetected dementia among community dwelling elderly subjects. J Neurol Neurosurg Psychiatry 70:821–, 2001

Meagher D, Trzepacz PT: Phenomenological distinctions needed in DSM-V: delirium, subsyndromal delirium, and dementias. J Neuropsychiatry Clin Neurosci 19:468–470, 2007

Meagher DJ, MacLullich AMJ, Laurila JV: Defining delirium for the International Classification of Diseases, 11th Revision. J Psychosom Res 65:207–214, 2008a

Meagher DJ, Moran M, Raju B, et al: Motor symptoms in 100 patients with delirium versus control subjects: comparison of subtyping methods. Psychosomatics 49:300–308, 2008b

Michaud L, Büla C, Berney A, et al: Delirium: guidelines for general hospitals. J Psychosom Res 62:371–383, 2007

Milisen K, Lemiengre J, Braes T, et al: Multicomponent intervention strategies for managing delirium in hospitalized older people: systematic review. J Adv Nurs 52:79–90, 2005

Minger SL, Esiri MM, McDonald B, et al: Cholinergic deficits contribute to behavioral disturbance in patients with dementia. Neurology 55:1460–1467, 2000

Minnick A, Leipzig RM, Johnson ME: Elderly patients' reports of physical restraint experiences in intensive care units. Am J Crit Care 10:168–171, 2001

Moretti R, Torre P, Antonello RM, et al: Cholinesterase inhibition as a possible therapy for delirium in vascular dementia: a controlled, open 24-month study of 246 patients. Am J Alzheimers Dis Other Demen 19:333–339, 2004

Mori E, Yamadori A: Acute confusional state and acute agitated delirium: occurrence after infarction in the right middle cerebral artery territory. Arch Neurol 44:1139–1143, 1987

Mulsant BH, Pollock BG, Kirshner M, et al: Serum anticholinergic activity in a community-based sample of older adults: relationship with cognitive performance. Arch Gen Psychiatry 60:198–203, 2003

Murphy BA: Delirium. Emerg Med Clin North Am 18:243–252, 2000

Mussi C, Ferrari R, Ascari S, et al: Importance of serum anticholinergic activity in the assessment of elderly patients with delirium. J Geriatr Psychiatry Neurol 12:82–86, 1999

Nakase-Thompson R, Sherer M, Yablon SA, et al: Acute confusion following traumatic brain injury. Brain Inj 18:131–142, 2004

Namba M, Morita T, Imura C, et al: Terminal delirium: families' experience. Palliat Med 21:587–594, 2007

Naughton BJ, Saltzman S, Ramadan F, et al: A multifactorial intervention to reduce prevalence of delirium and shorten hospital length of stay. J Am Geriatr Soc 53:18–23, 2005

O'Keefe ST, Lavan JN: Clinical significance of delirium subtypes in older people. Age Ageing 28:115–119, 1999

O'Malley G, Leonard M, Meagher D, et al: The delirium experience: a review. J Psychosom Res 65:223–228, 2008

Oldenbeuving AW, de Kort PLM, Jansen BP, et al: Delirium in acute stroke: a review. Int J Stroke 2:270–275, 2007

Ouimet S, Riker R, Bergeron N, et al: Subsyndromal delirium in the ICU: evidence for a disease spectrum. Intensive Care Med 33: 1007–1013, 2007

Overshott R, Karim S, Burns A: Cholinesterase inhibitors for delirium. Cochrane Database of Systematic Reviews 2008, Issue 1. Art. No.: CD005317. DOI: 10.1002/14651858.CD005317.pub2

Pandharipande P, Jackson J, Ely EW: Delirium: acute cognitive dysfunction in the critically ill. Curr Opin Crit Care 11:360–368, 2005

Pandharipande P, Cotton BA, Shintani A, et al: Motoric subtypes of delirium in mechanically ventilated surgical and trauma intensive care unit patients. Intensive Care Med 33:1726–1731, 2007
Peterson JF, Pun BT, Dittus RS, et al: Delirium and its motoric subtypes: a study of 614 critically ill patients. J Am Geriatr Soc 54: 479–484, 2006
Pisani MA, Murphy TE, Van Ness PH, et al: Characteristics associated with delirium in older patients in a medical intensive care unit. Arch Intern Med 167:1629–1634, 2007
Pisani MA, Murphy TE, Araujo KL, et al: Benzodiazepine and opioid use and the duration of intensive care unit delirium in an older population. Crit Care Med 37:177–183, 2009
Pitkälä KH, Laurila JV, Strandberg TE, et al: Multicomponent geriatric intervention for elderly inpatients with delirium: a randomized, controlled trial. J Gerontol A Biol Sci Med Sci 61:176–181, 2006
Pitkälä KH, Laurila JV, Strandberg TE, et al: Multicomponent geriatric intervention for elderly inpatients with delirium: effects on costs and health-related quality of life. J Gerontol A Biol Sci Med Sci 63:56–61, 2008
Prakanrattana U, Prapaitrakool S: Efficacy of risperidone for prevention of postoperative delirium in cardiac surgery. Anaesth Intensive Care 35:714–719, 2007
Pun BT, Ely EW: The importance of diagnosing and managing ICU delirium. Chest 132:624–636, 2007
Rahkonen T, Luukkainen-Markkula R, Paanila S, et al: Delirium episode as a sign of undetected dementia among community dwelling elderly subjects: a 2 year follow up study. J Neurol Neurosurg Psychiatry 69:519–521, 2000
Rahkonen T, Eloniemi-Sulkava U, Halonen P, et al: Delirium in the non-demented oldest old in the general population: risk factors and prognosis. Int J Geriatr Psychiatry 16:415–421, 2001
Rea RS, Battistone S, Fong JJ, et al: Atypical antipsychotics versus haloperidol for treatment of delirium in acutely ill patients. Pharmacotherapy 27:588–594, 2007
Reischies FM, Neuhaus AH, Hansen ML, et al: Electrophysiological and neuropsychological analysis of a delirious state: the role of the anterior cingulate gyrus. Psychiatry Res 138:171–181, 2005
Roche V: Etiology and management of delirium. Am J Med Sci 325:20–30, 2003
Sampson EL, Raven PR, Ndhlovu PN, et al: A randomized, double-blind, placebo-controlled trial of donepezil hydrochloride (Aricept) for reducing the incidence of postoperative delirium after elective total hip replacement. Int J Geriatr Psychiatry 22:343–349, 2007
Sandberg O, Gustafson Y, Brännström B, et al: Prevalence of dementia, delirium, and psychiatric symptoms in various care settings for the elderly. Scand J Soc Med 26:56–62, 1998
Saravay SM, Kaplowitz M, Kurek J, et al: How do delirium and dementia increase length of stay of elderly general medical inpatients? Psychosomatics 45:235–242, 2004
Schofield I: A small exploratory study of the reaction of older people to an episode of delirium. J Adv Nurs 25:942–952, 1997
Schuurmans MJ, Duursma SA, Shortridge-Baggett LM: Early recognition of delirium: review of the literature. J Clin Nurs 10:721–729, 2001
Schwartz TL, Masand PS: The role of atypical antipsychotics in the treatment of delirium. Psychosomatics 43:171–174, 2002
Siddiqi N, Holt R, Britton AM, et al: Interventions for preventing delirium in hospitalised patients. Cochrane Database of Systematic Reviews 2007, Issue 2. Art. No.: CD005563. DOI: 10.1002/14651858.CD005563.pub2
Siegal MD: Management of agitation in the intensive care unit. Clin Chest Med 24:713–725, 2003
Sirois F: Delirium: 100 cases. Can J Psychiatry 33:375–378, 1988
Soiza RL, Sharma V, Ferguson K, et al: Neuroimaging studies of delirium: a systematic review. J Psychosom Res 65:239–248, 2008
Stagno D, Gibson C, Breitbart W: The delirium subtypes: a review of prevalence, phenomenology, pathophysiology, and treatment response. Palliat Support Care 2:171–179, 2004
Swigart SE, Kishi Y, Thurber S, et al: Misdiagnosed delirium in patient referrals to a university-based hospital psychiatry department. Psychosomatics 49:104–108, 2008
Sylvestre M-P, McCusker J, Cole M, et al: Classification of patterns of delirium severity scores over time in an elderly population. Int Psychogeriatr 18:667–680, 2006
Thomason JWW, Shintani A, Peterson JF, et al: Intensive care unit delirium is an independent predictor of longer hospital stay: a prospective analysis of 261 non-ventilated patients. Crit Care 9: R375–R381, 2005
Trzepacz PT: The neuropathogenesis of delirium: a need to focus our research. Psychosomatics 35:374–391, 1994
Trzepacz PT: Update on the neuropathogenesis of delirium. Dement Geriatr Cogn Disord 10:330–334, 1999
Trzepacz PT, Dew MA: Further analyses of the delirium rating scale. Gen Hosp Psychiatry 17:75–79, 1995
Tune L: Serum anticholinergic activity levels and delirium in the elderly. Semin Clin Neuropsychiatry 5:149–153, 2000
Tune L: Anticholinergic effects of medication in elderly patients. J Clin Psychiatry 62 (suppl 21):11–14, 2001
Tune L: The role of antipsychotics in treating delirium. Curr Psychiatry Rep 4:209–212, 2002
Tune L: How acute is delirium in nursing homes: an observational study from Wesley Woods at Emory. Am J Geriatr Psychiatry 16:786, 2008
Tune LE, Bylsma FW: Benzodiazepine-induced and anticholinergic-induced delirium in the elderly. Int Psychogeriatr 3:397–408, 1991
Tune LE, Egeli S: Acetylcholine and delirium. Dement Geriatr Cogn Disord 10:342–344, 1999
Tune LE, Damlouji NF, Holland A, et al: Association of postoperative delirium with raised serum levels of anticholinergic drugs. Lancet 2(8248):651–653, 1981
Tune L, Carr S, Hoag E, et al: Anticholinergic effects of drugs commonly prescribed for the elderly: potential means for assessing risk of delirium. Am J Psychiatry 149:1393–1394, 1992
Tune L, Carr S, Cooper T, et al: Association of anticholinergic activity of prescribed medications with postoperative delirium. J Neuropsychiatry Clin Neurosci 5:208–210, 1993

Van Eijk MM, Kesecioglu J, Slooter AJ: Intensive care delirium monitoring and standardised treatment: a complete survey of Dutch Intensive Care Units. Intensive Crit Care Nurs 24:218–221, 2008

Van Eijk MM, Roes KC, Honing ML, et al: Effect of rivastigmine as an adjunct to usual care with haloperidol on duration of delirium and mortality in critically ill patients: a multicentre, double blind, placebo-controlled randomized trial. Lancet 376:1829–1837, 2010

Vollmer C, Rich C, Robinson S: How to prevent delirium: a practical protocol. Nursing 37:26–28, 2007

Wacker P, Nunes PV, Cabrita H, et al: Post-operative delirium is associated with poor cognitive outcome and dementia. Dement Geriatr Cogn Disord 21:221–227, 2006

Weber JB, Coverdale JH, Kunik ME: Delirium: current trends in prevention and treatment. Intern Med J 34:115–121, 2004

Webster R, Holroyd S: Prevalence of psychotic symptoms in delirium. Psychosomatics 41:519–522, 2000

White S, Calver BL, Newsway V, et al: Enzymes of drug metabolism during delirium. Age Ageing 34:603–608, 2005

Xie Z, Dong Y, Maeda U, et al: Isoflurane-induced apoptosis: a potential pathogenic link between delirium and dementia. J Gerontol A Biol Sci Med Sci 61:1300–1306, 2006

Yokota H, Ogawa S, Kurokawa A, et al: Regional cerebral blood flow in delirium patients. Psychiatry Clin Neurosci 57:337–339, 2003

Young J, Leentjens AF, George J, et al: Systematic approaches to the prevention and management of patients with delirium. J Psychosom Res 65:267–272, 2008

16

Alzheimer's Disease and the Frontotemporal Dementia Syndromes

John M. Ringman, M.D., M.S.
Harry V. Vinters, M.D.

An estimated 14% of the population ages 71 and older have dementia (Plassman et al. 2007), and with increasing longevity in the United States as well as worldwide, the absolute number of persons with dementia is certain to increase. In response to this impending epidemic, substantial resources have been invested in research into the nature and causes of dementia, and the last 20 years have seen significant advances in understanding of dementing disorders. In this chapter, we focus on Alzheimer's disease (AD) and the frontotemporal dementia (FTD) syndromes, arguably two of the most common neurodegenerative causes of dementia.

AD is usually considered a unitary disorder despite clinical, genetic, and pathological variability. In contrast, controversy exists over how to classify the clinically and pathologically diverse syndromes associated with progressive frontotemporal degeneration. Although categorization based on clinical features (e.g., behavioral variant of FTD, progressive nonfluent aphasia, semantic dementia) (Neary et al. 1998) is useful in characterizing a given patient's presentation, these classification schemes have repeatedly been shown to map only imperfectly onto the underlying neuropathology. For this reason, the heterogeneous pathological changes underlying progressive frontal and temporal lobe atrophy may be subsumed under the category of frontotemporal lobar degenerations (FTLDs). Genetic breakthroughs are improving our ability to categorize these diseases and understand the sequence of events leading to their manifestation. These findings are beginning to change understanding of the pathogenesis of these disorders, and ultimately they offer hope for the development of better therapies that will modify disease progression. In this chapter, we discuss AD and FTD and address the evolving understanding of their clinical, epidemiological, genetic, imaging, chemical, and pathological features, as well as their treatment.

Alzheimer's Disease

Clinical Features

AD is a clinicopathological entity, usually associated with advanced age, defined by the presence of an acquired dementia syndrome of gradual onset and progression, with specific neuropathological changes. The cognitive presentation typically begins with loss of recent episodic memory. Initially, persons with AD may be forgetful and repetitive, losing objects, repeating stories, and missing appointments. The amnestic syndrome in AD may be distinguished to some degree from memory complaints due to frontal or subcortical injury, in which contextual or other cues can augment recollection to a greater extent. Memory deficits are typically followed over months to years by deficits in executive function, visuospatial function, language, and praxis. At initial presentation, inquiries regarding the patient's ability to perform complex instrumental activities of daily living that involve multiple cognitive abilities (e.g., managing finances, driving) should be made. Visuospatial deficits may develop early, with deficits in navigation being a common early complaint. This can be manifested on bedside cognitive testing by difficulty copying the overlapping pentagons on the Mini-Mental State Examina-

John M. Ringman, M.D., and Harry V. Vinters, M.D., are supported by NIA P50 AG16570. Harry V. Vinters, M.D., is supported by the Daljit S. and Elaine Sarkaria Chair in Diagnostic Medicine at UCLA.

tion (Folstein et al. 1975) or on the clock-drawing task (Aprahamian et al. 2010). Word-finding difficulty is a common early complaint, and diminished verbal fluency may be detected using quantitative neuropsychological testing. A fluent aphasia may eventually emerge, associated with diminished comprehension (Cummings et al. 1985). Eventually, global cognitive deterioration ensues, difficulty with long-term memory occurs, and abilities to perform overlearned visuospatial tasks such as eating and dressing are lost.

There are many exceptions to this typical pattern of progression, however (Galton et al. 2000). Visuospatial deficits (Renner et al. 2004), language deficits (primary progressive aphasia; Li et al. 2000), or even asymmetrical motor deficits akin to those of corticobasal degeneration (Doran et al. 2003) can initially dominate the clinical picture. Behavioral changes are common; although they may be subtle in early AD, they become more prevalent and problematic as the disease progresses. Dysphoria, anxiety, and apathy (manifested as withdrawal from one's ordinary hobbies and social interactions) are common early features. Over time, irritability, verbal and physical agitation, and psychosis manifested as delusions and hallucinations become major concerns and impact caregiving. The psychosis of dementia is qualitatively distinct from that seen in schizophrenia; in dementia, the hallucinations are most commonly visual and the delusions commonly relate in some way to absent or false memories (e.g., confabulation, delusions of theft, Capgras syndrome) (Cummings et al. 1987). Neuropsychiatric changes are ultimately present in at least 88% of patients with AD (Mega et al. 1996) and represent a common cause of nursing home placement (Tun et al. 2007).

During the final stages of AD, patients are bedridden and unable to swallow or mobilize, so that death is often secondary to dehydration or sepsis. Estimates of survival duration after a diagnosis of AD vary from a median of ~5 years (Larson et al. 2004) to 10 years (Brookmeyer et al. 2002), with male gender and advanced age at the time of diagnosis predicting shorter survival times. The nature and quality of nursing care of the bedridden patient with AD also undoubtedly affect survival time.

Epidemiology

Approximately 5.2 million Americans had AD in 2008 (Alzheimer's Association 2008), of whom 200,000 were younger than age 65. It has been estimated that someone in America develops AD every 71 seconds (Alzheimer's Association 2008). By far the greatest risk factor for AD is aging, and the prevalence of AD rises with each decade of life. AD has a prevalence of approximately 6.2% over age 65, 20% over age 80, and 45% over age 95. The prevalence of AD and dementia in those over age 71 is clearly higher in women (16%) than in men (11%). This is at least partly explained by the fact that women live longer, and whether or not women have a higher risk independent of longevity is a matter of controversy (Fitzpatrick et al. 2004). AD was reported to be the seventh leading cause of death in people of all ages in the United States in 2005 and the fifth leading cause of death for people over age 65 (Alzheimer's Association 2008). This ranking probably underestimates the number of persons dying with the illness, however, because the presence of AD may not be documented on death certificates that tend to focus on proximate causes of death (e.g., cardiopulmonary arrest).

Multiple epidemiological studies have shown that having achieved a higher level of education and occupational attainment is associated with a decreased risk of both AD and dementia. Such findings are far from proof of a causative relationship, because variables associated with education, such as lifestyle, environmental exposures, overall health, and detection bias, can confound such studies. At least one study, however, in which vascular and lifestyle factors were controlled to some extent (Ngandu et al. 2007) again found a relationship between higher levels of education and reduced risk for AD.

Besides lower education level, other risk factors for clinically defined AD and dementia that have been identified are a history of head injury (McDowell 2001) and small head size (Schofield et al. 1997). Increasing evidence suggests that whether or not one manifests the symptoms of dementia depends in part on what has been termed one's "cognitive reserve." Neuropathological and more recently amyloid imaging studies (Kemppainen et al. 2008) have shown that the relationship between an individual's cognitive status and the extent of AD pathology present in the brain is far from direct, with some persons having extensive AD pathology without clinical manifestations. One possible explanation is that every individual has a unique capacity to absorb brain insults, such as AD pathology, before manifesting cognitive symptoms. This cognitive reserve is likely to be the result of genetic and environmental influences and to determine the threshold of neuropathology above which symptoms are manifested. In studies of dementia, part of the definition of the illness is performance on neuropsychological tests, which is clearly subject to socioeconomic, occupational, and educational influences. Although neuropsychologists attempt to control for these influences, such adjustment is always imperfect; therefore, having lower levels (or lower quality) of education might in itself increase the likelihood of being categorized as having impairment or dementia. In epidemiological studies, disentangling these influences can be difficult, and therefore it is possible that factors such as education level, history of education, and head size are not risk factors for AD pathology but rather for detectable cognitive impairment. Carefully controlled neuropathological or perhaps neuroimaging studies can address these questions more directly.

Genetics

Although much remains to be learned, since the 1990s, substantial advances have occurred in understanding the genetics of AD. A convergence of evidence, much of it genetic, supports the prevailing "amyloid hypothesis" of the etiology of AD. Specifically, the major protein constituent of the amyloid angiopathy and plaques characteristic of AD was identified to be β-amyloid (Aβ) (Glenner and Wong 1984), the precursor of which is amyloid precursor protein (APP). Alterations in the gene coding for APP on chromosome 21 were linked to young-onset autosomal-dominant AD (Goate et al. 1991). Furthermore, essentially all persons with Down syndrome due to triplication of chromosome 21 develop AD pathology in their brains and an accompanying behavioral syndrome if they live long enough.

Additional evidence that overproduction and decreased degradation of aberrant forms of Aβ are primary events in the etiology of AD was provided by the discovery that two additional genes that cause young-onset autosomal-dominant AD (*PSEN1* and *PSEN2*) lead to aberrant metabolism of APP, such that excessive amounts of the 42-amino-acid-length version of the peptide (Aβ42) is produced. Alterations in the *PSEN1* gene account for the majority (~65%) of autosomal-dominant cases, followed by *APP* and *PSEN2*. More recently, duplications of the *APP* gene have also been associated with young-onset autosomal-dominant AD (Rovelet-Lecrux et al. 2006). In a study by Lippa et al. (2000), mutations in *PSEN1* were found to have the youngest age at onset (44–46 years), followed by *APP* (49 years), and *PSEN2* (58–59 years). The neuropathology and clinical presentation of young-onset autosomal-dominant AD can be very similar to those of late-onset AD, although distinctive features can occur. Familial AD due to *APP*, *PSEN1*, or *PSEN2* mutations is more likely to feature spastic paraparesis, early myoclonus and seizures, headaches, and atypical cognitive presentations such as disproportionate language or frontal lobe dysfunction. Neuropathologically, some families feature large distinctive "cotton wool" plaques that are largely composed of Aβ42, tend to displace surrounding tissue, and are frequently associated with the spastic paraparesis phenotype. Although leading to substantial insights into the disease, alterations in the *APP*, *PSEN1*, and *PSEN2* genes account for 2% or less of AD cases. Screening for mutations in the *PSEN1*, *APP*, and *PSEN2* genes (and duplications in the case of *APP*) is commercially available but should be reserved for young-onset cases in which a strong family history consistent with an autosomal-dominant pattern of inheritance is evident (Rogaeva et al. 2001). Furthermore, appropriate genetic counseling is necessary to ensure that family members understand the implications of a positive test to themselves prior to testing.

In the early 1990s, an association was observed between polymorphisms of the apolipoprotein E gene (*APOE*) and risk of AD (Corder et al. 1993). In most populations, the ε3 allele is the most common (78% in whites), followed by the ε4 allele (14%), with the ε2 allele being least common (8%) (Utermann et al. 1980). An association between the ε4 allele and increased risk for and decreased onset age of AD was observed (Corder et al. 1993), with the presence of two copies of the ε4 allele conferring a greater risk than one copy. Although the ε4 version of the allele accounts for only 14% of *APOE* alleles in the general white population, among patients with AD, ~40% have the ε4 allele (Saunders et al. 1993). The ε3 allele confers a diminished risk and ε2 an even lower risk. This effect has been replicated in multiple populations (Murrell et al. 2006); however, some studies in nonwhite populations either failed to show this effect (Tang et al. 1998) or showed a weaker effect than is seen in whites (Harwood et al. 1999).

The mechanisms by which different apolipoprotein E (apoE) isoforms influence the risk of AD are not entirely clear. Although many studies suggest a direct effect on augmenting amyloid pathology (Bennett et al. 2005; Holtzman et al. 2000), apoE is a pleiotropic protein, and differential effects of apoE isoforms on neurotoxicity, tau phosphorylation, synaptic plasticity, and inflammation may be playing roles. Furthermore, clinical studies have provided evidence that the ε4 allele has effects on cognition (Wetter et al. 2005) and brain activation in normal young persons (Filippini et al. 2009) and that it confers a higher risk for cognitive sequelae in head trauma (Jordan et al. 1997), Parkinson's disease (Harhangi et al. 2000), and coronary bypass surgery (Newman et al. 1995). Although the association of the *APOE* ε4 allele and AD risk is well established, many *APOE* ε4 carriers do not develop AD, and therefore it is best thought of as a susceptibility gene. Therefore, although commercial *APOE* genotyping is available, it is not generally recommended in asymptomatic persons but can be informative in patients with relatively early-onset AD who are lacking an autosomal-dominant family history. A randomized clinical trial of disclosure (vs. nondisclosure) of *APOE* genotype (Green et al. 2009) did not demonstrate increased test-related distress in the *APOE* ε4–positive disclosure group, indicating that such testing may have a role in certain persons, especially when disease-modifying interventions are available.

After controlling for *APOE* status, investigators have found that many late-onset cases still appear to have a genetic contribution. It has been estimated that greater than 30% and possibly greater than 70% of the genetic variance in AD is due to genetic loci that have not yet been identified (Daw et al. 2000). Multiple large studies attempting to identify these additional genes have been performed and are ongoing. To date, no genes have been identified that have as large an effect on AD risk as the *APOE* gene; however, two genome-wide association studies have implicated polymorphisms in the genes for clusterin (*CLU*) or the apolipoprotein J gene on chromosome 8; phosphatidylinositol-binding clathrin assembly protein (*PICALM*) on chromosome 11; and complement component receptor 1 (*CR1*) on chromosome 1 (Harold et al. 2009; Lambert et al. 2009). Many other loci have also been implicated in individual studies, and the reader is referred to the Alzheimer Research Forum Web site for the most recent findings in Alzheimer's genetics (www.alzgene.org). Although the development of AD is clearly under genetic control, at least in part, these observations do not rule out the existence of environmental influences. Concordance for AD in identical twins is ~40%, and there can be a significant discrepancy between the ages at onset in twins concordant for the illness (Creasey et al. 1989).

Neuropathology

Neuropathological examination of the brain—either at autopsy or (less commonly) through biopsy—has continued to be the "gold standard" for the diagnosis of AD (Goedert and Ghetti 2007), even as neuroradiographic techniques are emerging that seem capable of detecting Aβ peptide or β-pleated sheet proteins in the brain while patients are alive or even completely asymptomatic (Mintun et al. 2006). The main neuropathological feature of the AD brain on gross examination is cortical atrophy, which is usually diffuse throughout the brain rather than being focally accentuated (as in the case of FTLDs). When the fixed brain is cut, the cortical atrophy is usually accompanied by enlargement of the ventricular system, or hydrocephalus ex vacuo. If the brain of a patient with dementia shows hydrocephalus out of proportion to the degree of cerebral cortical atrophy, the possibility of normal-pressure hydrocephalus must be considered, although microscopic lesions of AD should still be sought in such a brain. In practice, most experienced neuropathologists are struck by the variability in brain weights (normal adult range is 1,200–1,400 g), cerebral cortical atrophy, and hydrocephalus ex vacuo among individuals who eventually have the diagnosis of AD confirmed by light microscopy (Joachim et al. 1988).

The microscopic lesions that accumulate in the central nervous system (mainly cerebral cortex) of individuals with AD can, when prominent and abundant, be seen on sections of the brain stained with hematoxylin and eosin, but these lesions are much more easily demonstrated using special stains and (over the past 20+ years) by immunohistochemistry using highly specific primary antibodies. The special stains used to demonstrate the senile plaques (SPs) and neurofibrillary tangles (NFTs) seen in abundance in the cerebral cortex of a patient with end-stage AD historically have been silver impregnation techniques, usually the modified Bielschowsky and Bodian stains, and in more recent years, the Campbell-Switzer and Gallyas methods—the latter two used effectively in seminal studies of SP and NFT distribution by Heiko and Eva Braak (Braak and Braak 1995). SPs appear, on routine stains, as a faint coarsening of the neuropil (the "neuritic" component of the SP) centered on an amorphous eosinophilic "globule" of amyloid, the core of the SP. The relationship between the amyloid core of a mature SP and its neuritic corona (both seen well on the silver stains named above) has been debated for years and remains largely unresolved, but such mature neuritic SPs are thought to be more reflective of cortical injury than are the more diffuse SPs that are *lacking* a neuritic component. Although SPs (especially neuritic SPs) have a neuronal component, insofar as the neurites represent processes emerging from presumably damaged nerve cell bodies, they are substantially extraneuronal or located within the neuropil. Although SPs are found in elderly individuals without AD, their density is in general far less than that in patients with AD. That having been said, most neuropathologists have encountered autopsy brains from cognitively intact elderly individuals that contain abundant neuritic SPs.

NFTs, the other major lesion of AD, are dense intraneuronal cytoplasmic aggregates of filaments that include, on ultrastructural examination, characteristic paired helical filaments (also known as bifilar helices). NFTs are usually accompanied by neuropil threads in the adjacent neuropil (Braak et al. 1986). NFTs occur with many non-AD neurodegenerative conditions, including subacute sclerosing panencephalitis, dementia pugilistica, aluminum intoxication, postencephalitic parkinsonism, and the parkinsonism–amyotrophic lateral sclerosis–dementia complex of Guam (Wisniewski et al. 1979). Of interest, NFT-like neuronal cytoplasmic lesions are commonly encountered within the dysmorphic neuronal cell bodies of infants and children with epilepsy-associated cortical dysplasia or cortical tubers of tuberous sclerosis complex (Mischel et al. 1995). These NFTs, easily demonstrable on silver stains, are *not* composed of paired helical filaments by ultrastructural examination.

A third important, but often underappreciated, lesion of AD is cerebral amyloid angiopathy (CAA) (Vinters 1987). The reason that CAA has remained in the background in discussions of AD neuropathological features may be that it is extremely variable among patients with AD; however, when sought diligently, it is found (to some extent) in an estimated 90%–95% of AD brains. CAA describes a process whereby the media of parenchymal arterioles, normally composed of smooth muscle cells, undergoes progressive loss of these smooth muscle cells together with an accumulation of an eosinophilic hyaline material that has the staining properties of amyloid (i.e., positivity for thioflavin S or T) and congophilia (Vinters et al. 1994). When a brain with prominent CAA is stained with Congo red and polarized, the walls of affected arterioles will show characteristic yellow-green birefringence. CAA may also involve cortical parenchymal venules and capillaries. Meningeal arteries are often affected by CAA; when CAA occurs in these larger vessels, the amyloid deposits are usually adventitial rather than medial. CAA almost never involves the subcortical white matter, basal ganglia, brain stem, or spinal cord, but (in severe cases) it may involve the cerebellar meningeal and molecular layer (Vinters and Gilbert 1983). From a historical perspective, CAA played a major role in understanding of the molecular basis of AD; Glenner and Wong (1984) initially isolated the peptide now referred to as Aβ from amyloid-laden vessels removed from the brains of AD patients. CAA is also important as a cause of nontraumatic intracerebral hemorrhage within the brains of elderly individuals, including many who do not manifest overt features of a dementing illness at the time of their stroke (Vinters 1987). CAA-related intraparenchymal hematomas are usually lobar, unlike the centrencephalic bleeds seen with hypertensive microvascular disease (Vinters et al. 1998); these large and invariably symptomatic, sometimes fatal hematomas occur in a relatively small proportion of those with AD and severe CAA, but CAA-related microbleeds (detectable on high-resolution magnetic resonance imaging [MRI] scanning) are now accepted as a fairly reliable marker for the presence of CAA within the brain (Zhang-Nunes et al. 2006). More recently, severe CAA has also been associated with the occurrence of cerebral microinfarcts, lesions that may obviously worsen cognitive impairment in a patient already afflicted by AD (Soontornniyomkij et al. 2009).

Although SPs, NFTs, and CAA are the major microscopic lesions of AD and are widely distributed throughout the cortex, two others merit mention. Granulovacuolar degeneration of Simchowicz (GVD) describes a neuronal cytoplasmic lesion in which the neuronal cytoplasm of hippocampal pyramidal cells is replaced by vacuoles containing small basophilic granules. Hippocampi showing prominent GVD also often show eosinophilic hyaline rod-like structures in the adjacent neuropil—these are described as rod-like bodies of Hirano. Perhaps because of their limited distribution within the brains of AD patients and their rarity in the neocortex, GVDs and rod-like bodies of Hirano have been the subject of limited study in terms of assessing their possible contributions to AD pathogenesis and progression.

Although we have emphasized in this section the lesions commonly seen in AD brains—either focally or diffusely in the cortex—one of the most important findings, demonstrable biochemically or by immunohistochemistry in AD brain, is synapse loss. This is shown on sections of affected cortex when they are immunostained with antibodies against a synaptic protein, such as synaptophysin, and compared closely with a reference control specimen (Davidson and Blennow 1998). AD brains also frequently show comorbidity, not surprising given the many age-related diseases (e.g., cerebrovascular disease) that may impact the brain. Coexistent Parkinson's disease changes and evidence of infarcts or hemorrhage are common in AD brains (Gearing et al. 1995b). Indeed, the theme of comorbidity between ischemic brain lesions and AD microscopic changes—both common in the elderly—features prominently in modern dementia research, possibly because it represents a more real-world scenario than considering AD and multi-infarct/ischemic vascular dementia as "pure" entities (Vinters et al. 2000).

Immunohistochemical Features

The amyloid cores of SPs and CAA have a major component of Aβ protein. The immunohistochemical study of AD brain lesions began in earnest as soon as the peptide sequence of Aβ (then termed "A4") was first published; several groups prepared antibodies to synthetic peptides representing portions of the molecule (Vinters et al. 1988). Currently, numerous commercially available antibodies to Aβ, tau, ubiquitin, and alpha-synuclein (to detect Lewy bodies) are available to facilitate immunohistochemical characterization of a given necropsy brain specimen. SPs are more prominently immunoreactive for the 1–42 amino acid length of Aβ, whereas CAA immunolabels more strongly with antibodies to Aβ 1–40; however, there are striking exceptions to this "predominance" of a given Aβ length in one or the other lesion (Figures 16–1 and 16–2). Diffuse SPs are shown well by anti-Aβ antibodies incorporated into appropriate immunohistochemical protocols, as are the amyloid cores of mature SPs. The neuritic coronas of mature SPs are prominently immunolabeled with antibodies to phosphorylated tau, as are NFTs and neuropil threads (Figures 16–3 and 16–4). Anti-ubiquitin also stains NFTs and SPs but is not specific. In cases of severe CAA, gamma-trace may also be found in the affected vessel walls (Vinters et al. 1990).

"Staging" Alzheimer's Disease and Quantifying Lesions

Because essentially all AD lesions described in the "Neuropathology" section above may be encountered in the cerebral cortex of cognitively normal elderly individuals, it is important to quantify (or *semiquantify*) these lesions and to assess their topographical distribution. Correlations between lesion "load," severity of neuropathological findings, and (in vivo) neuropsychological symptoms in a given patient are crucial; however, they are especially difficult to make when examining the brain of an end-stage patient, and that patient may have experienced his or her maximal neurological deficit years before he or she passed (Galasko et al. 1994). Rare biopsies are carried out to confirm the diagnosis of AD, but in that situation only a small portion of the brain is available for examination. Nonetheless, small studies have described the

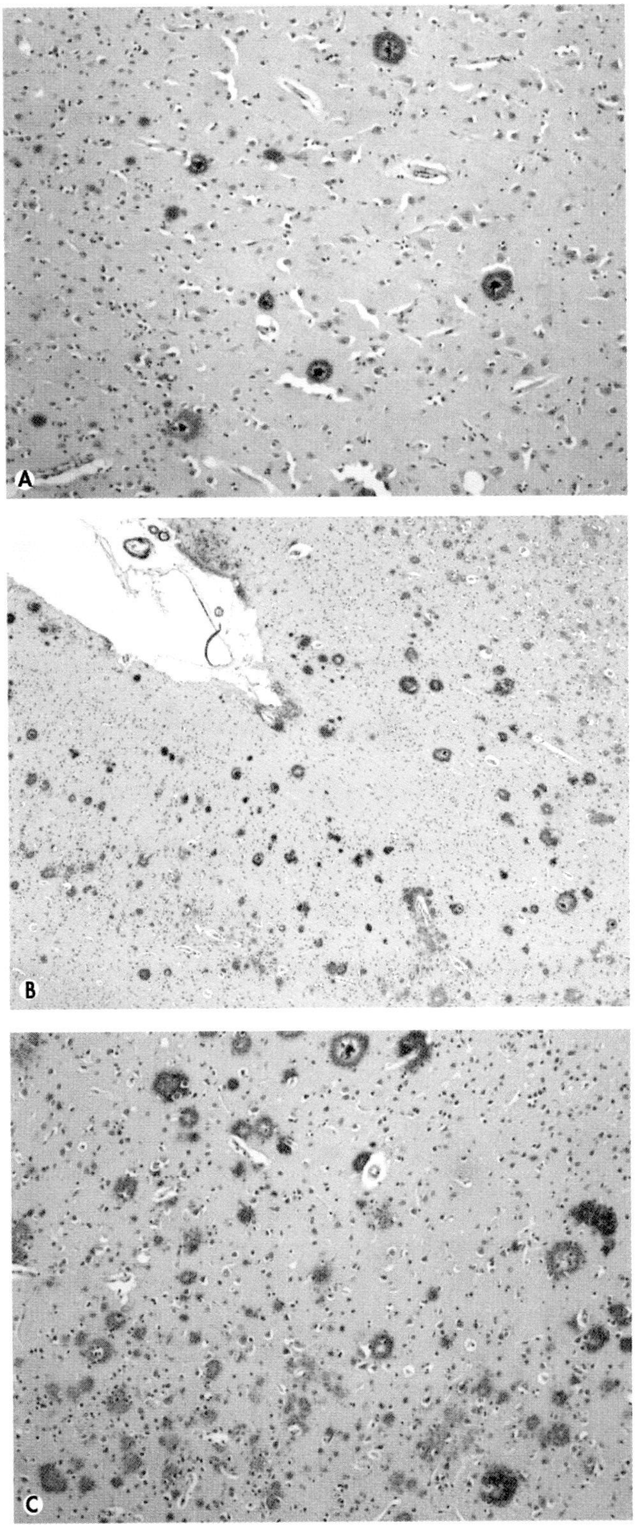

FIGURE 16–1. Sections of brain immunostained with anti-β-amyloid.

Panel A: Relatively sparse density of senile plaques (SPs), many of which contain a compact core and a "halo" of immunoreactivity. **Panels B and C:** High density of SPs, photographed at intermediate *(Panel B)* and high *(Panel C)* magnification. Both mature and diffuse SPs are identified.

progression of AD lesions over the years between biopsy and autopsy (Di Patre et al. 1999).

Many attempts have been made to standardize neuropathological diagnostic criteria for AD versus normal aging (Gearing et al. 1995b). A paper that resulted from a consensus conference in the mid-1980s resulted in the widely used Khachaturian criteria for the neuropathological diagnosis of AD (Khachaturian 1985). These were modified and updated by the Consortium to Establish a Registry for Alzheimer's Disease (CERAD; Gearing et al. 1995a). Braak criteria for AD severity (Braak and Braak 1995) assume a progression of neuropathological abnormalities (predominantly NFT accumulation) from the transentorhinal cortex (stages I and II) to the hippocampus (stages III and IV), with ultimate involvement of the neocortex/isocortex (stages V and VI). It has been argued that the neuropathological change of Braak stage III or IV AD is associated clinically with mild cognitive impairment but not overt dementia (Petersen et al. 2006). In the middle to late 1990s, the National Institute on Aging (NIA)–Reagan Institute criteria for the neuropathological diagnosis of AD came into widespread use, and these criteria have since been tested and operationalized by various groups (Newell et al. 1999). These criteria assign—based on thorough neuropathological examination of a brain specimen—a high, intermediate, or low likelihood that a given individual's dementia was due to AD neuropathological features. One excellent study not only found a good correlation between a high NIA-Reagan likelihood of AD and clinical dementia but ascertained that the older Khachaturian and CERAD criteria correlated fairly well with NIA-Reagan criteria (Newell et al. 1999). However, occasional cases arise, especially among the oldest old, in which Braak stage VI AD changes and an NIA-Reagan assessment of high likelihood of AD are clearly present in the brains of subjects who were known to be cognitively intact until shortly before death (Berlau et al. 2007). The quantification of AD neuropathological change is increasingly facilitated by the ability to digitize immunostained glass slides, retain the images as a permanent electronic record of a given autopsy (e.g., Figure 16–5), and if necessary use these digital images as a starting point for further quantitative morphometry of that specimen.

Clinical Evaluation

In patients presenting with overt cognitive or behavioral symptoms as described earlier in "Clinical Features," which are impacting the patients' abilities to perform their usual social and occupational activities, the diagnosis of dementia and AD in particular should be considered. Because current treatments for AD are of limited efficacy, the most important consideration continues to be the exclusion of more treatable causes of such impairment. After exclusion of overt causes of delirium (concurrent infection, medication effect), the most recent American Academy of Neurology recommendations are that

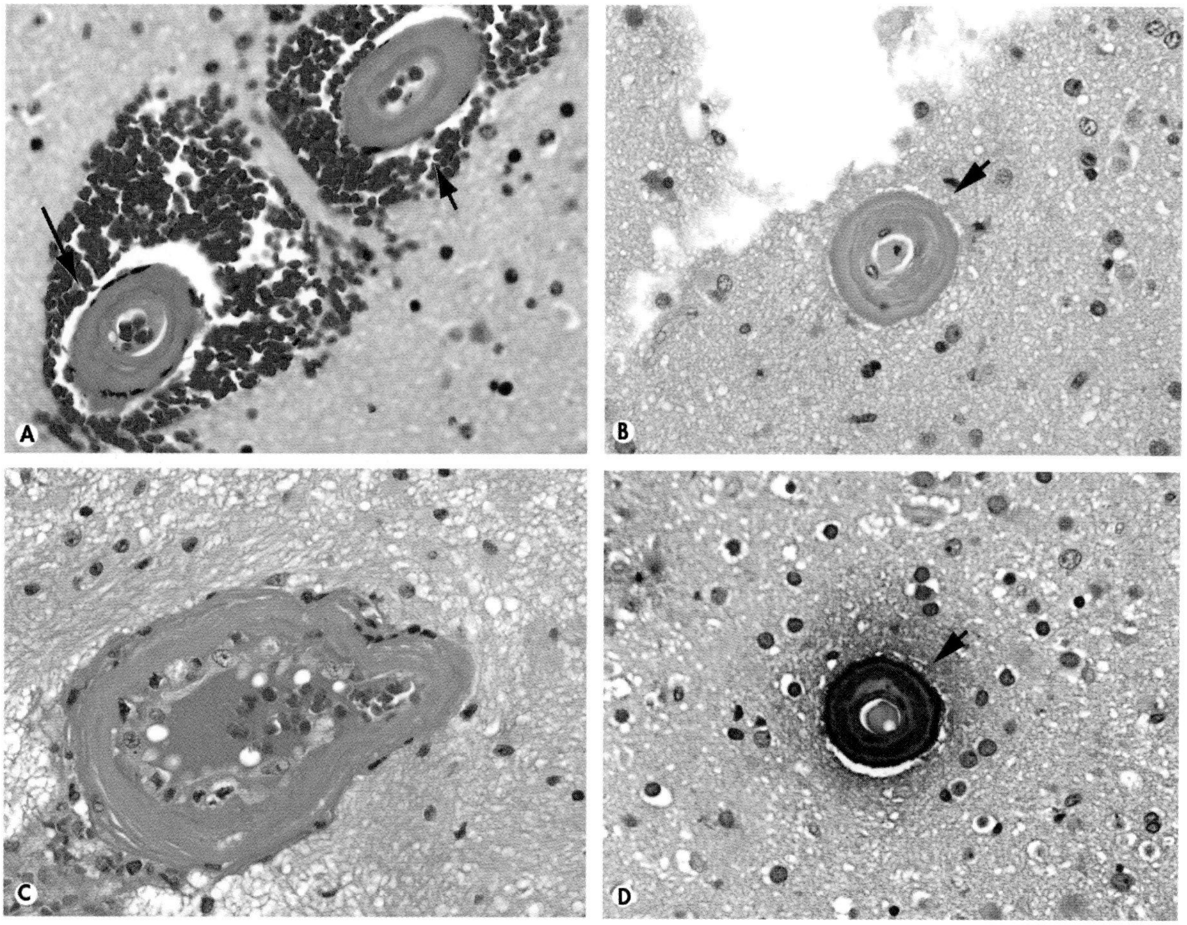

FIGURE 16–2. Sections of a biopsy specimen from a patient who had experienced lobar intracerebral hemorrhage.

Panels A, B, and C: Sections stained with hematoxylin and eosin. **Panel D:** Section immunostained with antibody to β-amyloid (Aβ). In all vessel profiles (*Panels A, B, and D* cut in cross-section, indicated by *arrows*), arterioles lack medial smooth muscle cells, which have been replaced by glassy/fibrillar eosinophilic material that has immunohistochemical properties of Aβ *(Panel D)*. *Panel C* shows an artery that has undergone fibrinoid necrosis, a "superimposed" microvascular abnormality that is thought to predispose to intracerebral hemorrhage.

hypothyroidism and hyperthyroidism as well as cobalamin deficiency be routinely ruled out with appropriate laboratory tests (Doody et al. 2001). Former recommendations included screening tests for syphilis and/or neurosyphilis; considering a physician's practice milieu, such testing may still be indicated. In addition, some form of neuroimaging is also recommended in the current guidelines. Although a computed tomography (CT) brain scan is usually adequate in ruling out significant cerebral pathology for which interventions may be indicated (occult brain tumor, hydrocephalus, large strokes), an MRI study can provide additional information regarding subtle white matter ischemic changes and regional cerebral atrophy pattern.

A greater challenge is presented by persons with more subtle cognitive or behavioral impairment in whom a diagnosis of dementia is not unequivocally present. A careful history from both the patient and an informant should be obtained, with particular attention to how the deficits impact the patient's daily activities. It is also important to screen for depression and other psychiatric morbidity; this is done in part to identify significant depression or anxiety that might contribute to or even be the sole cause of mild cognitive deficits. In addition, a subtle degree of depression and apathy is not uncommon in early AD, and other psychiatric symptoms (e.g., early hallucinations, delusions, disinhibition) may suggest other diagnoses. We also recommend a comprehensive bedside mental status examination, including but not limited to a quantitative screen, such as the Mini-Mental State Examination (Folstein et al. 1975) or the Montreal Cognitive Assessment (Nasreddine et al. 2005), and a reliable and valid test of delayed recall to help delineate the extent of a patient's deficits. If this testing is not possible or

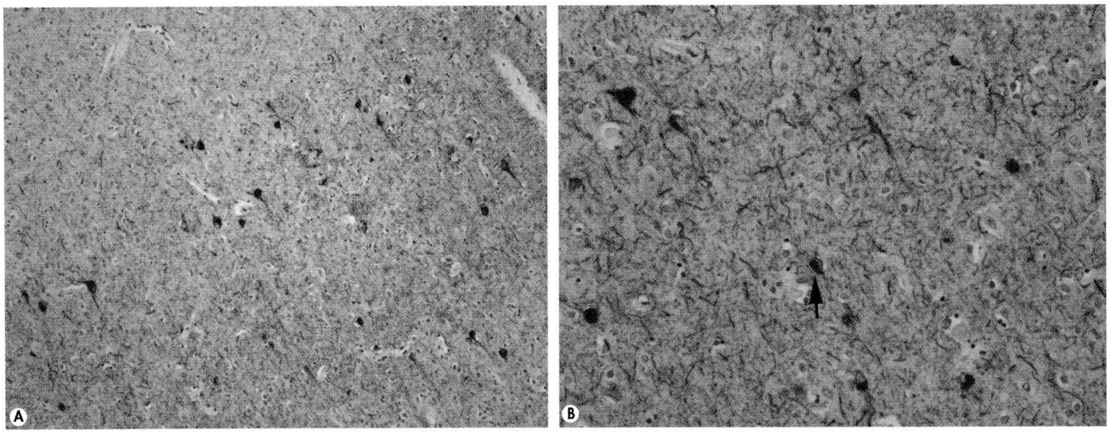

FIGURE 16–3. Section of brain (neocortex) from patient with Alzheimer's disease, immunostained with anti-tau and photographed at low (Panel A) and high (Panel B) magnification.

Abundant immunoreactive neuronal cell bodies (e.g., *arrow in Panel B*) are surrounded by numerous neuropil threads. With this density of neurofibrillary tangles in the neocortex/isocortex, the patient would have been described as having Braak stage VI Alzheimer's disease changes.

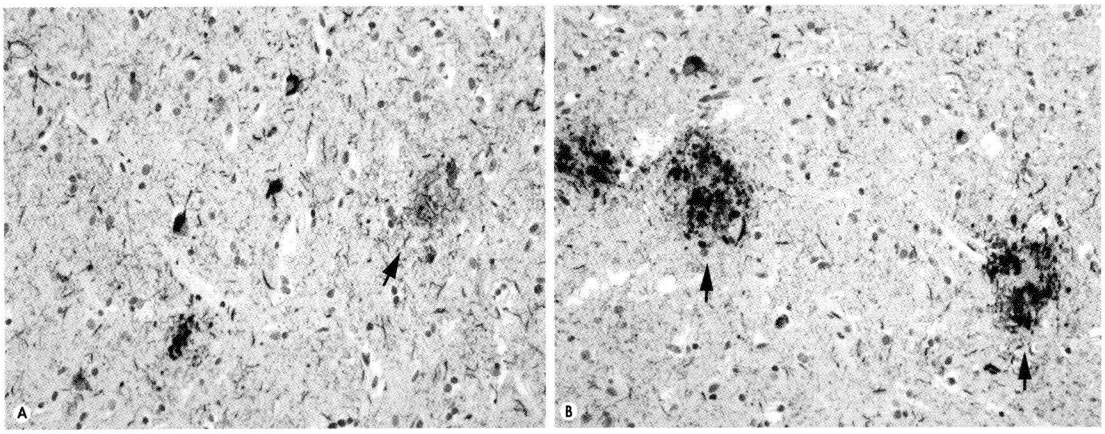

FIGURE 16–4. Sections of brain from patient with Alzheimer's disease, immunostained with anti-tau.

Panel A: Neurofibrillary tangles, a poorly formed senile plaque (SP) with a neuritic component *(arrow)*, and abundant neuropil threads. **Panel B:** SPs *(arrows)* with prominent neuritic components; the neurites are tau-immunoreactive.

when it does not provide adequate information, formal neuropsychological testing is recommended to delineate a patient's strengths and weaknesses relative to appropriate education-, age-, and gender-matched normative values.

Currently, the diagnostic schema employed at many academic dementia centers in the United States is that put forward by the National Institute of Neurological and Communicative Disorders and Stroke and the Alzheimer's Disease and Related Disorders Association (NINCDS-ADRDA; McKhann et al. 1984). The NINCDS-ADRDA criteria for definite AD depend on the availability of pathological (biopsy or autopsy) confirmation of plaques and tangles (see the section "Neuropathology" earlier in this chapter). To meet criteria for either probable or possible AD, dementia must be present. It is well recognized that the pathology of AD precedes clinical dementia by years or even decades; therefore, it should be possible to diagnose incipient AD in its preclinical state. Because delayed recall of episodic material is the most common early feature of AD, the condition of amnestic mild cognitive impairment (MCI) was defined, in which a significant memory deficit is present but other aspects of cognition and one's ability to perform functional activities are relatively intact. Follow-up of persons with MCI in various studies has demonstrated that such persons progress to diagnosable dementia at a rate of ~10%–15% per year (Petersen et al. 2001). Subsequently, other subtypes of MCI, which are defined by impairments in other

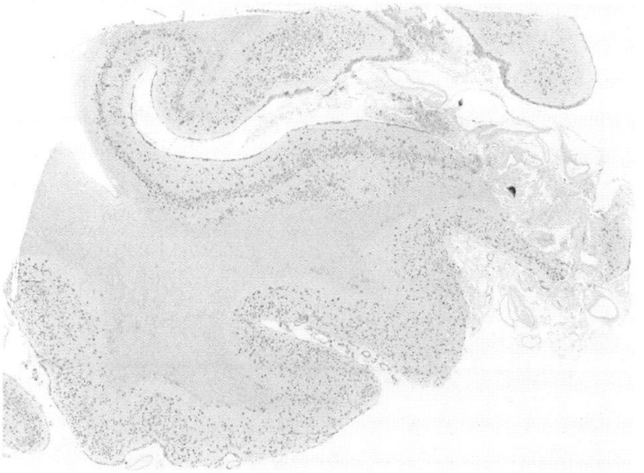

FIGURE 16–5. Section of cortex from patient with Alzheimer's disease, immunostained with primary antibody to β-amyloid (Aβ).

The entire section has been digitally scanned. Note very high density of senile plaques in the cortex, but none in the deep subcortical white matter. Such an image can be used to quantitatively assess Aβ "load" within the cortex, using appropriate microimaging software.

realms of cognition with or without memory impairment, have been delineated (Petersen 2004). Although the cognitively based classification of MCI has helped define a population at increased risk for AD, its implementation in different settings has been heterogeneous.

It is now well established that the pathological changes of AD begin to accumulate in the brain many years before the development of overt dementia (Price and Morris 1999). Because reversing advanced pathology, once present, is difficult and may prove to be impossible, there is increasing emphasis on identifying persons who are destined to develop symptoms in the future but in whom progression of pathology may be slowed or prevented. Due to tremendous advances in knowledge regarding antecedent imaging and biochemical markers in AD, there is now the possibility of diagnosing AD in this "predementia" phase (DuBois et al. 2007).

Biochemical Markers

Diverse molecules in the plasma and cerebrospinal fluid (CSF) have been studied as potential diagnostic markers for established and incipient AD (Frank et al. 2003). These include, but are not limited to, indices of inflammation (Ray et al. 2007), oxidative stress (Pratico et al. 2000), glial damage (Han et al. 2003), and neuronal damage (Sunderland et al. 2003). The ideal biochemical marker for the diagnosis of AD should be precise, reliable, inexpensive, and relatively noninvasive; be validated against autopsy-proven cases; and be able to detect a fundamental feature of the disease (Frank et al. 2003). In part due to the presence of Aβ and tau in the hallmark pathological features of AD, much attention has been devoted to their measurement in biological fluids. Aβ levels in plasma are highly variable and their association with disease is controversial (Graff-Radford et al. 2007), but decreased levels of Aβ42 in the CSF have consistently been shown to occur both in established AD (Sunderland et al. 2003) and in MCI that progresses to diagnosable AD (Mattsson et al. 2009). However, this finding is not entirely specific because such decreased levels of some Aβ peptides have also been described in Creutzfeldt-Jakob disease (Wiltfang et al. 2003) and in HIV-associated neurocognitive disorder (Clifford et al. 2009). Elevated levels of tau in CSF are also characteristic of AD but are thought to reflect neuronal damage in general and therefore are also elevated after stroke (Hesse et al. 2001) and head injury (Zetterberg et al. 2006). Because tau is abnormally phosphorylated in AD brain, elevated CSF levels of tau phosphorylated at various sites (e.g., p-tau_{181} or p-tau_{231}) are thought to be a finding more specific for AD (Hesse et al. 2001). The ratio of Aβ42 to tau measured in the CSF currently holds the most promise as a diagnostic marker for established and incipient AD (Mattsson et al. 2009). Although measurement of Aβ, t-tau, and p-tau in the CSF is now commercially available, their widespread use is precluded by 1) the variability in assay methods and results, 2) the perceived invasiveness of lumbar punctures, and 3) the paucity of effective preclinical interventions.

Neuroimaging

Neuroimaging techniques also show promise for improving the accuracy of the diagnosis of AD. CT helps to identify focal brain masses or hydrocephalus and detects many, but not all, previous strokes. AD leads to cerebral atrophy, particularly in the medial temporal lobes, although atrophy also occurs in elderly individuals without AD and in patients with non-AD degenerative dementias. Therefore, atrophy by itself is unreliable as a diagnostic marker for AD.

MRI is of higher resolution and therefore superior to CT in defining temporal lobe and cerebral anatomy in general. Being sensitive to water content of soft tissues, MRI is also better at identifying the tissue rarefaction seen with various cerebral insults, such as subcortical ischemia (Boone et al. 1992). However, as with CT, atrophy that can be seen on MRI, as conventionally performed in clinical practice, is not useful in itself to make a diagnosis of AD. Modern MRI techniques, in which the volume of the whole brain or various subregions is carefully quantified, are more accurate in both the diagnosis of established AD (Kesslak et al. 1991) and the identification of persons with MCI whose cognition is destined to worsen (Apostolova et al. 2006; Jack et al. 1999). Capitalizing on the predilection for pathology and atrophy in the hippocampus and other medial temporal structures, quantifying atrophy and change in these areas shows substantial promise in tracking the course of the disease and assessing response to putative disease-modifying agents.

Nuclear imaging techniques, including fluorodeoxyglucose positron emission tomography (FDG-PET) and single-photon emission computed tomography (SPECT), can define areas of brain that are dysfunctional in patients with AD despite comparatively preserved gross anatomy. With both FDG-PET (Benson et al. 1983) and SPECT (Jagust et al. 1987), deficits in metabolism or perfusion in the temporoparietal region can be seen. The presence of such a pattern has been reported to have sensitivities and specificities as high as 94% and 73%, respectively, in pathologically proven AD (Silverman et al. 2001). Conditions in which misclassification can occur include Parkinson's disease (Read et al. 1995), hypoxia, sleep apnea, and Creutzfeldt-Jakob disease. Because AD and FTD tend to have distinctive patterns of glucose hypometabolism, distinguishing between these entities is currently a Medicare-approved indication for FDG-PET. FDG-PET can also reveal the characteristic hypometabolic pattern of AD in early and possibly in presymptomatic disease. Asymptomatic carriers of the *APOE* ε4 allele have been demonstrated to show temporoparietal metabolic deficits (Reiman et al. 2004). In one study, the presence of this pattern predicted patients' conversion from MCI to AD with a sensitivity and specificity of 92% and 89%, respectively, over a mean period of 16 months (Drzezga et al. 2005). In part due to the limited amount of follow-up time in many studies, the true predictive value of this finding, however, remains to be fully defined.

In recent years, substantial progress has been made in the ability to detect amyloid pathology in the brain using positron emission tomography (PET) to detect amyloid-binding ligands. Although many such ligands are under investigation, the most developed to date is Pittsburgh compound B (PiB). Employing a carbon-11 (^{11}C) isotope, PiB has been demonstrated to differentiate patients with AD from controls (Klunk et al. 2004), inversely correlate with CSF Aβ42 levels (Fagan et al. 2006), and positively correlate with fibrillar amyloid deposits in postmortem brain specimens (Ikonomovic et al. 2008). In addition, substantial PiB binding is frequently seen in asymptomatic subjects (Mintun et al. 2006), and it has been shown to predict progression from cognitive normality to symptomatic AD (Morris et al. 2009) and overt dementia in some persons with MCI (Okello et al. 2009). Extremely encouraging as a marker for amyloid pathology, due to the poor correlation of amyloid pathology and clinical status, as well as documented cases of autopsy-proven AD in individuals who had negative PiB scans during life (Cairns et al. 2009; Leinonen et al. 2008), the ultimate role of PiB in the prediction and diagnosis of cognitive impairment in elderly individuals has yet to be determined. Also, due to the short half-life of ^{11}C, other ligands (e.g., those employing the fluorine-18 isotope) are being developed and will likely achieve more widespread use.

Treatment

In light of the limited efficacy of currently available pharmacological treatments for AD, a multidisciplinary approach, involving consultation regarding caregiving strategies and the availability of psychosocial support and other resources, is critical. In the United States, referral to the local chapter of the Alzheimer's Association can initiate access to many such resources. As important as prescribing medications to help with AD is the discontinuation of medications (e.g., benzodiazepines and medications with anticholinergic properties) that may be exacerbating cognitive decline and behavioral problems.

Interventions for AD might be conceptualized as symptomatic (i.e., addressing the cognitive or behavioral symptoms of AD without a presumed impact on the pathology underlying the disease) or disease modifying (i.e., ameliorating the responsible underlying pathology and therefore having an effect on disease onset or progression). To date, no treatments have been unequivocally demonstrated to be disease modifying. Currently in the United States, the standard for approval by the U.S. Food and Drug Administration (FDA) for a drug specifically for the treatment of AD requires demonstration of efficacy in cognition and on a global measure of functional status. Treatments approved by the FDA for the treatment of AD fall under two main categories: the acetylcholinesterase inhibitors (AChEIs) and memantine.

Development of the AChEIs was fueled by the demonstration that neurotransmitter pathways employing acetylcholine are disproportionately affected in the course of AD (Whitehouse et al. 1982). After multiple attempts at stimulating activity in these pathways, including administering acetylcholine precursors and direct acetylcholine receptor agonists, inhibiting the enzyme responsible for the degradation of acetylcholine ultimately led to medications that were safe and at least mildly efficacious. In the United States, three AChEIs are commonly used for AD: donepezil, galantamine, and rivastigmine. All three of these medications have been demonstrated in randomized, blinded, placebo-controlled studies to have an effect on cognition and global function. In studies typically lasting 6–12 months, treatment with these medications is associated with statistically significant differences between the placebo and medication-treated groups. The Cognitive subscale of the Alzheimer's Disease Assessment Scale (ADAS-Cog; Mohs et al. 1997) is frequently used to measure cognition. The ADAS-Cog is a 70-point scale, and differences seen between placebo and medication-treated groups typically average ~2–4 points, a difference largely accounted for by a greater degree of decline in the placebo-treated group. Although the clinical significance of such an impact has been argued (Courtney et al. 2004), the global effect and safety of these medications merit a trial of their use in most cases of mild to moderate AD. Side effects are typically those associated with increased cholinergic activity; a mild degree of nausea or loose stools is not uncommon. For persons unable to tolerate oral AChEIs, a transdermal formulation of rivastigmine appears to be better tolerated, due to its more gradual absorption (Winblad et al. 2007).

Memantine is a low-affinity antagonist of *N*-methyl-D-aspartate (NMDA) receptors and was developed as a treatment for AD due to a putative neuroprotective effect. It was demonstrated to have a modest effect on cognition and global function in moderately to severely affected patients with AD, both as monotherapy (Reisberg et al. 2003) and in conjunction with AChEIs (Tariot et al. 2004). Although developed as a potential disease-modifying agent, in light of the fact that a slight symptomatic improvement is sometimes seen, the mechanism of action responsible is yet to be completely defined. It is also generally well tolerated and therefore warrants a trial in most AD cases.

Management of behavioral problems in AD poses a particular challenge because the efficacy of standard treatments can be disappointing and the treatments have substantial risks. If behavioral changes are of acute onset, the clinician should always consider a precipitating medical illness, such as an infection, or an adverse effect of medication. Once such a confounding factor has been ruled out, the clinician can consider nonpharmacological environmental manipulations, such as removing aggravating stimuli, redirecting patients, or better controlling sleep-wake cycles. Improving control of patients' sleep-wake cycles might be achieved by decreasing their daytime naps, by changing ambient light, or if necessary, by giving a sleeping medication such as trazodone to help induce sleep at the appropriate time. If further pharmacological therapy is thought to be necessary, the AChEIs and memantine can have beneficial effects on some behaviors in some patients (Trinh et al. 2003). These medications are relatively safe and should be considered as first-line interventions. Because depression can be a factor contributing to agitation, consideration of treatment with a selective serotonin reuptake inhibitor (SSRI) might be attempted if depression is thought to be present. If these interventions are unsuccessful or if the behavioral disturbances are severe in degree, treatment with a typical or atypical neuroleptic medication might be beneficial. Risks of these medications, such as increased rate of stroke and myocardial infarction, as well as the possibility of worsening extrapyramidal symptoms in patients with dementia with Lewy bodies, need to be considered before starting such treatment.

Symptomatic treatments, although necessary, will not have an impact on the prevalence or incidence of the disease. Because the neuronal loss of AD may ultimately prove to be irreversible, slowing the disease and preventing it altogether are important goals. Due to the impending epidemic of dementia, multiple interventions designed to prevent AD or to have disease-modifying effects are in various stages of development. There have been many epidemiological studies regarding behavioral or environmental factors that are associated with a decreased risk for the illness, but to date none has been shown to have a preventative effect in prospective, randomized, blinded, controlled studies; this is due in part to logistical challenges to performing such studies. Such behavioral or environmental factors include, but are not limited to, dietary influences (e.g., consumption of fish or foods with antioxidant properties, moderate alcohol consumption), aerobic exercise, and mental exercise.

Frontotemporal Dementia

Clinical Features

The term *frontotemporal dementia* (FTD) encompasses a variety of clinical syndromes whose genetic and pathological substrates are currently an active area of discovery. In the field of neuropathology, the term *frontotemporal lobar degeneration* (FTLD) is used more commonly and usually includes progressive supranuclear palsy and corticobasal degeneration, neurodegenerative illnesses that typically involve a significant motor deficit. In this chapter, we focus on the FTD syndromes most frequently presenting with behavioral and cognitive manifestations. Estimates of the prevalence of FTD range from 3 to 15 cases per 100,000 persons (Ratnavalli et al. 2002; Rosso et al. 2003). Although generally rare, because age at onset of FTD tends to be in the 50s or 60s, it is thought to account for at least 8% (Barker et al. 2002) and possibly as high as 50% (Ratnavalli et al. 2002) of cases of presenile dementia.

In 1892, Arnold Pick described a combination of progressive aphasia, apraxia, and behavioral changes associated with atrophy of the frontal and temporal lobes on pathological examination, an illness that came to be known as Pick's disease. Other than rare case descriptions, including that of a progressive aphasia and apraxia in the French composer Maurice Ravel, this group of illnesses did not receive much attention in the medical literature until the 1990s. Since then, there has been a surge in publications regarding this set of illnesses, including several categorization schemes based on clinical presentation. One such classification attempt, published in 1998, defines three FTD subgroups: behavioral variant, progressive nonfluent aphasia, and semantic dementia (Neary et al. 1998). These guidelines put forth a set of core criteria common to all three entities and then specific symptoms characteristic of each subtype. The behavioral variant manifests primarily with disordered interpersonal conduct, disinhibition, apathy, stereotypical motor behaviors, and lack of personal awareness. Persons with progressive nonfluent aphasia have decreased speech output that with disease progression leads to mutism. Patients with semantic dementia demonstrate a loss of knowledge and have comprehension difficulties as well as prosopagnosia in some cases. Features of behavioral variant, progressive nonfluent aphasia, and semantic dementia frequently co-occur in individual patients. In addition to the cognitive and behavioral features, evidence of motor neuron disease and full-blown amyotrophic lateral sclerosis (ALS) frequently co-occurs with FTD, with up to 15% of FTD patients having evidence of motor neuron disease and 20% of ALS patients having FTD symptoms (Lomen-Hoerth et al. 2002).

Clinical characteristics may enable one to distinguish between AD and the FTLDs during life. FTD tends to have a young age at onset and more often features decline in social and personal conduct, hyperorality, and absence of memory or significant visuospatial deficits (Pachana et al. 1996; Rosen et al. 2002b). The emergence of disinhibition, apathy (Levy et al. 1996), stereotyped/perseverative behaviors, and progressive reduction of speech (Miller et al. 1997) also helps to differentiate FTD from AD and other neurodegenerative syndromes.

Nonetheless, it has been repeatedly demonstrated that correlations between clinical syndromes and the underlying pathology are imperfect. For example, in a series of patients with primary progressive aphasia, although nonfluent patients were more likely to have tau pathology and the fluent patients were more likely to have a ubiquitin-positive, tau-negative pathology, nearly one-third of both groups had AD as the most likely causative pathological diagnosis (Knibb et al. 2006). Furthermore, persons presenting with classic corticobasal degeneration have underlying AD pathology 29% of the time (Hu et al. 2009). In addition, neurodegenerative illnesses due to a common genetic mutation can have diverse clinical presentations, and multiple syndromes in a given family have been repeatedly described. For example, in a single family with a mutation in the microtubule-associated protein tau gene *MAPT*, the father presented with FTD, whereas the son's presentation was consistent with corticobasal degeneration (Bugiani et al. 1999). Clinical categorizations must therefore be considered descriptive, and caution should be exercised when attempting to relate them to the underlying genetic or neuropathological substrate.

Genetics

In probands presenting with FTD, a family history of a similar illness is common, being present 25%–40% of the time, depending on the phenotype used to define cases, with an autosomal-dominant pattern of inheritance being consistent in many families (Bird et al. 2003; Chow et al. 1999). Although the story is still incomplete, significant advances have been made in the understanding of the genetics underlying FTD.

Wilhelmsen et al. (1994) showed linkage of FTD to chromosome 17 in a large family with "disinhibition-dementia-parkinsonism and amyotrophy." Later, linkage to this region was also found in patients with progressive subcortical gliosis, multiple tauopathy, hereditary dysphasic dementia, pallido-pontonigral degeneration, and bilateral amygdala degeneration (Foster et al. 1997). In some families with chromosome 17 linkage, mutations in *MAPT* were identified (Reed et al. 2001); mutations in *MAPT* are thought to account for 10%–30% of familial FTD cases (Poorkaj et al. 2001). Both intronic and exonic alterations appear to cause FTD, and alteration in this protein critical for microtubule assembly implicates derangements of the cytoskeleton in the etiology of FTD.

A number of additional families with FTD had been genetically linked to a region in chromosome 17 near the *MAPT* gene, although no mutation in *MAPT* was identified. In 2006 (Baker et al. 2006; Cruts et al. 2006), mutations in the *PGRN* gene encoding progranulin, which lies near the *MAPT* gene, were identified in families with such linkage. Mutations in *PGRN* were subsequently identified in 10% of FTD cases and therefore appear to be as common as *MAPT* mutations as a cause of FTD (Gass et al. 2006). FTD due to mutations in *PGRN* can manifest as behavioral variant FTD, progressive nonfluent aphasia, corticobasal degeneration (Masellis et al. 2006), and possibly FTD with ALS (Spina et al. 2007), underscoring the clinical heterogeneity associated with alterations in a single gene. Progranulin functions as a mediator of wound healing and plays a role in development and tumorigenesis (He et al. 2003). Pathogenic mutations cause disease through haploinsufficiency and are associated with decreased plasma levels of progranulin.

Other rare mutations described in FTD families include mutations found in the charged multivesicular body protein 2b gene *CHMP2B* and the valosin-containing protein gene *VCP*. *VCP* mutations cause a distinctive phenotype characterized by inclusion body myopathy and Paget's disease of the bone, in addition to a frontal lobe degeneration.

Pathology

The morphoanatomical study of FTLD has become one of the most challenging areas of diagnostic neuropathology. Credit is due the Lund and Manchester groups for their seminal clinicopathological studies aimed at characterizing this interesting group of entities when they were first recognized and initially described as FTD (Neary et al. 1988). To many neuropathologists, the "paradigmatic" FTLD remains Pick's disease, characterized by severe (often "knife edge") but often asymmetrical atrophy of the frontal and temporal lobes, characteristic affliction of the middle and inferior temporal gyri with sparing of a portion of the superior temporal gyrus, and intraneuronal Pick bodies. Intraneuronal Pick bodies are found in abundance in the neocortex (Figure 16–6) and in the hippocampus (including pyramidal and granule cell layer neurons) (Figure 16–7). As noted early in studies of FTDs, many of the clinical entities described showed neuropathological similarities: brain weight was slightly to moderately reduced from normal; grossly, the brain showed mild to severe frontal and/or frontal and anterotemporal atrophy; neuronal loss, gliosis, and mild to moderate spongiform changes were found, primarily in the first three layers of the cortex; and gliosis (especially in regions of neuron loss) was easily visualized with immunohistochemical stains for glial fibrillary acidic protein. SPs and NFTs did not occur beyond what is seen in elderly individuals without FTD. Subcortical structures, such as the substantia nigra, were sometimes abnormal (e.g., depigmented).

The larger group of FTLDs now encompasses many disorders. Comprehending their pathogenesis has been revolutionized by key genetic and immunohistochemical discoveries that have intensified in recent years. Kumar-Singh and Van Broeckhoven (2007) presented an illuminating synthesis of the FTLDs, integrating their "core" clinical features and syndromes, preferential regions of brain involvement, biochemical and distinctive neuropathological features, and genetic etiology. There are prominent regions of clinical (and neuropathological) overlap among the entities, as well as many cases that are difficult to classify. Many FTLD patients show evidence of aphasia and behavioral abnormalities (including disinhibited behavior), extrapyramidal symptoms, and other motor disorders. Previously distinct nosological entities sometimes incorporated into the FTLD family include the following: FTLD with tau abnormalities (including FTD and parkinsonism linked to chromosome 17, Pick's disease, corticobasal ganglionic degeneration, progressive supranuclear palsy [Cairns et al. 2007], and argyrophilic grain disease), FTLD with ubiquitin abnormalities, dementia lacking distinctive histology (Knopman et al. 1990), and FTLD associated with motor neuron disease. Some investigators argue for the inclusion of the following additional entities under this umbrella, given the high frequency of tau pathology in the form of NFTs: NFT-predominant AD, dementia pugilistica, multiple-system tauopathy with dementia, and Parkinson-dementia complex of Guam. Cases in which evidence of aberrant tau processing is evident on pathology include those associated with *MAPT* mutations and are therefore often described using the term *tauopathies* (Hernandez and Avila 2007). The majority of FTLD cases feature evidence of either a tauopathy or excessive reactivity to ubiquitin, and therefore it had been suggested that all FTLDs be classified as either "tauopathies" or "ubiquitinopathies" (Bigio 2008). In most cases that stain negative for tau and positive for ubiquitin, excessive reactivity to TAR DNA-binding protein 43 (TDP-43) has been identified. Among such cases are FTD with motor neuron disease and those due to *PGRN* mutations. For a comprehensive classification scheme, the reader is referred to Cairns et al. (2007). However, it should be noted that this is a dynamic field, and even more recently, these criteria were modified (Mackenzie et al. 2009) to include findings regarding the identification of a new protein (fused in sarcoma, or FUS) found in the inclusions in most cases in which no specific protein had been identified. Mackenzie et al. (2009) recommend dividing FTLD into FTLD-tau, FTLD-TDP, FTLD-UPS (ubiquitin proteasome system), FTLD-FUS, and FTLD-ni (no inclusion) subtypes.

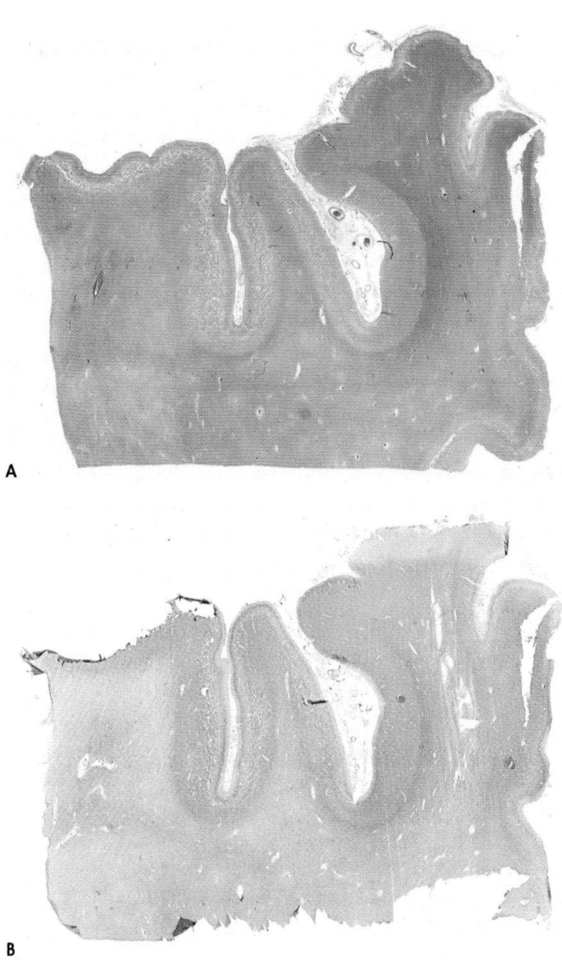

A

B

FIGURE 16–6. Sections of cortex from patient with Pick's disease.

Panel A: A low-magnification view (stained with hematoxylin and eosin) of frontal cortex with marked cortical atrophy. Pallor represents spongy change in the cortex. **Panel B:** A parallel section immunostained with anti-tau, showing prominent staining throughout the neocortex.

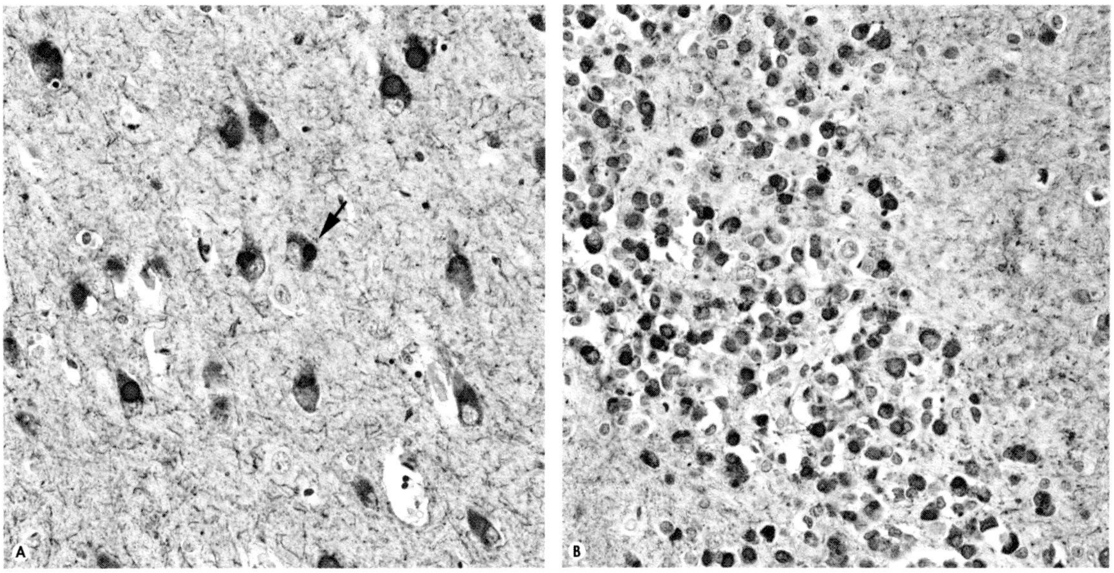

FIGURE 16–7. Tau-immunoreactive Pick bodies, noted in pyramidal cells (Panel A) and granule cells (Panel B) of hippocampus of brain of patient from Figure 16–6.

Pick bodies are spherical intensely tau-immunoreactive cytoplasmic inclusions (e.g., *arrow in Panel A*). In *Panel B*, the vast majority of neurons in the granule cell layer of the hippocampus contain Pick bodies.

As implied in the previous paragraph, the neuropathological workup of these entities is incomplete without detailed immunohistochemical study. The proteins tau, ubiquitin, and TDP-43 must be sought in brain tissue sections. TDP-43 often colocalizes with ubiquitin, and immunopositivity may be difficult to judge with absolute certainty, as it is "counted" when positive signal is noted in the cytoplasm *rather than* the nucleus of a given neuron. Clearly, these recommendations are likely to change with advances in the genetics and pathogenesis of these disorders.

Clinical Evaluation

Patients with FTD can frequently be identified through a careful history of the illness, including manifesting cognitive and behavioral changes; a careful family history; and a neurological examination focused on determining the presence of apraxia, parkinsonism, and motor neuron disease. In suspect cases of FTD, neuropsychological evaluation can also help in identifying the degrees to which executive function is affected and memory and visuospatial abilities are spared. The evaluation is otherwise similar to that for any person presenting with a potential neurodegenerative illness, with routine laboratory tests and structural imaging targeted at identifying reversible medical conditions.

Although structural imaging can help identify gross frontal or temporal atrophy and distinguish it from posterior atrophy more characteristic of AD, such changes are not always evident to the eye. Volumetric studies can help identify focal atrophy of FTD and the various FTD subtypes (Rosen et al. 2002a), but these techniques are not widely used clinically. In cases where the clinical assessment suggests features of both FTD and AD, FDG-PET scanning may be of utility in differentiating them (Foster et al. 2007), and this indication for FDG-PET is currently approved by Medicare in the United States.

Treatment

Treatment for FTD is currently symptomatic, and few controlled trials have been performed. SSRIs may be of benefit in treating the irritability, impulsivity, and compulsions frequently associated with the illness (Swartz et al. 1997), whereas trazodone and the atypical antipsychotics may be useful in managing agitation (Mendez 2009). Cholinesterase inhibitors do not seem to be helpful and can worsen irritability (Mendez et al. 2007). In that medical treatment is currently limited, behavioral interventions and education of caregivers become critical, and referral to the Alzheimer's Association (www.alz.org) and the Association for Frontotemporal Dementias (www.ftd-picks.org) is recommended. For a review of treatment options in FTD, the reader is referred to Mendez (2009). In light of the significant advances in understanding of the biology of these illnesses, there is significant hope for disease-modifying therapies in the future (Trojanowski et al. 2008).

Key Points

- AD is the most common cause of dementia in the elderly and features behavioral changes in addition to cognitive decline.
- The "amyloid hypothesis" of the cause of AD explains many of the scientific observations made regarding this illness.
- Advances in understanding the biochemical changes occurring in AD as well as in neuroimaging now allow us to diagnose the disease at an earlier stage.
- Currently available treatments for AD are of modest benefit, although they are safe and can sometimes improve behaviors as well as cognition.
- FTDs comprise a complex group of disorders, the genetics and pathology of which are becoming increasingly understood.

References

Alzheimer's Association: 2008 Alzheimer's disease facts and figures. Alzheimers Dement 4:110–133, 2008

Apostolova LG, Dutton RA, Dinov ID, et al: Conversion of mild cognitive impairment to Alzheimer disease predicted by hippocampal atrophy maps. Arch Neurol 63:693–699, 2006

Aprahamian I, Martinelli JE, Neri AL, et al: The accuracy of the Clock Drawing Test compared to that of standard screening tests for Alzheimer's disease: results from a study of Brazilian elderly with heterogeneous educational backgrounds. Int Psychogeriatr 22:64–71, 2010

Baker M, Mackenzie IR, Pickering-Brown SM, et al: Mutations in progranulin cause tau-negative frontotemporal dementia linked to chromosome 17. Nature 442:916–919, 2006

Barker WW, Luis CA, Kashuba A, et al: Relative frequencies of Alzheimer disease, Lewy body, vascular and frontotemporal dementia, and hippocampal sclerosis in the State of Florida Brain Bank. Alzheimer Dis Assoc Disord 16:203–212, 2002

Bennett DA, Schneider JA, Wilson RS, et al: Amyloid mediates the association of apolipoprotein E e4 allele to cognitive function in older people. J Neurol Neurosurg Psychiatry 76:1194–1199, 2005

Benson DF, Kuhl DE, Hawkins RA, et al: The fluorodeoxyglucose 18F scan in Alzheimer's disease and multi-infarct dementia. Arch Neurol 40:711–714, 1983

Berlau DJ, Kahle-Wrobleski K, Head E, et al: Dissociation of neuropathologic findings and cognition: case report of an apolipoprotein E epsilon2/epsilon2 genotype. Arch Neurol 64:1193–1196, 2007

Bigio EH: Update on recent molecular and genetic advances in frontotemporal lobar degeneration. J Neuropathol Exp Neurol 67:635–648, 2008

Bird T, Knopman D, VanSwieten J, et al: Epidemiology and genetics of frontotemporal dementia/Pick's disease. Ann Neurol 54(suppl): S29–S31, 2003

Boone KB, Miller BL, Lesser IM, et al: Neuropsychological correlates of white-matter lesions in healthy elderly subjects: a threshold effect. Arch Neurol 49:549–554, 1992

Braak H, Braak E: Staging of Alzheimer's disease-related neurofibrillary changes. Neurobiol Aging 16:271–278; discussion 278–284, 1995

Braak H, Braak E, Grundke-Iqbal I, et al: Occurrence of neuropil threads in the senile human brain and in Alzheimer's disease: a third location of paired helical filaments outside of neurofibrillary tangles and neuritic plaques. Neurosci Lett 65:351–355, 1986

Brookmeyer R, Corrada MM, Curriero FC, et al: Survival following a diagnosis of Alzheimer disease. Arch Neurol 59:1764–1767, 2002

Bugiani O, Murrell JR, Giaccone G, et al: Frontotemporal dementia and corticobasal degeneration in a family with a P301S mutation in tau. J Neuropathol Exp Neurol 58:667–677, 1999

Cairns NJ, Bigio EH, Mackenzie IR, et al: Neuropathologic diagnostic and nosologic criteria for frontotemporal lobar degeneration: consensus of the Consortium for Frontotemporal Lobar Degeneration. Acta Neuropathol 114:5–22, 2007

Cairns NJ, Ikonomovic MD, Benzinger T, et al: Absence of Pittsburgh compound B detection of cerebral amyloid beta in a patient with clinical, cognitive, and cerebrospinal fluid markers of Alzheimer disease: a case report. Arch Neurol 66:1557–1562, 2009

Chow TW, Miller BL, Hayashi VN, et al: Inheritance of frontotemporal dementia. Arch Neurol 56:817–822, 1999

Clifford DB, Fagan AM, Holtzman DM, et al: CSF biomarkers of Alzheimer disease in HIV-associated neurologic disease. Neurology 73:1982–1987, 2009

Corder EH, Saunders AM, Strittmatter WJ, et al: Gene dose of apolipoprotein E type 4 allele and the risk of Alzheimer's disease in late onset families. Science 261:921–923, 1993

Courtney C, Farrell D, Gray R, et al: Long-term donepezil treatment in 565 patients with Alzheimer's disease (AD2000): randomised double-blind trial. Lancet 363:2105–2115, 2004

Creasey H, Jorm A, Longley W, et al: Monozygotic twins discordant for Alzheimer's disease. Neurology 39:1474–1476, 1989

Cruts M, Gijselinck I, van der Zee J, et al: Null mutations in progranulin cause ubiquitin-positive frontotemporal dementia linked to chromosome 17q21. Nature 442:920–924, 2006

Cummings JL, Benson F, Hill MA, et al: Aphasia in dementia of the Alzheimer type. Neurology 35:394–397, 1985

Cummings JL, Miller B, Hill MA, et al: Neuropsychiatric aspects of multi-infarct dementia and dementia of the Alzheimer type. Arch Neurol 44:389–393, 1987

Davidsson P, Blennow K: Neurochemical dissection of synaptic pathology in Alzheimer's disease. Int Psychogeriatr 10:11–23, 1998

Daw EW, Payami H, Nemens EJ, et al: The number of trait loci in late-onset Alzheimer disease. Am J Hum Genet 66:196–204, 2000

Di Patre PL, Read SL, Cummings JL, et al: Progression of clinical deterioration and pathological changes in patients with Alzheimer disease evaluated at biopsy and autopsy. Arch Neurol 56:1254–1261, 1999

Doody RS, Stevens JC, Beck C, et al: Practice parameter: management of dementia (an evidence-based review). Report of the Quality Standards Subcommittee of the American Academy of Neurology. Neurology 56:1154–1166, 2001

Doran M, du Plessis DG, Enevoldson TP, et al: Pathological heterogeneity of clinically diagnosed corticobasal degeneration. J Neurol Sci 216:127–134, 2003

Drzezga A, Grimmer T, Riemenschneider M, et al: Prediction of individual clinical outcome in MCI by means of genetic assessment and (18)F-FDG PET. J Nucl Med 46:1625–1632, 2005

Dubois B, Feldman HH, Jacova C, et al: Research criteria for the diagnosis of Alzheimer's disease: revising the NINCDS-ADRDA criteria. Lancet Neurol 6:734–746, 2007

Fagan AM, Mintun MA, Mach RH, et al: Inverse relation between in vivo amyloid imaging load and cerebrospinal fluid Abeta42 in humans. Ann Neurol 59:512–519, 2006

Filippini N, MacIntosh BJ, Hough MG, et al: Distinct patterns of brain activity in young carriers of the APOE-epsilon4 allele. Proc Natl Acad Sci U S A 106:7209–7214, 2009

Fitzpatrick AL, Kuller LH, Ives DG, et al: Incidence and prevalence of dementia in the Cardiovascular Health Study. J Am Geriatr Soc 52:195–204, 2004

Folstein MF, Folstein SE, McHugh PR: "Mini-mental state": a practical method for grading the cognitive state of patients for the clinician. J Psychiatr Res 12:189–198, 1975

Foster NL, Wilhelmsen K, Sima AA, et al: Frontotemporal dementia and parkinsonism linked to chromosome 17: a consensus conference. Conference Participants. Ann Neurol 41:706–715, 1997

Foster NL, Heidebrink JL, Clark CM, et al: FDG-PET improves accuracy in distinguishing frontotemporal dementia and Alzheimer's disease. Brain 130:2616–2635, 2007

Frank R, Galasko D, Hampel H, et al: Biological markers for therapeutic trials in Alzheimer's disease: proceedings of the biological markers working group; the NIA initiative on neuroimaging in Alzheimer's disease. Neurobiol Aging 24:521–536, 2003

Galasko D, Hansen LA, Katzman R, et al: Clinical-neuropathological correlations in Alzheimer's disease and related dementias. Arch Neurol 51:888–895, 1994

Galton CJ, Patterson K, Xuereb JH, et al: Atypical and typical presentations of Alzheimer's disease: a clinical, neuropsychological, neuroimaging and pathological study of 13 cases. Brain 123 (Pt 3):484–498, 2000

Gass J, Cannon A, Mackenzie IR, et al: Mutations in progranulin are a major cause of ubiquitin-positive frontotemporal lobar degeneration. Hum Mol Genet 15:2988–3001, 2006

Gearing M, Mirra SS, Hedreen JC, et al: The Consortium to Establish a Registry for Alzheimer's Disease (CERAD), part X: neuropathology confirmation of the clinical diagnosis of Alzheimer's disease. Neurology 45:461–466, 1995a

Gearing M, Schneider JA, Rebeck GW, et al: Alzheimer's disease with and without coexisting Parkinson's disease changes: apolipoprotein E genotype and neuropathologic correlates. Neurology 45: 1985–1990, 1995b

Glenner GG, Wong CW: Alzheimer's disease: initial report of the purification and characterization of a novel cerebrovascular amyloid protein. Biochem Biophys Res Commun 120:885–890, 1984

Goate A, Chartier-Harlin MC, Mullan M, et al: Segregation of a missense mutation in the amyloid precursor protein gene with familial Alzheimer's disease. Nature 349:704–706, 1991

Goedert M, Ghetti B: Alois Alzheimer: his life and times. Brain Pathol 17:57–62, 2007

Graff-Radford NR, Crook JE, Lucas J, et al: Association of low plasma Abeta42/Abeta40 ratios with increased imminent risk for mild cognitive impairment and Alzheimer disease. Arch Neurol 64: 354–362, 2007

Green RC, Roberts JS, Cupples LA, et al: Disclosure of APOE genotype for risk of Alzheimer's disease. N Engl J Med 361:245–254, 2009

Han X, Fagan AM, Cheng H, et al: Cerebrospinal fluid sulfatide is decreased in subjects with incipient dementia. Ann Neurol 54:115–119, 2003

Harhangi BS, de Rijk MC, van Duijn CM, et al: APOE and the risk of PD with or without dementia in a population-based study. Neurology 54:1272–1276, 2000

Harold D, Abraham R, Hollingworth P, et al: Genome-wide association study identifies variants at CLU and PICALM associated with Alzheimer's disease. Nat Genet 41:1088–1093, 2009

Harwood DG, Barker WW, Loewenstein DA, et al: A cross-ethnic analysis of risk factors for AD in white Hispanics and white non-Hispanics. Neurology 52:551–556, 1999

He Z, Ong CH, Halper J, et al: Progranulin is a mediator of the wound response. Nat Med 9:225–229, 2003

Hernandez F, Avila J: Tauopathies. Cell Mol Life Sci 64:2219–2233, 2007

Hesse C, Rosengren L, Andreasen N, et al: Transient increase in total tau but not phospho-tau in human cerebrospinal fluid after acute stroke. Neurosci Lett 297:187–190, 2001

Holtzman DM, Bales KR, Tenkova T, et al: Apolipoprotein E isoform-dependent amyloid deposition and neuritic degeneration in a mouse model of Alzheimer's disease. Proc Natl Acad Sci U S A 97:2892–2897, 2000

Hu WT, Rippon GW, Boeve BF, et al: Alzheimer's disease and corticobasal degeneration presenting as corticobasal syndrome. Mov Disord 24:1375–1379, 2009

Ikonomovic MD, Klunk WE, Abrahamson EE, et al: Post-mortem correlates of in vivo PiB-PET amyloid imaging in a typical case of Alzheimer's disease. Brain 131:1630–1645, 2008

Jack CR Jr, Petersen RC, Xu YC, et al: Prediction of AD with MRI-based hippocampal volume in mild cognitive impairment. Neurology 52:1397–1403, 1999

Jagust WJ, Budinger TF, Reed BR: The diagnosis of dementia with single photon emission computed tomography. Arch Neurol 44:258–262, 1987

Joachim CL, Morris JH, Selkoe DJ: Clinically diagnosed Alzheimer's disease: autopsy results in 150 cases. Ann Neurol 24:50–56, 1988

Jordan BD, Relkin NR, Ravdin LD, et al: Apolipoprotein E epsilon4 associated with chronic traumatic brain injury in boxing. JAMA 278:136–140, 1997

Kemppainen NM, Aalto S, Karrasch M, et al: Cognitive reserve hypothesis: Pittsburgh Compound B and fluorodeoxyglucose positron emission tomography in relation to education in mild Alzheimer's disease. Ann Neurol 63:112–118, 2008

Kesslak JP, Nalcioglu O, Cotman CW: Quantification of magnetic resonance scans for hippocampal and parahippocampal atrophy in Alzheimer's disease. Neurology 41:51–54, 1991

Khachaturian ZS: Diagnosis of Alzheimer's disease. Arch Neurol 42:1097–1105, 1985

Klunk WE, Engler H, Nordberg A, et al: Imaging brain amyloid in Alzheimer's disease with Pittsburgh Compound-B. Ann Neurol 55:306–319, 2004

Knibb JA, Xuereb JH, Patterson K, et al: Clinical and pathological characterization of progressive aphasia. Ann Neurol 59:156–165, 2006

Knopman DS, Mastri AR, Frey WH II, et al: Dementia lacking distinctive histologic features: a common non-Alzheimer degenerative dementia. Neurology 40:251–256, 1990

Kumar-Singh S, Van Broeckhoven C: Frontotemporal lobar degeneration: current concepts in the light of recent advances. Brain Pathol 17:104–114, 2007

Lambert JC, Heath S, Even G, et al: Genome-wide association study identifies variants at CLU and CR1 associated with Alzheimer's disease. Nat Genet 41:1094–1099, 2009

Larson EB, Shadlen MF, Wang L, et al: Survival after initial diagnosis of Alzheimer disease. Ann Intern Med 140:501–509, 2004

Leinonen V, Alafuzoff I, Aalto S, et al: Assessment of beta-amyloid in a frontal cortical brain biopsy specimen and by positron emission tomography with carbon 11-labeled Pittsburgh Compound B. Arch Neurol 65:1304–1309, 2008

Levy ML, Miller BL, Cummings JL, et al: Alzheimer disease and frontotemporal dementias: behavioral distinctions. Arch Neurol 53: 687–690, 1996

Li F, Iseki E, Kato M, et al: An autopsy case of Alzheimer's disease presenting with primary progressive aphasia: a clinicopathological and immunohistochemical study. Neuropathology 20:239–245, 2000

Lippa CF, Swearer JM, Kane KJ, et al: Familial Alzheimer's disease: site of mutation influences clinical phenotype. Ann Neurol 48:376–379, 2000

Lomen-Hoerth C, Anderson T, Miller B: The overlap of amyotrophic lateral sclerosis and frontotemporal dementia. Neurology 59: 1077–1079, 2002

Mackenzie IR, Neumann M, Bigio EH, et al: Nomenclature and nosology for neuropathologic subtypes of frontotemporal lobar degeneration: an update. Acta Neuropathol 119:1–4, 2009

Masellis M, Momeni P, Meschino W, et al: Novel splicing mutation in the progranulin gene causing familial corticobasal syndrome. Brain 129:3115–3123, 2006

Mattsson N, Zetterberg H, Hansson O, et al: CSF biomarkers and incipient Alzheimer disease in patients with mild cognitive impairment. JAMA 302:385–393, 2009

McDowell I: Alzheimer's disease: insights from epidemiology. Aging (Milano) 13:143–162, 2001

McKhann G, Drachman D, Folstein M, et al: Clinical diagnosis of Alzheimer's disease: report of the NINCDS-ADRDA Work Group under the auspices of Department of Health and Human Services Task Force on Alzheimer's Disease. Neurology 34:939–944, 1984

Mega MS, Cummings JL, Fiorello T, et al: The spectrum of behavioral changes in Alzheimer's disease. Neurology 46:130–135, 1996

Mendez MF: Frontotemporal dementia: therapeutic interventions. Front Neurol Neurosci 24:168–178, 2009

Mendez MF, Shapira JS, McMurtray A, et al: Preliminary findings: behavioral worsening on donepezil in patients with frontotemporal dementia. Am J Geriatr Psychiatry 15:84–87, 2007

Miller BL, Ikonte C, Ponton M, et al: A study of the Lund-Manchester research criteria for frontotemporal dementia: clinical and single-photon emission CT correlations. Neurology 48:937–942, 1997

Mintun MA, Larossa GN, Sheline YI, et al: [11C]PIB in a nondemented population: potential antecedent marker of Alzheimer disease. Neurology 67:446–452, 2006

Mischel PS, Nguyen LP, Vinters HV: Cerebral cortical dysplasia associated with pediatric epilepsy: review of neuropathologic features and proposal for a grading system. J Neuropathol Exp Neurol 54:137–153, 1995

Mohs RC, Knopman D, Petersen RC, et al: Development of cognitive instruments for use in clinical trials of antidementia drugs: additions to the Alzheimer's Disease Assessment Scale that broaden its scope. The Alzheimer's Disease Cooperative Study. Alzheimer Dis Assoc Disord 11 Suppl 2:S13–S21, 1997

Morris JC, Roe CM, Grant EA, et al: Pittsburgh compound B imaging and prediction of progression from cognitive normality to symptomatic Alzheimer disease. Arch Neurol 66:1469–1475, 2009

Murrell JR, Price B, Lane KA, et al: Association of apolipoprotein E genotype and Alzheimer disease in African Americans. Arch Neurol 63:431–434, 2006

Nasreddine ZS, Phillips NA, Bedirian V, et al: The Montreal Cognitive Assessment, MoCA: a brief screening tool for mild cognitive impairment. J Am Geriatr Soc 53:695–699, 2005

Neary D, Snowden JS, Northen B, et al: Dementia of frontal lobe type. J Neurol Neurosurg Psychiatry 51:353–361, 1988

Neary D, Snowden JS, Gustafson L, et al: Frontotemporal lobar degeneration: a consensus on clinical diagnostic criteria. Neurology 51:1546–1554, 1998

Newell KL, Hyman BT, Growdon JH, et al: Application of the National Institute on Aging (NIA)-Reagan Institute criteria for the neuropathological diagnosis of Alzheimer disease. J Neuropathol Exp Neurol 58:1147–1155, 1999

Newman MF, Croughwell ND, Blumenthal JA, et al: Predictors of cognitive decline after cardiac operation. Ann Thorac Surg 59: 1326–1330, 1995

Ngandu T, von Strauss E, Helkala EL, et al: Education and dementia: what lies behind the association? Neurology 69:1442–1450, 2007

Okello A, Koivunen J, Edison P, et al: Conversion of amyloid positive and negative MCI to AD over 3 years: an 11C-PIB PET study. Neurology 73:754–760, 2009

Pachana NA, Boone KB, Miller BL, et al: Comparison of neuropsychological functioning in Alzheimer's disease and frontotemporal dementia. J Int Neuropsychol Soc 2:505–510, 1996

Petersen RC: Mild cognitive impairment as a diagnostic entity. J Intern Med 256:183–194, 2004

Petersen RC, Stevens JC, Ganguli M, et al: Practice parameter: early detection of dementia: mild cognitive impairment (an evidence-based review). Report of the Quality Standards Subcommittee of the American Academy of Neurology. Neurology 56:1133–1142, 2001

Petersen RC, Parisi JE, Dickson DW, et al: Neuropathologic features of amnestic mild cognitive impairment. Arch Neurol 63:665–672, 2006

Plassman BL, Langa KM, Fisher GG, et al: Prevalence of dementia in the United States: the aging, demographics, and memory study. Neuroepidemiology 29:125–132, 2007

Poorkaj P, Grossman M, Steinbart E, et al: Frequency of tau gene mutations in familial and sporadic cases of non-Alzheimer dementia. Arch Neurol 58:383–387, 2001

Pratico D, Clark CM, Lee VM, et al: Increased 8,12-iso-iPF2alpha-VI in Alzheimer's disease: correlation of a noninvasive index of lipid peroxidation with disease severity. Ann Neurol 48:809–812, 2000

Price JL, Morris JC: Tangles and plaques in nondemented aging and "preclinical" Alzheimer's disease. Ann Neurol 45:358–368, 1999

Ratnavalli E, Brayne C, Dawson K, et al: The prevalence of frontotemporal dementia. Neurology 58:1615–1621, 2002

Ray S, Britschgi M, Herbert C, et al: Classification and prediction of clinical Alzheimer's diagnosis based on plasma signaling proteins. Nat Med 13:1359–1362, 2007

Read SL, Miller BL, Mena I, et al: SPECT in dementia: clinical and pathological correlation. J Am Geriatr Soc 43:1243–1247, 1995

Reed LA, Wszolek ZK, Hutton M: Phenotypic correlations in FTDP-17. Neurobiol Aging 22:89–107, 2001

Reiman EM, Chen K, Alexander GE, et al: Functional brain abnormalities in young adults at genetic risk for late-onset Alzheimer's dementia. Proc Natl Acad Sci U S A 101:284–289, 2004

Reisberg B, Doody R, Stoffler A, et al: Memantine in moderate-to-severe Alzheimer's disease. N Engl J Med 348:1333–1341, 2003

Renner JA, Burns JM, Hou CE, et al: Progressive posterior cortical dysfunction: a clinicopathologic series. Neurology 63:1175–1180, 2004

Rogaeva EA, Fafel KC, Song YQ, et al: Screening for PS1 mutations in a referral-based series of AD cases: 21 novel mutations. Neurology 57:621–625, 2001

Rosen HJ, Gorno-Tempini ML, Goldman WP, et al: Patterns of brain atrophy in frontotemporal dementia and semantic dementia. Neurology 58:198–208, 2002a

Rosen HJ, Hartikainen KM, Jagust W, et al: Utility of clinical criteria in differentiating frontotemporal lobar degeneration (FTLD) from AD. Neurology 58:1608–1615, 2002b

Rosso SM, Donker Kaat L, Baks T, et al: Frontotemporal dementia in The Netherlands: patient characteristics and prevalence estimates from a population-based study. Brain 126:2016–2022, 2003

Rovelet-Lecrux A, Hannequin D, Raux G, et al: APP locus duplication causes autosomal dominant early onset Alzheimer disease with cerebral amyloid angiopathy. Nat Genet 38:24–26, 2006

Saunders AM, Strittmatter WJ, Schmechel D, et al: Association of apolipoprotein E allele epsilon 4 with late-onset familial and sporadic Alzheimer's disease. Neurology 43:1467–1472, 1993

Schofield PW, Logroscino G, Andrews HF, et al: An association between head circumference and Alzheimer's disease in a population-based study of aging and dementia. Neurology 49:30–37, 1997

Silverman DH, Small GW, Chang CY, et al: Positron emission tomography in evaluation of dementia: regional brain metabolism and long-term outcome. JAMA 286:2120–2127, 2001

Soontornniyomkij V, Lynch MD, Mermash S, et al: Cerebral microinfarcts associated with severe cerebral beta-amyloid angiopathy. Brain Pathol 20:459–467, 2009

Spina S, Murrell JR, Huey ED, et al: Clinicopathologic features of frontotemporal dementia with progranulin sequence variation. Neurology 68:820–827, 2007

Sunderland T, Linker G, Mirza N, et al: Decreased beta-amyloid1–42 and increased tau levels in cerebrospinal fluid of patients with Alzheimer disease. JAMA 289:2094–2103, 2003

Swartz JR, Miller BL, Lesser IM, et al: Frontotemporal dementia: treatment response to serotonin selective reuptake inhibitors. J Clin Psychiatry 58:212–216, 1997

Tang MX, Stern Y, Marder K, et al: The APOE-epsilon4 allele and the risk of Alzheimer disease among African Americans, whites, and Hispanics. JAMA 279:751–755, 1998

Tariot PN, Farlow MR, Grossberg GT, et al: Memantine treatment in patients with moderate to severe Alzheimer disease already receiving donepezil: a randomized controlled trial. JAMA 291: 317–324, 2004

Trinh NH, Hoblyn J, Mohanty S, et al: Efficacy of cholinesterase inhibitors in the treatment of neuropsychiatric symptoms and functional impairment in Alzheimer disease: a meta-analysis. JAMA 289:210–216, 2003

Trojanowski JQ, Duff K, Fillit H, et al: New directions for frontotemporal dementia drug discovery. Alzheimers Dement 4:89–93, 2008

Tun SM, Murman DL, Long HL, et al: Predictive validity of neuropsychiatric subgroups on nursing home placement and survival in patients with Alzheimer disease. Am J Geriatr Psychiatry 15:314–327, 2007

Utermann G, Langenbeck U, Beisiegel U, et al: Genetics of the apolipoprotein E system in man. Am J Hum Genet 32:339–347, 1980

Vinters HV: Cerebral amyloid angiopathy: a critical review. Stroke 18:311–324, 1987

Vinters HV, Gilbert JJ: Cerebral amyloid angiopathy: incidence and complications in the aging brain, II: the distribution of amyloid vascular changes. Stroke 14:924–928, 1983

Vinters HV, Pardridge WM, Yang J: Immunohistochemical study of cerebral amyloid angiopathy: use of an antiserum to a synthetic 28-amino-acid peptide fragment of the Alzheimer's disease amyloid precursor. Hum Pathol 19:214–222, 1988

Vinters HV, Nishimura GS, Secor DL, et al: Immunoreactive A4 and gamma-trace peptide colocalization in amyloidotic arteriolar lesions in brains of patients with Alzheimer's disease. Am J Pathol 137:233–240, 1990

Vinters HV, Secor DL, Read SL, et al: Microvasculature in brain biopsy specimens from patients with Alzheimer's disease: an immunohistochemical and ultrastructural study. Ultrastruct Pathol 18:333–348, 1994

Vinters HV, Natte R, Maat-Schieman ML, et al: Secondary microvascular degeneration in amyloid angiopathy of patients with hereditary cerebral hemorrhage with amyloidosis, Dutch type (HCHWA-D). Acta Neuropathol 95:235–244, 1998

Vinters HV, Ellis WG, Zarow C, et al: Neuropathologic substrates of ischemic vascular dementia. J Neuropathol Exp Neurol 59:931–945, 2000

Wetter SR, Delis DC, Houston WS, et al: Deficits in inhibition and flexibility are associated with the APOE-E4 allele in nondemented older adults. J Clin Exp Neuropsychol 27:943–952, 2005

Whitehouse PJ, Price DL, Struble RG, et al: Alzheimer's disease and senile dementia: loss of neurons in the basal forebrain. Science 215:1237–1239, 1982

Wilhelmsen KC, Lynch T, Pavlou E, et al: Localization of disinhibition-dementia-parkinsonism-amyotrophy complex to 17q21–22. Am J Hum Genet 55:1159–1165, 1994

Wiltfang J, Esselmann H, Smirnov A, et al: Beta-amyloid peptides in cerebrospinal fluid of patients with Creutzfeldt-Jakob disease. Ann Neurol 54:263–267, 2003

Winblad B, Cummings J, Andreasen N, et al: A six-month double-blind, randomized, placebo-controlled study of a transdermal patch in Alzheimer's disease: rivastigmine patch versus capsule. Int J Geriatr Psychiatry 22:456–467, 2007

Wisniewski K, Jervis GA, Moretz RC, et al: Alzheimer neurofibrillary tangles in diseases other than senile and presenile dementia. Ann Neurol 5:288–294, 1979

Zetterberg H, Hietala MA, Jonsson M, et al: Neurochemical aftermath of amateur boxing. Arch Neurol 63:1277–1280, 2006

Zhang-Nunes SX, Maat-Schieman ML, van Duinen SG, et al: The cerebral beta-amyloid angiopathies: hereditary and sporadic. Brain Pathol 16:30–39, 2006

17

Addiction

Elena Volfson, M.D., M.P.H.
David W. Oslin, M.D.

Substance abuse, particularly of alcohol and prescription drugs, among adults ages 60 and older presents a costly challenge for the health care system. As the number of older adults who have these disorders is increasing, the problem remains underestimated, underidentified, underdiagnosed, and undertreated (Blow 1998; Dowling et al. 2008; Simoni-Wastila and Yang 2006). Older adults have unique patterns of and health consequences from substance abuse and, therefore, require unique approaches to addiction, diagnosis, and treatment. In this chapter, we review problems related to alcohol abuse, nicotine dependence, prescription medication abuse, and illicit drug use among older adults, who for the purposes of this chapter are defined as persons ages 60 and older.

Epidemiology

Current and Projected Trends

In general, the prevalence of addiction is thought to decrease with age. Several reasons have been proposed to explain this reduction, such as successful treatment of addiction at a younger age, inability of older adults to carry out the activities necessary to engage in alcohol and drug abuse, and earlier death for addicted individuals. However, several studies show that substance abuse is on the rise among the current and emerging cohorts of older adults (Colliver et al. 2006; Gfroerer et al. 2002; McCabe et al. 2008). Compared with previous cohorts, the so-called baby boomers, born between 1946 and 1964, seem to have higher rates of alcoholism, prescription medication abuse, nicotine dependence, illicit drug abuse, and psychiatric comorbidities. One explanation rests on a recognized age cohort effect: the ready availability of certain drugs (e.g., crack cocaine) only to the newest generation of older adults. As evidence of a cohort effect in lifetime drug use, in 1995 half of the baby boomer cohort had used illicit drugs in their lifetime, compared with only 10% of adults ages 50 and older (Substance Abuse and Mental Health Services Administration 1996). Moreover, the population size of the baby boom generation is larger than any earlier cohorts.

According to statistical projections, the number of adults ages 60–69 with past-year substance use disorders is expected to more than triple from 0.6 million in 2002–2006 to 1.9 million in 2020 due both to population increase and to higher rates of substance use disorders in this age cohort (Han et al. 2009). These estimates indicate an urgent need to expand the treatment approaches and availability of substance abuse treatment services for older adults.

Barriers to Identification and Treatment

The available epidemiological data on elderly substance abuse most likely underestimate the true scope of the problem, because health care providers often overlook substance abuse and misuse among older adults. Diagnosis may be difficult because symptoms of substance abuse in older individuals often mimic symptoms of other common age-related general medical and neuropsychiatric disorders, such as diabetes, dementia, and depression. Nonspecific complaints, such as fatigue, irritability, insomnia, chronic pain, or impotence, may be caused or modified by alcohol or illicit drugs but are more often thought of as "normal aging." Finally, the DSM-IV-TR criteria for substance dependence (American Psychiatric Association 2000) may not apply readily to older adults. The recognition and diagnosis of substance dependence are heavily influenced by the presence of trouble at work, family problems, drinking while driving, and impairment in social activities. Many of these criteria are difficult to apply in a group enriched by retirement, widowhood, and contracted social circles. The net effect is that older patients are significantly less likely to have substance abuse problems identified during routine medical care, and even if a diagnosis of substance abuse is made, an older patient is less likely to have treatment recommended (Curtis et al. 1989). During short office visits, providers might not have enough time to discuss the issues of substance abuse while also having to address numerous general medical issues. Some providers may also believe that older persons with substance abuse do not benefit from treatment as much as younger patients do. Contrary to these misconceptions, research indicates that compared with younger patients, older adults are more likely to complete treatment and have outcomes that are as good as or better than those of younger adults (Oslin et al. 2002).

Special Populations

Several subpopulations of older adults deserve special mention. Elderly women who drink tend to do so at home and therefore are less likely to be identified. Elderly women also have less lean muscle mass than men, which leads to increased distribution of alcohol and other mood-altering substances in the body (Blow 1998). They are more likely to be prescribed psychoactive drugs, particularly benzodiazepines, and often take these medications chronically. Little is known about the role of race, ethnicity, or rural residence, but these groups often receive less preventive care and have less continuity with providers. Finally, many elderly patients are homebound and lack resources to seek health care or adhere to complex treatment visit schedules, or they do not have the social support necessary to engage in successful treatment.

Core Addiction Syndrome

Diagnostic criteria for addiction include a loss of control over drug intake; repeated unsuccessful attempts at quitting or reducing drug use; continued drug use despite negative consequences; a reduction in engagement in social, occupational, and recreational activities in lieu of drug-seeking or drug-administration behavior; and the emergence of symptoms of tolerance or withdrawal (American Psychiatric Association 2000). Addiction is associated with changes in the brain that are reflected in behaviors with two essential features: impaired ability to regulate the drive to obtain and use drugs, and reduced drive to obtain natural rewards. In other words, the reward circuitry of the brain becomes altered (Kalivas and O'Brien 2008). Increasing evidence points to neuroplastic changes that underlie a "core addiction syndrome" that develops in response to chronic administration of different substances of abuse. Although most of this research has been conducted in younger cohorts, where appropriate we comment on age-related changes in key neurotransmitter symptoms. Although older adults are often more responsive to treatment, the theoretical model of addiction does not seem to differ in older adults from that hypothesized in middle-aged adults.

Dopamine is a key neurotransmitter in addiction. Dopamine cells in the ventral tegmental area release dopamine in the prefrontal cortex (PFC), amygdala, and nucleus accumbens, regions that constitute reward circuitry. Dopamine in the mesolimbic pathway is involved in the acute reinforcing effects of alcohol and other drugs. With addictive substances, dopamine is released each time the drug is taken. With chronic use of drugs, a higher dosage is needed to achieve dopamine release, but it invariably occurs. Repeated use of drugs promotes increasing associations between the drug and life events or cues, and reinforces prior learning of drug-related behaviors. Thus, the addiction is "overlearned" (Kalivas and O'Brien 2008).

Dopamine release is modulated by γ-aminobutyric acid (GABA), glutamate, endogenous opioids, endocannabinoids, and a variety of neuropeptides and hormones. Figures 17–1 and 17–2 illustrate multiple pathways and neurotransmitters involved in reward circuitry. Once drug seeking is well learned, behaviors are thought to be maintained by glutamatergic connections between PFC and nucleus accumbens, and all addictive substances induce excessive glutamate release in cortical and subcortical circuits. Restoring (lowering) extracellular glutamate levels is one target for pharmacological interventions in chronic addicts.

Hypofrontality and Reduced Response to Biological Rewards

Glutamatergic neurotransmission from orbital PFC to motor circuits seems to be of critical importance for maintenance of addictive behavior and chronic relapse vulnerability. Once addictive behaviors are well established, subcortical glutamatergic connections to motor circuits assume primacy and reduce cortical control over the drug seeking, so that the behavior becomes automatic. The capacity of prefrontal circuitry to disrupt the drug seeking is impaired, consistent with neuroimaging studies that have demonstrated hypofrontality in individuals addicted to different substances (Kalivas et al. 2005; Volkow et al. 2004). However, drug-associated stimuli activate the PFC in a manner of excessive, uncontrolled responding to a drug, and there is poor or inappropriate response to biologically important stimuli (Kalivas and O'Brien 2008). One would hypothesize that age-associated decreases in cortical processing, neurodegenerative diseases such as Alzheimer's disease, and long-term exposure to neurotoxins such as alcohol would make hypofrontality a more prominent feature in elderly individuals with alcohol dependence. Indeed, evidence suggests that alcohol can cause substantial global cognitive deficits. However, no literature specifically demonstrates age-related increases in PFC deficits.

Craving

Craving, defined as "the desire to experience the effects of a previously used psychoactive substance" (World Health Organization 2010) is a common phenomenon for many substances of abuse. This desire can be driven by wanting to experience a high from a drug (positive reinforcement); by wanting to overcome a negative state, such as anxiety or withdrawal (negative reinforcement); or simply by having an urge or compulsion. Craving can occur even after long-term abstinence and is typically provoked by stress, conditioned substance-associated stimuli, and internal stimuli such as changes in mood (Vengeliene et al. 2008). Some researchers differentiate reward craving (positive reinforcement) and relief craving (negative reinforcement) (Heinz et al. 2003). This distinction is important for the treatment of craving, in that reward craving might result from dopamine-opioid dysregulation, whereas relief craving might result from either GABA/glutamatergic dysregulation or dysregulation in the corticotrophin-releasing factor (CRF) signaling pathway (Heilig and Koob 2007). Age-related illnesses such as stroke or neurodegenerative disorders may be hypothesized to affect craving. However, a study of craving failed to demonstrate an age-related decline in craving (Oslin et al. 2009). Indeed, about one-third of subjects in this older adult sample demonstrated persistence of craving despite abstinence.

Intoxication, Withdrawal, and Relapse

All drugs of abuse cause intoxication, which is manifested differently for each substance. Elderly patients are more sensitive to alcohol and other drugs and generally require a lower dose of a substance to result in intoxication.

All addictive substances cause specific discontinuation syndromes. Although withdrawal from many substances is unpleasant, only alcohol withdrawal is potentially life threatening. Elderly persons might be more sensitive to withdrawal due to the age-related changes in brain function and the presence of substantial concurrent illnesses, so inpatient detoxification might be preferred for older adults (Brower et al. 1994). Medical safety and removal of ongoing access to alcohol or drugs of abuse are primary considerations in this decision. Treatment of alcohol withdrawal is usually conducted with a cross-tolerant benzodiazepine such as oxazepam. However, agents that affect glutamate neurotransmission, such as acamprosate, gabapentin, topiramate, and memantine, as well as GABAergic anticonvulsants, such as carbamazepine and valproate, can also be used for alcohol withdrawal treatment (Nutt and Lingford-Hughes 2008). More recent evidence in older adults suggests that craving persists in about 25% of older adults, and its presence is associated with early relapse during the course of treatment (Oslin et al. 2009).

Relapse to drug use after a prolonged period of abstinence occurs commonly in addicted patients. This phenomenon presents a most significant problem for the long-term treatment of addicted individuals. One piece of good news is that elderly individuals engaged in treatment appear to have lower rates of relapse than younger individuals (Oslin et al. 2002).

Neurotransmission in the Aging Brain

Age-related neurophysiological changes in the central nervous system (CNS) are complex and not yet well defined (see Chapter 2, "Neurobiology of Aging"). It becomes especially challenging to superimpose substance-induced changes over the natural aging of the brain. Not only does brain volume shrink with aging (see Chapter 6, "Imaging the Structure of the Aging Human Brain"), but aging affects receptors, neurotransmitters, neurohormones, and neuromodulators. Elderly persons have significant alterations in most, but not all, neurotransmission systems, including the dopaminergic, serotonergic, noradrenergic, GABAergic, and glutamatergic systems. The net result of these various changes is the increased vulnerability of the brain as it ages. The reduced transmission of neuronal messages in the aging brain is thought to be associated with emotional, behavioral, and cognitive disorders in elderly persons. Finally, the ability of receptors to upregulate or downregulate in response to substances and medications decreases with age, which may account for the increased intoxication vulnerability to addictive substances and medications in elderly persons (Sunderland 2005).

Specific Neurotransmitter Systems Related to Treatment of Addiction

Modulators of dopaminergic and glutamatergic neurotransmission are the principal targets for pharmacological interventions for the treatment of addiction. The process of dopamine release is modulated by GABA, glutamate, serotonin, acetylcholine, endogenous opioids, endocannabinoids, and a variety of neuropeptides and hormones. Therefore, dopaminergic neurotransmission may be influenced either 1) directly by targeting the dopamine receptors, transporters, and enzymes; or 2) indirectly via changing the modulating effect of other neurotransmitter systems.

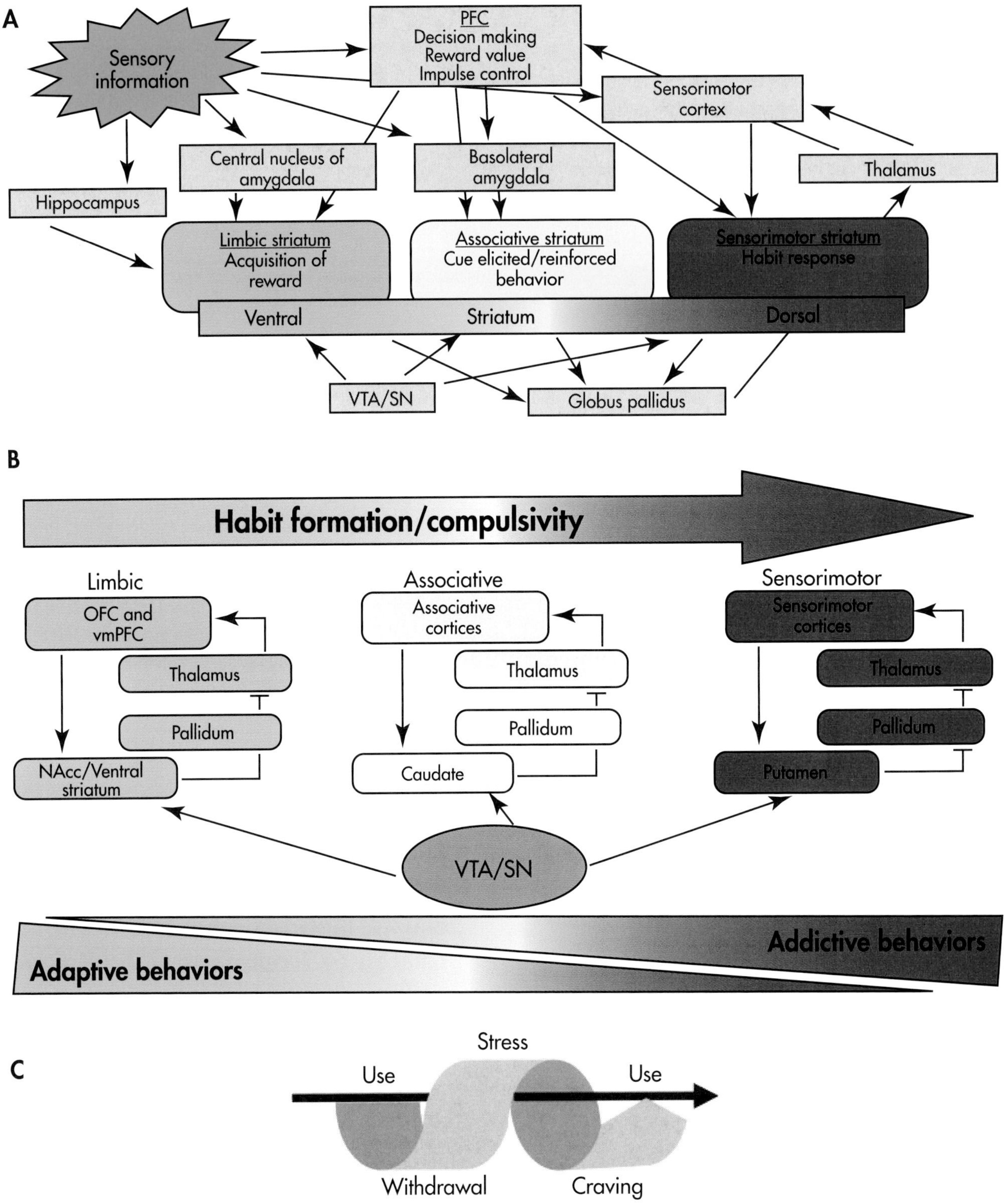
A
Sensory information
PFC
Decision making
Reward value
Impulse control
Sensorimotor cortex
Thalamus
Central nucleus of amygdala
Basolateral amygdala
Hippocampus
Limbic striatum
Acquisition of reward
Associative striatum
Cue elicited/reinforced behavior
Sensorimotor striatum
Habit response
Ventral
Striatum
Dorsal
VTA/SN
Globus pallidus
B
Habit formation/compulsivity
Limbic
Associative
Sensorimotor
OFC and vmPFC
Thalamus
Pallidum
NAcc/Ventral striatum
Associative cortices
Thalamus
Pallidum
Caudate
Sensorimotor cortices
Thalamus
Pallidum
Putamen
VTA/SN
Adaptive behaviors
Addictive behaviors
C
Stress
Use
Use
Withdrawal
Craving

FIGURE 17–1. Pathways and neurotransmitters involved in reward circuitry.

Panel A: Brain circuitry implicated in addiction. PFC=prefrontal cortex; SN=substantia nigra; VTA=ventral tegmental area. **Panel B:** Transition of activation of different corticostriatal networks with the formation of habit. Different colors reflect distinct corticostriatal circuits that underlie motivated and habitual behavior. The multicolored arrow represents the shift in involvement of these circuits as behavior becomes more habitual or compulsive in nature. Bottom triangles reflect hypothesized proportions of the motivational behavior repertoire that are devoted to adaptive and addictive behaviors, respectively, as involvement of more dorsal striatal circuits become more prominent and addictive behaviors become more severe. NAcc=nucleus accumbens; OFC=orbitofrontal cortex; SN=substantia nigra; vmPFC=ventromedial prefrontal cortex; VTA=ventral tegmental area. **Panel C:** Habit formation in addiction progression. Cyclical arrow represents pattern of behaviors posited as central to the addictive process. Straight arrow represents transition from acquisition to habitual/compulsive behaviors in addiction formation.

Source. Reprinted from Brewer JA, Potenza MN: "The Neurobiology and Genetics of Impulse Control Disorders: Relationships to Drug Addictions." *Biochemical Pharmacology* 25:63–75, 2008. Copyright © 2008, with permission from Elsevier.

Dopaminergic Neurotransmission

Five G-protein-coupled dopamine receptors have been identified. They are classified into two families: 1) D_1 and D_5 receptors, which stimulate production of cyclic adenosine monophosphate, and 2) D_2, D_3, and D_4 receptors, which inhibit the production of cyclic adenosine monophosphate. The functions of D_1, D_2, and D_3 receptors primarily concern motivation and reward, whereas D_4 and D_5 receptors are more involved with behavioral inhibition (Goodman 2008). As a person ages, dopamine neurotransmission decreases overall, and the ratio of D_1 to D_2 receptors increases, suggesting a qualitative change in dopamine neurotransmission (Sunderland 2005).

Relevance to Addictive Behavior

Haney et al. (2001) reported that long-term administration of a selective D_1 antagonist to human subjects enhanced both self-administration and subjective effects of cocaine, compared with placebo. Positron emission tomography (PET) and single-photon emission computed tomography (SPECT) neuroimaging studies of alcoholics, as well as cocaine, methamphetamine, and heroin addicts, have shown reductions in D_2 receptor density in the ventral striatum that persist long after detoxification (Volkow et al. 2001, 2004). For example, studies have found a correlation between the baseline availability of D_2 receptors in nonaddicted individuals and their subjective responses to alcohol and other addictive substances (Volkow et al. 1999; Yoder et al. 2005). A new area of interest is the genetic variability within each neurotransmitter system. For instance, the Al allele of the D_2 receptor gene *Taq1A* polymorphism has been associated with alcoholism, cocaine addiction, psychostimulant addiction, and cigarette smoking (Goodman 2008).

GABAergic Neurotransmission

GABA is the chief inhibitory neurotransmitter in the CNS. Three classes of GABA receptors have been identified: $GABA_A$, $GABA_B$, and $GABA_C$. $GABA_A$ and $GABA_C$ receptors are ionotropic receptors (ligand-gated ion channels), whereas $GABA_B$ receptors are metabotropic (G-protein-coupled) receptors that open transmembrane potassium channels, suppress calcium channels, and reduce the activity of adenylate cyclase (Goodman 2008). In addition to an active GABA binding site, $GABA_A$ receptors have specific allosteric sites that bind benzodiazepines, barbiturates, ethanol, neuroactive steroids, and other substances. In the case of GABA-benzodiazepine receptors, GABA potentiates binding of benzodiazepine molecules to the receptors, where benzodiazepines in turn sensitize GABA receptors to their ligand, thus enhancing GABA effect upon binding to its receptor. There is a paucity of information about age-related changes in GABAergic neurotransmission. PET scans have failed to show any age-related changes of the GABAergic system; however, that contradicts a clinically established hypersensitivity of the elderly to benzodiazepines (Sunderland 2005).

Relevance to Addictive Behavior

Because activation of GABA receptors on interneurons inhibits dopamine release, enhancing GABA neurotransmission has been a target for medication development. Medications that promote GABA transmission, such as vigabatrin (inhibitor of GABA transferase), gabapentin (mechanism unclear), and baclofen ($GABA_B$ agonist), were effective in small-scale clinical studies (O'Brien 2005). Anticonvulsants that affect the GABA system, such as valproate, tiagabine, and topiramate, have shown promise in treating psychostimulant misuse and

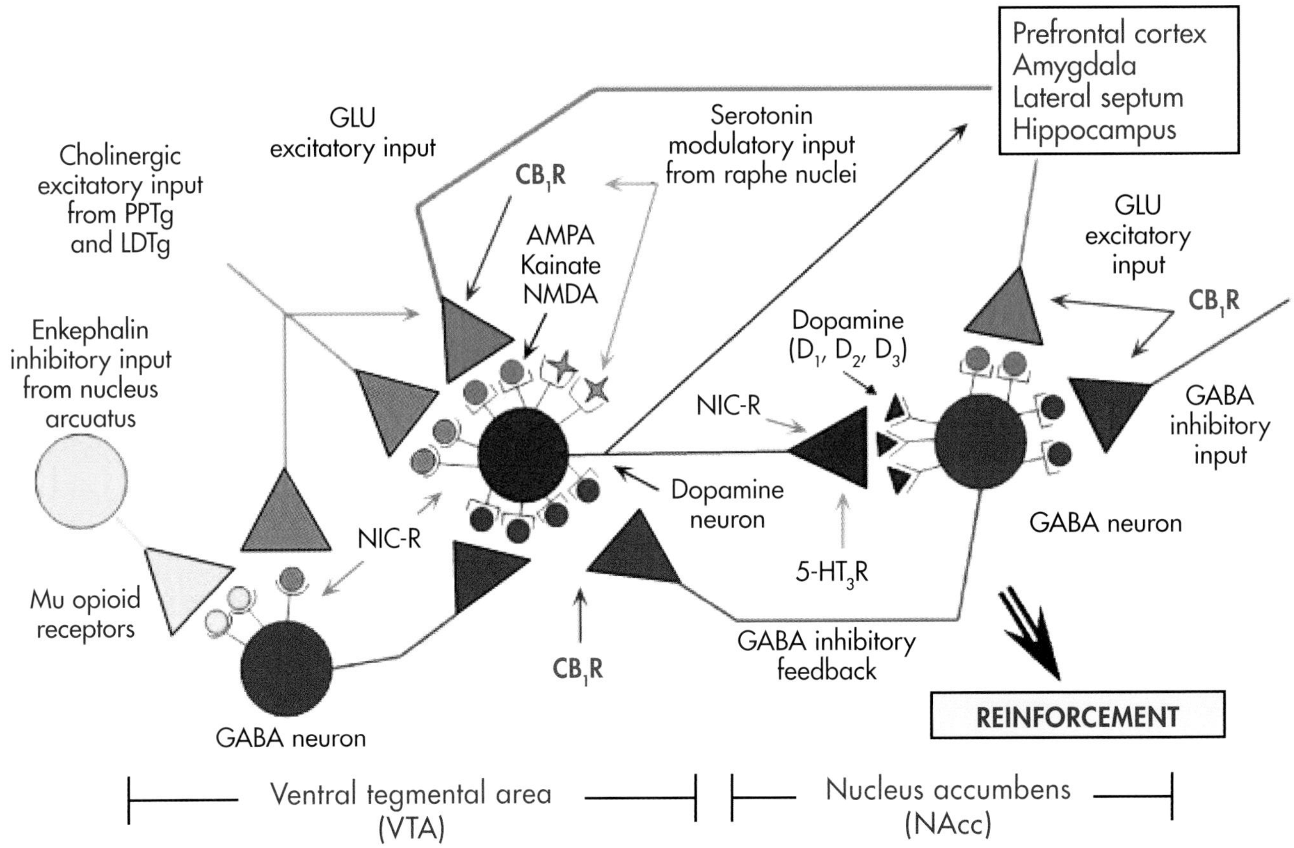

FIGURE 17–2. Neuronal pathways involved with the reinforcing effects of alcohol and other abused drugs.

Cholinergic inputs that arise from the caudal part of the pedunculopontine tegmental nucleus (PPTg) and laterodorsal tegmental nucleus (LDTg) can stimulate ventral tegmental area (VTA) dopamine neurons. The VTA dopamine neuron projection to the nucleus accumbens (NAcc) and cortex, the critical substrate for the reinforcing effects of abused drugs (including alcohol), is modulated by a variety of inhibitory (γ-aminobutyric acid [GABA] and opioid) and excitatory (nicotinic [NIC-R], glutamate [GLU], and cannabinoid-1 receptor [CB_1R]) inputs. The GLU pathways include those that express AMPA, kainate, and *N*-methyl-D-aspartate (NMDA) receptors. Serotonin-3 receptors (5-HT_3R) also modulate dopamine release in the NAcc.

Source. Reprinted from Johnson BA: "Update on Neuropharmacological Treatments for Alcoholism: Scientific Basis and Clinical Findings." *Biochemical Pharmacology* 75:34–56, 2008. Copyright © 2008, with permission from Elsevier.

alcoholism, although more research is necessary, and these medications have not been approved by the U.S. Food and Drug Administration (FDA) for treatment of addiction at this time (Johnson 2008). No studies to date have examined these medications specifically in older adults with addiction.

Glutamatergic Neurotransmission

Glutamate is the most abundant excitatory neurotransmitter in the brain, mediating as much as 70% of synaptic transmission within the CNS. Three different types of ionotropic glutamate receptors mediate fast excitatory neurotransmission: the *N*-methyl-D-aspartate (NMDA) receptor, the α-amino-3-hydroxy-5-methylisoxazole-4-propionic acid (AMPA) receptor, and the kainic acid (KA) receptor. Glutamate also binds to metabotropic receptors that mediate slow modulatory neurotransmission. Data are sparse on the changes in glutamatergic neurotransmission with aging. Instead of an absolute increase or decrease of glutamatergic activity, there are thought to be qualitative changes in glutamatergic-cholinergic, glutamatergic-serotonergic, and glutamatergic-hormonal interactions in the aging brain (Sunderland 2005). Older brains are likely to be more susceptible to the toxic effects of the increased extracellular glutamate levels caused by alcohol and drugs. In addition, increased glutamate levels are involved in the pathogenesis of neurodegenerative diseases and strokes. Thus, substance abuse may facilitate the development of and contribute to earlier onset of neurodegenerative conditions in the elderly.

Relevance to Addictive Behavior

Glutamatergic projections and neurons expressing glutamate receptors in reward circuitry modulate not only dopamine release but also synaptic plasticity, which is important in learning and memory. Glutamatergic medications, such as acamprosate (NMDA antagonist and modulator of metabotropic glutamate receptors), *N*-acetylcysteine (cystine-glutamate exchange modifier), modafinil (complex glutamatergic mechanism of action), topiramate (KA and AMPA antagonist), lamotrigine (glutamate release inhibitor), gabapentin (glutamate release inhibitor), and memantine (NMDA antagonist), have shown promise in treatment of various addictive disorders, but these medications have not been studied in elderly persons (Gass and Olive 2008; Johnson 2008).

Endogenous Opioid System

The endogenous opioid system includes a large number of opioid peptides that are ligands for numerous types of opioid receptors. Four distinct families of endogenous opioid peptides have been well characterized: endorphins, enkephalins, dynorphins, and endomorphins. These peptides have diverse physiological functions, one of which involves antinociception (pain control), and they can function as neurotransmitters, neuromodulators, or in some cases neurohormones. In the CNS, there are three primary opioid receptor types: mu, kappa, and delta. High densities of opioid receptors are located in the brain stem, medial thalamus, spinal cord, hypothalamus, and limbic system. A significant loss in availability and structure of endogenous opioid neurotransmitters has been observed with aging, including in the frontal lobes, hippocampus, and striatum (Sunderland 2005).

Relevance to Addictive Behavior

Both endogenous opioids and dopamine are released in response to rewarding stimuli, including natural reinforcers and substances of abuse, and there is interaction between the two systems. By binding to μ-opioid receptors on GABAergic interneurons, endorphins inhibit GABA and, therefore, promote dopamine release. In contrast, action of endogenous dynorphin on κ-opioid receptors inhibits the release of dopamine and generates dysphoria. Dynorphin also causes presynaptic inhibition of glutamate release. PET studies in recently abstinent cocaine, alcohol, and heroine addicts have shown the increased levels of μ-opioid receptors (Heinz et al. 2005; Williams et al. 2007).

Naltrexone, a μ-opioid receptor antagonist, has been shown in a number of clinical trials to reduce the risk of relapse in alcoholics (Pettinati and Rabinowitz 2005). The effectiveness of naltrexone varies between patients, which may be explained by μ-opioid receptor polymorphism (Anton et al. 2006b; Oslin et al. 2003). Interestingly, studies of naltrexone for the treatment of cocaine dependence have failed to show treatment efficacy. Naltrexone is well tolerated by elderly patients, helps modify drinking behavior (Oslin et al. 1997), and is the treatment of choice for alcohol dependence in older adults because of its safety and effectiveness.

Noradrenergic Neurotransmission

Norepinephrine is both a neurotransmitter produced primarily by the locus coeruleus in the brain stem and a hormone produced by the adrenal medulla. It is synthesized from dopamine by the enzyme dopamine β-hydroxylase. Both norepinephrine and epinephrine are ligands for adrenergic receptors, which are G-protein-coupled receptors, either α-adrenergic (subgroups α_1 and α_2) or β-adrenergic (subgroups β_1, β_2, and β_3) (Goodman 2008). Data regarding the effects of aging on the noradrenergic system are sparse and often contradictory. On the one hand, aging brains have reduced norepinephrine activity due to a decrease in the number of locus coeruleus neurons, as well as decreased activity of tyrosine hydroxylase and dopa decarboxylase, key enzymes in norepinephrine synthesis. Furthermore, both the concentration and activity of monoamine oxidase (MAO), the enzyme responsible for the presynaptic breakdown of norepinephrine, increase with age. On the other hand, concentration of norepinephrine in cerebrospinal fluid (CSF) has been shown to increase with age, and the concentration of norepinephrine metabolite 3-methoxy-4-hydroxyphenylglycol (MHPG) also increases in some areas of the aging brain (Sunderland 2005).

Relevance to Addictive Behavior

Noradrenergic neurotransmission modulates dopamine release in the reward circuitry and the prefrontal cortex. One treatment used as an adjunct in opioid detoxification is clonidine, an α_2-adrenergic receptor agonist. Disulfiram, used in the treatment of alcoholism and perhaps helpful in cocaine addiction, has been shown to block the enzyme dopamine β-hydroxylase, thereby reducing the availability of norepinephrine (Petrakis et al. 2000).

Serotonergic Neurotransmission

Serotonin (5-HT) activity is associated with behavioral inhibition, emotional stabilization, appetite modulation, sensory reactivity, pain sensitivity, sleep, sexual behavior, and cognitive function. At least 14 subtypes of 5-HT receptors have been cloned and identified. Postmortem studies indicate a decrease of 5-HT_2 receptors with aging in the cortex, but not in the hypothalamus or striatum. An age-related decrease in receptor activity in the caudate, putamen, and frontal cortex has been shown by PET. Age-related alterations in serotonin synthesis or receptor activity are believed to explain changes in sleep, appetite, and mood, as well as cognitive decline, in elderly persons (Sunderland 2005).

Relevance to Addictive Behavior

Even though serotonin is not directly involved in the rewarding effects of substances, it modulates the dopamine system and is important in behavioral inhibition. The 5-HT_{2C} receptor is the only receptor that, when stimulated, inhibits many addiction-related behaviors (Goodman 2008; Muller and Huston 2006). The 5-HT_{1B} receptor plays an especially significant role in motivational circuitry. GABA neurons in the mesolimbic system contain 5-HT_{1B} receptors that, when activated, inhibit GABA release, thereby potentiating dopamine release. Studies have determined that low levels of CSF 5-hydroxylindolacetic acid, a major metabolite of 5-HT and an indicator of 5-HT activity, are associated with impulsivity, aggression, depression, and early-onset alcoholism (Kreek et al. 2004). Pharmacological studies have shown that selective serotonin reuptake inhibitors (SSRIs), although well tolerated by elderly patients, have not been useful in the treatment of alcohol dependence (Johnson 2008). Ondansetron, a 5-HT_3 antagonist, has been shown to be effective for a subset of individuals with early-onset alcoholism, but this finding lacks replication (Johnson et al. 2000).

Endocannabinoids

Cannabinoid receptors are distributed throughout the CNS and peripheral tissues, including the immune system, reproductive and gastrointestinal tracts, sympathetic ganglia, endocrine glands, arteries, lungs, and heart. There are at least two types of G-protein-coupled cannabinoid receptors, CB_1 and CB_2. CB_1 receptors are located primarily on central and peripheral neurons, modulating neurotransmitter release. CB_1 receptors are the most abundant G-protein-coupled receptors in the brain. CB_2 receptors are present mainly on immune cells. Endogenous agonists for cannabinoid receptors (endocannabinoids) have also been discovered, the most important being arachidonoyl ethanolamide (anandamide), 2-arachidonoyl glycerol, and 2-arachidonyl glyceryl ether.

Relevance to Addictive Behavior

Activation of CB_1 receptors stimulates dopaminergic neurotransmission and increases rewarding effects of drugs of abuse and natural reinforcers. The endocannabinoid system is thought to reinforce both the motivation and the reward functions of the mesolimbic dopamine system. Genetic variants of CB_1 receptors have been identified as probable factors in a person's vulnerability to develop an addictive disorder (Zhang et al. 2004). During chronic alcohol exposure, endocannabinoid levels in the brain are elevated, and CB_1 receptor levels are reduced. 9-Tetrahydrocannabinol (THC), an active ingredient of marijuana, binds to CB_1 receptors and produces reinforcing effects. The CB_1 receptor blocker rimonabant modulates dopamine responses to administration of nicotine, ethanol, and cocaine (Cheer et al. 2007). Rimonabant has been used safely, with no dosage adjustment for elderly patients, for the treatment of obesity, but there is no available evidence at this time that rimonabant is efficacious for addictions.

Common Substances of Abuse in the Elderly

Alcohol

After tobacco, the substance most commonly abused by elderly people is alcohol. In 2007, rates of current alcohol use were 47.6% among people ages 60–64 and 38.1% among people ages 65 and older (Substance Abuse and Mental Health Services Administration 2008). Adults ages 65 and older had lower rates of binge drinking (7.6%) than adults in other age groups. The rate of heavy drinking among persons ages 65 and older was 1.4%. However, these numbers might be an underestimation, because multiple community prevalence studies have shown elderly people to have a wide range of problematic drinking, from 1% to 15% (Oslin 2004). Other indicators that the problem is larger come from data demonstrating that the percentage of persons driving under the influence of alcohol in the past year was 6.3% among people ages 60–64 and 2.4% among persons ages 65 and older (Substance Abuse and Mental Health Services Administration 2008).

Neurobiology of Alcohol Dependence

Alcohol affects multiple molecular targets, both directly and indirectly. Among those targets are the NMDA, $GABA_A$, glycine, serotonin 5-HT_3, and nicotinic acetylcholine (nACh) receptors, as well as ion channels (Vengeliene et al. 2008). Biological genetically influenced predisposition and environmental factors appear to play important roles in initiation of alcohol consumption and abuse. Furthermore, underlying individual differences in the reward system lead to different effects of alcohol. For instance, polymorphisms in $GABA_A$ receptor subunits have been linked to alcohol response in humans (Dick et al. 2006; Soyka et al. 2008). The innate hyperactivity of the CRF system and hypoactivity of the neuropeptide Y (NPY) system are known to promote alcohol consumption. Studies have reported associations between the onset of alcoholism and specific variants of the *NPY* gene (Mottagui-Tabar et al. 2005) and the CRF_1 receptor (Treutlein et al. 2006). Chronic alcohol consumption affects GABAergic, glutamatergic, dopaminergic, and opioidergic systems, as well as the endocannabinoid system and brain stress CRF and antistress NPY systems. Which particular changes are responsible for the switch to compulsive use is currently unknown. However, this switch is estimated to occur in 10%–15% of the drinking population and is believed to result from genetic and environmental vulnerabilities (Vengeliene et al. 2008). Also unknown is how aging affects the vulnerability or development of alcohol dependence. Although many older adults have had difficulty with drinking for years, other older adults become addicted only in late life after a lifetime of no more than social drinking.

Of the many factors that influence the initiation and maintenance of alcohol addiction, critical factors include reward and relief craving, loss of executive control, and affective dysregulation. For instance, evidence suggesting that a genetic polymorphism of the μ-opioid receptor may be associated with reward craving and predict treatment response to opioid antagonists (Anton et al. 2008; Oslin et al. 2003) has implications for only 25% of the European Americans who have this polymorphism. Similarly, despite high rates of psychiatric comorbidity, most alcohol-dependent persons do not have depressive syndromes, so treatment with mood stabilizers or antidepressants is relevant only for a subset of alcohol-dependent individuals.

Pharmacological Treatment of Alcohol Dependence

Pharmacological treatments have not traditionally played a major role in the long-term treatment of older alcohol-dependent adults. Until recently, disulfiram was the only medication approved for the treatment of alcohol dependence, but it was seldom used in older patients because of concerns related to adverse effects. In 1995, the opioid antagonist naltrexone was approved by the FDA for the treatment of alcohol dependence. Clinical practice guidelines from the National Institute on Alcohol Abuse and Alcoholism (2007) suggest that pharmacotherapy should be used as part of the initial treatment of alcohol dependence. In particular, naltrexone and acamprosate are considered first-line treatments for alcohol dependence. However, pharmacotherapy should be considered an adjunct to a psychosocial treatment plan including therapies such as cognitive-behavioral therapy, group therapies, or 12-step programs.

Naltrexone. In 1994, the opioid antagonist naltrexone was approved by the FDA for the treatment of alcohol dependence based on its demonstrated efficacy in middle-aged adults. Oslin et al. (1997) subsequently demonstrated the safety and efficacy of naltrexone in elderly patients, although nausea is reported as significant in up to 15% of patients. In multiple studies, naltrexone was found useful in preventing relapse and reducing the craving for alcohol, especially in patients with familial loading for alcoholism. However, the effect size of naltrexone appears to be modest, with a corresponding number needed to treat of seven (Johnson 2008). To address the issues of noncompliance and adverse events and to provide steady-state levels of medication, depot naltrexone formulations in injectable intramuscular form or as subcutaneous implants have been developed and used with good clinical outcomes (Johnson et al. 2004). The injectable forms provide steady levels of medication for about 30 days, whereas naltrexone implants are effective for up to several months. However, their usefulness might be limited in elderly patients because of 1) a high prevalence of chronic pain conditions requiring the use of opioid medications and 2) the substantial costs of depot formulations. Naltrexone is straightforward to use at 50 mg/day. Most adults, including elderly patients, can start at 50 mg/day, and occasionally raising the dosage to 100 mg/day increases effectiveness. The effect of naltrexone or acamprosate, unlike antidepressants, should occur rapidly. If patients are failing to curb or eliminate drinking within 8 weeks, the treatment plan should be reviewed. There are no contraindications to using naltrexone in the frail elderly or patients with dementia or common medical problems of late life.

Acamprosate. Acamprosate (calcium acetylhomotaurine) is a derivative of homotaurine (a nonspecific GABA agonist). Acamprosate was developed in Europe in the 1980s as a pharmacological agent to reduce alcohol consumption, craving, and relapse in alcoholic patients. Since then, acamprosate has demonstrated moderate efficacy in reducing overall alcohol consumption and subjective measures of alcohol craving, as well as in promoting abstinence. Acamprosate indirectly increases GABAergic neurotransmission by blocking inhibitory presynaptic $GABA_B$ autoreceptors and by increasing extracellular levels of taurine, an endogenous sulfonated amino acid that can potentiate $GABA_A$ receptor–mediated chloride influx (Gass and Olive 2008; Johnson 2008). It acts on both metabotropic and ionotropic glutamate receptors. Acamprosate is believed to restore the imbalance between excitatory and inhibitory neurotransmission caused by chronic alcohol exposure.

Most of the clinical evidence for the efficacy of acamprosate in the treatment of alcohol dependence comes from a series of European studies (Mann et al. 2004). In contrast, a number of studies in the United States failed to find any therapeutic benefit of acamprosate compared with placebo on any drinking outcome measures (Anton et al. 2006a). From the European studies, acamprosate appears to benefit individuals with alcohol dependence who are females and who have increased levels of anxiety, physiological dependence, a negative family history, and late age at onset (Verheul et al. 2005). Acamprosate is complicated to use because it requires dosing three to four times per day. There are no recommended dosage adjustments for older adults. Patients with chronic renal failure should not take acamprosate.

Disulfiram. Disulfiram is an FDA-approved medication that has been used for treating alcoholism since the 1940s. Its principal mode of action is as an aversive agent. Disulfiram inhibits aldehyde dehydrogenase and prevents the metabolism of alcohol's primary metabolite, acetaldehyde. If alcohol is ingested, the accumulation of acetaldehyde in the blood causes unpleasant effects, including sweating, headache, dyspnea, lowered blood pressure, flushing, sympathetic overactivity, palpitations, nausea, and vomiting. The association of these symptoms with drinking discourages further consumption of alcohol. Serious side effects have also been reported and include hepatitis, hepatotoxicity, depression, and psychotic reactions, making use of disulfiram unacceptable in frail elderly patients. Furthermore, disulfiram has no significant effect on craving for alcohol, and poor compliance is common. In older adults the disulfiram reaction may complicate preexisting general medical problems, such as heart disease, and the medication should be used with caution in the frail elderly.

Serotonergic medications. In general, serotonergic agents have not been found useful for treating addiction. However, growing evidence suggests that SSRIs are of therapeutic benefit for a specific group of individuals with alcoholism. For clinical and research purposes, two subtypes of alcoholic individuals have been identified by Cloninger (1987). Type A alcoholics, characterized by a later age at onset of problem drinking (typically after age 25), a preponderance of psychosocial morbidity, and low familial loading for alcohol dependence, can experience improved drinking outcomes after SSRI treatment. Type B alcoholics, characterized by an early age at onset of problem drinking, high familial loading, and a range of impulsive or antisocial traits, do not improve with SSRI treatment and may actually worsen or experience relapse with SSRI exposure. Allelic variation at the 5-HT transporter might account in part for this difference (Johnson 2008).

Other potential agents. Topiramate, lamotrigine, gabapentin, modafinil, and *N*-acetylcysteine have shown some promise in treatment of alcohol dependence in younger populations but have not been studied in alcohol-dependent older adults (Gass and Olive 2008; Johnson 2008).

Tobacco

Tobacco dependence is a significant problem in the elderly population. In the United States, tobacco is used more widely than illicit drugs, and it is implicated in more deaths each year than alcohol and illicit drugs combined. In a study by the Substance Abuse and Mental Health Services Administration (2008), the reported rates of past-month cigarette use were 18.8% among persons ages 60–64 and 9.0% among persons ages 65 and older. The past-month rates of nicotine dependence among the past-month cigarette users were reported to be 69.1% among persons ages 50–64 and 57.3% among those ages 65 and older. In addition to well-established tobacco-related health problems, a high comorbidity with other substance use disorders and psychiatric disorders has been established. In general, compared with younger smokers, older smokers are less educated, have a lower socioeconomic status, and are more likely to be female (Andrews et al. 2004).

Older adults can be as successful in quitting their tobacco use as their younger counterparts and can experience physical, social, and psychological benefits from cessation (Andrews et al. 2004). In a large-sample study examining the trends in current smoking and the prevalence of smoking cessation among older adults (>12,000 individuals ages 65 and older), Husten et al. (1997) found that among older adults, the prevalence of cessation rose with increasing educational attainment and was consistently higher for men than for women and for whites than for blacks. In a more recent study, Sachs-Ericsson et al. (2009) reported that smoking cessation behavior of older adults is best explained by higher levels of distress and health problems, regardless of race or gender. The presence of current drinking problems and depressive symptoms predicts lower likelihood of smoking cessation in older adult smokers (Kenney et al. 2009). Unlike alcohol addiction, initiating and becoming addicted to nicotine for the first time in late life are relatively uncommon for older adults.

Neurobiology of Tobacco Dependence

Upon inhalation of cigarette smoke, nicotine quickly crosses the blood-brain barrier and binds to $\alpha_4\beta_2$ nACh receptors in the brain. It stimulates dopamine release in the mesocorticolimbic system. Presynaptic α_7 nACh receptors activate glutamatergic projections, which enhances the excitatory input. Dopamine release is inhibited by nACh receptors on GABAergic interneurons. Although nACh receptors are primary targets of nicotine, other neurotransmitter systems are closely involved in the maintenance of nicotine addiction. Other components of tobacco smoke thought to be associated with tobacco dependence include ammonia, compounds with MAO inhibitory properties, acetaldehyde, salsolinol, and harman.

Pharmacological Treatment of Nicotine Dependence

Medications commonly prescribed to assist in smoking cessation include nicotine replacement therapy (NRT), such as the nicotine patch, nicotine gum, nicotine nasal spray, nicotine inhaler, and nicotine lozenge. Other agents include varenicline and bupropion. Studies focused specifically on elderly persons are lacking, but there is no a priori reason that use of NRT should differ in older adults.

Nicotine replacement therapy. The aim of NRT is to temporarily replace nicotine from cigarettes to reduce both motivation to smoke and nicotine withdrawal symptoms, thus easing the transition from cigarette smoking to abstinence. Stead et al. (2008) reviewed the effectiveness of NRT in a meta-analysis of 132 trials with over 40,000 participants. The risk ratio of abstinence after at least 6 months of follow-up for any form of NRT relative to control was 1.58 (95% confidence interval [CI], 1.50–1.66). The effects were largely independent of the duration of therapy, the intensity of additional support provided, or the setting in which NRT was offered. NRTs increased the rate of quitting by 50%–70%, regardless of setting. The use of NRT has been shown to be safe and efficacious among older smokers with cardiovascular disease (Doolan and Froelicher 2008).

Nicotine receptor partial agonist (varenicline). Varenicline is a partial agonist of $\alpha_4\beta_2$ nACh receptors. This medication may help people to stop smoking through a combination of maintaining moderate levels of dopamine to counteract withdrawal symptoms (acting as an agonist) and reducing smoking satisfaction (acting as an antagonist). In a meta-analysis (Cahill et al. 2010) that included nine trials with 7,267 participants, the pooled risk ratio for continuous abstinence with varenicline versus placebo at 6 months was 2.33 (95% CI, 1.95–2.80), versus bupropion at 1 year was 1.52 (95% CI, 1.22–1.88), and versus NRT at 1 year was 1.31 (95% CI, 1.01–1.71). The main adverse effect of varenicline was nausea, which was mostly at mild to moderate levels and usually subsided over time. Postmarketing safety data suggest that varenicline may be associated with depressed mood, agitation, and suicidal behavior or ideation, which caused the FDA to issue a warning. In one study, varenicline has been safely used in elderly patients (Burstein et al. 2006).

Bupropion. Bupropion is an antidepressant that has been used safely in elderly patients. It is helpful in the treatment of tobacco dependence, and before the approval of varenicline, it was the only pharmacological agent available (Hughes et al. 2007). Immediate-release, sustained-release, and extended-release formulations of bupropion are available. The recommended daily dosage range for smoking cessation in elderly patients is 150–300 mg.

Opioids

Prescription analgesics are among the most commonly used medications by elderly persons. Chronic pain due to neurological and cerebrovascular diseases, osteoarthritis, cancer, and other conditions is a very common phenomenon in this patient population. The most recently available report indicates that 14.9% of community-dwelling older adults were prescribed more than one controlled opioid analgesic in 1999 (Simoni-Wastila et al. 2005). Although timely and adequate management of acute and chronic pain is paramount in providing adequate quality of life, clinicians should be cognizant of potential deleterious effects of analgesics in elderly patients. The sense of euphoria and well-being produced by opioid analgesics contributes to their addictive potential. Conservative estimates of patients prescribed long-term opioids who develop some sort of addictive disorder usually range from 2% to 6% (Fields 2007); however, this estimate can be higher in persons with a substance abuse history. Most of the opioid medications used in the United States are full μ-opioid agonists, with the exception of buprenorphine, which is a partial μ-opioid agonist. Sublingual buprenorphine and oral methadone are FDA approved for the detoxification and the treatment of opioid dependence.

Older patients are more vulnerable than their younger counterparts to respiratory depression and cardiovascular toxicity associated with full μ-opioid agonists. Also, elderly persons may become overly sedated and cognitively impaired with prolonged opioid use. For all opioid medications except buprenorphine, half-life of the active drug and metabolites is increased in elderly persons. Compared with the full μ-opioid agonists, buprenorphine is less likely to induce respiratory depression, immunosuppression, and hyperalgesia (paradoxical increase in pain) with chronic use (Pergolizzi et al. 2008); therefore, this medication is an attractive option for pain management and treatment of opioid dependence in elderly patients.

Benzodiazepines

Abuse of benzodiazepine medications by elderly persons is another well-established clinical problem. According to Simoni-Wastila et al. (2005), 10.4% of community-dwelling older adults were prescribed more than one anxiolytic or sedative-hypnotic in 1999. Although high-dose addiction is rather rare in elderly persons, low-dose dependence is estimated to occur in about half of regular benzodiazepine consumers (Förster and Thomas 2009). In one study of over 1,000 individuals ages 65 and older, 5.5% of men and 9.8% of women were found to be benzodiazepine users. Users were significantly more likely than nonusers to be female and less educated, report more depressive and anxiety symptoms, use more prescription medications, have lower self-rated health, have difficulty maintaining sleep, and be less likely to consume alcohol (Stowell et al. 2008). In another research study, Simoni-Wastila and Yang (2006) estimated that up to 11% of elderly women misuse benzodiazepines. In other studies, major predictors of benzodiazepine use in the elderly were reported to be female gender, dysthymia, alcohol dependence, anxiety, somatoform disorder, borderline personality, and widowhood (Petrovic et al. 2002; Simoni-Wastila and Yang 2006; Stowell et al. 2008).

The use of benzodiazepines in geriatric patients should be limited to 4 months' duration (Blow 1998). If benzodiazepine therapy is indicated, short-acting types and the types that do not require liver metabolism (e.g., lorazepam, oxazepam) should be used to avoid dependence. Furthermore, multiple adverse reactions, such as residual sedation, decreased attention span, impairment of memory and cognition, and increased risk of falls or motor vehicle accidents, are reduced with short-acting agents.

Conclusion and Future Directions

The goal of substance abuse treatment for elderly patients is the same as for their younger counterparts: to promote and maintain long-term abstinence. As understanding of the complex neurobiology of addictions increases, more effective treatments for abuse and dependence can be developed. Currently, very few of the new pharmacological treatment approaches are used in elderly patients. With the projected significant increase in the number of older adults with substance abuse problems in the near future, more data are urgently needed on the epidemiology, neurobiology, and psychopharmacology of substance abuse disorders in elderly persons. In addition, more research is needed on specific diagnostic instruments and psychosocial treatments for the elderly. Substance use disorders, like other chronic illnesses, require early and timely interventions and ongoing care. The future management of substance use disorders in the elderly population will likely shift more into primary care settings, requiring appropriate training of those providers.

Key Points

- The aging baby boomers' cohort greatly outnumbers and has higher rates of substance abuse disorders than previous cohorts.
- Elderly people are more sensitive than younger people to the neurotoxic effects of substances.
- The complicated neurobiology of substance use disorders is superimposed on age-related changes in the brain.
- More research is needed on the epidemiology, neurobiology, and psychopharmacology of substance abuse disorders in elderly patients to provide more effective treatment in the future.

Recommended Readings and Web Sites

Bartels SJ, Blow FC, Brockman LM, et al: Substance Abuse and Mental Health Among Older Americans: The State of the Knowledge and Future Directions. August 11, 2005. Rockville, MD, Older American Substance Abuse and Mental Health Technical Assistance Center, Substance Abuse and Mental Health Services Administration. Available at: http://www.samhsa.gov/OlderAdultsTAC/SA_MH_%20AmongOlderAdultsfinal102105.pdf. Accessed June 18, 2010.

Gass JT, Olive MF: Glutamatergic substrates of drug addiction and alcoholism. Biochem Pharmacol 1:218–265, 2008

Goodman A: Neurobiology of addiction: an integrative review. Biochem Pharmacol 75:266–322, 2008

Han B, Gfroerer JC, Colliver JD, et al: Substance use disorders among older adults in the United States in 2020. Addiction 204:88–96, 2009

Johnson BA: Update on neuropharmacological treatments for alcoholism: scientific basis and clinical findings. Biochem Pharmacol 75:34–56, 2008

Kalivas P, O'Brien C: Drug addiction as a pathology of staged neuroplasticity. Neuropsychopharmacology 33:166–180, 2008

Nutt D, Lingford-Hughes A: Addiction: the clinical interface. Br J Pharmacol 154:397–405, 2008

Oslin D: Late-life alcoholism: issues relevant to the geriatric psychiatrist. Am J Geriatr Psychiatry 12:571–583, 2004

Substance Abuse and Mental Health Services Administration, Office of Applied Studies: Results from the 2007 National Survey on Drug Use and Health: National Findings. 2008. Available at: http://www.oas.samhsa.gov/nsduh/2k7nsduh/2k7Results.cfm. Accessed June 18, 2010.

The following Web sites provide excellent resources for both clinicians and their patients:

National Institute on Alcohol Abuse and Alcoholism: www.niaaa.nih.gov/guide

Substance Abuse and Mental Health Services Administration: www.samhsa.gov

References

American Psychiatric Association: Diagnostic and Statistical Manual of Mental Disorders, 4th Edition, Text Revision. Washington, DC, American Psychiatric Association, 2000

Andrews J, Heath J, Graham-Garcia J: Management of tobacco dependence in older adults. J Gerontol Nurs 30:13–24, 2004

Anton RF, O'Malley SS, Ciraulo DA, et al: Combined pharmacotherapies and behavioral interventions for alcohol dependence (the COMBINE study): a randomized controlled trial. JAMA 295: 2003–2017, 2006a

Anton RF, O'Malley S, Couper D, et al: Does a common variant of the mu opiate receptor gene predict response to naltrexone in the treatment of alcoholism? Results from the COMBINE study. Neuropsychopharmacology 31 (suppl 1):S24, 2006b

Anton RF, Oroszi G, O'Malley S, et al: An evaluation of mu-opioid receptor (OPRM1) as a predictor of naltrexone response in the treatment of alcohol dependence: results from the Combined Pharmacotherapies and Behavioral Interventions for Alcohol Dependence (COMBINE) study (see comment). Arch Gen Psychiatry 65:135–144, 2008

Blow F: Substance Abuse Among Older Americans: Treatment Improvement Protocol (C.f.S.A. Treatment). Washington, DC, U.S. Government Printing Office, 1998

Brower KJ, Mudd S, Blow FC, et al: Severity and treatment of alcohol withdrawal in elderly versus younger patients. Alcohol Clin Exp Res 18:196–201, 1994

Burstein A, Fulleron T, Clark DJ, et al: Pharmacokinetics, safety and tolerability after single and multiple oral doses of varenicline in elderly smokers. J Clin Pharmacol 46:1234–1240, 2006

Cahill K, Stead L, Lancaster T: Nicotine receptor partial agonists for smoking cessation. Cochrane Database of Systematic Reviews 2010, Issue 12. Art. No.: CD006103. DOI: 10.1002/14651858.CD006103.pub4

Cheer J, Wassum K, Sombers LA, et al: Phasic dopamine release evoked by abused substances requires cannabinoid receptor activation. J Neurosci 27:791–795, 2007

Cloninger CR: Neurogenetic adaptive mechanisms in alcoholism. Science 236:410–416, 1987

Colliver JD, Compton WM, Gfroerer JC, et al: Projecting drug use among aging baby boomers in 2020. Ann Epidemiol 16:257–265, 2006

Curtis J, Geller G, Stokes EJ, et al: Characteristics, diagnosis, and treatment of alcoholism in elderly patients. J Am Geriatr Soc 37:310–316, 1989

Dick D, Plunkett J, Weatherill LF, et al: Association between GABRA1 and drinking behaviors in the collaborative study on the genetics of alcoholism sample. Alcohol Clin Exp Res 30:1101–1110, 2006

Doolan DM, Froelicher ES: Smoking cessation interventions and older adults. Prog Cardiovasc Nurs 23:119–127, 2008

Dowling GJ, Weiss SR, Condon TP: Drugs of abuse and the aging brain. Neuropsychopharmacology 33:209–218, 2008

Fields H: Should we be reluctant to prescribe opioids for chronic non-malignant pain? Pain 129:233–234, 2007

Förster M, Thomas C: Aspects of substance dependence in old age from a geriatric-gerontopsychiatric perspective [in German]. Suchttherapie 10:12–16, 2009

Gass JT, Olive MF: Glutamatergic substrates of drug addiction and alcoholism. Biochem Pharmacol 1:218–265, 2008

Gfroerer JC, Penne MA, Pemberton MR, et al: "The Aging Baby Boom Cohort and Future Prevalence of Substance Abuse," in Substance Use by Older Adults: Estimates of Future Impact on the Treatment System. Rockville, MD, Substance Abuse and Mental Health Services Administration, Office of Applied Studies, 2002

Goodman A: Neurobiology of addiction: an integrative review. Biochem Pharmacol 75:266–322, 2008

Han B, Gfroerer JC, Colliver JD, et al: Substance use disorder among older adults in the United States in 2020. Addiction 104:88–96, 2009

Haney M, Ward AS, Foltin RW, et al: Effects of ecopipam, a selective dopamine D_1 antagonist, on smoked cocaine self-administration by humans. Psychopharmacology 155:330–337, 2001

Heilig M, Koob G: A key role for corticotropin-releasing factor in alcohol dependence. Trends Neurosci 30:399–406, 2007

Heinz A, Lober S, Georgi A, et al: Reward craving and withdrawal relief craving: assessment of different motivational pathways to alcohol intake. Alcohol Alcohol 38:35–39, 2003

Heinz A, Siessmeier T, Wrase J, et al: Correlation of alcohol craving with striatal dopamine synthesis capacity and D2/3 receptor availability: a combined [18F]DOPA and [18F]DMFP PET study in detoxified alcoholic patients. Am J Psychiatry 162:1515–1520, 2005

Hughes JR, Stead LF, Lancaster T: Antidepressants for smoking cessation. Cochrane Database of Systematic Reviews 2007, Issue 1. Art. No.: CD000031. DOI: 10.1002/14651858.CD000031.pub3

Husten C, Shelton D, Chrismon JH, et al: Cigarette smoking and smoking cessation among older adults: United States, 1965–1994. Tobacco Control 6:175–180, 1997

Johnson B: Update on neuropharmacological treatments for alcoholism: scientific basis and clinical findings. Biochem Pharmacol 75:34–56, 2008

Johnson B, Roache J, Javors MA, et al: Ondansetron for reduction of drinking among biologically predisposed alcoholic patients: a randomized controlled trial. JAMA 284:1016–1017, 2000

Johnson B, Ait-Daoud N, Aubin HJ, et al: A pilot evaluation of the safety and tolerability of repeat dose administration of long-acting injectable naltrexone (Vivitrex) in patients with alcohol dependence. Alcohol Clin Exp 28:1356–1361, 2004

Kalivas P, O'Brien C: Drug addiction as a pathology of staged neuroplasticity. Neuropsychopharmacology 33:166–180, 2008

Kalivas P, Volkow N, Seamans J: Unmanageable motivation in addiction: a pathology of prefrontal-accumbens glutamate transmission. Neuron 45:647–650, 2005

Kenney BA, Holahan CJ, Holahan CK, et al: Depressive symptoms, drinking problems, and smoking cessation in older smokers. Addict Behav 34:548–553, 2009

Kreek MJ, Schlussman SD, Bart G, et al: Evolving perspectives on neurobiological research on the addictions: celebration of the 30th anniversary of NIDA. Neuropharmacology 47:324–344, 2004

Mann K, Lehert P, Morgan MY: The efficacy of acamprosate in the maintenance of abstinence in alcohol-dependent individuals: results of a meta-analysis. Alcohol Clin Exp Res 28:51–63, 2004

McCabe SE, Cranford JA, West BT: Trends in prescription drug abuse and dependence, co-occurrence with other substance use disorders, and treatment utilization: results from two national surveys. Addict Behav 33:1297–1305, 2008

Mottagui-Tabar S, Prince J, Wahlestedt C, et al: A novel single nucleotide polymorphism of the neuropeptide Y (NPY) gene associated with alcohol dependence. Alcohol Clin Exp Res 29:702–707, 2005

Muller C, Huston J: Determining the region-specific contributions of 5-HT receptors to the psychostimulant effects of cocaine. Trends Pharmacol Sci 27:105–112, 2006

National Institute on Alcohol Abuse and Alcoholism: Helping Patients Who Drink Too Much: A Clinician's Guide, Updated 2005 Edition. January 2007. Available at: http://pubs.niaaa.nih.gov/publications/Practitioner/CliniciansGuide2005/clinicians_guide.htm. Accessed July 14, 2010.

Nutt D, Lingford-Hughes A: Addiction: the clinical interface. Br J Pharmacol 154:397–405, 2008

O'Brien CP: Anticraving medications for relapse prevention: a possible new class of psychoactive medications. Am J Psychiatry 162:1423–1431, 2005

Oslin D: Late-life alcoholism: issues relevant to the geriatric psychiatrist. Am J Geriatr Psychiatry 12:571–583, 2004

Oslin D, Liberto JG, O'Brien J, et al: Tolerability of naltrexone in treating older, alcohol-dependent patients. Am J Addict 6:266–270, 1997

Oslin D, Pettinati H, Volpicelli JR: Alcoholism treatment adherence: older age predicts better adherence and drinking outcomes. Am J Geriatr Psychiatry 10:740–747, 2002

Oslin D, Berrettini W, Kranzler HR, et al: A functional polymorphism of the mu-opioid receptor gene is associated with naltrexone response in alcohol-dependent patients. Neuropsychopharmacology 28:1546–1552, 2003

Oslin D, Cary M, Slaymaker V, et al: Daily ratings measures of alcohol craving during an inpatient stay define subtypes of alcohol addiction that predict subsequent risk for resumption of drinking. Drug Alcohol Depend 103:131–136, 2009

Pergolizzi J, Böger R, Budd K, et al: Opioids and the management of chronic severe pain in the elderly: consensus statement of an International Expert Panel with focus on the six clinically most often used World Health Organization step III opioids (buprenorphine, fentanyl, hydromorphone, methadone, morphine, oxycodone). Pain Pract 8:287–313, 2008

Petrakis I, Carroll K, Nich C, et al: Disulfiram treatment for cocaine dependence in methadone-maintained opioid addicts. Addiction 95:219–228, 2000

Petrovic M, Vandierendonck A, Mariman A, et al: Personality traits and socio-epidemiological status of hospitalised elderly benzodiazepine users. Int J Geriatr Psychiatry 17:733–738, 2002

Pettinati HM, Rabinowitz AR: Recent advances in the treatment of alcoholism. Clin Neurosci Res 5:151–159, 2005

Sachs-Ericsson N, Schmidt NB, Zvolensky MJ, et al: Smoking cessation behavior in older adults by race and gender: the role of health problems and psychological distress. Nicotine Tob Res 11:433–443, 2009

Simoni-Wastila L, Yang HK: Psychoactive drug abuse in older adults. Am J Geriatr Pharmacother 4:380–394, 2006

Simoni-Wastila L, Zhuckerman I, Singhal PK, et al: National estimates of exposure to prescription drugs with addiction potential in the community-dwelling elders. Subst Abuse 26:33–42, 2005

Soyka M, Preuss U, Hesselbrock V, et al: GABA-A2 receptor subunit gene (GABRA2) polymorphisms and risk for alcohol dependence. J Psychiatr Res 42:184–191, 2008

Stead L, Perera R, Bullen C, et al: Nicotine replacement therapy for smoking cessation. Cochrane Database of Systematic Reviews 2008, Issue 1. Art. No.: CD000146. DOI: 10.1002/14651858.CD000146.pub3

Stowell K, Chang C, Bilt J, et al: Sustained benzodiazepine use in a community sample of older adults. J Am Geriatr Soc 56:2285–2291, 2008

Substance Abuse and Mental Health Services Administration: Preliminary Estimates from 1995 National Household Survey on Drug Abuse. Rockville, MD, Substance Abuse and Mental Health Services Administration, 1996

Substance Abuse and Mental Health Services Administration: National Survey on Drug Use and Health 2007. Rockville, MD, Substance Abuse and Mental Health Services Administration, 2008

Sunderland T: Neurotransmission in the aging central nervous system, in Clinical Geriatric Psychopharmacology, 4th Edition. Edited by Salzman C. Philadelphia, PA, Lippincott Williams & Wilkins, 2005, pp 63–85

Treutlein J, Kissling C, Frank J, et al: Genetic association of the human corticotropin releasing hormone receptor 1 (CRHR1) with binge drinking and alcohol intake patterns in two independent samples. Mol Psychiatry 11:594–602, 2006

Vengeliene V, Bilbao A, Molander A, et al: Neuropharmacology of alcohol addiction. Br J Pharmacol 154:299–315, 2008

Verheul R, Lehert P, Geerlings PJ, et al: Predictors of acamprosate efficacy: results from a pooled analysis of seven European trials including 1485 alcohol-dependent patients. Psychopharmacology (Berl) 178:167–173, 2005

Volkow N, Wang GL, Fowler JS, et al: Prediction of reinforcing responses to psychostimulants in humans by brain dopamine D2 receptor levels. Am J Psychiatry 156:1440–1443, 1999

Volkow N, Chang L, Wang GJ, et al: Low level of brain dopamine D2 receptors in methamphetamine abusers: association with metabolism in the orbitofrontal cortex. Am J Psychiatry 158:2015–2021, 2001

Volkow N, Fowler J, Wang GJ, et al: Dopamine in drug abuse and addiction: results from imaging studies and treatment implications. Mol Psychiatry 9:557–569, 2004

Williams JW Jr, Gerrity M, Holsinger T, et al: Systematic review of multifaceted interventions to improve depression care. Gen Hosp Psychiatry 29:91–116, 2007

World Health Organization: Lexicon of alcohol and drug terms published by the World Health Organization. Available at: http://www.who.int/substance_abuse/terminology/who_lexicon/en. Accessed April 23, 2010.

Yoder KK, Kareken DA, Seyoum RA, et al: Dopamine D(2) receptor availability is associated with subjective responses to alcohol. Alcohol Clin Exp Res 29:965–970, 2005

Zhang P, Ishiguro H, Ohtsuki T, et al: Human cannabinoid receptor 1: 5′ exons, candidate regulatory regions, polymorphisms, haplotypes and association with polysubstance abuse. Mol Psychiatry 9:916–931, 2004

18

Sleep Disorders

Alon Y. Avidan, M.D., M.P.H.

Sleep complaints and difficulty are common among older adults, as evident from a large-scale National Institute on Aging study in which over 50% of the more than 9,000 participants ages 65 older reported at least one chronic sleep complaint (Foley et al. 1999). Sleep disturbances in older persons are multifactorial and ubiquitous, and old age presents a number of risk factors that impair a person's ability to sleep. Sleep disturbances may be caused and potentiated by expected age-related physiological changes, comorbid medical and psychiatric diseases, changes in the endogenous circadian rhythm, retirement, and loss of spouse.

As aging commences, it is the impaired ability of a person to sleep, rather than reduced sleep need or aging per se, that causes disrupted sleep (Ancoli-Israel and Kripke 1991; Ancoli-Israel et al. 2005, 2008; Ayalon et al. 2004). Older adults are at risk for a wide spectrum of sleep disturbances, including insomnia; sleep apnea; motor disorders of sleep, such as restless legs syndrome (RLS); and a general advancement of circadian rhythm timing (Avidan 2005b; Bachman 1992; Bloom et al. 2009; Flamer 1996; Johnston 1994; Mazza et al. 2004; Neubauer 1999; Wolkove et al. 2007a, 2007b; Wooten 1992). Clinical sequelae of impaired sleep include excessive daytime sleepiness (or hypersomnolence), disturbed cognition, confusion, psychomotor retardation, and increased risk of injury, any of which may compromise quality of life and create social and economic burdens for caregivers (Ancoli-Israel et al. 2008). Appropriate evaluation and effective management may result in optimization of daytime alertness and improvements in cognitive impairments.

In this chapter, I discuss normal and predictable age-related physiological changes in sleep and the common sleep pathologies in the older person through a case vignette format. Diagnostic criteria, clinical presentation, sleep study (polysomnographic) features, and treatment options are presented for each of the sleep disorders discussed, which include insomnia, obstructive sleep apnea, restless legs syndrome and periodic leg movement disorder of sleep, advanced sleep phase disorder, and rapid eye movement sleep behavior disorder.

Physiological Sleep Changes Associated With Aging

Older adults undergo expected age-related changes in sleep physiology. Sleep architecture becomes more fragmented, resulting in reduced sleep efficiency and decreased quality of sleep. Slow-wave (delta) sleep is reduced, and the amplitude of this brain wave activity is attenuated. The older person also spends more time in the lighter stages of sleep and experiences increased fragmentations of the sleep-wake cycle (Phillips and Ancoli-Israel 2001; Shochat et al. 2001). The latency to the first rapid eye movement (REM) period decreases, and the individual experiences an overall reduction in the total amount of REM sleep as well as an overall reduction in total nocturnal sleep time (Williams et al. 1974). Sleep stage changes expected over a lifetime are illustrated in Figure 18–1. Older adults often take a longer time to initiate sleep, resulting in increased sleep latency; have a reduced total sleep time, leading to reduced sleep efficiency; experience early morning awakening; and have an increased need to nap during the daytime (Dement et al. 1985; McGheie and Russel 1962). Typical sleep architectural changes are depicted in Figure 18–2, which shows the sleep hypnogram of a young person's sleep (Panel A) compared with that of an older person's sleep (Panel B).

Older adults experience more frequent napping behaviors, with prevalence rates of napping ranging from 25% to 80% (Prinz 1977; Wauquier et al. 1992). This observed tendency to nap during the day has been previously demonstrated objectively by the Multiple Sleep Latency Test, a test useful in evaluating physiological sleep tendency. When given the opportunity, older patients tend to fall asleep faster during the day than do younger patients (Dement and Carskadon

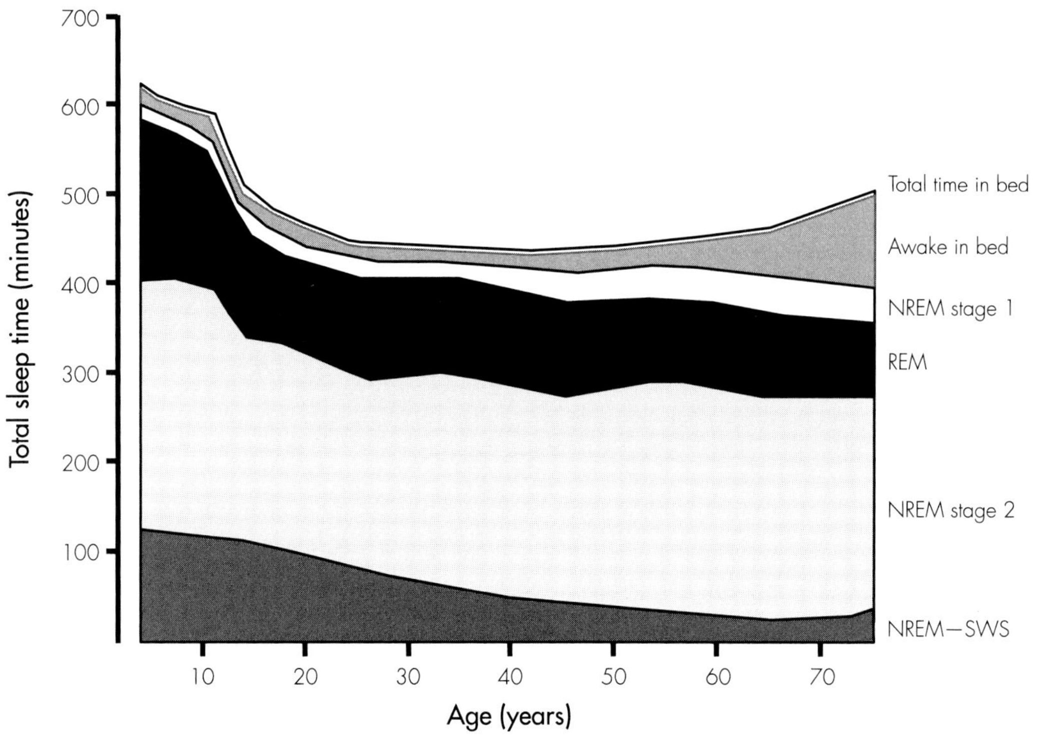

FIGURE 18–1. Sleep architectural changes with aging.

From adolescence to middle age to aging, delta sleep diminishes and lighter sleep staging increases. Rapid eye movement (REM) sleep percentage decreases, and sleep efficiency and continuity decrease.
NREM=non–rapid eye movement; SWS=slow-wave sleep.

Source. Adapted from Williams et al. 1974.

1982; Dement et al. 1985). This observation provides further evidence that older adults experience persistent excessive daytime sleepiness. These data suggest that older adults lack sufficient restorative sleep at night rather than that they have a reduced need for sleep; therefore, it is their ability to sleep well that is altered rather than the need for sleep (Ancoli-Israel 1997).

Gender differences in the sleep of healthy older adult cohorts reveal that women maintain sleep better with aging than do men (Rediehs et al. 1990). However, data on the effects of menopause on sleep revealed subjective complaints of insomnia. Objectively, menopause is associated with decreased total sleep time, prolonged sleep latency, and reduced percentage of time spent in REM sleep. Treatment with estrogen replacement therapy has been shown to potentially alleviate these problems (Wooten 1994).

Clinical Sleep History

The clinical evaluation and assessment of sleep disorders in older patients should involve a comprehensive multidisciplinary approach. Essential components include a history of present illness, detailed account of the sleep complaint inventory, past sleep history, list of current medications, evaluation of the upper airway size (using the Mallampati classification), neck circumference, and neurological evaluation. Sleep history, which should ideally be conducted in the presence of one's sleeping partner, helps to establish or guide the clinician toward the correct diagnosis of sleep apnea (indicated by snoring and gasping for air) or motor disorders of sleep, such as REM sleep behavior disorder (dream enactment) or periodic leg movement disorder of sleep (frequent leg jerks). Inquiry regarding the social history should focus on use of tobacco, alcohol (which may exacerbate sleep apnea), and caffeine (which is known to exacerbate insomnia). Review of medications, including dosage and timing, is often useful in the assessment of underlying causes for insomnia (decongestants) or hypersomnolence (sedating antidepressants).

The following key questions are important when obtaining the sleep history:

1. Do you have difficulties initiating sleep?
2. Do you feel that you are excessively sleepy during the daytime?

3. What is your sleep-wake schedule?
4. How many hours do you sleep per night?
5. How long does it take you to fall asleep?
6. How many times do you wake up during a typical night?
7. How long does it take you to "get going" after you get out of bed?
8. Do you (or have you been told that you) snore or stop breathing at night?
9. Do you have crawling or uncomfortable sensations in your legs in the evenings or when trying to fall asleep?
10. Do you (or have you been told that you) kick or twitch your limbs during sleep?
11. Have you been told that you "act out" your dreams by punching, kicking, flailing arms, or screaming while sleeping?
12. Are you currently using caffeine to help keep you going during the day?
13. Are you currently using any substances to help you fall asleep, such as alcohol and over-the-counter or prescription drugs?

This inventory is ideally supplemented by having the patient keep a careful sleep diary for several weeks.

The sleep clinical visit allows an opportunity for inquiry about other key possible causes of daytime sleepiness, such as psychiatric factors (e.g., depression, anxiety), poor sleep hygiene and insufficient sleep, abnormal movement disorders, and circadian rhythm disorders such as advanced sleep phase disorder. A sleep diary kept for several weeks is often helpful. The patient's sleeping partner may offer additional insight, especially in regard to the patient's daytime behaviors and functioning; the patient's propensity to fall asleep at inappropriate or dangerous times (e.g., during conversations, while driving a car); and any snoring, gasp awakenings, apneic spells, unusual nocturnal events, or periodic leg jerks. For older adults who have no spouse or sleeping partner, the clinical evaluation can be somewhat challenging.

Patients should be asked to bring a complete medication list to their initial appointment. It should include all prescription medications, dietary supplements (e.g., melatonin, tryptophan), and over-the-counter agents. Patients should also be asked about caffeine, alcohol, and nicotine use. While in the waiting room, the patient may be asked to complete the Epworth Sleepiness Scale (Johns 1991), an eight-item inventory asking patients to rate their propensity to fall asleep in multiple situations (e.g., while sitting and reading, while watching TV) on a scale from 0 (*no chance of dozing*) to 3 (*high chance of dozing off*). The maximum score is 24; patients with total scores of 10 and higher are considered to have a degree of clinically significant daytime sleepiness, and those with scores over 15 have severe daytime sleepiness. However, the utility and validity of the scale have not been widely tested in older cohorts.

Laboratory Evaluation of Sleep Disorders

Objective assessment of sleep disorders is conducted using sleep studies (polysomnography), which is critical in the assessment of sleep-disordered breathing, motor disorders of sleep, quantification of hypersomnolence, and evaluation of unusual nocturnal behaviors. The Multiple Sleep Latency Test can be used as an objectively verifiable indicator in the assessment of excessive daytime somnolence. The use of video manometry during polysomnography may be useful when evaluating patients with abnormal nocturnal spells, such as REM sleep behavior disorder (RBD) and nocturnal seizures.

Sleep Disorders in Older Adults

Insomnia

Case Vignette 1

A 71-year-old woman presents to the sleep disorders clinic complaining that she has had difficulties initiating and maintaining sleep over the past 5 years. She generally retires to bed between 9 and 10 P.M. and watches TV, while in bed, until about midnight. She describes difficulties with sleep initiation and feeling "worried" about not being able to fall asleep. She stays in bed and feels frustrated, becomes anxious as the hours pass, and finally falls asleep at 2–3 A.M. She has difficulties waking at the same time as her husband, who is typically up at 6 A.M. During the daytime, she drinks up to five cups of coffee to "get her energy back" and often takes 2- to 3-hour naps between noon to 5 P.M. The clinician asks her to keep a sleep log (Figure 18–3). The patient is diagnosed with psychophysiological/conditioned insomnia.

Insomnia is the most common sleep complaint reported by older patients. It is defined as the inability to either initiate or maintain sleep, or as early morning awakening associated with disturbed daytime functioning (National Institutes of Health 2005). Epidemiological data have shown a higher prevalence of insomnia in older persons than in younger individuals (Klink et al. 1992), and Miles and Dement (1980) determined that up to 40% of people over age 60 may experience insomnia, frequent awakening, and light and disrupted sleep. Older adults are also more likely to experience sleep maintenance insomnia (difficulty remaining asleep) and early morning awakening (waking early in the morning with the inability to reinitiate sleep).

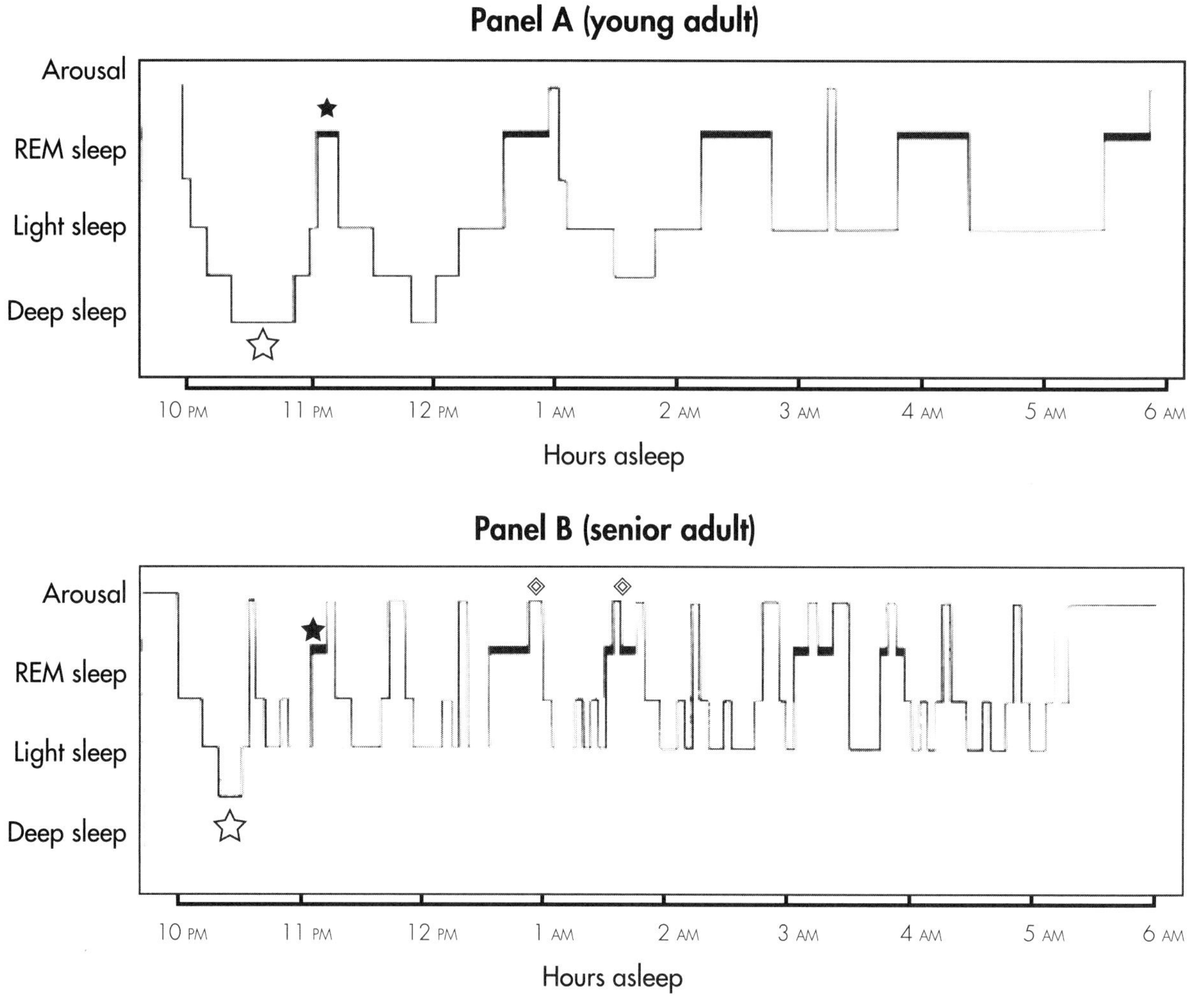

FIGURE 18–2. Sleep hypnograms depicting sleep laboratory recordings over a sleep period of 8 hours for a 15-year-old patient (Panel A) and a 75-year-old patient (Panel B).

Each hypnogram demonstrates organization of a night's sleep for a given patient. The y-axis shows the various stages of non–rapid eye movement sleep alternating with rapid eye movement (REM) sleep (within the *bold line [solid star]*), with most slow-wave sleep (SWS) occurring in the first part of the night and most REM sleep occurring in the last part. These hypnograms demonstrate maturation of sleep with aging: REM sleep becomes more fragmented and is decreased with advancing age. This is also true regarding SWS *(open star)*, which is maximal in children and is diminished or absent in elderly individuals. Older patients also have more frequent arousals *(diamonds)*.

In a survey of over 9,000 adults ages 65 and older (Foley et al. 1995), 28% of respondents reported difficulty with falling asleep, and 42% reported difficulty with both falling asleep and maintaining sleep. Sleep complaints in this cohort were associated with an increasing number of physical disabilities, respiratory symptoms, depressive symptoms, nonprescription medications, and poorer self-perceived health.

When insomnia is present in older patients, the etiology may be multifactorial and is often related to underlying medical and psychiatric illnesses and polypharmacy. The first step in the clinical evaluation of insomnia should be a detailed medical and sleep history taking, as described previously. Sleep logs, like the one shown in Figure 18–3, are often instrumental in the evaluation. A sleep log is a record of an individual's sleeping and waking times, usually tabulated over a period of several weeks. A patient is frequently instructed to record the following data:

1. Amount of time required to fall asleep
2. Time patient thinks he or she fell asleep
3. Number, time, and length of any nocturnal awakenings
4. Any meals or drinks used (e.g., snacks, alcohol)

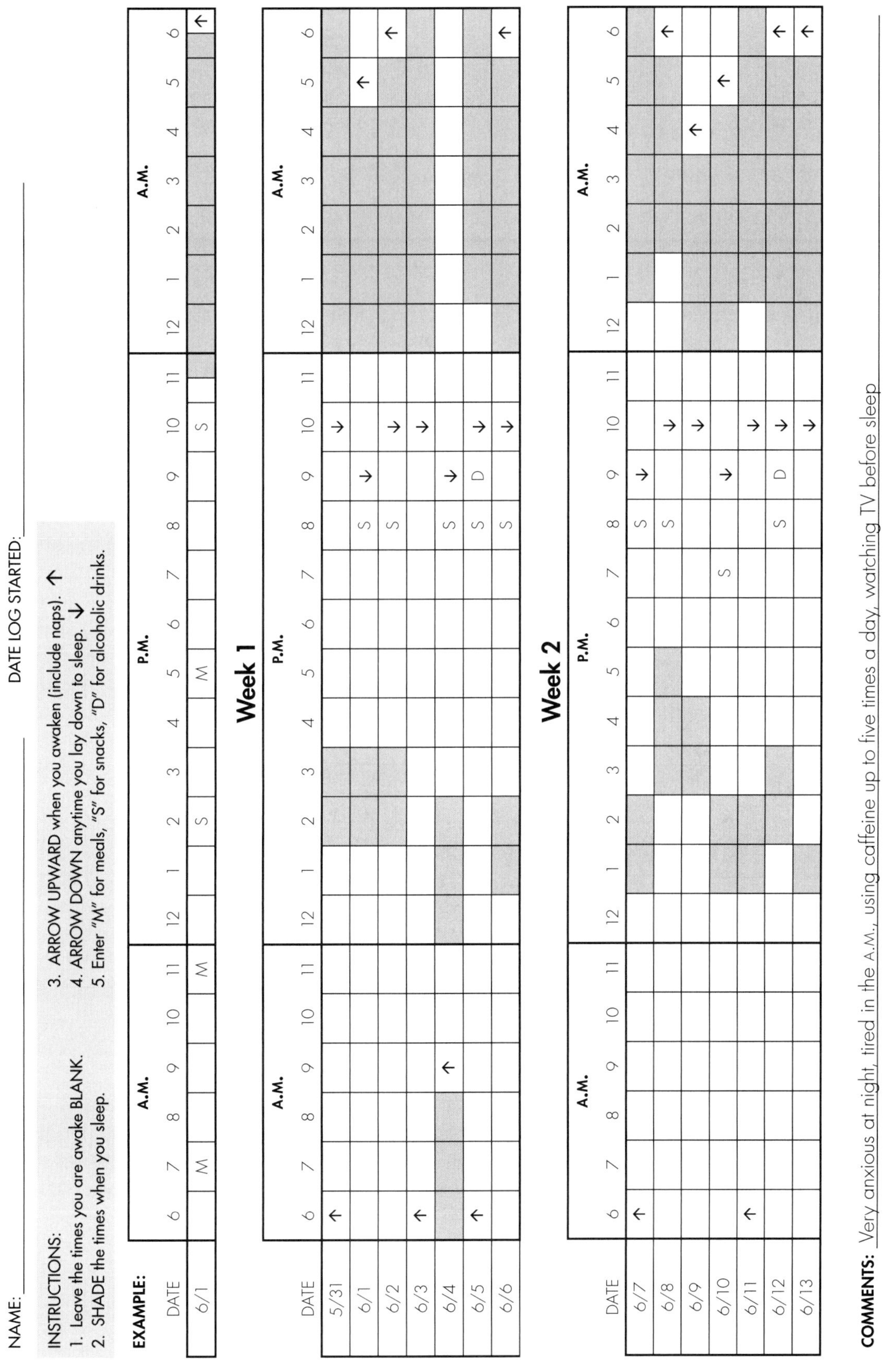

SLEEP LOG
NAME:
DATE LOG STARTED:
INSTRUCTIONS:
1. Leave the times you are awake BLANK.
2. SHADE the times when you sleep.
3. ARROW UPWARD when you awaken (include naps). ↑
4. ARROW DOWN anytime you lay down to sleep. ↓
5. Enter "M" for meals, "S" for snacks, "D" for alcoholic drinks.
EXAMPLE:
DATE
A.M.
P.M.
Week 1
Week 2
COMMENTS: Very anxious at night, tired in the A.M., using caffeine up to five times a day, watching TV before sleep

FIGURE 18–3. Sleep log demonstrating psychophysiological/conditioned insomnia.

This record shows sleeping and waking times for 71-year-old woman described in Case Vignette 1.

5. Final wake-up time
6. Time patient got out of bed
7. Time patient had wanted to wake up
8. How patient felt during the day
9. Start and end times of any daytime naps
10. Potential medications used
11. Other comments

These self-reported subjective measures provide for an easy calculation of total time in bed, total sleep time, and sleep efficiency and help corroborate subjective reports from patients (Gillin and Byerley 1990). For the patient in Case Vignette 1, the sleep log helped corroborate her complaints and visually demonstrate her poor sleep hygiene (e.g., watching TV, as shown in Figure 18–3).

Evaluation

Sleep studies are unnecessary in the initial evaluation of most patients who present with insomnia. A single sleep study may not be representative of a patient's sleep at home and may fail to detect clinically significant insomnia that is present on a nightly basis. Sleep studies are sometimes helpful when the patient is suspected of having other underlying conditions, such as sleep apnea, RBD, or periodic leg movement disorder of sleep (Edinger et al. 1989). Formal polysomnography may also be useful in diagnosing a patient when traditional therapy of insomnia fails and the possibility of an underlying primary sleep disturbance persists (Lichstein and Reidel 1994). Besides polysomnograms and sleep logs, another tool in laboratory evaluation of insomnia is the actigraph, a noninvasive accelerometer device worn on the wrist to record human rest (sleep) and activity (wake) cycles. It provides a useful objective measure that can be used in conjunction with the sleep log (Hauri and Wisbey 1992).

Older patients with underlying psychiatric conditions, neurodegenerative disorders, pulmonary disease, and pain can present with comorbid insomnia. Psychiatric pathologies are important contributors to disruption of the sleep architecture. Up to 90% of patients with depression have abnormal sleep architecture (Reynolds 1989); the most striking polysomnographic features of depression are a characteristic decreased REM-sleep latency and early morning awakening (Benca et al. 1992).

Management

Substance use. In the sleep medicine practice, it is not uncommon for older patients with insomnia to report the use of alcohol as a sleeping aid. Its effect on sleep is profound and includes the initial therapeutic benefit of decreased sleep latency; however, later during the night, it induces frequent arousals, fragmentation of sleep architecture, REM-sleep deprivation, and REM-sleep rebound. Alcohol, when consumed by geriatric patients, has a longer half-life because its metabolism is slower in people of advanced age, and it therefore has more potent sedating effects (Dufour et al. 1992) and conceivably worsens sleep-disordered breathing in susceptible patients.

Other commonly used substances affect sleep. Stimulants (e.g., nicotine, caffeine) are notorious causes of insomnia and should be avoided (Espie 1991). Caffeine use is associated with increased sleep latency (insomnia), decreased sleep efficiency, and spontaneous arousals. Caffeine withdrawal is associated with depression, irritability, and hypersomnolence.

Hypnotic therapy. The role of polypharmacy is a critical consideration in assessments of older persons with sleep disorders. Elderly patients are often treated by multiple physicians, who may prescribe multiple medications with deleterious effects on patients' sleep (e.g., anticholinergics, antihypertensives, psychiatric agents).

Treatment of insomnia by pharmacological agents in the older person may be challenging due to age-related changes in pharmacokinetics and pharmacodynamics (Hicks et al. 1981). Some medications used as sleep aids, particularly those with longer half-lives, have multiple side effects in older persons, including hypersomnolence and sleep architectural disturbances (reduced REM and slow-wave sleep), and an increased association with accidents (Roth et al. 1988). Another major concern with the longer-acting hypnotics is tolerance, which is the need for higher drug dosage to achieve the same clinical efficacy, resulting in undesirable rebound insomnia.

When hypnotics are administered in the older patient, they need to be prescribed at the lowest effective dosage and for the shortest time period. Shorter-acting hypnotics are preferable, and patients need to be followed up carefully and closely. Possible adverse effects of hypnotics with short to intermediate half-lives include anterograde amnesia and rebound insomnia. All hypnotics will inevitably improve insomnia if given at the appropriate dosages. The ultimate goal is to use these agents to result in clinical improvement until other nonpharmacological therapies, such as cognitive and behavioral therapy, gain momentum.

The currently available newer hypnotics may have fewer undesirable side effects and may be safer in the geriatric patient. Examples include zaleplon (a nonbenzodiazepine hypnotic from the pyrazolopyrimidine class selective for the benzodiazepine-1 receptor), zolpidem (a nonbenzodiazepine hypnotic of the imidazopyridine class selective for the type 1 γ-aminobutyric acid [GABA] type A–benzodiazepine receptor), and eszopiclone (a nonbenzodiazepine agent that is a pyrrolopyrazine derivative of the cyclopyrrolone class) (Ancoli-Israel et al. 2005; Doghramji 2001; Finucane 2002; Kamel and Gammack 2006; McCall 2004; Melton et al. 2005). Zolpidem tartrate extended-release tablets are available for the treatment of sleep maintenance insomnia (the drug consists of a coated two-layer tablet: one layer releases its drug content immediately, and another layer allows a slower release of additional drug content) (Moen and Plosker 2006; Neubauer 2006; Owen 2006b). In 2005, another drug class, the melatonin receptor agonist ramelteon, became available for the management of sleep initiation insomnia, with the advantage of being a nonscheduled agent with no evidence of abuse or tolerance. This agent selectively binds to the melatonin type 1 and 2 receptors at the level of the suprachiasmatic nucleus (SCN), leading to the attenuation of the alerting signal generated by the SCN, which is thought to facilitate the onset of sleep (Laustsen and Andersen 2006; McGechan and Wellington 2005; Owen 2006a; Pandi-Perumal et al. 2005). In 2010, doxepin (a selective histamine H_1 antagonist) also became available for treatment of chronic sleep onset and sleep maintenance insomnia. Table 18–1 lists these hypnotic agents.

In research investigating the risk of falls associated with hypnotics or insomnia, evidence suggests that successful amelioration of insomnia may be protective against falls in some circumstances. In a cross-sectional survey of 1,526 community-dwelling older adults, insomnia but not psychoactive medication was associated with falls within the past year (Brassington et al. 2000). Results from a large, well-controlled longitudinal study of institutionalized older adults in Michigan (Avidan et al. 2004) indicated that hypnotic use did not predict future falls or hip fractures, whereas underlying insomnia predicted falls. Although the treatment of underlying causes of insomnia is often preferable, data demonstrate that strategic use of hypnotics may help protect against future falls by preventing insomnia.

Sleep hygiene. Pharmacological management with a hypnotic alone is sometimes not enough to eradicate chronic insomnia. Drug therapy should be combined with educational, behavioral, and cognitive interventions aimed at introducing adaptive behaviors. Figure 18–4 lists common sleep hygiene instructions. One of the most important educational approaches for insomnia is to modify disadvantageous sleep hygiene habits that patients may have adopted over the years (Hauri 2003). Originally developed by Hauri (1979, 1998), the basic elements of better sleep hygiene include limiting naps to <30 minutes per day, avoiding stimulants and sedatives, limiting liquids at bedtime, keeping a regular sleep-wake schedule, and incorporating light exposure and moderate exercise into the daily routines. Stimulus-control therapy, originally suggested by Bootzin and Nicassio (1978), proposes that sleep disturbances are behaviorally conditioned and thus need to be reconditioned. The aim of this intervention is to recondition the bed and bedroom as cues for sleep. Patients are instructed to go to bed only when tired, to get out of bed after 20 minutes of being unable to fall asleep, and to return to bed when sleepy. They are also instructed to avoid looking at the clock, shorten daytime naps, use the bed only for sleep, and get up at a consistent time in the morning (Espie 1991, 2002; Schneider 2002).

Sleep restriction therapy, proposed by Spielman et al. (1987), has among its merits the need to curtail time awake in bed to provide for improved sleep efficiency. Curtailing time in bed and total sleep time may initially lead to a state of sleep deprivation. The technique works by preventing patients from becoming frustrated by restricting the time spent in bed. Other common therapeutic modalities for insomnia include cognitive intervention, which helps patients gain insight into maladaptive beliefs and attitudes toward sleep, and a combination of relaxation techniques and biofeedback, which helps patients lower the degree of anxiety and arousal associated with insomnia (Bootzin and Nicassio 1978).

Obstructive Sleep Apnea

Case Vignette 2

An obese 66-year-old man with a history of loud snoring that repeatedly awakens his spouse presents for an evaluation at the sleep disorders clinic. In addition, he reports memory difficulties, severe daytime sleepiness, and frequent daytime napping, often exceeding 2 hours despite obtaining 8 hours of sleep. He has gained nearly 13.6 kg since a hip fracture 5 years earlier, and his shirts feel tight around his neck. The patient had a nocturnal polysomnogram. Figure 18–5 shows a typical example from his study, demonstrating key aspects of obstructive sleep apnea.

Obstructive sleep apnea (OSA) is characterized by repetitive upper airway obstruction, electroencephalogram (EEG) arousals, and a decrease in oxygen saturations. OSA is one of the most critical sleep disturbances in the older person because it diminishes quality of life by adversely affecting almost every organ system. Patients affected by OSA most commonly complain of hypersomnolence, snoring, and impairment of cognition. Epidemiological studies demonstrate sleep apnea prevalence rates to be as high as 4% for older women and 13% for older men. The prevalence of snoring was even higher, at 19% for women and 33% for men (Enright et al. 1996; Shochat and Pillar 2003). For older patients (>65 years of age), prevalence of OSA is particularly high (Shochat and Pillar 2003). Data from a large sample of randomly selected older adults demonstrated sleep apnea prevalence of 28% in men and 19% in women (Ancoli-Israel et al. 1991). In women, menopause seems to play a pivotal role in modulating both the presence and the severity of OSA (Resta et al. 2003). Data from a pop-

TABLE 18–1. Medication chart: newer hypnotic agents for treating insomnia

Medication	Indication	Half-life (hours)	Sleep initiation	Sleep maintenance	Approved dosage (mg)
Zaleplon	Short-term management of insomnia (improves sleep latency)	1	✓		5
Zolpidem	Short-term management of insomnia (improves sleep latency and increases total sleep time)	2.5	✓		5
Zolpidem CR	Insomnia characterized by difficulties with sleep onset and/or sleep maintenance	2.8	✓	✓	6.25
Eszopiclone	Short- and long-term management of insomnia (improves sleep latency and increases total sleep time)	6	✓	✓	1–2
Ramelteon	Insomnia characterized by difficulty with sleep initiation (improves sleep latency and increases total sleep time)	1–2.6	✓		8
Doxepin	Short- and long-term management of insomnia (improves sleep latency and increases total sleep time)	15	✓	✓	3, 6

Note. CR=controlled release.
Source. *Physicians' Desk Reference*, 60th Edition. New York, Thomson Reuters, 2005.

ulation-based Wisconsin Sleep Cohort Study demonstrated that passage into menopause has a significant association with OSA, independent of other known confounding factors (Young et al. 2003). Therefore, evaluation for sleep-disordered breathing should be a critical review of system domain in the assessment of menopausal women who report symptoms of daytime somnolence, snoring, gasping arousals, or unrefreshing sleep (Young et al. 2003).

Compared with the diagnosis of OSA in younger patients, the diagnosis in older patients is often delayed because many have atypical clinical presentations, and their sleep-related complaints are often mistakenly considered by clinicians to be inherent to the normal aging process. Performing sleep studies in older adults can sometimes be challenging from a technical standpoint. This is especially true in patients with nocturnal agitation who have dementia as a comorbidity (Janssens et al. 2000). The apnea-hypopnea index (AHI) is an objectively verifiable indicator of the number of apneas (breathing cessation for a period of 10 seconds or longer) and hypopneas (30% reduction of effort or airflow lasting 10 seconds or greater) per hour of sleep. The AHI is used in sleep medicine practice to establish the significance and severity of underlying OSA. Unfortunately, to date, normative geriatric AHI data are lacking because most studies applying the AHI to clinical use have not been conducted in older cohorts and the applicability of this index in geriatric practice is still an unsettled issue.

The respiratory tree undergoes key anatomical and physiological changes with aging, which may impact sleep-disordered breathing. The anticipated anatomical changes include reduction in airway size due to changes in the supporting connective tissue (Chan and Welsh 1998). Histological changes in the elastin:collagen ratio contribute to reduction in oxygen diffusion capacity (expressed by D_LCO, which stands for the diffusion lung capacity for carbon monoxide). Premature airway closure due to changes in tissue composition also leads to ventilation-perfusion mismatch (Chan and Welsh 1998). Rib cage rigidity, caused by calcification of intercostal cartilage, arthritis of the costovertebral joints, and age-related kyphoscoliosis, leads to a decrement in vital capacity and dependence on diaphragmatic and abdominal breathing. Senescence leads to a decline in the patient's ability to interpret information from peripheral and central chemoreceptors to generate an appropriate ventilatory response to hypercapnia and hypoxemia (Janssens et al. 2000; Kronenberg 1973).

Frequent and repeated brain wave arousals due to respiratory arousals and hypoxemia result in significant sleep fragmentation leading to hypersomnolence, one of the principal and most debilitating symptoms of OSA, in addition to dis-

Incorporating good sleep habits may be useful in the treatment of many sleep disorders. In patients with insomnia and circadian rhythm sleep disorders, increasing the drive for nocturnal sleep and improving the regularity of the sleep and wake cycle are essential components of behavioral therapy.

Below are some useful tips for better sleep:

Increase drive for sleep at night

1. Avoid excessive napping, except a brief "power nap" (20–30 minutes) during the day (preferably in the afternoon).
2. Avoid spending too much time in bed awake.
3. Get regular exercise each day for about 40 minutes in duration and preferably 4 hours before bedtime.
4. Take a hot bath within 2 hours of bedtime.

Improve the regularity of sleep-wake schedule

1. Keep a regular bedtime and wake time 7 days a week.
2. Avoid excessive bright light if you have to get up at night.
3. Increase exposure to bright light during the early part of the day, particularly in the morning.
4. Exercise at a regular time each day.

Manage medication and drug effects

1. Avoid tobacco.
2. Avoid caffeinated beverages after 10:00 A.M. (because caffeine can be found in a wide variety of beverages, please review nutrition labels).
3. Restrict alcoholic beverage consumption. Alcohol may promote sleep initially, but it can cause significant sleep fragmentation during the second half of sleep.
4. Review medications to determine which could be stimulating or sedating.

Reduce arousal in sleep setting

1. Keep the clock face turned away, and do not find out what time it is when you wake up at night.
2. Avoid vigorous exercise in the evenings.
3. Do not eat or drink heavily for 3 hours before bedtime. A light bedtime snack may help.
4. If you have gastric reflux, avoid heavy meals and spices in the evening.
5. Do not retire too hungry or too full.
6. Keep your room dark, quiet, well ventilated, and at a comfortable temperature throughout the night.
7. Use a bedtime ritual. Reading before lights-out may be helpful if it is relaxing.
8. Set aside a worry time; make a list of problems for the following day.
9. Learn simple relaxation skills to use if you awaken at night.
10. Use stress management in the daytime.
11. Avoid unfamiliar sleep environments.
12. Use the bed for sleep and intimacy only.
13. Be sure mattress is not too soft or too firm; use pillow of proper height and firmness.

FIGURE 18–4. Sleep hygiene instructions.

These instructions are provided to patients at their initial clinic visit.

turbances and a decline in concentration, memory, and neurocognitive functions (Findley et al. 1986; Greenberg et al. 1987; Shochat and Pillar 2003).

The clinical diagnosis of sleep-related breathing disorder is suspected when patients present with snoring, witnessed apneas, and hypersomnolence. Phenotypic features suspicious for OSA include a crowded oropharyngeal inlet as exemplified by a high Mallampati score, obesity (body mass index [BMI] >30 kg/m^2), a thick neck (neck circumference >16 inches in women and >17 inches in men), and the presence of retrognathia (maxilla or mandible that has abnormal posterior displacement) and micrognathia (undersized jaw). It is a good idea to screen patients for endocrinopathies, such as acromegaly and hypothyroidism, and to obtain measurements of vital signs, such as blood pressure and pulse rate, because sleep apnea can often exacerbate hypertension.

Data regarding the management of OSA in older patients are lacking, and practice guidelines about specific therapies with continuous positive airway pressure (CPAP), oral appliances, or surgery have not been uniformly formalized. It is possible that the severity of the disorder against the underlying comorbidities rather than the advancing age per se should be the leading factor when considering treatment. Treatment of OSA in older patients is rewarding in that it may help improve neurocognitive disturbances and ameliorate other chronic conditions such as hypertension (Shochat et al. 2000).

Management of OSA can be divided into conservative and nonconservative (surgical) approaches. CPAP is at present the most commonly accepted conservative mode of therapy. Treatment with CPAP should be viewed as a symptomatic rather than a curative therapy because patients need to use it nightly as long as sleep apnea is present, which for most patients means indefinitely (Shochat and Pillar 2003). When OSA is mild or occurs mainly in the supine position, additional treatments include weight loss and avoiding sleeping on the back. Weight reduction in obese patients with OSA improves the upper airway cross-sectional area (Rubinstein et al. 1988). However, the use of pharmacotherapy to achieve weight loss is discouraged in older patients due to insufficient data and increased risk associated with using these drugs with older patients (Shochat and Pillar 2003).

CPAP is probably the most effective option for treating OSA in the older patient, but compliance rates are low, ranging between 46% and 80% (Kribbs et al. 1993; Pepin et al. 1999). Poor adherence is often related to claustrophobia and inability to wear the nasal mask due to nasal congestion; however, with older patients, compliance issues may also be related to problems with dexterity, maintaining and cleaning the equipment, and remembering to place the mask on and off when getting up. Older patients with neurodegenerative dis-

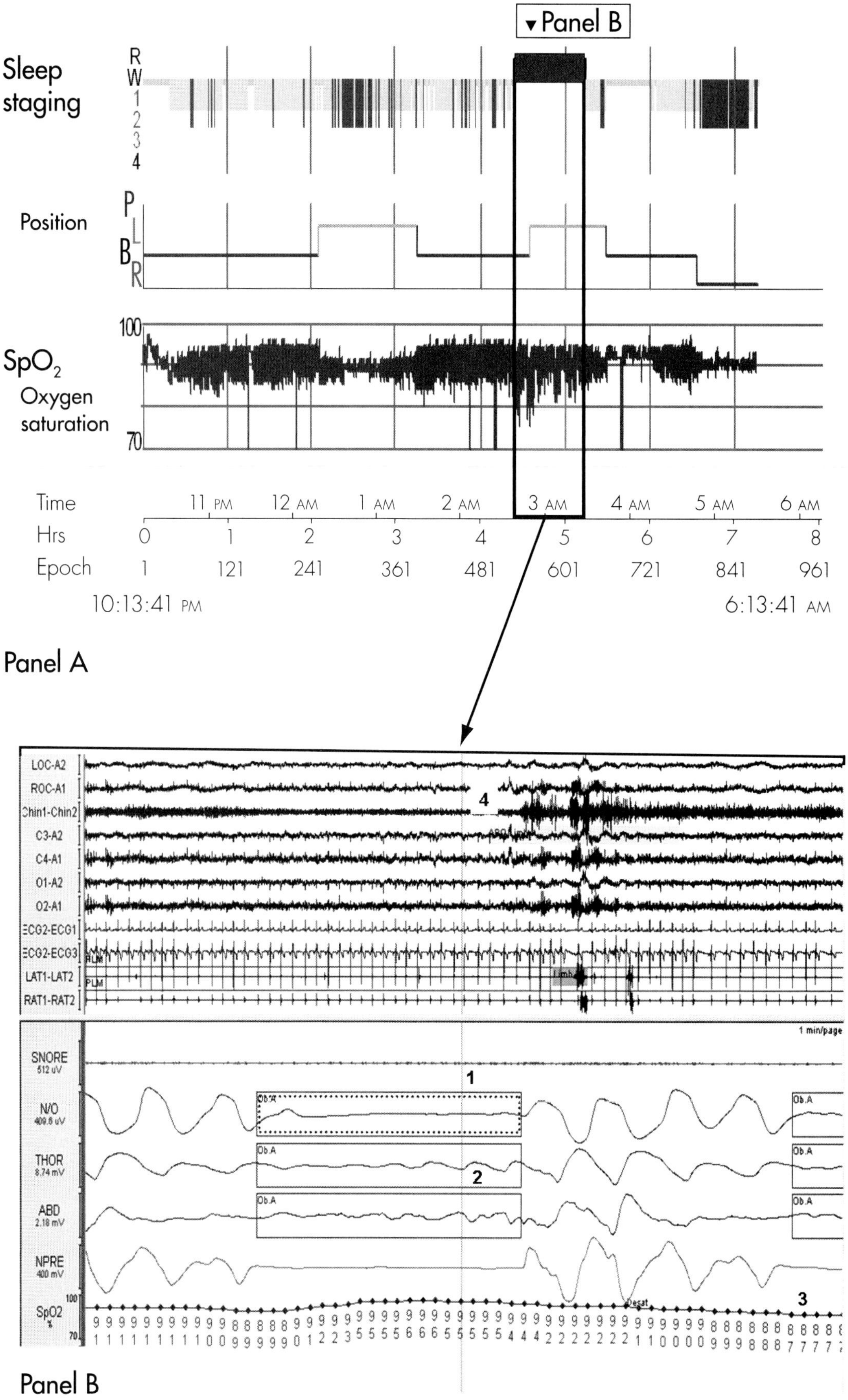
Panel B
Sleep staging
R
W
1
2
3
4
Position
P
L
B
R
SpO2
Oxygen saturation
100
70
Time
11 PM
12 AM
1 AM
2 AM
3 AM
4 AM
5 AM
6 AM
Hrs
0
1
2
3
4
5
6
7
8
Epoch
1
121
241
361
481
601
721
841
961
10:13:41 PM
6:13:41 AM
Panel A
LOC-A2
ROC-A1
Chin1-Chin2
C3-A2
C4-A1
O1-A2
O2-A1
ECG2-ECG1
ECG2-ECG3
LAT1-LAT2
RAT1-RAT2
PLM
4
1 min/page
SNORE
N/O
THOR
ABD
NPRE
SpO2
Ob.A
1
2
3
Panel B

FIGURE 18–5. Polysomnographic illustration of obstructive sleep apnea (OSA).

Panel A: Hypnogram from a polysomnogram of the 66-year-old man with snoring, memory difficulties, and daytime somnolence in Case Vignette 2. Hypnogram shows severe sleep fragmentations (sleep staging) and worsening sleep apnea and hypoxemia (shown by SpO_2 [oxygen saturation measured by pulse oximetry]) during rapid eye movement (REM) sleep, at about 3 A.M., as shown by the box from which Panel B is derived. **Panel B:** A 1-minute epoch from the baseline portion of the diagnostic polysomnogram. Obstructive sleep apnea (OSA) is characterized by (1) nasal oral (N/O) breathing cessation in the presence of (2) persistent respiratory effort, (3) oxygen desaturation, and (4) arousals. The diagnosis of OSA is established with a polysomnogram demonstrating an apnea-hypopnea index of more than five events per hour of sleep associated with one or more of the following: bradytachycardia, frequent arousals from sleep, and arterial oxygen desaturation.
From top to bottom, channels are as follows: electrooculogram (left: LOC-A2; right: ROC-A1); chin electromyography (Chin1-Chin2); electroencephalography (left central: C3-A2; right central: C4-A1; left occipital: O1-A2; right occipital: O2-A1); electrocardiogram (ECG2-ECG1 and ECG2-ECG3); limb electromyography (left leg: LAT1-LAT2; right leg: RAT1-RAT2); snoring (SNORE); nasal-oral airflow (N/O); respiratory effort (thoracic [THOR], abdominal [ABD]); nasal pressure (NPRE); and oxygen desaturation (SpO_2).

orders have underlying neurocognitive difficulties that limit comprehension when first learning to use the mask. A close therapeutic relationship with the provider is encouraged, and education is essential, especially during the initial period of therapy. Participation and involvement of spouse and family can sometimes ameliorate these obstacles.

Another option for managing OSA is the use of oral appliances (mandibular repositioning devices). Considered by many as useful for the treatment of snoring and mild to moderate sleep apnea, oral appliances work by repositioning the mandible anteriorly and expanding the upper airway space at the hypopharyngeal level. Some older patients are edentulous (lack teeth), which may preclude the use of these devices.

The prevalence of OSA in women increases after menopause, probably due to a decline of progesterone and estrogen levels. Progesterone functions as a respiratory stimulant, and estrogen affects body fat distribution; a decline in these hormones is believed to predispose women to sleep-disordered breathing after menopause. The Sleep Heart Health Study evaluated the significance of hormone replacement therapy in sleep-disordered breathing in women ages 50 and older (Shahar et al. 2003). The prevalence of sleep-disordered breathing among patients using hormone replacement therapy was reported to be approximately half that of nonusers. An earlier study found that postmenopausal women had a significantly higher mean AHI compared with premenopausal women and that this significant difference persisted even after controlling for such potential confounders as BMI and neck circumference (Dancey et al. 2001). The authors suggested that physiological differences rather than upper airway anatomy may be responsible for the observed differences in the prevalence and severity of OSA between premenopausal and postmenopausal women (Dancey et al. 2001).

Sleep-Related Movement Disorders

Sleep-related movement disorders include a wide spectrum of clinical syndromes. These include RLS, periodic leg movement disorder (PLMD), and sleep-related legs cramps (American Academy of Sleep Medicine 2005a).

Restless Legs Syndrome

Epidemiology. The prevalence of RLS in older populations is estimated at between 9% and 35% (Milligan and Chesson 2002; Spiegelhalder and Hornyak 2008).

Clinical presentation. As established during the National Institutes of Health workshop with members of the International Restless Legs Syndrome Study Group (IRLSSG), four criteria are necessary for the diagnosis of RLS (Allen et al. 2003; Chaudhuri et al. 2004): 1) an urge to move the legs that is usually accompanied by or caused by uncomfortable or unpleasant sensations in the legs; 2) the urge to move or the unpleasant sensation begins or worsens during periods of rest or inactivity, such as lying or sitting; 3) the urge to move or the unpleasant sensation is partially or totally relieved by movement, such as walking or stretching, at least as long as the activity continues; and 4) the urge to move or the unpleasant sensation is worse in the evening or night than during the day or occurs only in the evening or night. Supportive features of uncertain significance have also been established: 1) presence of a family history among first-degree relatives, 2) response to dopaminergic therapy, and 3) periodic leg movements during wakefulness or sleep.

Patients with RLS are most bothered by the irresistible and profound urge to move their legs, often contributing to sleep initiation insomnia and prolonged awakenings, which lead to significantly reduced sleep time (Allen and Earley 2000). RLS symptoms are present at rest, with significant worsening before the patient's sleep period (Gamaldo and Earley 2006). Patients have a hard time concisely describing their sensory complaints; they often use terms such as "creepy-crawly," "tingling," "creeping," "electric," "burning," "crawling," "pulling," "prickling," or "itching." RLS symptoms improve when patients engage in challenging activities.

The majority of patients experience symptoms that involve the legs, but when the condition is severe, the arms and trunk may also be affected. Typical spells last a few minutes to several hours, most often distributed bilaterally rather than unilaterally, but spells may be asymmetric in both severity and frequency. Most patients with RLS experience symptoms during the day, but the general trend is for severe exacerbation as evening approaches and during times of prolonged inactivity, particularly in a confining space such as an airplane or car while traveling long distances. Patients with RLS score low on quality-of-life measures and demonstrate scores comparable to or even worse than scores of patients with serious conditions such as hypertension, cardiovascular conditions, and diabetes (Abetz et al. 2004; Berger et al. 2004; Saletu et al. 2002). Data also indicate that the symptoms of RLS exceed those of depression or anxiety and that the severity of mood symptoms relates to the severity of RLS symptoms (Becker 2006).

Pathophysiology. The evening-time exacerbation of symptoms in patients with RLS corresponds with the timing of the falling phase of the core temperature circadian cycle, during which the amplitude of circadian rhythm of dopaminergic function is increased with a hypofunction at night (Garcia-Borreguero et al. 2002a, 2002b). These observations, in addition to data showing that RLS responds to treatment with dopamine and is exacerbated by dopamine antagonists, fuel the hypothesis that dopamine dysfunction is the central dogma of RLS pathophysiology. Additional data implicate a deficiency of brain iron storage in RLS (Earley et al. 2000) and reduced cerebrospinal fluid iron content (Earley et al. 1999) compared with normal controls, suggesting that brain iron as well as dopaminergic dysfunction may be central to the pathophysiology of RLS. The iron-dopamine model suggests that iron deficiency in the brain induces an abnormality in the dopaminergic system that causes RLS (Miyamoto et al. 2009).

RLS has two forms with separate etiologies and onset ages (Karroum et al. 2008). Of concern to this discussion of geriatric-related sleep disorders is late-onset RLS, which typically begins after age 45 and is more frequent in older adults, is more severe, has a more rapid rate of progression, has an equal male:female ratio, tends to affect patients daily, has little or no family history association, and is more frequently associated with underlying medical conditions such as neuropathy, radiculopathy, and myelopathy (Berger et al. 2004; Smith and Tolson 2008; Whittom et al. 2007).

Comorbidities in older age. RLS is very frequent in patients with renal failure requiring hemodialysis, who experience prevalence rates ranging between 20% and 53%, and maybe even higher (Al-Jahdali et al. 2009; Hui et al. 2000, 2002; Kim et al. 2008). Higher prevalence rates of RLS have also been reported in patients with other neurological conditions, such as Parkinson's disease (Krishnan et al. 2003; Ondo et al. 2002), spinocerebellar ataxia type 3 (Abele et al. 2001; Schols et al. 1998), low back pain, myelopathy, and arthropathy (Banno et al. 2000). Medications that are associated with and exacerbate RLS include dopamine antagonists (particularly the antiemetics); antihistamines (histamine H_1 antagonists); antidepressants, such as tricyclic antidepressants (TCAs); selective serotonin reuptake inhibitors (SSRIs); serotonin-norepinephrine reuptake inhibitors (SNRIs), particularly venlafaxine, which worsen periodic leg movements; and neuroleptics (Agargun et al. 2002; Bakshi 1996; Hargrave and Beckley 1998; Sanz-Fuentenebro et al. 1996).

Most patients with RLS (about 80%) present with periodic leg movements (Hening et al. 2007a, 2007b; Karatas 2007; Lesage and Earley 2004; Santos et al. 2008; Tan and Ondo 2000; Yee et al. 2009); however, the minority of patients with periodic leg movements (20%–30%) actually have RLS. RLS patients with periodic leg movements often experience psychosocial disturbances such as anxiety and depression. Patients with RLS often seek medical attention due to severe insomnia, psychological disturbance, and depression rather than the RLS symptoms per se.

Differential diagnosis. Many other disorders can be confused with RLS. Some can be ruled out by careful history and clinical examination, lack of circadian evening exacerbation, aggravating factors, and associated psychiatric, medical, and neurological comorbidities (Hening et al. 2007a, 2007b; Lesage and Hening 2004). The differential diagnosis of RLS and other potential conditions seen in older patients is shown in Table 18–2.

Diagnostic evaluation. Patients who fulfill the core IRLSSG essential criteria (Allen et al. 2003; Chaudhuri et al. 2004) may be helped from review of medications known to exacerbate RLS and a screening neurological evaluation for underlying peripheral neuropathy. Sleep studies are not needed to establish RLS diagnosis when the clinical diagnostic criteria have been met (Chesson et al. 1997; Littner et al. 2003). Polysomnography may be helpful in patients with RLS in whom conventional therapy does not yield positive results and in patients suspected of having underlying primary sleep disorders such as sleep apnea. Serum ferritin measurement is essential in all patients with RLS, and those with a level <45 μg/L are at a higher risk of having RLS and should be managed with iron

TABLE 18–2. Differential diagnosis of restless legs syndrome

Restless legs syndrome (RLS)	Awake symptom diagnosis is made by clinical history. Symptoms include uncomfortable, deep, creepy-crawling sensation at time of inactivity or rest (sitting and lying); immediate relief, either complete or partial, with movement; symptomatic relief that persists as long as movement continues; and presence of circadian pattern.
Periodic leg movement disorder (PLMD)	This sleep phenomenon is diagnosed through sleep study. No sensory symptoms, such as urge to move or paresthesias, are present while awake. Patient may have sleep disturbance and complaint of daytime fatigue and sleepiness. Other causes of PLMD, including sleep-disordered breathing, must be excluded.
Nocturnal leg cramps	Despite coming on at night and being relieved with stretching, these leg cramps or "charley horse" cramps are experienced as a usually painful muscular contraction, unlike RLS sensations.
Painful peripheral neuropathy	Sensory symptoms are commonly reported as numbness, burning, and pain. These descriptors are not as common in RLS. Although the sensory symptoms can increase at night, they usually are present throughout the day. Complete and persistent relief is not obtained while walking or during sustained movement.
Hypotensive akathisias	Feeling of restlessness, which may be localized in legs, is brought on by sitting still. Symptoms should not occur while lying down but might be relieved with movement. Symptoms occur in individuals with orthostatic hypotension.
Arthritis of lower limb	Discomfort is centered more in joints, and prominent circadian pattern seen in RLS is uncommon.
Volitional movements (e.g., foot tapping, leg rocking)	Movements occur in individuals who fidget, especially when bored or anxious. Fidgeting is usually not accompanied by sensory symptoms, discomfort, or conscious urge to move. A circadian pattern is usually lacking.
Positional discomfort	Discomfort often comes on with prolonged sitting or lying in the same position but is usually relieved by a simple change in position, unlike RLS which often returns when change of position, movement, or walking is not continued.
Neuroleptic-induced akathisia	Usually discomfort is felt throughout whole body rather than only in limbs. Patient has no pronounced circadian pattern, less associated sensations, and often no relief with movement. History of specific medication exposure is useful, particularly dopamine antagonists.
Burning or painful feet and moving toes	Usually patients have continuous, slow writhing or repetitive movements of toes. No circadian pattern is present.

Source. Adapted from Lesage and Hening 2004.

supplementation (see Figure 18–4) and followed up and observed closely to avoid the development of iron overload (O'Keeffe et al. 1994; Sun et al. 1998).

Treatment. Treatment for RLS is reviewed in Table 18–3. These suggestions are based on previously published data (Adler 1997; Ahmed 2002; Akpinar 1987; Albanese and Filippini 2003; Allen and Earley 1996; Hening 2004; Hening et al. 2004b; Silber et al. 2003). Management ranges from nonpharmacological to pharmacological measures and depends on severity and frequency of the symptoms' impact on quality of life and contribution to sleep disturbance, such as insomnia (Gamaldo and Earley 2006; Yee et al. 2009). Not every patient who has clinical symptoms suggestive of RLS needs to be placed on daily medications, and management depends on a patient's interest in medications, weighed against the risks of side effects and the degree to which sleep and quality of life are affected by RLS (Gamaldo and Earley 2006; Trenkwalder et al. 2008).

As an initial step, it is vital to assess a patient for an iron-deficient state, which may be the primary focus of subsequent treatment (Lesage and Hening 2004; Schapira 2004; Smith

TABLE 18–3. Medication chart: treatment of restless legs syndrome in the older adult

Drug class (generic/brand)	Dosage	Potential side effects
Dopamine agonists		
Pramipexole (Mirapex)[a]	0.125–1.5 mg, 1–2 hours before symptoms Start low and increase slowly	Significant daytime sleepiness, sleep attacks, nausea, compulsive behaviors (compulsive hypersexuality, hallucinations)
Ropinirole (Requip)[a]	0.5–4 mg 1–2 hours before symptoms Start low and increase slowly	
Iron		
Ferrous sulfate	325 mg bid/tid with vitamin C 100–200 mg Recommended when ferritin <45 µg/L	Gastrointestinal side effects, constipation
Dopamine precursors		
Levodopa/carbidopa (Sinemet)	25/200 mg: 0.5–3 tablets 30 minutes before onset of symptoms	Augmentation, rebound, nausea, sleepiness, insomnia, gastrointestinal disturbances
Anticonvulsants		
Gabapentin (Neurontin)	100–1,800 mg/day divided tid	Daytime sleepiness, nausea
Benzodiazepines		
Temazepam (Restoril)	7.5	Drowsiness, dizziness, sedation, amnesia, ataxia, gastrointestinal symptoms
Triazolam (Halcion)	0.125–0.25	
Benzodiazepine agonists		
Zaleplon (Sonata)	5 mg 15–30 minutes before bedtime	Drowsiness, dizziness, sedation, amnesia, ataxia, gastrointestinal symptoms
Zolpidem (Ambien)		
Opiates		
Codeine	30 mg	Nausea, vomiting, restlessness, constipation Addiction and tolerance may be possible
Darvocet[b]; Darvocet-N[c]	300 mg/day	
Propoxyphene (Darvon)	65–135 mg at bedtime	

[a]Only treatment indicated by U.S. Food and Drug Administration for moderate to severe restless legs syndrome.
[b]Propoxyphene and acetaminophen.
[c]Propoxyphene napsylate and acetaminophen.
Source. Adler 1997; Ahmed 2002; Akpinar 1987; Albanese and Filippini 2003; Allen and Earley 1996; Hening 2004; Hening et al. 2004b; Silber et al. 2003.

and Tolson 2008). Patients with serum ferritin levels <45 µg/L should begin iron replacement therapy (O'Keeffe et al. 1994) with iron sulfate and vitamin C (to facilitate gastrointestinal absorption; see Figure 18–4). When iron stores are normal, the dopamine (D_3) agonists ropinirole and pramipexole are available for treatment of moderate to severe RLS (Gamaldo and Earley 2006; Trenkwalder et al. 2009).

Dopamine agonists in general are preferred because they control RLS symptoms throughout the night (Silber et al. 2003). As of August 2009, ropinirole and pramipexole are the only two therapies approved by the U.S. Food and Drug Administration (FDA) for RLS. Alternative agents include benzodiazepines such as clonazepam or temazepam (Mitler et al. 1986), levodopa/carbidopa (Kaplan et al. 1993), and benzodiazepine receptor agonists (e.g., flurazepam, triazolam, temazepam). Both dopamine precursors (levodopa) and dopamine agonists improve RLS symptoms, reduce periodic leg movement, and improve sleep (Byrne et al. 2006; Gamaldo and Earley 2006; Hening et al. 1999, 2004b; Yee et al. 2009). Therapy with a dopamine precursor has unique advantages: the ability to improve symptoms quickly—and it may be used "on demand" in anticipation situations, such as before sitting through a long show, prolonged flight, or lengthy car ride. Two potential drawbacks of levodopa therapy are the potential for augmentation—that is, the development of an increased symptom severity earlier in the day (Allen and Earley 1996)—and rebound—that is, the delay and worsening of symptoms to later in the night or early morning.

The anticonvulsants carbamazepine and gabapentin have been suggested as treatments; of the two, more data are available about gabapentin improving leg movements (Garcia-Borreguero et al. 2002a, 2002b). Pregabalin has been suggested as an innovative approach for the management of secondary RLS for patients with neuropathic pain (Sommer et al. 2007). Refractory cases may respond more effectively to opiates, but these drugs are reserved as a treatment of last resort (Kavey et al. 1988).

Nonpharmacological therapies may consist of hot or cold baths, rubbing of the limbs before sleep, exercise before RLS symptoms, or vibratory or electrical stimulation of the distal lower limbs before bedtime (Adler 1997; Ahmed 2002; Akpinar 1987; Albanese and Filippini 2003; Allen and Earley 1996; Hening et al. 2004a, 2004b; Silber et al. 2003).

Periodic Leg Movement Disorder

Case Vignette 3

A 71-year-old woman is bothered by the irresistible need to constantly move her legs and significant daytime sleepiness. She experiences difficulties remaining still during shows and long flights, and her family members describe her as "very jumpy and restless as the day progresses." During the evening, her symptoms become very intolerable. She is observed to be engaging in vigorous massaging, stretching, and flexing of her legs, all of which she claims help improve her condition. Her husband reports that during the night she "kicked him periodically." Because the leg movements were severely disrupting his sleep, he had to move to a different bed a few months ago. Figure 18–6 is from a nocturnal polysomnogram of the patient, illustrating these nocturnal movements. The patient's periodic leg movements of sleep were treated with pramipexole, a dopamine agonist, which alleviated her symptoms.

Definitions. The term *periodic leg movements* (PLM) refers to a series of four or more stereotyped leg movements that recur periodically (5- to 90-second intervals) in any sleep or wake state (at a typical rate of 0.5 to 5- or 10-second duration) (Gamaldo and Earley 2006; "Recording and Scoring Leg Movements: The Atlas Task Force" 1993). The polysomnographic recording shown in Figure 18–6 indicated characteristic PLM during sleep (PLMS). Although diagnoses of PLM, PLMS, and PLM during wakefulness imply polysomnographic findings, PLMD refers to a specific sleep disorder in patients who experience PLM (usually >15 movements/hour of sleep) with an associated underlying sleep complaint (insomnia, hypersomnia) that cannot be otherwise explained (Gamaldo and Earley 2006).

Epidemiology. PLMS is estimated to occur in 4%–11% of adults (Hornyak et al. 2006), and it is very common in a variety of sleep disorders, including RLS (in 80%–90% of cases) and RBD (in ~70% of cases) (Wetter and Pollmacher 1997). The prevalence of PLMD is 3.9% in the general population (Ohayon and Roth 2002) and increases dramatically in older adults, occurring in over 50% of the population (Dickel and Mosko 1990; Ferri et al. 2009; Youngstedt et al. 1998).

Clinical manifestations. PLM implies the existence of periodic, stereotyped, and repetitive limb movements that occur during sleep and are documented on the polysomnogram. The movements usually occur in the lower extremities and are visualized as extension of the big toe along with partial flexion of the ankle or knee. Although most patients are unaware of the limb movements or the frequent sleep disruption, their bed partners often succumb to the kicking from the patients and move to sleep in separate beds. PLM may be an incidental finding on routine sleep studies, but these electrographic findings should lead clinicians to question patients about any underlying daytime sleepiness or insomnia and to determine whether these movements occur in isolation or as part of a clinically significant sleep disorder that may benefit from further management (e.g., PLMD).

Diagnostic evaluation. Polysomnography reveals repetitive electromyography (EMG) contractions of the anterior tibialis muscle lasting from 0.5 to 5 or 10 seconds, with more than 15 leg movements per hour of sleep captured in adults. Four or more consecutive movements are required, and the interval between movements is typically 20–40 seconds. The movements should appear in a sequence of four or more, separated by an interval of >5 seconds and <90 seconds, and should have an amplitude of ≥25% of toe dorsiflexion during the biocalibration (American Academy of Sleep Medicine 2005b).

Management. Management of PLMD is similar to that of RLS (see Figure 18–6). Only a few studies have evaluated the efficacy of specific medications in eradicating or reducing PLMS in patients with PLMD (Hornyak et al. 2006). Compared with therapy of RLS, treatment of PLMD relies more heavily on sedative-hypnotics and dopamine precursors (Lesage and Hening 2004). Another important consideration when treating PLMD is that many patients may have coexistent OSA (Ancoli-Israel et al. 1985; Carelli et al. 1999); therefore, agents that may worsen sleep apnea (e.g., long-acting benzodiazepines such as clonazepam) should be used with caution (Ancoli-Israel et al. 1993).

Sleep-Related Leg Cramps

Nocturnal leg cramps are painful muscular contractions, usually involving the calf or foot, that occur exclusively during the

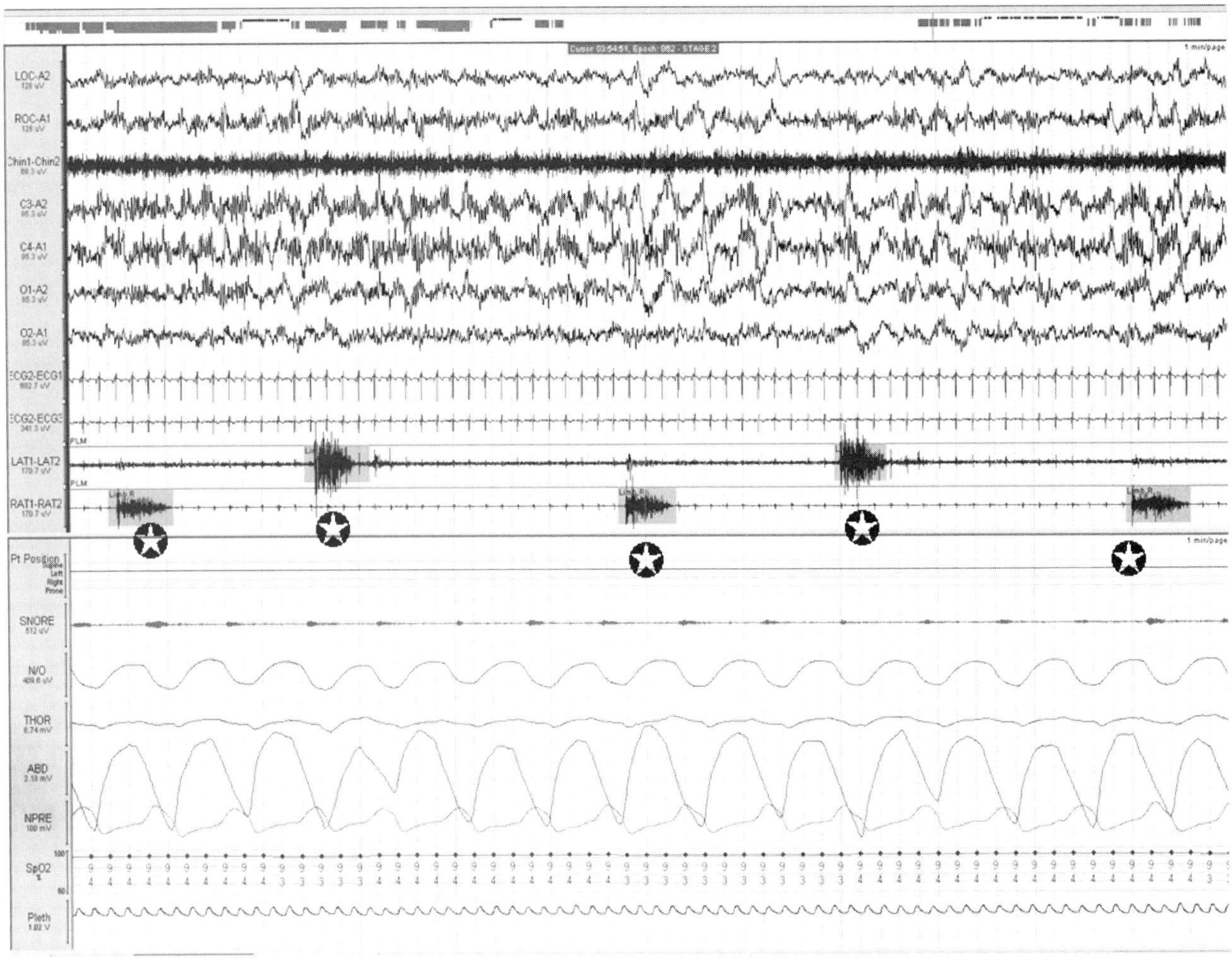

FIGURE 18–6. A 1-minute epoch of stage 2 sleep from a diagnostic polysomnogram illustrating periodic leg movements of sleep.

The 71-year-old woman in Case Vignette 3 had a history of "leg discomfort," most notably during the evening hours, and a history of frequent leg jerks noted at night by her husband. This epoch demonstrates a succession of five leg movements *(stars)*. From top to bottom, channels are as follows: electrooculogram (left: LOC-A2; right: ROC-A1); chin electromyography (Chin1-Chin2); electroencephalography (left central: C3-A2; right central: C4-A1; left occipital: O1-A2; right occipital: O2-A1); electrocardiogram (ECG2-ECG1 and ECG2-ECG3); limb electromyography (left leg: LAT1-LAT2; right leg: RAT1-RAT2); patient (Pt) position; snoring (SNORE); nasal-oral airflow (N/O); respiratory effort (thoracic [THOR], abdominal [ABD]); nasal pressure (NPRE); and oxygen desaturation measures: oxygen saturation measured by pulse oximetry (SpO_2) and plethysmography (Pleth).

night (Manila 2009; "Nocturnal Leg Cramps" 2002). The condition, which arises after vigorous exercise, has an increased incidence among older patients. The peak onset is usually in middle-age adults but may be seen for the first time in old age. Underlying predisposing factors include diabetes mellitus, arthritis, fluid and electrolyte disturbances, and metabolic disorders (Butler et al. 2002; Kelly 1995; Manila 2009; "Nocturnal Leg Cramps" 2002). The major complications include insomnia and sleepiness due to interruptions in sleep.

Quinine, which was widely used in the past for this condition, has significant hepatic side effects (Brasic 2001; Crum and Gable 2000); therefore, use of quinine should be avoided in nocturnal leg cramps (Mandal et al. 1995). Therapy with diltiazam, and possibly newer anticonvulsant agents, is suggested when conservative management fails (Butler et al. 2002; Del Mar et al. 2001; Guay 2008; Voon and Sheu 2001). Mild stretching exercise and heat therapy may also be effective as conservative therapy.

Circadian Rhythm Sleep Disorders and Abnormalities

Advanced Sleep Phase Disorder

Case Vignette 4

A 77-year-old man presents to the sleep disorders clinic complaining of a 5-year history of early morning awakening. He feels "extremely tired" in the early evening hours and goes to bed between 8:30 and 9:30 P.M. but does not fall asleep until about 10:30 or 11:00 P.M. When he decides to fall asleep ("lights out"), he has a sleep latency of 5 minutes. He wakes up at 3:00 A.M. and is unable to obtain any further sleep. He lies in bed for 60–90 minutes and eventually gets up between 4:00 and 4:30 A.M. He takes 3-hour late morning naps four or five times per week. The patient's sleep log is shown in Figure 18–7.

Located in the anterior hypothalamus is the body's master circadian modulator, the suprachiasmatic nucleus (SCN), which generates the endogenous sleep-wake cycle. Light is the most powerful exogenous circadian cue and is critical in synchronizing the circadian rhythms (Baker and Zee 2000; Reid and Zee 2004). Circadian rhythm sleep disturbances are caused by a mismatch or a misalignment between one's sleep and the 24-hour social and physical environment (Jacobs et al. 1989). Normal aging is associated with reduced input to the SCN, which degrades the normal physiological neuronal activation that generates the endogenous 24-hour rhythm (Van Someren 2000). This deactivation is probably reversible, because supplementation of stimuli that act as circadian cues at the level of the SCN can reactivate these neurons and help ameliorate sleep-wake rhythm disturbances (Van Someren 2000).

Advanced sleep phase disorder (ASPD) is a circadian rhythm sleep disturbance common among older adults, occurring in roughly 7.4% of middle-aged and older patients (Ando et al. 2002). Patients with ASPD demonstrate stable advancement of the major sleep period and are distinguished by habitual sleep onset and wake periods that are several hours earlier relative to conventional times (American Academy of Sleep Medicine 2005b). Complaints of early evening sleepiness are common, and patients typically wake early (3–4 A.M., as in Case Vignette 4) and have difficulties reinitiating sleep, resulting in a persistent state of sleep deprivation (Ancoli-Israel 1997). Typical patients become sleepy in the evening hours but sometimes try to remain awake until a more socially acceptable time, such as 10–11 P.M.

Bright light therapy (Figure 18–8) is the most effective way of ameliorating ASPD because light is the strongest cue for synchronizing circadian rhythms. Delay in sleep initiation and realignment of sleep-wake time are expected when patients are exposed to about 2,500 lux of light exposure in the early evening hours at approximately 1 meter distance at eye level (Campbell et al. 1988, 1995; Czeisler et al. 1989). Treatment with light therapy in older patients should be applied carefully because it may worsen macular degeneration and may not be efficacious in patients with cataracts.

The neurohormone melatonin, which is produced by the pineal gland, is potent in helping reset sleep onset by synchronization of the internal circadian clock (Dawson and Encel 1993). Because melatonin levels decrease with advancing age, some interest was prompted in melatonin replacement therapy for a variety of sleep disturbances, including management of insomnia in old age (Reiter 1995). In 1995, Haimov et al. showed a positive correlation between lower peak level of melatonin and poor sleep efficiency in older patients who have insomnia. Melatonin treatment early in the morning has been suggested for ASPD; however, data are lacking to substantiate this claim. (More data exist for using melatonin in the evening for treating delayed sleep phase disorder, which is common in adolescents.) Currently, more data are needed to improve understanding of the appropriate dosage, pharmacological properties, indications, safety, and efficacy of melatonin. Because the FDA does not regulate melatonin, care must be exercised when using it.

Parasomnias in Older Age

Parasomnias are undesirable and nondeliberate events that accompany sleep or wake-sleep transition. These nocturnal spells typically occur during entry into sleep or during arousals from sleep and may be augmented by the sleep state. Parasomnias may be extremely undesirable to some individuals, but may be of no concern to others. They often include abnormal movements, behaviors, emotions, perceptions, dream mentation, and autonomic activity (Broughton 1998). The most important parasomnia to consider in the geriatric population is RBD.

REM Sleep Behavior Disorder

Case Vignette 5

A 75-year-old man has experienced nocturnal spells for the past 5 years. His wife describes frequent arousals characterized by yelling, screaming, grunting, speaking, and hitting the pillows. These episodes consistently occur during the first 3 hours of the night. Over the past 12 months, these nocturnal events have become more dramatic. In one such episode, he broke his nose when he hit his face on the wall while fighting. His wife urged him to seek medical attention after one of these episodes, when he hit her face, resulting in a nosebleed and ecchymoses. She moved to a separate sleeping quarter after that event. The patient's neurologist had confirmed a diagnosis of Parkinson's disease 9 months ear-

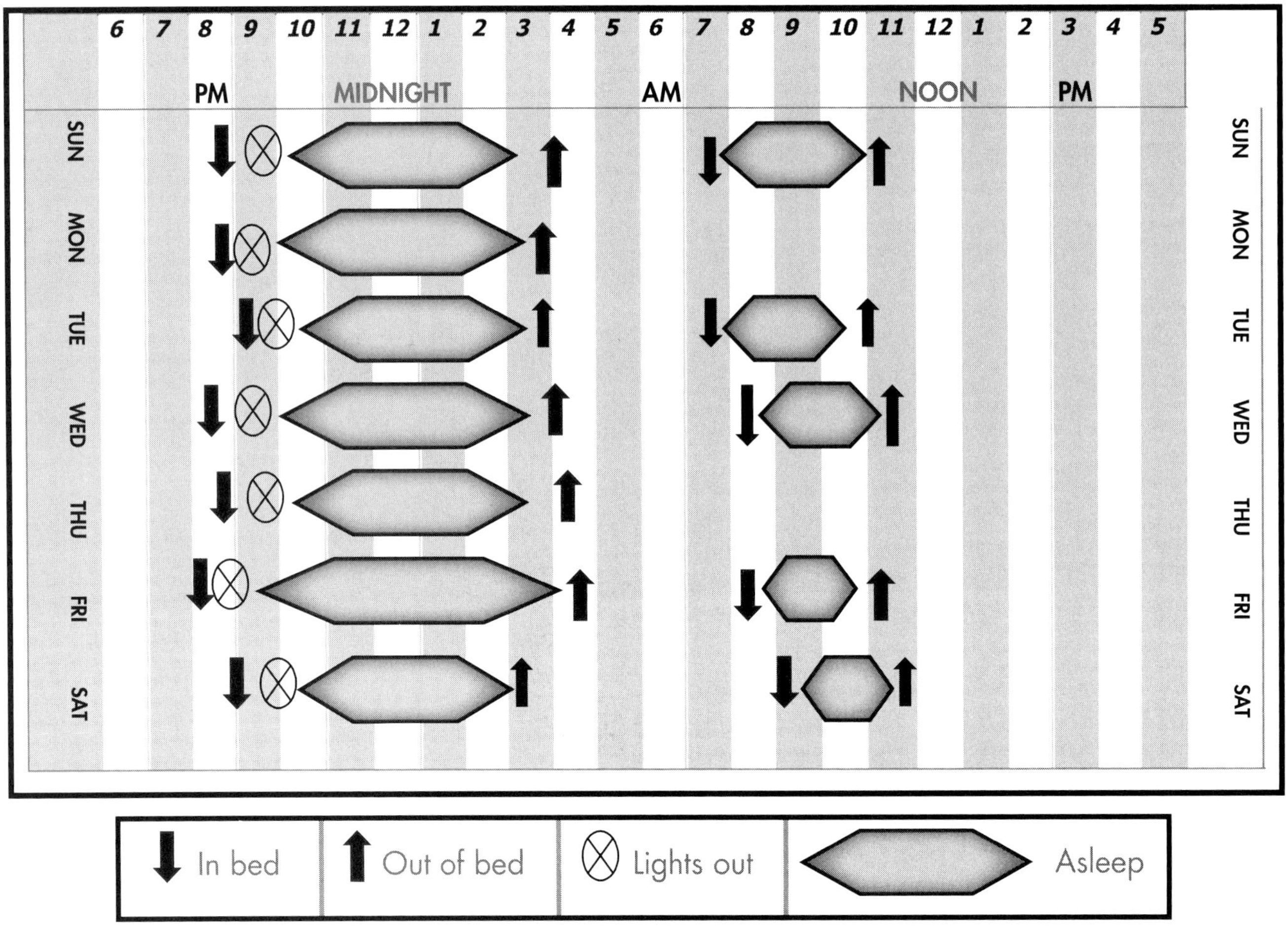

FIGURE 18–7. Sleep log demonstrating advanced sleep phase disorder.

This record shows the sleeping and waking times for the 77-year-old man who presents to a sleep disorders clinic complaining of a 5-year history of early morning awakening, as described in Case Vignette 4.

lier. Neurological examination confirms the presence of resting tremor, hypomimia, bradykinesia, and cogwheel rigidity. Figure 18–9 shows the sleep hypnogram and a 1-minute sample during REM sleep when this patient experienced one of his typical spells.

The prevalence of RBD is ~0.5% (Ohayon et al. 1997). The disorder has an increased predilection to affect men (9:1 male:female ratio) and has a higher prevalence in adults ages 50 and older. About one-quarter of patients with parkinsonism have dream enactment behaviors suggestive of RBD, and about 47% of Parkinson's patients who experience sleep disturbances are confirmed to have RBD based on sleep studies (Comella et al. 1998; Eisehsehr et al. 2001).

RBD is distinguished by abnormal elevation of limb or chin EMG tone during REM sleep and by complex and elaborate movements associated with the patient's dream mentation. Patients demonstrate a wide spectrum of abnormal dream experiences, ranging from simple vocalization, singing, yelling, shouting, and screaming to more exaggerated and complex motor phenomena such as running, walking, punching, kicking, jumping, and dramatic and sometimes violent agitated behaviors that correlate with the reported dream imagery. The injury associated with the spells often brings the patient or bed partner to medical attention.

Case Vignette 6

A 65-year-old man presented with violent and complex dreams reported by his spouse. His dreams had become extremely violent in the last few months before presentation for sleep medicine evaluation. He was witnessed as being aggressive during the night and injuring himself as a result. After sustaining a serious facial injury during one episode, he designed a set of handcuffs and placed a seat belt over his mattress to prevent himself from moving and hurting himself and his wife (Figure 18–10).

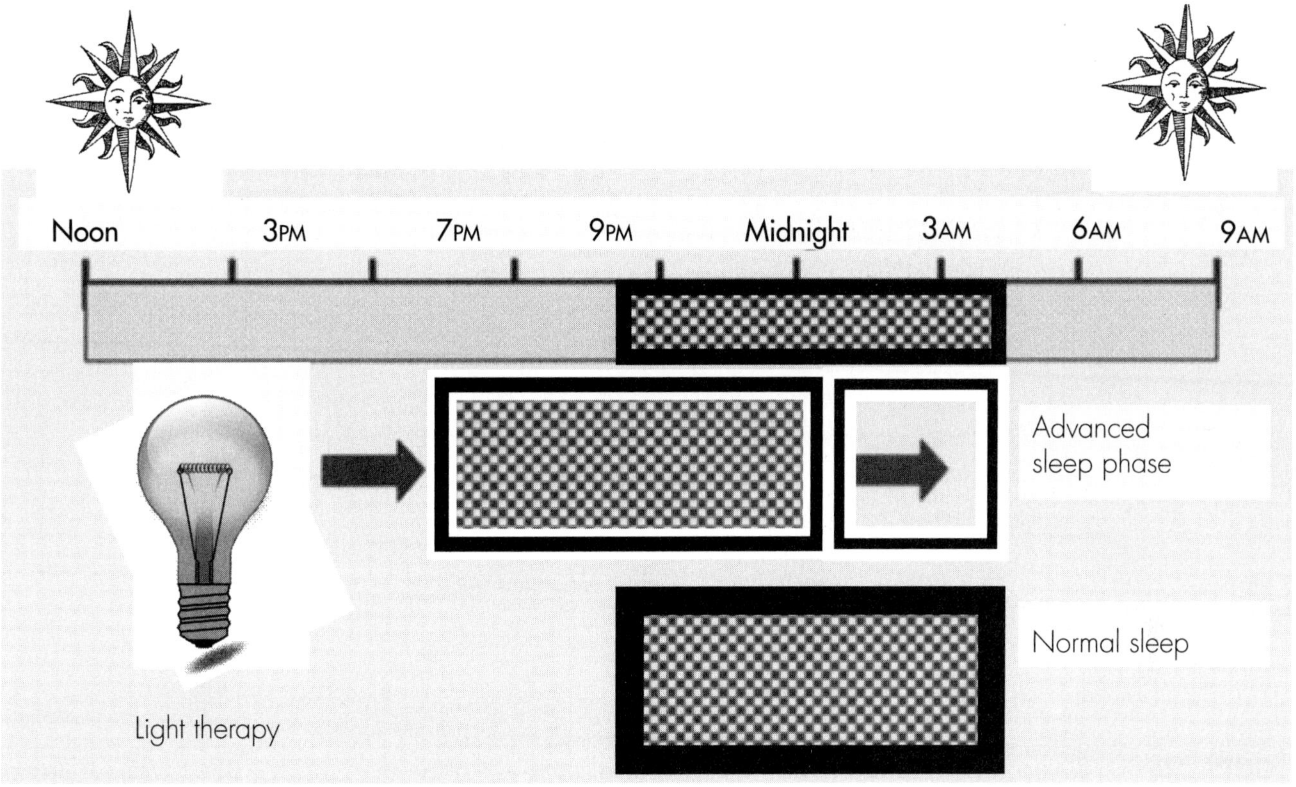

FIGURE 18–8. Advanced sleep phase disorder (ASPD) and management with evening light therapy.
This figure illustrates several options in the management of patients with ASPD. These include chronotherapy, timed bright light exposure in the evening, and pharmacotherapy with hypnotics to maintain sleep during the early morning. The most commonly used treatment for ASPD is bright light therapy for 2 hours in the evening, typically between 7–9 P.M., which improves sleep efficiency and delays the phase of circadian rhythms. Melatonin treatment early in the morning theoretically may be used for ASPD.

Patients with RBD typically experience spells as soon as they enter REM sleep (e.g., typically 90 minutes after sleep onset) and more commonly during the second half of the night. The frequency of spells varies greatly, occurring as rarely as a few times during the year to once a month to nightly episodes; patients with more frequent spells experience greater sleep disruption and are more likely to be referred. RBD has two forms: acute and chronic. The acute form is commonly seen in the setting of toxic or metabolic derangements and in association with certain drugs or substances. The most commonly seen drug-related form includes abrupt discontinuation of sedative-hypnotic agents (which results in REM rebound) and exposure to TCAs, monoamine oxidase inhibitors (MAOIs), biperiden, cholinergic agents, and SSRIs, which induce a characteristic state of loss of REM atonia (Akindele et al. 1970; Bental et al. 1979; Besset 1978; Carlander et al. 1996; Guilleminault et al. 1976; Passouant et al. 1972; Ross and Shua-Haim 1998; Schenck et al. 1992; Schutte and Doghramji 1996; Shimizu et al. 1985; Tachibana et al. 1975). Rapid withdrawal from alcohol and excessive use of caffeine (in the form of chocolate) have been implicated (Stolz and Aldrich 1991; Vorona and Ware 2002). Acute neurological derangements, such as brain stem lesions due to multiple sclerosis, subarachnoid hemorrhage, pontine stroke, and brain stem neoplasm, have all been implicated in the acute form of RBD (Plazzi and Montagna 2002; Schenck and Mahowald 2005; Schenck et al. 1987; Xi and Luning 2009).

Older age is a predisposing factor for the chronic and idiopathic form of RBD, which is more common than acute RBD, has an onset later in life, and progresses over time and often stabilizes. The majority of RBD cases, roughly 60%, are idiopathic; the remaining cases are comorbid with underlying neurodegenerative disorders commonly occurring in synucleinopathies, such as olivopontocerebellar atrophy and dementia with Lewy bodies, which have characteristic α-synuclein inclusions in nerve cell bodies. The condition has also been associated with Machado-Joseph disease (spinocerebellar ataxia type 3) and Guillain-Barré syndrome (Friedman 2002; Schenck et al. 1987).

RBD typically begins around ages 60–70 and may precede clinical manifestation of the underlying neuropathological lesion process by several years, even decades (Boeve et al. 2001,

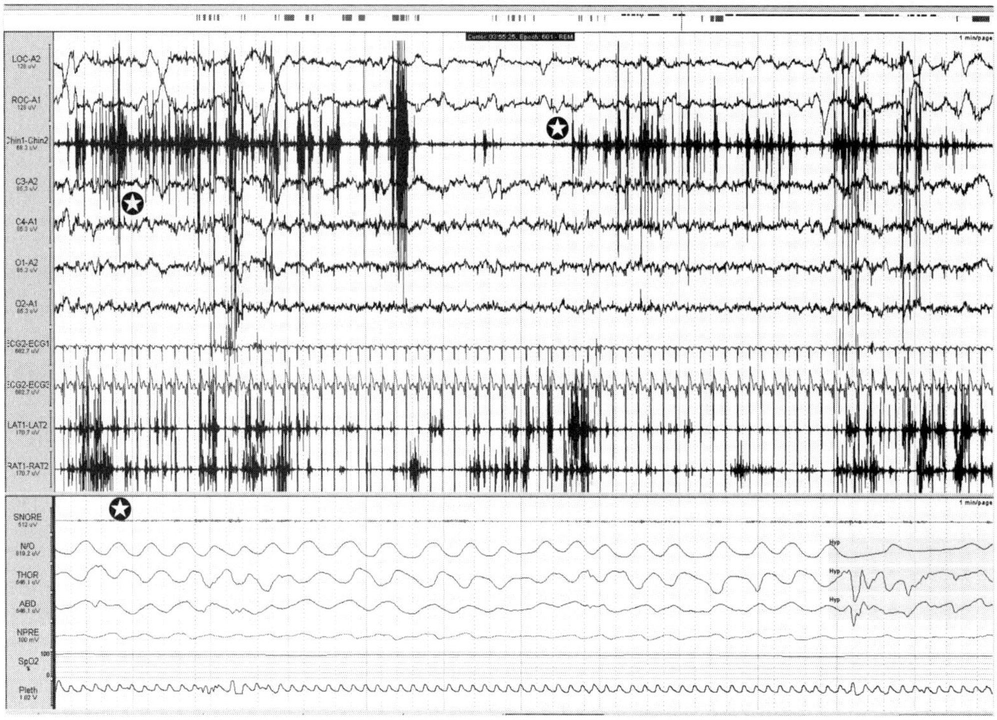

FIGURE 18–9. Polysomnographic recording illustrating rapid eye movement (REM) sleep without atonia in a patient with REM sleep behavior disorder.

This 75-year-old patient had a history of Parkinson's disease and dream enactment behavioral spells as described in Case Vignette 5. The baseline polysomnogram was recorded during REM sleep, as shown by the rapid eye movements in left and right outer canthi referenced to the ear electrodes (A1, A2). During the study, the patient was documented to yell, punch, kick, jump from bed, and have arm flailing movements. When awakened, he described trying to protect himself against an intruder. This 1-minute epoch demonstrated abnormal augmentation of REM sleep tone *(stars).*

From top to bottom, channels are as follows: electrooculogram (left: LOC-A2; right: ROC-A1); chin electromyography (Chin1-Chin2); electroencephalography (left central: C3-A2; right central: C4-A1; left occipital: O1-A2; right occipital: O2-A1); electrocardiogram (ECG2-ECG1 and ECG2-ECG3); limb electromyography (left leg: LAT1-LAT2; right leg: RAT1-RAT2); snoring (SNORE); nasal-oral airflow (N/O); respiratory effort (thoracic [THOR], abdominal [ABD]); nasal pressure (NPRE); and oxygen desaturation measures: oxygen saturation measured by pulse oximetry (SpO_2) and plethysmography (Pleth).

2003; Montplaisir et al. 1997; Pareja et al. 1996; Schenck et al. 1996). As noted earlier, RBD is much more predominant in males than in females, although the reason for this gender predilection is unclear (Abad and Guilleminault 2004; Ozekmekci et al. 2005; Schenck et al. 1987).

The underlying pathophysiology may be related to abnormal brain stem control of medullary inhibitory regions (Figure 18–11; Avidan 2005a). An identical syndrome was reported in cats with a preparation of bilateral lesions in the pontine regions adjacent to the locus coeruleus, causing absence of the REM-related atonia and abnormal motor behaviors during sleep (Jouvet and Delorme 1965). The condition was eventually characterized by Schenck et al. (1986) as a new parasomnia in a classic report of a series of mainly older male humans with aggressive nocturnal behaviors. The possible underlying RBD mechanism is related to either a reduction of REM atonia or an abnormal augmentation of locomotor intermittent excitatory influences during REM sleep, or both (Mahowald and Schenck 2000; Paparrigopoulos 2005).

Neuroimaging studies using single-photon emission computed tomography (SPECT) have demonstrated dopaminergic abnormalities showing decreased striatal dopaminergic innervations as well as reduced striatal dopamine transporters (Albin et al. 2000; Eisensehr et al. 2000, 2003). Positron emission tomography and SPECT studies in patients with multiple-system atrophy and RBD have further confirmed reduced nigrostriatal dopaminergic projections (Gilman et al. 2003). RBD is believed to be mediated via complex multiple neurotransmitter dysfunction involving GABAergic, glutamatergic, and monoaminergic systems, and it is probably not a product of isolated or direct abnormal α-synuclein inclusions or striatonigral dopaminergic deficiency alone (Iranzo et al.

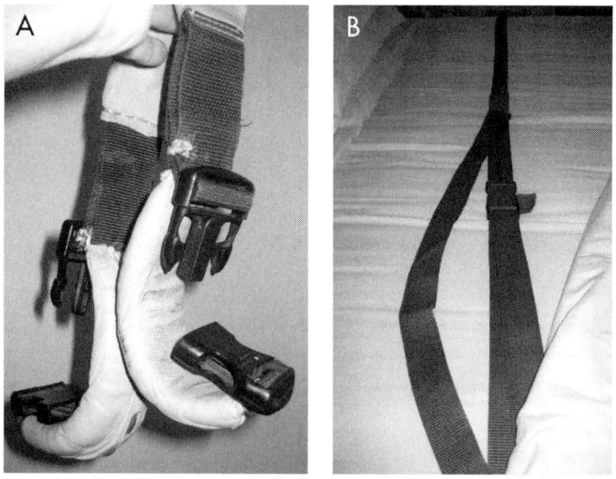

FIGURE 18–10. Restraints fabricated by man with a history of violent and aggressive dream enactment, as described in Case Vignette 6.

Panel A: Handcuffs patient used to tie his hands. **Panel B:** Seat belt patient used to restrain himself in bed.

2009). In patients with idiopathic RBD, impaired cortical activation as determined by EEG spectral analysis supports the relationship between RBD and neurodegenerative disorders (Fantini et al. 2003b).

Diagnostic Evaluation

RBD is characterized by abnormal EMG augmentation during REM sleep (see Figure 18–9). Typical spells are described as complex (involving both limbs and trunk movements) and consist of repeated kicking, punching, and yelling, often associated with emotionally charged utterances (Mahowald 2004; Schenck and Mahowald 2002). Some patients have preservation of dream content when awakened from their episodes and provide vivid reports of their dream content that correlate with the observed behaviors. The need to conduct more detailed neurological testing, such as computed tomography or magnetic resonance imaging, depends on the results of the neurological history and examination, the age of the patient, the underlying acute neurological process (stroke, demyelination), or the presence of a structural lesion. Further neurological testing is especially important if the episodes do not adhere to the typical demographic characteristics (i.e., younger patients and women), are acute, or have a temporal association with neurological injury (Bonakis et al. 2009; Plazzi and Montagna 2002; Stores 2008).

Differential Diagnosis

The differential diagnosis of RBD includes nocturnal seizures, posttraumatic stress disorder, and non-REM parasomnias, such as confusional arousals, sleepwalking, sleep terrors, and nightmares. Non-REM parasomnias and frontal lobe nocturnal seizures are much more common in children and adolescents, making distinction from RBD easier. RBD is also distinguished by the complex nature of the episodes, onset later in the night when REM density is higher, and the characteristic demographics—that is, older men.

Management

Meticulous attention to safety measures for patients with RBD is critical, especially in those who experience displacement from bed and aggressive spells. When the potential for injury to patient and/or bed partner is high, pharmacological and safety interventions should be instituted without delay. Safety measures such as sleeping on the ground floor in a sleeping bag and barricading the windows with curtains should be recommended until the episodes are fully managed. Pharmacotherapy for RBD is very effective, with clonazepam (0.25–1 mg orally at bedtime) achieving improvement in most (90%) patients with little evidence of tolerance or abuse (Mahowald and Ettinger 1990; Mahowald and Schenck 1994; Schenck and Mahowald 1990). Clonazepam does not reinstate normal limb-EMG tone but prevents the arousals associated with the REM-sleep dissociation. Management with melatonin may restore REM-sleep atonia and is also very effective, controlling RBD spells in 87% of patients taking 3–12 mg at bedtime (Boeve 2001; Takeuchi et al. 2001). However, as discussed in the management of circadian rhythm disorders, melatonin is a dietary supplement, is not approved by the FDA, has poorly regulated pharmacological preparation, and is not supported by careful studies measuring side effects, especially in older adults. Other agents that may be helpful for RBD include the TCA imipramine (25 mg orally at bedtime), carbamazepine (100 mg orally twice daily), and the dopaminergic agents pramipexole and levodopa (Fantini et al. 2003a; Schmidt et al. 2006; Tan et al. 1996). One study described successful amelioration of RBD with sodium oxybate (an agent approved for the management of narcolepsy and cataplexy) when other treatments are ineffective or poorly tolerated (Shneerson 2009). This response also suggests that RBD and cataplexy may in part share a common pathophysiology (Shneerson 2009).

Conclusion

Sleep transforms dramatically in older age. Both subjective and objective measurements of sleep demonstrate an increase in disturbances of sleep, including fragmented sleep, less deep sleep, and more early morning awakening. When older patients present with sleep disorders, they often report insomnia, hypersomnia, or abnormal movements. In making the appropriate

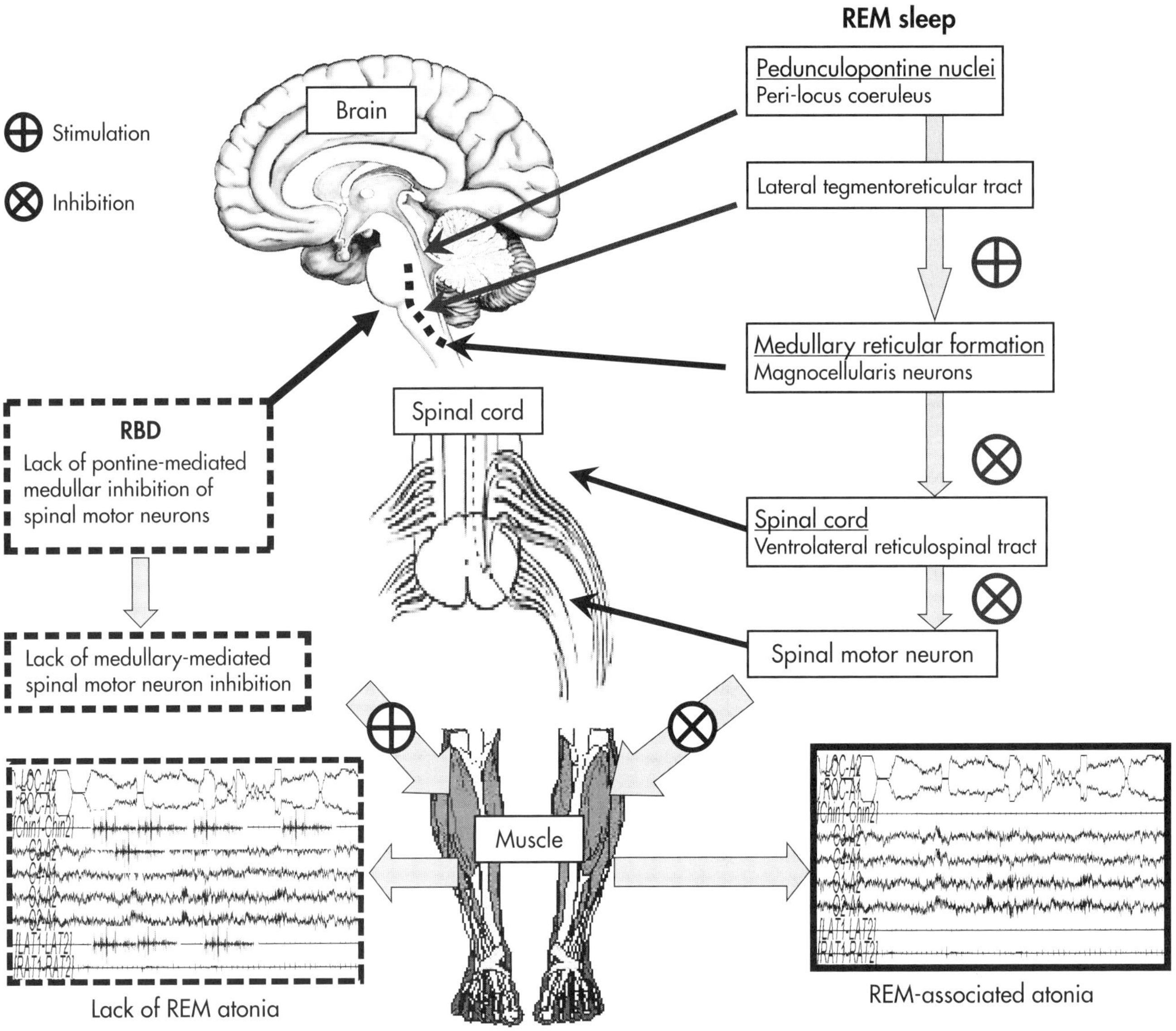

FIGURE 18–11. Underlying pathophysiology of rapid eye movement (REM) sleep (right panel, solid boxes) and REM sleep behavior disorder (RBD) (left panel, dotted boxes).

Normally, generalized muscle atonia during REM sleep results from pontine-mediated peri–locus coeruleus inhibition of motor activity. This pontine activity exerts an excitatory influence on medullary reticular formation (magnocellularis neurons) via the lateral tegmentoreticular tract. These neuronal groups, in turn, hyperpolarize the spinal motor neuron postsynaptic membranes via the ventrolateral reticulospinal tract. This normal activity is shown in solid boxes at right of figure. In RBD (shown in dotted boxes at left), the brain stem mechanisms generating the muscle atonia normally seen in REM sleep may be disrupted. The pathophysiology of RBD in humans is based on the cat model, in which bilateral pontine lesions result in a persistent absence of REM atonia associated with prominent motor activity during REM sleep. The pathophysiology of the idiopathic form of RBD in humans is still not very well understood but may be related to reduction of striatal presynaptic dopamine transporters.

Source. Adapted from Avidan (2005a).

diagnosis, the psychiatrist should review the patient's medical and psychiatric history, medications, underlying medical illnesses, and sleep-wake schedule pattern. The aging process itself does not directly lead to sleep problems, and sleep requirements do not decrease with advanced age. Insomnia, sleep-related breathing disorder, PLMD, and RLS increase in prevalence with aging and may lead to poorer sleep quality. Because many sleep disorders are potentially reversible, it is the physician's responsibility to screen for these problems. Furthermore, a carefully planned clinical decision-making process when encountering a sleep disturbance in the elderly patient can greatly enhance the patient's quality of life and daytime function.

Key Points

- Untreated sleep disturbances lead to decreased sleep at night, resulting in difficulties with cognitive disturbances, concentration and memory difficulties, and overall poorer quality of life.
- The most ubiquitous sleep complaint of older adults is insomnia, characterized as difficulties initiating or maintaining sleep.
- Sleep apnea is one of the most dangerous sleep disorders; it often remains underdiagnosed and untreated in patients who would significantly benefit from carefully orchestrated management.
- Circadian rhythm disorders in older patients are attributed to disruption in the endogenous circadian clock in the brain and are exacerbated by insufficient light exposure.
- Motor disorders of sleep are sometimes unappreciated by physicians who may not be familiar with them, yet treatment is exceptionally useful, especially for conditions such as restless legs syndrome and REM sleep behavior disorders.
- Sleep disturbances in older adults should not be viewed as an inevitable part of aging. It is the responsibility of the geriatric neurologist or psychiatrist to screen, evaluate, and treat these disorders, because many are frequently comorbid with or secondary to neurological, medical, and psychiatric disease or are a result of polypharmacy.

Recommended Readings and Web Sites

Ancoli-Israel S: Sleep and aging: prevalence of disturbed sleep and treatment considerations in older adults. J Clin Psychiatry 66(suppl):24–30; quiz 42–23, 2005

Ancoli-Israel S, Alessi C: Sleep and aging. Am J Geriatr Psychiatry 13: 341–343, 2005

Avidan AY: Clinical neurology of insomnia in neurodegenerative and other disorders of neurological function. Rev Neurol Dis 4:21–34, 2007

Avidan AY, Alessi CA (eds): Geriatric Sleep Medicine. New York, Informa Healthcare, 2008

Bloom HG, Ahmed I, Alessi CA, et al: Evidence-based recommendations for the assessment and management of sleep disorders in older persons. J Am Geriatr Soc 57:761–789, 2009

Dijk DJ: Sleep of aging women and men: back to basics. Sleep 29:12–13, 2006

Espiritu JR: Aging-related sleep changes. Clin Geriatr Med 24:1–14, v, 2008

Floyd JA: Sleep and aging. Nurs Clin North Am 37:719–731, 2002

Kryger M: Sleep, health, and aging. Geriatrics 59:23, 2004

Professional Sleep Associations and Societies

American Academy of Sleep Medicine: www.aasmnet.org

National Institutes of Health, National Institute on Aging Senior Health (Sleep and Aging): http://nihseniorhealth.gov/sleepandaging/toc.html#skip2

National Sleep Foundation: www.sleepfoundation.org

Sleep Research Society: www.sleepresearchsociety.org

Patient Educational Resources

American Sleep Apnea Association: www.sleepapnea.org

National Heart, Lung and Blood Institute Sleep Disorders Information: www.nhlbi.nih.gov/health/public/sleep/index.htm

Restless Legs Syndrome Foundation: www.rls.org

References

Abad VC, Guilleminault C: Review of rapid eye movement behavior sleep disorders. Curr Neurol Neurosci Rep 4:157–163, 2004

Abele M, Burk K, Laccone F, et al: Restless legs syndrome in spinocerebellar ataxia types 1, 2, and 3. J Neurol 248:311–314, 2001

Abetz L, Allen R, Follet A, et al: Evaluating the quality of life of patients with restless legs syndrome. Clin Ther 26:925–935, 2004

Adler CH: Treatment of restless legs syndrome with gabapentin. Clin Neuropharmacol 20:148–151, 1997

Agargun MY, Kara H, Ozbek H, et al: Restless legs syndrome induced by mirtazapine. J Clin Psychiatry 63:1179, 2002

Ahmed I: Ropinirole in restless leg syndrome. Mo Med 99:500–501, 2002

Akindele MO, Evans JI, Oswald I: Monoamine oxidase inhibitors, sleep and mood. Electroencephalogr Clin Neurophysiol 29:47–56, 1970

Akpinar S: Restless legs syndrome treatment with dopaminergic drugs. Clin Neuropharmacol 10:69–79, 1987

Albanese A, Filippini G: Gabapentin improved sensory and motor symptoms in the restless legs syndrome. ACP J Club 139:17, 2003

Albin RL, Koeppe RA, Chervin RD, et al: Decreased striatal dopaminergic innervation in REM sleep behavior disorder. Neurology 55:1410–1412, 2000

Al-Jahdali HH, Al-Qadhi WA, Khogeer HA, et al: Restless legs syndrome in patients on dialysis. Saudi J Kidney Dis Transpl 20:378–385, 2009

Allen RP, Earley CJ: Augmentation of the restless legs syndrome with carbidopa/levodopa. Sleep 19:205–213, 1996

Allen RP, Earley CJ: Defining the phenotype of the restless legs syndrome (RLS) using age-of-symptom-onset. Sleep Med 1:11–19, 2000

Allen RP, Picchietti D, Hening WA, et al: Restless legs syndrome: diagnostic criteria, special considerations, and epidemiology: a report from the Restless Legs Syndrome Diagnosis and Epidemiology Workshop at the National Institutes of Health. Sleep Medicine 4:101–119, 2003

American Academy of Sleep Medicine: The International Classification of Sleep Disorders. Westchester, IL, American Academy of Sleep Medicine, 2005a

American Academy of Sleep Medicine: International Classification of Sleep Disorders, Diagnostic and Coding Manual, 2nd Edition. Westchester, IL, American Academy of Sleep Medicine, 2005b

Ancoli-Israel S: Sleep problems in older adults: putting myths to bed. Geriatrics 52:20–30, 1997

Ancoli-Israel S, Kripke DF: Prevalent sleep problems in the aged. Biofeedback Self Regul 16:349–359, 1991

Ancoli-Israel S, Kripke DF, Mason W, et al: Sleep apnea and periodic movements in an aging sample. J Gerontol 40:419–425, 1985

Ancoli-Israel S, Kripke DF, Klauber MR, et al: Sleep-disordered breathing in community-dwelling elderly. Sleep 14:486–495, 1991

Ancoli-Israel S, Bliwise DL, Mant A: Sleep and breathing in the elderly, in Sleep and Breathing. Edited by Saunders NA, Sullivan CE. New York, Marcel Dekker, 1993, pp 673–693

Ancoli-Israel S, Richardson GS, Mangano RM, et al: Long-term use of sedative hypnotics in older patients with insomnia. Sleep Med 6:107–113, 2005

Ancoli-Israel S, Ayalon L, Salzman C: Sleep in the elderly: normal variations and common sleep disorders. Harv Rev Psychiatry 16:279–286, 2008

Ando K, Kripke DF, Ancoli-Israel S: Delayed and advanced sleep phase symptoms. Isr J Psychiatry Relat Sci 39:11–18, 2002

Avidan AY: Sleep disorders in the older patient. Prim Care 32:563–586, 2005a

Avidan AY: Sleep in the geriatric patient population. Semin Neurol 25:52–63, 2005b

Avidan AY, James ML, Kristina MA, et al: Insomnia and hypnotic use as predictors of falls and hip fractures in older nursing home residents. Sleep 27:A122, 2004

Ayalon L, Liu L, Ancoli-Israel S: Diagnosing and treating sleep disorders in the older adult. Med Clin North Am 88:737–750, ix–x, 2004

Bachman DL: Sleep disorders with aging: evaluation and treatment. Geriatrics 47:53–56, 59–61, 1992

Baker SK, Zee PC: Circadian disorders of the sleep-wake cycle, in Principles and Practice of Sleep Medicine. Edited by Kryger MH, Roth T, Dement WC. Philadelphia, PA, WB Saunders, 2000, pp 606–614

Bakshi R: Fluoxetine and restless legs syndrome. J Neurol Sci 142: 151–152, 1996

Banno K, Delaive K, Walld R, et al: Restless legs syndrome in 218 patients: associated disorders. Sleep Med 1:221–229, 2000

Becker PM: The biopsychosocial effects of restless legs syndrome (RLS). Neuropsychiatr Dis Treat 2:505–512, 2006

Benca RM, Obermeyer WH, Thisted RA, et al: Sleep and psychiatric disorders: a meta-analysis. Arch Gen Psychiatry 49:651–668; discussion 669–670, 1992

Bental E, Lavie P, Sharf B: Severe hypermotility during sleep in treatment of cataplexy with clomipramine. Isr J Med Sci 15:607–609, 1979

Berger K, Luedemann J, Trenkwalder C, et al: Sex and the risk of restless legs syndrome in the general population. Arch Intern Med 164: 196–202, 2004

Besset A: Effect of antidepressants on human sleep. Adv Biosci 21: 141–148, 1978

Bloom HG, Ahmed I, Alessi CA, et al: Evidence-based recommendations for the assessment and management of sleep disorders in older persons. J Am Geriatr Soc 57:761–789, 2009

Boeve BF: Melatonin for treatment of REM sleep behavior disorder: response in 8 patients. Sleep 24(suppl):A35, 2001

Boeve BF, Silber MH, Ferman JT, et al: Association of REM sleep behavior disorder and neurodegenerative disease may reflect an underlying synucleinopathy. Mov Disord 16:622–630, 2001

Boeve BF, Silber MH, Parisi JE, et al: Synucleinopathy pathology often underlies REM sleep behavior disorder and dementia or parkinsonism. Neurology 61:40–45, 2003

Bonakis A, Howard RS, Ebrahim IO, et al: REM sleep behaviour disorder (RBD) and its associations in young patients. Sleep Med 10:641–645, 2009

Bootzin R, Nicassio P: Behavioral treatments for insomnia, in Progress in Behavior Modification. Edited by Hersen M, Eisler R, Miller P. New York, Academic Press, 1978, pp 1–45

Brasic JR: Quinine-induced thrombocytopenia in a 64-year-old man who consumed tonic water to relieve nocturnal leg cramps. Mayo Clin Proc 76:863–864, 2001

Brassington GS, King AC, Bliwise DL: Sleep problems as a risk factor for falls in a sample of community-dwelling adults aged 64–99 years. J Am Geriatr Soc 48:1234–1240, 2000

Broughton R: Behavioral parasomnias, in Sleep Disorders Medicine. Edited by Chokroverty S, Daroff RB. Boston, MA, Butterworth-Heinemann, 1998, pp 635–660

Butler JV, Mulkerrin EC, O'Keeffe ST: Nocturnal leg cramps in older people. Postgrad Med J 78:596–598, 2002

Byrne R, Sinha S, Chaudhuri KR: Restless legs syndrome: diagnosis and review of management options. Neuropsychiatr Dis Treat 2:155–164, 2006

Campbell SS, Kripke DF, Gillin JC, et al: Exposure to light in healthy elderly subjects and Alzheimer's patients. Physiol Behav 42:141–144, 1988

Campbell SS, Terman M, Lewy A, et al: Light treatment for sleep disorders: consensus report, V: age-related disturbances. J Biol Rhythms 10:151–154, 1995

Carelli G, Krieger J, Calvi-Gries F, et al: Periodic limb movements and obstructive sleep apneas before and after continuous positive airway pressure treatment. J Sleep Res 8:211–216, 1999

Carlander B, Touchon J, Ondze B, et al: REM sleep behavior disorder induced by cholinergic treatment in Alzheimer's disease. J Sleep Res 5(suppl):28, 1996

Chan ED, Welsh CH: Geriatric respiratory medicine. Chest 114: 1704–1733, 1998

Chaudhuri KR, Forbes A, Grosset D, et al: Diagnosing restless legs syndrome (RLS) in primary care. Curr Med Res Opin 20:1785–1795, 2004

Chesson AL Jr, Ferber RA, Fry JM, et al: The indications for polysomnography and related procedures. Sleep 20:423–487, 1997

Comella CL, Nardine TM, Diederich NJ, et al: Sleep-related violence, injury, and REM sleep behavior disorder in Parkinson's disease. Neurology 51:526–529, 1998

Crum NF, Gable P: Quinine-induced hemolytic-uremic syndrome. South Med J 93:726–728, 2000

Czeisler CA, Kronauer RE, Allan JS, et al: Bright light induction of strong (type 0) resetting of the human circadian pacemaker. Science 244:1328–1332, 1989

Dancey DR, Hanly PJ, Soong C, et al: Impact of menopause on the prevalence and severity of sleep apnea. Chest 120:151–155, 2001

Dawson D, Encel N: Melatonin and sleep in humans (review). J Pineal Res 15:1–12, 1993

Del Mar CB, Glasziou PP, Spinks AB, et al: Treatment alternatives for nocturnal leg cramps. Med J Aust 174:540, 2001

Dement W, Carskadon M: "White paper" on sleep and aging. J Am Geriatr Soc 30:25–50, 1982

Dement W, Richardson G, Prinz P, et al: Changes of sleep and wakefulness with age, in Handbook of the Biology of Aging, 2nd Edition. Edited by Finch CE, Schneider EL. New York, Van Nostrand Reinhold, 1985, pp 692–717

Dickel MJ, Mosko SS: Morbidity cut-offs for sleep apnea and periodic leg movements in predicting subjective complaints in seniors. Sleep 13:155–166, 1990

Doghramji PP: Treatment of insomnia with zaleplon, a novel sleep medication. Int J Clin Pract 55:329–334, 2001

Dufour MC, Archer L, Gordis E: Alcohol and the elderly. Clin Geriatr Med 8:127–141, 1992

Earley CJ, Connors JR, Allen RP: RLS patients have abnormally reduced CSF ferritin compared to normal controls. Neurology 52(suppl):A111–A112, 1999

Earley CJ, Allen RP, Beard JL, et al: Insight into the pathophysiology of restless legs syndrome. J Neurosci Res 62:623–628, 2000

Edinger JD, Hoelscher TJ, Webb MD, et al: Polysomnographic assessment of DIMS: empirical evaluation of its diagnostic value. Sleep 12:315–322, 1989

Eisensehr I, Linke R, Noachtar S, et al: Reduced striatal dopamine transporters in idiopathic rapid eye movement sleep behavior disorder: comparison with Parkinson's disease and controls. Brain 123:1155–1160, 2000

Eisehsehr I, Parrino L, Noachtar S, et al: Sleep in Lennox-Gastaut syndrome: the role of the cyclic alternating pattern (CAP) in the gate control of clinical seizures and generalized polyspikes. Epilepsy Res 46:241–250, 2001

Eisehsehr I, Linke R, Tatsch K, et al: Increased muscle activity during rapid eye movement sleep correlates with decrease of striatal presynaptic dopamine transporters: IPT and IBZM SPECT imaging in subclinical and clinically manifest idiopathic REM sleep behavior disorder, Parkinson's disease, and controls. Sleep 26: 507–512, 2003

Enright PL, Newman AB, Wahl PW, et al: Prevalence and correlates of snoring and observed apneas in 5201 older adults. Sleep 19: 531–538, 1996

Espie CA: The Psychological Treatment of Insomnia. Chichester, UK, Wiley, 1991

Espie CA: Insomnia: conceptual issues in the development, persistence, and treatment of sleep disorder in adults. Annu Rev Psychol 53:215–243, 2002

Fantini ML, Gagnon JF, Filipini D, et al: The effects of pramipexole in REM sleep behavior disorder. Neurology 61:1418–1420, 2003a

Fantini ML, Gagnon JF, Petit D, et al: Slowing of electroencephalogram in rapid eye movement sleep behavior disorder. Ann Neurol 53:774–780, 2003b

Ferri R, Gschliesser V, Frauscher B, et al: Periodic leg movements during sleep and periodic limb movement disorder in patients presenting with unexplained insomnia. Clin Neurophysiol 120: 257–263, 2009

Findley LJ, Barth JT, Powers DC, et al: Cognitive impairment in patients with obstructive sleep apnea and associated hypoxemia. Chest 90:686–690, 1986

Finucane TE: Treatment for insomnia. Lancet 359:1434, author reply 1434, 2002

Flamer HE: Sleep disorders in the elderly. Aust N Z J Med 26:96–104, 1996

Foley DJ, Monjan AA, Brown SL, et al: Sleep complaints among elderly persons: an epidemiologic study of three communities. Sleep 18:425–432, 1995

Foley DJ, Monjan A, Simonsick EM, et al: Incidence and remission of insomnia among elderly adults: an epidemiologic study of 6,800 persons over three years. Sleep 22(suppl):S366–S372, 1999

Friedman JH: Presumed rapid eye movement behavior disorder in Machado-Joseph disease (spinocerebellar ataxia type 3). Mov Disord 17:1350–1353, 2002

Gamaldo CE, Earley CJ: Restless legs syndrome: a clinical update. Chest 130:1596–1604, 2006

Garcia-Borreguero D, Larrosa O, de la Llave Y: Circadian aspects in the pathophysiology of the restless legs syndrome. Sleep Med 3(suppl):S17–21, 2002a

Garcia-Borreguero D, Larrosa O, de la Llave Y, et al: Treatment of restless legs syndrome with gabapentin: a double-blind, cross-over study. Neurology 59:1573–1579, 2002b

Gillin JC, Byerley WF: The diagnosis and management of insomnia. N Engl J Med 322:239–248, 1990

Gilman S, Koeppe RA, Chervin R, et al: REM sleep behavior disorder is related to striatal monoaminergic deficit in MSA. Neurology 61:29–34, 2003

Greenberg DG, Watson RK, Deptula D: Neuropsychological dysfunction in sleep apnea. Sleep 10:254–262, 1987

Guay DR: Are there alternatives to the use of quinine to treat nocturnal leg cramps? Consult Pharm 23:141–156, 2008

Guilleminault C, Raynal D, Takahashi S, et al: Evaluation of short-term and long-term treatment of the narcolepsy syndrome with clomipramine hydrochloride. Acta Neurol Scand 54:71–87, 1976

Haimov I, Lavie P, Laudon M, et al: Melatonin replacement therapy of elderly insomniacs. Sleep 18:598–603, 1995

Hargrave R, Beckley DJ: Restless leg syndrome exacerbated by sertraline. Psychosomatics 39:177–178, 1998

Hauri PJ: Behavioral treatment of insomnia. Med Times 107:36–47, 1979

Hauri PJ: Insomnia. Clin Chest Med 19:157–168, 1998

Hauri PJ: Advances in the behavioral treatment of insomnia. Sleep Med Rev 7:201–202, 2003

Hauri PJ, Wisbey J: Wrist actigraphy in insomnia. Sleep 15:293–301, 1992

Hening W: The clinical neurophysiology of the restless legs syndrome and periodic limb movements, part I: diagnosis, assessment, and characterization. Clin Neurophysiol 115:1965–1974, 2004

Hening W, Allen R, Earley C, et al: The treatment of restless legs syndrome and periodic limb movement disorder: an American Academy of Sleep Medicine review. Sleep 22:970–999, 1999

Hening W, Allen RP, Earley CJ, et al: An update on the dopaminergic treatment of restless legs syndrome and periodic limb movement disorder: an American Academy of Sleep Medicine Interim Review. Sleep 27:560–583, 2004a

Hening W, Walters AS, Allen RP, et al: Impact, diagnosis and treatment of restless legs syndrome (RLS) in a primary care population: the REST (RLS Epidemiology, Symptoms, and Treatment) primary care study. Sleep Med 5:237–246, 2004b

Hening W, Allen RP, Chaudhuri KR, et al: Clinical significance of RLS. Mov Disord 22(suppl):S395–S400, 2007a

Hening W, Allen RP, Tenzer P, et al: Restless legs syndrome: demographics, presentation, and differential diagnosis. Geriatrics 62:26–29, 2007b

Hicks R, Dysken MW, Davis JM, et al: The pharmacokinetics of psychotropic medication in the elderly: a review. J Clin Psychiatry 42:374–385, 1981

Hornyak M, Feige B, Riemann D, et al: Periodic leg movements in sleep and periodic limb movement disorder: prevalence, clinical significance and treatment. Sleep Med Rev 10:169–177, 2006

Hui D, Wong TY, Ko FW, et al: Prevalence of sleep disturbances in Chinese patients with end-stage renal failure on continuous ambulatory peritoneal dialysis. Am J Kidney Dis 36:783–788, 2000

Hui D, Wong T, Li T, et al: Prevalence of sleep disturbances in Chinese patients with end stage renal failure on maintenance hemodialysis. Med Sci Monit 8:CR331–CR336, 2002

Iranzo A, Santamaria J, Tolosa E: The clinical and pathophysiological relevance of REM sleep behavior disorder in neurodegenerative diseases. Sleep Med Rev 13:385–401, 2009

Jacobs D, Ancoli-Israel S, Parker L, et al: Twenty-four-hour sleep-wake patterns in a nursing home population. Psychol Aging 4: 352–356, 1989

Janssens JP, Hilleret H, Michel J-P: Sleep disordered breathing in the elderly. Aging Clin Exp Res 12:417–429, 2000

Johns MW: A new method for measuring daytime sleepiness: the Epworth Sleepiness Scale. Sleep 14:540–545, 1991

Johnston JE: Sleep problems in the elderly. J Am Acad Nurse Pract 6:161–166, 1994

Jouvet M, Delorme F: Locus coeruleus et sommeil paradoxal. CR Soc Biol 159:895–899, 1965

Kamel NS, Gammack JK: Insomnia in the elderly: cause, approach, and treatment. Am J Med 119:463–469, 2006

Kaplan P, Allen RP, Buchholz DW, et al: A double-blind, placebo-controlled study of the treatment of periodic limb movements in sleep using carbidopa/levodopa and propoxyphene. Sleep 16:717–723, 1993

Karatas M: Restless legs syndrome and periodic limb movements during sleep: diagnosis and treatment. Neurologist 13:294–301, 2007

Karroum E, Konofal E, Arnulf I: Restless-legs syndrome [in French]. Rev Neurol (Paris) 164:701–721, 2008

Kavey N, Walters AS, Hening W, et al: Opioid treatment of periodic movements in sleep in patients without restless legs. Neuropeptides 11:181–184, 1988

Kelly J: Nocturnal leg cramps in the elderly. N Z Med J 108:207, 1995

Kim JM, Kwon HM, Lim CS, et al: Restless legs syndrome in patients on hemodialysis: symptom severity and risk factors. J Clin Neurol 4:153–157, 2008

Klink ME, Quan SF, Kaltenborn WT, et al: Risk factors associated with complaints of insomnia in a general adult population: influence of previous complaints of insomnia. Arch Intern Med 152:1634–1637, 1992

Kribbs NB, Pack AI, Kline LR, et al: Objective measurement of patterns of nasal CPAP use by patients with obstructive sleep apnea. Am Rev Respir Dis 147:887–895, 1993

Krishnan PR, Bhatia M, Behari M: Restless legs syndrome in Parkinson's disease: a case-controlled study. Mov Disord 18:181–185, 2003

Kronenberg R: Attenuation of the ventiatory and heart rate responses to hypoxia and hypercapnia with aging in normal man. Am Rev Respir Dis 52:1812–1819, 1973

Laustsen G, Andersen M: Ramelteon (Rozerem) a novel approach for insomnia treatment. Nurse Pract 31:52–55, 2006

Lesage S, Earley CJ: Restless legs syndrome. Curr Treat Options Neurol 6:209–219, 2004

Lesage S, Hening WA: The restless legs syndrome and periodic limb movement disorder: a review of management. Semin Neurol 24:249–259, 2004
Lichstein KL, Reidel BW: Behavioral assessment and treatment of insomnia: a review with an emphasis on clinical application. Behav Ther 15:659–688, 1994
Littner M, Hirshkowitz M, Kramer M, et al: Practice parameters for using polysomnography to evaluate insomnia: an update. Sleep 26:754–760, 2003
Mahowald MW: Parasomnias. Med Clin North Am 88:669–678, ix, 2004
Mahowald MW, Ettinger MG: Things that go bump in the night: the parasomnias revisited. J Clin Neurophysiol 7:119–143, 1990
Mahowald MW, Schenck CH: REM sleep behavior disorder, in Principles and Practice of Sleep Medicine. Edited by Kryger MH, Roth T, Dement WC. Philadelphia, PA, WB Saunders, 1994, pp 574–588
Mahowald MW, Schenck C: REM sleep parasomnias, in Principles and Practice of Sleep Medicine. Edited by Kryger MH, Roth T, Dement WC. Philadelphia, PA, WB Saunders, 2000, pp 724–737
Mandal AK, Abernathy T, Nelluri SN, et al: Is quinine effective and safe in leg cramps? J Clin Pharmacol 35:588–593, 1995
Manila MN: Leg cramps in relation to metabolic syndrome. Georgian Med News Jan:51–54, 2009
Mazza M, Della Marca G, De Risio S, et al: Sleep disorders in the elderly. Clin Ter 155:391–394, 2004
McCall WV: Sleep in the elderly: burden, diagnosis, and treatment. Prim Care Companion J Clin Psychiatry 6:9–20, 2004
McGechan A, Wellington K: Ramelteon. CNS Drugs 19:1057–1065; discussion 1066–1057, 2005
McGheie A, Russel S: The subjective assessment of normal sleep patterns. J Ment Sci 108:642–654, 1962
Melton ST, Wood JM, Kirkwood CK: Eszopiclone for insomnia. Ann Pharmacother 39:1659–1665, 2005
Miles L, Dement WC: Sleep and aging. Sleep 3:119–220, 1980
Milligan SA, Chesson AL: Restless legs syndrome in the older adult: diagnosis and management. Drugs Aging 19:741–751, 2002
Mitler MM, Browman CP, Menn SJ, et al: Nocturnal myoclonus: treatment efficacy of clonazepam and temazepam. Sleep 9:385–392, 1986
Miyamoto M, Miyamoto T, Iwanami M, et al: The pathophysiology of restless legs syndrome [in Japanese]. Brain Nerve 61:523–532, 2009
Moen MD, Plosker GL: Zolpidem extended release in insomnia: profile report. Drugs Aging 23:843–846, 2006
Montplaisir J, Petit D, Decary A, et al: Sleep and quantitative EEG in patients with progressive supranuclear palsy. Neurology 49:999–1003, 1997
National Institutes of Health: NIH State-of-the-Science Conference Statement on Manifestations and Management of Chronic Insomnia in Adults. NIH Consens State Sci Statements 22:1–30, 2005
Neubauer DN: Sleep problems in the elderly. Am Fam Physician 59:2551–2558, 2559–2560, 1999
Neubauer DN: New approaches in managing chronic insomnia. CNS Spectr 11:1–13, 2006
Nocturnal leg cramps. Postgrad Med 111:125–126, 2002
Ohayon MM, Roth T: Prevalence of restless legs syndrome and periodic limb movement disorder in the general population. J Psychosom Res 53:547–554, 2002
Ohayon MM, Caulet M, Priest RG: Violent behavior during sleep. J Clin Psychiatry 58:369–376; quiz 377, 1997
O'Keeffe ST, Gavin K, Lavan JN: Iron status and restless legs syndrome in the elderly. Age Ageing 23:200–203, 1994
Ondo WG, Vuong KD, Jankovic J: Exploring the relationship between Parkinson disease and restless legs syndrome. Arch Neurol 59:421–424, 2002
Owen RT: Extended-release zolpidem: efficacy and tolerability profile. Drugs Today (Barc) 42:721–727, 2006a
Owen RT: Ramelteon: profile of a new sleep-promoting medication. Drugs Today (Barc) 42:255–263, 2006b
Ozekmekci S, Apaydin H, Kilic E: Clinical features of 35 patients with Parkinson's disease displaying REM behavior disorder. Clin Neurol Neurosurg 107:306–309, 2005
Pandi-Perumal SR, Zisapel N, Srinivasan V, et al: Melatonin and sleep in aging population. Exp Gerontol 40:911–925, 2005
Paparrigopoulos TJ: REM sleep behaviour disorder: clinical profiles and pathophysiology. Int Rev Psychiatry 17:293–300, 2005
Pareja JA, Caminero AB, Masa JF, et al: A first case of progressive supranuclear palsy and pre-clinical REM sleep behavior disorder presenting as inhibition of speech during wakefulness and somniloquy with phasic muscle twitching during REM sleep. Neurologia 11:304–306, 1996
Passouant P, Cadilhac J, Ribstein M: Sleep privation with eye movements using antidepressive agents [in French]. Rev Neurol (Paris) 127:173–192, 1972
Pepin JL, Krieger J, Rodenstein D, et al: Effective compliance during the first 3 months of continuous positive airway pressure: a European prospective study of 121 patients. Am J Respir Crit Care Med 160:1124–1129, 1999
Phillips B, Ancoli-Israel S: Sleep disorders in the elderly. Sleep Med 2:99–114, 2001
Physicians' Desk Reference, 60th Edition. New York, Thomson Reuters, 2005
Plazzi G, Montagna P: Remitting REM sleep behavior disorder as the initial sign of multiple sclerosis. Sleep Med 3:437–439, 2002
Prinz P: Sleep patterns in the healthy aged: relationship with intellectual function. J Gerontol 32:179–185, 1977
Recording and scoring leg movements: The Atlas Task Force. Sleep 16:748–759, 1993
Rediehs MH, Reis JS, Creason NS: Sleep in old age: focus on gender differences. Sleep 13:410–424, 1990
Reid KJ, Zee PC: Circadian rhythm disorders. Semin Neurol 24:315–325, 2004
Reiter RJ: The pineal gland and melatonin in relation to aging: a summary of the theories and of the data. Exp Gerontol 30:199–212, 1995

Resta O, Caratozzolo G, Pannacciulli N, et al: Gender, age and menopause effects on the prevalence and the characteristics of obstructive sleep apnea in obesity. Eur J Clin Invest 33:1084–1089, 2003

Reynolds CF III: Sleep in affective disorders, in Principles and Practice of Sleep Medicine. Edited by Kryger MH, Roth T, Dement WC. Philadelphia, PA, Saunders, 1989, pp 413–415

Ross JS, Shua-Haim JR: Aricept-induced nightmares in Alzheimer's disease: 2 case reports. J Am Geriatr Soc 46:119–120, 1998

Roth T, Roehrs T, Zorick F: Pharmacological treatment of sleep disorders, in Sleep Disorders: Diagnosis and Treatment. Edited by Williams RL, Karacan I, Moore CA. New York, Wiley, 1988, pp 373–395

Rubinstein I, Colapinto N, Rotstein LE, et al: Improvement in upper airway function after weight loss in patients with obstructive sleep apnea. Am Rev Respir Dis 138:1192–1195, 1988

Saletu M, Anderer P, Saletu B, et al: EEG mapping in patients with restless legs syndrome as compared with normal controls. Psychiatry Res 115:49–61, 2002

Santos B, Oliveira AS, Canhao C, et al: Restless legs syndrome [in Portuguese]. Acta Med Port 21:359–366, 2008

Sanz-Fuentenebro FJ, Huidobro A, Tejadas-Rivas A: Restless legs syndrome and paroxetine. Acta Psychiatr Scand 94:482–484, 1996

Schapira AH: Restless legs syndrome: an update on treatment options. Drugs 64:149–158, 2004

Schenck CH, Mahowald MW: Polysomnographic, neurologic, psychiatric, and clinical outcome report on 70 consecutive cases with REM sleep behavior disorder (RBD): sustained clonazepam efficacy in 89.5% of 57 treated patients. Cleve Clin J Med 57(suppl):S9–S23, 1990

Schenck CH, Mahowald MW: REM parasomnias. Neurol Clin 14:697–720, 1996

Schenck CH, Mahowald MW: REM sleep behavior disorder: clinical, developmental, and neuroscience perspectives 16 years after its formal identification in SLEEP. Sleep 25:120–138, 2002

Schenck CH, Mahowald MW: Rapid eye movement sleep parasomnias. Neurol Clin 23:1107–1126, 2005

Schenck CH, Bundlie SR, Ettinger MG, et al: Chronic behavioral disorders of human REM sleep: a new category of parasomnia. Sleep 9:293–308, 1986

Schenck CH, Bundlie SR, Patterson AL, et al: Rapid eye movement sleep behavior disorder: a treatable parasomnia affecting older adults. JAMA 257:1786–1789, 1987

Schenck CH, Mahowald MW, Kim SW, et al: Prominent eye movements during NREM sleep and REM sleep behavior disorder associated with fluoxetine treatment of depression and obsessive-compulsive disorder. Sleep 15:226–235, 1992

Schenck CH, Bundlie SR, Mahowald MW: Delayed emergence of a parkinsonian disorder in 38% of 29 older men initially diagnosed with idiopathic rapid eye movement sleep behavior disorder. Neurology 46:388–393, 1996

Schmidt MH, Koshal VB, Schmidt HS: Use of pramipexole in REM sleep behavior disorder: results from a case series. Sleep Med 7:418–423, 2006

Schneider DL: Insomnia: safe and effective therapy for sleep problems in the older patient. Geriatrics 57:24–26, 29, 32, 2002

Schols L, Haan J, Riess O, et al: Sleep disturbance in spinocerebellar ataxias: is the SCA3 mutation a cause of restless legs syndrome? Neurology 51:1603–1607, 1998

Schutte S, Doghramji K: REM behavior disorder seen with venlafaxine (Effexor). Sleep Res 25:364, 1996

Shahar E, Redline S, Young T, et al: Hormone replacement therapy and sleep-disordered breathing. Am J Respir Crit Care Med 167:1186–1192, 2003

Shimizu T, Ookawa M, Iijuma S, et al: Effect of clomipramine on nocturnal sleep of normal human subjects. Ann Rev Pharmacopsychiat Res Found 16:138, 1985

Shneerson JM: Successful treatment of REM sleep behavior disorder with sodium oxybate. Clin Neuropharmacol 32:158–159, 2009

Shochat T, Pillar G: Sleep apnoea in the older adult: pathophysiology, epidemiology, consequences and management. Drugs Aging 20:551–560, 2003

Shochat T, Cohen-Zion M, Ancoli-Israel S: The effects of CPAP treatment on cognitive function in dementia: a pilot study (abstract). Sleep 23 (suppl 2):A218, 2000

Shochat T, Loredo J, Ancoli-Israel S: Sleep disorders in the elderly. Curr Treat Options Neurol 3:19–36, 2001

Silber MH, Girish M, Izurieta R: Pramipexole in the management of restless legs syndrome: an extended study. Sleep 26:819–821, 2003

Smith JE, Tolson JM: Recognition, diagnosis, and treatment of restless legs syndrome. J Am Acad Nurse Pract 20:396–401, 2008

Sommer M, Bachmann CG, Liebetanz KM, et al: Pregabalin in restless legs syndrome with and without neuropathic pain. Acta Neurol Scand 115:347–350, 2007

Spiegelhalder K, Hornyak M: Restless legs syndrome in older adults. Clin Geriatr Med 24:167–180, ix, 2008

Spielman AJ, Saskin P, Thorpy MJ: Treatment of chronic insomnia by restriction of time in bed. Sleep 10:45–56, 1987

Stolz SE, Aldrich MS: REM sleep behavior disorder associated with caffeine abuse. Sleep Res 20:341, 1991

Stores G: Rapid eye movement sleep behaviour disorder in children and adolescents. Dev Med Child Neurol 50:728–732, 2008

Sun ER, Chen CA, Ho G, et al: Iron and the restless legs syndrome. Sleep 21:371–377, 1998

Tachibana M, Tanaka K, Hishikawa Y, et al: A sleep study of acute psychotic states due to alcohol and meprobamate addiction. Advances in Sleep Research 2:177–205, 1975

Takeuchi N, Uchimura N, Hashizume Y, et al: Melatonin therapy for REM sleep behavior disorder. Psychiatry Clin Neurosci 55:267–269, 2001

Tan A, Salgado M, Fahn S: Rapid eye movement sleep behavior disorder preceding Parkinson's disease with therapeutic response to levodopa. Mov Disord 11:214–216, 1996

Tan EK, Ondo W: Restless legs syndrome: clinical features and treatment. Am J Med Sci 319:397–403, 2000

Trenkwalder C, Hening WA, Montagna P, et al: Treatment of restless legs syndrome: an evidence-based review and implications for clinical practice. Mov Disord 23:2267–2302, 2008

Trenkwalder C, Hogl B, Winkelmann J: Recent advances in the diagnosis, genetics and treatment of restless legs syndrome. J Neurol 256:539–553, 2009

Van Someren EJ: Circadian and sleep disturbances in the elderly. Exp Gerontol 35:1229–1237, 2000

Voon WC, Sheu SH: Diltiazem for nocturnal leg cramps. Age Ageing 30:91–92, 2001

Vorona RD, Ware JC: Exacerbation of REM sleep behavior disorder by chocolate ingestion: a case report. Sleep Med 3:365–367, 2002

Wauquier A, van Sweden B, Lagaay AM, et al: Ambulatory monitoring of sleep-wakefulness patterns in healthy elderly males and females (greater than 88 years): the "Senieur" protocol. J Am Geriatr Soc 40:109–114, 1992

Wetter TC, Pollmacher T: Restless legs and periodic leg movements in sleep syndromes. J Neurol 244:S37–S45, 1997

Whittom S, Dauvilliers Y, Pennestri MH, et al: Age-at-onset in restless legs syndrome: a clinical and polysomnographic study. Sleep Med 9:54–59, 2007

Williams RL, Karacan I, Hursch CJ: Electroencephalography (EEG) of Human Sleep: Clinical Applications. New York, Wiley, 1974

Wolkove N, Elkholy O, Baltzan M, et al: Sleep and aging, 1: sleep disorders commonly found in older people. CMAJ 176:1299–1304, 2007a

Wolkove N, Elkholy O, Baltzan M, et al: Sleep and aging, 2: management of sleep disorders in older people. CMAJ 176:1449–1454, 2007b

Wooten V: Sleep disorders in geriatric patients. Clin Geriatr Med 8:427–439, 1992

Wooten V: Medical causes of insomnia, in Principles and Practice of Sleep Medicine. Edited by Kryger MH, Roth T, Dement WC. Philadelphia, WB Saunders, 1994, pp 456–475

Xi Z, Luning W: REM sleep behavior disorder in a patient with pontine stroke. Sleep Med 10:143–146, 2009

Yee B, Killick R, Wong K: Restless legs syndrome. Aust Fam Physician 38:296–300, 2009

Young T, Finn L, Austin D, et al: Menopausal status and sleep-disordered breathing in the Wisconsin Sleep Cohort Study. Am J Respir Crit Care Med 167:1181–1185, 2003

Youngstedt SD, Kripke DF, Klauber MR, et al: Periodic leg movements during sleep and sleep disturbances in elders. J Gerontol A Biol Sci Med Sci 53:M391–M394, 1998

19

Mood Disorders

M. Justin Coffey, M.D.
C. Edward Coffey, M.D.

It ought to be generally known that the source of our pleasure, merriment, laughter and amusement, as of our grief, pain, anxiety and tears, is none other than the brain.

—The Hippocratic writers

If old age brings with it a "decline in physical strength, in mental alertness, in earning capacity, in prestige at home and in society, combined with economic deprivation, the loss of significant others, social isolation, and the prospect of death...why is not every old person in a profound state of depression?" (Jarvik 1976, p. 325). The answer to this resonating question is not entirely clear. What is clear is that *depression* means many things, that the majority of older persons are *not* clinically depressed, and that mood disorders are *not* a part of normal aging.

Nevertheless, depression is an illness that remains underdiagnosed and undertreated, especially in the elderly population (Unutzer 2007). As the number of elderly persons continues to rise, the number of these persons with a mood disorder will also rise. These demographics call attention to the need for the neuropsychiatric clinician to consider mood disorders high on the differential diagnosis whenever an older person presents with a functional decline or behavioral change. Depression is highly responsive to proper treatment, and without treatment depressed individuals suffer poor quality of life, poor functioning, heavy general medical burden, increased morbidity, and increased mortality, including suicide.

Our goal in this chapter is to improve the quality of care for elderly persons with mood disorders by offering clinicians a strategy to care for these patients. We begin by defining terms and providing a neural network model of the neurobiology of emotion. Then we describe the mood syndromes for clinicians to recognize and distinguish, and we discuss the differential diagnosis of mood disturbances in elderly patients, a list that includes primary psychiatric disorders and common neurological conditions. Our discussion of treatment recommendations is meant to guide clinicians at the bedside based on questions we often encounter in clinical practice. Our goal is to simplify the clinical approach to mood disturbances in the elderly population without oversimplifying the complexity of patients, their lives, and their illnesses.

Definitions

Mood refers to the feeling state that an individual is experiencing at a particular moment in time. Its qualities can be either positive (e.g., happiness, relief) or negative (e.g., sadness, anger, fear, disgust). The term *mood* is not synonymous with the term *affect,* which refers to the behavioral domain in which the mood is expressed. Affect can be conceptualized 1) quantitatively by the range (flat or restricted to wide), intensity (shallow to deep), and stability (rigid or labile) of the mood; and 2) qualitatively by the appropriateness (congruence with the situation or thought content) and relatedness of the mood. Mood is to affect as weather is to climate.

Emotion may be defined as the moods, affects, and related physiological states associated with specific thoughts, ideas, or stimuli (particularly reinforcing stimuli). Emotions have many functions, including interpersonal (e.g., communication, social bonding), cognitive (e.g., affecting a perception, facilitating storage or recall of a memory), and motivational (e.g., preparation for action, including elicitation of autonomic and endocrinological responses). Each function has survival value.

Moods, affects, and emotions may be normal or pathological. *Normal mood* undulates in positive and negative directions. Positive mood states (e.g., elation, exaltation, euphoria, ecstasy) are normal when life is going well or when major goals are achieved, as well as in states of love, sexual pleasure, and religious fervor or transcendence. Negative mood states (e.g., feeling sad, blue, down, unhappy, or "depressed") are normal when life is not going well and commonly follow a loss or disappointment. Other negative mood states often occur in response to stress; these include irritability, anger, anxiety, indifference, and dysphoria (being "ill at ease" or dissatisfied). These positive and negative variations in normal mood typically last only hours to days and do not involve significant derangement in other organ systems.

Abnormal mood reflects dysregulated emotional perception, expression, or both (see the section "Neurobiology of Emotion" below). The resulting collection of behavioral symptoms (features elicited in the history) and signs (features identified on examination) constitutes a specific clinical *syndrome*. Mood syndromes are more than extremes of normal mood. They are sustained, maladaptive, or distressing, and they may respond to specific treatments. A single occurrence of a clinical mood syndrome is referred to as a *mood episode*. The term *mood disorder* implies either recurrent mood episodes (e.g., major depressive disorder, bipolar disorder) or a single yet unremitting mood episode (e.g., dysthymic disorder).

Neurobiology of Emotion

As noted in the "Definitions" section above, an emotion involves a subjective experience or feeling state and the related goal-directed behavior, both of which occur in response to emotionally salient stimuli from the external or internal (thoughts or memories) environments that signal danger or reward. The *primary emotions* of fear, anger, happiness, and sadness are seen in all social mammals; are felt to be elicited by the immediate primary appraisal of the stimulus; and have obvious survival value, such as by alerting the animal for fight or flight (fear, anger) or by maintaining social structures and hierarchies (as with fear, happiness, sadness). The *secondary* or *social emotions* may be unique to humans and are presumably elicited by a second cognitive appraisal that is heavily influenced by culture (left hemisphere appraisal) and personal experience and memory (limbic system). As with the primary emotions, these secondary emotions may provide an evolutionary advantage—for example, by strengthening bonding and socialization (the emotion of gratitude) or by reinforcing the acquisition (the emotion of pride) or protection (the emotion of jealousy) of valuable resources.

How the brain mediates emotional experience is not fully understood. Several converging lines of research with animals and humans (including studies of patients with mood disorders or focal brain lesions) suggest a *neural network model*, wherein specific aspects of emotional behavior (e.g., perception and arousal, appraisal, response, and system regulation) are mediated by distinct but bidirectionally interconnected neural systems (Dalgleish 2004; LeDoux 2000; Mayberg et al. 2005; Phillips et al. 2003a, 2003b). In this model, a *ventral system* mediates the covert (medial temporal, amygdala, ventral basal ganglia, and midbrain) and overt (medial frontal, orbitofrontal, and perigenual anterior cingulate cortices) cognitive and emotional processing of the emotional stimuli. This system receives sensory input from the thalamus, identifies the emotional salience of the stimulus, and coordinates the autonomic, endocrine, and skeletomotor responses (i.e., arousal) that are mediated by subgenual anterior cingulate cortex, anterior insula, and hypothalamus. Disruption of any part of these circuits is intrinsic to mood (and anxiety) disorders. In such disorders, emotions may be overexpressed or emerge without provocation, and emotional perception may be distorted or lost altogether.

A *dorsal system* regulates the emotional state; this system includes the hippocampus and dorsal prefrontal, dorsal anterior cingulate, posterior cingulate, and parietal cortices. Isolated dysfunction of the dorsal system may result in avolition or disinhibition syndromes that may mimic melancholia or mania. When disruption of both the ventral and dorsal systems occurs simultaneously, normal emotional experience is severely deranged.

Consistent with this neural network model of emotion, functional brain imaging studies suggest that clinical depression is characterized by dysfunction in these networks. Specifically, reduced activity occurs in frontal cortical areas (particularly the subgenual cingulate cortex), and hyperactivity occurs in the amygdala and related limbic areas (Drevets 1999; Mayberg et al. 1999).

Communication between and within these dorsal and ventral emotion networks is accomplished primarily by *chemical neurotransmission*. The relative activity of the various neurotransmitters may affect the emotional state through mediation of arousal (norepinephrine), motivation and reward (dopamine), and mood and impulsivity (serotonin). Although there is evidence to support the involvement of nearly all of the major neurotransmitters in the pathophysiology of major depression and mania (not surprising given the multitude of symptoms constituting the mood syndromes), most of the scientific focus has been on these three major monoamine systems (Belmaker and Agam 2008). In general, the research shows that depressed mood is typically (but not always) associated with decreased functional activity (variously measured, and in various brain regions) of norepinephrine, dopamine, or serotonin and that drugs or procedures that increase the activity of these three transmitters have antidepressant properties. The potential relation between elevated plasma homocysteine (an amino acid necessary for the production of monoamine neurotransmitters) and depression in older patients is consistent with this view of decreased functional neurotransmitter activity (Almeida et al. 2006). More recent investigations have begun to focus on the downstream effects of these neurotransmitter systems on neuronal plasticity and resilience, with evidence that these processes might be impaired in severe mood states and that they might be promoted by effective antidepressant treatments. Less is known about the relation of these neurotransmitters to mania.

What determines an individual's threshold for developing a mood disorder? A potential answer lies in the substantial *genetic vulnerability* to the illness. Roughly 30%–40% of the risk for developing depressive illness comes from genetic factors (Merikangas et al. 2002), although the search continues for specific genes or genetic abnormalities that confer this risk. One's genetic vulnerability interacts with one's environment, which presumably accounts for the remaining variability in risk (Rutter et al. 2009). Early, severe, and chronic stressful experiences increase the likelihood that a genetic vulnerability will be expressed as a mood disorder (Risch et al. 2009). Acute stress can also precipitate illness recurrence (the stress-diathesis model). The response to stress is mediated by the hypothalamic-pituitary-adrenal (HPA) axis (in particular, corticotrophin-releasing hormone neural circuits), and the panoply of clinical and neurobiological manifestations of a major mood disorder are consistent with an abnormal stress response characterized by a hypercortisol state (Vreeburg et al. 2009).

Patients with depression also exhibit evidence of systemic inflammation, and such changes are associated with many of the signs and symptoms of depression, including sleep, fatigue, and cognitive dysfunction. A potential mechanism linking depression and inflammation is suggested by the observed relations between peripheral markers of inflammation (e.g., inflammatory cytokines) and the pathophysiological domains of neurotransmitter metabolism, neuroendocrine function, and neural plasticity (Miller et al. 2009).

Mood disorders may thus be conceptualized as prototypical complex diseases resulting from gene-environment interactions, although no candidate genes have been identified that might mediate the relations between environmental stress, the HPA axis, and depression (Risch et al. 2009; Rutter et al. 2009). Early reports that this relation may be mediated by polymorphisms in the serotonin transporter gene remain controversial (Risch et al. 2009; Rutter et al. 2009).

It is unclear whether or how *age-related changes in brain structure and function* (see Chapter 2, "Neurobiology of Aging"; Chapter 6, "Imaging the Structure of the Aging Human Brain"; and Chapter 7, "Molecular Imaging in Neuropsychiatry") might affect the complex neural systems that mediate emotional experience. Certainly, depressive illness is *not* a part of normal aging. Age is not a risk factor for primary mood disorders, and most data taken together indicate a decline in prevalence of major depression with age (Ernst and Angst 1995). In addition, the phenomenology of depressive or manic episodes within individuals appears not to change with aging.

On the other hand, research from our laboratory and others indicates that patients with mood disorders exhibit changes in brain structure and function, some of which are consistent with a pattern suggestive of "accelerated" brain aging (e.g., more severe frontal and medial temporal atrophy, ventricular enlargement, and microvascular disease, all of which are seen to a lesser degree in "normal" aging) (Kempton et al. 2008; Sheline 2003). In addition, age is associated with suicide mortality, as well as with certain general medical (e.g., cardiovascular disease) and neurological (e.g., stroke, dementia, other degenerative brain diseases) conditions that are commonly comorbid with mood disturbances. Insults from these age-related illnesses may damage the neural circuits that modulate mood, cognition, and behavior, leaving the brain vulnerable either to a recurrence of a preexisting mood disorder or to a new-onset mood syndrome. Not all older persons with neurological diseases develop depressive illness, however, and younger persons with certain neurological conditions (e.g., epilepsy; see Chapter 27, "Epilepsy") can develop mood disorders early in life. Thus, one theory is that the presence of certain illnesses or insults—independent of age—modifies the threshold for depressive illness (Alexopoulos et al. 2005).

Identifying the Mood Disturbance

At the cornerstone of safe and effective care of elderly patients with mood symptoms is an accurate clinical diagnosis. Identifying the specific mood disturbance leads directly to evidence-based care decisions.

For the most part, the mood disturbance becomes evident through the patient's history. The key is to describe the mood state. This information then guides the determinations of whether the mood is normal or abnormal and whether the patient actually has a disturbance in emotional experience (e.g., depression, anxiety, dysphoria, anhedonia) rather than motivation (e.g., apathy) or cognition (e.g., dementia) alone. (See Chapter 4, "Neuropsychiatric Assessment," for a more detailed discussion of the neuropsychiatric evaluation.)

Table 19–1 lists the important mood disturbances in elderly patients. We include mood disturbances recognized by

TABLE 19–1. Mood disturbances in the elderly population

Major depressive episode, with melancholia or psychosis
Dysthymia and minor depressive episode
Adjustment disorder
Bereavement
Demoralization
Apathy
Pathological laughing and crying
Mania
Affective lability

TABLE 19–2. Key features of melancholia

1. Apprehensive, dysphoric, gloomy, or apathetic mood
2. Cognitive impairment (in processing speed, concentration, and working memory)
3. Psychomotor retardation (from reluctance to complete activities of daily living to withdrawal and inactivity severe enough to become stupor) or agitation (from restlessness and hand-wringing to purposeless hyperactivity severe enough to become frenzy)
4. Vegetative signs (e.g., reduced total sleep time and sleep efficiency, increased sleep latency, decreased rapid eye movement latency, early morning awakening, loss of appetite and weight, loss of interest in family activities and self-care, loss of libido, immune system compromise, generalized analgesia)

current classification systems—DSM-IV-TR (American Psychiatric Association 2000) and ICD-10 (World Health Organization 1992)—as well as those identified as important foci of clinical attention in neuropsychiatry. Because states of low mood are more prevalent in the elderly population and have a longer differential diagnosis, we discuss them first. We then turn to mania and related syndromes of elated mood.

Major Depressive Episode

The clinical syndrome of major depressive episode is defined by either *abnormal* sadness or loss of interest or pleasure, occurring most of the time for at least 2 weeks, together with four or more of the following symptoms: changes in appetite (or weight loss), sleep, or psychomotor behavior; fatigue or loss of energy; feelings of worthlessness or inappropriate guilt; impaired concentration and thinking; and recurrent thoughts of death or suicide. All these symptoms must cause clinically significant distress or functional impairment to reach the threshold for diagnosis.

Approximately 20% of adult patients with a major depressive episode will present with *melancholic features* (Taylor and Fink 2006; Table 19–2), which include a unique quality to the depressed mood together with "vegetative" signs indicative of midbrain (neuroendocrine and autonomic nervous system) dysfunction. The patient with melancholia suffers from anhedonia, guilt, and a relentless and profound gloominess that are experienced as unique (i.e., unlike sadness following typical life events) and totally unresponsive to positive stimuli. The vegetative features of melancholia include profound reductions in appetite, sleep, and sexual functioning, as well as alterations in circadian rhythms, including matinal worsening of mood and psychomotor behavior. Approximately 15% of adult patients with melancholia also experience psychotic symptoms (Taylor and Fink 2006), which may or may not be congruent with the depressed mood. Melancholia is a medical emergency and demands aggressive treatment (see the section "Treatment" later in this chapter).

The clinical phenomenology of major depressive episodes is similar in patients with early onset and those with late-age onset (i.e., after age 60) (Baldwin and Tomenson 1995). As a group, however, elderly persons tend to display more vegetative signs (disturbances in sleep, hunger, digestion, and libido) and cognitive disturbances, as well as less subjective dysphoria, than younger patients. Depressed older persons may also be more likely to exhibit melancholic features (Parker et al. 2001).

As discussed in more detail later in this chapter (see the section "Differential Diagnosis of the Mood Syndromes"), a major depressive episode has a broad differential diagnosis, including episodes secondary to a general medical (including neurological) condition or substance or those occurring in the setting of a primary mood disorder, such as major depressive disorder or bipolar disorder.

Dysthymia and Minor Depressive Episode

Some patients experience an attenuated, low-grade depression that does not meet diagnostic criteria for a major depressive episode. When these symptoms persist for at least 2 years, the syndrome is called *dysthymia.* Dysthymia is seen in approximately 2% of community-dwelling elderly persons (compared with the 1% prevalence of major depressive disorder) and is frequently comorbid with major depression (so-called "double depression"). By definition, dysthymia is not a sequel to a major depressive episode (i.e., it is not chronic depressive disorder), and in most cases patients report having felt depressed nearly all their lives. Onset of dysthymia after age 50 is rare (Devanand et al. 1994).

Other elderly persons in the community (4%–13%) report a variety of depressive symptoms that do not meet the severity or duration criteria for major depressive episode or dysthymia (Bellino et al. 2000). These mood syndromes (given the DSM-IV-TR diagnosis of depressive disorder not otherwise specified) are labeled "minor depression" and "recurrent brief depression."

Controversy exists over whether these subthreshold affective conditions are distinct depressive subtypes, part of a continuum of more pathological mood states, or reflective of temperament or personality traits (Akiskal 1994). Family history data do not support such categories (Akiskal and Cassano 1997). Nonetheless, they have functional and clinical outcomes similar to those for major depression and therefore warrant treatment (Howland et al. 2008). Selective serotonin reuptake inhibitors (SSRIs) are the preferred treatment on the basis of controlled studies including large mixed-age samples and a small literature on older adults (Bellino et al. 2000). Treatment should continue for at least 2 years. The evidence supporting psychotherapy is limited and suggests only modest efficacy, if any, compared with medications (Imel et al. 2008; Markowitz 1994).

Adjustment Disorder

The term *adjustment disorder* refers to a stress-related disturbance in mood and behavior that is disproportionate to the precipitating event or life change. Some examples of potential stressors for older persons include health problems, marital conflict, difficulties with children, or the myriad changes sometimes associated with retirement, including financial insecurity, relocation, and loss of social role and purpose. Adjustment disorder is not diagnosed in the context of bereavement (discussed in the next section) and must be distinguished from demoralization (see the section "Demoralization" later in this chapter). The core feature of adjustment disorder is that the psychological reaction to a stressor is *excessive* or *disproportionate*, although no criteria exist to guide this determination (Bonelli and Bugram 2000). Overall, the diagnosis has clinical utility but poor phenomenological rigor (Strain and Diefenbacher 2008).

The mood disturbance in adjustment disorder is "subthreshold" in that its symptoms do not meet criteria for a mood disorder (defined in "Differential Diagnosis of the Mood Syndromes" later in this chapter), although it significantly impairs functioning. Patients may have depressed, anxious, irritable, or labile mood states. The mood fluctuates in valence and maintains some reactivity to pleasurable circumstances. Vegetative signs are not prominent, and bodily functions remain normal. Psychosis is not present. Patients exhibit minimal psychomotor dysfunction, although they may have emotionally dramatic presentations. These clinical features do not vary between age groups. The diagnosis of adjustment disorder is less common in older than in younger populations.

Symptom onset typically occurs within 3 months of the stressful event, and in adults symptoms and impairment typically improve within 6 months of the stressor's resolving. The vast majority of adults diagnosed with adjustment disorder are well at follow-up (Andreasen and Hoenk 1982). Adjustment disorders appear to have a poorer outcome (e.g., prolonged symptoms or development of a mental disorder) in children and adolescents, particularly if associated with a general medical disorder. A chronic form may occur in patients with premorbid maladaptive personality traits.

It is important to recognize that some patients with adjustment disorder may be in the early stages of a full mood episode or other major psychiatric disorder. During the acute phase of adjustment disorder, patients are at increased risk of suicide (see the section "Assessing Patient Safety" later in this chapter). The interval between symptom onset and suicidal behavior appears, at least in younger populations, to be shorter in adjustment disorder than in major depression, borderline personality disorder, and schizophrenia (Jones et al. 1999; Polyakova et al. 1998).

Bereavement

Bereavement is the loss of a loved one through death. *Grief* (a term often used interchangeably with *bereavement*) is the normal, involuntary emotional and behavioral response to bereavement. The expression of grief may include a sense of disbelief or affective numbing, feelings of anger or despair, intrusive thoughts of or pining for the deceased, nondisturbing visual and auditory hallucinations of the deceased, tearfulness, or recurrent pangs of intense sadness (Parkes 1998). Although each of these expressions of grief may occur at any time, formal studies of the course of grief identify three stages: "numbness," lasting hours to weeks; "depression" (a stage characterized by irritability, crying, and restlessness), lasting weeks to years; and "recovery," lasting months (Clayton 1982; Clayton et al. 1968, 1971). In 80% of individuals, the features of grief begin to resolve spontaneously after approximately 6 months, although sadness and longing for the deceased may persist indefinitely. Grief is associated with excess risk of mortality (primarily from decrements in general medical health) in the first few weeks or months after the loss, but the vast majority of individuals do not die as a result of their loss (Stroebe 2008).

Approximately 10%–20% of bereaved individuals develop "complicated (or traumatic) grief," a recently proposed syndrome characterized by prolonged (longer than 2 months) and unusually intense symptoms, including intrusive, distressing preoccupation with the deceased (Prigerson et al. 1999). Thus defined, the syndrome may be debilitating and associated with negative health outcomes. Factor analysis studies indicate that complicated grief resembles but may be distinct from the core features of major depression or posttraumatic stress disorder. However, the high rates of co-occurrence (20%–50%) of these syndromes call attention to the need for further empirical validation of complicated grief, a distinct clinical syndrome.

Bereavement is a significant life stressor that increases the risk that a psychiatric disorder (e.g., mood, anxiety, substance use, or personality disorder) may be expressed. The challenge for the neuropsychiatric clinician is to recognize depressive illness when it occurs in the context of bereavement, because many of the signs and symptoms of a major depressive episode may be seen in bereavement. The key to this challenge is to assess for features of melancholia (see the section "Major Depressive Episode" earlier in this chapter). If melancholic features exist, the patient is at substantial risk of morbidity and mortality, and he or she thus requires immediate treatment of the major depressive episode (see the section "Treatment" later in this chapter).

Demoralization

Persons with a severe general medical or neuropsychiatric illness may experience not only dysphoria but also a sense of existential despair. This state is referred to as *demoralization* and is characterized by a persistent inability to cope, together with feelings of helplessness ("I don't know what to do"), hopelessness, meaninglessness, subjective incompetence, and diminished self-esteem (Frank 1974). Features of demoralization may emerge at any point during the precipitating illness, and the severity of symptoms may fluctuate with the course and treatment of that illness. Not all patients with severe illness become demoralized. Risk factors are unknown but may include the type or severity of illness (e.g., paralyzing, disfiguring, intensely painful, incurable), premorbid personality traits challenged by the new illness (e.g., perfectionism), and the individual's interpersonal relationships and social support system (Slavney 1999).

Although neuropsychiatric clinicians commonly encounter such patients, demoralization as a construct is controversial (Clarke and Kissane 2002; Slavney 1999). For example, there is debate about whether demoralization should be considered a "normal" reaction to the stressor (distinct from the "abnormal" reaction of an adjustment disorder) or an "understandable but always abnormal" reaction. Similarly, should demoralization be excluded (trumped) by major depression, or can the two coexist?

Apathy

Apathy refers to a lack of motivation that is not attributable to intellectual impairment, emotional distress, or diminished arousal. Apathy is a common symptom in many neuropsychiatric disorders (Duffy and Campbell 1994; Marin 1991; van Reekum et al. 2005), including primary psychiatric disorders (e.g., dementias, delirium, mood disorders, anxiety disorders, psychotic disorders, substance use disorders, personality disorders) and neurological disorders (e.g., stroke, traumatic brain injury [TBI], anoxia, degenerative brain disease, multiple sclerosis), as well as in general medical conditions (e.g., hypothyroidism, hypotestosteronism, sleep apnea). Apathy may also appear as a side effect of medications, including SSRIs, dopamine-blocking drugs (e.g., antipsychotics, metoclopromide), and felbamate.

Although the neurobiology of apathy is not fully understood, apathy is a common symptom following disruption of frontal-subcortical circuits, particularly the anterior cingulate circuit. Motivation appears to depend on dopamine and glutamate neurotransmission, which may mediate motivational valence and intensity of the behavioral response, respectively. The motivational response may be modulated, in turn, by cholinergic (approach behavior) and serotonergic (avoidance or inhibitory) neurotransmission.

Some authors have proposed that apathy is a syndrome as well as a symptom, and they have proposed criteria for the former (Marin 1991, 1996). Research is under way to validate this concept. Regardless, the presence of apathy may have important prognostic implications (van Reekum et al. 2005). For example, in studies of patients with Alzheimer's disease (see Chapter 16, "Alzheimer's Disease and the Frontotemporal Dementia Syndromes"), apathy is associated with functional impairment and with more rapid cognitive and functional decline. Apathy predicts a poorer prognosis in patients with major depression. In patients with schizophrenia (see Chapter 21, "Psychosis"), apathy is associated with poor medication adherence and lack of benefit from social skills training.

Pathological Laughing and Crying

Patients with pathological laughing and crying (PLC) exhibit emotional expression that is disconnected from emotional experience. This condition takes various forms and has been known by many terms (e.g., pseudobulbar affect, emotional incontinence, involuntary emotional expression disorder). Patients may laugh or cry excessively in a situation that is not consistent with the quality or intensity of the emotional reaction and, when questioned, will deny feeling the emotion itself or the emotional intensity they are displaying. Laughing or crying may occur at socially inappropriate times and cause the patient embarrassment and distress. Unless they have dementia, patients with PLC also exhibit no cognitive deficits and retain insight into their condition.

Patients with PLC may exhibit a depressed mood, but the paroxysmal nature of PLC distinguishes it from the pervasive, sustained, nonreactive emotional state of a mood disorder. PLC is distinguished from affective lability (see the section "Affective

Lability" later in this chapter) by the incongruence between the patient's mood and affective displays. Paroxysms of intense emotion that are incongruent with the situation or the patient's mood may also represent complex partial seizures (Blumer et al. 2004; Trimble 2002) (see Chapter 27, "Epilepsy").

The pathophysiology of PLC is not known. PLC can be a feature of amyotrophic lateral sclerosis, multiple system atrophy, stroke, multiple sclerosis, Parkinson's disease (PD), TBI, dementia, and other brain disorders (Parvizi et al. 2006). Historically, PLC has been attributed to failure of voluntary control over emotional expression due to bilateral damage to the descending corticobulbar tracts (so-called pseudobulbar affect). A more recent alternative hypothesizes that descending information from the cortex to cerebellum is intact and that the PLC is a result of disturbed modulation of emotional expression by the cerebellum (Parvizi et al. 2009).

Mania

The clinical syndrome of a *manic episode* is defined by *abnormally* elevated, expansive, or irritable mood lasting for at least 1 week, together with three or more of the following symptoms: inflated self-esteem or grandiosity, flight of ideas or racing thoughts, distractibility, increased psychomotor activity, and excessive involvement in pleasurable activities. All these symptoms must cause clinically significant distress or functional impairment. Hospitalization is typically necessary.

A manic episode may manifest in any of its three described stages (Carlson and Goodwin 1973):

1. An early milder form referred to as *hypomania,* which involves feelings of intense well-being
2. Acute mania, in which behavior involves impulsivity, carelessness, and risk taking and in which mood is either predominantly elated or euphoric but can be swiftly replaced by moments of intense hostility, gloom, and despair (*mixed state*)
3. A *psychotic stage*, in which grandiose or religious delusions accompany increasing psychomotor agitation and hyperactivity and extreme emotional lability

Mania should be distinguished from two related syndromes, delirium (see Chapter 15, "Delirium") and behavioral disinhibition (see Chapter 16, "Alzheimer's Disease and the Frontotemporal Dementia Syndromes," and Chapter 26, "Traumatic Brain Injury").

Late-age-onset mania is rare (Tohen et al. 1994). Clinical descriptions of mania in old age often portray it as involving less elation or euphoria and more irritability, dysphoria, and paranoia than mania earlier in life. Prospective data do not support this view and instead indicate that the clinical features of mania are consistent across age groups (Broadhead and Jacoby 1990; Young et al. 2007). As with late-onset major depressive episodes, late-onset mania is associated with more microvascular brain changes, more cognitive impairment, and less family history of mood disorder (Evans et al. 1995; Stone 1989; Young and Klerman 1992).

As discussed in "Differential Diagnosis of the Mood Syndromes" later in this chapter, a manic episode has a broad differential diagnosis, including 1) episodes secondary to a general medical (including neurological) condition or substance use and 2) those occurring in the setting of a primary mood disorder, such as bipolar disorder.

Affective Lability

When patients exhibit dramatic fluctuations in mood within a wide range of emotional expression, they are said to have *affective lability*. This condition is common in patients with bipolar disorder, even during periods of euthymia (Henry et al. 2008). Affective lability is also seen in patients with personality disorder, dementia, mental retardation, or dysfunction of the midbrain or frontal lobe (see Chapter 16, "Alzheimer's Disease and the Frontotemporal Dementia Syndromes"). Patients with affective lability typically have an irritable mood and may shift rapidly from positive (e.g., happiness or euphoria) to negative (e.g., sadness or anger) mood states. These emotional outbursts are usually short lived, and the affect is congruent with the mood (e.g., the patient both appears and feels angry, and he or she behaves accordingly).

Differential Diagnosis of the Mood Syndromes

After identifying the patient's acute mood *disturbance* from the neuropsychiatric history and examination, the clinician must next confirm the underlying *disorder* causing the mood disturbance. The first step is to rule out so-called *secondary mood disorders*—that is, mood syndromes due to a general medical (including neurological) condition or a substance (e.g., medication, toxin, or drug of abuse). All other mood disorders (e.g., the major depressive disorders and bipolar disorders) do not have a currently defined etiology and are thus considered idiopathic. These *primary mood disorders* are essentially diagnoses of exclusion.

Mood Disorders Associated With Substances or General Medical Conditions

Every older person presenting with a behavioral change or decline in function should be actively assessed for mood and behavioral symptoms associated with many general medical conditions (see Chapter 23, "Pain," and Chapter 28, "Neoplas-

TABLE 19–3. General medical conditions associated with mood disorders

Endocrinopathies (e.g., thyroid disease, hyperparathyroidism, Cushing's disease, Addison's disease)
Cancers (all types)
Cardiovascular disease (e.g., myocardial infarction, congestive heart failure, stroke)
Infection (e.g., viral)
Metabolic disorders (e.g., folate deficiency, B_{12} deficiency, electrolyte imbalance)
Chronic renal disease
Rheumatic disease (e.g., systemic lupus erythematosus)
Neurological disease (e.g., seizure disorders, traumatic brain injury)

tic, Demyelinating, Infectious, and Inflammatory Brain Disorders") and their therapies (see Chapter 29, "Neuropsychiatric Disorders Associated With General Medical Therapies"). Table 19–3 lists general medical conditions common in elderly patients that may be associated with mood disturbances. These secondary mood disorders usually involve a single episode of the mood disturbance, may have atypical features, and may have a later age at onset (making them particularly important considerations when evaluating an elderly patient). There is usually no personal or family history of significant mood symptoms.

Diagnosing a secondary mood disorder is often challenging, because many of the symptoms of a potential mood disorder (e.g., fatigue, low energy, disturbed sleep and appetite) may be the result of the general medical disorder. An additional diagnostic challenge relates to the assessment of symptoms that require verbal expression (e.g., sadness, hopelessness) in patients who cannot speak (e.g., due to an aphasia). The key to addressing these challenges is to assess for features of melancholia or mania (see the "Major Depressive Episode" and "Mania" sections earlier in this chapter). If either is present, the patient is at substantial risk of morbidity and mortality and thus should receive immediate treatment of the major depressive episode.

Certain laboratory studies (Table 19–4) may be useful to *confirm* the presence of a general medical, neurological, or substance use disorder, as suggested by the history and examination (Baldwin et al. 2002).

Older patients taking multiple medications are at risk for adverse effects from polypharmacy (see Chapter 9, "Geriatric Neuropsychopharmacology"). Many prescribed medications

TABLE 19–4. Clinical relevance to mood disorders of selected laboratory tests

Complete blood count	Anemia can cause fatigue, apathy; leukocytosis and thrombocytosis are signs of a stress response and can indicate acute infection or severe mood disorder; cancer may cause depression.
Serum chemistries	Sodium, potassium, and acid-base imbalance can cause fatigue, apathy, listlessness, delirium.
Renal function	Renal insufficiency can cause fatigue, apathy, listlessness, delirium; renal function may affect drug metabolism.
Glucose	Hypoglycemia or hyperglycemia may cause fatigue, irritability, psychosis, delirium.
Calcium	Hypocalcemia or hypercalcemia can cause fatigue, depression, apathy, irritability, delirium.
Liver function	Hepatic encephalopathy may cause listlessness, apathy, fatigue, bradykinesia; liver function may affect drug metabolism.
Thyroid stimulation hormone	Hypothyroidism or hyperthyroidism may mimic depressive illness.
Vitamin B_{12}, folate	Deficiencies can cause reversible cognitive impairment.

can cause changes in mood (see Chapter 29, "Neuropsychiatric Disorders Associated With General Medical Therapies"). Table 19–5 lists some offending agents commonly used in elderly patients. Discontinuation of the offending agents (when clinically appropriate) typically brings about resolution of the mood disorder within five half-lives of the medication.

Aside from nicotine, alcohol is the most commonly abused substance among older persons with mood symptoms. The prevalence of alcohol use in elderly persons is three to four times greater among depressed individuals than their nondepressed counterparts (Grant and Harford 1995). Discerning any causal relationship between alcohol abuse and mood disorders is difficult but very important because the presence of alcohol use affects depression outcomes in older persons (Devanand 2002). (See Chapter 17, "Addiction," for a more detailed discussion.)

TABLE 19–5. Medications associated with substance-induced mood disorder

Cardiovascular	Beta-blockers, propranolol, hydralazine, clonidine, nifedipine, reserpine, quinidine, procainamide, lidocaine, methyldopa
Hormonal	Corticosteroids, estrogens, progestational agents
Antineoplastic	Vincristine, vinblastine, tamoxifen
Antibiotics	Penicillins, mycins
Sedatives/analgesics	Benzodiazepines, alcohol, dextropropoxyphene, baclofen
Histamine receptor (H_2) blockers	Cimetidine, ranitidine
Anticonvulsants	Phenytoin, barbiturates, ethosuximide
Others	Interferon beta, disulfiram, cyproheptadine, methysergide

Alzheimer's Disease

Alzheimer's disease (AD) is associated with a variety of mood disturbances, including apathy syndromes (prevalence of 45%–90%), depression (prevalence of 15%–50%), or both (Table 19–6). (See Chapter 16, "Alzheimer's Disease and the Frontotemporal Dementia Syndromes," for a more detailed discussion.)

Apathy and depression syndromes typically occur earlier in the course of AD than do psychosis, agitation, or motor symptoms (Craig et al. 2005). Both apathy and major depression may reflect a prodromal phase of AD (Robert et al. 2006) or even be a harbinger of more aggressive AD (Mizrahi and Starkstein 2007; Starkstein et al. 2006). As in patients with stroke, the presence of apathy in persons with AD predicts a depressive disorder, although depression does not appear to predict apathy (Starkstein et al. 2006). In patients with AD, the apolipoprotein E ε4 allele (*APOE*E4*) is associated with apathy (Monastero et al. 2006).

The presence of either an apathy syndrome or a depressive disorder in a patient with AD is associated with greater physical and cognitive impairment (and hence earlier placement in higher levels of care), increased mortality and (in depression) suicide, and greater caregiver burden (Benoit et al. 2008; Cummings 2004; Landes et al. 2005). Effectively treating these mood disturbances may therefore reduce mortality and improve the functional status of these patients.

Cognitive inefficiency and impairment are common in patients with mood disorders. When severe, this depression-related cognitive dysfunction (historically referred to as "pseudodementia") may be difficult to distinguish from dementia (Table 19–7) (Ballard et al. 1996a). In general, patients with depression-related cognitive dysfunction tend to report greater impairment and to exert less effort on testing, whereas patients with dementia may not recognize their cognitive impairment (particularly if insight is impaired) and yet may also exhibit other signs of cortical involvement (e.g., aphasia, agnosia, apraxia) on examination.

Stroke

Stroke is associated with a variety of mood disturbances in the weeks and months following the insult, including demoralization and "catastrophic reactions" (5%–20%), emotional lability and PLC (20%), apathy with (10%) or without (10%) depression, major (10%) or minor (10%–40%) depression, and mania (rare). These mood disturbances are discussed in greater detail in Chapter 25, "Cerebrovascular Disease."

TABLE 19–6. Prevalence of mood disturbances in the elderly population

Population	MDD	Apathy	PLC	Demoralization	Mania
General elderly population	1%–4%	—	—	—	<1%
Alzheimer's disease	15%–50%	45%–90%	—	Unlikely	—
Stroke	20%–40%	20%–25%	10%–25%	5%–20%	1%
Parkinson's disease	Up to 25%	30%–50%	5%	—	Rare

Note. MDD=major depressive disorder; PLC=pathological laughing and crying.

TABLE 19–7. Distinguishing depressive pseudodementia from Alzheimer's dementia

Clinical feature	Depressive pseudodementia	Alzheimer's disease
Mood	Melancholic	Apathetic, avolitional
Cognition	Bradyphrenia, executive dysfunction, recall deficits, false-negative errors, some benefit from serial presentation, less behavioral consistency	Visuospatial deficits, executive dysfunction, recall deficits, false-negative errors, no benefit from serial presentation, more behavioral consistency
Insight	Exaggeration of problems	Minimization of problems
Course	Episodic; more discrete onset	Progressive; insidious onset with mild cognitive impairment
Personal history	Mood disorder	None
Family history	Mood disorder	Dementia

Poststroke depression is associated with poorer quality of life, cognitive impairment, greater impairment in activities of daily living, and greater (three to five times) long-term mortality. The diagnosis may be difficult, however, both in the overlap of depressive symptoms with stroke symptoms and in patients with aphasia, denial/neglect, or severe dementia. Information from caregivers may greatly assist diagnosis. Care should be taken to rule out hypothyroidism. Several studies have examined whether medications or psychotherapy can *prevent* poststroke depression (Almeida et al. 2006; Chen et al. 2007; Palomäki et al. 1999; Rasmussen et al. 2003; Robinson et al. 2008). A Cochrane review concluded that antidepressants were not effective prophylaxis but that psychotherapy had a small positive effect (Hackett et al. 2008a).

Distinguishing apathy from depression in patients with stroke can be challenging. Poststroke apathy (Starkstein and Manes 2000) has features of anergia, amotivation, indifference toward stroke-related disabilities, and bradykinesia. Although these patients are not typically agitated or anxious, they may be helpless to change their circumstances. They do not complain about or exaggerate their troubles, however, as is characteristic of patients with melancholia. Poststroke apathy is not characterized by psychosis or suicidality.

Parkinson's Disease

Disturbances of mood are common in patients with PD and include depression (40%–50%, up to half of whom may experience major depression), apathy (30%–50%), PLC (5%), and rarely mania (see also Chapter 24, "Parkinson's Disease and Movement Disorders"). Risk factors for comorbid depressive illness include greater cognitive impairment, the presence of psychosis, and personal or family history of mood disorder. Women and persons developing PD before age 65 may be at the greatest risk for depressive illness (Slaughter et al. 2001). Data suggest an increased risk for depressive symptoms in persons with PD who have elevated plasma homocysteine levels or the low-activity allele of the serotonin-transporter-linked polymorphic region (5-HTTLPR) (McDonald et al. 2003).

In persons with PD, depressive illness is associated with greater personal suffering, faster progression of physical symptoms, greater disability, and greater decline in both cognitive skills and ability for self-care (Weintraub et al. 2004). The risk of suicide in depressed patients with PD has not been defined, although suicide does not occur more frequently in patients with PD than in the general population (Slaughter et al. 2001). Effective treatment of depression may improve the functional status of patients with PD (Norman et al. 2002). Apathy in PD is also associated with greater cognitive impairment and poorer functional status (Pedersen et al. 2009; Richard 2007). It remains unclear whether apathy in patients with PD predisposes them to depressive illness.

Several considerations are important in the assessment of mood disturbances in patients with PD:

1. The incidence of hypothyroidism is increased in persons with PD (perhaps due to inhibited release of thyrotropin-releasing hormone by levodopa stimulation of the pituitary) and may contribute to apathy, low mood, and cognitive symptoms.
2. Testosterone deficiency, present in up to 25% of men over age 60, may contribute to low mood, fatigue, and other nonmotor symptoms in patients with PD, although this finding is controversial (Kenangil et al. 2009; Ready et al. 2004).
3. Deep brain stimulation of the subthalamic nucleus for the motor features of PD may be linked to subsequent depression, apathy, mania, aggression, and cognitive impairment, although this is controversial (Deuschl 2009); in some cases, deep brain stimulation improves symptoms of depression, apathy, and obsessive-compulsive disorder.

4. Patients should be assessed for demoralization, apathy, or adjustment disorder and treated accordingly.
5. Psychotic symptoms may be a manifestation of PD or its treatment and should be distinguished from psychotic depression.

Major Depressive Disorder

Major depressive disorder (MDD) is defined by one or more episodes of major depression. MDD is the most common mood disorder, with a lifetime prevalence in the community of 10%–25% for women and 5%–12% for men and with a current (1-year) prevalence rate of ~6% for women and ~3% for men (Blazer 2003). Prevalence rates are substantially lower in persons over age 45 years; in the elderly population, the current prevalence of major depression is ~1% (similar for both genders), although methodological issues confound such estimates (Ernst and Angst 1995) (see Table 19–6). The occurrence of major depression is much higher among elderly patients in hospital or long-term-care facilities (20%–25%).

MDD may manifest either as a single episode that never recurs (~25%–33% of patients) or as recurrent episodes (~67%–75% of patients). At least half of all patients with MDD experience their first episode before age 60. Those with the *nonrecurrent* form of the disorder tend to be older and less likely to have a family history of mood disorders, and their episode tends to be more protracted (1–2 years in duration). The *recurrent* form of the disorder is more likely in younger individuals, in patients with dysthymia (see the section "Dysthymia and Minor Depressive Episode" earlier in this chapter) or a "depressive" temperament, and in those with a family history of mood disorders. Patients with the recurrent disorder will experience, on average, five to six episodes over the course of a lifetime, the duration of which is on average approximately 6–9 months. New episodes tend to be similar to prior ones in terms of duration and clinical presentation. Most episodes will remit spontaneously, but 10%–20% may remain chronic. The interval between episodes varies but is typically years, and there may be varying degrees of residual symptoms between episodes. Some evidence suggests that the interval between episodes shortens with age (Kessing 2008; Mitchell and Subramaniam 2005).

The prognosis for elderly patients is similar to that for younger patients, as long as the former do not have comorbid medical illness or cognitive or functional impairment. Additional factors associated with a good outcome include strong social support, an absence of psychiatric comorbidity, less severe depression, and a history of recovery from previous episodes.

Major depression in elderly persons is associated with a number of problems that may predispose, trigger, or perpetuate the mood disorder, including cognitive and functional impairment, comorbid general medical illness, pain (see Chapter 23, "Pain"), and comorbid psychiatric illness. Cognitive impairment and functional decline are common manifestations of a major depressive episode in elderly persons, yet both can also trigger or worsen depressive symptoms. Both typically improve as the depression resolves. Depressed elderly patients (particularly those with cognitive impairment) are at increased risk (1.6-fold) of developing AD (see Chapter 16, "Alzheimer's Disease and the Frontotemporal Dementia Syndromes") (Green et al. 2003), particularly if they possess the *APOE*E4* allele (7-fold) (Irie et al. 2008). Depression also complicates the course and outcome of dementia.

As discussed earlier (see the section "Neurobiology of Emotion"), depression in elderly persons is associated with a number of changes in brain structure, function, and chemistry, including reduced volumes of certain frontal, medial temporal, and subcortical regions, as well as increased severity and prevalence of microvascular disease. Some of these changes appear to be more extensive in elderly patients with late-age onset of the mood disorder than in those with an earlier age at onset, suggesting potential pathways to late-life depression (Ballmaier et al. 2004, 2008). Some of these changes may also adversely impact course of illness and treatment response.

The elderly population has a high rate of general medical illness (e.g., cardiovascular disease, diabetes, osteoporosis and hip fracture), which has a bidirectional relation to major depression. Of particular interest is the relation between depression and cardiovascular disease (depression complicating cerebrovascular disease was discussed earlier), in that depression is both an independent risk factor for development of ischemic heart disease and a predictor of poorer outcome after myocardial infarction (Carney and Freedland 2007; Glassman and Bigger 2007). The mechanism for this interesting relation is unclear but may include reduced heart rate variability, increased platelet clotting (a phenomenon linked to the serotonin transporter polymorphism discussed earlier), and increased systemic inflammation.

Major depression is frequently comorbid with a number of other mental disorders, particularly substance abuse (see Chapter 17, "Addiction"), other mood disorders (e.g., dysthymia; see Chapter 19, "Mood Disorders"), anxiety disorders (see Chapter 20, "Anxiety Disorders"), and personality disorders (see Chapter 22, "Contemporary Personality Psychology"), any of which worsens the prognosis.

Major depression is associated with substantial mortality, both from suicide and from all causes. Although suicidal ideation decreases with age, *suicide attempts* are twice as frequent in the elderly population (five times as frequent in white males) than in the general population, and they are more lethal (violent methods are more common). Mood disorders (particularly if severe) and substance use disorders are independent risk factors for suicide (the former is the most common diagnosis in elderly suicide victims, whereas the latter—usually comorbid with depression—is the most common diagnosis in nonelderly victims), as are disruption of social ties and the availability of firearms. Physical illness and disability also increase the risk, an effect mediated through depression. Depression is also associated with an increased (two- to fourfold) rate of *all-cause mortality* in patients (particularly men) with comorbid general medical illness.

Bipolar Disorder

Late-onset mania is rare and necessitates a thorough evaluation for underlying causes, including stroke (especially right hemisphere lesions; see Chapter 25, "Cerebrovascular Disease"), medications (see Table 19–5) or toxins, TBI, and HIV (Evans et al. 1995; Shulman 1997; Starkstein et al. 1991). Most cases of mania in elderly persons occur in the setting of bipolar disorder.

Bipolar disorder is defined by one or more episodes of mania or hypomania. There are three recognized bipolar disorders: 1) bipolar disorder with manic (type I) or hypomanic (type II) episodes (usually with a history of major depressive episodes as well), 2) cyclothymic disorder (characterized by at least a 2-year history of numerous hypomanic episodes and depressed mood that does not meet diagnostic criteria for major depression), and 3) bipolar disorder not otherwise specified.

The clinical literature on mania, hypomania, and bipolar disorder in older adults is scarce and consists mainly of clinical case series and case reports. Prevalence rates of bipolar disorder in community samples range from 0.1% to 0.5% of seniors (no gender differences) (see Table 19–6), lower than estimates among younger adults (1.2%–1.4%) (Benedetti et al. 2008; Depp and Jeste 2004). However, bipolar disorder accounts for similar proportions of psychiatric hospitalizations among both older adults and younger adults (5%–19%). The prevalence of bipolar disorder in long-term-care settings ranges from 3% to 10% (Depp and Jeste 2004).

The pathophysiology of mania is not understood, and most of what is known is similar to that described for depression (see the section "Neurobiology of Emotion" earlier in this chapter). Bipolar I disorder is among the most heritable of psychiatric disorders, with genetic factors accounting for roughly 80% of the risk of developing the disorder. Despite ongoing research efforts, investigators have discovered no single gene or genotype-phenotype relationship. Brain imaging studies indicate that small prefrontal brain changes may occur early in the illness or even predate it, whereas other changes may develop within and between mood episodes (Strakowski et al. 2005).

Bipolar disorder is a highly recurrent illness that typically begins in the teenage years and whose subsequent course varies widely among patients (Goodwin et al. 2007). In ~50% of patients, depression is the initial manifestation of the illness, and most patients experience more (up to three times more) depressed than manic episodes. In some patients the illness follows a classic pattern of psychotic manias followed by melancholic depressions, whereas other individuals have depressive episodes for many years before experiencing the first manic episode. The episodes of mania or depression tend to occur in clusters. A minority of patients experience only manic episodes. The duration of depressive episodes tends to be somewhat shorter than in MDD. Prospective studies indicate that recurrence of mania does not decrease with age and that the illness does not "burn out" (Angst and Preisig 1995a, 1995b).

Adults with bipolar disorder frequently experience psychiatric comorbidity (particularly substance abuse, anxiety disorders, and personality disorders), but whether these same relations hold in elderly persons with bipolar disorder is not known. Indeed, substance abuse may actually be less common in elderly than nonelderly patients with bipolar disorder (Depp and Jeste 2004). Cognitive impairment may be associated with bipolar disorder in elderly persons and may be associated with poorer outcomes, but it appears that few patients progress to frank dementia (Shulman 1996). Elderly persons with bipolar disorder have a high rate of general medical illness, including diabetes and neurological illness (particularly among patients with an onset of the disorder in late life). The relation of this comorbidity to bipolar disorder has not been well studied (Beyer et al. 2005).

Elderly patients with bipolar disorder have higher all-cause mortality than individuals without psychiatric illness. Acute mania can be especially dangerous for elderly persons, who are susceptible to the adverse effects of dehydration and falls. Some elderly patients with bipolar disorder never achieve full functional recovery, and these patients may be at even higher risk of nonsuicide mortality than those with MDD (Shulman et al. 1992; Tohen et al. 2004).

Assessing Patient Safety

Upon completion of the neuropsychiatric assessment, the clinician must next evaluate the safety of the patient. This assessment must include an ongoing evaluation of the patient's risk to self or others, as well as a determination of the appropriate treatment setting (e.g., whether hospitalization is required).

Suicide is *the* primary medical emergency for the neuropsychiatric health care provider. Mood disorders and psychotic disorders are major risk factors for suicide, with estimated lifetime risks of death by suicide of 15%–20% for patients with bipolar disorder and 10% for patients with major depression, other mood disorders, and schizophrenia.

These risks are increased by the presence of other diagnoses, most notably substance abuse (see Chapter 17, "Addiction") and panic disorder (see Chapter 20, "Anxiety Disorders").

Age is positively correlated with suicide mortality, and this age effect is greater in women (3.2 times greater in older women than younger women) than in men (2 times greater in older men than younger men). The relation between increasing age and suicide mortality has lessened with recent age cohorts. In contrast to patients with major depression, the prevalence of suicide in patients with bipolar disorder tends to decrease with age (Depp and Jeste 2004), although this finding may reflect a survivor cohort.

Suicide in the elderly population is closely linked to depressive illness (Reza et al. 2001). Tragically, <25% of elderly suicide victims were receiving antidepressant medications at the time of their death (Abrams et al. 2009). Depressed persons are at highest risk for suicide when their illness is severe, melancholic, or psychotic; involves severe anxiety or agitation; or involves mild to moderate (but not severe) cognitive impairment (Busch et al. 2003; Coryell and Young 2005; Grunebaum et al. 2004). First onset of the mood disorder late in life also increases risk for suicide (Ahearn et al. 2001). The most important acute risk factor, however, is access to firearms (Hemenway and Miller 2002).

The clinician should determine and continually reassess the treatment setting (inpatient vs. partial hospital vs. outpatient) based on the assessment of the patient's safety, clinical status, available support systems, ready availability of weapons and means to commit suicide, and ability to care adequately for self and cooperate with treatment. Although not all suicides can be predicted, the risks may be reduced for populations (e.g., through gun and poison control) and individuals (e.g., through better treatment for depression). Indeed, the authors have developed a model of care that has achieved and sustained dramatic reductions in suicide rate among patients in a large health maintenance organization population through an extensive redesign of depression care that leverages formal suicide prevention guidelines and a commitment to "zero suicides" (Coffey 2007). A detailed discussion of the assessment and treatment of patients with suicidal behavior is beyond the scope of this chapter; however, guidelines exist to inform such management (American Psychiatric Association 2003).

Treatment

Guidelines have been published to inform the care of elderly persons with a mood disorder (Alexopoulos et al. 2001; Baldwin et al. 2002; Eastham et al. 1998; Young et al. 2004). In general, treatment is similar to that for younger patients, with a few notable exceptions relating to the older patients' high occurrence of comorbid general medical and neuropsychiatric illness and their increased sensitivity to the side effects of somatic treatments (medications, electroconvulsive therapy [ECT]). Elsewhere in this text, detailed descriptions are provided of the principles and practice of psychotherapy (Chapter 8, "Psychosocial Therapies"), psychopharmacology (Chapter 9, "Geriatric Neuropsychopharmacology), and neuromodulatory therapies (Chapter 10, "Electroconvulsive Therapy and Related Treatments").

In this section, we discuss treatment of each of the specific mood disturbances identified earlier in the chapter, paying particular attention, where relevant, to differences in the management of the mood syndrome based on the underlying disorder. Regardless of the mood disturbance, effective treatment begins with the following steps:

1. *Define full remission as the goal of treatment. Acute phase treatment* serves to resolve the present episode; *continuation treatment* to maintain remission, restore quality of life, and prevent relapse; and *maintenance treatment* to reduce the risk of recurrence.
2. *Optimize the patient's general medical health* and ensure that all underlying general medical and neurological disorders have been optimally treated, including the provision of pain management. Aging is associated with an increase in medical burden, and a number of these general medical disorders (e.g., hypothyroidism, cerebrovascular disease, degenerative brain disease; see Table 19–3) may produce mood disturbances (see Chapter 29, "Neuropsychiatric Disorders Associated With General Medical Therapies"). Some clinical literature suggests that elderly persons may be particularly prone to the mood-altering effects of some of these conditions.
3. *Review all the patient's current medications.* Drugs of abuse (see Chapter 17, "Addiction") as well as various medications (see Table 19–5; see also Chapter 29) and toxins may be associated with mood disturbances in elderly persons. It is not known whether elderly persons as a group are more prone to substance-induced mood disorders than other age groups, but they are susceptible to medication side effects. Treatment of these disorders involves careful removal of the offending substance. Even severe symptoms (including, e.g., a full-blown major depressive episode) improve dramatically within days to weeks of abstinence or of resolution of withdrawal. Some residual milder symptoms (dysthymia, cyclothymia) may persist for longer periods, but these too usually diminish and remit over time.
4. *Address functional impairments* and optimize the patient's environment and lifestyle, including the promotion of regular exercise, a healthy diet, and sleep hygiene. It is also

important to evaluate and address the patient's key interpersonal relationships. Caregivers should be supported and educated, particularly about *behavioral management* of the patient's symptoms, the importance of *treatment adherence*, and the early signs of *relapse*.

5. *Coordinate the patient's care among all providers.* Elderly patients often receive care from multiple clinicians (e.g., psychotherapist, primary care physician, neurologist, neurosurgeon, physical medicine and rehabilitation specialist, speech therapist)—and coordinating the patient's care among these providers is imperative.

Major Depressive Episode

In this section, we discuss in turn the treatment of MDD, bipolar depression, and depression in patients with stroke, AD, or PD.

Major Depressive Disorder

Acute phase treatment. Decisions regarding acute phase treatment depend on the presence or absence of melancholia or other severe forms of the disorder. Patients with melancholia, psychotic depression, depression with catatonic features, or other signs of severity (e.g., acutely suicidal, refusing to eat) should be considered for ECT. ECT is the treatment of choice when 1) a patient with a severe mood disorder is gravely ill and in need of a rapid and definitive treatment response, 2) medications have failed or are poorly tolerated, 3) the patient has a history of a good response to ECT, or 4) the patient prefers ECT (Weiner 2001) (see Chapter 10, "Electroconvulsive Therapy and Related Treatments"). Response rates among mixed-age samples range from 65% to 90% depending on a number of factors, with response rates highest for patients with psychotic depression. For patients with depressive illness, response rates generally increase with age (Abrams 2002; O'Connor et al. 2001). ECT is very safe, even in the elderly patient with comorbid general medical disorders. Modifications in the ECT technique may be required, however, based on the patient's general medical or neurological status and concerns about cognitive side effects (see Chapter 10).

Although some guidelines call for the use of combined drug therapy (antidepressant plus antipsychotic) for patients with psychotic symptoms, limited data have been reported on this issue in elderly patients (Meyers et al. 2009). We try to avoid antipsychotic agents given their motor, metabolic, and vascular risks in elderly persons. For patients with psychotic depression, ECT is generally a safer and more effective alternative.

Pharmacotherapy is recommended for patients with severe depression who are unable to receive ECT, as well as for patients with less severe, nonmelancholic forms of depression (American Psychiatric Association 2010). Multiple medications have been approved by the U.S. Food and Drug Administration (FDA) for treatment of depression in elderly patients (Unutzer 2007). Controlled trials confirm the efficacy of antidepressant medication in older (including elderly) adults in both outpatient and institutional settings (Andreescu et al. 2008; Mottram et al. 2006; Nelson et al. 2008), although such treatment may be less successful (slower, less robust, associated with higher risk of relapse) than in younger patients (Dew et al. 2007). Notably, although the use of antidepressant medications may increase suicidality in youths and young adults, these medications may actually exert a protective effect in older adults (Kuehn 2007). As discussed in Chapter 9, "Geriatric Neuropsychopharmacology," these drugs do not differ in their overall effectiveness or speed of response. As such, the choice of agent is based on its safety profile (e.g., side effects, potential for drug interactions), ease of use, costs, and patient preference. Considering these factors, we typically treat initially with citalopram (Mottram et al. 2006). Nortriptyline, venlafaxine, and mirtazapine are reasonable second-line alternatives. The dosage of the first-choice agent should be maximized as swiftly as possible on the basis of its tolerability (using the maxim "start low, go slow, and don't stop"). A medication trial should last 4–6 weeks at adequate dosage, but if by this time there has not been at least a partial response (e.g., 25% reduction in symptom severity), then an alternative treatment is indicated. The patient's intolerance of the side effects of the medications may also dictate a switch to an alternative treatment. The clinician has three reasonable options: 1) ECT; 2) augmenting with lithium, an agent with established safety and efficacy in melancholia (Alvarez et al. 1997); and 3) switching classes of medications.

In addition to ECT, two newer brain stimulation procedures have been approved by the FDA for the treatment of depression: vagus nerve stimulation (VNS) and rapid (or repetitive) transcranial magnetic stimulation (rTMS) (see Chapter 11, "Brain Stimulation Therapies"). VNS was approved in July 2005 as an adjunctive long-term treatment of chronic or recurrent depression for patients ages 18 years and older who are experiencing a major depressive episode and have not had an adequate response to four or more adequate antidepressant treatments. In February 2007, however, the Centers for Medicare and Medicaid issued a decision not to cover the procedure (citing lack of efficacy), and other insurers quickly followed (VNS remains a covered benefit for treatment of epilepsy). Therefore, very few seniors are likely to use this procedure. rTMS was approved in 2008 for treatment of adults with a major depressive episode that has been refractory to one adequate trial of pharmacotherapy. The procedure appears to be remarkably safe and may offer an alternative to medications (and their troublesome side effects) in persons with mild to moderate depression. Only a few studies have examined the efficacy of rTMS in elderly persons with depression, and results are conflicting (George et al. 2009). Similar to VNS, rTMS is not currently covered by insurance, an issue that may further limit its availability to most seniors.

We use benzodiazepines judiciously in older persons due to their adverse cognitive and behavioral side effects (Gray et al. 2006; Landi et al. 2005; Paterniti et al. 2002).

When used alone, psychotherapy (cognitive-behavioral therapy, interpersonal therapy, or problem-solving therapy) that is brief and structured is generally effective for inducing symptom remission in elderly patients with mild to moderately severe depression (Alexopoulos et al. 2008; Areán et al. 2010; Cuijpers et al. 2007a, 2007b) (see Chapter 8, "Psychosocial Therapies"). Psychotherapy may also help to increase adherence to somatic therapies, as well as to reduce the psychosocial consequences of the mood disorder (e.g., family discord, occupational functioning). Combining psychotherapy with somatic therapy may be particularly useful in patients with severe or chronic illness (Pinquart et al. 2006).

Although the use of complementary and alternative medicines (CAMs) decreases with age, almost 5% of adults reported having used some form of CAM in the previous 12 months for mood symptoms (Barnes et al. 2004). St. John's wort (SJW) is a CAM used to treat depressive disorders. A Cochrane review concluded that in mixed-aged samples, SJW is well tolerated and its effectiveness is similar to that of most antidepressant medications in patients with mild to moderate depression (Linde et al. 2008). Current evidence is insufficient to establish whether SJW is as effective as conventional antidepressant treatments for severe depression. In addition, use of SJW is potentially problematic, in that the effects of other medications might be compromised. Older persons in particular are susceptible to herb-mediated changes in cytochrome P450 activity, especially those induced by SJW (Gurley et al. 2005). Finally, the neurobiological effects of CAMs may impact the course and outcome of more effective antidepressant treatments such as ECT (Patra and Coffey 2004). For all these reasons, in our practice we recommend against the use of any CAM for older persons being treated for mood disorders.

Continuation treatment. Successful acute phase treatment should be continued for at least 9–12 months to prevent a relapse of the episode of illness. A longer duration should be considered for patients with psychotic symptoms. For continuation ECT, the frequency of treatments is tapered over this time course. If medications were used for acute phase treatment, they are continued at the fully effective dosage. At the end of the continuation phase, and if maintenance treatment (see discussion below) is not indicated, the continuation treatment should be gradually tapered before discontinuation, and the patient should be followed closely for several months to ensure euthymia.

Psychotherapy may be continued throughout the continuation treatment phase and may take the form of ongoing psychoeducation. The Internet is an increasingly used resource for mental health information, with roughly 20% of older persons using the Internet for some health-related question or concern (Fox 2004). Clinicians should be aware, however, that the quality of information about depression is generally poor (Ferreira-Lay and Miller 2008) and that online interventions (e.g., Internet-based psychotherapy) are still being developed and evaluated (Andersson et al. 2005; Christensen et al. 2004; Griffiths et al. 2004).

Maintenance treatment. To prevent recurrences, maintenance treatment is indicated in all patients who have experienced multiple (at least two or three) episodes of illness. Treatment modality (ECT, pharmacotherapy) and "dosage" are generally the same as during the continuation treatment phase. Close collaboration between the clinician and patient (and/or his or her significant others) is required to support adherence, treat symptom breakthrough, manage the care during the development of an intercurrent general medical disorder (e.g., stroke, dementia), and make decisions about the duration of treatment. Limited data exist to guide decisions regarding the duration of maintenance treatment, but in general, the more recurrent the patient's illness and the more serious the depressive episodes, the more aggressive we are in extending the maintenance phase.

Bipolar Disorder ("Bipolar Depression")

Acute phase treatment. As in younger adults with bipolar disorder, the mainstays of acute treatment in older adults with bipolar depression are ECT or combination pharmacotherapy. ECT should be considered whenever a patient with bipolar depression is severely ill (e.g., psychotic, melancholic) or in need of a rapid, definitive treatment response (e.g., actively suicidal) (Eastham et al. 1998). Use of ECT in these patients is often complicated, however, by the presence of maintenance medications that may contribute to ECT side effects (e.g., lithium) or that may lessen the efficacy of the treatment by interfering with the induction of a therapeutic seizure (e.g., anticonvulsants, benzodiazepines).

Combination pharmacotherapy may be considered for patients who are not candidates for ECT and for those who have less severe bipolar depression. Treatment consists of optimizing a mood stabilizer (lithium, valproate), followed by the addition of an antidepressant medication in select cases. The data are conflicting, however, concerning the efficacy of antidepressant medications in this setting, and these medications may trigger a "switch" into mania. Minimal controlled data are available for elderly patients (Belmaker 2007; Ghaemi et al. 2007; Sachs et al. 2007).

In our practice, we base the choice of medication regimen for the acute treatment of bipolar depression in part on the patient's clinical history. After ensuring that the mood stabilizer is optimized, we add an antidepressant medication for patients who have a history of mild manic episodes but severe or lengthy depressive episodes. We prefer bupropion or citalopram, because they may have less risk of inducing mania than do tricyclics or other noradrenergic reuptake inhibitors. We almost never add an antidepressant medication in patients with a history of life-threatening mania. Lamotrigine is another option in that some (but not all) data support its efficacy in this setting, and it appears to have a low risk of inducing mania. Other mood stabilizers (e.g., valproate) may also be considered.

Psychotherapy for patients with bipolar depression follows the same principles as those discussed earlier for patients with major depression and is effective as an adjunctive treatment (Miklowitz et al. 2007b).

Maintenance treatment. Although patients with bipolar disorder clearly require prophylaxis against future episodes, there is a paucity of controlled data to guide the choice of maintenance treatment. Knowledge is even more limited for elderly patients. Treatment recommendations are based on the small number of controlled studies in adults, and most of these focus on maintenance treatment after episodes of mood elevation (Suppes et al. 2005b).

As a general recommendation, effective and well-tolerated acute phase treatment should be continued for maintenance, with an effort to simplify the treatment regimen whenever possible. If ECT was used acutely for bipolar depression, it may be employed as maintenance treatment, for a minimum of 9–12 months. The frequency of treatments is slowly tapered, and treatments are spaced as far apart as possible without breakthrough of symptoms. During this maintenance ECT course, we generally continue to withhold mood-stabilizing agents (e.g., lithium, anticonvulsants) to avoid their potential complications. On the other hand, some clinicians, who are concerned that breakthrough mood syndromes may occur as the frequency of the maintenance ECT treatments is decreased, prefer to administer a mood stabilizer between treatments, holding the dose a few days before a scheduled ECT treatment to avoid potential complications. Some clinical literature and our own experience suggest that ECT may be used indefinitely (alone or in combination with psychotropic medication variously prescribed) as successful maintenance therapy in some patients who require long-term maintenance and who tolerate the procedure and related logistical issues well. Other clinicians attempt to transition patients to mood-stabilizing pharmacotherapy after a course of maintenance ECT.

Psychotherapy during maintenance treatment for bipolar disorder in adults may improve understanding of the illness and its treatment, improve social functioning, improve adherence to the maintenance treatment, and reduce the need for hospitalization (Bauer 2001; Miklowitz et al. 2007a). However, limited data are available on this issue in elderly patients (see Chapter 8, "Psychosocial Therapies").

Stroke

In patients with poststroke depression, ECT should be considered for those who are severely depressed, melancholic, psychotic, or otherwise in need of rapid clinical improvement. A small uncontrolled (primarily retrospective) clinical literature supports the safety, tolerability, and efficacy of ECT in such patients (Currier et al. 1992; Murray et al. 1986), although randomized controlled data are lacking. ECT should generally take place several weeks after an acute infarct so that fragile vasculature is allowed to heal before receiving the increased cerebral blood flow associated with ECT. Other modifications in ECT technique may be required based on the patient's medical status and concerns about cognitive side effects.

In patients with less severe depression, antidepressant medications may be considered. No medications have been approved by the FDA for poststroke depression, and the results of several controlled trials are mixed, although results are limited by several methodological concerns (Hackett et al. 2008b). The medications studied are associated with an increased incidence of side effects, however, which contribute to a high dropout rate in these studies. Still, the potential for these medications to improve stroke recovery, cognitive impairment, and mortality supports their use in most patients. We treat initially with citalopram on the basis of its safety, tolerability, and costs, as well as its efficacy as demonstrated in two small controlled trials (Hackett et al. 2008b). Sertraline is a reasonable alternative. It should be noted that all serotonin reuptake inhibitors should be used with caution in patients with subarachnoid hemorrhage (where these medications have been associated with vasospasm) and in patients receiving antiplatelet or anticoagulant medications (where they may potentiate the risk of bleeding). Nortriptyline is a reasonable second-line agent, provided that the patient has no contraindications (e.g., heart block, cardiac arrhythmia, narrow-angle glaucoma; note that the tricyclics may potentiate the effects of warfarin). A small trial found left prefrontal rTMS to be effective for poststroke depression, but more research is needed (Jorge et al. 2004).

Successful acute treatment, with ECT or medication, should be continued for at least 9–12 months. Antidepressant treatment of poststroke depression is associated with a lower mortality over the ensuing 9 years.

Only a few controlled investigations of psychotherapy for poststroke depression have been reported, and these have not demonstrated efficacy (Hackett et al. 2008b). In our experience, however, psychotherapy may be useful to help patients cope with and manage their cerebrovascular disease and related functional impairments. Brief structured psychotherapy (e.g., cognitive-behavioral therapy or interpersonal therapy) can be considered for patients who have mild to moderate severe depression and who are able to participate in the treatment.

Alzheimer's Disease

As a first step in treatment of patients with AD who have a mood disturbance, clinicians should optimize the use of cholinesterase inhibitors. Controlled data suggest that these agents may improve neuropsychiatric symptoms (including apathy and depression) and functional status (Coffey et al. 2007).

ECT should be considered for use in patients with AD who are severely depressed, melancholic, psychotic, or otherwise in need of rapid clinical improvement. Findings from a small uncontrolled (primarily retrospective) clinical literature suggest that ECT in depressed patients with dementia is safe and effective (Rao and Lyketsos 2000). ECT does not appear to worsen the underlying dementing disorder, although some patients with dementia may be at increased risk for developing more persistent disorientation, cognitive impairment, and interictal electroencephalogram (EEG) slowing with ECT. These adverse effects may be minimized with modifications in ECT technique.

In patients with less severe depression, antidepressant medications may be considered. No medications have been approved by the FDA for depression in patients with AD, and the few existing randomized controlled trials report mixed results (Lyketsos and Olin 2002), perhaps due in part to a variety of methodological issues. We typically start with citalopram because of its safety, tolerability, demonstrated efficacy (Gottfries et al. 1992), and low cost (Pollock et al. 2002). Venlafaxine is a reasonable second-line agent. The limited controlled data do not support the efficacy of cyclic antidepressants. In addition, medications with anticholinergic side effects (e.g., tricyclic antidepressants) should be used cautiously, because they may worsen memory impairment. Antipsychotic medications should be used sparingly given their small risk of stroke and death in elderly persons.

Successful acute therapy should be continued for at least 9–12 months.

Certain types of psychosocial therapies may be effective for the treatment of depression (major and minor) in patients with dementia, in both outpatient and residential settings (see Chapter 8, "Psychosocial Therapies"). Such treatment can also positively improve the mood of the caregiver. Caregivers should be trained in the behavioral management of the patient's behavioral problems, which can help reduce depression in both patient and caregiver. Caregivers themselves should also be monitored for depressive symptoms (Ballard et al. 1996b).

Parkinson's Disease

ECT should be considered for use in patients with PD who are severely depressed, melancholic, psychotic (but see next paragraph), or otherwise in need of rapid clinical improvement. A small uncontrolled (primarily retrospective) clinical literature supports the safety, tolerability, and efficacy of ECT in such patients, although randomized controlled data are lacking. Modifications in ECT technique may be required, however, based on the patient's neurological status and concerns about cognitive side effects. Of note, controlled studies indicate that ECT may also temporarily improve the motor symptoms of PD, irrespective of its effect on mood.

The treatment of concomitant psychotic symptoms in patients with PD is complex. Treatment decisions should be based on a thorough assessment of the potential causative factors (e.g., medication-induced depression vs. depression with psychotic features vs. dementia with Lewy bodies). Psychotic depression should be treated aggressively with ECT. We generally avoid antipsychotic medications, given their potential to worsen motor symptoms and their small risk of stroke and death in elderly patients.

In patients with less severe depression, antidepressant medications are commonly used. No medications have been approved by the FDA for depression in patients with PD. In a Cochrane review, Ghazi-Noori et al. (2003) reported that the few available controlled data were not sufficient to determine the safety or effectiveness of antidepressant medications in these patients. A later meta-analysis of controlled studies found that although antidepressant medications were generally well tolerated by patients with PD, large effect sizes were observed for both antidepressant medications and placebo, with no difference between the two (Weintraub et al. 2005).

Many clinicians favor SSRIs, but we typically begin pharmacotherapy with nortriptyline, based on its demonstrated superiority to placebo and controlled-release paroxetine (Menza et al. 2009), its safety and tolerability, and its cost. In addition, nortriptyline's anticholinergic properties may ameliorate the tremor and salivation that occur in PD. These benefits must be carefully weighed against nortriptyline's potential to worsen orthostatic hypotension and cognitive impairment. Nortriptyline is contraindicated in patients with heart block, cardiac arrhythmia, and narrow-angle glaucoma. Bupropion is a reasonable second choice, given its dopaminergic properties and its relatively lower incidence of sexual side effects, but it may also induce psychotic symptoms. We generally avoid amoxapine and lithium because they may worsen the movement disorder, although it remains unclear whether SSRIs do in fact worsen the movement disorder (see Chapter 24, "Parkinson's Disease and Movement Disorders"). In addition, the SSRIs may induce apathy and may rarely result in serotonin toxicity or hypertensive crisis in patients receiving selegiline or rasagiline (monoamine oxidase type B inhibitors) for PD.

Adjustment Disorder

No controlled data have been reported on the treatment of adjustment disorders in elderly persons (Strain and Diefenbacher 2008). In mixed-age samples, there have been two randomized controlled trials of psychotherapeutic interventions (Gonzales-Jaimes and Turnbull-Plaza 2003; van der Klink et al. 2003) and two randomized controlled trials of plant extracts (Bourin et al. 1997; Volz and Kieser 1997). Other data are extrapolated from studies that included subjects with adjustment disorder in larger cohorts of depressive or anxiety disorders. Treatment is generally supportive and focused on psychosocial efforts to identify the stressor, minimize its impact, and enhance the patient's problem-solving skills and support system (Strain and Diefenbacher 2008). Clinicians may consider adding a medication to psychotherapy for specific symptoms of anxiety or insomnia (Schatzberg 1990).

Bereavement

By definition, grief is normal. No empirical evidence supports the effectiveness of routine psychosocial interventions to "treat" grief, and indeed such interventions given soon after bereavement may actually interfere with the normal grieving process (Schut and Stroebe 2005). Clinicians may facilitate healthy grieving, however, by carefully evaluating which patients and families may benefit from social support and education about the normal grieving process (Jordan and Neimeyer 2003).

When depressive illness is recognized during bereavement, treatment is warranted and should follow the previously described recommendations for patients with MDD. If melancholic features exist, the patient's risk of psychiatric morbidity increases the longer the illness goes untreated. Treatment studies of major depression specifically in the context of bereavement support antidepressant treatments generally known to be effective for major depression in other contexts. One double-blind controlled trial demonstrated efficacy for nortriptyline (particularly in combination with interpersonal psychotherapy), but not for interpersonal psychotherapy alone, for bereavement-related depression in adults ages 50 and older (Reynolds et al. 1999). Open-label studies in mixed-age adult samples suggest that in addition to nortriptyline, desipramine and sustained-release bupropion may also be effective against bereavement-related depression (Hensley 2006).

As mentioned earlier in "Identifying the Mood Disturbance," a syndrome of complicated grief has been proposed. As with other forms of nonmelancholic depression, randomized controlled trials of adults (including seniors) support the effectiveness of psychotherapy (particularly a combination of cognitive-behavioral therapy focusing on loss, together with interpersonal therapy focusing on restoration), but response rates are only around 50% (Shear et al. 2005). Treatment for bereavement-related depression does not appear to be effective against complicated grief.

Demoralization

Regardless of the conceptual issues surrounding demoralization (discussed earlier in "Identifying the Mood Disturbance"), hopelessness, a core feature of demoralization, has been linked to poor outcomes from both general medical and psychiatric illnesses (Clarke and Kissane 2002). Therefore, treatment is indicated and consists of symptomatic treatment (e.g., of pain or distressing mental symptoms such as anxiety), together with the provision of information, support (informal or formal), and psychotherapy (e.g., cognitive-behavioral therapy). The patient should be assessed carefully for emerging signs of melancholia. If a demoralization reaction does not resolve shortly after resolution of the general medical or neurological condition (e.g., the stroke), then the clinician should reassess the patient for melancholia and treat accordingly.

Apathy

The treatment of apathy begins with optimizing the patient's general medical health (including the endocrine status) and eliminating, when possible, any medications that may cause or worsen apathy (as noted earlier in "Identifying the Mood Disturbance"). The treatment of any comorbid neuropsychiatric disorder (e.g., depression, delirium, substance abuse) should also be optimized. In this regard, controlled studies have demonstrated a beneficial effect of acetylcholinesterase inhibitors on apathy in patients with dementia. A small uncontrolled clinical study suggests that psychostimulants, amantadine, and dopamine agonists may improve apathy in patients with dementia or TBI (van Reekum et al. 2005). A small number of controlled studies of treatment options for apathy specifically following stroke support a trial of a psychostimulant (e.g., methylphenidate) (Starkstein and Manes 2000; Watanabe et al. 1995) or the nootropic nefiracetam (Robinson et al. 2009). A sparse clinical literature also supports the merits of psychostimulants (methylphenidate, D-amphetamine), dopaminergic agents (bromocriptine, amantadine, and bupropion), and various psychosocial adjunctive strategies in the treatment of apathy in patients with AD (Boyle and Malloy 2004) and PD (Chatterjee and Fahn 2002; Pluck and Brown 2002; Richard 2007). Psychosocial approaches may be helpful (although they have not been formally studied) and include the provision of a structured repetitive daily routine and an environment with low expressed emotion.

Pathological Laughing and Crying

No somatic treatments have been approved by the FDA for PLC, and only a few studies have examined this issue prospectively. Both nortriptyline and citalopram have been found to be effective in small randomized controlled trials of PLC following stroke (see Chapter 25, "Cerebrovascular Disease"). Amitriptyline was found effective for PLC in a randomized controlled trial of 12 patients with multiple sclerosis (Schiffer et al. 1985). Two more recent controlled clinical trials found that AVP-39 (a combination of quinidine 30 mg and dextromethorphan 30 mg orally) was effective in relieving PLC and improving quality of life in patients with amyotrophic lateral sclerosis (Brooks et al. 2004) and in patients with multiple sclerosis (Panitch et al. 2006). This compound is under review for approval by the FDA. Case reports also support the use of tricyclic antidepressants, serotonin reuptake inhibitors, levodopa, and mood stabilizers for PLC in various neurological disorders.

Mania

There is a dearth of controlled data regarding the management of older patients with bipolar disorder (Eastham et al. 1998; McDonald and Wermager 2002; Young et al. 2004). Treatment generally follows that for younger persons, but with caution due to the dangers of acute mania in frail and elderly persons, the high rate of comorbid general medical illness, and the sensitivity of older patients to treatment side effects. Age at onset does not appear to predict treatment response (Young et al. 2004).

Acute Treatment

Acute mania is a medical emergency, and many patients require hospitalization while treatment is being initiated. As in younger adults with bipolar disorder, the mainstays of treatment in older adults with acute mania are ECT or pharmacotherapy. ECT should be considered when a patient with acute mania is severely ill (e.g., psychotic, aggressive); when the patient is in need of a rapid, definitive treatment response (e.g., catatonia, malignant hyperthermia); or when psychopharmacology is unsafe or intolerable for the patient. Use of ECT in these patients is often complicated, however, by the presence of maintenance medications that may either contribute to ECT side effects (e.g., lithium) or lessen the efficacy of the treatment by interfering with the induction of a therapeutic seizure (e.g., anticonvulsants, benzodiazepines).

In patients with less severe mania, treatment begins with monopharmacotherapy with a mood stabilizer (lithium, valproate) (American Psychiatric Association 2002; Belmaker 2004). Among the mood stabilizers, lithium is recommended for euphoric or irritable mania, whereas the anticonvulsants are generally used for patients who have a history of rapid cycling or who do not respond to lithium. Valproic acid may be preferred over lithium for secondary mania, perhaps due to its more favorable side-effect profile in such patients (Evans et al. 1995). Because the mood-stabilizing agents may be somewhat slow to work against acute mania, they may be combined with a benzodiazepine (e.g., lorazepam) or antipsychotic for control of the patient's agitation, insomnia, aggression, dysphoria, or panic.

Antipsychotic drugs may be used as monotherapy (Suppes et al. 2005a), although we prefer to employ them as second-line antimanic agents. Among the antipsychotic agents, the atypical agents are generally preferred over the classic antipsychotic agents for antimanic monotherapy (Chengappa et al. 2004), given the antipsychotic agents' lower risk of acute extrapyramidal side effects and greater acceptance by most patients. (There are five FDA-approved agents: olanzapine, risperidone, quetiapine, ziprasidone, and aripiprazole.) Typical antipsychotic agents (neuroleptics) should be considered for patients who had a good response to them in the past.

Psychotherapy typically has limited value during acute mania.

Maintenance Therapy

If pharmacotherapy was used successfully for acute treatment of patients with mania, it may be employed as maintenance therapy. Lithium or valproate is recommended for patients with frequent, recent, or severe mania. The safe use of these two agents (e.g., drug-drug interactions, metabolism in elderly persons, common side effects) is reviewed in detail in Chapter 9, "Geriatric Neuropsychopharmacology."[1] Lamotrigine monotherapy may be an alternative in patients without frequent or severe mania. Adjunctive antipsychotic medication should be tapered and discontinued as soon as clinically possible to avoid the cardiovascular risk and long-term complications such as tardive dyskinesia (patients with bipolar disorder appear to be particularly prone to this adverse effect). Various guidelines exist to inform the maintenance treatment if these initial recommendations are not effective (American Psychiatric Association 2002; Suppes et al. 2005b).

---

[1] Recently the FDA issued an alert advising clinicians to monitor patients taking anticonvulsants for increased suicidality. A review of clinical trials of anticonvulsant medications found a twofold increased risk of suicidal ideation or behavior, compared with placebo. The risk was particularly high among patients with "psychiatric disorders."

Although several of the atypical antipsychotics have received FDA approval for treatment of acute mania (olanzapine, risperidone, quetiapine, ziprasidone, and aripiprazole), for bipolar depression (olanzapine/fluoxetine, quetiapine), and for maintenance therapy of bipolar disorder (olanzapine, aripiprazole), their many untoward side effects (e.g., motor, metabolic, and cardiovascular) make them undesirable as first-line agents in elderly patients.

Affective Lability

No medications have been approved by the FDA for affective lability, and no controlled studies have been reported. Treatment involves managing the underlying illness (e.g., dementia, bipolar disorder). Most clinicians employ the same medications used for PLC (Brousseau et al. 2005).

Key Points

- Depressive illness is *not* a normal part of aging.
- Mood disorders are highly recurrent illnesses with early onset; first onset late in life is rare. However, the number of elderly patients with mood disorders is increasing because the number of elderly individuals is increasing.
- Mood disturbances are common in neuropsychiatric disorders, and many increase in prevalence and incidence with age.
- The etiology of mood disorders is heterogeneous. The pathophysiology is not fully understood but reflects a severely abnormal stress response.
- Distinguishing depression from bereavement, demoralization, apathy, and other mood disturbances sets the stage for safe and effective treatment.
- Once depressive illness is diagnosed, the presence or absence of melancholic or psychotic features determines treatment strategies.
- The treatment of mood disorders late in life generally follows evidence-based recommendations for the biopsychosocial treatment of younger adults.
- ECT is safe and effective in elderly persons and should be considered whenever an older patient with a mood disorder is severely ill or in need of a rapid, definitive treatment response.
- Pharmacotherapy can be safe and effective for elderly patients when clinicians follow the mantra "start low, go slow, and don't stop."
- Mania in an older person is a potentially life-threatening condition and should be treated aggressively.

Recommended Readings and Web Sites

Baldwin RC, Chiu E, Katona C, et al: Guidelines on Depression in Older People: Practicing the Evidence. London, Martin Dunitz, 2002

Coffey CE, McAllister TW, Silver JM: Guide to Neuropsychiatric Therapeutics. Philadelphia, PA, Lippincott Williams & Wilkins, 2007

Eastham JH, Jeste DV, Young RC: Assessment and treatment of bipolar disorder in the elderly. Drugs Aging 12:205–224, 1998

Mottram PG, Wilson K, Strobl JJ: Antidepressants for depressed elderly. Cochrane Database of Systematic Reviews 2006, Issue 1. Art. No.: CD003491. DOI: 10.1002/14651858.CD003491.pub2

Taylor MA, Fink M: Melancholia: The Diagnosis, Pathophysiology, and Treatment of Depressive Illness. New York, Cambridge University Press, 2006

Young RC, Gyulai L, Mulsant BH, et al: Pharmacotherapy of bipolar disorder in old age: review and recommendations. Am J Geriatr Psychiatry 12:342–357, 2004

Geriatric Mental Health Foundation: www.gmhfonline.org/gmhf. A resource established by the American Association for Geriatric Psychiatry to raise awareness of psychiatric and mental health disorders affecting the elderly, eliminate the stigma of mental illness and treatment, promote healthy aging strategies, and increase access to quality mental health care for the elderly.

References

Abrams R: Electroconvulsive Therapy, 4th Edition. New York, Oxford University Press, 2002

Abrams RC, Leon AC, Tardiff K, et al: Antidepressant use in elderly suicide victims in New York City: an analysis of 255 cases. J Clin Psychiatry 70:312–317, 2009

Ahearn EP, Jamison KR, Steffens DC, et al: MRI correlates of suicide attempt history in unipolar depression. Biol Psychiatry 50:266–270, 2001

Akiskal HS: Dysthymia: clinical and external validity. Acta Psychiatr Scand Suppl 383:19–23, 1994

Akiskal HS, Cassano GB: Dysthymia and the Spectrum of Chronic Depressions. New York, Guilford, 1997

Alexopoulos GS, Katz IR, Reynolds CF III, et al: The expert consensus guideline series: pharmacotherapy of depressive disorders in older patients. Postgrad Med (Spec No):1–86, 2001

Alexopoulos GS, Schultz SK, Lebowitz BD: Late-life depression: a model for medical classification. Biol Psychiatry 58:283–289, 2005

Alexopoulos GS, Raue PJ, Kanellopoulos D, et al: Problem solving therapy for the depression-executive dysfunction syndrome of late life. Int J Geriatr Psychiatry 23:782–788, 2008

Almeida OP, Waterreus A, Hankey GJ: Preventing depression after stroke: results from a randomized placebo-controlled trial. J Clin Psychiatry 67:1104–1109, 2006

Alvarez E, Perez-Sola V, Perez-Blanco J, et al: Predicting outcome of lithium added to antidepressants in resistant depression. J Affect Disord 42:179–186, 1997

American Psychiatric Association: Diagnostic and Statistical Manual of Mental Disorders, 4th Edition, Text Revision. Washington, DC, American Psychiatric Association, 2000

American Psychiatric Association: Practice guideline for the treatment of patients with major depressive disorder, third edition. Am J Psychiatry 167(suppl):1–118, 2010. Available at: http://www.psychiatryonline.com/pracGuide/pracGuideTopic_7.aspx. Accessed December 22, 2010.

American Psychiatric Association: Practice guideline for the treatment of patients with bipolar disorder (revision). Am J Psychiatry 159 (suppl 4):1–50, 2002. Available at: http://www.psychiatryonline.com/pracGuide/pracGuideTopic_8.aspx. Accessed October 4, 2010.

American Psychiatric Association: Practice guideline for the assessment and treatment of patients with suicidal behaviors. Am J Psychiatry 160(suppl):1–60, 2003. Available at: http://www.psychiatryonline.com/pracGuide/pracGuideTopic_14.aspx. Accessed July 7, 2010.

Andersson G, Bergstrom J, Hollandare F, et al: Internet-based self-help for depression: randomised controlled trial. Br J Psychiatry 187:456–461, 2005

Andreasen NC, Hoenk PR: The predictive value of adjustment disorders: a follow-up study. Am J Psychiatry 139:584–590, 1982

Andreescu C, Mulsant BH, Houck PR, et al: Empirically derived decision trees for the treatment of late-life depression. Am J Psychiatry 165:855–862, 2008

Angst J, Preisig M: Course of a clinical cohort of unipolar, bipolar and schizoaffective patients: results of a prospective study from 1959 to 1985. Schweiz Arch Neurol Psychiatr 146:5–16, 1995a

Angst J, Preisig M: Outcome of a clinical cohort of unipolar, bipolar and schizoaffective patients: results of a prospective study from 1959 to 1985. Schweiz Arch Neurol Psychiatr 146:17–23, 1995b

Areán PA, Raue P, Mackin RS, et al: Problem-solving therapy and supportive therapy in older adults with major depression and executive dysfunction. Am J Psychiatry 167:1391–1398, 2010

Baldwin RC, Tomenson B: Depression in later life: a comparison of symptoms and risk factors in early and late onset cases. Br J Psychiatry 167:649–652, 1995

Baldwin RC, Chiu E, Katona C, et al: Guidelines on Depression in Older People: Practicing the Evidence. London, Martin Dunitz, 2002

Ballard C, Bannister C, Solis M, et al: The prevalence, associations and symptoms of depression amongst dementia sufferers. J Affect Disord 36:135–144, 1996a

Ballard C, Eastwood C, Gahir M, et al: A follow up study of depression in the carers of dementia sufferers. BMJ 312:947, 1996b

Ballmaier M, Toga AW, Blanton RE, et al: Anterior cingulate, gyrus rectus, and orbitofrontal abnormalities in elderly depressed patients: an MRI-based parcellation of the prefrontal cortex. Am J Psychiatry 161:99–108, 2004

Ballmaier M, Narr KL, Toga AW, et al: Hippocampal morphology and distinguishing late-onset from early onset elderly depression. Am J Psychiatry 165:229–237, 2008

Barnes PM, Powell-Griner E, McFann K, et al: Complementary and alternative medicine use among adults: United States 2002. Adv Data 27:1–19, 2004

Bauer MS: An evidence-based review of psychosocial treatments for bipolar disorder. Psychopharmacol Bull 35:109–134, 2001

Bellino S, Bogetto F, Vaschetto P, et al: Recognition and treatment of dysthymia in elderly patients. Drugs Aging 16:107–121, 2000

Belmaker RH: Bipolar disorder. N Engl J Med 351:476–486, 2004

Belmaker RH: Treatment of bipolar depression. N Engl J Med 356:1771–1773, 2007

Belmaker RH, Agam G: Major depressive disorder. N Engl J Med 358:55–68, 2008

Benedetti A, Scarpellini P, Casamassima F, et al: Bipolar disorder in late life: clinical characteristics in a sample of older adults admitted for manic episode. Clin Pract Epidemiol Ment Health 4:22, 2008

Benoit M, Andrieu S, Lechowski L, et al: Apathy and depression in Alzheimer's disease are associated with functional deficit and psychotropic prescription. Int J Geriatr Psychiatry 23:409–414, 2008

Beyer J, Kuchibhatla M, Gersing K, et al: Medical comorbidity in a bipolar outpatient clinical population. Neuropsychopharmacology 30:401–404, 2005

Blazer DG: Depression in late life: review and commentary. J Gerontol A Biol Sci Med Sci 58:249–265, 2003

Blumer D, Montouris G, Davies K: The interictal dysphoric disorder: recognition, pathogenesis, and treatment of the major psychiatric disorder of epilepsy. Epilepsy Behav 5:826–840, 2004

Bonelli RM, Bugram R: Additional A-criterion for adjustment disorders? Can J Psychiatry 45:763, 2000

Bourin M, Bougerol T, Guitton B, et al: A combination of plant extracts in the treatment of outpatients with adjustment disorder with anxious mood: controlled study versus placebo. Fundam Clin Pharmacol 11:127–132, 1997

Boyle PA, Malloy PF: Treating apathy in Alzheimer's disease. Dement Geriatr Cogn Disord 17:91–99, 2004

Broadhead J, Jacoby R: Mania in old age: a first prospective study. Int J Geriatr Psychiatry 5:215–222, 1990

Brooks BR, Thisted RA, Appel SH, et al: Treatment of pseudobulbar affect in ALS with dextromethorphan/quinidine: a randomized trial. Neurology 63:1364–1370, 2004

Brousseau K, Arciniegas D, Harris S: Pharmacologic management of anxiety and affective lability during recovery from Guillain-Barre syndrome: some preliminary observations. Neuropsychiatr Dis Treat 1:145–149, 2005

Busch KA, Fawcett J, Jacobs DG: Clinical correlates of inpatient suicide. J Clin Psychiatry 64:14–19, 2003

Carlson GA, Goodwin FK: The stages of mania: a longitudinal analysis of the manic episode. Arch Gen Psychiatry 28:221–228, 1973

Carney RM, Freedland KE: Does treating depression improve survival after acute coronary syndrome? Invited commentary on effects of antidepressant treatment following myocardial infarction. Br J Psychiatry 190:467–468, 2007

Chatterjee A, Fahn S: Methylphenidate treats apathy in Parkinson's disease. J Neuropsychiatry Clin Neurosci 14:461–462, 2002

Chen Y, Patel NC, Guo JJ, et al: Antidepressant prophylaxis for post-stroke depression: a meta-analysis. Int Clin Psychopharmacol 22:159–166, 2007

Chengappa KN, Suppes T, Berk M: Treatment of bipolar mania with atypical antipsychotics. Expert Rev Neurother 4 (suppl 2):S17–S25, 2004

Christensen H, Griffiths KM, Jorm AF: Delivering interventions for depression by using the internet: randomised controlled trial. BMJ 328:265, 2004

Clarke DM, Kissane DW: Demoralization: its phenomenology and importance. Aust N Z J Psychiatry 36:733–742, 2002

Clayton P: Bereavement, in Handbook of Affective Disorders. Edited by Paykel E. New York, Guilford, 1982, pp 403–415

Clayton P, Desmarais L, Winokur G: A study of normal bereavement. Am J Psychiatry 125:168–178, 1968

Clayton P, Halikes JA, Maurice WL: The bereavement of the widowed. Dis Nerv Syst 32:597–604, 1971

Coffey CE: Building a system of perfect depression care in behavioral health. Jt Comm J Qual Patient Saf 33:193–199, 2007

Coffey CE, McAllister TW, Silver JM: Guide to Neuropsychiatric Therapeutics. Philadelphia, PA, Lippincott Williams & Wilkins, 2007

Coryell W, Young EA: Clinical predictors of suicide in primary major depressive disorder. J Clin Psychiatry 66:412–417, 2005

Craig D, Mirakhur A, Hart DJ, et al: A cross-sectional study of neuropsychiatric symptoms in 435 patients with Alzheimer's disease. Am J Geriatr Psychiatry 13:460–468, 2005

Cuijpers P, van Straten A, Warmerdam L: Behavioral activation treatments of depression: a meta-analysis. Clin Psychol Rev 27:318–326, 2007a

Cuijpers P, van Straten A, Warmerdam L: Problem solving therapies for depression: a meta-analysis. Eur Psychiatry 22:9–15, 2007b

Cummings JL: Alzheimer's disease. N Engl J Med 351:56–67, 2004

Currier MB, Murray GB, Welch CC: Electroconvulsive therapy for post-stroke depressed geriatric patients. J Neuropsychiatry Clin Neurosci 4:140–144, 1992

Dalgleish T: The emotional brain. Nat Rev Neurosci 5:583–589, 2004

Depp CA, Jeste DV: Bipolar disorder in older adults: a critical review. Bipolar Disord 6:343–367, 2004

Deuschl G: Neurostimulation for Parkinson disease. JAMA 301:104–105, 2009

Devanand DP: Comorbid psychiatric disorders in late life depression. Biol Psychiatry 52:236–242, 2002

Devanand DP, Nobler MS, Singer T, et al: Is dysthymia a different disorder in the elderly? Am J Psychiatry 151:1592–1599, 1994

Dew MA, Whyte EM, Lenze EJ, et al: Recovery from major depression in older adults receiving augmentation of antidepressant pharmacotherapy. Am J Psychiatry 164:892–899, 2007

Drevets WC: Prefrontal cortical-amygdalar metabolism in major depression. Ann N Y Acad Sci 877:614–637, 1999

Duffy JD, Campbell JJ III: The regional prefrontal syndromes: a theoretical and clinical overview. J Neuropsychiatry Clin Neurosci 6:379–387, 1994

Eastham JH, Jeste DV, Young RC: Assessment and treatment of bipolar disorder in the elderly. Drugs Aging 12:205–224, 1998

Ernst C, Angst J: Depression in old age: is there a real decrease in prevalence? A review. Eur Arch Psychiatry Clin Neurosci 245: 272–287, 1995

Evans DL, Byerly MJ, Greer RA: Secondary mania: diagnosis and treatment. J Clin Psychiatry 56(suppl):31–37, 1995

Ferreira-Lay P, Miller S: The quality of internet information on depression for lay people. Psychiatr Bull 32:170–173, 2008

Fox S: Older Americans and the Internet. Washington, DC, Pew Internet and American Life Project, 2004

Frank JD: Psychotherapy: the restoration of morale. Am J Psychiatry 131:271–274, 1974

George MS, Padberg F, Schlaepfer TE, et al: Controversy: repetitive transcranial magnetic stimulation or transcranial direct current stimulation shows efficacy in treating psychiatric diseases. Brain Stimulat 2:14–21, 2009

Ghaemi SN, Gilmer WS, Goldberg JF, et al: Divalproex in the treatment of acute bipolar depression: a preliminary double-blind, randomized, placebo-controlled pilot study. J Clin Psychiatry 68:1840–1844, 2007

Ghazi-Noori S, Chung TH, Deane K, et al: Therapies for depression in Parkinson's disease. Cochrane Database of Systematic Reviews 2003, Issue 3. Art. No.: CD003465. DOI: 10.1002/14651858.CD003465

Glassman AH, Bigger JT Jr: Antidepressants in coronary heart disease: SSRIs reduce depression, but do they save lives? JAMA 297:411–412, 2007

González-Jaimes EI, Turnbull-Plaza B: Selection of psychotherapeutic treatment for adjustment disorder with depressive mood due to acute myocardial infarction. Arch Med Res 34:298–304, 2003

Goodwin FK, Jamison KR, Ghaemi SN: Manic-Depressive Illness: Bipolar Disorders and Recurrent Depression, 2nd Edition. New York, Oxford University Press, 2007

Gottfries CG, Karlsson I, Nyth AL: Treatment of depression in elderly patients with and without dementia disorders. Int Clin Psychopharmacol 6(suppl):55–64, 1992

Grant BF, Harford TC: Comorbidity between DSM-IV alcohol use disorders and major depression: results of a national survey. Drug Alcohol Depend 39:197–206, 1995

Gray SL, LaCroix AZ, Hanlon JT, et al: Benzodiazepine use and physical disability in community-dwelling older adults. J Am Geriatr Soc 54:224–230, 2006

Green RC, Cupples LA, Kurz A, et al: Depression as a risk factor for Alzheimer disease: the MIRAGE Study. Arch Neurol 60:753–759, 2003

Griffiths KM, Christensen H, Jorm AF, et al: Effect of web-based depression literacy and cognitive-behavioural therapy interventions on stigmatising attitudes to depression: randomised controlled trial. Br J Psychiatry 185:342–349, 2004

Grunebaum MF, Galfalvy HC, Oquendo MA, et al: Melancholia and the probability and lethality of suicide attempts. Br J Psychiatry 184:534–535, 2004

Gurley BJ, Gardner SF, Hubbard MA, et al: Clinical assessment of effects of botanical supplementation on cytochrome P450 phenotypes in the elderly: St John's wort, garlic oil, Panax ginseng and Ginkgo biloba. Drugs Aging 22:525–539, 2005

Hackett ML, Anderson CS, House A, et al: Interventions for preventing depression after stroke. Cochrane Database of Systematic Reviews 2008a, Issue 3. Art. No.: CD003689. DOI: 10.1002/14651858.CD003689.pub3

Hackett ML, Anderson CS, House A, et al: Interventions for treating depression after stroke. Cochrane Database of Systematic Reviews 2008b, Issue 4. Art. No.: CD003437. DOI: 10.1002/14651858.CD003437.pub3

Hemenway D, Miller M: Association of rates of household handgun ownership, lifetime major depression, and serious suicidal thoughts with rates of suicide across U.S. census regions. Inj Prev 8:313–316, 2002

Henry C, Van den Bulke D, Bellivier F, et al: Affective lability and affect intensity as core dimensions of bipolar disorders during euthymic period. Psychiatry Res 159:1–6, 2008

Hensley PL: Treatment of bereavement-related depression and traumatic grief. J Affect Disord 92:117–124, 2006

Howland RH, Schettler PJ, Rapaport MH, et al: Clinical features and functioning of patients with minor depression. Psychother Psychosom 77:384–389, 2008

Imel ZE, Malterer MB, McKay KM, et al: A meta-analysis of psychotherapy and medication in unipolar depression and dysthymia. J Affect Disord 110:197–206, 2008

Irie F, Masaki KH, Petrovitch H, et al: Apolipoprotein E epsilon4 allele genotype and the effect of depressive symptoms on the risk of dementia in men: the Honolulu-Asia Aging Study. Arch Gen Psychiatry 65:906–912, 2008

Jarvik LF: Aging and depression: some unanswered questions. J Gerontol 31:324–326, 1976

Jones R, Yates WR, Williams S, et al: Outcome for adjustment disorder with depressed mood: comparison with other mood disorders. J Affect Disord 55:55–61, 1999

Jordan JR, Neimeyer RA: Does grief counseling work? Death Stud 27:765–786, 2003

Jorge RE, Robinson RG, Tateno A, et al: Repetitive transcranial magnetic stimulation as treatment of poststroke depression: a preliminary study. Biol Psychiatry 55:398–405, 2004

Kempton MJ, Geddes JR, Ettinger U, et al: Meta-analysis, database, and meta-regression of 98 structural imaging studies in bipolar disorder. Arch Gen Psychiatry 65:1017–1032, 2008

Kenangil G, Orken DN, Ur E, et al: The relation of testosterone levels with fatigue and apathy in Parkinson's disease. Clin Neurol Neurosurg 111:412–414, 2009

Kessing LV: Severity of depressive episodes during the course of depressive disorder. Br J Psychiatry 192:290–293, 2008

Kuehn BM: FDA panel seeks to balance risks in warnings for antidepressants. JAMA 297:573–574, 2007

Landes AM, Sperry SD, Strauss ME: Prevalence of apathy, dysphoria, and depression in relation to dementia severity in Alzheimer's disease. J Neuropsychiatry Clin Neurosci 17:342–349, 2005

Landi F, Onder G, Cesari M, et al: Psychotropic medications and risk for falls among community-dwelling frail older people: an observational study. J Gerontol A Biol Sci Med Sci 60:622–626, 2005

LeDoux JE: Emotion circuits in the brain. Annu Rev Neurosci 23:155–184, 2000

Linde K, Berner MM, Kriston L: St. John's wort for major depression. Cochrane Database of Systematic Reviews 2008, Issue 4. Art. No.: CD000448. DOI: 10.1002/14651858.CD000448.pub3

Lyketsos CG, Olin J: Depression in Alzheimer's disease: overview and treatment. Biol Psychiatry 52:243–252, 2002

Marin RS: Apathy: a neuropsychiatric syndrome. J Neuropsychiatry Clin Neurosci 3:243–254, 1991

Marin RS: Apathy: concept, syndrome, neural mechanisms, and treatment. Semin Clin Neuropsychiatry 1:304–314, 1996

Markowitz JC: Psychotherapy of dysthymia. Am J Psychiatry 151:1114–1121, 1994

Mayberg HS, Liotti M, Brannan SK, et al: Reciprocal limbic-cortical function and negative mood: converging PET findings in depression and normal sadness. Am J Psychiatry 156:675–682, 1999

Mayberg HS, Lozano AM, Voon V, et al: Deep brain stimulation for treatment-resistant depression. Neuron 45:651–660, 2005

McDonald WM, Wermager J: Pharmacologic treatment of geriatric mania. Curr Psychiatry Rep 4:43–50, 2002

McDonald WM, Richard IH, DeLong MR: Prevalence, etiology, and treatment of depression in Parkinson's disease. Biol Psychiatry 54:363–375, 2003

Menza M, Dobkin RD, Marin H, et al: A controlled trial of antidepressants in patients with Parkinson disease and depression. Neurology 72:886–892, 2009

Merikangas KR, Chakravarti A, Moldin SO, et al: Future of genetics of mood disorders research. Biol Psychiatry 52:457–477, 2002

Meyers BS, Flint AJ, Rothschild AJ, et al: A double-blind randomized controlled trial of olanzapine plus sertraline vs. olanzapine plus placebo for psychotic depression. Arch Gen Psychiatry 66:838–847, 2009

Miklowitz DJ, Otto MW, Frank E, et al: Intensive psychosocial intervention enhances functioning in patients with bipolar depression: results from a 9-month randomized controlled trial. Am J Psychiatry 164:1340–1347, 2007a

Miklowitz DJ, Otto MW, Frank E, et al: Psychosocial treatments for bipolar depression: a 1-year randomized trial from the Systematic Treatment Enhancement Program. Arch Gen Psychiatry 64: 419–426, 2007b

Miller AH, Maletic V, Raison CL: Inflammation and its discontents: the role of cytokines in the pathophysiology of major depression. Biol Psychiatry 65:732–741, 2009

Mitchell AJ, Subramaniam H: Prognosis of depression in old age compared to middle age: a systematic review of comparative studies. Am J Psychiatry 162:1588–1601, 2005

Mizrahi R, Starkstein SE: Epidemiology and management of apathy in patients with Alzheimer's disease. Drugs Aging 24:547–554, 2007

Monastero R, Mariani E, Camarda C, et al: Association between apolipoprotein E epsilon4 allele and apathy in probable Alzheimer's disease. Acta Psychiatr Scand 113:59–63, 2006

Mottram P, Wilson K, Strobl J: Antidepressants for depressed elderly. Cochrane Database of Systematic Reviews 2006, Issue 1. Art. No.: CD003491. DOI: 10.1002/14651858.CD003491.pub2

Murray GB, Shea V, Conn DK: Electroconvulsive therapy for poststroke depression. J Clin Psychiatry 47:258–260, 1986

Nelson JC, Delucchi K, Schneider LS: Efficacy of second generation antidepressants in late-life depression: a meta-analysis of the evidence. Am J Geriatr Psychiatry 16:558–567, 2008

Norman S, Troster AI, Fields JA, et al: Effects of depression and Parkinson's disease on cognitive functioning. J Neuropsychiatry Clin Neurosci 14:31–36, 2002

O'Connor MK, Knapp R, Husain M, et al: The influence of age on the response of major depression to electroconvulsive therapy: a C.O.R.E. report. Am J Geriatr Psychiatry 9:382–390, 2001

Palomäki H, Kaste M, Berg A, et al: Prevention of poststroke depression: 1 year randomised placebo controlled double blind trial of mianserin with 6 month follow up after therapy. J Neurol Neurosurg Psychiatry 66:490–494, 1999

Panitch HS, Thisted RA, Smith RA, et al: Randomized, controlled trial of dextromethorphan/quinidine for pseudobulbar affect in multiple sclerosis. Ann Neurol 59:780–787, 2006

Parker G, Roy K, Hadzi-Pavlovic D, et al: The differential impact of age on the phenomenology of melancholia. Psychol Med 31: 1231–1236, 2001

Parkes CM: Bereavement in adult life. BMJ 316:856–859, 1998

Parvizi J, Arciniegas DB, Bernardini GL, et al: Diagnosis and management of pathological laughter and crying. Mayo Clin Proc 81:1482–1486, 2006

Parvizi J, Coburn K, Shillcutt S, et al: Neuroanatomy of pathological laughing and crying: a report of the American Neuropsychiatric Association Committee on Research. J Clin Neuropsychiatry Clin Neurosci 21:75–87, 2009

Paterniti S, Dufouil C, Alperovitch A: Long-term benzodiazepine use and cognitive decline in the elderly: the Epidemiology of Vascular Aging Study. J Clin Psychopharmacol 22:285–293, 2002

Patra KK, Coffey CE: Implications of herbal alternative medicine for electroconvulsive therapy. J ECT 20:186–194, 2004

Pedersen KF, Larsen JP, Alves G, et al: Prevalence and clinical correlates of apathy in Parkinson's disease: a community-based study. Parkinsonism Relat Disord 15:295–299, 2009

Phillips ML, Drevets WC, Rauch SL, et al: Neurobiology of emotion perception, I: the neural basis of normal emotion perception. Biol Psychiatry 54:504–514, 2003a

Phillips ML, Drevets WC, Rauch SL, et al: Neurobiology of emotion perception, II: implications for major psychiatric disorders. Biol Psychiatry 54:515–528, 2003b

Pinquart M, Duberstein PR, Lyness JM: Treatments for later-life depressive conditions: a meta-analytic comparison of pharmacotherapy and psychotherapy. Am J Psychiatry 163:1493–1501, 2006

Pluck GC, Brown RG: Apathy in Parkinson's disease. J Neurol Neurosurg Psychiatry 73:636–642, 2002

Pollock BG, Mulsant BH, Rosen J, et al: Comparison of citalopram, perphenazine, and placebo for the acute treatment of psychosis and behavioral disturbances in hospitalized, demented patients. Am J Psychiatry 159:460–465, 2002

Polyakova I, Knobler HY, Ambrumova A, et al: Characteristics of suicidal attempts in major depression versus adjustment reactions. J Affect Disord 47:159–167, 1998

Prigerson HG, Shear MK, Jacobs SC, et al: Consensus criteria for traumatic grief: a preliminary empirical test. Br J Psychiatry 174:67–73, 1999

Rao V, Lyketsos CG: The benefits and risks of ECT for patients with primary dementia who also suffer from depression. Int J Geriatr Psychiatry 15:729–735, 2000

Rasmussen A, Lunde M, Poulsen DL, et al: A double-blind, placebo-controlled study of sertraline in the prevention of depression in stroke patients. Psychosomatics 44:216–221, 2003

Ready RE, Friedman J, Grace J, et al: Testosterone deficiency and apathy in Parkinson's disease: a pilot study. J Neurol Neurosurg Psychiatry 75:1323–1326, 2004

Reynolds CF III, Miller MD, Pasternak RE, et al: Treatment of bereavement-related major depressive episodes in later life: a controlled study of acute and continuation treatment with nortriptyline and interpersonal psychotherapy. Am J Psychiatry 156: 202–208, 1999

Reza A, Mercy JA, Krug E: Epidemiology of violent deaths in the world. Inj Prev 7:104–111, 2001

Richard IH: Depression and apathy in Parkinson's disease. Curr Neurol Neurosci Rep 7:295–301, 2007

Risch N, Herrell R, Lehner T, et al: Interaction between the serotonin transporter gene (5-HTTLPR), stressful life events, and risks of depression: a meta-analysis. JAMA 301:2462–2471, 2009

Robert PH, Berr C, Volteau M, et al: Apathy in patients with mild cognitive impairment and the risk of developing dementia of Alzheimer's disease: a one-year follow-up study. Clin Neurol Neurosurg 108:733–736, 2006

Robinson RG, Jorge RE, Moser DJ, et al: Escitalopram and problem-solving therapy for prevention of poststroke depression: a randomized controlled trial. JAMA 299:2391–2400, 2008

Robinson RG, Jorge RE, Clarence-Smith K, et al: Double-blind treatment of apathy in patients with poststroke depression using nefiracetam. J Neuropsychiatry Clin Neurosci 21:144–151, 2009

Rutter M, Thapar A, Pickles A: Gene-environment interactions. Arch Gen Psychiatry 66:1287–1289, 2009

Sachs GS, Nierenberg AA, Calabrese JR, et al: Effectiveness of adjunctive antidepressant treatment for bipolar depression. N Engl J Med 356:1711–1722, 2007

Schatzberg AF: Anxiety and adjustment disorder: a treatment approach. J Clin Psychiatry 51(suppl):20–24, 1990. Erratum in: J Clin Psychiatry 52:140, 1991.

Schiffer RB, Herndon RM, Rudick RA: Treatment of pathologic laughing and weeping with amitriptyline. N Engl J Med 312:1480–1482, 1985

Schut H, Stroebe MS: Interventions to enhance adaptation to bereavement. J Palliat Med 8(suppl):S140–S147, 2005

Shear K, Frank E, Houck PR, et al: Treatment of complicated grief: a randomized controlled trial. JAMA 293:2601–2608, 2005

Sheline YI: Neuroimaging studies of mood disorder effects on the brain. Biol Psychiatry 54:338–352, 2003

Shulman KI: Recent developments in epidemiology, comorbidity, and outcome of old age. Rev Clin Gerontol 6:249–254, 1996

Shulman KI: Disinhibition syndromes, secondary mania and bipolar disorder in old age. J Affect Disord 46:175–182, 1997

Shulman KI, Tohen M, Satlin A, et al: Mania compared with unipolar depression in old age. Am J Psychiatry 149:341–345, 1992

Slaughter JR, Slaughter KA, Nichols D, et al: Prevalence, clinical manifestations, etiology, and treatment of depression in Parkinson's disease. J Neuropsychiatry Clin Neurosci 13:187–196, 2001

Slavney PR: Diagnosing demoralization in consultation psychiatry. Psychosomatics 40:325–329, 1999

Starkstein SE, Manes F: Apathy and depression following stroke. CNS Spectr 5:43–50, 2000

Starkstein SE, Fedoroff P, Berthier ML, et al: Manic-depressive and pure manic states after brain lesions. Biol Psychiatry 29:149–158, 1991

Starkstein SE, Jorge R, Mizrahi R, et al: A prospective longitudinal study of apathy in Alzheimer's disease. J Neurol Neurosurg Psychiatry 77:8–11, 2006

Stone K: Mania in the elderly. Br J Psychiatry 155:220–224, 1989

Strain JJ, Diefenbacher A: The adjustment disorders: the conundrums of the diagnoses. Compr Psychiatry 49:121–130, 2008

Strakowski SM, Delbello MP, Adler CM: The functional neuroanatomy of bipolar disorder: a review of neuroimaging findings. Mol Psychiatry 10:105–116, 2005

Stroebe MS: Handbook of Bereavement Research and Practice: Advances in Theory and Intervention. Washington, DC, American Psychological Association, 2008

Suppes T, Dennehy EB, Hirschfeld RM, et al: The Texas implementation of medication algorithms: update to the algorithms for treatment of bipolar I disorder. J Clin Psychiatry 66:870–886, 2005a

Suppes T, Kelly DI, Perla JM: Challenges in the management of bipolar depression. J Clin Psychiatry 66(suppl):11–16, 2005b

Taylor MA, Fink M: Melancholia: The Diagnosis, Pathophysiology, and Treatment of Depressive Illness. New York, Cambridge University Press, 2006

Tohen M, Shulman KI, Satlin A: First-episode mania in late life. Am J Psychiatry 151:130–132, 1994

Tohen M, Chengappa KN, Suppes T, et al: Relapse prevention in bipolar I disorder: 18-month comparison of olanzapine plus mood stabiliser v. mood stabiliser alone. Br J Psychiatry 184:337–345, 2004

Trimble MR: Clinical presentations in neuropsychiatry. Semin Clin Neuropsychiatry 7:11–17, 2002

Unutzer J: Clinical practice: late-life depression. N Engl J Med 357: 2269–2276, 2007

van der Klink JJ, Blonk RW, Schene AH, et al: Reducing long term sickness absence by an activating intervention in adjustment disorders: a cluster randomised controlled design. Occup Environ Med 60:429–437, 2003

van Reekum R, Stuss DT, Ostrander L: Apathy: why care? J Neuropsychiatry Clin Neurosci 17:7–19, 2005

Volz HP, Kieser M: Kava-kava extract WS 1490 versus placebo in anxiety disorders—a randomized placebo-controlled 25-week outpatient trial. Pharmacopsychiatry 30:1–5, 1997

Vreeburg SA, Hoogendijk WJG, van Pelt J, et al: Major depressive disorder and hypothalamic-pituitary-adrenal axis activity. Arch Gen Psychiatry 66:617–626, 2009

Watanabe MD, Martin EM, DeLeon OA, et al: Successful methylphenidate treatment of apathy after subcortical infarcts. J Neuropsychiatry Clin Neurosci 7:502–504, 1995

Weiner RD (ed): The Practice of Electroconvulsive Therapy: Recommendations for Treatment, Training, and Privileging. A Task Force Report of the American Psychiatric Association, 2nd Edition. Washington, DC, American Psychiatric Association, 2001

Weintraub D, Moberg PJ, Duda JE, et al: Effect of psychiatric and other nonmotor symptoms on disability in Parkinson's disease. J Am Geriatr Soc 52:784–788, 2004

Weintraub D, Morales KH, Moberg PJ, et al: Antidepressant studies in Parkinson's disease: a review and meta-analysis. Mov Disord 20:1161–1169, 2005

World Health Organization: International Statistical Classification of Diseases and Related Health Problems, 10th Revision. Geneva, World Health Organization, 1992

Young RC, Klerman GL: Mania in late life: focus on age at onset. Am J Psychiatry 149:867–876, 1992

Young RC, Gyulai L, Mulsant BH, et al: Pharmacotherapy of bipolar disorder in old age: review and recommendations. Am J Geriatr Psychiatry 12:342–357, 2004

Young RC, Kiosses D, Heo M, et al: Age and ratings of manic psychopathology. Bipolar Disord 9:301–304, 2007

20

Anxiety Disorders

Eric J. Lenze, M.D.
Julie Loebach Wetherell, Ph.D.
Carmen Andreescu, M.D.

Anxiety disorders are common in older adults and cause considerable distress and functional impairment. Due to demographic shifts and inadequate management, geriatric anxiety disorders will become an increasing human and economic burden. Despite their obvious public health importance, they are typically not assessed or managed properly, and many unanswered questions remain regarding their underlying neurobiology and sources of variability in treatment response. Therefore, in this chapter, we review four key issues related to geriatric anxiety disorders: 1) epidemiology and course; 2) neurobiology, neuropsychology, and stress biology; 3) treatment outcome studies; and 4) guidelines for assessment and management.

Anxiety disorders in the geriatric population differ in important ways from anxiety disorders in younger adults. First, they are more detrimental to health and cognition in individuals who, by virtue of age, experience higher rates of medical illness and cognitive decline. As we describe in more detail in this chapter, aging increases vulnerability to adverse health impacts of stress, including cognitive decline. Second, anxiety disorders may be more treatment resistant in older adults than in younger adults. We describe results of recent studies with antidepressant treatment and with psychotherapy that indicate this reduced and/or delayed response to treatment. These observations suggest the need for a more intensive examination of the sources of treatment response variability in geriatric patients with anxiety.

Epidemiology and Course

Epidemiology

Epidemiological studies have produced wide variation in prevalence estimates of anxiety disorders in elderly persons. A review of this topic found 28 published epidemiological studies—19 in community samples and 9 in various clinical samples—of anxiety symptoms or disorders in older adults (Bryant et al. 2008). The review's authors concluded that the prevalence of anxiety disorders ranges from 1.2% to 15% in community samples and from 1% to 28% in medical settings. The prevalence of clinically relevant anxiety symptoms ranges from 15% to 52% in community samples and from 15% to 56% in medical settings.

Such ranges in estimates may be inevitable given the methodological differences across epidemiological studies. However, some authors have questioned whether diagnostic criteria and the methods used to observe them are adequate in detecting mental disorders in older adults (Jeste et al. 2005). This issue may be particularly relevant for anxiety disorders, because disorders may manifest differently (Bryant et al. 2008; Flint 2005), measures developed for young adults may not capture fear or anxiety as reported by older adults (Kogan and Edelstein 2004), and somatic symptoms could be attributed by older adults to medical conditions rather than anxiety (Lenze et al. 2005a).

Another relevant point is that existing diagnostic categories for anxiety disorders are not necessarily valid from a neurobiological standpoint. The high comorbidity of anxiety disorders with each other and with unipolar depression (see Chapter 19, "Mood Disorders") underscores the inability of such diagnostic boundaries to adequately capture clinical anxiety. This inadequacy of the current diagnostic system may be particularly relevant for older adults, in whom anxiety symptoms frequently do not conform to current diagnostic criteria (Bryant et al. 2008). Thus, a system based more closely on neurobiology than on diagnostic taxonomy may be particularly helpful in geriatric anxiety, especially given the close linkage of fear and anxiety behaviors to neurobiological substrates (Mobbs et al. 2007; Paulus 2008). Therefore, more collaboration between geriatric mental health researchers and basic science researchers is needed to ensure that advances in anxiety assessment and treatment apply to older age groups.

With these caveats, Table 20–1 shows prevalence estimates from several large epidemiological studies that focused on elderly persons. As a whole, the studies suggest that generalized anxiety disorder (GAD) is the most common anxiety disorder and is as common in older as in younger adults, and that other anxiety disorders are less common, although the concerns about being able to properly diagnose problems such as panic attacks in this age group are noted.

Late-Onset Anxiety

Etiology

Anxiety disorders, particularly social phobia and panic disorder, are usually considered to have onset in childhood or early adulthood. Age-related changes in brain structure or function (see Chapter 2, "Neurobiology of Aging"; Chapter 6, "Imaging the Structure of the Aging Human Brain"; and Chapter 7, "Molecular Imaging in Neuropsychiatry") may reduce the propensity for panic or other highly autonomic responses (Flint et al. 2002). Some have suggested that the onset of anxiety in old age is rare and likely due to an underlying medical problem, such as hyperthyroidism (Flint 2005). On the other hand, a number of anxiogenic stressors—chronic illness and disability, caregiver status, bereavement, or worries related to intractable financial issues—are associated with aging, and a few clinical studies of elderly patients with anxiety disorder have reported that many of the patients had late onset of illness (Lenze et al. 2005b; Le Roux et al. 2005; Sheikh et al. 2004b).

The difficulty of retrospective evaluation of age at onset of mental disorders has been noted (Wiener et al. 1997), however, and the nature of late-onset anxiety may prevent its detection by standard diagnostic measures, which typically require insight into the excessiveness of the fear and avoidance (Bryant et al. 2008). As an example, fear of falling is a common geriatric syndrome—probably the most frequent anxiety reported by older adults (Howland et al. 1993)—and it is marked by high levels of fear and avoidance. Nevertheless, when Gagnon et al. (2005) used a diagnostic measure to examine 48 older adults with fear of falling, only 1 believed the fear to be excessive, a requirement in diagnosing phobia. The one anxiety disorder that seems to manifest commonly in late life is GAD: several studies have suggested that approximately one-half of older adults with GAD have onset later in life (Chou 2009; Lenze et al. 2005b; Le Roux et al. 2005).

Another issue is that many common conditions in older adults could exacerbate anxiety. Dementia can cause anxiety, often manifesting as agitation (Mintzer and Brawman-Mintzer 1996), hoarding syndrome (Saxena et al. 2002), or other atypical symptoms (Starkstein et al. 2007). Many common medical conditions are highly anxiogenic, such as heart disease (Todaro et al. 2007), lung disease (Yohannes et al. 2006), and neurological disease such as Parkinson's disease. Comorbid anxiety is extremely common with late-life depression (Beekman et al. 2000; Lenze et al. 2000). Also, the decline of function that occurs with aging, creating frailty and gait instability, can result in fear of falling (Gagnon et al. 2005; Nagaratnam et al. 2005) or agoraphobic-like behavior, which may not be discerned by standard epidemiological assessments or methodology.

Assessment

Late-onset anxiety disorders usually require a clinical search for a medical or medication-related pathogenesis. Anxiety can be induced by some prescription medications, including frequently prescribed psychiatric medications (e.g., psychostimulants, antidepressants), or can be caused by withdrawal from medications (e.g., sedative-hypnotics, antidepressants). In our experience, ambulatory elderly persons usually know (or sometimes overinterpret) that a medication they are taking causes anxiety; however, hospitalized, institutionalized, or cognitively impaired elderly are much less likely to be aware of medication changes and, therefore, to have insight into a medication-related cause of anxiety. Clinicians should also note that elderly persons are likely to have polypharmacy and that combinations of fairly benign medications might result in cumulative or interactive effects (e.g., combination of several anticholinergics, or one drug inhibiting the metabolism of another).

Course

Anxiety disorders are among the most chronic and persistent syndromes in mental health. Findings from the few longitudinal studies of older adults with anxiety suggest that anxiety is similarly persistent in this age group (Schuurmans et al. 2005). Between 60% and 70% of anxious older adults in epidemiological and treatment-seeking samples retrospectively report an onset in or before early adulthood (Blazer et al. 1991; Lenze et al. 2005b; Le Roux et al. 2005; Sheikh et al. 1991).

Like depression, anxiety has a strong and bidirectional relationship with disability in older adults (Lenze et al. 2001). Anxiety's association with disability is greater with increasing age (Brenes et al. 2008). Anxiety increases disability (Brenes et al. 2005) and potentially elevates mortality risk (Brenes et al. 2007). Significant quality-of-life impairment has been noted in older adults with GAD, similar to that seen in older adults with late-life depression (Porensky et al. 2009; Wetherell et al. 2004).

TABLE 20–1. Prevalence of anxiety disorders in elderly persons in six community studies

	LASA (Beekman et al. 1998)	ECA (Flint 1994)	AMSTEL (Schoevers et al. 2003)	NMHWS (Trollor et al. 2007)	CCHS (Cairney et al. 2008)	NCS-R (Gum et al. 2009)
N	3,107	5,702	4,051	1,792	12,792	1,461
Age	55–85	65+	65–84	65+	55+	65+
Any anxiety disorder	10.2%	5.5%	NA	4.4%	NA	7.0%
GAD	7.3%	1.9%[a]	3.2%	2.4%	NA	1.2%
Any phobia	3.1%	4.8%	NA	NA	NA	4.7%[b]
Social phobia	NA	NA	NA	0.6%	1.3%	2.3%
Agoraphobia	NA	NA	NA	0.8%[c]	0.6%	0.4%
Panic disorder	1.0%	0.1%	NA	0.8%[c]	0.8%	0.7%
OCD	0.6%	0.8%	NA	0.1%	NA	NA
PTSD	0.9%	NA	NA	1.0%	NA	0.4%

Note. AMSTEL=Amsterdam Study of the Elderly; CCHS=Canadian Community Health Survey; ECA=Epidemiologic Catchment Area; GAD=generalized anxiety disorder; LASA=Longitudinal Aging Study Amsterdam; NA=not assessed; NCS-R=National Comorbidity Study–Replication; NMHWS=Australian National Mental Health and Well-Being Survey; OCD=obsessive-compulsive disorder; PTSD=posttraumatic stress disorder.

[a]Prevalence estimate of GAD in ECA is from one site only.

[b]Prevalence estimate from NCS-R is for specific phobia.

[c]Prevalence estimate from NMHWS is for panic disorder and/or agoraphobia.

Comorbid Anxiety and Depression

Elderly patients with comorbid depression and anxiety have greater somatic symptoms, greater likelihood of suicidal ideation (Jeste et al. 2006; Lenze et al. 2000), a higher risk of suicide (Allgulander and Lavori 1993), and a delayed or diminished response to antidepressants (see Chapter 19, "Mood Disorders"). Longitudinally, anxiety symptoms appear to be more stable over time than depressive symptoms and more likely to lead to depressive symptoms than vice versa (Wetherell et al. 2001). Anxiety disorders could be a risk factor for late-life depression, as has been suggested in young adults (Hettema et al. 2006). Conversely, the combination of anxiety and depression may appear simultaneously (Lenze et al. 2005b), as has been reported in young adults; in this case, anxiety symptoms often persist after remission of depression and increase risk for depressive relapse (Dombrovski et al. 2007; Flint and Rifat 1997b). Thus, it may be the greater persistence over time of anxiety symptoms that leads to the poorer outcomes in comorbid late-life depression and anxiety.

Many studies have demonstrated a longer time to depression treatment response and/or a reduced response rate in patients with comorbid anxiety symptoms or disorders (Andreescu et al. 2007; Flint and Rifat 1997a; Steffens and McQuoid 2005), although other research disputes these findings (Nelson et al. 2009). Additionally, some preliminary research suggests that comorbid anxiety predicts greater decline in memory during long-term follow-up of late-life depression (DeLuca et al. 2005).

On the whole, these studies support the conceptualization of anxious depression as a severe treatment-relevant subtype of late-life depression. A key gap in this literature, then, is an understanding of what exactly this comorbidity reflects. Further research must determine whether "anxious depression" reflects diagnostic or dimensional phenotypic overlap; or a common neurobiological, behavioral, and/or psychological underpinning (e.g., rumination and worry); or some additional illness entirely. Studies must also clarify whether anxious depression is particularly relevant in geriatrics (e.g., by causing more severe cognitive decline).

Neuropsychiatry of Anxiety in Older Adults

Neurobiology of Anxiety

Understanding the neuropsychiatry of anxiety in older adults requires comprehension of the underlying structural and functional neuroanatomy of geriatric anxiety, much of which is yet uncharted. Most of the evidence is adopted from midlife neurobiological studies and includes amygdala hyperactivation in panic disorders and specific phobias; insula hyperactivation in GAD, phobias, and posttraumatic stress disorder (PTSD); and right prefrontal hyperactivation and altered coupling of the amygdala-prefrontal circuit in anxious arousal (Bishop 2007; R.J. Davidson 2002; LeDoux 2000; Stein et al. 2007). However, the neural network abnormalities described in younger adults might not be entirely translatable into older adults, given the various anatomical and pathophysiological changes observed in the aging brain (Smith et al. 2007) (see Chapter 2, "Neurobiology of Aging").

The amygdala-prefrontal circuitry is centrally involved in the neurobiology of anxiety throughout the life span (Figure 20–1). This circuit enables both representations of salient emotions and implementation of top-down control mechanisms to influence interpretative processes (Bishop 2007). Disruption of this circuitry, including deficient recruitment of prefrontal control mechanisms and amygdala hyperresponsivity to threat, leads to a sustained threat-related processing bias in anxious individuals (Bishop 2007). Excessive anxiety triggers various anxiety-regulation strategies, ranging from simple attentional control to higher-level cognitive restructuring used to modulate emotion perception and response (Ochsner and Gross 2005). Most often anxiety-regulation strategies involve higher-level cognitive restructuring through the medial prefrontal cortex (mPFC) (Amodio and Frith 2006; R.J. Davidson et al. 1999; Erk et al. 2006). Top-down conscious reinterpretation reappraises potentially threatening stimuli as less threatening (Bishop 2007; Simmons et al. 2008) through the activation of the cingulate cortex and the mPFC (Bishop 2007; LeDoux 2000; Simmons et al. 2008). From the large area of the mPFC involved in the top-down reappraisal of threatening stimuli, some reports have delineated the subgenual anterior cingulate cortex (sACC) (the affective division of the ACC) as a key region in assessing the salience of emotional information and the regulation of emotional response (Bissiere et al. 2008; Bush et al. 2000).

Inappropriate recruitment of the sACC during emotional events is one of the functional neuroanatomical bases of clinical anxiety (Bissiere et al. 2008; Simmons et al. 2008). One other brain region frequently described in anxiety-related studies is the insula, which is associated with the discomfort of one's own physiological responses to emotionally salient stimuli (Amodio and Frith 2006). Several reports have described increased insula activation in young anxiety-prone adults (Arce et al. 2008; Stein and Stein 2008; Stein et al. 2007). Abnormalities in the prefrontal and limbic-paralimbic cortex likely exist in anxiety disorders, although it is not clear if these findings are disorder specific and/or reflect common etiological and vulnerability factors that result in common pathophysiological profiles that span through all anxiety disorders (Deckersbach et al. 2006).

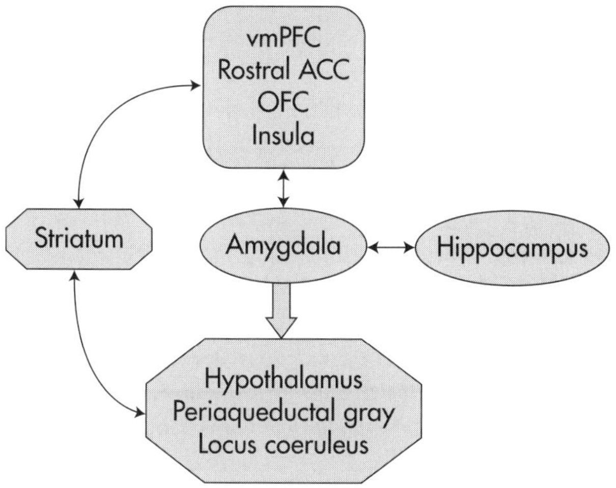

FIGURE 20–1. The neural circuitry of anxiety.
ACC=anterior cingulate cortex; OFC=orbitofrontal cortex; vmPFC=ventromedial prefrontal cortex.

Degeneration in brain regions associated with adaptive responses to anxiety (e.g., the dorsolateral prefrontal cortex) may reduce the individual's ability to modulate the anxious response, thereby undermining protective factors such as cognitive control of affect that otherwise kept an anxiety disorder from manifesting earlier.

Neuropsychiatric Conditions Associated With Anxiety in Older Adults

In patients with neurodegenerative disease that results in pathological anxiety, the pathophysiology is likely to be network dysregulation, including centrally the dysregulation of the sACC-amygdala axis (Bissiere et al. 2008). Given this disconnectivity hypothesis, neuropsychiatric conditions that affect subcortical white matter, or the functioning of cortical and subcortical components of this network, are likely to be anxiogenic. Of course, the anxiety that frequently arises in stroke and other medical conditions may also reflect their status as anxiogenic life stressors (e.g., leading to sudden or chronic loss of control).

Parkinson's disease (see Chapter 24, "Parkinson's Disease and Movement Disorders") may be a particularly anxiogenic neurodegenerative illness because of its association not only with subcortical disease, but also with autonomic dysfunction (potentially leading to panic attacks or similar autonomic symptoms), and the uncontrollability over basic movements and activities it causes (Lauterbach et al. 2003; Marsh 2000; Richard et al. 1996). Huntington's disease (also discussed in Chapter 24) is another subcortical neurodegenerative disease with a high prevalence of anxiety symptoms (Paulsen et al. 2001). Traumatic brain injury (TBI; see Chapter 26) can result in diffuse axonal injury, likely leading to the high observed prevalence of post-TBI anxiety symptoms (Jorge et al. 1993).

Stroke (see Chapter 25, "Cerebrovascular Disease") can cause anxiety symptoms (De Wit et al. 2008), GAD (Astrom 1996; Castillo et al. 1995), or obsessive-compulsive disorder (Swoboda and Jenike 1995). As with depression, some evidence suggests that left hemisphere lesions may be more likely to cause anxiety (Barker-Collo 2007), although the pathophysiology underlying this link is unclear.

Dementing illness (see Chapter 16, "Alzheimer's Disease and the Frontotemporal Dementia Syndromes") can cause anxiety symptoms (Ballard et al. 2000; Lyketsos et al. 2002) or GAD (Starkstein et al. 2007). Consistent with the disconnectivity hypothesis is evidence that amyloid binding in the posterior cingulate region is associated with increased anxiety symptoms in older adults without dementia (Lavretsky et al. 2009). Finally, epilepsy (see Chapter 27) is associated with anxiety (Marsh and Rao 2002).

The link between chronic anxiety and neuropsychiatric disorders of aging (e.g., Alzheimer's disease, cerebrovascular disease) is also likely bidirectional, with anxiety causing or exacerbating these disorders. Anxiety symptoms or disorders in elderly adults are associated with accelerated cognitive decline (DeLuca et al. 2005; Palmer et al. 2007; Sinoff and Werner 2003). This is particularly true in older adults, because aging increases vulnerability to adverse effects of stress, due to diminished homeostatic mechanisms that in younger people prevent an excessive biological stress response and its deleterious effects (Lenze and Wetherell 2009; Urry et al. 2006). As a result, pathological anxiety in late life is associated with activation of the hypothalamic-pituitary-adrenal (HPA) axis, leading to higher cortisol levels (Mantella et al. 2008). Aging individuals are likely more susceptible to such elevations and their putative toxic effects, because homeostatic control is reduced (in the brain and systemically). Research shows increases in β-amyloid 42 peptide ($A\beta_{42}$) production and tau hyperphosphorylation attributable to excessive HPA activation (mediated via corticotropin-releasing factor-1 [CRF1]), suggesting a direct link between chronic stress, increased CRF production, and the putative pathogenic steps in Alzheimer's disease (Csernansky et al. 2006; Green et al. 2006; Kang et al. 2007).

Vascular disease, including cerebrovascular disease, is increasingly recognized as the main cause of premature mortality in patients with mental illness (Newcomer and Hennekens 2007), and more recent research has elucidated mechanisms between anxiety in elderly patients and in cerebrovascular disease via insulin resistance, endothelial reactivity, and impaired autonomic function (Narita et al. 2008). Elevated blood pressure in anxious older adults improves with the treatment of the anxiety disorder (Lenze et al. 2009). Research in stress and cellular aging (Epel et al. 2004, 2006) has given rise to the hypothesis that chronic affective disorders lead, via oxidative stress, to decreased telomerase activity and telomere shrinkage (Simon et al. 2006), another mechanism by which chronic anxiety may be accelerating the aging process. Finally, altering serotonin function in an aging model modifies not only stress responsivity but also age-related neurodegeneration (Sibille et al. 2007).

Neuropsychological Impairments in Late-Life Anxiety

Neuropsychological impairments are common and clinically significant components of late-life emotional disorders, particularly in domains of memory, attention, and executive function. A review of cognitive impairment in late-life anxiety concluded that anxiety and cognitive impairment have a consistent and bidirectional relationship in older adults (Beaudreau and O'Hara 2008). Particularly in older adults, anxiety impairs working memory, attention, and problem-solving ability (Cohen et al. 1980; Deptula et al. 1993; Hogan 2003). Other investigations have extended these observations to clinical samples, describing poorer short-term memory in geriatric patients with GAD (Mantella et al. 2007) and poorer working memory in those with greater GAD symptoms (Caudle et al. 2007). Anxiety symptoms appear to predict cognitive decline in older adults (Wetherell et al. 2002). Geriatric GAD is associated with mild impairments in immediate and delayed recall, working memory, and executive function (Caudle et al. 2007; Mantella et al. 2007; Mohlman and Gorman 2005), as contrasted with geriatric depression, in which more widespread cognitive deficits are noted (Mantella et al. 2007).

Cognitive performance was examined as a predictor of psychotherapy outcome in a pooled sample of data from cognitive-behavioral therapy (CBT) studies for geriatric GAD (Caudle et al. 2007). In this analysis, errors in temporal orientation predicted poorer maintenance of treatment gains at 6-month follow-up. There was a trend toward poorer 6-month maintenance among those with poorer working memory. These data suggest that mild cognitive impairment may reduce the efficacy of CBT for geriatric GAD, particularly as a maintenance treatment.

It is possible that psychotherapy response is more sensitive than pharmacotherapy response to the relatively subtle pattern of cognitive deficits associated with geriatric GAD. Because the ability to engage in learning-based psychotherapy is contingent upon intact memory and executive function, neuropsychological impairment may moderate the efficacy of CBT. Cognitive impairment, particularly executive dysfunction, is associated with poorer response to pharmacotherapy and to psychotherapy for geriatric depression (Alexopoulos et al. 2008); however, it remains unclear whether this same relationship is seen with medication for anxiety.

Despite the wealth of research in the stress, immunology, and aging fields that could be applied to elucidate these connections, to our knowledge no longitudinal research has been done examining long-term consequences of chronic pathological anxiety in late life. Nevertheless, the research discussed above generates the hypothesis that treating late-life anxiety would slow down or prevent neuropsychiatric complications of aging, via the mechanisms described.

Treatment Studies

Treatments for young adults with anxiety disorders may not have the same benefits or risks in older adults and, in the case of psychotherapy, typically need to be adapted for this age group (Knight 2004; Lenze and Wetherell 2009). In this section, we summarize treatment literature in geriatric anxiety disorders and then distill this literature into a set of management guidelines.

Although both psychotherapy and pharmacotherapy appear to be effective treatment options in older adults (Wetherell et al. 2005b), a meta-analysis and one direct randomized comparison of pharmacotherapy and psychotherapy found medications to be more effective than CBT in the acute phase of treatment (Pinquart and Duberstein 2007; Schuurmans et al. 2006). Given the paucity of overall treatment research, particularly long-term studies, however, there is at this point insufficient evidence to support a consensus about whether psychotherapy or medication should be first-line treatment. Likely, a patient's and provider's preferences will decide.

Regarding long-term management of GAD, naturalistic follow-up studies of older patients treated with CBT have demonstrated maintenance of gains for up to 1 year following discontinuation of treatment (Stanley et al. 2003). Benefits of CBT relative to supportive counseling were greater at 1 year follow-up than immediately following treatment in a sample of patients who had been treated for at least 3 months with medications before receiving CBT, suggesting that sustained or increasing gains are possible for older adults receiving CBT for anxiety following an acute course of pharmacotherapy (Barrowclough et al. 2001).

Psychotherapy

It remains unclear whether CBT is superior to other psychotherapy approaches in treating late-life anxiety disorders; however, CBT is presently the dominant and most widely available formal psychotherapy for anxiety disorders. CBT might be particularly effective for anxiety disorders in older adults who are able to learn new skills in therapy and use them

TABLE 20–2. Example of a modular cognitive-behavioral therapy (CBT) protocol for late-life anxiety disorders

Module	Description
Education/monitoring (2 sessions)	Introduce biopsychosocial model of anxiety; goals and requirements of CBT, including need for daily practice; motivational interviewing techniques, addressing ambivalence about the work involved; discussion of the patient's anxiety symptoms, stressors, and coping repertoire; and the purpose and practice of symptom monitoring.
Relaxation training (3 sessions)	Provide instruction in diaphragmatic breathing, progressive muscle relaxation, and guided imagery.
Problem-solving skills training (3 sessions)	Tackle a major life problem by breaking down the problem-solving process into a series of steps: identify a specific aspect of the problem to be addressed; brainstorm possible solutions; and evaluate, select, and implement a solution.
Cognitive therapy (3 sessions)	Identify cognitive distortions and underlying schema; challenge overestimation of risk and catastrophization.
Skills practice (up to 5 sessions)	Discuss potentially problematic future situations, reviewing skills and strategies that can be applied to manage anxiety in those situations.
Optional modules	**Description**
Family (1 session)	Educate close family member about anxiety; elicit support for patient's participation in treatment program; obtain objective information about patient's anxiety symptoms and behaviors.
Sleep hygiene (1 session)	Introduce good sleep guidelines (e.g., setting a regular schedule for going to bed and waking up, limiting naps).
Behavioral activation (2 sessions)	Encourage identification and scheduling of pleasant events and engaging in them regardless of motivation level.
Exposure (2 sessions)	Develop a fear-avoidance hierarchy, then use systematic desensitization to decrease fear and avoidance.

effectively (Wetherell et al. 2005a). Therefore, consideration of a patient's cognition, motivation, and ability to practice skills should be part of an evaluation for psychotherapy.

Similar to treatment of anxiety in younger adults (Stanley et al. 2004), CBT for late-life anxiety typically involves psychoeducation, relaxation, cognitive therapy, problem-solving skills training, exposure exercises (i.e., exposure and habituation to anxiogenic situations), and sleep hygiene when necessary for the common problem of insomnia (Brenes et al. 2009). In elderly persons, the most effective ingredient of CBT may be relaxation (Thorp et al. 2009). CBT has been shown to be effective in the primary care setting (Stanley et al. 2009), although the lack of highly skilled CBT therapists with experience treating late-life anxiety may at present be a barrier to widespread implementation.

Modular treatment reflects a new approach in psychotherapy research, consistent with personalized medicine in the pharmacological domain. In modular treatment, the patient's presenting problems or symptoms are used to guide the specific components of treatment (Chorpita et al. 2005; Lang et al. 2006). This patient-centered process appears to increase engagement and reduce attrition (Wetherell et al. 2005c, 2009). An example of a modular treatment protocol for older adults with anxiety disorders is shown in Table 20–2.

Booster sessions to prevent loss of efficacy during maintenance treatment are particularly important for older adults, because aging is associated with poorer performance on attention and memory tasks for which internally generated and maintained strategies are required (Prull et al. 2006). Booster sessions are also responsive to life events, which appear to play a role in long-term outcomes from late-life GAD (Wetherell et al. 2009). Booster therapy sessions use the same format as is used for general skills practice during CBT, with an emphasis on skills most applicable to the situation the patient is currently facing. When patients are scheduled for a follow-up booster session, they are assigned at-home practice to complete between sessions.

Adaptations for older adults include using a slower pace with increased repetition, employing less abstract cognitive-restructuring techniques (and correspondingly applying more focus on behavioral change and health-related problems), and incorporating a family session reflecting the importance of engaging the family in geriatric mental health treatment. In addition to in-session discussions and a written summary of material, we audiotape sessions for participants to consolidate their learning. We emphasize problem solving on the basis of the observation that older patients with GAD often employ a perseverative or avoidant problem-solving style (Wetherell et al. 2009) and on the finding that worry about minor matters may be less prominent among older adults with GAD than among younger patients with GAD, relative to excessive and uncontrollable worry about more substantial problems (Wetherell et al. 2003b). Another possible adaptation is the integration of religion into CBT, particularly for older adults who may have more of a spiritual than cognitive view of their emotional lives (Paukert et al. 2009).

One other psychotherapy treatment, often overlooked, is bibliotherapy (Brenes et al. 2010). A study of late-life anxiety and depression prevention found that a stepped-care approach, in which the first intervention was bibliotherapy, was effective at preventing anxiety and depressive episodes (van't Veer-Tazelaar et al. 2009). Many self-help workbooks exist for anxiety disorders, although none to our knowledge are focused on older adults. Also, many patients are using the Internet as a guide for treatment, but it is unknown how much this is the case for older adults.

Pharmacotherapy

The evidence base for pharmacotherapy in older adults is limited and consists mainly of several small clinical trials, many quite old and in mixed populations. Benzodiazepines are the most commonly used pharmacological treatment for geriatric anxiety (Benitez et al. 2008), despite the association of these medications with falls (Landi et al. 2005), disability (Gray et al. 2006), and cognitive impairment and decline (Paterniti et al. 2002).

Two small randomized controlled trials (RCTs) (Lenze et al. 2005c; Schuurmans et al. 2006) and a full-scale RCT (Lenze et al. 2009) demonstrated the efficacy of selective serotonin reuptake inhibitors (SSRIs) in the acute treatment of older adults with anxiety disorders, predominantly GAD. Lenze et al. (2009) randomly assigned 177 older adults with GAD to either escitalopram or placebo and found that escitalopram was superior to placebo in cumulative response (69% vs. 51%). Additionally, escitalopram produced improvements in measures of anxiety symptoms, role function, and blood pressure. The effect sizes for most outcome measures in that study were in the low to medium range.

With respect to serotonin-norepinephrine reuptake inhibitors (SNRIs), a retrospective examination of phase 3 extended-release venlafaxine data found the drug to be efficacious in adults ages 60 and older, with an effect size (drug-placebo difference) and side-effect profile similar to those of younger adults (Katz et al. 2002). Similar findings have been reported with duloxetine (J. Davidson et al. 2008). Additionally, a large-scale study found pregabalin to be efficacious in geriatric GAD (Montgomery et al. 2008). The mechanism of action of pregabalin for anxiety is unknown; it binds to auxiliary subunit voltage-gated calcium channels and is thought to reduce the synaptic release of several neurotransmitters. It should be noted that pregabalin has not been approved by the U.S. Food and Drug Administration (FDA) to treat anxiety disorders.

These studies have found side effects in elderly persons that are similar to those in younger adults; however, the studies were not designed to determine some of the more recently reported potential risks of SSRIs in the elderly population, including gait impairment, which increases the risk for falls (Laghrissi-Thode et al. 1995); gastrointestinal bleeding (Yuan et al. 2006); bone loss (Diem et al. 2007); and hyponatremia (Fabian et al. 2004). Such reports suggest that the risk-benefit ratio for acute and long-term SSRI use by older patients is not the same as that for younger adults. These additional concerns require closer monitoring of geriatric patients, particularly when frail or medically ill.

Although most of the pharmacotherapy research has focused on geriatric GAD, some other medication studies should be noted. In research involving patients with PTSD, one study supported the use of citalopram (English et al. 2006), another supported superiority of mirtazapine over an SSRI (Chung et al. 2004), and a third found evidence that the α-adrenergic antagonist prazosin is efficacious for sleep-related concerns in PTSD, although not for other PTSD symptoms (Raskind et al. 2007). In studies of patients with late-life panic disorder, Rampello et al. (2006) found evidence for the superiority of escitalopram over citalopram in time-to-treatment response, and a small open-label study found evidence of benefit from sertraline (Sheikh et al. 2004a). Finally, in the only study to our knowledge testing pharmacotherapy for GAD in the context of stroke, Kimura et al. (2003) found that nortriptyline was efficacious; it should be noted that this was a merged data set of several RCTs of poststroke depression in which patients with comorbid GAD were analyzed.

The only published augmentation study of patients with late-life anxiety disorders was a small study with risperidone (Morinigo et al. 2005). The use of atypical antipsychotics in elderly patients is problematic given concerns about higher mortality with antipsychotics than with placebo in older patients with dementia. It remains unclear whether these risks apply to elderly patients without dementia. No data exist on the efficacy and safety of complementary and alternative medications for anxiety in older adults. This is an important issue because many patients appear to be using such treatments, often without informing their doctors.

Thus, based on these studies, SSRIs and SNRIs are appropriate as first-line pharmacological treatment in late-life anxiety disorders. Benzodiazepines should be used only temporarily, and their use should be accompanied by information about associated risks. The long-term or maintenance treatment of late-life anxiety with medication has not been studied, and no augmentation strategies can be recommended with confidence.

Combining Medication and Psychotherapy

The inadequacy of monotherapy is widely noted in mood and anxiety disorders, and combination treatments may be more effective, particularly antidepressants and CBT (Fava et al. 2005), which have different mechanisms and may be able to treat different components of the illness (Arce et al. 2008; McNally 2007). Fava et al. (2006) suggested that such combination treatment be sequential rather than of simultaneous onset. The advantages of a sequential approach are that 1) it allows the patient and provider to focus sequentially on different aspects of treatment rather than divide focus among multiple treatments and components of illness at once; 2) it is likely more reflective of real clinical practice, in which providers will examine a patient's response to one therapeutic option before adding another; and 3) it allows for one treatment to be a catalyst for the next. In GAD, for example, SSRI treatment can reduce acute distress and somatic symptoms, whereas CBT can be used to teach worry control skills, address cognitive distortions, and improve coping skills. Thus, with two treatments targeting the different facets of the illness, persistent residual features and relapse are less likely.

A final reason for sequenced treatment is that older patients with anxiety disorder often do not wish to continue medications indefinitely (Wetherell and Unutzer 2003). Thus, adding psychotherapy for anxiety control may provide durable improvements, even if medication treatment is then discontinued. A review of meta-analyses concluded that psychotherapies involving cognitive and behavioral strategies for GAD are 1) superior to nondirective therapy and pill placebo and 2) equivalent to pharmacotherapy in the acute phase of treatment, with robust effects extending as long as 10 years following discontinuation of treatment (Butler et al. 2006).

The strategy of sequencing medication with CBT is not without controversy, however, particularly in treating anxiety disorders (Foa et al. 2002; Westra and Stewart 1998). Concerns that have been cited include the following: pharmacotherapy might interfere with the development of self-efficacy or with the successful challenging of catastrophic beliefs during psychotherapy; individuals treated with medications may be less motivated to engage in psychotherapy; and psychotherapy in the context of medications may result in state-dependent learning that does not persist when the medication is discontinued (Barlow et al. 2000; Raffa et al. 2008). Because of this controversy, it will be important to examine the strategy of sequenced medication and CBT within a controlled study design.

For the treatment of anxiety, many patients use complementary medicines, particularly kava, valerian, passionflower, and chamomile (Werneke et al. 2006). A small literature supports anxiolytic (kava, passionflower) or sedative (valerian) properties for some of these agents. The safety and effectiveness of these and related treatments have not been rigorously studied in elderly persons, however. Indeed, kava was recently withdrawn from the United Kingdom market because of concerns about liver toxicity.

Looking Forward: Research in Geriatric Anxiety Disorders

Many questions remain unanswered in geriatric anxiety. How do basic processes of anxiety—fear conditioning, extinction, and attentional bias toward threat—play out in an aging individual (Fox and Knight 2005)? Are genetic and environmental influences different from those in younger adults? What neurobiological paradigms, such as neural circuit connectivity, underlie the development and maintenance of anxiety in older adults?

Regarding treatments, little to nothing is known about what are the optimal long-term strategies or who should receive which treatments. No maintenance studies have examined the long-term benefits of pharmacotherapy in older adults with anxiety disorder. Studies of geriatric anxiety patients treated with CBT have suggested some maintenance of gains for up to 1 year, but carefully controlled maintenance studies are needed (Barrowclough et al. 2001; Stanley et al. 2003; Wetherell et al. 2003a). Such treatment studies should also clarify putative mechanistic links between chronic anxiety and its long-term adverse consequences (such as cognitive decline).

Regarding community-based or implementation research, primary care physicians are the main providers who see geriatric patients with anxiety disorder (Ettner and Hermann 1997; Tolin et al. 2005), yet these physicians typically prescribe benzodiazepines—or no treatment (Benitez et al. 2008; Harman et al. 2002). What is urgently needed, then, are evidence-based and practicable treatment strategies so that primary care physicians can provide or refer their patients to these treatments. Little is known, however, about the barriers to detecting and managing late-life anxiety disorders in patients who present to primary care or other settings (Ettner

TABLE 20–3. Principles of effective management of geriatric anxiety disorders

1. Measure severity and provide objective criteria for assessing response. Additionally, assess comorbidity, prior treatment, cognitive status, and need for a medical workup.
2. Avoid knee-jerk benzodiazepine prescription.
3. Provide psychoeducation about anxiety and treatment, including potential health benefits.
4. Determine first-line treatment according to patient preference, provider preference and competence, and treatment availability.
5. Provide frequent follow-up, particularly within the first month of treatment or dosage change, to encourage adherence and monitor treatment response.
6. With medications, start low, go slow, but *go*—as aggressively as required to treat symptoms to remission.
7. Consider augmentation treatment and refer to experts if necessary.
8. Provide maintenance treatment; evaluate the need for such if treatment is discontinued.

and Hermann 1997). Unlike the many collaborative care studies in late-life depression, no such efforts have focused on late-life anxiety disorders.

Despite, or perhaps because of, these unanswered questions, geriatric anxiety disorders are an ideal "laboratory" for examining neurobiology and treatment surrounding the interrelationship of stress, health, and aging (Lenze and Wetherell 2009). Research on basic behavioral processes in anxiety disorders—such as attentional bias toward threat, abnormal fear conditioning and extinction, and evaluation of ambiguous stimuli—has been greatly augmented by neuroimaging research, specifically functional magnetic resonance imaging of limbic-prefrontal-insular interactions (Bishop 2007). Additionally, the fields of stress neurobiology and aging research intersect in late-life anxiety.

Principles of Effective Management

Eight principles of effective management of geriatric anxiety disorders are discussed below. Table 20–3 provides a summary of these principles.

1. *Measure severity and provide objective criteria for assessing response. Additionally, assess comorbidity, prior treatment, cognitive status, and need for a medical workup.* Detecting anxiety is a necessary precursor to managing it, yet assessment of anxiety is often overlooked by geriatric mental health providers. Older adults often conceptualize anxiety differently than younger adults and may not find terms such as *anxiety* or even *worry* to be relevant, preferring words like *concern*. They may assert that anxiety is a realistic response to their environment or current stressors. A helpful introduction to the topic is to ask about stress (e.g., "Older adults often deal with stress. How do you feel in times of stress?"). Patients who describe symptoms suggestive of anxiety or worry can then be further queried. Of note, asking directly if anxiety or worry is "excessive" or "uncontrollable" is unhelpful. Clinicians should use nondirective questioning to determine the severity of anxiety symptoms. Geriatric anxiety disorders are defined, in presence and severity, by the following: a) level of distress (often detected by asking how much the anxiety symptoms bother the patient, how much he or she thinks about it, and what strategies the patient is trying in order to control or avoid it); b) the amount of time the patient feels worried or tries to manage those feelings; and c) avoidance. Although avoidance is a key component of all anxiety disorders and is one of the most disabling components for older adults, it often is not recognized or is described subtly by patients. For example, older adults may rationalize that changes in behavior patterns are due to perceived poor health, even when their health status is objectively good. Paradoxically, avoidance may also take the form of excessive engagement in activities as a form of distraction or intrusive overinvolvement with family members as an attempt to decrease perceived loss of control.

   Inquiring about somatic symptoms is helpful, because these are often a source of distress. For example, patients may not endorse "panic attacks" but may admit to brief periods with multiple physical symptoms (particularly autonomic symptoms such as palpitations). Likewise, patients with GAD may downplay the effects of worrying on their lives but more readily complain about distress from sleep disturbance or difficulty concentrating (regarding the latter, patients typically interpret this as a memory problem, and anxious elderly patients often have concerns about Alzheimer's disease).

Assessment tools recommended for older adults include the 21-item Beck Anxiety Inventory (Beck et al. 1988) and the 8-item short form of the Penn State Worry Questionnaire (Hopko et al. 2003). Other instruments appropriate for assessment of anxiety in older adults include the clinician-administered Anxiety Disorders Interview Schedule for DSM-IV (DiNardo et al. 1994), Structured Clinical Interview for DSM-IV Axis I Disorders (First et al. 1996), Hamilton Anxiety Scale (Hamilton 1959), and Generalized Anxiety Disorder Severity Scale (Shear et al. 2006). Recommended self-report measures include the Geriatric Anxiety Inventory (Boddice and Pachana 2008), Worry Scale for Older Adults (Wisocki et al. 1986), State-Trait Anxiety Inventory (Stanley et al. 1996), and Zung Self-Rated Anxiety Scale (Zung 1971). The 14-item Hospital Anxiety and Depression Scale (HADS; Zigmond and Snaith 1983) and the 18-item form of the Brief Symptom Inventory (BSI-18; Derogatis 2000) are multidimensional instruments that include anxiety as well as depression; the HADS deliberately excludes symptoms that can reflect underlying medical conditions, and the BSI-18 includes those symptoms in a separate Somatization subscale.

High in the minds of most psychiatrists will be differentiating anxiety from depression. In our experience, patients fail to appreciate the importance we place on this diagnostic distinction. Clinically, the clinician will often have to deal with anxiety as well as depression in a patient, often concurrently.

Only 30%–40% of anxious older adults present with a recent onset of symptoms. Many older adults who present with an anxiety disorder, even of recent onset, describe some long-term, often lifelong, anxiety vulnerability or proneness. This pattern fits with the conceptualization of anxiety vulnerability as hardwired in a neurodevelopmental fashion. As such, a report that "I was never an anxious person, until just recently" should elicit consideration of a medical workup. The medical differentiation of late-onset anxiety is long but generally should consider the following:

- Depression
- Cognitive impairment (dementia, delirium)
- Anxiety-inducing medications (or recent discontinuation of sedatives)
- Common and rare medical conditions that could masquerade as an anxiety disorder; these include thyroid disease, vitamin B_{12} deficiency, hypoxia, ischemia, metabolic changes (e.g., hypercalcemia or hypoglycemia), arrhythmia, or that iconic zebra, pheochromocytoma

2. *Avoid knee-jerk benzodiazepine prescription.* Two studies have demonstrated the acute efficacy of benzodiazepines in reducing symptoms of late-life anxiety (Bresolin et al. 1988; Koepke et al. 1982). However, their use is already common in this age group (van Balkom et al. 2000). Benzodiazepines, like any sedatives, have a poorer risk-benefit ratio in elderly persons than in young adults. As previously noted, they are associated with an increased risk of falling in elderly persons, who already are the age group in which falls and fall-related injuries are most relevant. Using medications with shorter half-lives and less complicated elimination (e.g., lorazepam rather than diazepam) is a widely prescribed recommendation in geriatrics but has not been demonstrated to reduce the risk of falls or fall-related injuries. Furthermore, benzodiazepines appear to cause cognitive impairment, particularly involving recall, in this age group (Pomara et al. 1989, 1998a, 1998b). This cognitive problem is more likely with higher dosages of benzodiazepines and in elderly persons who already have a predisposition for cognitive impairment. Therefore, long-term use of benzodiazepines appears unfavorable in this age group. At a minimum, as part of the informed consent process, patients should be warned about the potential risks associated with these medications.

   Benzodiazepines may provide a fast anxiolytic action; a common recommendation is to use these medications at low dosage as a short-term adjunct, in which case they may provide some early relief and improve adherence to the treatment regimen. Even this short-term adjunctive use of benzodiazepines is typically unnecessary and can reinforce an inappropriate message to patients that anxiety must be immediately relieved, which is akin to an avoidance response. Because many patients will require psychotherapy at some point, sending this contradictory message with benzodiazepine use should be minimized. If a benzodiazepine is coprescribed, a 6-week maximum is recommended, with explanation of this to the patient at the initiation of treatment.
3. *Provide psychoeducation about anxiety and treatment, including potential health benefits.* Psychoeducation may be the most important management step, because most older adults, even those with a lifelong history of anxiety, have never received the diagnosis before. Providers should inform patients that they have a treatable condition and should address stigma, misinformation, and other common and entirely remediable barriers to treatment. Of paramount importance (because psychoeducation will improve treatment adherence) are the implications of treating anxiety for improving the patient's quality of life, health, and cognition.
4. *Determine first-line treatment according to patient preference, provider preference and competence, and treatment availability.* This chapter represents the view that the evidence supporting medication over psychotherapy as a first-line treatment is

still too limited to justify a definitive recommendation. Therefore, it is better that the patient's preference and the provider's competence should decide first-line treatment. First-line options include one or more of the following: SSRI, relaxation training, and/or CBT. Bibliotherapy can be recommended alongside any of these options.

5. *Provide frequent follow-up, particularly within the first month of treatment or dosage change, to encourage adherence and monitor treatment response.* The patient's anxiety will affect his or her views about treatment, particularly with antidepressants, which can initially have a stimulating or mildly anxiogenic effect. Older adults with anxiety disorders often report that they are sensitive to or intolerant of antidepressant medications, comments that appear to stem from their anticipatory concern about side effects, their vigilance toward interoceptive stimuli, and their tendency to catastrophize about any interoceptive sensations they detect (even if unrelated to the antidepressant). In other words, the manifestations of the anxiety itself interfere in many ways with acceptance of and adherence to pharmacotherapy.

   Elderly persons vary from young adults in terms of increased comorbid medical conditions, pharmacokinetic changes, frailty, drug interactions, and side effects. In particular, older and frailer or medically ill individuals need close monitoring (e.g., of gait, vital signs, or any incident medical issues that arise in the context of treatment and the potential role of the antianxiety medication in these problems).

   Overcoming patients' fears related to the medication's potentially negative effects is not an easy task. This task is made more difficult by a medication's laundry list of potential side effects, many of which sound frightening (e.g., hallucinations) or are symptoms that the patient already has (e.g., fatigue, insomnia). Often patients will have refused treatment in the past because of such fears. The management of this fear, as part of the process of engaging the patient in treatment, involves describing how such antidepressant medications have established efficacy and high tolerability. Also, the health care provider should describe his or her own experience in prescribing this medication; specifically state that although side effects are possible, no particular side effect is inevitable; indicate that most patients taking the medication either will have no side effects or will have brief, self-limited side effects that subside in a few weeks; and emphasize that the medication is unlikely to be incapacitating. If a patient appears to be focusing on the list of side effects before or immediately after starting the drug, the clinician should explain that this is a list of all side effects that patients in trials for this medication have described, however infrequently, and that the medication does not necessarily cause these side effects. When patients mention that "I already have that symptom," the clinician should assure them that they are not more likely to have increased symptoms as a side effect. In our experience, physical symptoms tend to decrease rather than increase over the course of treatment (Blank et al. 2006).

   Family involvement can help with adherence. The clinician should take time to address patients' and families' concerns about medication during an initial visit. Nevertheless, patients often have additional concerns between when the medication is prescribed and when they take the first dose (or even when they fill the prescription). The clinician can address this potentiality in several ways: a) by explicitly stating to patients and families that it is natural for patients to have questions, encouraging patients to call at any time to discuss their concerns, and providing 24-hour contact information (typically they do not call but benefit from the knowledge that they can); b) by calling the patient a day or two after the medication is started to ask about and address any questions; and c) by scheduling weekly or biweekly visits, with interim telephone contacts, for the first month of treatment and the month subsequent to a dosage increase, because these are times when patients are most likely to develop concerns about side effects.

   Follow-up includes interviewing patients closely for any concerns about perceived side effects. In our experience, patients frequently have symptoms that they misperceive as side effects, even though the symptom often predates the start of medication or is clearly a symptom of the disorder. For patients with anxiety, adherence issues stem from vigilance to perceived side effects and subsequent catastrophizing. If such an issue is noted (even if the patient does not bring it up spontaneously or expresses that he or she does not think it is "important"), an immediate contact by the treating psychiatrist should be made, usually as a same-day phone call. This reassures the patient that he or she is being monitored closely by experts and that the medication is not causing some sort of severe or worsening problem. We have found that this oversight is helpful in reducing premature discontinuation of pharmacotherapy.

   Geriatric patients with anxiety disorder usually get better, but given the fluctuating nature of the disorders and the issues with insight, they often do not realize they are improving unless clinical management includes following objective treatment targets, such as severity, frequency, and level of avoidance. Repeated assessment with an objective measure can be helpful in demonstrating improvement to the patient, particularly in the early phase of treatment.

6. *With medications, start low, go slow, but go—as aggressively as required to treat symptoms to remission.* A main goal of follow-up care is to keep the patient on a treatment of suf-

ficient intensity and duration to alleviate symptoms. Patients will frequently report that they have received no benefit from a medication trial when it turns out that they have been maintained for long periods on a minimal or even subclinical dosage. In our experience, the problem of inadequate treatment is at least as significant as the problem of medication intolerance (and in fact, as described above in Principle 5, medication "intolerance" may represent insufficiently well-treated anxiety symptoms rather than true medication side effects).

7. *Consider augmentation treatment and refer to experts if necessary.* Monotherapy is usually inadequate, and persistence is required. If a good trial does not help enough, add another. If the clinician has exhausted the options that he or she is comfortable providing, the patient should be referred to someone with expertise in geriatrics or other empirically supported forms of treatment for anxiety (e.g., generalist psychiatrists might consider referral to a geriatric psychiatrist, whereas psychiatrists who focus on pharmacotherapy might consider referral to a psychotherapist skilled at treating anxiety disorders; most members of the Association for Behavioral and Cognitive Therapies are well versed in anxiety treatment, and the organization's Web site includes a therapist locator: www.abct.org/Home).
8. *Provide maintenance treatment; evaluate the need for such if treatment is discontinued.* Because anxiety is chronic and waxes and wanes, treatment will probably need to be long term (e.g., maintenance medication, booster therapy). Maintenance pharmacotherapy tends to be simpler, in that the patient has already overcome any fears or initial side effects of medication. Less frequent oversight is necessary, although continued monitoring of vital signs, side effects, changes in coprescribed medications, and patient concerns is necessary.

A patient who chooses to taper off a medication should be informed that he or she may need to resume treatment at some future point. If a taper is performed, it should be very gradual to avoid rebound anxiety symptoms. Long-term monitoring for recurrence is essential; in our experience, relapse following discontinuation of a medication typically occurs within the first 3 months, whereas relapse following discontinuation of psychotherapy is often conditional upon stressful life events coupled with the failure to continue practicing anxiety management skills. In short, management does not have an end point, even when the patient is no longer receiving treatment.

Conclusion

Significant advances have been made in the understanding of anxiety disorders in older adults. The close and reciprocal relationships of anxiety with cognitive impairment and with disability, as well as the high prevalence of these syndromes, highlight the importance of these disorders for public health. Understanding of the neuropsychiatry of late-life anxiety is in its infancy, but it suggests a strong bidirectional link between anxiety and neurodegenerative changes in aging. Effective treatments include antidepressants and psychotherapy, but much more needs to be learned about the most effective ways to use these treatments and to ensure widespread implementation of their effective and appropriate use. Nevertheless, by following simple management strategies, as outlined in this chapter, clinicians can more effectively manage their older patients with anxiety disorders and minimize the use of ineffective or unsafe treatments. Finally, the future looks bright for research in this "ideal laboratory" for examining the interplay of stress, health, and aging.

Key Points

- Anxiety disorders are common and impairing in older adults.
- The most common manifestation appears to be generalized anxiety disorder. However, existing epidemiological instruments may be insufficient to detect anxiety disorders in this age group.
- Treatment for anxiety disorders in older adults includes serotonergic antidepressants and CBT. Benzodiazepines are not recommended for chronic treatment given their risks in this age group.
- The ability to modulate anxiety in the elderly is undermined by age-related structural changes in the prefrontal-limbic network.
- Careful clinical management is essential and is more important than the specific pharmacotherapeutic agent chosen.

Recommended Readings

Beaudreau SA, O'Hara R: Late-life anxiety and cognitive impairment: a review. Am J Geriatr Psychiatry 16:790–803, 2008

Bishop SJ: Neurocognitive mechanisms of anxiety: an integrative account. Trends Cogn Sci 11:307–316, 2007

Bryant C, Jackson H, Ames D: The prevalence of anxiety in older adults: methodological issues and a review of the literature. J Affect Disord 109:233–250, 2008

Hendriks GJ, Oude Voshaar RC, Keijsers GP, et al: Cognitive-behavioural therapy for late-life anxiety disorders: a systematic review and meta-analysis. Acta Psychiatr Scand 117:403–411, 2008

Lenze EJ, Wetherell JL: Bringing the bedside to the bench, and then to the community: a prospectus for intervention research in late-life anxiety disorders. Int J Geriatr Psychiatry 24:1–14, 2009

Lenze EJ, Rollman BL, Shear MK, et al: Escitalopram for older adults with generalized anxiety disorder: a placebo-controlled trial. JAMA 301:296–303, 2009

Stanley MA, Wilson NL, Novy DM, et al: Cognitive behavior therapy for generalized anxiety disorder among older adults in primary care: a randomized clinical trial. JAMA 301:1460–1467, 2009

van't Veer-Tazelaar PJ, van Marwijk HW, van Oppen P, et al: Stepped-care prevention of anxiety and depression in late life: a randomized controlled trial. Arch Gen Psychiatry 66:297–304, 2009

Wetherell JL, Lenze EJ, Stanley MA: Evidence-based treatment of geriatric anxiety disorders. Psychiatr Clin North Am 28:871–896, ix, 2005

References

Alexopoulos GS, Murphy CF, Gunning-Dixon FM, et al: Microstructural white matter abnormalities and remission of geriatric depression. Am J Psychiatry 165:238–244, 2008

Allgulander C, Lavori PW: Causes of death among 936 elderly patients with "pure" anxiety neurosis in Stockholm County, Sweden, and in patients with depressive neurosis or both diagnoses. Compr Psychiatry 34:299–302, 1993

Amodio DM, Frith CD: Meeting of minds: the medial frontal cortex and social cognition. Nat Rev Neurosci 7:268–277, 2006

Andreescu C, Lenze EJ, Dew MA, et al: Effect of comorbid anxiety on treatment response and relapse risk in late-life depression: controlled study. Br J Psychiatry 190:344–349, 2007

Arce E, Simmons AN, Lovero KL, et al: Escitalopram effects on insula and amygdala BOLD activation during emotional processing. Psychopharmacology (Berl) 196:661–672, 2008

Astrom M: Generalized anxiety disorder in stroke patients: a 3-year longitudinal study. Stroke 27:270–275, 1996

Ballard C, Neill D, O'Brien J, et al: Anxiety, depression and psychosis in vascular dementia: prevalence and associations. J Affect Disord 59:97–106, 2000

Barker-Collo SL: Depression and anxiety 3 months post stroke: prevalence and correlates. Arch Clin Neuropsychol 22:519–531, 2007

Barlow DH, Gorman JM, Shear MK, et al: Cognitive-behavioral therapy, imipramine, or their combination for panic disorder: a randomized controlled trial. JAMA 283:2529–2536, 2000

Barrowclough C, King P, Colville J, et al: A randomized trial of the effectiveness of cognitive-behavioral therapy and supportive counseling for anxiety symptoms in older adults. J Consult Clin Psychol 69:756–762, 2001

Beaudreau SA, O'Hara R: Late-life anxiety and cognitive impairment: a review. Am J Geriatr Psychiatry 16:790–803, 2008

Beck AT, Epstein N, Brown G, et al: An inventory for measuring clinical anxiety: psychometric properties. J Consult Clin Psychol 56:893–897, 1988

Beekman AT, Bremmer MA, Deeg DJ, et al: Anxiety disorders in later life: a report from the Longitudinal Aging Study Amsterdam. Int J Geriatr Psychiatry 13:717–726, 1998

Beekman AT, de Beurs E, van Balkom AJ, et al: Anxiety and depression in later life: co-occurrence and communality of risk factors. Am J Psychiatry 157:89–95, 2000

Benitez CI, Smith K, Vasile RG, et al: Use of benzodiazepines and selective serotonin reuptake inhibitors in middle-aged and older adults with anxiety disorders: a longitudinal and prospective study. Am J Geriatr Psychiatry 16:5–13, 2008

Bishop SJ: Neurocognitive mechanisms of anxiety: an integrative account. Trends Cogn Sci 11:307–316, 2007

Bissiere S, Plachta N, Hoyer D, et al: The rostral anterior cingulate cortex modulates the efficiency of amygdala-dependent fear learning. Biol Psychiatry 63:821–831, 2008

Blank S, Lenze EJ, Mulsant BH, et al: Outcomes of late-life anxiety disorders during 32 weeks of citalopram treatment. J Clin Psychiatry 67:468–472, 2006

Blazer D, George KL, Hughes D: The epidemiology of anxiety disorders: an age comparison, in Anxiety in the Elderly: Treatment and Research. Edited by Salzman CLB. New York, Springer, 1991, pp 17–30

Boddice G, Pachana NA: The clinical utility of the geriatric anxiety inventory in older adults with cognitive impairment. Nurs Older People 20:36–39; quiz 40, 2008

Brenes GA, Guralnik JM, Williamson JD, et al: The influence of anxiety on the progression of disability. J Am Geriatr Soc 53:34–39, 2005

Brenes GA, Kritchevsky SB, Mehta KM, et al: Scared to death: results from the Health, Aging, and Body Composition study. Am J Geriatr Psychiatry 15:262–265, 2007

Brenes GA, Penninx BW, Judd PH, et al: Anxiety, depression and disability across the lifespan. Aging Ment Health 12:158–163, 2008

Brenes GA, Miller ME, Stanley MA, et al: Insomnia in older adults with generalized anxiety disorder. Am J Geriatr Psychiatry 17: 465–472, 2009

Brenes GA, McCall WV, Williamson JD, et al: Feasibility and Acceptability of Bibliotherapy and Telephone Sessions for the Treatment of Late-life Anxiety Disorders. Clin Gerontol 33:62–68, 2010

Bresolin N, Monza G, Scarpini E, et al: Treatment of anxiety with ketazolam in elderly patients. Clin Ther 10:536–542, 1988

Bryant C, Jackson H, Ames D: The prevalence of anxiety in older adults: methodological issues and a review of the literature. J Affect Disord 109:233–250, 2008

Bush G, Luu P, Posner MI: Cognitive and emotional influences in anterior cingulate cortex. Trends Cogn Sci 4:215–222, 2000

Butler AC, Chapman JE, Forman EM, et al: The empirical status of cognitive-behavioral therapy: a review of meta-analyses. Clin Psychol Rev 26:17–31, 2006

Cairney J, Corna LM, Veldhuizen S, et al: Comorbid depression and anxiety in later life: patterns of association, subjective well-being, and impairment. Am J Geriatr Psychiatry 16:201–208, 2008

Castillo CS, Schultz SK, Robinson RG: Clinical correlates of early onset and late-onset poststroke generalized anxiety. Am J Psychiatry 152:1174–1179, 1995

Caudle DD, Senior AC, Wetherell JL, et al: Cognitive errors, symptom severity, and response to cognitive behavior therapy in older adults with generalized anxiety disorder. Am J Geriatr Psychiatry 15:680–689, 2007

Chorpita BF, Daleiden EL, Weisz JR: Modularity in the design and application of therapeutic interventions. Appl Prev Psychol 11: 141–156, 2005

Chou KL: Age at onset of generalized anxiety disorder in older adults. Am J Geriatr Psychiatry 17:455–464, 2009

Chung MY, Min KH, Jun YJ, et al: Efficacy and tolerability of mirtazapine and sertraline in Korean veterans with posttraumatic stress disorder: a randomized open label trial. Hum Psychopharmacol 19:489–494, 2004

Cohen D, Eisdorfer C, Vitaliano PP, et al: The relationship of age, anxiety, and serum immunoglobulins with crystallized and fluid intelligence. Biol Psychiatry 15:699–709, 1980

Csernansky JG, Dong H, Fagan AM, et al: Plasma cortisol and progression of dementia in subjects with Alzheimer-type dementia. Am J Psychiatry 163:2164–2169, 2006

Davidson J, Allgulander C, Pollack MH, et al: Efficacy and tolerability of duloxetine in elderly patients with generalized anxiety disorder: a pooled analysis of four randomized, double-blind, placebo-controlled studies. Hum Psychopharmacol 23:519–526, 2008

Davidson RJ: Anxiety and affective style: role of prefrontal cortex and amygdala. Biol Psychiatry 51:68–80, 2002

Davidson RJ, Abercrombie H, Nitschke JB, et al: Regional brain function, emotion and disorders of emotion. Curr Opin Neurobiol 9:228–234, 1999

Deckersbach T, Dougherty DD, Rauch SL: Functional imaging of mood and anxiety disorders. J Neuroimaging 16:1–10, 2006

DeLuca AK, Lenze EJ, Mulsant BH, et al: Comorbid anxiety disorder in late life depression: association with memory decline over four years. Int J Geriatr Psychiatry 20:848–854, 2005

Deptula D, Singh R, Pomara N: Aging, emotional states, and memory. Am J Psychiatry 150:429–434, 1993

Derogatis LR: Brief Symptom Inventory 18 (BSI-18): Administration, Scoring and Procedures Manual. Minneapolis, MN, National Computer Systems, 2000

De Wit L, Putman K, Baert I, et al: Anxiety and depression in the first six months after stroke: a longitudinal multicentre study. Disabil Rehabil 30:1858–1866, 2008

Diem SJ, Blackwell TL, Stone KL, et al: Use of antidepressants and rates of hip bone loss in older women: the study of osteoporotic fractures. Arch Intern Med 167:1240–1245, 2007

DiNardo PA, Brown TA, Barlow DH: Anxiety Disorders Interview Schedule for DSM-IV. Boston, MA, Center for Stress and Anxiety Related Disorders, Boston University, 1994

Dombrovski AY, Mulsant BH, Houck PR, et al: Residual symptoms and recurrence during maintenance treatment of late-life depression. J Affect Disord 103:77–82, 2007

English BA, Jewell M, Jewell G, et al: Treatment of chronic posttraumatic stress disorder in combat veterans with citalopram: an open trial. J Clin Psychopharmacol 26:84–88, 2006

Epel ES, Blackburn EH, Lin J, et al: Accelerated telomere shortening in response to life stress. Proc Natl Acad Sci U S A 101:17312–17315, 2004

Epel ES, Lin J, Wilhelm FH, et al: Cell aging in relation to stress arousal and cardiovascular disease risk factors. Psychoneuroendocrinology 31:277–287, 2006

Erk S, Abler B, Walter H: Cognitive modulation of emotion anticipation. Eur J Neurosci 24:1227–1236, 2006

Ettner SL, Hermann RC: Provider specialty choice among Medicare beneficiaries treated for psychiatric disorders. Health Care Financ Rev 18:43–59, 1997

Fabian TJ, Amico JA, Kroboth PD, et al: Paroxetine-induced hyponatremia in older adults: a 12-week prospective study. Arch Intern Med 164:327–332, 2004

Fava GA, Ruini C, Rafanelli C: Sequential treatment of mood and anxiety disorders. J Clin Psychiatry 66:1392–1400, 2005

Fava GA, Park SK, Sonino N: Treatment of recurrent depression. Expert Rev Neurother 6:1735–1740, 2006

First MB, Spitzer RL, Gibbon M: Structured Clinical Interview for DSM-IV Axis I Disorders (SCID), Clinician Version: Administration Booklet. Washington, DC, American Psychiatric Press, 1996

Flint AJ: Epidemiology and comorbidity of anxiety disorders in the elderly. Am J Psychiatry 151:640–649, 1994

Flint AJ: Anxiety and its disorders in late life: moving the field forward. Am J Geriatr Psychiatry 13:3–6, 2005

Flint AJ, Rifat SL: Anxious depression in elderly patients: response to antidepressant treatment. Am J Geriatr Psychiatry 5:107–115, 1997a

Flint AJ, Rifat SL: Two-year outcome of elderly patients with anxious depression. Psychiatry Res 66:23–31, 1997b

Flint A, Bradwejn J, Vaccarino F, et al: Aging and panicogenic response to cholecystokinin tetrapeptide: an examination of the cholecystokinin system. Neuropsychopharmacology 27:663–671, 2002

Foa EB, Franklin ME, Moser J: Context in the clinic: how well do cognitive-behavioral therapies and medications work in combination? Biol Psychiatry 52:987–997, 2002

Fox LS, Knight BG: The effects of anxiety on attentional processes in older adults. Aging Ment Health 9:585–593, 2005

Gagnon N, Flint AJ, Naglie G, et al: Affective correlates of fear of falling in elderly persons. Am J Geriatr Psychiatry 13:7–14, 2005

Gray SL, LaCroix AZ, Hanlon JT, et al: Benzodiazepine use and physical disability in community-dwelling older adults. J Am Geriatr Soc 54:224–230, 2006

Green KN, Billings LM, Roozendaal B, et al: Glucocorticoids increase amyloid-beta and tau pathology in a mouse model of Alzheimer's disease. J Neurosci 26:9047–9056, 2006

Gum AM, King-Kallimanis B, Kohn R, et al: Prevalence of mood, anxiety, and substance abuse disorders for older Americans in the National Comorbidity Survey–Replication. Am J Geriatr Psychiatry 17:769–781, 2009

Hamilton M: The assessment of anxiety states by rating. Br J Med Psychol 32:50–55, 1959

Harman JS, Rollman BL, Hanusa BH, et al: Physician office visits of adults for anxiety disorders in the United States, 1985–1998. J Gen Intern Med 17:165–172, 2002

Hettema JM, Kuhn JW, Prescott CA, et al: The impact of generalized anxiety disorder and stressful life events on risk for major depressive episodes. Psychol Med 36:789–795, 2006

Hogan MJ: Divided attention in older but not younger adults is impaired by anxiety. Exp Aging Res 29:111–136, 2003

Hopko DR, Stanley MA, Reas DL, et al: Assessing worry in older adults: confirmatory factor analysis of the Penn State Worry Questionnaire and psychometric properties of an abbreviated model. Psychol Assess 15:173–183, 2003

Howland J, Peterson EW, Levin WC, et al: Fear of falling among the community-dwelling elderly. J Aging Health 5:229–243, 1993

Jeste DV, Blazer DG, First M: Aging-related diagnostic variations: need for diagnostic criteria appropriate for elderly psychiatric patients. Biol Psychiatry 58:265–271, 2005

Jeste ND, Hays JC, Steffens DC: Clinical correlates of anxious depression among elderly patients with depression. J Affect Disord 90:37–41, 2006

Jorge RE, Robinson RG, Starkstein SE, et al: Depression and anxiety following traumatic brain injury. J Neuropsychiatry Clin Neurosci 5:369–374, 1993

Kang JE, Cirrito JR, Dong H, et al: Acute stress increases interstitial fluid amyloid-beta via corticotropin-releasing factor and neuronal activity. Proc Natl Acad Sci U S A 104:10673–10678, 2007

Katz IR, Reynolds CF III, Alexopoulos GS, et al: Venlafaxine ER as a treatment for generalized anxiety disorder in older adults: pooled analysis of five randomized placebo-controlled clinical trials. J Am Geriatr Soc 50:18–25, 2002

Kimura M, Tateno A, Robinson RG: Treatment of poststroke generalized anxiety disorder comorbid with poststroke depression: merged analysis of nortriptyline trials. Am J Geriatr Psychiatry 11:320–327, 2003

Knight BG: Psychotherapy With Older Adults. Thousand Oaks, CA, Sage, 2004

Koepke HH, Gold RL, Linden ME, et al: Multicenter controlled study of oxazepam in anxious elderly outpatients. Psychosomatics 23:641–645, 1982

Kogan JN, Edelstein BA: Modification and psychometric examination of a self-report measure of fear in older adults. J Anxiety Disord 18:397–409, 2004

Laghrissi-Thode F, Pollock BG, Miller MC, et al: Double-blind comparison of paroxetine and nortriptyline on the postural stability of late-life depressed patients. Psychopharmacol Bull 31:659–663, 1995

Landi F, Onder G, Cesari M, et al: Psychotropic medications and risk for falls among community-dwelling frail older people: an observational study. J Gerontol A Biol Sci Med Sci 60:622–626, 2005

Lang AJ, Norman GJ, Casmar PV: A randomized trial of a brief mental health intervention for primary care patients. J Consult Clin Psychol 74:1173–1179, 2006

Lauterbach EC, Freeman A, Vogel RL: Correlates of generalized anxiety and panic attacks in dystonia and Parkinson disease. Cogn Behav Neurol 16:225–233, 2003

Lavretsky H, Siddarth P, Kepe V, et al: Depression and anxiety symptoms are associated with cerebral FDDNP-PET binding in middle-aged and older nondemented adults. Am J Geriatr Psychiatry 17:493–502, 2009

LeDoux JE: Emotion circuits in the brain. Annu Rev Neurosci 23: 155–184, 2000

Lenze EJ, Wetherell JL: Bringing the bedside to the bench, and then to the community: a prospectus for intervention research in late-life anxiety disorders. Int J Geriatr Psychiatry 24:1–14, 2009

Lenze EJ, Mulsant BH, Shear MK, et al: Comorbid anxiety disorders in depressed elderly patients. Am J Psychiatry 157:722–728, 2000

Lenze EJ, Rogers JC, Martire LM, et al: The association of late-life depression and anxiety with physical disability: a review of the literature and prospectus for future research. Am J Geriatr Psychiatry 9:113–135, 2001

Lenze EJ, Karp JF, Mulsant BH, et al: Somatic symptoms in late-life anxiety: treatment issues. J Geriatr Psychiatry Neurol 18:89–96, 2005a

Lenze EJ, Mulsant BH, Mohlman J, et al: Generalized anxiety disorder in late life: lifetime course and comorbidity with major depressive disorder. Am J Geriatr Psychiatry 13:77–80, 2005b

Lenze EJ, Mulsant BH, Shear MK, et al: Efficacy and tolerability of citalopram in the treatment of late-life anxiety disorders: results from an 8-week randomized, placebo-controlled trial. Am J Psychiatry 162:146–150, 2005c

Lenze EJ, Rollman BL, Shear MK, et al: Escitalopram for older adults with generalized anxiety disorder: a placebo-controlled trial. JAMA 301:295–303, 2009

Le Roux H, Gatz M, Wetherell JL: Age at onset of generalized anxiety disorder in older adults. Am J Geriatr Psychiatry 13:23–30, 2005

Lyketsos CG, Lopez O, Jones B, et al: Prevalence of neuropsychiatric symptoms in dementia and mild cognitive impairment: results from the cardiovascular health study. JAMA 288:1475–1483, 2002

Mantella RC, Butters MA, Dew MA, et al: Cognitive impairment in late-life generalized anxiety disorder. Am J Geriatr Psychiatry 15:673–679, 2007

Mantella RC, Butters MA, Amico JA, et al: Salivary cortisol is associated with diagnosis and severity of late-life generalized anxiety disorder. Psychoneuroendocrinology 33:773–781, 2008

Marsh L: Neuropsychiatric aspects of Parkinson's disease. Psychosomatics 41:15–23, 2000

Marsh L, Rao V: Psychiatric complications in patients with epilepsy: a review. Epilepsy Res 49:11–33, 2002

McNally RJ: Mechanisms of exposure therapy: how neuroscience can improve psychological treatments for anxiety disorders. Clin Psychol Rev 27:750–759, 2007

Mintzer JE, Brawman-Mintzer O: Agitation as a possible expression of generalized anxiety disorder in demented elderly patients: toward a treatment approach. J Clin Psychiatry 57(suppl):55–63; discussion 73–55, 1996

Mobbs D, Petrovic P, Marchant JL, et al: When fear is near: threat imminence elicits prefrontal-periaqueductal gray shifts in humans. Science 317:1079–1083, 2007

Mohlman J, Gorman JM: The role of executive functioning in CBT: a pilot study with anxious older adults. Behav Res Ther 43:447–465, 2005

Montgomery S, Chatamra K, Pauer L, et al: Efficacy and safety of pregabalin in elderly people with generalised anxiety disorder. Br J Psychiatry 193:389–394, 2008

Morinigo A, Blanco M, Labrador J, et al: Risperidone for resistant anxiety in elderly persons. Am J Geriatr Psychiatry 13:81–82, 2005

Nagaratnam N, Ip J, Bou-Haidar P: The vestibular dysfunction and anxiety disorder interface: a descriptive study with special reference to the elderly. Arch Gerontol Geriatr 40:253–264, 2005

Narita K, Murata T, Hamada T, et al: Associations between trait anxiety, insulin resistance, and atherosclerosis in the elderly: a pilot cross-sectional study. Psychoneuroendocrinology 33:305–312, 2008

Nelson JC, Delucchi K, Schneider LS: Anxiety does not predict response to antidepressant treatment in late life depression: results of a meta-analysis. Int J Geriatr Psychiatry 24:539–544, 2009

Newcomer JW, Hennekens CH: Severe mental illness and risk of cardiovascular disease. JAMA 298:1794–1796, 2007

Ochsner KN, Gross JJ: The cognitive control of emotion. Trends Cogn Sci 9:242–249, 2005

Palmer K, Berger AK, Monastero R, et al: Predictors of progression from mild cognitive impairment to Alzheimer disease. Neurology 68:1596–1602, 2007

Paterniti S, Dufouil C, Alperovitch A: Long-term benzodiazepine use and cognitive decline in the elderly: the Epidemiology of Vascular Aging Study. J Clin Psychopharmacol 22:285–293, 2002

Paukert AL, Phillips L, Cully JA, et al: Integration of religion into cognitive-behavioral therapy for geriatric anxiety and depression. J Psychiatr Pract 15:103–112, 2009

Paulsen JS, Ready RE, Hamilton JM, et al: Neuropsychiatric aspects of Huntington's disease. J Neurol Neurosurg Psychiatry 71:310–314, 2001

Paulus MP: The role of neuroimaging for the diagnosis and treatment of anxiety disorders. Depress Anxiety 25:348–356, 2008

Pinquart M, Duberstein PR: Treatment of anxiety disorders in older adults: a meta-analytic comparison of behavioral and pharmacological interventions. Am J Geriatr Psychiatry 15:639–651, 2007

Pomara N, Deptula D, Medel M, et al: Effects of diazepam on recall memory: relationship to aging, dose, and duration of treatment. Psychopharmacol Bull 25:144–148, 1989

Pomara N, Tun H, DaSilva D, et al: The acute and chronic performance effects of alprazolam and lorazepam in the elderly: relationship to duration of treatment and self-rated sedation. Psychopharmacol Bull 34:139–153, 1998a

Pomara N, Tun H, DaSilva D, et al: Benzodiazepine use and crash risk in older patients. JAMA 279:113–114; author reply 115, 1998b

Porensky EK, Dew MA, Karp JF, et al: The burden of late life generalized anxiety disorder: effects on disability, health-related quality of life, and healthcare utilization. Am J Geriatr Psychiatry 17:473–482, 2009

Prull MW, Dawes LL, Martin AM III, et al: Recollection and familiarity in recognition memory: adult age differences and neuropsychological test correlates. Psychol Aging 21:107–118, 2006

Raffa SD, Stoddard JA, White KS, et al: Relapse following combined treatment discontinuation in a placebo-controlled trial for panic disorder. J Nerv Ment Dis 196:548–555, 2008

Rampello L, Alvano A, Raffaele R, et al: New possibilities of treatment for panic attacks in elderly patients: escitalopram versus citalopram. J Clin Psychopharmacol 26:67–70, 2006

Raskind MA, Peskind ER, Hoff DJ, et al: A parallel group placebo controlled study of prazosin for trauma nightmares and sleep disturbance in combat veterans with post-traumatic stress disorder. Biol Psychiatry 61:928–934, 2007

Richard IH, Schiffer RB, Kurlan R: Anxiety and Parkinson's disease. J Neuropsychiatry Clin Neurosci 8:383–392, 1996

Saxena S, Maidment KM, Vapnik T, et al: Obsessive-compulsive hoarding: symptom severity and response to multimodal treatment. J Clin Psychiatry 63:21–27, 2002

Schoevers RA, Beekman AT, Deeg DJ, et al: Comorbidity and risk-patterns of depression, generalised anxiety disorder and mixed anxiety-depression in later life: results from the AMSTEL study. Int J Geriatr Psychiatry 18:994–1001, 2003

Schuurmans J, Comijs HC, Beekman AT, et al: The outcome of anxiety disorders in older people at 6-year follow-up: results from the Longitudinal Aging Study Amsterdam. Acta Psychiatr Scand 111:420–428, 2005

Schuurmans J, Comijs H, Emmelkamp PM, et al: A randomized, controlled trial of the effectiveness of cognitive-behavioral therapy and sertraline versus a waitlist control group for anxiety disorders in older adults. Am J Geriatr Psychiatry 14:255–263, 2006

Shear K, Belnap BH, Mazumdar S, et al: Generalized anxiety disorder severity scale (GADSS): a preliminary validation study. Depress Anxiety 23:77–82, 2006

Sheikh JI, King RJ, Taylor CB: Comparative phenomenology of early-onset versus late-onset panic attacks: a pilot survey. Am J Psychiatry 148:1231–1233, 1991

Sheikh JI, Lauderdale SA, Cassidy EL: Efficacy of sertraline for panic disorder in older adults: a preliminary open-label trial. Am J Geriatr Psychiatry 12:230, 2004a

Sheikh JI, Swales PJ, Carlson EB, et al: Aging and panic disorder: phenomenology, comorbidity, and risk factors. Am J Geriatr Psychiatry 12:102–109, 2004b

Sibille E, Su J, Leman S, et al: Lack of serotonin1B receptor expression leads to age-related motor dysfunction, early onset of brain molecular aging and reduced longevity. Mol Psychiatry 12:1042–1056, 1975, 2007

Simmons A, Matthews SC, Feinstein JS, et al: Anxiety vulnerability is associated with altered anterior cingulate response to an affective appraisal task. Neuroreport 19:1033–1037, 2008

Simon NM, Smoller JW, McNamara KL, et al: Telomere shortening and mood disorders: preliminary support for a chronic stress model of accelerated aging. Biol Psychiatry 60:432–435, 2006

Sinoff G, Werner P: Anxiety disorder and accompanying subjective memory loss in the elderly as a predictor of future cognitive decline. Int J Geriatr Psychiatry 18:951–959, 2003

Smith GS, Gunning-Dixon FM, Lotrich FE, et al: Translational research in late-life mood disorders: implications for future intervention and prevention research. Neuropsychopharmacology 32:1857–1875, 2007

Stanley MA, Beck JG, Zebb BJ: Psychometric properties of four anxiety measures in older adults. Behav Res Ther 34:827–838, 1996

Stanley MA, Beck JG, Novy DM, et al: Cognitive-behavioral treatment of late-life generalized anxiety disorder. J Consult Clin Psychol 71:309–319, 2003

Stanley MA, Diefenbach GJ, Hopko DR: Cognitive behavioral treatment for older adults with generalized anxiety disorder: a therapist manual for primary care settings. Behav Modif 28:73–117, 2004

Stanley MA, Wilson NL, Novy DM, et al: Cognitive behavior therapy for generalized anxiety disorder among older adults in primary care: a randomized clinical trial. JAMA 301:1460–1467, 2009

Starkstein SE, Jorge R, Petracca G, et al: The construct of generalized anxiety disorder in Alzheimer disease. Am J Geriatr Psychiatry 15:42–49, 2007

Steffens DC, McQuoid DR: Impact of symptoms of generalized anxiety disorder on the course of late-life depression. Am J Geriatr Psychiatry 13:40–47, 2005

Stein MB, Stein DJ: Social anxiety disorder. Lancet 371:1115–1125, 2008

Stein MB, Simmons AN, Feinstein JS, et al: Increased amygdala and insula activation during emotion processing in anxiety-prone subjects. Am J Psychiatry 164:318–327, 2007

Swoboda KJ, Jenike MA: Frontal abnormalities in a patient with obsessive-compulsive disorder: the role of structural lesions in obsessive-compulsive behavior. Neurology 45:2130–2134, 1995

Thorp SR, Ayers CR, Nuevo R, et al: Meta-analysis comparing different behavioral treatments for late-life anxiety. Am J Geriatr Psychiatry 17:105–115, 2009

Todaro JF, Shen BJ, Raffa SD, et al: Prevalence of anxiety disorders in men and women with established coronary heart disease. J Cardiopulm Rehabil Prev 27:86–91, 2007

Tolin DF, Robison JT, Gaztambide S, et al: Anxiety disorders in older Puerto Rican primary care patients. Am J Geriatr Psychiatry 13:150–156, 2005

Trollor JN, Anderson TM, Sachdev PS, et al: Prevalence of mental disorders in the elderly: the Australian National Mental Health and Well-Being Survey. Am J Geriatr Psychiatry 15:455–466, 2007

Urry HL, van Reekum CM, Johnstone T, et al: Amygdala and ventromedial prefrontal cortex are inversely coupled during regulation of negative affect and predict the diurnal pattern of cortisol secretion among older adults. J Neurosci 26:4415–4425, 2006

van Balkom AJ, Beekman AT, de Beurs E, et al: Comorbidity of the anxiety disorders in a community-based older population in the Netherlands. Acta Psychiatr Scand 101:37–45, 2000

van't Veer-Tazelaar PJ, van Marwijk HW, van Oppen P, et al: Stepped-care prevention of anxiety and depression in late life: a randomized controlled trial. Arch Gen Psychiatry 66:297–304, 2009

Werneke U, Turner T, Priebe S: Complementary medicines in psychiatry. Br J Psychiatry 188:109–121, 2006

Westra HA, Stewart SH: Cognitive behavioural therapy and pharmacotherapy: complementary or contradictory approaches to the treatment of anxiety? Clin Psychol Rev 18:307–340, 1998

Wetherell JL, Unutzer J: Adherence to treatment for geriatric depression and anxiety. CNS Spectr 8:48–59, 2003

Wetherell JL, Gatz M, Pedersen NL: A longitudinal analysis of anxiety and depressive symptoms. Psychol Aging 16:187–195, 2001

Wetherell JL, Reynolds CA, Gatz M, et al: Anxiety, cognitive performance, and cognitive decline in normal aging. J Gerontol B Psychol Sci Soc Sci 57:P246–P255, 2002

Wetherell JL, Gatz M, Craske MG: Treatment of generalized anxiety disorder in older adults. J Consult Clin Psychol 71:31–40, 2003a

Wetherell JL, Le Roux H, Gatz M: DSM-IV criteria for generalized anxiety disorder in older adults: distinguishing the worried from the well. Psychol Aging 18:622–627, 2003b

Wetherell JL, Thorp SR, Patterson TL, et al: Quality of life in geriatric generalized anxiety disorder: a preliminary investigation. J Psychiatr Res 38:305–312, 2004

Wetherell JL, Hopko DR, Diefenbach GJ, et al: Cognitive-behavioral therapy for late-life generalized anxiety disorder: who gets better? Behav Ther 36:147–156, 2005a

Wetherell JL, Lenze EJ, Stanley MA: Evidence-based treatment of geriatric anxiety disorders. Psychiatr Clin North Am 28:871–896, ix, 2005b

Wetherell JL, Sorrell JT, Thorp SR, et al: Psychological interventions for late-life anxiety: a review and early lessons from the CALM study. J Geriatr Psychiatry Neurol 18:72–82, 2005c

Wetherell JL, Ayers CR, Sorrell JT, et al: Modular psychotherapy for anxiety in older primary care patients. Am J Geriatr Psychiatry 17:483–492, 2009

Wiener P, Alexopoulos GS, Kakuma T, et al: The limits of history-taking in geriatric depression. Am J Geriatr Psychiatry 5:116–125, 1997

Wisocki P, Handen B, Morse C: The Worry Scale as a measure of anxiety among homebound and community active elderly. Behavior Therapist 9:91–95, 1986

Yohannes AM, Baldwin RC, Connolly MJ: Depression and anxiety in elderly patients with chronic obstructive pulmonary disease. Age Ageing 35:457–459, 2006

Yuan Y, Tsoi K, Hunt RH: Selective serotonin reuptake inhibitors and risk of upper GI bleeding: confusion or confounding? Am J Med 119:719–727, 2006

Zigmond AS, Snaith RP: The hospital anxiety and depression scale. Acta Psychiatr Scand 67:361–370, 1983

Zung WW: A rating instrument for anxiety disorders. Psychosomatics 12:371–379, 1971

21

Psychosis

D.P. Devanand, M.D.

Elderly adults make up approximately 12% of the current U.S. population, a percentage that is expected to increase to 20% by the year 2030 (Broadway and Mintzer 2007). Accordingly, psychotic disorders in the elderly are likely to increase in prevalence. In elderly subjects, although psychosis can occur in the context of a variety of disorders, psychosis in dementia is the most common type because the prevalence of dementia greatly exceeds that of primary psychotic disorders. Psychosis and behavioral dyscontrol occur in the majority of patients with dementia during their course of illness (Devanand et al. 1997; Lyketsos et al. 2000). Consequently, the use of antipsychotic medications in patients with dementia is greater than in elderly patients with schizophrenia (Colenda et al. 2002), even though antipsychotics are not approved by the U.S. Food and Drug Administration (FDA) for the treatment of psychosis in dementia. Other causes of psychosis in late life include affective disorders (see Chapter 19, "Mood Disorders"), schizophrenia, schizoaffective disorder, psychosis induced by prescription and other medications (see Chapter 29, "Neuropsychiatric Disorders Associated With General Medical Therapies"), delirium (see Chapters 15), and brief psychotic disorder.

Definition

The broad definition of *psychosis* is a mental disorder in which a key feature is being out of touch with reality. This term is typically restricted to describing patients with delusions (disorders of thought content) or hallucinations (disorders of perception). A *delusion* is defined as a false belief that is not altered by presentation of the facts and is not in keeping with the subject's cultural or religious background. This classical definition was developed after careful observations of patients with schizophrenia. However, in many elderly patients with dementia, delusions may be amenable to change upon presentation of the facts, but only temporarily. Therefore, delusions in dementia may be chronic or intermittent, which distinguishes them from the invariably chronic delusions in schizophrenia.

A *hallucination* is defined as a false sensory perception in the absence of a real stimulus to evoke that sensation. In dementia, patients may have vague or unclear hallucinations (e.g., a patient is talking to an empty chair [phantom boarder syndrome] but upon inquiry denies that there is anyone in the chair). Both auditory and visual hallucinations occur in dementia. Based on the presence of these types of clinical features, diagnostic criteria for psychosis in Alzheimer's disease (AD) have been developed (Jeste and Finkel 2000). Considerable variability in psychotic symptoms also occurs in patients with other types of cognitive impairment (e.g., in delirium, disorientation is a cardinal feature). In contrast, the classical symptoms of psychosis—for example, complex systematized delusions and command auditory hallucinations—are present in elderly patients with schizophrenia, schizoaffective disorder, and bipolar disorder regardless of age at onset. Psychotic symptoms in patients with depression, including somatic delusions and delusions of guilt, are similar to those observed in young adults with psychotic depression.

Epidemiology

In the community-dwelling elderly, psychotic disorders range in prevalence from <1% to 5%, and in nursing home residents, the prevalence may be as high as 10%–63% (Zayas and Grossberg 1998). In the elderly, the population prevalence of schizophrenia remains <1%, whereas the prevalence of dementia is approximately 2%–5% for people above age 60 and 15%–40% for people above age 85 (Thomas et al. 2001). In elderly patients with schizophrenia, approximately 75% have a psychotic illness that began in adolescence or young adulthood, and only a minority have late-onset schizophrenia with the first episode occurring after age 45–50 (Jeste et al. 1999; Koenig et al. 1994).

Approximately 10%–20% of the elderly population will experience psychosis, primarily due to dementia (Jeste and Finkel 2000; Koenig et al. 1994). AD and dementia with Lewy bodies (DLB) account for most cases of psychosis in patients with dementia, but psychotic symptoms can also occur in vascular dementia. Psychosis in Parkinson's disease (PD) is usually iatrogenic (i.e., caused by dopamine-enhancing medications).

After dementia, the second most common cause of psychosis in geriatric patients is depression (unipolar and bipolar illness), which accounts for one-fifth of psychosis cases in elderly patients (Holroyd and Laurie 1999) (see also Chapter 19, "Mood Disorders"). The prevalence of psychotic symptoms in unipolar and bipolar affective disorder is similar to that in young adults. Late-onset depression with psychotic features is characterized by delusions, but hallucinations are rare, hence the term *delusional depression*. In contrast, hallucinations can occur in young adults with depression and are more likely to occur in bipolar depressive or manic episodes than in unipolar depression (Nelson et al. 1978).

Late-life delusional disorder (i.e., delusions in the absence of other psychotic features) is rare, and consequently reliable prevalence estimates are lacking. For other causes of psychosis in the elderly, systematic data on population prevalence and incidence estimates are limited, largely because their rates are relatively low.

History of Illness

The time course of illness development is important. In a patient with cognitive decline, a history of gradual deterioration suggests dementia, episodic cognitive deficits with confusion suggest delirium, and focal neurological symptoms or signs suggest cerebrovascular disease. Current age and age at onset of symptoms are critical variables in the elderly patient. Late-onset schizophrenia differs in some ways from early-onset schizophrenia, with a greater preponderance of females, greater prevalence of the paranoid subtype, and some differences in neuropsychological test profiles. Patients with late-onset major depression (i.e., onset after age 50–60) are less likely to have a positive family history of affective disorder and more likely to have evidence of cerebrovascular disease and cerebral atrophy than elderly patients with early-onset depressive illness (see Chapter 19, "Mood Disorders").

On the basis of the clinical presentation, inquiry should focus on pertinent symptoms to make a DSM-IV-TR (American Psychiatric Association 2000) diagnosis of an Axis I or Axis II disorder. Symptom review should include depressed mood; suicidal thoughts; lack of interest; agitation, aggression, or impulsivity; delusions; and hallucinations. In patients with cognitive impairment, the temporal relationship between psychotic and cognitive symptoms may help establish the diagnosis. If psychosis clearly preceded cognitive impairment by several years, a primary psychotic disorder (e.g., schizophrenia or mood disorders) is likely. If psychosis developed after the onset of cognitive impairment, a diagnosis of dementia, possibly AD or DLB, should be considered.

In elderly persons, there is a high rate of delirium after admission to a hospital. This high rate may be related to the lower "cognitive reserve" of older compared to young adults, and hallucinations and delusions are common in delirium. If delirium is suspected, potential risk factors should be evaluated, including fever, urinary tract infection, urinary retention, or fecal impaction (see Chapter 15, "Delirium"). Visual and hearing deficits contribute to an increased likelihood of late-onset psychosis of all types.

Direct questions should be asked about alcohol or substance abuse (discussed below), history of head trauma, infections such as meningitis or syphilis, stroke, seizure disorder, and other neurological conditions, all of which can be associated with hallucinations and delusions. In working with a patient with impaired cognition, it is necessary to obtain detailed history from an informant, often separately, because patients often deny the presence of hallucinations, delusions, or behavioral changes of agitation or aggression.

Elderly patients typically have several comorbid medical illnesses and take a large number of medications (see Chapter 29, "Neuropsychiatric Disorders Associated With General Medical Therapies"). Benzodiazepines, corticosteroids, and anticholinergic medications can lead to cognitive impairment and even delirium. Levodopa and dopamine agonists prescribed for PD, as well as steroids for multiple indications, can lead to psychosis.

Alcohol abuse is not uncommon in older adults, and explicit inquiry is often needed to elicit this history (see Chapter 17, "Addiction"). Even when alcohol consumption has been constant in amount for many decades, it can lead to cognitive decline in susceptible patients as they grow older, perhaps because of decreased cognitive reserve. Acute alcohol intoxication or withdrawal can lead to hallucinations. Abuse of other substances is less common in elderly patients, but some subjects in recent cohorts have reported regular marijuana use. Use of benzodiazepines and other hypnotics is fairly widespread. Patients with chronic pain (see Chapter 23, "Pain") may be dependent on narcotics that can give rise to a variety of psychiatric symptoms, although these drugs generally do not induce psychosis in the absence of delirium.

Neurobiology of Psychosis

The original theory of excess dopamine leading to psychosis has undergone several modifications but remains largely intact. There are serotonin and dopamine interactions that may be explanatory, and several atypical antipsychotics affect both neurotransmitter systems (Richtand and McNamara 2008).

During the process of aging, changes in neurobiology affect the symptom manifestation of psychosis (see Chapter 2, "Neurobiology of Aging"). Dopamine neurons degenerate with aging, particularly after age 70. Degeneration and loss of dopaminergic neurons occur in the substantia nigra, leading to bradykinesia and an increased prevalence of minimal parkinsonian signs (Louis and Bennett 2007). The reduction in the number of available dopaminergic receptors lowers the tolerance of elderly patients to antipsychotics, thereby increasing the likelihood of extrapyramidal symptoms (EPS) and tardive dyskinesia (TD). Furthermore, the number of cholinergic receptors decreases in patients with AD (Davies and Maloney 1976; Perry et al. 1977), indirectly affecting the manifestation of neurological side effects of antipsychotics that may be related to the relative levels of available dopamine and acetylcholine. Preliminary evidence suggests that glutamate/*N*-methyl-D-aspartate (NMDA) receptor abnormalities may underlie the manifestations of psychosis in schizophrenia (Labrie and Roder 2010).

Etiology and Pathophysiology

Psychotic disorders in the elderly broadly fall into three categories: 1) early-onset psychosis extending into the patient's old age, 2) late-onset psychosis without an underlying medical/neurological etiology, and 3) late-onset psychosis with an underlying medical/neurological etiology. The first two categories are discussed in this section; the third category is discussed in the following section, "Clinical Features and Diagnosis."

Most studies of early-onset psychosis have focused on schizophrenia. Several lines of evidence point to a neurodevelopmental disorder with genetic loading, possible prenatal insult (poor nutrition, viral infection), and structural and functional brain abnormalities. Aberrant structural changes, including loss of gray matter, are prominent in the prefrontal and temporal brain regions, and these changes may be present in high-risk patients before they manifest the illness clinically (Pantelis et al. 2007). Structural and functional brain abnormalities in limbic regions, particularly the amygdala, have been reported in patients with mood disorders, particularly bipolar disorder (see Chapter 19, "Mood Disorders").

The degeneration of catecholaminergic and cholinergic neurons that occurs in the brain with aging is present in patients with both early-onset and late-onset schizophrenia, as well as in patients with mood disorders.

In patients with AD, psychosis may be associated with specific genetic and neurobiological abnormalities (Forstl et al. 1993), and there may be specific subtypes of psychosis (Cook et al. 2003). Higher levels of norepinephrine in the substantia nigra (Zubenko et al. 1991) and higher levels of β-adrenergic receptors (Russo-Neustadt and Cotman 1997) in multiple brain regions have been reported in psychotic compared with nonpsychotic patients with AD. These data suggest an enhanced responsiveness of catecholamines that may be associated with increased psychosis in AD (Raskind and Peskind 1994).

Homozygosity of the 1 and 2 alleles of the dopamine receptor *DR3* gene (Holmes et al. 2001; Sweet et al. 1998) and homozygosity for the C102 allele of the serotonin 2A receptor gene may be associated with psychosis in AD (Nacmias et al. 2001). A decrease in serotonin in the prosubiculum of the cerebral cortex has been reported in psychotic compared to nonpsychotic patients with AD (Lawlor et al. 1995; Zubenko et al. 1991). Blockade of dopamine D_2 receptors is believed to be the primary mechanism of action of antipsychotics. Atypical antipsychotics are more potent antagonists at the serotonin type 2a receptor ($5\text{-}HT_{2a}$) than at the D_2 receptor, less frequently resulting in EPS and TD when compared with typical antipsychotics (Jeste et al. 1999). Nonetheless, the precise pathophysiology underlying psychosis in AD is still unknown. Decrease in acetylcholine has been correlated with increase in thought disorder (Sunderland et al. 1997). Cholinergic agents, including the acetylcholinesterase inhibitors (donepezil, rivastigmine, galantamine) that are used to treat the cognitive impairment in AD, may also improve apathy and other behavioral symptoms (Bodick et al. 1997; Gauthier et al. 2002; Kaufer et al. 1996; Raskind 1999), but specific antipsychotic effects have not been established (Grimmer and Kurz 2006).

Clinical Features and Diagnosis

Schizophrenia

Schizophrenia is a neurodevelopmental disorder associated with perceptual, behavioral, and cognitive abnormalities (Table 21–1). These abnormalities are less clear in patients with late-onset schizophrenia, who comprise approximately 25% of elderly patients with schizophrenia (Jeste et al. 1999). The International Late-Onset Schizophrenia Group concluded that the diagnoses of late-onset schizophrenia (onset after age 40) and very-late-onset schizophrenia (onset after age 60) have face validity and clinical utility (Howard et al. 2000). Late-onset schizophrenia is more common in women and is characterized by a predominance of positive symptoms rather than negative symptoms; there is no increase in family history of schizophrenia. In contrast, in early-onset schizophrenia, sex distribution is equal, family history of schizophrenia is increased compared with the general population, and delusions are often complex and persecutory (Jeste et al. 1997; Paulsen et al. 2000).

TABLE 21–1. Features of psychosis and clinical course in different disorders in the elderly

Diagnosis in the elderly	Features of psychosis	Clinical course	Other clinical features
Alcohol intoxication or withdrawal	Auditory hallucinations	Clinical course depends on abstinence from alcohol use	Short-term memory loss
Alzheimer's disease	Isolated delusions and hallucinations, often intermittent; paranoid delusions of someone stealing things, spouse's infidelity, or home not being one's own	Psychotic features may or may not persist over time; agitation and aggression often present; response to antipsychotics limited by side effects	Progressive memory loss with decline in instrumental and basic activities of daily living with disease progression
Bipolar disorder, mania	Euphoria or irritability, grandiosity, flight of ideas, excessive spending, hypersexuality	Responsive to lithium, anticonvulsants	May be secondary to medical disorders or medication toxicity
Brief psychotic disorder	Variable delusional thinking and hallucinations	Variable course, often resolves within days to weeks	Stressors are common antecedents
Delirium	Markedly fluctuating psychotic features	Resolves rapidly after identifying and treating the underlying cause	Disorientation, specific medical etiology
Delusional disorder	Persecutory, erotomanic, or somatic delusions	Difficult to treat, partial response to antipsychotics	Not accompanied by hallucinations
Frontotemporal dementia	Symptoms of disinhibition resembling hypomania; clear-cut delusions and hallucinations are uncommon	Memory preserved through the early part of the illness; frontal lobe release signs and executive function deficits	Impulsivity in the verbal, motor, sexual, and appetite domains; apathy more common in later stages
Lewy body dementia	Prominent visual hallucinations	Fluctuating course short term, rapidly progressive dementia longer term	Extrapyramidal signs worsen markedly with most antipsychotics
Parkinson's disease	Hallucinations and delusions	Psychosis typically related to levodopa or dopamine agonist use and diminishes with dosage reduction	Extrapyramidal signs worsen with most antipsychotics
Psychotic depression	Somatic delusions, delusions of guilt, rare hallucinations	Responsive to electroconvulsive therapy, antipsychotic plus antidepressant treatment	Major depression present; late-onset patients do not have increased family history of affective disorder
Schizophrenia	Complex systematized delusions, command hallucinations	Positive symptoms may respond to antipsychotics; negative symptoms difficult to treat	Late onset: more females, positive symptoms, auditory and visual hallucinations, family history not common
Vascular dementia	Psychotic features overlap with those of Alzheimer's disease	Stepwise progression, focal neurological signs, depression and executive function deficits common	Vascular risk factors: obesity, hypertension, hypercholesterolemia, smoking, family history

Brief Psychotic Disorder

Brief psychotic disorder used to be called "brief reactive psychosis." Patients with this disorder usually experience a stressor, psychological or medical, and the symptoms of psychosis can be highly varied in presentation. Symptoms can include delusions, hallucinations, formal thought disorder with incoherence at times, and changes in behavior that may include catatonia. Severe stress is often antecedent to such symptoms. This syndrome occurs less frequently in elderly adults than in young adults, and hence its prevalence in the elderly population has not been determined (Pillmann et al. 2003).

Schizoaffective Disorder

As in young adults, schizoaffective disorder that has late onset is characterized by symptoms of both schizophrenia and mood disorder. However, new-onset schizoaffective disorder is rare in elderly persons. The depressed subtype of schizoaffective disorder is more common in elderly patients, whereas the bipolar subtype is more common in young adults. Schizoaffective disorder may be more common in women, who generally have a later age at onset than men (Khouzam and Emes 2007).

Delusional Disorder

Delusional disorder is characterized by persistent delusions (Khouzam and Emes 2007), and patients typically have no hallucinations. The population prevalence of delusional disorder is very low (<0.1%), and the age at onset ranges from 10 to 90 years. Delusions in delusional disorder can be persecutory, erotomanic, somatic, or of other types. There is some overlap with schizophrenia, and in the British literature, the term *paraphrenia* has been used to describe new-onset late-life psychosis.

Psychotic Depression

Psychosis in patients with major depression typically manifests as delusional depression, and hallucinations are rare. In contrast, hallucinations are less uncommon in patients with bipolar disorder who develop an episode of psychotic depression. Prominent symptoms of depression in delusional depression include excessive guilt and somatization, both of which can be near-delusional or delusional in nature, and these symptoms may occur more commonly in elderly patients (Meyers et al. 2001). The delusion is typically mood congruent, and the presence of mood-incongruent delusions can occur but should raise the possibility of an alternative diagnosis. Neurovegetative signs of disturbances in sleep, appetite, and libido are common in patients with psychotic depression who typically meet criteria for melancholia. The diagnosis of psychotic depression appears to be associated with an increased risk of recurring episodes and suicide (Meyers et al. 2001).

Bipolar Disorder

Bipolar disorder in late life is defined as manic and/or depressive episodes in the absence of concomitant medical or related causative factors (see Chapter 19, "Mood Disorders"). Secondary mania or depression can occur (i.e., the illness is caused by concomitant medical or neurological disorders, medication toxicity, or related factors) (Jorgensen et al. 1997). The majority of elderly patients with bipolar disorder have onset of illness early in life. Symptoms of mania in elderly patients are similar to those in young adults, but excessive psychomotor activity is less prominent. Among elderly patients with late age at onset of bipolar disorder, secondary causes need to be investigated thoroughly. Crucial parts of the evaluation are a metabolic workup to rule out endocrine or other metabolic abnormalities; structural brain imaging (magnetic resonance imaging [MRI] or computed tomography [CT]) to rule out neoplastic, vascular, and other causes; and evaluation of possible medication toxicity (e.g., corticosteroid use). Rare causes (e.g., frontal lobe tumor) may be discovered with appropriate investigation. Bipolar disorder, regardless of age group, is associated with an increased risk of suicide.

Dementia

Psychosis in dementia is typically accompanied by behavioral changes such as agitation, irritability, and aggression. The reverse is *not* true; that is, many dementia patients with behavioral changes do not manifest psychotic features (Devanand et al. 1998). Psychosis can occur in many types of dementia, although most studies have been done in patients with AD because it is the most common type of dementia.

Alzheimer's Disease

Psychotic symptoms are common in AD, with the prevalence ranging from 10% to 50% across studies (Devanand et al. 1997; Lyketsos et al. 2000; Reisberg et al. 1989). Isolated delusions are more common than diagnosable psychotic disorders, and paranoid delusions of theft and suspicion are the most frequent types of delusions. Systematized complex delusions and grandiose delusions are relatively rare in AD and other dementias. Delusional processes in dementia can be chronic or intermittent, a feature that distinguishes them from delusions in schizophrenia. Hallucinations, which can be visual or auditory, occur in 5%–15% of patients with dementia. In AD, a typical hallucination is the idea that someone else is in the house (i.e., phantom boarder syndrome). Based on these clinical features, diagnostic criteria have been developed for psychosis in AD (Jeste and Finkel 2000).

Rating Scales for Assessment of Psychopathology in Alzheimer's Disease

The marked cognitive decline intrinsic to AD, as well as other dementias, has led to most rating scales being developed as informant-based interviews. Commonly used rating scales to measure neuropsychiatric symptoms of AD include the Neuropsychiatric Inventory (NPI; Cummings et al. 1994), NPI–Nursing Home version (Wood et al. 2000), Behavioral Pathology in Alzheimer's Disease Rating Scale (Reisberg et al. 1987), Consortium to Establish a Registry for Alzheimer's Disease's CERAD Behavior Rating Scale (Tariot et al. 1995), Cohen-Mansfield Agitation Inventory (Cohen-Mansfield et al. 1989), and Columbia University Scale for Psychopathology in Alzheimer's Disease (Devanand et al. 1992). Currently, the NPI, which uses a time-efficient decision-tree approach, is the most widely used scale to evaluate the effects of antipsychotic treatment in patients with dementia.

Dementia With Lewy Bodies

DLB is a progressive dementia that develops in patients age 50–90 years old and is characterized by intracellular inclusions in brain cells termed *Lewy bodies,* which contain a protein called α-synuclein (see Chapter 16, "Alzheimer's Disease and the Frontotemporal Dementia Syndromes"). This disorder overlaps with AD and PD. Dementing features in DLB include progressive loss of memory and other cognitive functions, and functional impairment. Classical features of PD are usually present: rigidity, tremor, and bradykinesia with slow shuffling gait. The disease is characterized by fluctuating levels of alertness over short intervals, as well as by visual hallucinations that can be the main manifesting feature of psychosis. Delusions similar to those observed in patients with AD may also be present. Patients who have DLB are particularly sensitive to the side effects of benzodiazepines and antipsychotics. Typical antipsychotics, and to a lesser extent atypical antipsychotics, can markedly worsen EPS present in this condition and lead to falls, with further complications.

Parkinson's Disease

Psychosis occurs rarely in patients with untreated PD. Treatments for this disorder that increase dopamine in the brain are particularly prone to lead to a frank psychosis with hallucinations and delusions. This psychosis is difficult to treat because the antidopaminergic effects of antipsychotics can worsen the movement disorder of PD.

Vascular Dementia

In vascular dementia, prominent cerebrovascular lesions are considered to be the primary cause of the dementia. Depression is common, and psychosis may also occur. Because a large number of patients over ages 75–80 years have both cerebrovascular and AD pathology, it is not uncommon for patients to have "mixed" dementia with both types of brain pathology. In such cases, the clinical manifestations overlap. Partly because of this problem of overlap, psychotic and related symptoms in vascular dementia and AD can be difficult to distinguish.

Delirium and Other Medical Conditions

Psychosis that is due to an identifiable cause can occur in delirium and other medical conditions. Diagnostically, the hallucinations and delusions tend to be poorly formed and transient, and occur in the presence of disorientation. A thorough mental status examination is usually sufficient to make the diagnosis, and delirium typically resolves over time when the underlying medical disorder remits. Psychosis can also occur in patients with brain tumors, seizure disorder, and traumatic brain injury (TBI). Manifestations of psychosis tend to vary depending on the site and location of the lesion, and symptoms of anhedonia and psychomotor retardation are common in patients with TBI. Although laterality of lesion has been associated with depression, the associations between laterality and psychosis are not established.

Other Psychoses in the Elderly

Several prescription, over-the-counter, and alternative medications have been associated with the precipitation of psychosis. Alcohol dependence with Wernicke's encephalopathy or Korsakoff's syndrome can be associated with psychosis, as can alcohol withdrawal. Depression, anxiety, and disorientation are common concomitants in these patients.

Medical conditions that are considered part of the aging process can be associated with psychosis. Macular degeneration and other forms of vision loss can be associated with visual hallucinations that are typically well formed. The Charles Bonnet syndrome refers to visual hallucinations in the absence of other psychopathology. Correction of hearing and visual impairments may lead to improvement in psychotic symptoms.

Pathology and Laboratory Examination

Alzheimer's patients with psychosis have been found to have significantly more plaques and tangles in the medial temporal prosubicular area and the middle frontal cortex (Zubenko et al. 1991), and four to five times higher levels of abnormal paired helical filament–tau protein in the entorhinal and temporal cortices (Mukaetova-Ladinska et al. 1993). Pathologically, there are concomitant changes in catecholamine neurotransmitter concentrations (Bondareff 1996; Zubenko et al. 1991).

In comparisons of AD patients with and without psychosis, positron emission tomography (PET) has shown regional glucose metabolism differences (Mega et al. 2000; Sultzer et al. 2003). Although the specific associations between these abnormalities and symptom manifestations and treatment response have not been established, it is clear that the loss of dopaminergic, noradrenergic, and serotonergic neurons increases the likelihood of side effects with psychotropic medications. Consequently, antipsychotics and benzodiazepines, in particular, need to be prescribed in elderly patients in dosages that are small fractions of the dosages used in young adults.

Differential Diagnosis

In the differential diagnosis of late-life psychosis, there are two key questions: 1) Is the illness of early onset with a recurrent or chronic history, or is it a new-onset disorder in late life? 2) Is there a possible medical etiology for the psychosis? Addressing these two questions is essential in the differential diagnosis of every patient with late-life psychosis.

For patients with chronic or recurrent psychotic illness that began early in life, the diagnosis is straightforward—that is, the patient with long-standing schizophrenia presenting in late life in all probability still has the same illness, and a patient with a long-standing major affective disorder with recurrent episodes likely still has the same illness. Additional history from treatment records and informants may be needed if patients cannot communicate clearly about their history. Assessment of mood and cognition is important to help clarify the diagnosis in elderly patients. In all cases, evaluation of possible stressors and medical etiologies that can exacerbate the illness and precipitate hospitalization is critical, because the goal of treatment is to address such causes in addition to the treatment of the underlying mental disorder. Assessment may include an evaluation of vision and hearing because deficits in these areas can predispose to hallucinations.

For patients with new-onset psychosis in late life, a thorough medical workup is indicated. The metabolic workup should include complete blood count, glucose levels, renal and liver function tests, thyroid function tests, and vitamin B_{12} and folate levels. CT or MRI scan should be done to rule out the possibility of a cerebrovascular event (lacune or infarct) or tumor or other space-occupying lesion. Electroencephalography (EEG) should be done if the symptoms suggest possible seizure disorder. After a structural brain scan to rule out a brain mass, lumbar puncture with spinal fluid examination may need to be considered if there is cognitive impairment with suspicion of neoplastic metastases, infection, or immunological disorders. In elderly patients, assessment and treatment of psychosis should occur after reversible medical conditions (e.g., occult urinary tract infection, metabolic imbalance, iatrogenic or medication-induced symptoms) have been identified and treated.

If mood-congruent somatic delusions or delusions of guilt occur in the presence of depressed mood and the absence of cognitive impairment, the diagnosis of psychotic depression is likely. Hypomanic and manic symptoms rarely occur in patients with AD but can be present in patients with frontotemporal dementia, in whom the euphoric and disinhibited symptoms may not be mood congruent. Frontotemporal dementia is characterized by an absence of a history of bipolar disorder and the presence of executive function deficits with frontal lobe release signs on neurological examination that are typically not present in bipolar disorder. Euphoria can also occur in delirium, in which concomitant disorientation and confusion will clarify the diagnosis.

Unlike brief psychotic disorder, delirium is characterized by disorientation and by other cognitive deficits in several domains. The etiology and boundaries of brief psychotic disorder are not well defined, and a clinician should exclude all other potential causes of psychosis before making this diagnosis.

In patients with schizophrenia, early-onset illness is characterized by positive (hallucinations, delusions) and negative (apathy, lack of interest) symptoms, positive family history, poor premorbid psychosocial functioning, and schizoid or schizotypal personality traits. Late-onset schizophrenia is characterized by greater female preponderance, more prominent hallucinations and paranoia, less prominent negative symptoms, lower likelihood of a positive family history, and relatively good premorbid psychosocial functioning (marriage, work history) (Jeste et al. 1997; Paulsen et al. 2000).

In contrast to the persistent psychotic symptoms in schizophrenia, the symptoms of psychosis in dementia may be intermittent and are often accompanied by psychomotor agitation, and in some cases, aggressive behavior. Delusions have characteristic content (e.g., someone is stealing things, the house is not one's home, the spouse is unfaithful).

The clinical history and urine or blood drug toxicology screen are important in distinguishing drug-induced psychosis from other psychotic disorders. In elderly patients, hallucinations or delusions related to alcohol use or withdrawal can occur, but psychosis induced by other drugs (e.g., lysergic acid diethylamide [LSD], phencyclidine [PCP], amphetamine, cocaine) is rare. Occasionally, over-the-counter medications, prescription medications, and herbal or alternative agents can precipitate psychosis in elderly people. The lack of information regarding the components of these alternative medications (e.g., their anticholinergic properties) can make the diagnosis difficult.

Course and Prognosis

The clinical course and prognosis of elderly patients with long-standing psychotic disorders (see Table 21–1) are not dissimilar to those of young adults, with negative symptoms becoming more prominent with aging. The few differences that occur as a function of age are a consequence of three factors: 1) elderly patients with early-onset psychosis are the "survivors" in that they have not succumbed to suicide, poor medical care, or other causes of death that occur in adults with psychosis; 2) social supports have generally stabilized for patients with psychosis by the time they reach old age; and 3) intervening medical and neurological disorders can alter the symptoms and subsequent clinical course. Therefore, a patient with early-onset schizophrenia who has no major cognitive deficits, a strong social support system, and sound medical care is likely to remain clinically more stable than is a patient with early-onset schizophrenia who does not have a permanent residence or strong social supports and has significant cognitive impairment. This type of cognitive impairment is fairly specific for schizophrenia. Of note, the type of cognitive impairment seen in patients with schizophrenia does not appear to increase the risk of developing dementia (Purohit et al. 1998).

In patients with mood disorders who develop psychotic features, the clinical course in elderly patients is similar to that in young adults. Patients who survive into old age may be those who are more likely to be compliant with medications, thereby reducing the risk of relapse and repeated hospitalizations. Low dosages of psychotropic medications are important in decreasing the likelihood of long-term side effects of antipsychotics (TD) and lithium (thyroid and renal dysfunction).

In patients with dementia who develop psychosis, the clinical course has been studied extensively. In a series of 235 patients with mild to moderate AD who were followed prospectively for up to 5 years, approximately half the patients with paranoid delusions or hallucinations were likely to manifest the same symptoms 6 months later (Devanand et al. 1997), a finding consistent with other reports (Ballard et al. 1997; Paulsen et al. 2000). However, paranoid delusions or hallucinations occurred in ≥3 of 4 consecutive visits (2 years) in only 10%–15% of patients, which raises the question of how long patients need to continue taking psychotropic medications after treatment response. As the dementia progresses, patients are more likely to become apathetic or occasionally aggressive, and the greatest prevalence of agitation and aggression in patients with AD is in nursing homes (Cohen-Mansfield 2008). In severe dementia, it is often difficult to assess psychosis because of the decline in the patient's ability to communicate.

In patients with vascular dementia, depression and mood lability are features that may accompany psychosis. In patients with DLB, the progression of illness may be more rapid than in those with AD, and hallucinations may persist through the illness course. The impulsive behaviors of frontotemporal dementia are dominant in the early to middle stages of the illness, and apathy becomes more frequent in the later stages.

Management

Principles

Because antipsychotics are associated with a wide range of side effects, psychosocial interventions should be considered to the maximum extent possible. Cognitive-behavioral therapy and behavioral management may be useful in addressing negative symptoms in elderly patients with schizophrenia and related psychotic disorders; however, controlled data from systematic studies are lacking for elderly patients. For psychosis in patients with dementia, psychosocial interventions focus more on the caregiver than on the patient because the degree of dementia markedly impacts the patient's ability to recall the input from psychotherapy or related psychosocial interventions. Despite face validity for psychoeducational efforts with caregivers to improve their understanding and ability to cope with the symptoms of psychosis and other consequences of progressive illness in the patient with dementia, controlled data to support such an approach are sparse.

Antipsychotics remain the first-line treatment for schizophrenia and other psychotic disorders across the life span. Although not explicitly approved by the FDA for this purpose, the published studies suggest that these medications are useful in the treatment of psychosis and behavioral disinhibition in AD and possibly other types of dementia. While elderly patients are taking antipsychotics, the clinician should closely monitor target symptoms, somatic side effects including mobility and drowsiness, potential drug interactions, cognition, and activities of daily living as necessary. Patients and families need to be informed about the potential serious side effects of antipsychotics before they are prescribed, and the transmission of this information needs to be documented in the patient's chart. Daily dosages for antipsychotics commonly used in the elderly are included in Table 21–2. Evidence supporting the efficacy of other classes of medications to treat elderly patients with primary psychotic disorders or psychosis in dementia is very limited.

Drug Therapies

Efficacy of Antipsychotics in Schizophrenia

The majority of elderly patients with schizophrenia are first diagnosed as young adults, and only a minority are first diagnosed with schizophrenia later in life. Although age at onset

TABLE 21–2. Daily dosages of antipsychotics commonly used for psychosis in elderly patients with schizophrenia and dementia

	Daily dosage			
Antipsychotic	Schizophrenia and related disorders	Alzheimer's disease and other dementias	Efficacy	Main side effects
Aripiprazole	5–30 mg	2–15 mg	Moderate efficacy in schizophrenia Equivocal findings of efficacy in dementia	Sedation in some patients, little weight gain
Clozapine	300–900 mg	25–300 mg (no dose comparison study in dementia)	Most effective in schizophrenia Likely effective in dementia but not well studied because of side effects	Blood dyscrasias including agranulocytosis, weight gain and metabolic syndrome, sedation
Haloperidol	2–10 mg	0.5–2 mg	Established in schizophrenia Some efficacy in dementia	Extrapyramidal signs, tardive dyskinesia
Olanzapine	10–30 mg	2.5–10 mg	Established in schizophrenia Some evidence of efficacy in Alzheimer's and Lewy body dementia	Weight gain and metabolic syndrome, sedation
Paliperidone	3–12 mg	Unknown; 1–4 mg used clinically	Established in schizophrenia Little data in dementia	Extrapyramidal signs highly dose dependent, moderate weight gain and sedation
Quetiapine	200–600 mg	25–600 mg (lack of dose comparison studies)	Low efficacy in schizophrenia Minimal to no efficacy in dementia	Sedation, weight gain
Risperidone	1–6 mg	0.5–2 mg	Established in schizophrenia Some efficacy in dementia	Extrapyramidal signs highly dose dependent, moderate weight gain and sedation
Ziprasidone	80–160 mg	Unknown; 40–160 mg used clinically	Established in schizophrenia No data in dementia	Prolonged QTc on electrocardiogram, no weight gain

impacts the clinical presentation to some extent (Sable and Jeste 2002), it does not impact appreciably on the likelihood of response to antipsychotics or the occurrence of side effects, although the elderly are more prone to neurological side effects.

Most elderly patients with young-adult-onset schizophrenia have already been taking antipsychotics for many years, often decades, when they enter old age. Tapering and stopping antipsychotics in patients with schizophrenia is associated with a high risk of relapse (Csernansky and Schuchart 2002), making it difficult to conduct placebo-controlled trials in elderly patients with schizophrenia (Sable and Jeste 2002). However, because many of these patients develop EPS and/or TD over time, attempts are often made to switch from a typical to an atypical antipsychotic to reduce the neurological toxicity profile. Switching from typical antipsychotics to risperidone has been reported to be effective and well tolerated (Barak et al. 2002). A study of veterans suggested that adherence to atypical antipsychotics is slightly higher than adherence to typical antipsychotics (Dolder et al. 2002).

Comparisons of antipsychotics. In mixed-age samples of patients with schizophrenia, among the atypical antipsychotics only clozapine showed a clear advantage (Kane et al. 1988). The National Institute of Mental Health's Clinical Antipsychotic Trials of Intervention Effectiveness (CATIE) study of adults with schizophrenia showed minimal superiority for the effectiveness of olanzapine compared with typical and other atypical antipsychotics (Lieberman et al. 2005). In the United Kingdom, the Cost Utility of the Latest Antipsychotic Drugs in Schizophrenia Study of 227 adults with schizophrenia did not show any differences in treatment response for atypical versus typical antipsychotics (Jones et al. 2006). The CATIE studies also showed that although quetiapine is well tolerated, it lacks clinically meaningful efficacy in patients with schizophrenia or AD (Lieberman et al. 2005; Schneider et al. 2006).

In all age groups, it has been difficult to show that the atypical antipsychotics approved for use in the United States improve negative symptoms, such as anhedonia and apathy, even though this putative effect was a key factor driving the development of these compounds. However, amisulpride, an antipsychotic approved in Europe, was shown in a controlled study to be efficacious in improving the negative symptoms of schizophrenia (Möller 2001).

Antipsychotic treatment issues. In elderly patients with schizophrenia, antipsychotic treatment may need to be combined with psychosocial intervention when appropriate (Sable and Jeste 2002). The dosages of typical antipsychotics used in elderly patients with schizophrenia should be lower than the dosages used in young adults (Jeste and Finkel 2000), but there is a lack of published dosage-comparison studies of individual antipsychotics in these patients. Abrupt withdrawal of atypical antipsychotics, particularly quetiapine, has not been shown to cause major adverse effects; nonetheless, gradual withdrawal over a few days is advisable for all antipsychotics (Cutler et al. 2002). Atypical antipsychotics can be safely combined with cholinesterase inhibitors for their putative cognitive-enhancing properties, although little objective evidence backs this approach. When such an approach is used, little change in treatment response of psychotic symptoms is likely (Friedman and Fernandez 2002).

Efficacy of Antipsychotics in Other Psychotic Disorders

Late-onset delusional disorder is uncommon and difficult to treat, and the delusions often do not remit even with adequate antipsychotic treatment. In psychotic depression, antipsychotics combined with antidepressants are the treatment of choice, but electroconvulsive therapy is still considered the most effective treatment for this disorder (Mulsant and Pollock 1998; Sackeim et al. 1995; Spiker et al. 1985). Initial evidence suggests that antidepressants alone may be comparable to combined antipsychotic-antidepressant continuation treatment following improvement in the acute episode in elderly patients (Meyers et al. 2001). More data from controlled studies using typical or atypical antipsychotics in older adults are needed before this approach can be recommended for standard clinical practice.

Antipsychotics are used widely in the treatment of the manic phase of bipolar disorder across the life span (Levine et al. 2000). Lithium's toxicity, particularly in the neurological domain, is problematic in elderly patients (McDonald 2000). Hence, anticonvulsants and atypical antipsychotics are used frequently to treat mania in elderly patients. In the absence of controlled data, however, the optimal choice of antipsychotic and the optimal dosage to use in elderly patients with bipolar disorder are unresolved issues that are still being addressed in research.

Efficacy of Antipsychotics in Dementia

The neurological side effects of typical antipsychotics, particularly in nursing home patients with dementia, led to the Omnibus Budget Reconciliation Act (OBRA) of 1987 (Elon and Pawlson 1992), which became effective in 1990. OBRA requires identification of target symptoms, justification for the use of antipsychotics, and mandatory attempts to decrease or stop the antipsychotic medication every 3 months. In spite of this increased regulatory burden, drug utilization studies show one-third to one-half of elderly institutionalized patients are taking antipsychotics (Giron et al. 2001; Lantz et al. 1990).

The results of an earlier meta-analysis of placebo-controlled treatment trials indicated that typical antipsychotic treatment in patients with dementia was significantly more efficacious than placebo and that the magnitude of the advantage over placebo averaged 18% (Schneider et al. 1990). In subsequent placebo-controlled clinical trials using typical or atypical antipsychotics, the response rates varied between 45% and 60% for active medication and between 20% and 45% for placebo (De Deyn et al. 1999; Devanand et al. 1998; Katz et al. 1999; Street et al. 2000), and the overall advantage for antipsychotic over placebo was in the range of 18%–26% (Kindermann et al. 2002; Lanctot et al. 1998). Differences in response have been moderate on average, and clinically, a complete "cure" of the target psychotic and behavioral symptoms is uncommon. In patients with dementia, placebo-controlled studies consistently show comparable advantages for antipsychotics over placebo for symptoms of both psychosis and agitation or aggression (Brodaty et al. 2003; De Deyn et al. 1999; Devanand et al. 1998; Katz et al. 1999; Street et al. 2000).

Typical antipsychotics and selective serotonin reuptake inhibitors in dementia. Studies of antipsychotics and selective serotonin reuptake inhibitors (SSRIs) in dementia have invariably included patients with psychosis or with agitation or aggression. In a double-blind, placebo-controlled, randomized comparison of haloperidol 2–3 mg/day and 0.5–0.75 mg/day in 71 outpatients with AD (Devanand et al. 1998), haloperidol 2–3 mg/day was efficacious and significantly better than either low-dosage haloperidol or placebo on the Brief Psychiatric Rating Scale (BPRS) psychosis factor and psychomotor agitation. EPS tended to be greater for patients in the haloperidol 2–3 mg/day condition than for those in the other two conditions, primarily because of a subgroup (20%) that developed moderate to severe EPS. Low-dosage haloperidol did not differ from placebo on any measure of efficacy or side effects. The results indicated a favorable therapeutic profile for haloperidol in dosages of 2–3 mg/day, even though the subgroup did develop moderate to severe EPS (Devanand et al. 1998). In contrast, a multicenter study showed no significant advantage for haloperidol over either trazodone or placebo in 149 patients with AD (Teri et al. 2000). However, that study had several methodological flaws, including the assignment of a subset of patients at only some of the sites to receive behavioral treatment that was not administered in a double-blind manner (Teri et al. 2000). In another study that compared citalopram to perphenazine and placebo, citalopram was comparable to perphenazine in efficacy and significantly superior to placebo, with an advantageous side-effect profile (Pollock et al. 2002), but independent replication in larger samples is needed before SSRIs can be recommended. Furthermore, even if SSRIs may help in treating behavioral dyscontrol, it is unlikely that they will be effective in treating psychosis specifically.

Atypical antipsychotics in dementia. Atypical antipsychotics can be safely administered with cognition-enhancing agents that are currently available to treat dementia and that have been FDA approved for the treatment of AD (i.e., cholinesterase inhibitors [donepezil, rivastigmine, galantamine] and memantine). Clozapine, risperidone (and paliperidone), olanzapine, quetiapine, ziprasidone, and aripiprazole are the atypical antipsychotics that are currently available in the United States.

Clozapine. Clozapine may be more efficacious than other antipsychotics in schizophrenia, and there is essentially no risk of developing TD (Kane et al. 1988). Circulating levels of clozapine rise with dosage and age and may be slightly higher in women than in men; orthostatic hypotension and sedation are common; and seizure potential is elevated (Centorrino et al. 1994; Kurz et al. 1998). Clozapine's anticholinergic properties can lead to dry mouth and constipation and can adversely impact cognition in elderly patients. Also, there is a need for intensive monitoring for blood dyscrasias that are not uncommon, particularly the serious condition of agranulocytosis, which is reported to occur in 0.4% of patients (Kane et al. 1988). Partly because of these safety concerns, no double-blind, placebo-controlled trials have been done using clozapine to treat behavioral complications in dementia, and the few reported case series indicate moderate efficacy with significant adverse events, suggesting very low tolerability (Chengappa et al. 1995; Oberholzer et al. 1992; Pitner et al. 1995). Therefore, clozapine is considered a last-line treatment. Of note, clozapine is the only antipsychotic shown to be efficacious in the treatment of psychosis in patients with PD.

Risperidone. Compared with the other atypical antipsychotics, risperidone may be more likely to lead to EPS and TD, although this risk is considerably lower than with typical antipsychotics such as haloperidol (Jeste and Finkel 2000). In 255 elderly institutionalized patients with dementia and without baseline TD who were treated with risperidone at an average dosage of 0.96 (SD 0.53) mg/day, the 1-year cumulative incidence of persistent emergent TD was a relatively low 2.6% (Jeste and Finkel 2000). Risperidone is mildly sedating and has the potential to cause orthostatic hypotension; however, the latter effect is uncommon when low dosages are used in the elderly (Katz et al. 1999).

In a multicenter study, 625 nursing home patients with dementia (mean age 83 years; 73% with AD) who had behavioral complications were randomly assigned to receive risperidone 0.5 mg/day, risperidone 1 mg/day, risperidone 2 mg/day, or placebo for 12 weeks (Katz et al. 1999). At end point, placebo and 0.5 mg/day showed similar response rates (33%), whereas 1-mg (45%) and 2-mg dosages (50%) showed significantly superior response rates to either placebo or 0.5 mg. Patients receiving risperidone 2 mg/day were more likely to develop EPS and sedation than were patients receiving risperidone 0.5 or 1 mg/day, suggesting a relatively narrow therapeutic window (Katz et al. 1999). Therefore, a risperidone starting dosage of 0.5 mg/day with gradual, upward dosage titration to 1–2 mg/day is recommended. This range is lower than the optimal risperidone dosage of 6 mg/day in adults with schizophrenia (Chouinard et al. 1993). In a meta-analysis of four large-scale placebo-controlled trials, risperidone was found to be superior to placebo in treating psychosis and agitation, particularly in severely disturbed patients with dementia (Katz et al. 2007).

Paliperidone, or 9-hydroxyrisperidone, is a metabolite of risperidone that has been approved for the treatment of schizophrenia. Paliperidone extended-release (ER) tablets need to be prescribed once daily. There is a lack of data on paliperidone's efficacy and side-effect profile in elderly patients with dementia.

Olanzapine. In an 8-week double-blind, randomized treatment trial of 238 elderly outpatients (mean age 78.6 years) with AD and behavioral complications, olanzapine at an average dosage of 2.4 mg/day was not superior to placebo. The lack of efficacy, however, may have been due to the dosage of olanzapine being too low (Satterlee and Sussman 1998). In another double-blind, placebo-controlled multicenter clinical trial, 206 nursing home patients with AD with behavioral complications were randomly assigned to placebo or fixed-dose olanzapine 5 mg/day, 10 mg/day, or 15 mg/day for 6 weeks. A dosage of 5 mg/day was significantly more efficacious than placebo, but the 10-mg/day and 15-mg/day dosages were not superior. The side effects of sedation and weight gain were limiting factors at the higher dosages (Street et al. 2000). If olanzapine is used in elderly patients with dementia, a starting dosage of 2.5 mg/day with gradual upward dosage titration is recommended.

Quetiapine. In a study of 284 elderly patients with dementia, quetiapine (average dosage 97 mg) and haloperidol (average dosage 2 mg) were indistinguishable from placebo on most measures of efficacy, although haloperidol led to more EPS (Tariot et al. 2006). Unfortunately, the optimal dosage for quetiapine is undetermined because dosage-comparison studies have not been conducted in elderly patients with schizophrenia or dementia. Wide dosage ranges, from 25 to 600 mg/day, are used in clinical practice. Physicians often prescribe quetiapine because of its relatively benign side-effect profile, other than sedation.

Ziprasidone. Ziprasidone is an antipsychotic that is used in dosages of 80–160 mg/day in adults (Arato et al. 2002). Unlike the other atypical antipsychotics, it causes little weight gain, produces minimal to no EPS, and has no anticholinergic side effects (Arato et al. 2002). However, ziprasidone can cause prolongation of the QTc interval on the electrocardiogram, and the need for serial monitoring limits its use in elderly patients with cardiovascular disease. Not surprisingly, published data on the use of ziprasidone in elderly patients are limited.

Aripiprazole. A placebo-controlled study of aripiprazole in 208 outpatients with AD who had behavioral complications showed no advantage for aripiprazole on the main outcome measure (NPI score), but superiority was demonstrated on secondary outcome measures (BPRS psychosis and core scores). The average dosage used was 10 mg/day, and it was generally well tolerated (De Deyn et al. 2005). These limited data suggest that aripiprazole, which may have dopamine-enhancing properties at low dosages and dopamine-blocking properties at higher dosages, may be used as a second-line atypical antipsychotic in patients with AD who have psychosis.

Comparisons of antipsychotics. Head-to-head comparison studies show few differences in efficacy among typical antipsychotics (Barnes et al. 1982; Carlyle et al. 1993; Petrie et al. 1982; Smith et al. 1974; Tsuang et al. 1971) and between typical and atypical antipsychotics (Chan et al. 2001; De Deyn et al. 1999; Suh et al. 2004) in the treatment of psychosis and agitation/aggression in dementia. The main difference is in the propensity to cause neurological side effects, which are less common with atypical antipsychotics.

In the 421 elderly patients with psychosis or agitation/aggression who participated in the CATIE Alzheimer's study that compared risperidone, olanzapine, quetiapine, and placebo (initial randomized phase), there were no significant differences in time to discontinuation because the superior efficacy of risperidone and olanzapine was compromised by their increased propensity to side effects; quetiapine was indistinguishable from placebo (Schneider et al. 2006). Thus, efficacy must be weighed against side effects when prescribing risperidone or olanzapine in a patient with dementia, and quetiapine may not be effective.

Choice of antipsychotic for patients with dementia. Given the relative lack of differences in efficacy among antipsychotics (except the possible lower efficacy for quetiapine) for treating psychosis or behavioral dyscontrol in dementia, the potential side-effect profile should determine the choice for individual patients (Ellingrod et al. 2002). Patients prone to orthostatic hypotension (e.g., patients receiving beta-blockers) may develop this side effect when taking risperidone or olanzapine, although this side effect is uncommon at low dosages (Katz et al. 1999; Street et al. 2000). Olanzapine causes weight gain and is strongly sedating, but the latter side effect may be advantageous in patients with prominent insomnia. Quetiapine is generally well tolerated but can be sedating. Risperidone is more likely to cause EPS, so olanzapine or quetiapine should be preferred for elderly patients who have parkinsonian features. In a study of 35 agitated patients with dementia who were switched from haloperidol to risperidone, the crossover was generally safe and effective (Lane et al. 2002).

Optimal dosing strategy. In patients with AD, risperidone should be started at 0.25–0.5 mg/day at bedtime (or twice-daily dosing), with a 0.5-mg/day increase per week to a maximum of 2 (possibly 3) mg/day. The starting dosage for olanzapine should be 2.5 mg/day or 5 mg/day at bedtime, slowly increased to a targeted dosage of 5–10 mg/day. Quetiapine should be started at 25 mg twice daily, with doses increased as tolerated up to 300 mg twice daily based solely on clinical response and side effects because the optimal dosage range for quetiapine has not been identified. If a typical antipsychotic is used, a starting dose equivalent to haloperidol 0.5 mg/day is suggested, with subsequent individualized dosage titration.

Concomitant psychotropics. Anticholinergic agents to treat EPS should be avoided, particularly in patients with AD, in whom the cholinergic deficit is believed to underlie much of the cognitive impairment. In some patients, the concomitant use of a hypnotic (e.g., zolpidem 5–10 mg, zaleplon 5–10 mg) may be required. Trazodone in dosages of 25–200 mg/day can also be used as a hypnotic in these patients.

Optimal duration of antipsychotic treatment. A trial of 6–12 weeks in duration is usually sufficient to determine the outcome of an antipsychotic treatment trial. There is conflicting evidence regarding how long these patients should continue taking antipsychotics. Early studies indicated a moderate to high rate of relapse after discontinuation (Avorn et al. 1992; Fitz and Mallya 1992; Horwitz et al. 1995), but more recent reports suggest that antipsychotics can be discontinued in nursing home patients with dementia without increased risk of relapse (Ballard 2009; Cohen-Mansfield et al. 1999). The common flaw in these studies is that patients already receiving antipsychotics were identified and those medications were discontinued, and therefore it remains unclear if these patients actually needed to be treated with antipsychotics in the first place.

Effects on cognition and activities of daily living. The anticholinergic activity of antipsychotics may further compromise cholinergic cognitive deficits in patients with AD. The level of cognitive impairment may be increased by the use of antipsychotics with strong anticholinergic properties or by the addition of anticholinergic agents to treat drug-induced EPS. Therefore, if EPS develop following antipsychotic treatment in a patient with dementia, switching to an antipsychotic that is less likely to cause EPS is strongly preferable to adding an anticholinergic medication to treat EPS. At another level, the sedation produced by antipsychotics may worsen the degree of disorientation and cognitive impairment in patients with AD.

Benzodiazepines and Anticonvulsants

Benzodiazepines and anticonvulsants are not used specifically to treat psychosis in dementia but have been studied as potential treatments for behavioral dyscontrol. Early studies comparing antipsychotics to benzodiazepines showed few differences and suffered from methodological flaws, particularly in sample selection and study design (Burgio et al. 1992; Covington 1975; Kirven and Montero 1973; Stotsky 1984; Tewfik et al. 1970). Benzodiazepines have deleterious effects on learning and memory in normal subjects (Ghoneim et al. 1981; Jones et al. 1978; Liljequist et al. 1978), particularly in elderly persons (Pomara et al. 1989). Benzodiazepines can lead to tolerance and dependence, and worsening of cognition is a concern. Therefore, benzodiazepines should be used in low dosages and restricted to short-term crisis management of agitated and anxious behaviors if antipsychotics or other medications are ineffective.

A small sample study suggested that carbamazepine was effective in the treatment of behavioral complications of AD (Tariot et al. 1995), and valproate was efficacious in a single-site study by the same research group (Porsteinsson et al. 2001). However, valproate at an average dosage of 800 mg/day did not show superiority over placebo in a larger study of 153 nursing home patients who participated in a double-blind, placebo-controlled trial (Tariot et al. 2006).

Antipsychotics in Other Neurodegenerative Disorders

Antipsychotic efficacy has not been systematically compared in different subtypes of dementia (e.g., AD and vascular dementia). The antipsychotic treatment trials that included patients with vascular, mixed, and other forms of dementia did not reveal any differences in treatment response among the diagnostic subtypes of dementia (De Deyn et al. 1999; Katz et al. 1999). The recommendations for the use of antipsychotics in AD generally apply to their use in other types of dementia, except DLB and PD. A post hoc analysis of the olanzapine dosage comparison study in patients with AD suggested that olanzapine was safe and effective for the subgroup that met diagnostic criteria for DLB (Cummings et al. 2002).

Patients with PD can develop iatrogenic psychosis caused by the levodopa or dopamine agonists. Lowering the dosage of the dopaminergic agent may lead to improvement in psychotic symptoms, but patients may experience an unacceptable increase in parkinsonian symptoms (Breier et al. 2002). In such cases, antipsychotics with a very low propensity to cause EPS can be considered. Clozapine, but not olanzapine, may be of some value in treating the psychosis of PD (Breier et al. 2002; Friedman and Fernandez 2002).

In patients with delirium, a standard treatment strategy is short-term administration of antipsychotics, particularly antipsychotics with low anticholinergic properties such as haloperidol (Tune 2002). Atypical antipsychotics are useful in the management of delirium, and olanzapine has been reported to be safe and efficacious for the treatment of symptoms of delirium in hospitalized patients (Breitbart et al. 2002).

Side Effects of Antipsychotic Medications

Older patients are more sensitive to the side effects of antipsychotics, which can cause a variety of side effects in all age groups: sedation; cardiac effects including tachycardia and orthostatic hypotension; anticholinergic side effects including dry mouth, blurred vision, constipation and urinary retention, and in severe cases confusion and disorientation; neuroleptic malignant syndrome with hyperpyrexia; autonomic instability and tachycardia; pigmentary retinopathy; weight gain and associated metabolic changes; allergic reactions; and seizures (Arana 2000). In elderly patients, particularly important risks are orthostatic hypotension leading to falls and fractures, anticholinergic side effects, and neurological side effects of EPS and TD.

The antipsychotics most likely to cause orthostatic hypotension are low-potency conventional antipsychotics such as chlorpromazine and thioridazine, and the atypical antipsychotics clozapine, risperidone, olanzapine, and quetiapine (Tandon 1998). Low-potency conventional antipsychotics and clozapine have the most significant anticholinergic effects. At comparable dosages, low-potency conventional antipsychotics are less likely to cause EPS than high-potency antipsychotics such as haloperidol, but up to 50% of all patients between ages 60 and 80 receiving typical antipsychotics develop either EPS or TD (Jeste et al. 1999; Saltz et al. 1991). Besides increasing age, other risk factors for TD include early development of EPS, cumulative use of antipsychotics, duration of antipsychotic treatment, and history of alcohol abuse or dependence (Lohr et al. 2002). Atypical antipsychotics have a lower potential for TD compared to typical antipsychotics (Jeste and Finkel 2000).

Metabolic Syndrome

The metabolic syndrome with glucose dysregulation is a potential side effect of all antipsychotics, to varying degrees. New-onset type 2 diabetes mellitus or diabetic ketoacidosis may be more common with clozapine and olanzapine than with other antipsychotics, and blood glucose levels need to be monitored in elderly patients (Jin et al. 2004). In a meta-analysis of 11 studies of typical and atypical antipsychotics, the relative risk of diabetes in patients with schizophrenia prescribed one of the second-generation antipsychotics (only clozapine, olanzapine, risperidone, and quetiapine had sufficient data to be included in the analysis) versus first-generation antipsychotics was 1.32 (95% confidence interval, 1.15–1.51). Therefore, the increase in risk of diabetes by using second-generation versus first-generation antipsychotics was not large (Smith et al. 2008). Overall, the issue of weight gain, with the consequent risk of the metabolic syndrome, needs to be considered in all patients, particularly those who are overweight before starting antipsychotic medication.

Mortality Risk

The use of antipsychotics is associated with an increased risk of sudden cardiac death (Ray et al. 2009). Among the typical antipsychotics, thioridazine appears to carry the highest risk of sudden, unexplained death that is believed to be due to cardiac causes (Reilly et al. 2002). Prolongation of the QTc interval, which is associated with the development of torsades de pointes and sudden death, is also known to occur with most atypical antipsychotics, but aripiprazole may reduce rather than increase the QTc interval (Goodnick et al. 2002).

On the basis of a review of 17 double-blind, placebo-controlled trials of atypical antipsychotics in patients with dementia (over 5,000 patients, average age 81 years, two-thirds received drug over a 6–12 week period), the FDA concluded that there was a significantly greater mortality risk (1.5–1.7 times) for patients treated with these medications than for those treated with placebo. Separately, in an observational study of patients in a pharmacy benefit program for the elderly, all-cause mortality for patients taking typical or conventional antipsychotics was similar to that of patients taking atypical antipsychotic drugs (Wang et al. 2005). As a result, all typical and atypical antipsychotics carry a black box warning about increased mortality risk (Jeste et al. 2008).

At this time, there is no definite pathophysiological explanation as to why elderly patients with dementia who take these medications have an increased mortality risk. There appears to be a small increase in the risk of stroke (Brodaty et al. 2003), for which the mechanism has not been identified (Jeste et al. 2008). However, this increase in stroke risk does not by itself account for the increased mortality risk (Jeste et al. 2008), and most deaths in the 17 studies evaluated by the FDA were due to cardiac or infectious causes, which generally are among the most common causes of death for patients with dementia. One possible pathophysiological explanation is that excessive sedation increases the risk of aspiration and subsequent pneumonia.

Psychosocial Intervention

For patients with schizophrenia and other primary psychotic disorders, the psychosocial interventions used with young adults can also be used with elderly patients. Preliminary evidence suggests that a combination of skills training and cognitive-behavioral therapy may be helpful for elderly patients (Berry and Barrowclough 2009). This type of intervention is helpful in treating the social and cognitive symptoms of schizophrenia, but it is unlikely that positive psychotic symptoms are influenced by these forms of therapy. The difficulties faced by patients with schizophrenia with respect to effective functioning and quality of life are compounded by the advent of medical illnesses and changes in social support that occur with aging.

For patients with AD, psychosocial interventions have focused on the caregiver primarily because patients with moderate to severe dementia typically develop psychosis and behavioral disinhibition, and their severe cognitive impairment limits their ability to use psychotherapeutic intervention. One study of behavioral intervention with caregivers found it to be comparable to haloperidol, trazodone, and placebo, but all groups did poorly, and the behavioral intervention was conducted in a nonrandomized, unblinded subgroup, thereby limiting its interpretation (Teri et al. 2000).

Prevention Strategies and Environmental Manipulation

Because the etiology of psychosis in elderly patients is not fully understood, specific preventive strategies have not yet been identified. After the illness begins, it is important to reduce exposure to stressors that can exacerbate symptoms, to educate caregivers and individuals in the social support network, and to ensure adequate treatment with systematic follow-up to promote adherence. In this context, improving the psychosocial environment is important, and a variety of efforts may be effective. For example, one suggestion has been that introducing pets may decrease agitation and aggression in patients in nursing homes, but systematic controlled data are lacking.

Key Points

- Psychotic disorders in the elderly broadly fall into three categories: early onset, late onset, and psychosis secondary to medical or neurological disorders. Diagnosis, estimation of prognosis, and treatment differ as a function of these categories.
- Antipsychotics remain the first-line treatment for schizophrenia and other primary psychotic disorders across the life span. Although not explicitly approved by the FDA for this purpose, the extant studies suggest that these medications are also useful in the treatment of psychosis and behavioral dyscontrol in Alzheimer's disease and other types of dementia.
- For elderly patients, low dosages of antipsychotics should be used. Close monitoring of target symptoms, somatic side effects including mobility and drowsiness, potential drug interactions, cognition, and activities of daily living is necessary.
- Psychosocial treatments, including educational strategies, behavioral interventions, and cognitive therapy with patients or caregivers, may have some utility, but controlled studies in elderly patients with psychosis are lacking.

Recommended Readings and Web Sites

Blazer DG, Steffens D (eds): The American Psychiatric Publishing Textbook of Geriatric Psychiatry, 4th Edition. Washington, DC, American Psychiatric Publishing, 2009

Salzman C: Clinical Geriatric Psychopharmacology, 4th Edition. Baltimore, MD, Lippincott Williams & Wilkins, 2004

Alzheimer's Association: www.alz.org/index.asp. Provides information on the latest Alzheimer's disease care strategies, research findings, and advocacy initiatives.

National Alliance on Mental Illness: www.nami.org. This is a nonprofit, grassroots, self-help, support, and advocacy organization of consumers, families, and friends of people suffering from mental illness.

References

American Psychiatric Association: Diagnostic and Statistical Manual of Mental Disorders, 4th Edition, Text Revision. Washington, DC, American Psychiatric Association, 2000

Arana GW: An overview of side effects caused by typical antipsychotics. J Clin Psychiatry 61(suppl):5–11; discussion 12–13, 2000

Arato M, O'Connor R, Meltzer HY: A 1-year, double-blind, placebo-controlled trial of ziprasidone 40, 80, and 160 mg/day in chronic schizophrenia: the Ziprasidone Extended Use in Schizophrenia (ZEUS) study. Int Clin Psychopharmacol 17:207–215, 2002

Avorn J, Soumerai SB, Everitt DE, et al: A randomized trial of a program to reduce the use of psychoactive drugs in nursing homes. N Engl J Med 327:168–173, 1992

Ballard C: Atypical antipsychotics fail to improve functioning or quality of life in people with Alzheimer's disease. Evid Based Ment Health 12:20, 2009

Ballard C, O'Brien J, Coope B, et al: A prospective study of psychotic symptoms in dementia sufferers: psychosis in dementia. Int Psychogeriatr 9:57–64, 1997

Barak Y, Shamir E, Weizman R: Would a switch from typical antipsychotics to risperidone be beneficial for elderly schizophrenic patients? A naturalistic, long-term, retrospective, comparative study. J Clin Psychopharmacol 22:115–120, 2002

Barnes R, Veith R, Okimoto J, et al: Efficacy of antipsychotic medications in behaviorally disturbed dementia patients. Am J Psychiatry 139:1170–1174, 1982

Berry K, Barrowclough C: The needs of older adults with schizophrenia: implications for psychological interventions. Clin Psychol Rev 29:68–76, 2009

Bodick NC, Offen WW, Shannon HE, et al: The selective muscarinic agonist xanomeline improves both the cognitive deficits and behavioral symptoms of Alzheimer disease. Alzheimer Dis Assoc Disord 11(suppl):S16–S22, 1997

Bondareff W: Neuropathology of psychotic symptoms in Alzheimer's disease. Int Psychogeriatr 8(suppl):233–237; discussion 269–272, 1996

Breier A, Sutton VK, Feldman PD, et al: Olanzapine in the treatment of dopamimetic-induced psychosis in patients with Parkinson's disease. Biol Psychiatry 52:438–445, 2002

Breitbart W, Tremblay A, Gibson C: An open trial of olanzapine for the treatment of delirium in hospitalized cancer patients. Psychosomatics 43:175–182, 2002

Broadway J, Mintzer J: The many faces of psychosis in the elderly. Curr Opin Psychiatry 20:551–558, 2007

Brodaty H, Ames D, Snowdon J, et al: A randomized placebo-controlled trial of risperidone for the treatment of aggression, agitation, and psychosis of dementia. J Clin Psychiatry 64:134–143, 2003

Burgio LD, Reynolds CF III, Janosky JE, et al: A behavioral microanalysis of the effects of haloperidol and oxazepam in demented psychogeriatric inpatients. Int J Geriatr Psychiatry 7: 253–262, 1992

Carlyle W, Ancill RJ, Sheldon L: Aggression in the demented patient: a double-blind study of loxapine versus haloperidol. Int Clin Psychopharmacol 8:103–108, 1993

Centorrino F, Baldessarini RJ, Kando JC, et al: Clozapine and metabolites: concentrations in serum and clinical findings during treatment of chronically psychotic patients. J Clin Psychopharmacol 14:119–125, 1994

Chan WC, Lam LC, Choy CN, et al: A double-blind randomised comparison of risperidone and haloperidol in the treatment of behavioural and psychological symptoms in Chinese dementia patients. Int J Geriatr Psychiatry 16:1156–1162, 2001

Chengappa KN, Baker RW, Kreinbrook SB, et al: Clozapine use in female geriatric patients with psychoses. J Geriatr Psychiatry Neurol 8:12–15, 1995

Chouinard G, Jones B, Remington G, et al: A Canadian multicenter placebo-controlled study of fixed doses of risperidone and haloperidol in the treatment of chronic schizophrenic patients. J Clin Psychopharmacol 13:25–40, 1993

Cohen-Mansfield J: Agitated behavior in persons with dementia: the relationship between type of behavior, its frequency, and its disruptiveness. J Psychiatr Res 43:64–69, 2008

Cohen-Mansfield J, Marx MS, Rosenthal AS: A description of agitation in a nursing home. J Gerontol 44:M77–M84, 1989

Cohen-Mansfield J, Lipson S, Werner P, et al: Withdrawal of haloperidol, thioridazine, and lorazepam in the nursing home: a controlled, double-blind study. Arch Intern Med 159:1733–1740, 1999

Colenda CC, Mickus MA, Marcus SC, et al: Comparison of adult and geriatric psychiatric practice patterns: findings from the American Psychiatric Association's Practice Research Network. Am J Geriatr Psychiatry 10:609–617, 2002

Cook SE, Miyahara S, Bacanu SA, et al: Psychotic symptoms in Alzheimer disease: evidence for subtypes. Am J Geriatr Psychiatry 11:406–413, 2003

Covington JS: Alleviating agitation, apprehension, and related symptoms in geriatric patients: a double-blind comparison of a phenothiazine and a benzodiazepine. South Med J 68:719–724, 1975

Csernansky JG, Schuchart EK: Relapse and rehospitalisation rates in patients with schizophrenia: effects of second generation antipsychotics. CNS Drugs 16:473–484, 2002

Cummings JL, Mega M, Gray K, et al: The Neuropsychiatric Inventory: comprehensive assessment of psychopathology in dementia. Neurology 44:2308–2314, 1994

Cummings JL, Street J, Masterman D, et al: Efficacy of olanzapine in the treatment of psychosis in dementia with Lewy bodies. Dement Geriatr Cogn Disord 13:67–73, 2002

Cutler AJ, Goldstein JM, Tumas JA: Dosing and switching strategies for quetiapine fumarate. Clin Ther 24:209–222, 2002

Davies P, Maloney AJ: Selective loss of central cholinergic neurons in Alzheimer's disease. Lancet 2:1403, 1976

De Deyn PP, Rabheru K, Rasmussen A, et al: A randomized trial of risperidone, placebo, and haloperidol for behavioral symptoms of dementia. Neurology 53:946–955, 1999

De Deyn P, Jeste DV, Swanink R, et al: Aripiprazole for the treatment of psychosis in patients with Alzheimer's disease: a randomized, placebo-controlled study. J Clin Psychopharmacol 25:463–467, 2005

Devanand DP, Miller L, Richards M, et al: The Columbia University Scale for Psychopathology in Alzheimer's disease. Arch Neurol 49:371–376, 1992

Devanand DP, Jacobs DM, Tang MX, et al: The course of psychopathologic features in mild to moderate Alzheimer disease. Arch Gen Psychiatry 54:257–263, 1997

Devanand DP, Marder K, Michaels KS, et al: A randomized, placebo-controlled dose-comparison trial of haloperidol for psychosis and disruptive behaviors in Alzheimer's disease. Am J Psychiatry 155:1512–1520, 1998

Dolder CR, Lacro JP, Dunn LB, et al: Antipsychotic medication adherence: is there a difference between typical and atypical agents? Am J Psychiatry 159:103–108, 2002

Ellingrod VL, Schultz SK, Ekstam-Smith K, et al: Comparison of risperidone with olanzapine in elderly patients with dementia and psychosis. Pharmacotherapy 22:1–5, 2002

Elon R, Pawlson LG: The impact of OBRA on medical practice within nursing facilities. J Am Geriatr Soc 40:958–963, 1992

Fitz D, Mallya A: Discontinuation of a psychogeriatric program for nursing home residents: psychotropic medication changes and behavioral reactions. J Appl Gerontol 11:50–63, 1992

Forstl H, Besthorn C, Geiger-Kabisch C, et al: Psychotic features and the course of Alzheimer's disease: relationship to cognitive, electroencephalographic and computerized tomography findings. Acta Psychiatr Scand 87:395–399, 1993

Friedman JH, Fernandez HH: Atypical antipsychotics in Parkinson-sensitive populations. J Geriatr Psychiatry Neurol 15:156–170, 2002

Gauthier S, Feldman H, Hecker J, et al: Efficacy of donepezil on behavioral symptoms in patients with moderate to severe Alzheimer's disease. Int Psychogeriatr 14:389–404, 2002

Ghoneim MM, Mewaldt SP, Berie JL, et al: Memory and performance effects of single and 3-week administration of diazepam. Psychopharmacology (Berl) 73:147–151, 1981

Giron MS, Forsell Y, Bernsten C, et al: Psychotropic drug use in elderly people with and without dementia. Int J Geriatr Psychiatry 16:900–906, 2001

Goodnick PJ, Jerry J, Parra F: Psychotropic drugs and the ECG: focus on the QTc interval. Expert Opin Pharmacother 3:479–498, 2002

Grimmer T, Kurz A: Effects of cholinesterase inhibitors on behavioural disturbances in Alzheimer's disease: a systematic review. Drugs Aging 23:957–967, 2006

Holmes C, Smith H, Ganderton R, et al: Psychosis and aggression in Alzheimer's disease: the effect of dopamine receptor gene variation. J Neurol Neurosurg Psychiatry 71:777–779, 2001

Holroyd S, Laurie S: Correlates of psychotic symptoms among elderly outpatients. Int J Geriatr Psychiatry 14:379–384, 1999

Horwitz GJ, Tariot PN, Mead K, et al: Discontinuation of antipsychotics in nursing home patients with dementia. Am J Geriatr Psychiatry 3:290–299, 1995

Howard R, Rabins PV, Seeman MV, et al: Late-onset schizophrenia and very-late-onset schizophrenia-like psychosis: an international consensus. The International Late-Onset Schizophrenia Group. Am J Psychiatry 157:172–178, 2000

Jeste DV, Finkel SI: Psychosis of Alzheimer's disease and related dementias: diagnostic criteria for a distinct syndrome. Am J Geriatr Psychiatry 8:29–34, 2000

Jeste DV, Symonds LL, Harris MJ, et al: Nondementia nonpraecox dementia praecox? Late-onset schizophrenia. Am J Geriatr Psychiatry 5:302–317, 1997

Jeste DV, Lacro JP, Palmer B, et al: Incidence of tardive dyskinesia in early stages of low-dose treatment with typical neuroleptics in older patients. Am J Psychiatry 156:309–311, 1999

Jeste DV, Blazer D, Casey D, et al: ACNP white paper: update on use of antipsychotic drugs in elderly persons with dementia. Neuropsychopharmacology 33:957–970, 2008

Jin H, Meyer JM, Jeste DV: Atypical antipsychotics and glucose dysregulation: a systematic review. Schizophr Res 71:195–212, 2004

Jones DM, Lewis MJ, Spriggs TL: The effects of low doses of diazepam on human performance in group administered tasks. Br J Clin Pharmacol 6:333–337, 1978

Jones PB, Barnes TR, Davies L, et al: Randomized controlled trial of the effect on Quality of Life of second- vs first-generation antipsychotic drugs in schizophrenia: Cost Utility of the Latest Antipsychotic Drugs in Schizophrenia Study (CUtLASS 1). Arch Gen Psychiatry 63:1079–1087, 2006

Jorgensen P, Bennedsen B, Christensen J, et al: Acute and transient psychotic disorder: a 1-year follow-up study. Acta Psychiatr Scand 96:150–154, 1997

Kane J, Honigfeld G, Singer J, et al: Clozapine for the treatment-resistant schizophrenic: a double-blind comparison with chlorpromazine. Arch Gen Psychiatry 45:789–796, 1988

Katz I, Jeste DV, Mintzer JE, et al: Comparison of risperidone and placebo for psychosis and behavioral disturbances associated with dementia: a randomized, double-blind trial. Risperidone Study Group. J Clin Psychiatry 60:107–115, 1999

Katz I, de Deyn PP, Mintzer J, et al: The efficacy and safety of risperidone in the treatment of psychosis of Alzheimer's disease and mixed dementia: a meta-analysis of 4 placebo-controlled clinical trials. Int J Geriatr Psychiatry 22:475–484, 2007

Kaufer DI, Cummings JL, Christine D: Effect of tacrine on behavioral symptoms in Alzheimer's disease: an open-label study. J Geriatr Psychiatry Neurol 9:1–6, 1996

Khouzam HR, Emes R: Late life psychosis: assessment and general treatment strategies. Compr Ther 33:127–143, 2007

Kindermann SS, Dolder CR, Bailey A, et al: Pharmacological treatment of psychosis and agitation in elderly patients with dementia: four decades of experience. Drugs Aging 19:257–276, 2002

Kirven LE, Montero EF: Comparison of thioridazine and diazepam in the control of nonpsychotic symptoms associated with senility: double-blind study. J Am Geriatr Soc 21:546–551, 1973

Koenig HG, George LK, Schneider R: Mental health care for older adults in the year 2020: a dangerous and avoided topic. Gerontologist 34:674–679, 1994

Kurz M, Hummer M, Kemmler G, et al: Long-term pharmacokinetics of clozapine. Br J Psychiatry 173:341–344, 1998

Labrie V, Roder JC: The involvement of the NMDA receptor D-serine/glycine site in the pathophysiology and treatment of schizophrenia. Neurosci Biobehav Rev 34:351–372, 2010

Lanctot KL, Best TS, Mittmann N, et al: Efficacy and safety of neuroleptics in behavioral disorders associated with dementia. J Clin Psychiatry 59:550–561; quiz 562–563, 1998

Lane HY, Chang YC, Chiu CC, et al: Association of risperidone treatment response with a polymorphism in the 5-HT(2A) receptor gene. Am J Psychiatry 159:1593–1595, 2002

Lantz MS, Louis A, Lowenstein G, et al: A longitudinal study of psychotropic prescriptions in a teaching nursing home. Am J Psychiatry 147:1637–1639, 1990

Lawlor BA, Ryan TM, Bierer LM, et al: Lack of association between clinical symptoms and postmortem indices of brain serotonin function in Alzheimer's disease. Biol Psychiatry 37:895–896, 1995

Levine J, Chengappa KN, Brar JS, et al: Psychotropic drug prescription patterns among patients with bipolar I disorder. Bipolar Disord 2:120–130, 2000

Lieberman JA, Stroup TS, McEvoy JP, et al: Effectiveness of antipsychotic drugs in patients with chronic schizophrenia. N Engl J Med 353:1209–1223, 2005

Liljequist R, Linnoila M, Mattila MJ: Effect of diazepam and chlorpromazine on memory functions in man. Eur J Clin Pharmacol 13:339–343, 1978

Lohr JB, Caligiuri MP, Edson R, et al: Treatment predictors of extrapyramidal side effects in patients with tardive dyskinesia: results from Veterans Affairs Cooperative Study 394. J Clin Psychopharmacol 22:196–200, 2002

Louis ED, Bennett DA: Mild Parkinsonian signs: an overview of an emerging concept. Mov Disord 22:1681–1688, 2007

Lyketsos CG, Steinberg M, Tschanz JT, et al: Mental and behavioral disturbances in dementia: findings from the Cache County Study on Memory in Aging. Am J Psychiatry 157:708–714, 2000

McDonald WM: Epidemiology, etiology, and treatment of geriatric mania. J Clin Psychiatry 61(suppl):3–11, 2000

Mega MS, Lee L, Dinov ID, et al: Cerebral correlates of psychotic symptoms in Alzheimer's disease. J Neurol Neurosurg Psychiatry 69:167–171, 2000

Meyers BS, Klimstra SA, Gabriele M, et al: Continuation treatment of delusional depression in older adults. Am J Geriatr Psychiatry 9:415–422, 2001

Möller HJ: Amisulpride: efficacy in the management of chronic patients with predominant negative symptoms of schizophrenia. Eur Arch Psychiatry Clin Neurosci 251:217–224, 2001

Mukaetova-Ladinska EB, Harrington CR, Roth M, et al: Biochemical and anatomical redistribution of tau protein in Alzheimer's disease. Am J Pathol 143:565–578, 1993

Mulsant BH, Pollock BG: Treatment-resistant depression in late life. J Geriatr Psychiatry Neurol 11:186–193, 1998

Nacmias B, Tedde A, Forleo P, et al: Association between 5-HT(2A) receptor polymorphism and psychotic symptoms in Alzheimer's disease. Biol Psychiatry 50:472–475, 2001

Nelson JC, Charney DS, Vingiano AW: False-positive diagnosis with primary-affective-disorder criteria. Lancet 2:1252–1253, 1978

Oberholzer AF, Hendriksen C, Monsch AU, et al: Safety and effectiveness of low-dose clozapine in psychogeriatric patients: a preliminary study. Int Psychogeriatr 4:187–195, 1992

Pantelis C, Velakoulis D, Wood SJ, et al: Neuroimaging and emerging psychotic disorders: the Melbourne ultra-high risk studies. Int Rev Psychiatry 19:371–381, 2007

Paulsen JS, Salmon DP, Thal LJ, et al: Incidence of and risk factors for hallucinations and delusions in patients with probable AD. Neurology 54:1965–1971, 2000

Perry EK, Gibson PH, Blessed G, et al: Neurotransmitter enzyme abnormalities in senile dementia: choline acetyltransferase and glutamic acid decarboxylase activities in necropsy brain tissue. J Neurol Sci 34:247–265, 1977

Petrie WM, Ban TA, Berney S, et al: Loxapine in psychogeriatrics: a placebo- and standard-controlled clinical investigation. J Clin Psychopharmacol 2:122–126, 1982

Pillmann F, Balzuweit S, Haring A, et al: Suicidal behavior in acute and transient psychotic disorders. Psychiatry Res 117:199–209, 2003

Pitner JK, Mintzer JE, Pennypacker LC, et al: Efficacy and adverse effects of clozapine in four elderly psychotic patients. J Clin Psychiatry 56:180–185, 1995

Pollock BG, Mulsant BH, Rosen J, et al: Comparison of citalopram, perphenazine, and placebo for the acute treatment of psychosis and behavioral disturbances in hospitalized, demented patients. Am J Psychiatry 159:460–465, 2002

Pomara N, Deptula D, Medel M, et al: Effects of diazepam on recall memory: relationship to aging, dose, and duration of treatment. Psychopharmacol Bull 25:144–148, 1989

Porsteinsson AP, Tariot PN, Erb R, et al: Placebo-controlled study of divalproex sodium for agitation in dementia. Am J Geriatr Psychiatry 9:58–66, 2001

Purohit DP, Perl DP, Haroutunian V, et al: Alzheimer disease and related neurodegenerative diseases in elderly patients with schizophrenia: a postmortem neuropathologic study of 100 cases. Arch Gen Psychiatry 55:205–211, 1998

Raskind MA: Evaluation and management of aggressive behavior in the elderly demented patient. J Clin Psychiatry 60(suppl):45–49, 1999

Raskind MA, Peskind ER: Neurobiologic bases of noncognitive behavioral problems in Alzheimer disease. Alzheimer Dis Assoc Disord 8(suppl):54–60, 1994

Ray WA, Chung CP, Murray KT, et al: Atypical antipsychotic drugs and the risk of sudden cardiac death. N Engl J Med 360:225–235, 2009

Reilly JG, Ayis SA, Ferrier IN, et al: Thioridazine and sudden unexplained death in psychiatric in-patients. Br J Psychiatry 180:515–522, 2002

Reisberg B, Borenstein J, Salob SP, et al: Behavioral symptoms in Alzheimer's disease: phenomenology and treatment. J Clin Psychiatry 48(suppl):9–15, 1987

Reisberg B, Ferris SH, de Leon MJ, et al: The stage specific temporal course of Alzheimer's disease: functional and behavioral concomitants based upon cross-sectional and longitudinal observation. Prog Clin Biol Res 317:23–41, 1989

Richtand NM, McNamara RK: Serotonin and dopamine interactions in psychosis prevention. Prog Brain Res 172:141–153, 2008

Russo-Neustadt A, Cotman CW: Adrenergic receptors in Alzheimer's disease brain: selective increases in the cerebella of aggressive patients. J Neurosci 17:5573–5580, 1997

Sable JA, Jeste DV: Antipsychotic treatment for late-life schizophrenia. Curr Psychiatry Rep 4:299–306, 2002

Sackeim HA, Devanand DP, Nobler M: Electroconvulsive therapy, in Psychopharmacology: The Fourth Generation of Progress. Edited by Bloom F, Kupfer D. New York, Raven, 1995, pp 1123–1141

Saltz BL, Woerner MG, Kane JM, et al: Prospective study of tardive dyskinesia incidence in the elderly. JAMA 266:2402–2406, 1991

Satterlee JS, Sussman MR: Unusual membrane-associated protein kinases in higher plants. J Membr Biol 164:205–213, 1998

Schneider LS, Pollock VE, Lyness SA: A meta-analysis of controlled trials of neuroleptic treatment in dementia. J Am Geriatr Soc 38:553–563, 1990

Schneider LS, Tariot PN, Dagerman KS, et al: Effectiveness of atypical antipsychotic drugs in patients with Alzheimer's disease. N Engl J Med 355:1525–1538, 2006

Smith GR, Taylor CW, Linkous P: Haloperidol versus thioridazine for the treatment of psychogeriatric patients: a double-blind clinical trial. Psychosomatics 15:134–138, 1974

Smith M, Hopkins D, Peveler RC, et al: First- v. second-generation antipsychotics and risk for diabetes in schizophrenia: systematic review and meta-analysis. Br J Psychiatry 192:406–411, 2008

Spiker DG, Weiss JC, Dealy RS, et al: The pharmacological treatment of delusional depression. Am J Psychiatry 142:430–436, 1985

Stotsky B: Multicenter study comparing thioridazine with diazepam and placebo in elderly, nonpsychotic patients with emotional and behavioral disorders. Clin Ther 6:546–559, 1984

Street JS, Clark WS, Gannon KS, et al: Olanzapine treatment of psychotic and behavioral symptoms in patients with Alzheimer disease in nursing care facilities: a double-blind, randomized, placebo-controlled trial. The HGEU Study Group. Arch Gen Psychiatry 57:968–976, 2000

Suh GH, Son HG, Ju YS, et al: A randomized, double-blind, crossover comparison of risperidone and haloperidol in Korean dementia patients with behavioral disturbances. Am J Geriatr Psychiatry 12:509–516, 2004

Sultzer DL, Brown CV, Mandelkern MA, et al: Delusional thoughts and regional frontal/temporal cortex metabolism in Alzheimer's disease. Am J Psychiatry 160:341–349, 2003

Sunderland T, Molchan SE, Little JT, et al: Pharmacologic challenges in Alzheimer disease and normal controls: cognitive modeling in humans. Alzheimer Dis Assoc Disord 11(suppl):S23–S26, 1997

Sweet RA, Nimgaonkar VL, Kamboh MI, et al: Dopamine receptor genetic variation, psychosis, and aggression in Alzheimer disease. Arch Neurol 55:1335–1340, 1998

Tandon R: Impact of antipsychotic treatment on long-term course of schizophrenic illness: an introduction. J Psychiatr Res 32:119–120, 1998

Tariot PN, Mack JL, Patterson MB, et al: The Behavior Rating Scale for Dementia of the Consortium to Establish a Registry for Alzheimer's Disease: The Behavioral Pathology Committee of the Consortium to Establish a Registry for Alzheimer's Disease. Am J Psychiatry 152:1349–1357, 1995

Tariot PN, Schneider L, Katz IR, et al: Quetiapine treatment of psychosis associated with dementia: a double-blind, randomized, placebo-controlled clinical trial. Am J Geriatr Psychiatry 14:767–776, 2006

Teri L, Logsdon RG, Peskind E, et al: Treatment of agitation in AD: a randomized, placebo-controlled clinical trial. Neurology 55: 1271–1278, 2000

Tewfik GI, Jain VK, Harcup M, et al: Effectiveness of various tranquilisers in the management of senile restlessness. Gerontol Clin (Basel) 12:351–359, 1970

Thomas VS, Darvesh S, MacKnight C, et al: Estimating the prevalence of dementia in elderly people: a comparison of the Canadian Study of Health and Aging and National Population Health Survey approaches. Int Psychogeriatr 13(suppl):169–175, 2001

Tsuang MM, Lu LM, Stotsky BA, et al: Haloperidol versus thioridazine for hospitalized psychogeriatric patients: double-blind study. J Am Geriatr Soc 19:593–600, 1971

Tune L: The role of antipsychotics in treating delirium. Curr Psychiatry Rep 4:209–212, 2002

Wang PS, Schneeweiss S, Avorn J, et al: Risk of death in elderly users of conventional vs. atypical antipsychotic medications. N Engl J Med 353:2335–2341, 2005

Wood S, Cummings JL, Hsu MA, et al: The use of the Neuropsychiatric Inventory in nursing home residents: characterization and measurement. Am J Geriatr Psychiatry 8:75–83, 2000

Zayas EM, Grossberg GT: The treatment of psychosis in late life. J Clin Psychiatry 59(suppl):5–10; discussion 11–12, 1998

Zubenko GS, Moossy J, Martinez AJ, et al: Neuropathologic and neurochemical correlates of psychosis in primary dementia. Arch Neurol 48:619–624, 1991

22

Contemporary Personality Psychology

Paul T. Costa Jr., Ph.D.
Robert R. McCrae, Ph.D.

Personality may seem to be too vague and metaphysical a topic to belong in a modern textbook of neuropsychiatry, but in fact it connects squarely with that discipline on two levels. First, it has become increasingly clear since the 1990s that personality traits have a biological basis. Although convincing theories of the specific neurobiological mechanisms involved are still lacking, strong collateral evidence indicates that such mechanisms must exist. Second, personality is directly relevant to the thoughts, feelings, and behaviors of patients, caregivers, and physicians. Forms of psychopathology, medical compliance, symptom reporting, caregiver burden (Hooker et al. 1998), and the physician's bedside manner are all influenced to a substantial degree by the pervasive and enduring characteristics that define personality.

The personality of patients with neuropsychiatric disorders is often ignored because of the belief that neuropsychological assessment is sufficient to understand a patient (Cahn and Gould 1996). When personality is considered, it is typically conceptualized either in terms of personality disorders—such as when the premorbid personality of an individual with late-life-onset psychosis is described as paranoid or schizoid (Pearlson and Petty 1994)—or as a catalog of traits discerned by clinical judgment (Todes and Lees 1985). In this chapter, we present a contemporary model of general personality traits and discuss their relevance to geriatric neuropsychiatry.

The questions of most interest to neuropsychiatrists are likely to be 1) whether there are distinctive personality profiles associated with different neuropsychiatric disorders (e.g., "Parkinson's personality," "epileptic personality") and 2) whether such distinctive traits are precursors—either causes or early markers—or consequences of the disorder. The history of research on personality and Parkinson's disease (PD) illustrates the difficulty of addressing these topics without the benefit of contemporary views. As long ago as 1913, Camp highlighted the industriousness and moralistic attitude toward life in people with PD. In 1942, Sands described a "masked personality" in those prone to PD: they appeared calm and prudent to naive observers, but concealed beneath was a sense of brooding and panic. It was the strain of repressing these emotions that was thought to contribute to the development of parkinsonism. Should credence be given to such dynamic psychosomatic theories? More modern theoretical guidance came from Cloninger (1988), whose biosocial theory of personality linked temperament to neurotransmitter systems. Menza et al. (1990) reported that concurrent and retrospective self-reports suggested that patients with PD had always been low on a trait called novelty seeking, which Cloninger argued was related to the dopaminergic system. However, subsequent studies seeking to confirm a dopamine-related low-novelty-seeking personality type in people with PD failed to replicate that finding (Jacobs et al. 2001; Resh 1998). Neuroimaging studies (see Kaasinen et al. 2001) have suggested that the problem is in the theoretical association of novelty seeking with dopamine functioning. A case control study of 55 patients with essential tremor and 61 controls by Chatterjee et al. (2004) failed to find a significant difference in novelty seeking but did for harm avoidance, a trait related to anxiety and depression.

A rare prospective study by Ishihara-Paul et al. (2008) suggested that the premorbid personality of patients with PD was characterized by anxiety and depression, but unfortunately

This research was supported entirely by the Intramural Research Program, National Institutes of Health, National Institute on Aging. Paul T. Costa Jr. and Robert R. McCrae receive royalties from the Revised NEO Personality Inventory. The authors thank Jamie Berry, Jeffrey Herbst, and Jason Thayer for assistance in the preparation of this chapter.

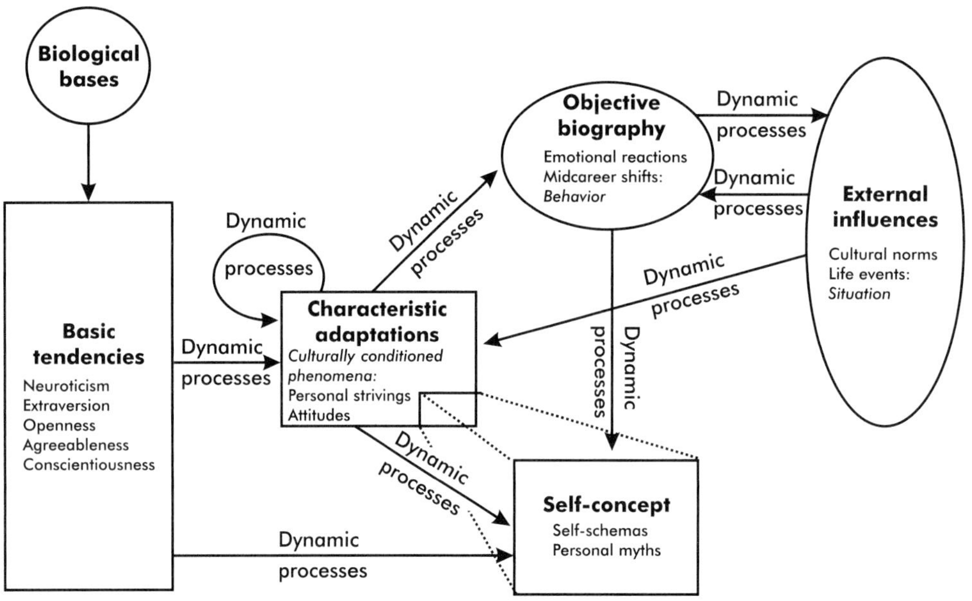

FIGURE 22–1. A model of the personality system, showing the major components of the system and the principal paths by which they are related.

Italicized words in the figure are exemplars of the personality system components.

Source. Adapted from McCrae and Costa 2008b.

their study did not assess other important traits, such as generosity and rigidity, which have also been associated with premorbid PD (Hubble et al. 1993). What traits ought to be included in prospective analyses? Depression—often untreated—is a common feature of early PD (Ravina et al. 2007), but depression is found in many neuropsychiatric disorders (e.g., stroke; Storor and Byrne 2006). Are other, more distinctive traits involved in PD? Perhaps the most consistent findings have compared current with retrospective reports of personality; they have shown that the development of PD is associated with perceived declines in emotional stability, extraversion, openness to experience, agreeableness, and conscientiousness (Glosser et al. 1995; Hubble et al. 1993; Mendelsohn et al. 1995). Are such perceptions of personality change accurate? Data are now available to answer that question. Although researchers are still far from a full understanding of personality and PD, they have a better idea of which traits need to be assessed and how best to assess them. A systematic approach to personality and geriatric neuropsychiatry is now possible.

Definition and Measurement of Personality

Although a textbook of personality theories can offer a bewildering array of definitions of its subject matter, two common and complementary approaches are in use. The first considers personality as a system that organizes and directs the behavior of the individual in ways that allow the satisfaction of needs and the expression of the self. Figure 22–1 provides a contemporary example of this type of model. In this view of the personality system, biologically based basic tendencies interact over time with external influences to create a repertoire of characteristic adaptations (skills, habits, attitudes, preferences, roles, relationships, etc.). These adaptations in turn interact with the immediate situation to determine what the individual does and experiences at a particular moment (McCrae and Costa 2008b).

Some such model of the personality system is required to understand how human beings function. For example, Figure 22–1 calls attention to the biological bases of personality dispositions, consistent with a wealth of literature on the heritability of most personality traits (Loehlin 1992; Riemann et al. 1997). However, the system approach is limited as a definition of personality because it applies equally to everyone.

The second approach commonly used to define personality calls attention to individual differences. Personality traits are ubiquitous in laypersons' descriptions of themselves and others, and traitlike constructs have been measured by psychologists for decades. Needs, temperaments, characters, folk concepts, cognitive styles, and a variety of personality disorders have all been proposed as the basic units of personality psychology. For many years, one of the central problems in the field was that so many individual difference variables had been identified that little progress could be made in understanding any of them.

It was clear, however, that all these different constructs were heavily redundant: poor ego strength was akin to low psychological resiliency and to general anxiety and negative affectivity (Watson and Clark 1984). Factor analysts such as Cattell (1973) and Eysenck (1960) attempted to summarize the redundancy in terms of a few broad personality factors or dimensions. After years of research and debate, a general (if not universal) consensus has emerged that most specific traits can be understood in terms of five broad factors, usually labeled openness to experience, conscientiousness, extraversion, agreeableness, and neuroticism (Digman 1990; McCrae and Costa 2008a); the acronym OCEAN is a handy mnemonic for these factors.

The Five-Factor Model of personality provides a systematic and comprehensive approach to personality and geriatric neuropsychiatry, and the traits described in the model are relevant to the DSM-IV-TR Axis I and Axis II disorders. These five factors were initially identified in studies based on English-language trait adjectives, but they were soon replicated in a variety of theoretically based personality questionnaires. One of the first inventories designed specifically to measure the Five-Factor Model was the Revised NEO Personality Inventory (NEO-PI-R; Costa and McCrae 1992a); Table 22–1 lists the 30 facets that define the five factors and gives some indication of their scope and nature. For example, the table shows that individuals high in openness to experience have an active fantasy life, appreciate art and beauty, are keenly aware of their feelings and emotions, prefer variety and novelty, are intellectually curious, and have liberal value systems.

The Five-Factor Model has proven to be generalizable not only over a wide range of personality instruments but also over many different populations. Similar factor structures are found in young and old adults, men and women, and white and nonwhite subsamples (Costa et al. 1991). Perhaps more important, the structure has also been replicated in studies using translations of the NEO-PI-R into such languages as Portuguese, Korean, and Filipino (McCrae and Costa 1997; McCrae et al. 2005). These cross-cultural replications suggest that personality traits are a species-wide characteristic. Finally, studies in psychiatric samples (Bagby et al. 1999; Yang et al. 1999) have reported the same structure as that found in psychiatrically healthy samples.

Personality trait assessment has been the topic of extensive research for decades. Because traits are abstract constructs that must be inferred from patterns of behavior and experience, no single method or instrument is perfect, but several approaches yield reasonably accurate assessments. Most common are self-report questionnaires or checklists (e.g., Costa and McCrae 1992a; Trapnell and Wiggins 1990) that ask respondents to describe their own interests, behaviors, and feelings. More familiar to psychiatrists are structured interviews (Trull and Widiger 1997), in which self-reports are elicited and evaluated by a trained professional. Informant ratings have also been shown to be valid alternatives to self-reports, especially valuable in situations in which self-reports may not be trustworthy (McCrae and Weiss 2007). For example, considerable research has been done on personality in patients with dementia by using ratings from spouses or caregivers (Glosser et al. 1995; Siegler et al. 1991).

TABLE 22–1. Revised NEO Personality Inventory facet scales defining the five basic personality factors

Neuroticism	**Agreeableness**
Anxiety	Trust
Angry hostility	Straightforwardness
Depression	Altruism
Self-consciousness	Compliance
Impulsiveness	Modesty
Vulnerability to stress	Tender-mindedness
Extraversion	**Conscientiousness**
Warmth	Competence
Gregariousness	Order
Assertiveness	Dutifulness
Activity	Achievement striving
Excitement seeking	Self-discipline
Positive emotions	Deliberation
Openness to experience	
Fantasy	
Aesthetics	
Feelings	
Actions	
Ideas	
Values	

Personality and Aging

Personality development from infancy through adolescence has been a major focus of personality theory and research for over a century. From the time of Sigmund Freud on, however, most psychologists assumed that personality development had ended by adulthood. Until Erikson's (1950) influential epigenetic model extended psychosocial development into old age, little attention was paid to adult personality. Erikson's stage model has received only partial support (e.g., Van de Water and McAdams 1989), but it stimulated cross-sectional and longitudinal research that has led to a clear and consistent picture of what happens to personality in the normal course of aging.

Two important and distinct questions need to be asked about personality and aging. The first concerns the preservation of individual differences; the second involves stability or change in mean levels. Examining differential stability requires assessment at different points in time and is usually addressed by longitudinal studies that measure the same group of individuals on multiple occasions separated by intervals of years or decades. Questions about mean levels can also be addressed by longitudinal data, but they are often approached through cross-sectional comparisons of different age groups.

By definition, traits are enduring dispositions, so if they exist at all, they must show some stability of rank order over a period of months or years. But traits might well change across longer portions of the life span, and most researchers have anticipated that life events, changes in physical health, and changing roles and responsibilities would each have profound impact on personality traits. That view is tenable during the first part of adulthood (Siegler et al. 1990); personality scores at age 30 are only moderately predictable from scores at age 18. After age 30, however, evidence shows impressive predictability and thus stability. Longitudinal studies covering periods of up to 40 years (Terracciano et al. 2006) find substantial stability in rank order for traits from all five factors. Costa and McCrae (1992b), for example, reported retest correlations ranging from 0.61 to 0.71 over a 24-year interval for a set of 10 traits. In the normal course of aging, extraverts at age 40 are still likely to be relatively extraverted at age 70; conscientious people remain conscientious across the adult life span.

Retest correlations, however, reflect only relative standing; they do not reflect developmental trends that may be common to an entire age group. It is entirely possible to show high retest correlations even when there are dramatic changes in mean level, and reasons have been suggested to hypothesize a number of changes in personality that might accompany aging. Popular stereotypes suggest that old age brings depression, withdrawal, rigidity, and crankiness—although popular stereotypes also suggest that it brings mellowness and wisdom. If predictable age changes in personality do exist, that fact is of considerable importance. Rival disengagement (Cumming and Henry 1961) and activity (Maddox 1963) theories of aging led to public policy debates on how society should deal with the elderly (Neugarten 1982): Should they be allowed to fade away with dignity, or should they be surrounded with opportunities and incentives for social interaction?

The major finding from subsequent research is one of predominant stability: most cross-sectional studies of adults over age 30 reported only a small age difference across long portions of the life span (Costa et al. 1986), and longitudinal studies confirm that changes are quite modest (Löckenhoff et al. 2008). Stereotypes about depression, withdrawal, and rigidity are myths, applicable, if at all, to only a small percentage of the elderly.

Coupled with the findings of stability in rank order, predominant mean level stability implies that personality traits are more or less constant across the adult life span. The same range of individual differences is found in older men and women as in younger men and women. Persons involved in the care of older adults, such as geriatric physicians, cannot prepare for the "typical" old person; they must learn to appreciate and respond to the full range of individual differences.

Although the major lesson from studies of adult personality development is that personality changes little, more recent research has confirmed that the little it changes is predictable. Between ages 18 and 30, moderately large changes—on the order of one-half standard deviation—are found in the mean levels of all five traits. The pattern, seen in both men and women, makes considerable sense: neuroticism, extraversion, and openness to experience decline, and agreeableness and conscientiousness increase—changes that collectively might be described as an increase in psychological maturity. Further, these same trends continue, at a slow rate, after age 30 (Terracciano et al. 2005).

So small are these changes that they can usually be detected only with very large samples observed across very long intervals. It would be easy to dismiss such small effects as meaningless were it not for the fact that similar trends are found in Germany, Croatia, South Korea, Portugal, and Italy (McCrae et al. 1999, 2005). Despite differences in language, culture, and recent history, the same developmental pattern appears everywhere. One interpretation of this phenomenon is that personality development is not so much the result of life experience as it is an intrinsic maturational process common to all people.

Normal and Abnormal Personality

Neuropsychiatrists are likely to be most familiar with personality in the form of DSM-IV-TR Axis II personality disorders (American Psychiatric Association 2000). Personality disorders—including borderline, paranoid, and antisocial disorders—are said to be marked by extreme and inflexible styles of behaving and experiencing and to cause personal distress or social impairment. DSM-IV-TR currently catalogues 10 specific personality disorders—antisocial, avoidant, borderline, dependent, histrionic, narcissistic, obsessive-compulsive, paranoid, schizoid, and schizotypal—along with a category for personality disorders not otherwise specified.

Personality disorders clearly represent significant clinical conditions to which neuropsychiatrists ought to attend. For many reasons, however, Axis II is not an optimal system for describing personality (McCrae 1994). The selection of disorders is based on no clear rationale—indeed, several disorders have come and gone in successive editions of DSM. Many individuals meet criteria for several personality disorder diagnoses—the problem of comorbidity—whereas most people receive no Axis II diagnosis at all and can be characterized only as "normal." Little empirical evidence exists to indicate that the defining symptoms cohere as syndromes (Livesley et al. 1989) or to substantiate the postulated categorical breaks between normal and abnormal personalities (Trull et al. 1990).

Since the 1990s, many psychiatrists and psychologists have become convinced that the traditional categorical model needs to be replaced by a dimensional model of personality disorders, in which the degree of psychopathology is graded. Furthermore, abundant evidence now indicates that individuals diagnosed with personality disorders manifest the same personality traits found in normal populations—the traits of the Five-Factor Model (Costa and Widiger 2002). The impairments these individuals experience are not reflections of distinct, diseased personality traits, but rather of the development of maladaptive ways of expressing personality traits common to everyone.

From this perspective, personality disorders can be viewed as personality-related problems, the kinds of affective, cognitive, and interpersonal difficulties toward which different personality traits predispose people. Most people have problems and all people have personalities, so the limited applicability of Axis II diagnoses is avoided in this approach. Instead, through personality assessment the clinician can obtain useful insight into the strengths and weaknesses of all patients. Widiger and Trull (2007) have argued for a new approach to Axis II diagnosis in DSM-5 based on these insights.

Normal personality traits are also relevant to a number of Axis I disorders (Widiger and Trull 1992). For example, low extraversion is associated with major depression (Bagby et al. 1995), low conscientiousness with substance abuse (Brooner et al. 1993), and high neuroticism with posttraumatic stress disorder (Hyer et al. 1994). Personality traits may predispose individuals to the development of certain forms of psychopathology, or they may themselves result from neuropsychiatric disorders. More recent evidence (Wilson et al. 2007) suggests that conscientiousness may be a protective factor for the development of Alzheimer's disease (AD); in a later section, "Personality in Geriatric Neuropsychiatry," we review a body of literature on the effects of that disorder on personality traits.

Biological Basis of Personality

Figure 22–1 presents a model of the personality system in which both biology and the environment play prominent shaping roles, reflecting the truism that personality is the result of both nature and nurture. That model, however, differs fundamentally from most earlier conceptualizations of personality by presuming that, as basic tendencies, personality traits themselves are endogenous and that the environment (except insofar as it modifies the underlying biology—e.g., through brain trauma) affects only their expression in acquired habits, tastes, attitudes, and so on. Doubtless the model oversimplifies, but it rests on a rapidly growing body of information on the biological basis of personality.

A long tradition links personality traits directly to neurophysiology. Perhaps most influential is the work of Hans Eysenck (1967), whose theories of the biological basis of neuroticism and extraversion have stimulated many programs of research. More recently, Cloninger (1988) proposed that personality traits (or at least those related to temperament) reflect activity of the serotonergic, dopaminergic, and noradrenergic systems. Some evidence supports these claims. For example, Cloninger linked dopamine to a set of traits he calls novelty seeking, and both novelty seeking (Cloninger et al. 1994) and dopamine D_2 receptors (Roth and Joseph 1994) decline with age.

The human brain is extraordinarily complex, however, and personality-brain associations are not readily amenable to experimental study, so it is perhaps not surprising that, at the present time, overall support for Eysenck's and Cloninger's theories is weak (Amelang and Ullwer 1991; Ebstein et al. 1997; Herbst et al. 2000). However, a wealth of evidence shows that personality is firmly rooted in biology and thus that the neurophysiological mechanisms are there to be discovered eventually.

Perhaps the most persuasive evidence comes from adoption and twin studies that have conclusively demonstrated the importance of genetic influences on all five personality factors (Bouchard 1994; Riemann et al. 1997) and on the specific traits that define them (Jang et al. 1998). By contrast, shared environmental influences, such as social class, parental role models, and religious training, appear to have little or no influence on adult personality traits, although they clearly have major effects on characteristic adaptations. Many attempts have been made to identify specific genes associated with personality traits (Benjamin et al. 1996); so far, these findings have not proven to be replicable (Malhotra et al. 1996; Terracciano et al. 2009). It seems likely that a large number of genes influence each trait, so the effects of any single gene are small and difficult to detect.

A second line of evidence for the biological basis of personality comes from cross-cultural studies. Both personality structure (McCrae and Costa 1997) and personality development (McCrae et al. 1999) appear to follow universal patterns that transcend language, culture, and history. Although such universal patterns might be attributable to shared experiences—for example, humans everywhere are aware of their own mortality—it is more plausible to see these as results of a common biology.

That argument is even stronger when comparisons are made not across cultures but across species. Research on both nonhuman primates (Weiss et al. 2006) and nonprimates

(Gosling et al. 2003) shows that personality characteristics resembling those found in humans can be reliably observed in other animal species. Some personality factors—notably conscientiousness—are absent or difficult to detect, but stable individual differences in aggressiveness, activity level, and shyness are easily demonstrated. Whatever their evolutionary function (Figueredo et al. 2005), personality traits appear to be a part of human beings' mammalian heritage.

Personality Assessment in Neuropsychiatric Populations

A final source of evidence on the neurological basis of personality comes from studies of neuropsychiatric disorders. It has long been recognized that both dementia and traumatic brain injury could affect such characteristics as motivation, mood, and impulse control. However, adequate descriptions of personality changes associated with these conditions were impeded by the lack of a comprehensive model of personality to guide systematic study and by difficulties in personality assessment among impaired patients. Recent advances associated with the Five-Factor Model have resolved both these problems.

Self-report questionnaires are the mainstay of personality assessment for both normal and psychiatric samples, but the validity of such instruments for individuals with cognitive impairments is questionable. Instead, most personality assessments of individuals with dementia or those who are otherwise incapacitated have relied on clinician ratings. Although these are of considerable value in describing a patient's current functioning, they are of limited use in assessing personality changes because clinicians rarely know the individual's premorbid status. Instead of a consequence, personality traits might be long-term predictors of the neuropsychiatric condition in question.

In the first of a series of papers, Siegler et al. (1991) asked caregiver informants (spouses and children) to provide personality ratings of 35 patients with memory impairment. Informants described both premorbid and current personality characteristics using the observer-rating version of the original NEO-PI (a version that measured all five factors but identified specific facets for only the first three). Premorbid personality profiles showed slightly lower than average levels of openness to experience, but otherwise mean scores were in the normal range. By contrast, current ratings depicted patients as being high in neuroticism, especially vulnerability to stress; low in extraversion; and very low in conscientiousness. These results were clearly replicated in three other studies (Chatterjee et al. 1992; Siegler et al. 1994; Welleford et al. 1995). Results (expressed as difference between premorbid and current ratings) from all four studies are plotted in Figure 22–2.

These dramatic and remarkably consistent findings are the basis for a number of conclusions. First, they clearly demonstrate that neuropsychiatric status can have profound effects on rated personality—in clear contrast to the general absence of effects from such physical conditions as heart disease and cancer (Costa et al. 1994). The widespread clinical belief that personality changes are among the more important signs of dementing disorders is apparently well founded and may be particularly important as indicators of early-stage disease (Duchek et al. 2007).

Next, these data point to specific traits and factors that are likely to change. At the facet level, the greatest change for patients with AD is in vulnerability, an inability to deal effectively with stress. At the factor level, these patients became higher in neuroticism and lower in extraversion, but they changed relatively little in openness to experience or agreeableness. The largest changes are in conscientiousness, a factor defined by such traits as competence, order, achievement striving, and self-discipline. Impairment in purposeful, goal-directed striving most characterized these individuals.

In hindsight, that finding seems intuitively reasonable because even individuals with mild dementia have difficulty in organizing and directing their lives. However, the importance of conscientiousness could not have been predicted from the prior literature. Most attention had been paid to memory loss and other forms of cognitive decline, but conscientiousness is not related to cognitive ability (McCrae and Costa 1985), and neuropsychiatrists should not assume that they can infer levels of conscientiousness from cognitive tests such as measures of executive function. Closer to personality, in the PsycLIT database, of more than 4,000 articles involving AD that were published between 1991 and 1997, a total of 464 included the word "depression," but only 4 included "conscientiousness"—all from studies informed by the Five-Factor Model. One of the chief advantages of a comprehensive model of personality is that it allows systematic exploration of personality correlates, including traits that might otherwise have been overlooked.

Finally, these studies suggest that informant ratings may be useful in the assessment of personality in other neuropsychiatric conditions, such as multiple sclerosis (Benedict et al. 2008). Studies by Strauss and colleagues (Strauss and Pasupathi 1994; Strauss et al. 1993) have shown that retrospective ratings by knowledgeable informants are consensually valid and temporally stable and that successive ratings are sensitive to the progression of AD. Standardized questionnaires provide an effective way to enlist the aid of caregivers in the comprehensive assessment of a patient. However, some studies have also shown that self-reports from neuropsychiatric patients can be valid (Kurtz and Putnam 2006; Mendelsohn et al. 1995). Assessments including both informant ratings and self-reports are probably optimal.

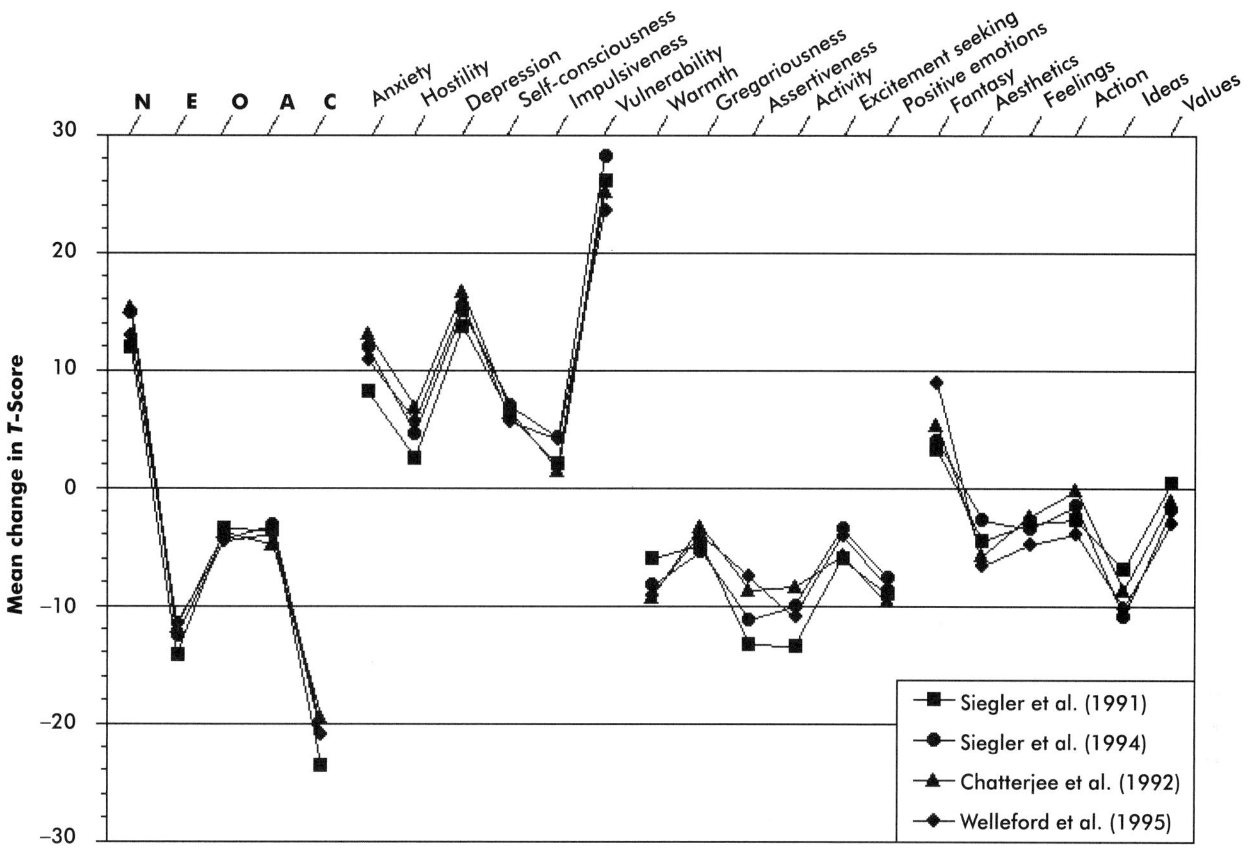

FIGURE 22–2. Mean changes from premorbid to current personality ratings in four studies of patients with Alzheimer's disease.

N=neuroticism; E=extraversion; O=openness to experience; A=agreeableness; C=conscientiousness.

Self-reports are commonly used in geriatric neuropsychiatry, but informant reports perhaps less so. Instead, psychiatrists are accustomed to making their own clinical judgments based on patient observation. Although such judgments are an invaluable part of the total assessment, in the case of personality traits, they may not be optimal. Lyons et al. (2004) assessed the skill of health professionals in decoding personality traits from the observation of behavior—in this case, taped interviews of patients with PD. They found that practitioners were able to correctly identify cues of three of the factors—openness to experience, agreeableness, and conscientiousness—but not of neuroticism and extraversion. This study is a useful reminder that trained professionals are not infallible sources of personality judgments; laypersons who are well acquainted with the target may sometimes provide superior ratings, provided that validated instruments are used to quantify their knowledge.

Personality in Geriatric Neuropsychiatry

The methods and findings of contemporary personality psychology are potentially useful at two levels: 1) in research on the causes and consequences of neuropsychiatric disorders, and 2) in understanding and helping patients and their families. A study by Storor and Byrne (2006) serves as an example of research on causes of neuropsychiatric disorders. They used informants' ratings on the NEO-PI-R to describe the personality of stroke patients 10 years before the stroke and found that high premorbid neuroticism scores conferred a twofold to fivefold greater risk of depression in the period immediately following a stroke. By contrast, age, gender, site of the stroke lesion, and physical and cognitive functioning were unrelated to depression. In this study at least, poststroke depression appeared to be a function of the patient's personality rather than the extent or location of the stroke itself.

Research on personality correlates of disease is valuable for several reasons. First, patterns such as those shown in Figure 22–2 may offer insights into brain-behavior relationships; for example, something about the neurochemical and neuroanatomical changes that accompany the progression of AD profoundly affects planning and goal-directed behavior while leaving intact the quality of interpersonal orientation (agreeableness vs. antagonism). Second, distinctive personality profiles or distinctive patterns of personality change may be helpful in formulating a clinical diagnosis. Third, understanding the personality of patients can aid in managing care. Indeed, knowledge of the individual's unique personality profile may enable caregivers to anticipate difficult management issues in the progression and treatment of the disease.

The quest for patterns of premorbid personality traits unique to different neuropsychiatric disorders is still in the early stages. In a review, Ishihara and Brayne (2006) found some consistent evidence that patients with PD were generally nervous, cautious, and conventional before clinical diagnosis of the disorder, but concluded that this might be an effect of an early stage of the disease. Prospective studies are needed that cover the full range of traits in the Five-Factor Model and that assess traits years or decades before the disease clinically manifests.

Cross-sectional studies of personality are easier and more promising. Many neuropsychiatric conditions, including AD, stroke, PD, and traumatic brain injury, are associated with increased levels of neuroticism (Costa 1996). It appears that diffuse brain damage, with or without cognitive impairment, leads to predictable patterns of personality change associated with anxiety, depression, and vulnerability. Some studies, however, also point to disorder-specific patterns of change on other personality factors. Figure 22–2 shows that AD has relatively little impact on openness to experience, whereas two studies involving PD patients (Glosser et al. 1995; Mendelsohn et al. 1995) found that openness to experience declined.

Such information has important clinical implications. Changes in personality can be detected by lay observers and can provide early signs of dementing disorders (Duchek et al. 2007). Because changes are progressive in AD (Strauss and Pasupathi 1994), their recognition can help caregivers anticipate how the patient is likely to change over the course of the disease. Memory loss is not the only, or even necessarily the most troubling, effect of AD; loss of purposefulness and vulnerability to stress also present problems with which the caregiver may have to deal. Those who care for patients with PD may note and should be prepared for a pattern of personality changes that includes a narrowing of interests and increasing apathy.

In addition to personality and behavioral changes associated with the natural history or progression of a disease, recently increased clinical attention has been given to problems that result from treating neuropsychiatric diseases, such as dopamine dysregulation syndrome (DDS) in patients with PD. DDS is a recently described iatrogenic neurobehavioral disorder that can complicate long-term symptomatic treatment of PD. As described by O'Sullivan et al. (2009), PD patients with DDS have a pattern of self-administering abnormally high dosages of dopamine replacement therapy, which develops into an addictive pattern resembling cocaine addiction. DDS is also characterized by a variety of impulse-control disorders, such as hypersexuality, pathological gambling, compulsive shopping, and compulsive eating. Only 3%–4% of patients with PD develop DDS; those with early-onset PD, with a previous history of alcohol or illicit drug use, and with impulsive sensation-seeking traits are more likely to develop DDS. Interestingly, premorbid personality traits related to impulsivity and sensation seeking (or novelty seeking) have also been related to drug dependence and substance abuse (Terracciano and Costa 2004). Mesolimbic dopaminergic systems are thought to mediate the links between impulsive personality traits and the vulnerability to develop DDS.

DDS nevertheless goes unrecognized for a variety of reasons. Patients enter treatment with a vast array of different premorbid personality traits, a situation that complicates the identification of patients most in need of scrutiny and alternative treatments. It is possible that having a comprehensive personality profile of the patient would be of diagnostic value to the neuropsychiatrist or other clinician. Further research employing comprehensive personality models and measures is needed to identify at-risk groups, making early intervention possible.

At a broader level, information on personality can be valuable to geriatric neuropsychiatrists because all patients have personality traits that influence their interactions with physicians (Stone and McCrae 2007). Individuals high in neuroticism are prone to exaggerate medical complaints, whereas those who are low in neuroticism may minimize them. Extraverts are talkative and, compared with introverts, may more readily volunteer information about their medical condition or ask questions about treatment. Open individuals are unconventional and willing to experiment; they may prefer innovative or nontraditional medical therapies. Disagreeable people are suspicious, demanding, and frequently dissatisfied with the medical treatment they receive (Roter and Hall 1992). Conscientious people have better health habits to begin with and comply more diligently with prescribed medical regimens. Those persons who are chronically low in conscientiousness, including those whose initial levels of conscientiousness are decreased by dementing disorders, may require extra assistance from family caregivers. For all these reasons, physicians are better equipped to understand, diagnose, and treat their patients if they appreciate the role of enduring individual differences.

Key Points

- The Five-Factor Model of personality provides a systematic and comprehensive approach to personality and geriatric neuropsychiatry.
- Almost all specific personality traits can be understood in terms of the five broad factors of the Five-Factor Model: openness to experience, conscientiousness, extraversion, agreeableness, and neuroticism (OCEAN).
- The traits described in the Five-Factor Model are relevant to the DSM-IV-TR Axis I and Axis II disorders.
- Stereotypes depicting old age as bringing increased depression, withdrawal, rigidity, and crankiness are not empirically supported.
- Predominant stability of both relative standing and mean level is the rule rather than the exception.
- Personality changes—especially vulnerability to stress and decreases in purposeful and goal-directed striving—are among the most prominent effects of dementing disorders on personality.
- A comprehensive personality profile is of clinical value to neuropsychiatrists and other clinicians who are helping to understand, diagnose, and treat their patients.

Recommended Readings

Costa PT Jr, Widiger TA (eds): Personality Disorders and the Five-Factor Model of Personality, 2nd Edition. Washington, DC, American Psychological Association, 2002—*Summarizes research and theory on personality and personality disorders*

Hooker K, Monahan DJ, Bowman SR, et al: Personality counts for a lot: predictors of mental and physical health of spouse caregivers in two disease groups. J Gerontol B Psychol Sci Soc Sci 53B:P73–P85, 1998—*Discusses the importance of personality for caregiver burden*

McCrae RR, Costa PT Jr: Personality in Adulthood: A Five-Factor Theory Perspective, 2nd Edition. New York, Guilford, 2003—*Provides a nontechnical introduction to personality traits in adulthood*

Siegler IC, Welsh KA, Dawson DV, et al: Ratings of personality change in patients being evaluated for memory disorders. Alzheimer Dis Assoc Disord 5:240–250, 1991—*A classic paper that illustrates the use of informant ratings in the study of memory disorders*

Stone SV, McCrae RR: Personality and health, in Cambridge Handbook of Psychology, Health and Medicine, 2nd Edition. Edited by Ayers S, Baum C, McManus S, et al. Cambridge, UK, Cambridge University Press, 2007, pp 151–155—*Surveys the field of personality and health and describes some ways to tailor treatment to individual patients*

References

Amelang M, Ullwer U: Correlations between psychometric measures and psychophysiological as well as experimental variables in studies on extraversion and neuroticism, in Explorations in Temperament: International Perspectives on Theory and Measurement. Edited by Strelau J, Angleitner A. New York, Plenum, 1991, pp 287–316

American Psychiatric Association: Diagnostic and Statistical Manual of Mental Disorders, 4th Edition, Text Revision. Washington, DC, American Psychiatric Association, 2000

Bagby RM, Joffe RT, Parker JDA, et al: Major depression and the Five-Factor Model of personality. J Pers Disord 9:224–234, 1995

Bagby RM, Costa PT Jr, McCrae RR, et al: Replicating the Five-Factor Model of personality in a psychiatric sample. Pers Individ Dif 27:1135–1140, 1999

Benedict RHB, Hussein S, Englert J, et al: Cortical atrophy and personality in multiple sclerosis. Neuropsychology 22:432–441, 2008

Benjamin J, Li L, Patterson C, et al: Population and familial association between the D4 dopamine receptor gene and measures of novelty seeking. Nat Genet 12:81–84, 1996

Bouchard TJ: Genes, environment, and personality. Science 264: 1700–1701, 1994

Brooner RK, Herbst JH, Schmidt CW, et al: Antisocial personality disorder among drug abusers: relations to other personality diagnoses and the Five-Factor Model of personality. J Nerv Ment Dis 181:313–319, 1993

Cahn G, Gould RE: Understanding head injury and intellectual recovery from brain damage: is IQ an adequate measure? Bull Am Acad Psychiatry Law 24:135–142, 1996

Camp CD: Paralysis agitans, multiple sclerosis and their treatment, in Modern Treatment of Nervous and Mental Disease. Edited by White WA, Jelliffe SE, Kimpton H. Philadelphia, PA, Lea and Febiger, 1913, pp 651–667

Cattell RB: Personality and Mood by Questionnaire. San Francisco, CA, Jossey-Bass, 1973

Chatterjee A, Strauss ME, Smyth KA, et al: Personality changes in Alzheimer's disease. Arch Neurol 49:486–491, 1992

Chatterjee A, Jurewicz, EC, Applegate, LM, et al: Personality in essential tremor: further evidence of non-motor manifestations of the disease. J Neurol Neurosurg Psychiatry 75:958–961, 2004

Cloninger CR: A unified biosocial theory of personality and its role in the development of anxiety states: a reply to commentaries. Psychiatr Dev 2:83–120, 1988

Cloninger CR, Przybeck TR, Svrakic DM, et al: The Temperament and Character Inventory (TCI): A Guide to Its Development and Use. St. Louis, MO, Washington University, 1994

Costa PT Jr: Personality assessment of neurologically impaired patients using Form R of the Revised NEO Personality Inventory (NEO-PI-R). Paper presented at the midwinter meeting of the Society for Personality Assessment, Denver, CO, March 1996

Costa PT Jr, McCrae RR: Revised NEO Personality Inventory (NEO-PI-R) and NEO Five-Factor Inventory (NEO-FFI) Professional Manual. Odessa, FL, Psychological Assessment Resources, 1992a

Costa PT Jr, McCrae RR: Trait psychology comes of age, in Nebraska Symposium on Motivation: Psychology and Aging. Edited by Sonderegger T. Lincoln, NE, University of Nebraska Press, 1992b, pp 169–204

Costa PT Jr, Widiger TA (eds): Personality Disorders and the Five-Factor Model of Personality, 2nd Edition. Washington, DC, American Psychological Association, 2002

Costa PT Jr, McCrae RR, Zonderman AB, et al: Cross-sectional studies of personality in a national sample, 2: stability in neuroticism, extraversion, and openness. Psychol Aging 1:144–149, 1986

Costa PT Jr, McCrae RR, Dye DA: Facet scales for agreeableness and conscientiousness: a revision of the NEO Personality Inventory. Pers Individ Dif 12:887–898, 1991

Costa PT Jr, Metter EJ, McCrae RR: Personality stability and its contribution to successful aging. J Geriatr Psychiatry 27:41–59, 1994

Cumming E, Henry W: Growing Old. New York, Basic Books, 1961

Digman JM: Personality structure: emergence of the Five-Factor Model. Annu Rev Psychol 41:417–440, 1990

Duchek JM, Balota DA, Storandt M et al: The power of personality in discriminating between healthy aging and early stage Alzheimer's disease. J Gerontol Psychol Sci 62B:P353–P361, 2007

Ebstein RP, Gritsenko I, Nemanov L, et al: No association between the serotonin transporter gene regulatory region polymorphism and the tridimensional personality questionnaire (TPQ) temperament of harm avoidance. Mol Psychiatry 2:224–226, 1997

Erikson EH: Childhood and Society. New York, WW Norton, 1950

Eysenck HJ: The Structure of Human Personality. London, Methuen, 1960

Eysenck HJ: The Biological Basis of Personality. Springfield, IL, Charles C Thomas, 1967

Figueredo AJ, Sefcek JA, Vasquez G, et al: Evolutionary personality psychology, in Handbook of Evolutionary Psychology. Edited by Buss DM. Hoboken, NJ, Wiley, 2005, pp 851–877

Glosser G, Clark C, Freundlich B, et al: A controlled investigation of current and premorbid personality: characteristics of Parkinson's disease patients. Mov Disord 10:201–206, 1995

Gosling SD, Kwan VSY, John OP: A dog's got personality: a cross-species comparative approach to personality judgments in dogs and humans. J Pers Soc Psychol 85:1161–1169, 2003

Herbst JH, Zonderman AB, McCrae RR et al: Do the dimensions of the Temperament and Character Inventory map a simple genetic architecture? Evidence from molecular genetics and factor analysis. Am J Psychiatry 157:1285–1290, 2000

Hooker K, Monahan DJ, Bowman SR, et al: Personality counts for a lot: predictors of mental and physical health of spouse caregivers in two disease groups. J Gerontol B Psychol Sci Soc Sci 53B:P73–P85, 1998

Hubble JP, Venkatesh R, Hassanein RES, et al: Personality and depression in Parkinson's disease. J Nerv Ment Dis 181:657–662, 1993

Hyer L, Braswell L, Albrecht B, et al: Relationship of NEO-PI to personality styles and severity of trauma in chronic PTSD victims. J Clin Psychol 50:699–707, 1994

Ishihara L, Brayne C: What is the evidence for a premorbid Parkinsonian personality: a systematic review. Mov Disord 21:1066–1072, 2006

Ishihara-Paul L, Wainwright NWJ, Khaw KT, et al: Prospective association between emotional health and clinical evidence of Parkinson's disease. Eur J Neurol 15:1148–1154, 2008

Jacobs H, Heberlein I, Vieregge A, et al: Personality traits in young patients with Parkinson's disease. Acta Neurol Scand 13:82–87, 2001

Jang KL, McCrae RR, Angleitner A, et al: Heritability of facet-level traits in a cross-cultural twin study: support for a hierarchical model of personality. J Pers Soc Psychol 74:1556–1565, 1998

Kaasinen V, Nurmi E, Bergman J, et al: Personality traits and brain dopaminergic function in Parkinson's disease. Proc Natl Acad Sci U S A 98:13272–13277, 2001

Kurtz JE, Putnam SH: Patient-informant agreement on personality ratings and self-awareness after head injury. Clin Neuropsychol 20:453–468, 2006

Livesley WJ, Jackson DN, Schroeder ML: A study of the factorial structure of personality pathology. J Pers Disord 3:292–306, 1989

Löckenhoff CE, Terracciano A, Bienvenu OJ, et al: Ethnicity, education, and the temporal stability of personality traits in the East Baltimore Epidemiologic Catchment Area study. J Res Pers 42: 577–598, 2008

Loehlin JC: Genes and Environment in Personality Development. Newbury Park, CA, Sage, 1992

Lyons KD, Tickle-Degnen L, Henry A, et al: Impressions of personality in Parkinson's disease: can rehabilitation practitioners see beyond the symptoms? Rehabil Psychol 49:328–333, 2004

Maddox GL: Activity and morale: a longitudinal study of selected elderly subjects. Soc Forces 42:195–204, 1963

Malhotra AK, Virkkunen M, Rooney W, et al: The association between the dopamine D4 receptor (D4DR) 16 amino acid repeat polymorphism and novelty seeking. Mol Psychiatry 1:388–391, 1996

McCrae RR: A reformulation of Axis II: personality and personality-related problems, in Personality Disorders and the Five-Factor Model of Personality. Edited by Costa PT Jr, Widiger TA. Washington, DC, American Psychological Association, 1994, pp 303–310

McCrae RR, Costa PT Jr: Updating Norman's "adequate taxonomy": intelligence and personality dimensions in natural language and in questionnaires. J Pers Soc Psychol 49:710–721, 1985

McCrae RR, Costa PT Jr: Personality trait structure as a human universal. Am Psychol 52:509–516, 1997

McCrae RR, Costa PT Jr: Empirical and theoretical status of the Five-Factor Model of personality traits, in Sage Handbook of Personality Theory and Assessment, Vol 1. Edited by Boyle G, Matthews G, Saklofske D. Los Angeles, CA, Sage, 2008a, pp 273–294

McCrae RR, Costa PT Jr: The five-factor theory of personality, in Handbook of Personality: Theory and Research, 3rd Edition. Edited by John OP, Robins RW, Pervin LA. New York, Guilford, 2008b, pp 157–180

McCrae RR, Weiss A: Observer ratings of personality, in Handbook of Research Methods in Personality Psychology. Edited by Robins RW, Fraley RC, Krueger RF. New York, Guilford, 2007, pp 259–272

McCrae RR, Costa PT Jr, Lima MP, et al: Age differences in personality across the adult lifespan: parallels in five cultures. Dev Psychol 35:466–477, 1999

McCrae RR, Terracciano A; Personality Profiles of Culture Project: Universal features of personality traits from the observer's perspective: data from 50 cultures. J Pers Soc Psychol 88:547–561, 2005

Mendelsohn GA, Dakof GA, Skaff M: Personality change in Parkinson's disease patients: chronic disease and aging. J Pers 63:233–257, 1995

Menza MA, Forman NE, Goldstein HS, et al: Parkinson's disease, personality, and dopamine. J Neuropsychiatry Clin Neurosci 2:282–287, 1990

Neugarten BL (ed): Age or Need? Public Policies for Older People. Beverly Hills, CA, Sage, 1982

O'Sullivan SS, Evans AH, Lees AJ: Dopamine dysregulation syndrome: an overview of its epidemiology, mechanisms and management. CNS Drugs 23:157–170, 2009

Pearlson GD, Petty RG: Late-life-onset psychoses, in The American Psychiatric Press Textbook of Geriatric Neuropsychiatry. Edited by Coffey CE, Cummings JL. Washington, DC, American Psychiatric Press, 1994, pp 261–277

Ravina B, Camicioli R, Como PG, et al: The impact of depressive symptoms in early Parkinson disease. Neurology 69:342–347, 2007

Resh RJ: Personality and neuropsychological functioning in nondemented patients with Parkinson's disease. Dissertation Abstracts International 58:5654, 1998

Riemann R, Angleitner A, Strelau J: Genetic and environmental influences on personality: a study of twins reared together using the self- and peer report NEO-FFI scales. J Pers 65:449–475, 1997

Roter DL, Hall JA: Doctors Talking With Patients/Patients Talking With Doctors: Improving Communication in Medical Visits. Westport, CT, Auburn House, 1992

Roth GS, Joseph JA: Age-related changes in transcriptional and post-transcriptional regulation of the dopaminergic system. Life Sci 55:2031–2035, 1994

Sands IJ: The type of personality susceptible to Parkinson disease. J Mt Sinai Hosp N Y 9:792–794, 1942

Siegler IC, Zonderman AB, Barefoot JC, et al: Predicting personality in adulthood from college MMPI scores: implications for follow-up studies in psychosomatic medicine. Psychosom Med 52:644–652, 1990

Siegler IC, Welsh KA, Dawson DV, et al: Ratings of personality change in patients being evaluated for memory disorders. Alzheimer Dis Assoc Disord 5:240–250, 1991

Siegler IC, Dawson DV, Welsh KA: Caregiver ratings of personality change in Alzheimer's disease patients: a replication. Psychol Aging 9:464–466, 1994

Stone SV, McCrae RR: Personality and health, in Cambridge Handbook of Psychology, Health and Medicine, 2nd Edition. Edited by Ayers S, Baum C, McManus S, et al. Cambridge, UK, Cambridge University Press, 2007, pp 151–155

Storor DL, Byrne GJA: Pre-morbid personality and depression following stroke. Int Psychogeriatr 18:457–469, 2006

Strauss ME, Pasupathi M: Primary caregivers' descriptions of Alzheimer patients' personality traits: temporal stability and sensitivity to change. Alzheimer Dis Assoc Disord 8:166–176, 1994

Strauss ME, Pasupathi M, Chatterjee A: Concordance between observers in descriptions of personality change in Alzheimer's disease. Psychol Aging 8:475–480, 1993

Terracciano A, Costa PT Jr: Smoking and the Five-Factor Model of personality. Addiction 99:472–481, 2004

Terracciano A, McCrae RR, Brant LJ, et al: Hierarchical linear modeling analyses of NEO-PI-R scales in the Baltimore Longitudinal Study of Aging. Psychol Aging 20:493–506, 2005

Terracciano A, Costa PT Jr, McCrae RR: Personality plasticity after age 30. Pers Soc Psychol Bull 32:999–1009, 2006

Terracciano A, Balaci L, Thayer J, et al: Variants of the serotonin transporter gene and NEO-PI-R Neuroticism: no association in the BLSA and SardiNIA samples. Am J Med Genet B Neuropsychiatr Genet 150B:1070–1077, 2009

Todes CJ, Lees AJ: The premorbid personality of patients with Parkinson's disease. J Neurol Neurosurg Psychiatry 48:97–100, 1985

Trapnell PD, Wiggins JS: Extension of the Interpersonal Adjective Scales to include the big five dimensions of personality. J Pers Soc Psychol 59:781–790, 1990

Trull TJ, Widiger TA: Structured Interview for the Five-Factor Model of Personality (SIFFM) Professional Manual. Odessa, FL, Psychological Assessment Resources, 1997

Trull TJ, Widiger TA, Guthrie P: The categorical versus dimensional status of borderline personality disorder. J Abnorm Psychol 99: 40–48, 1990

Van de Water D, McAdams DP: Generativity and Erikson's "belief in the species." J Res Pers 23:435–449, 1989

Watson D, Clark LA: Negative affectivity: the disposition to experience aversive emotional states. Psychol Bull 96:465–490, 1984

Weiss A, King JE, Perkins L: Personality and subjective well-being in orangutans (Pongo pygmaeus and Pongo abelii). J Pers Soc Psychol 90:501–511, 2006

Welleford EA, Harkins SW, Taylor JR: Personality change in dementia of the Alzheimer's type: relation to caregiver personality and burden. Exp Aging Res 21:295–314, 1995

Widiger TA, Trull TJ: Personality and psychopathology: an application of the Five-Factor Model. J Pers 60:363–393, 1992

Widiger TA, Trull TJ: Plate tectonics in the classification of personality disorder: shifting to a dimensional model. Am Psychol 62:71–83, 2007

Wilson RS, Schneider JA, Arnold SE, et al: Conscientiousness and the incidence of Alzheimer disease and mild cognitive impairment. Arch Gen Psychiatry 64:1204–1212, 2007

Yang J, McCrae RR, Costa PT Jr, et al: Cross-cultural personality assessment in psychiatric populations: the NEO-PI-R in the People's Republic of China. Psychol Assess 11:359–368, 1999

23

Pain

Michael R. Clark, M.D., M.P.H.

Definition and Assessment

Pain is a complex experience that integrates affective, cognitive, and behavioral factors with an extensive neurobiology. *Pain* has been defined by the International Association for the Study of Pain as "an unpleasant sensory and emotional experience associated with actual or potential tissue damage, or described in terms of such damage" (Merskey et al. 1986). Pain is the most common reason a patient presents to a physician for evaluation (Kroenke et al. 1990). This physician is rarely a neuropsychiatrist. However, if the patient has chronic pain (i.e., pain persisting on a daily basis for a month beyond what would be considered the usual time for healing of underlying pathology), then many specialists are likely to be involved in the care of the patient. Older persons are disproportionately represented in every aspect of the problems associated with chronic pain, including undetected high prevalence; inadequate assessment; multiple comorbidities; significant psychosocial problems; and poor access to treatment, which usually results in unacceptable outcomes (Charette and Ferrell 2007; Gibson 2007).

Pain is difficult to assess, especially in patients with terminal illnesses, cognitive impairments, and other chronic degenerative diseases of the brain. Pain rating scales attempt to measure the severity and intensity of pain. Even the simplest self-report measures to record the presence of pain cannot be effectively used by many elderly individuals. The elderly often have deficits in abstract ability that make it difficult for them to rate pain using a visual analog scale or a verbal descriptor scale that includes terms such as "discomforting," "distressing," and "excruciating." Increased age is associated with a greater frequency of incorrect responses on the visual analog scale, which may be primarily related to a decline in executive functioning (Oosterman et al. 2009). In a comparison study of several pain rating scales, the verbal descriptor scale was rated as the preferred, easiest, and best assessment tool for rating pain by the elderly (Herr and Mobily 1993).

Alternative tools for evaluating pain, such as pain drawings or maps and observations of pain behaviors, have been studied with positive results, but these methods are limited by reliance on an outside observer. The Geriatric Pain Measure short form is a 12-item, self-administered questionnaire targeted at community-dwelling elders to improve assessment of pain intensity, pain with ambulation, and disengagement because of pain (Blozik et al. 2007; Clough-Gorr et al. 2008). Good interrater reliability has been demonstrated for the Pain Assessment Checklist for Seniors With Limited Ability to Communicate (Cheung and Choi 2008), a tool that is used by caregivers to rate pain-related behaviors and that can be readministered to track detection of pain problems, prompt earlier treatment of pain in patients with dementia, and monitor response to therapies.

Epidemiology

In the community-dwelling elderly population, 25%–50% will suffer from pain (Gagliese and Melzack 1997). In people ages 65 and older, musculoskeletal pain is associated with three times the likelihood of significant difficulty performing three or more physical activities (Scudds and McD Robertson 1998). In a community sample of individuals over age 70, chronic pain was present in 52%, and obesity was associated with a twofold to fourfold increase in risk of having chronic pain (McCarthy et al. 2009). In persons over age 75, over two-thirds reported pain, almost half reported pain in multiple sites, and one-third rated pain as severe in at least one location (Brattberg et al. 1997). Sixty-six percent of nursing home residents over age 65 reported chronic pain, which was not detected by physicians in 34% of these residents (Stein and Ferrell 1996). The Study to Understand Prognoses and Preferences for Outcomes and Risks of Treatments (SUPPORT) has demonstrated that pain, dyspnea, and fatigue are the most prevalent symptoms experienced by patients with terminal illnesses at the end of life (Lynn et al. 1997).

Acute Pain Management

Acute pain management in elderly patients will usually be successful with straightforward strategies such as relaxation, immobilization, pharmacological agents (aspirin, acetaminophen, nonsteroidal anti-inflammatory drugs, opioids), massage, and transcutaneous electrical nerve stimulation (Institute for Clinical Systems Improvement 2008). Acute pain management initiated as early as possible and focused on preventing occurrence and reemergence of pain may allow for lower total dosages of analgesics. Sleep deprivation and anxiety may intensify the sensation of pain and increase requests for more medication. In acute pain management, psychiatric consultation is requested when a patient requires more analgesia than expected or has a history of substance abuse. Patients with an active or recent history of opioid addiction and those receiving methadone maintenance therapy have increased tolerance to opioids and may require up to 50% higher opioid doses than would usually be prescribed.

Psychiatric Comorbidity

Pain Disorder and Somatization

When a somatic cause for pain cannot be identified, many clinicians seek psychological causes. Pain "caused" by emotional factors was first classified in DSM-II (American Psychiatric Association 1968) under psychophysiological disorders, and DSM-III (American Psychiatric Association 1980) introduced the psychogenic pain disorder diagnosis. The lifetime prevalence of somatoform pain disorder (DSM-III-R; American Psychiatric Association 1987) in the general population is 34%, and the 6-month prevalence is 17% (Grabe et al. 2003). Applying the DSM-IV (American Psychiatric Association 1994) requirement of "significant distress or psychosocial impairment due to somatoform pain" reduced the lifetime prevalence of pain disorder to 12%, with a 6-month prevalence of 5% (Grabe et al. 2003). Injured workers with somatoform pain disorder, compared to those without, had more sites of pain with greater radiation of pain beyond the area of original injury, more opioid and benzodiazepine use, and higher rates of compensation claims and litigation (Streltzer et al. 2000). Neuroimaging studies of patients with pain disorder have shown significant decreases in gray matter density in prefrontal, cingulate, and insular cortex, which modulate the subjective experience of pain (Valet et al. 2009).

Although somatization disorder is rare in patients with chronic pain, the presence of multiple unexplained symptoms affects 4%–18% of primary care patients and is associated with higher rates of health care utilization and persistent somatic complaints (Jackson and Kroenke 2008). These patients are more likely to exhibit catastrophic thinking, believe the cause of their pain to be a mystery, have feelings of losing control, and think that physicians believe their pain is imaginary. Patients with chronic pain and medically unexplained symptoms are at risk for iatrogenic consequences of excessive diagnostic tests, inappropriate medications, unneeded surgery, functional disability, and role impairment.

Substance Abuse and Dependence

The prevalence of substance dependence or addiction in patients with chronic pain is estimated to range from 3% to 19% (McWilliams et al. 2003). Results from the Researched Abuse, Diversion and Addiction-Related Surveillance (RADARS) program indicate that prescription opioid abuse significantly increased over the course of the study (Cicero et al. 2007). Although the elderly are much more likely than other age groups to be prescribed these medications, screening instruments for prescription drug abuse have not been validated for this population (Culberson and Ziska 2008). Reliance on medications that provide pain relief can result in a number of stereotyped patient behaviors that can be mistaken for addiction. These actions may represent pseudoaddiction that results from therapeutic dependence and current or potential undertreatment, but not actual addiction (Kirsh et al. 2002). These behaviors, such as taking more medication than prescribed or obtaining medications from more than one doctor, abate with adequate analgesic therapy, and patient functioning subsequently improves.

Patients have concerns about medications that result in several patterns of nonadherence to or misuse of prescribed medications (McCracken et al. 2006). During the first 5 years after the onset of a chronic pain problem, patients are at increased risk for developing new drug-use problems and disorders. The risk is highest among those with a history of drug-use disorder or psychiatric comorbidity. Aberrant drug-related behaviors are common in patients with chronic pain who take prescribed chronic opioid analgesics, especially in patients with a history of substance abuse (Passik et al. 2006). The Pain Assessment and Documentation Tool has been used as an effective means to standardize follow-up care and decrease the risk of poor outcome with opioid therapy (Passik et al. 2005). Only 10% of occurrences of aberrant drug-taking behavior were determined to be a manifestation of addiction or diversion.

In a more recent comprehensive review, a calculated rate of abuse/addiction in patients with chronic pain was only 3.3% (Fishbain et al. 2008a). In the subgroup of patients with chronic pain who had no prior history of substance abuse, this rate dropped to 0.2%. However, as expected, aberrant drug-related behaviors and abnormal urine toxicology results were significantly more common in patients with chronic pain than in patients without chronic pain, reinforcing the need for risk screening and monitoring. Risk-prediction instruments, such as the Screener and Opioid Assessment for Patients With Pain, Opioid Risk Tool, and Current Opioid Misuse Measure, offer valuable guidance but have significant limitations (Chou et al. 2009). Strategies to optimize outcome and minimize abuse require careful analysis of the behavior of both patients and physicians (Clark et al. 2008; Passik and Kirsh 2008).

Depression and Affective Distress

Approximately 60% of patients with depression report pain symptoms at diagnosis. In the World Health Organization's data from 14 countries on five continents, 69% (range 45%–95%) of patients with depression presented with only somatic symptoms, of which pain complaints were most common (Simon et al. 1999). A survey of almost 19,000 Europeans found a fourfold increase in the prevalence of chronic painful conditions in subjects with major depression (Ohayon and Schatzberg 2003). A depressive disorder doubles the risk of developing chronic musculoskeletal pain, headache, and chest pain up to 13 years later (Larson et al. 2004). Older adults with depression are at increased risk for chronic neck, back, and hip pain. In patients with early inflammatory arthritis, baseline symptoms of depression predicted future pain better than did initial ratings of pain and disease activity (Schieir et al. 2009).

Individuals with chronic physical complaints have higher rates of lifetime major depression. The prevalence of major depression in patients with chronic low back pain is over three times the rate in the general population. In a study of late-onset depression in elderly patients, joint pain was one of the most important predictors of incident depression 5 years later (Hein et al. 2003). In general medical outpatients, the prevalence of depression was 12% in individuals with three or more pain complaints compared with only 1% in those with one or no pain complaints (Dworkin et al. 1990). In groups of patients with medically unexplained symptoms such as back pain and dizziness, two-thirds of patients have a history of recurrent major depression, compared with <20% of medically ill control groups (Sullivan and Katon 1993). In a review article, Dersh et al. (2002) reported that one-third to over one-half of patients presenting to chronic pain clinics met criteria for a current major depression.

In patients with chronic pain, depression is associated with greater pain intensity, more pain persistence, application for early retirement, and greater interference from pain, including more pain behaviors observed by others (Hasenbring et al. 1994). If pain resulted in a loss of independence or mobility that decreased an individual's participation in activities, the risk of depression was significantly increased (Williamson and Schulz 1992). However, depression is a better predictor of disability than are pain intensity and duration. Primary care patients with musculoskeletal pain complicated by depression were significantly more likely to use medications daily, in combinations, and to take sedative-hypnotics (Mantyselka et al. 2002). In patients with rheumatoid arthritis, depressive symptoms were significantly associated with negative health and functional outcomes, as well as increased health services utilization (Katz and Yelin 1993). In older adults with chronic pain, depression may be characterized by the absence of self-blame and may manifest as catastrophizing and maladaptive coping styles (Lopez-Lopez et al. 2008).

Patients with chronic pain syndromes also have increased rates of suicidal ideation, suicide attempts, and suicide completion. For example, patients with migraine, chronic abdominal pain, and orthopedic pain syndromes report increased rates of suicidal ideation and suicide attempts (Magni et al. 1998). The decrease in self-efficacy experienced by patients with chronic pain is highly associated with depressive symptoms that result in feelings of hopelessness (Rahman et al. 2008). Although other psychosocial variables play a role, depression is the most consistent and strongest predictor of suicidal ideation and behaviors in patients with chronic pain (Braden and Sullivan 2008). Pain is more likely to be an independent risk factor for suicide in patients with head or multiple types of pain (Ilgen et al. 2008). In patients who attempted suicide, 52% had a somatic disease and 21% were taking analgesics daily for pain (Stenager et al. 1994). Patients with chronic pain completed suicide at two to three times the rate in the general population.

Oncology patients with pain who also had depression were significantly more likely to request assistance in committing suicide as well as to take steps to end their lives, such as seeking information about suicide plans or hoarding medications. However, even if in pain, patients were unlikely to request the interventions of euthanasia and physician-assisted suicide when depression was not present (Emanuel et al. 1996). Depressive symptoms and poor self-reported health status predict worsening pain in community-dwelling older adults (Rosso et al. 2008). In patients over age 60 years with arthritis, antidepressants and/or problem-solving-oriented psychotherapy not only reduced depressive symptoms but also improved pain, functional status, and quality of life (Lin et al. 2003). In addition to having greater efficacy for the treatment of neuropathic pain, serotonin-norepinephrine reuptake inhibitors (SNRIs) and tricyclic antidepressants (TCAs) are associated with faster rates of improvement of depressive symptoms and lower rates of relapse of major depressive disorder (Rosenzweig-Lipson et al. 2007).

Anxiety, Fear, and Catastrophizing

Almost 50% of patients with chronic pain report anxiety symptoms, and up to 30% of patients have an anxiety disorder, such as generalized anxiety disorder, panic disorder, agoraphobia, and posttraumatic stress disorder (PTSD) (Dersh et al. 2002; McWilliams et al. 2003). One prospective study of 1,007 young adults found that a baseline history of migraine was significantly associated with an increased risk (odds ration [OR]=12.8) of first-incidence panic disorder (Breslau and Davis 1993). In patients with noncardiac chest pain, the presence of panic disorder significantly worsened health-related quality of life (Dammen et al. 2008). PTSD is increasingly recognized as a comorbid condition with significant consequences for patients with medical illnesses, especially chronic pain disorders (Liebschutz et al. 2007). Over half of fibromyalgia patients reported clinically relevant PTSD-like symptoms that were significantly associated with greater levels of pain, emotional distress, interference, and disability (Sherman et al. 2000). Compared with accident-related factors, PTSD symptoms and other psychological factors were the strongest predictors of the development of chronic pain in people who had experienced severe accidents 3 years earlier (Jenewein et al. 2009).

Conversely, anxiety symptoms and disorders are associated with high levels of somatic preoccupation and physical symptoms. Pain intensity in patients with rheumatoid arthritis was significantly increased by the presence of anxiety, even after controlling for disease activity (Smedstad et al. 1995). Almost two-thirds of patients with panic disorder reported at least one current pain symptom (Schmidt et al. 2002). Pain severity, pain-related disability, and health-related quality of life were significantly worse in patients with chronic musculoskeletal pain and comorbid anxiety or depression (Bair et al. 2008).

Fear of pain, movement, reinjury, and other negative consequences that result in the avoidance of activities promotes the transition to and sustaining of chronic pain and its associated disabilities (Greenberg and Burns 2003). Patients with chronic low back pain who restricted their activities developed physiological changes (muscle atrophy, weight gain), and functional deterioration attributed to deconditioning (Verbunt et al. 2003). This process is reinforced by low self-efficacy, catastrophic interpretations, and increased expectations of failure regarding attempts to engage in rehabilitation (Leeuw et al. 2007). Catastrophizing intensifies the experience of pain and increases emotional distress as well as self-perceived disability (Sullivan et al. 2001). Early treatment catastrophizing and feelings of helplessness in patients attending a 4-week multidisciplinary pain program predicted late-treatment outcomes, predicted disability due to new-onset low back pain 6 months later, and has been shown to be a predictor of suicidal ideation independent of depressive symptoms and pain severity (Burns et al. 2003; Edwards et al. 2006; Picavet et al. 2002).

Neurobiology of Pain

The neurobiology of pain is complex and reviewed by numerous authors (e.g., Clark and Treisman 2004; Leknes and Tracey 2008). Dynamic interactions take place throughout the peripheral and central nervous systems. Changes in peripheral nerves, spinal cord structures, spinal glia, and supraspinal structures contribute to sensory/discriminative abnormalities, such as hyperalgesia and allodynia, as well as affective/limbic pathophysiology, such as depression and suffering (Cao and Zhang 2008). Ongoing nociceptive or neuropathic stimulation causes sensory neurons to become electrically hyperexcitable and generate ectopic impulses. These changes are manifested as spontaneous firing and abnormal responsiveness of neuronal structures (e.g., neuroma end bulbs, regenerating sprouts, dorsal root ganglia, areas of demyelination, local uninjured axons) to a variety of stimuli. Extensive overlap exists between the neurobiology of pain and pleasure/reward, with mutual inhibitory effects and important modulating influences from the opioid and dopamine systems (Leknes and Tracey 2008).

Pathophysiological mechanisms contributing to chronic pain include the remodeling of voltage-sensitive ion channels, transducer molecules, and receptors in the cell membrane; activation of intracellular second messenger systems; gene induction leading to changes in protein synthesis; long-term potentiation of synaptic transmission; monoamine modulation; loss of inhibitory mechanisms; and apoptotic cell death (Pace et al. 2006). Continuing neurobiological discoveries generate new ideas for the design of novel pharmacological therapies. For example, modulation of synaptic transmission and membrane excitability could be achieved with sodium channel subtype antagonists, selective *N*-methyl-D-aspartate (NMDA) receptor antagonists, subtype-selective agents for γ-aminobutyric acid (GABA), adenosine A_1 receptor antagonists, nitric oxide synthase inhibitors, cholecystokinin receptor antagonists, cannabinoids, protein kinase C inhibitors, aldose reductase inhibitors, lipoic acid, oxytocin, vanilloid VR_1 receptor modulators, dronabinol, and cyclo-oxygenase-2 inhibitors (Gidal 2006; Knabl et al. 2008).

Ultimately, pharmacological treatments attempt to alleviate symptoms by targeting the pathophysiological mechanisms producing pain. Combinations of medications should employ a rational approach to polypharmacy through the utilization of synergistic effects to produce enhanced antinociception, adding medications to address the incremental contribution of an untreated mechanism, and strategies to minimize the risk of treatment failures (e.g., adverse events, toxicities, tolerance, dependence). Novel neuroimaging technologies and translational biomarkers may reveal neuroinflammation dynamics and targets for treatment based on cellular processes including genetics (Stephenson and Arneric 2008). Acetyl-L-carnitine has been studied as a means of inducing regeneration of peripheral nerves, minimizing the effects of oxidative stress, facilitating deoxyribonucleic acid (DNA) synthesis in mitochondria, and increasing the concentrations of nerve growth factors in peripheral neuropathies, such as those caused by diabetes and medications used to treat HIV infection and cancer (Vanotti et al. 2007).

Chronic Pain Conditions in the Elderly

Postherpetic Neuralgia

Postherpetic neuralgia (PHN) is defined as pain persisting or recurring at the site of shingles at least 3 months after the onset of the acute varicella zoster viral rash. PHN occurs in about 10% of patients with acute herpes zoster. More than half of patients over age 65 who have shingles develop PHN, and it is more likely to occur in patients with cancer, diabetes mellitus, and immunosuppression. Other risk factors include longer duration of prodromal symptoms, greater acute pain and rash severity, sensory impairment, and psychological distress (Volpi et al. 2008). Most cases gradually improve over time, with only about 25% of patients with PHN experiencing pain at 1 year after diagnosis. Studies have suggested the role of both peripheral and central mechanisms resulting from the loss of large-caliber neurons and subsequent central sensitization or adrenergic receptor activation and alterations in C-fiber activity (Truini et al. 2008). Early treatment of varicella zoster with low-dose amitriptyline reduced the prevalence of pain at 6 months by 50% (Johnson 1997). TCAs, anticonvulsants, and opioids are the most common effective treatments for PHN and may have potential for its prevention (Zin et al. 2008). Topical lidocaine has been approved by the U.S. Food and Drug Administration for treatment of PHN. A live attenuated varicella vaccine decreased the incidence of herpes zoster and PHN, as well as the burden of illness, in adults over age 60 (Harpaz et al. 2008; Johnson et al. 2008).

Peripheral Neuropathy Pain

Sensory neurons are damaged by many diseases, both directly and indirectly. The most common cause of painful peripheral neuropathy is diabetes mellitus (Veves et al. 2008; Zochodne 2008). Approximately 25% of patients with diabetes mellitus will experience painful diabetic neuropathy, with duration of illness and poor glycemic control increasing this risk factor (Tavakoli and Malik 2008). If C-fiber input is preserved but large-fiber input is lost, paresthesias and pain become the predominant sensory experiences. The pain of a peripheral neuropathy ranges from a constant burning to an episodic, paroxysmal, and lancinating quality. These phenomena are primarily the result of axonal degeneration, segmental demyelination, ectopic impulse generation, and increases in the magnitude and frequency of action potentials (Tomlinson and Gardiner 2008). The paroxysms of pain that result from stimulation of hyperexcitable damaged neurons and subsequent recruitment of nearby undamaged sensory afferents may be explained by central sensitization that amplifies and sustains neuronal activity by a variety of mechanisms, such as reduced inhibition of dorsal horn cells and glutamate release (Carozzi et al. 2008). Pharmacological treatments are almost identical to those used in the treatment of PHN (Jain 2008; Jensen and Finnerup 2007).

Parkinson's Disease

Pain is the most common sensory manifestation of Parkinson's disease (PD). Recent studies suggest that the majority of patients with PD, especially women, suffer from pain (Beiske et al. 2009). The pain is typically described as cramping and aching, located in the lower back and extremities, but not associated with muscle contraction or spasm. All forms of chronic pain are represented, including musculoskeletal, neuropathic (radicular, central), and dystonic pain. These pains often decrease when the patient is treated with levodopa, which suggests a central origin, such as the loss of dopaminergic input. Dopamine is now consistently implicated as having a role in the endogenous pain modulation system (Potvin et al. 2009; Wood 2008). In a review of French health system data, 82% of patients with PD were prescribed analgesics (Brefel-Courbon et al. 2009). Subthalamic deep brain stimulation may offer relief to patients refractory to other therapies (Kim et al. 2008).

Central Poststroke Pain and Spinal Cord Injury

Pain associated with lesions of the central nervous system is common after stroke (8%) or spinal cord trauma (60%–70%) (Finnerup 2008; Ullrich 2007). Symptoms of spinal cord injury pain or central poststroke pain are often poorly localized, vary over time, and include allodynia (>50% of patients with central poststroke pain), hyperalgesia, dysesthesias, lancinating pain, and muscle and visceral pain regardless of sensory deficits. Pain is described as burning, aching, lacerating, or pricking. Radiographic lesions are present in the thalamus, although other sites are often involved, such as the spinothalamic tracts, especially in spinal cord injury (Hari et al. 2009). A variety of mechanisms have been postulated, including increased voltage-gated sodium channel expression, microglial activation, and production of reactive oxygen species (Hains and Waxman 2007; Hulsebosch et al. 2009). Excitatory amino acids are likely involved in the development of central sensitization associated with this syndrome, and the onset of pain can occur more than a month after the stroke, suggesting multiple processes. Randomized clinical trials have demonstrated efficacy for amitriptyline and other drugs that reduce neuronal hyperexcitability, including lidocaine (intravenous), mexiletine, lamotrigine, fluvoxamine, and gabapentin, but not carbamazepine, phenytoin, opioids, or topiramate (Frese et al. 2006). In contrast, patients with spinal cord injury experience reductions in continuous and evoked pain with ketamine, μ-opioid receptor agonists, and intravenous lidocaine, suggesting different mechanisms. Morphine may decrease allodynia but not other components of central pain syndromes (Nicholson 2004). More recent reviews support the efficacy of amitriptyline, gabapentin, and pregabalin for the neuropathic pain associated with spinal cord injury (Baastrup and Finnerup 2008; Tzellos et al. 2008).

Migraine and Chronic Daily Headache

The peak incidence of migraine occurs between the third and sixth decades of life and then decreases with age (Silberstein et al. 2007). Over the life span, 18% of women and 6% of men experience migraine (Lipton et al. 2007). Theories of pathogenesis include the trigeminovascular system and plasma protein extravasation, antagonism of serotonin receptors, modulation of central aminergic control mechanisms, membrane-stabilizing effects through action at voltage-sensitive calcium channels, and release of substance P (Goadsby et al. 2009). Migraine is a unilateral pulsatile headache, which may be associated with other symptoms such as nausea, vomiting, photophobia, phonophobia, visual prodromal symptoms, or neurological deficits (Lipton et al. 2007). Placebo-controlled clinical trials suggest nonsteroidal anti-inflammatory drugs and triptans for acute treatment of migraine attacks (Mulleners and Chronicle 2008). In general, calcium channel blockers, beta-blockers, antidepressants, and anticonvulsants are the classes of choice for prophylaxis (Evers et al. 2006; Silberstein 2008). Behavioral treatments such as cognitive-behavioral psychotherapy and biofeedback/relaxation training are effective abortive and preventative therapies (Holroyd and Drew 2006).

Chronic daily headache affects about 5% of the population and is composed of constant (transformed) migraine, medication-overuse headache, chronic tension-type headache, new-onset daily persistent headache, and hemicrania continua (Dodick 2006). Patients with chronic daily headache are more likely to overuse medication, leading to rebound headache; to have psychiatric comorbidity such as depression and anxiety; to report functional disability; and to experience stress-related headache exacerbations (Penas and Schoenen 2009). Patients with transformed migraine have poor quality of life, with the worst Medical Outcome Study—Short Form (SF-36) profile compared with patients with episodic migraine or chronic tension-type headache (Wang et al. 2001). Chronic tension-type headaches typically manifest as daily pain that is difficult to manage and unresponsive to many treatments. Placebo-controlled clinical trials are few but support the use of amitriptyline, gabapentin, topiramate, and botulinum toxin type A (Dodick 2006). As with other chronic pain syndromes, empirical support exists for treating patients with other agents such as the SNRIs, TCAs, and anticonvulsants. Combined medication and cognitive-behavioral psychotherapy are more effective than either treatment alone.

Fibromyalgia

Fibromyalgia is a chronic pain syndrome characterized by chronic widespread musculoskeletal pain, subjective stiffness, and exaggerated tenderness. These symptoms are usually accompanied by poor sleep, cognitive difficulties, depression, and fatigue. Fibromyalgia is diagnosed in 3.4% of women and 0.5% of men and is clustered in families (Arnold et al. 2004). Current research suggests that fibromyalgia may be the result of dysfunctional central pain processing precipitated by a variety of mechanisms, including infection, physical trauma, psychological traits, and psychopathology (Abeles et al. 2007). Guidelines for fibromyalgia treatment recommend multidisciplinary treatment regimens (Carville et al. 2008; Hauser et al. 2009). Placebo-controlled trials suggest pain reduction with cyclobenzaprine, milnacipran, gabapentin, pregabalin, duloxetine, and tramadol (Crofford 2008; Mease et al. 2009; Tofferi et al. 2004).

Phantom Limb Pain

Phantom limb pain occurs in 50%–80% of amputees within a year of the amputation (Schley et al. 2008). This neuropathic pain is described as stabbing, throbbing, burning, or cramping and is more intense in the distal portion of the phantom limb. Although TCAs, gabapentin, and carbamazepine are considered first-line treatments for phantom pain, there are no controlled trials to support their use. Newer antidepressants and anticonvulsants with generally fewer side effects may result in greater effectiveness if higher dosages can be tolerated by patients. However, morphine, calcitonin, and ketamine have been shown to reduce phantom pain in controlled studies (Wu et al. 2008).

Orofacial Pain

Trigeminal Neuralgia

Trigeminal neuralgia (tic douloureux) is a chronic pain syndrome with severe, paroxysmal, recurrent, lancinating pain, with a unilateral distribution of cranial nerve V, most commonly the mandibular division (Obermann and Katsarava

2009; Prasad and Galetta 2009). Sensory or motor deficits are not usually present. Less commonly, the facial or glossopharyngeal nerve is involved, with pain in the ear, posterior pharynx, tongue, or larynx. Episodes of pain can be spontaneous or evoked by nonpainful stimuli to trigger zones, activities such as talking or chewing, or environmental conditions. Between episodes, patients are typically pain free. The majority of patients with classical trigeminal neuralgia show evidence of trigeminal nerve root compression by blood vessels (85%), mass lesions, or other diseases (multiple sclerosis, herpes zoster, PHN) that cause demyelination and hyperactivity of the trigeminal nucleus (Love and Coakham 2001). Pharmacological treatment includes anticonvulsants, antidepressants, baclofen, mexiletine, lidocaine, and opioids (Cruccu et al. 2008). Placebo-controlled trials identify carbamazepine as first-line treatment. When pharmacological treatments fail, a variety of surgical procedures, such as microvascular decompression, percutaneous gangliolysis, and stereotactic radiosurgery, may be undertaken (Gronseth et al. 2008; Miller et al. 2009).

Temporomandibular Disorder

Temporomandibular disorder (TMD) refers to complaints that involve the temporomandibular joint, muscles of mastication, and other orofacial musculoskeletal structures. Pain most commonly arises from the muscles of mastication and is precipitated by jaw function such as opening the mouth or chewing. Associated symptoms include feelings of muscle fatigue, weakness, and tightness, as well as changes in bite (malocclusion) or the inability to open or close the jaw. In contrast, temporomandibular joint dysfunction causes sharp, sudden, and intense pain, with joint movement that is often localized to the preauricular area. Psychological distress is common in patients with TMD. Patients with pain of muscular origin are usually more distressed and depressed and have greater levels of disability than those with temporomandibular joint pain. In treatment trials for patients with TMD, multidisciplinary treatment produced improvements in pain intensity, interference, catastrophizing, depression, and negative thoughts (Sherman and Turk 2001).

Burning Mouth Syndrome

Burning mouth syndrome (BMS) is characterized as pain in oral and pharyngeal cavities, especially the tongue, and is often associated with dryness and taste alterations. The oral mucosa is usually normal. The condition mainly affects middle-aged and postmenopausal women. Most cases are idiopathic, but BMS may coincide with a plethora of conditions, such as bruxism, poorly fitting dentures, oral candidiasis, xerostomia, malnutrition, food allergies and contact dermatitis, gastroesophageal reflux disease, diabetes mellitus, hypothyroidism, neoplasia, menopause, and psychiatric conditions such as depression, anxiety, and somatization (Drage and Rogers 2003). Psychological factors, such as severe life events, have been associated with the condition. Theories of etiology and pathogenesis include brain stem pathology, hyperactivity of sensory and motor components of the trigeminal nerve following loss of central inhibition that resulted from damage to the chorda tympani or glossopharyngeal nerves, disorders of the dopaminergic system, and small sensory fiber dysfunction. Potential underlying etiologies, such as depression and/or anxiety, nutritional deficiencies (iron, folate, vitamin B_{12}, and other B vitamins), maladaptive oral habits, and iatrogenic causes such as medications, should be identified and treated (Pinto et al. 2003). Treatment with antidepressants, anticonvulsants, benzodiazepines, topical analgesics, soft desensitizing oral appliances, vitamin and hormonal supplements, and habit awareness counseling may be helpful.

Low Back Pain

Low back pain (LBP) is one of the most common physical symptoms and the most expensive condition when considering health care costs and lost productivity (Deyo et al. 2009). Psychological factors, including distress, depressed mood, and somatization, are highly correlated with LBP and predict the transition from acute to chronic LBP (Pincus et al. 2002). A minority of patients with acute LBP will develop chronic LBP with disproportionate distress and disability. On the other hand, two-thirds of patients with chronic LBP at 3 months exhibited functional disability at 22 months (Pincus et al. 2002). The most powerful predictor of chronicity was poor functional status 4 weeks after seeking treatment.

The presence of a depressive disorder increases the risk of developing chronic musculoskeletal pain. In a 13-year follow-up study, depressive disorder was a significant risk factor for incident LBP (Larson et al. 2004). In another prospective analysis, participants who did not have current LBP were followed for 12 months (Croft et al. 1996). Patients with higher levels of distress at baseline were almost twice as likely to report a new episode of back pain. As much as 16% of LBP in the general population may be attributable to psychological distress. In contrast, chronic disabling occupational spinal disorders result in high levels of psychopathology that compromise outcomes and decrease benefits of treatment (Dersh et al. 2007).

The treatment of chronic LBP has been pursued with multiple modalities alone and in combination. A study of physiotherapy for chronic LBP showed that physiotherapist-led pain management classes offered a cost-effective alternative to outpatient physiotherapy and spinal stabilization classes, with greater reductions in health care use and similar improvements in pain, quality of life, and time off from work (Critchley et al. 2007). Behavioral therapies have been found to be more effective than waitlist or no-treatment controls, but their effectiveness is less convincing when these therapies are compared with usual treatment for chronic LBP (van Tulder et al. 2001). Interdisciplinary rehabilitation programs usually offer the best outcomes for reducing pain and pain-related disability; however, they are the most expensive treatment, and high-quality randomized controlled trials are still needed to document long-term efficacy (Huge et al. 2006).

Pharmacological Treatment

A number of drug classes are employed in the treatment of chronic pain, usually neuropathic pain (Moulin et al. 2007). Medications target mechanisms of peripheral and central nervous system sensitization, such as sodium and calcium channel upregulation, spinal hyperexcitability, descending modulation, and aberrant sympathetic-somatic nervous system interactions. Antidepressants and anticonvulsants are the best studied and are recommended as first-line therapies (Dworkin et al. 2007). Unfortunately, these medications are underutilized and underdosed. In one study of patients with neuropathic pain, 73% complained of inadequate pain control, but 72% had never received anticonvulsants, 60% had never received TCAs, 41% had never received opioids, and 25% had never received any of these medications (Gilron et al. 2002). No medication algorithm can provide a simple, straightforward approach to the complexities encountered during the treatment of patients with chronic pain. Rational combinations should be designed to optimize pharmacological synergies and minimize liabilities.

Opioids

Opioids reduce the sensory and affective components of pain by interacting with μ-, δ-, and κ-opiate receptors located from the periphery to central areas modulating pain transmission. They are potent analgesics for all types of neuropathic and nociceptive pain. Controversy surrounds the long-term use of opioids for chronic nonmalignant pain (Noble et al. 2008). Opioids should be slowly tapered and discontinued if the risks (side effects, toxicities, aberrant drug-related behaviors) outweigh the objective benefits (analgesia, functional improvements). The most common side effect of chronic opioid therapy is decreased gastrointestinal motility, causing constipation, vomiting, and abdominal pain (Tassinari et al. 2008). Long-term opiate administration may result in analgesic tolerance or opioid-induced hyperalgesia (Mitra 2008). When tolerance develops, coadministration of other analgesics, opioid rotation to a more potent agonist, or intermittent cessation of certain agents may restore analgesic effect (Dumas and Pollack 2008; Vorobeychik et al. 2008).

Guidelines have been established for the use of opioids in chronic pain (American Academy of Pain Medicine and the American Pain Society 2008). Suitable patients are those with moderate or severe pain persisting for > 3 months and adversely affecting function or quality of life. Before initiating opioid therapy, additional factors such as the patient's specific pain syndrome, response to other therapies, and potential for aberrant drug-related behaviors (misuse, abuse, addiction, diversion) should be considered (Ballantyne and LaForge 2007). A patient's suitability for chronic opioid therapy can be assessed with standardized questionnaires such as the Opioid Risk Tool (ORT); the Diagnosis, Intractability, Risk, Efficacy (DIRE) Inventory; and the Screener and Opioid Assessment for Patients with Pain (SOAPP). Treatment outcomes, including analgesia, activities of daily living, adverse events, and potential aberrant drug-related behaviors, can be assessed with the Pain Assessment and Documentation Tool (PADT). The Current Opioid Misuse Measure (COMM) evaluates patients who are taking opioids for concurrent signs or symptoms of intoxication, emotional volatility, poor response to medications, addiction, health care use patterns, and problematic medication behaviors. These scales can be downloaded from the Pain Treatment Topics Web site (http://pain-topics.org/opioid_rx/risk.php#).

Morphine, because of its hydrophilicity, has poor oral bioavailability (22%–48%), delayed central nervous system access, and slower onset of action compared with more lipophilic opioids. This delay prolongs the analgesic effect of morphine relative to its plasma half-life, which decreases the potential for accumulation and toxicity. Morphine is a more effective epidural spinal analgesic than oxycodone. *Oxycodone* has high oral bioavailability (>60%), a faster onset of action, and more predictable plasma levels than morphine. Oxycodone, compared with morphine, has similar analgesic efficacy, releases less histamine, and causes fewer hallucinations (Riley et al. 2008). *Hydrocodone* is similar to oxycodone, with rapid oral absorption and onset of analgesia. Hydrocodone is metabolized by *N*-demethylation to hydromorphone, which has properties similar to morphine but lower rates of side effects. *Fentanyl* is highly lipophilic, with affinity for neuronal tissues and the potential for transdermal or transmucosal delivery. *Methadone* warrants special consideration in the treatment of chronic pain because of its low cost, high bioavailability, rapid onset of action, slow hepatic clearance, multiple receptor affinities, lack of neurotoxic metabolites, and incomplete cross-tolerance with other opioids. However, compared with other opioids, methadone has a significantly greater risk of overdose attributed to a longer time for adaptation with oral use and a greater variation in plasma half-life (15–120 hours) (Sandoval et al. 2005). Extensive tissue distribution and prolonged half-life prevent withdrawal symptoms when a patient takes one dose per day. However, elimination is biphasic, and the more rapid elimination phase equates with the duration of analgesia that is limited to approximately 6 hours. Repeated dosing, with accumulation in tissue, may increase analgesia duration to 8–12 hours (Peng et al. 2008b).

Antidepressants

The analgesic properties of antidepressants are still underappreciated. The neurobiology of pain suggests that all antidepressants would be effective for treatment of chronic pain (McCleane 2008). TCAs and SNRIs in particular are effectively used for many chronic pain syndromes, including diabetic neuropathy, PHN, central pain, poststroke pain, tension-type headache, migraine, and orofacial pain, but not nonspecific LBP (Saarto and Wiffen 2007; Verdu et al. 2008). The analgesic effect of antidepressants is independent of their antidepressant effect and is primarily mediated by the blockade of reuptake of norepinephrine and serotonin, thereby increasing their levels and enhancing the activation of descending inhibitory neurons in the dorsal horn of the spinal cord (McCleane 2008; Mico et al. 2006). However, antidepressants may produce antinociceptive effects through a variety of pharmacological mechanisms, including monoamine modulation, interactions with opioid systems, and inhibition of ion channel activity and NMDA, histamine, and cholinergic receptors (Dick et al. 2007).

Tricyclic Antidepressants

TCAs have been shown in controlled trials to effectively treat central poststroke pain, PHN, painful diabetic and nondiabetic polyneuropathy, and postmastectomy pain syndrome, but not spinal cord injury pain, phantom limb pain, or pain in HIV neuropathy. A meta-analysis that focused on fibromyalgia found positive but diminishing effect comparing classes of antidepressants: TCAs > monoamine oxidase inhibitors (MAOIs) > selective serotonin reuptake inhibitors (SSRIs) = SNRIs (Hauser et al. 2009). Although they are equally effective for pain, secondary amine TCAs (e.g., nortriptyline) are better tolerated than tertiary agents (e.g., amitriptyline) (Dworkin et al. 2007). Antidepressants generally produce analgesia at lower dosages and with earlier onset of action than expected for the treatment of depression (Rojas-Corrales et al. 2003). However, the lack of analgesic effect in individuals and in studies of certain pain syndromes, such as spinal cord injury pain, may be due to inadequate dosing. A U.S. health insurance claims database found that the average daily dosage of TCAs for the treatment of neuropathic pain in patients ages 65 and older was only 23 mg (Berger et al. 2006). Patients in a multidisciplinary pain center study were typically prescribed ≤50 mg of amitriptyline, suggesting unrealized potential for additional pain relief.

Serotonin-Norepinephrine Reuptake Inhibitors

The SNRIs duloxetine, venlafaxine, desvenlafaxine, and milnacipran inhibit the presynaptic reuptake of serotonin, norepinephrine, and to a lesser extent dopamine, with fewer side effects than TCAs. Compared with venlafaxine, duloxetine more potently blocks serotonin (5-HT) and norepinephrine transporters (Berrocoso and Mico 2008). Milnacipran has antihyperalgesic effects mediated by monoamine and opioid systems, and clinical trials show its efficacy for treatment of fibromyalgia. Desvenlafaxine will likely be studied in models of nociception and neuropathic pain. SNRIs produce better analgesic efficacy than do SSRIs, even with the latter in combination with selective noradrenergic reuptake inhibitors (NRIs) (Jones et al. 2006). Venlafaxine significantly prevents migraine and decreases allodynia and hyperalgesia in both neuropathic pain and atypical facial pain (Yucel et al. 2005). Response improved with higher dosages attributable to increased reuptake inhibition of norepinephrine. In a study of painful diabetic neuropathy, 150–225 mg/day of venlafaxine produced a greater percentage reduction in pain (50%) than did 75 mg/day (32%) (Rowbotham et al. 2004). Duloxetine possesses analgesic efficacy in fibromyalgia and painful diabetic neuropathy (Wernicke et al. 2006). Guidelines for the treatment of neuropathic pain recommend duloxetine as a first-line treatment (Argoff et al. 2006). The efficacy of duloxetine in painful diabetic neuropathy was greater in patients with more severe pain but was not related to the severity of diabetes or neuropathy (Ziegler et al. 2007). Although patients with depression and painful somatic symptoms experienced relief when treated with duloxetine, the analgesic effects were independent of antidepressant actions (Perahia et al. 2006).

Selective Serotonin Reuptake Inhibitors

In clinical trials, the efficacy of SSRIs in chronic pain syndromes has been inconsistent and disappointing, especially in the treatment of neuropathic pain (Finnerup et al. 2005). A Cochrane review found SSRIs no more efficacious than placebo for migraine and less efficacious than TCAs for tension-type headache (Moja et al. 2005). Citalopram improved irritable bowel syndrome symptoms, independent of effects on anxiety and depression (Tack et al. 2006). Patients with DSM-IV-TR (American Psychiatric Association 2000) pain disorder experienced significant analgesic effects, independent of changes in depression, with citalopram but not the NRI reboxetine (Aragona et al. 2005). Paroxetine and citalopram, but not fluoxetine, have shown benefit for painful diabetic peripheral neuropathy in controlled studies. In another comparison study of gabapentin, paroxetine, and citalopram for painful diabetic peripheral neuropathy, patients reported better satisfaction, compliance, and mood with SSRIs, but similar efficacy of the three drugs for pain (Giannopoulos et al. 2007).

Overall, although not recommended as a first-line therapy for chronic pain, SSRIs are a recommended alternative to TCAs or SNRIs, with a favorable risk-benefit profile.

Anticonvulsants

Anticonvulsants inhibit excessive neuronal activity by blocking voltage-gated sodium channels, modulating calcium channels, inhibiting excitatory amino acid neurotransmission, or enhancing GABA-mediated inhibitory neurotransmission (Stefan and Feuerstein 2007). Anticonvulsants may produce better compliance compared with antidepressants because of fewer adverse effects. Anticonvulsants are effective for trigeminal neuralgia, diabetic neuropathy, PHN, and migraine recurrence. Anticonvulsants have better compliance compared with TCAs because of fewer adverse effects (Finnerup et al. 2005). Phenytoin was first reported as a successful treatment for trigeminal neuralgia in 1942. Carbamazepine is the most widely studied anticonvulsant effective for neuropathic pain. Valproic acid is most commonly used in the prophylaxis of migraine but is also effective for neuropathic pain. Sodium valproate was effective as a prophylactic treatment in over two-thirds of patients with migraine and almost three-fourths of those with cluster headache (Gallagher et al. 2002).

Pregabalin and gabapentin modulate the influx of calcium and decrease the release of neurotransmitters (Han et al. 2007; Taylor et al. 2007). They also activate the descending noradrenergic inhibitory system of nociception (Tanabe et al. 2008). Pregabalin and gabapentin are effective for the treatment of painful diabetic neuropathy, PHN, fibromyalgia, postamputation phantom limb pain, and central neuropathic pain associated with spinal cord injury (Tassone et al. 2007). Patients with chronic pain were more likely to respond to gabapentin if they experienced allodynia. In patients with PHN, flexible dosing strategies, compared with fixed-dose schedules, resulted in fewer discontinuations, higher final dosage, and slightly better pain relief (Stacey et al. 2008). Lamotrigine has multiple pharmacological actions and produced positive results for pain associated with HIV-related neuropathy and central poststroke pain, but it was disappointing for other neuropathic pain (Wiffen and Rees 2007). Dosages above 300 mg/day with serum levels below 15 mg/L were more effective for the treatment of painful diabetic neuropathy (Vinik et al. 2007). Topiramate offers the advantages of minimal hepatic metabolism and unchanged renal excretion, few drug interactions, a long half-life, and the unusual side effect of weight loss. Topiramate was found effective for migraine prophylaxis (Silberstein et al. 2006), and it decreased pain from chronic LBP, lumbar radiculopathy, and painful diabetic neuropathy (Muehlbacher et al. 2006; Silberstein et al. 2006; Van Passel et al. 2006).

Oxcarbazepine is a carbamazepine derivative with an improved safety and tolerability profile. Oxcarbazepine for refractory PHN decreased pain, with rapid onset of action and improvements in function and quality of life (Nasreddine and Beydoun 2007). A randomized, placebo-controlled trial for painful diabetic neuropathy found that about 35% of patients treated with oxcarbazepine experienced >50% improvement in their pain (Dogra et al. 2005). Tiagabine reduced pain by comparable amounts to gabapentin but showed significantly greater improvements in sleep quality (Todorov et al. 2005). Despite multiple mechanisms of action, zonisamide shows mixed results for the treatment of neuropathic pain (Kothare and Kaleyias 2008). Riluzole (sodium channel blocker), retigabine (potassium channel opener), ethosuximide (T-type calcium channel blocker), and levetiracetam attenuate nociceptive responses in animals (Munro et al. 2007). Lacosamide is a functionalized amino acid that selectively enhances slow inactivation of voltage-gated sodium channels and is under study for painful diabetic neuropathy (Beyreuther et al. 2007).

Combinations of anticonvulsants with complementary mechanisms of action may increase effectiveness and decrease adverse effects of treatment. Patients with multiple sclerosis or trigeminal neuralgia who had failed treatment with carbamazepine or lamotrigine at therapeutic dosages due to intolerable side effects benefited from gabapentin as an augmentation agent (Solaro et al. 2000). When anticonvulsants were combined with tramadol, synergistic effects were found for inhibiting allodynia and blocking nociception (Codd et al. 2008). Carbamazepine or oxcarbazepine combined with clonidine produced a synergistic antihyperalgesic effect on inflammatory pain (Vuckovic et al. 2006).

Benzodiazepines

Benzodiazepines are commonly prescribed for insomnia, anxiety, and spasticity, but no studies demonstrate any benefit for these target symptoms, and the drugs may be counterproductive in patients with chronic pain. Benzodiazepines decreased pain in only a limited number of chronic pain conditions, such as trigeminal neuralgia, tension headache, and TMD (Dellemijn and Fields 1994). Clonazepam may provide long-term relief for the episodic lancinating variety of phantom limb pain (Bartusch et al. 1996). Benzodiazepines cause sedation and cognitive impairment, especially in elderly people (Buffett-Jerrott and Stewart 2002). In patients with chronic pain, the use of benzodiazepines, but not opioids, was associated with decreased activity levels, higher rates of health care visits, increased domestic instability, depression, and more disability days (Ciccone et al. 2000). Combining benzodiazepines with opioids may be countertherapeutic and potentially dangerous. Benzodiazepines may exacerbate pain and interfere with opioid analgesia (Gear et al. 1997). These effects appear to be the result of activating supraspinal $GABA_A$ receptors known to antagonize opioid analgesia. Studies of methadone-related mortality found high rates of benzodiazepine use, with the cause of death being attributed to a combination of drug effects, especially in patients receiving methadone for chronic pain (Caplehorn and Drummer 2002).

Antipsychotics

Increasing evidence supports the effectiveness of antipsychotics in treating patients with diabetic neuropathy, PHN, headache, facial pain, pain associated with acquired immune deficiency syndrome (AIDS) and cancer, and musculoskeletal pain (Fishbain et al. 2004). In a meta-analysis of 11 controlled trials, Seidel et al. (2008) reported that some antipsychotics have been found to have analgesic efficacy in headache (haloperidol) and trigeminal neuralgia (pimozide). Other trials have focused on fibromyalgia, because evidence suggests dopaminergic D_2 receptor hypersensitivity and decreased release of dopamine from the basal ganglia in response to pain (Wood et al. 2007). An open-label study of the addition of quetiapine to patients' existing but ineffective fibromyalgia treatment regimen did not decrease pain but produced significant improvements on the Fibromyalgia Impact Questionnaire and quality-of-life measures (Hidalgo et al. 2007). Studies of ziprasidone and olanzapine showed beneficial effects but low response rates and poor tolerability (Calandre et al. 2007). Results are difficult to interpret because comorbid depressive, anxiety, and sleep disorders in patients with fibromyalgia might respond to treatment with atypical antipsychotics.

Psychological Treatments

Cognitive-Behavioral Models

Many psychological interventions have been effective in reducing pain and its associated distress (Molton et al. 2007). Psychological treatment for chronic pain was pioneered by Fordyce et al. (1973) using an operant conditioning behavioral model. The behavioral approach is based on an understanding of pain as it occurs in a social context. If pain behaviors receive reinforcement, the behavioral model assumes that pain and disability will continue and increase. In treatment, productive behaviors are targeted for reinforcement and pain behaviors for extinction. The cognitive-behavioral model of chronic pain assumes that individual beliefs, attitudes, and expectations affect emotional and behavioral reactions to life experiences. Pain and the resultant pain behaviors are influenced by biomedical, psychological, and socioenvironmental variables. If patients believe that pain, depression, and disability are inevitable and uncontrollable, then they will experience more negative affective responses, increased pain, and even more impaired physical and psychosocial functioning. Although physical disability was correlated with beliefs about pain interfering with function, patients also endorsed the belief that pain signifies injury and that therefore activity should be avoided. A change in perceived control over pain was the most significant predictor of beneficial effects of cognitive-behavioral therapies (CBTs) for chronic TMD pain (Turner et al. 2007).

The components of CBT, such as relaxation, guided imagery, biofeedback, meditation, hypnosis, motivational interviewing, external reinforcement, cognitive restructuring, and coping self-statement training, interrupt this cycle of disability. The goals of CBT, regardless of techniques employed, focus the patient on self-control and self-management to increase activity, independence, and resourcefulness (Turk et al. 2008). Patients are taught to become active participants in the management of their pain through the use of methods that minimize distressing thoughts and feelings. Specifically, elderly patients benefit from CBT that presents information in concrete, well-organized, and brief formats (Manetto and McPherson 1996). Outcome studies of CBT in patients with a variety of chronic pain syndromes have demonstrated significant improvements in pain intensity, pain behaviors, distress, depression, and coping. Pain reduction and improved physical function have continued up to 6 months after active CBT (Keefe et al. 1990).

Adjustment and Acceptance

The success of CBT in chronic pain treatment has led to focused attention on many elements of the chronic pain experience, including such concepts as psychological resilience and illness adaptation (Karoly and Ruehlman 2006). *Adjustment* is defined as the ability to carry out normal physical and psychosocial activities. Three dimensions of adjustment have been defined: social functioning, morale, and somatic health (Lazarus and Folkman 1984). Examples of these domains include pain intensity, medication use, depression, anxiety, employment, health care utilization, and functional ability. *Acceptance* of chronic pain is a two-factor construct (activity engagement and pain willingness), associated with multiple domains of the experience of chronic pain (Vowles et al. 2008b). Acceptance of pain was found to be associated with reports of lower pain intensity, less pain-related anxiety and avoidance, less depression, less physical and psychosocial disability, more daily uptime, and better work status (McCracken 1998). Acceptance has been found to mediate the effects of catastrophizing on depression, avoidance, and functioning in patients with chronic pain (Vowles et al. 2008a). In general, acceptance predicts adjustment to chronic pain and is independent from catastrophizing, coping strategies, and pain-related cognitions (Esteve et al. 2007; Vowles et al. 2007).

Coping

Coping is defined as "a person's cognitive and behavioral efforts to manage the internal and external demands of the person-environment transaction that is appraised as taxing or exceeding the person's resources" (Folkman et al. 1986, p. 571). Higher levels of disability were found in persons who remain passive or use maladaptive coping strategies of catastrophizing, ignoring or reinterpreting pain sensations, diverting attention from pain, and praying or hoping for relief. In a 6-month follow-up study of patients completing an inpatient pain treatment program, improvement was associated with decreases in the use of passive coping strategies and beliefs about pain being an illness (Jensen et al. 1994).

The effectiveness of particular coping strategies, with improved adjustment to chronic pain, is dependent on many aspects of a patient's experience with illness. For example, reinterpreting pain sensations as not being signs of ongoing injury has been typically formulated as useful for reducing the effects of experimentally induced pain. However, in a study of amputees with phantom limb pain, this coping strategy was not associated with reduced pain levels but instead with greater psychosocial dysfunction (Hill et al. 1995). Attempting to reinterpret pain sensations may not be an appropriate technique for individuals with persistent pain because it requires greater amounts of time spent focusing on pain and disability. This may prevent patients from engaging in social activities. Catastrophic thinking about pain has been attributed to the amplification of threatening information and interference with the attentional focus needed to help patients remain involved with productive instead of pain-related activities. Some evidence suggests that older patients with chronic pain use different patterns of coping strategies. In a study by Corran et al. (1994), older patients were more likely to use passive strategies, such as praying and hoping for relief from pain; less likely to ignore pain; and benefited most from coping self-statements that emphasize an ability to actively manage pain. In contrast, younger patients were more likely to benefit from ignoring pain. According to Keefe et al. (1990), training older adults to use adaptive coping strategies resulted in lower levels of pain and psychological disability.

Interdisciplinary Rehabilitation

Patients with chronic pain experience dramatic reductions in physical, psychological, and social well-being, and they rate health-related quality of life lower than do patients with almost all other medical conditions (Skevington 1998). Educational programs led by nonprofessional laypeople have shown short-term gains in self-efficacy, cognitive symptom management, and frequency of exercise (Foster et al. 2007). Collaborative care initiatives providing pain specialist assistance to primary care practitioners significantly improved pain-related outcomes (Dobscha et al. 2009). Self-management programs for elderly people with chronic pain demonstrate significant reductions in pain intensity and disability (Reid et al. 2008). An intervention trial combining pain assessment with physical therapy and physician-based analgesic protocols decreased rates of chronic pain and use of analgesics for older adults 6 months after orthopedic surgery (Morrison et al. 2009).

Evidence-based practice guidelines for patients with pain emphasize interdisciplinary rehabilitation, integrated treatment, and patient selection criteria (Sanders et al. 2005). The interdisciplinary pain rehabilitation program provides the full range of treatments for the most difficult pain syndromes, including those afflicting elderly patients, within a framework of collaborative ongoing communication among team members, patients, and other interested parties (Stanos and Houle 2006). Unfortunately, there is considerable variability in the type of practitioners and scope of practice of so-called multidisciplinary pain clinics (Peng et al. 2008a). A more recent survey in North Carolina found only 7% of such clinics met the criteria of having a medical physician, registered nurse, physical therapist, and mental health specialist (Castel et al. 2009).

Substantial evidence indicates that interdisciplinary pain rehabilitation programs improve functioning in a number of areas for patients with various chronic pain syndromes, even for patients with severe disabilities (Angst et al. 2006; Lake et al. 2009; McCracken et al. 2007; Van Wilgen et al. 2009). In a seminal review, a meta-analysis of 65 studies evaluated the efficacy of treatments in patients who attended multidisciplinary pain clinics (Flor et al. 1992). Although there were limitations to the study designs and descriptions, the authors concluded that multidisciplinary pain clinics are efficacious, a finding that has been supported by more recent reviews. Combination treatments were superior to unimodal treatments or no treatment; treatment effects were maintained over a period of up to 7 years; and improvements were found on both subjective and objective measures of effectiveness, such as return to work and decreased health care utilization. Current smoking status has been associated with poorer treatment outcome from multidisciplinary treatment, suggesting that these patients should receive targeted or more intensive treatments (Fishbain et al. 2008b). Analyses of interdisciplinary programs that use comprehensive assessments, severity-adapted or stepped-care treatments, and rehabilitation goals demonstrate significant reductions in pain along with functional and quality-of-life improvements (Kainz et al. 2006; Marnitz et al. 2008). Multidisciplinary outcome studies of elderly patients with chronic pain demonstrate a variety of benefits from treatment (Gibson et al. 1996; Middaugh et al. 1988). Ultimately, the goal of treating patients with chronic pain is to end disability and return people to work or other productive activities.

Conclusion

Chronic pain is a significant public health problem and frustrating to everyone affected by it, especially elderly patients who feel that health care has failed them but who wish to remain in their own homes, live independently, and avoid becoming a burden to others. Neuropsychiatrists functioning as medical specialists should take an active role in the care of these patients. They can offer pharmacological and psychological treatments that are recognized as effective in the management of chronic pain.

Key Points

- Chronic pain is very common in the elderly.
- Depression, not addiction, is the most common psychiatric condition in patients with chronic pain.
- Antidepressants offer independent efficacy for major depression and neuropathic pain in patients with chronic pain conditions.
- Psychotherapy and interdisciplinary rehabilitation programs offer incremental benefits to patients with refractory chronic pain.

Recommended Web Sites

American Chronic Pain Association: www.theacpa.org
American Pain Foundation: www.painfoundation.org
American Pain Society: www.ampainsoc.org
American Society of Pain Educators: www.paineducators.org
Chronic Pain Information Page, National Institute of Neurological Disorders and Stroke: www.ninds.nih.gov/disorders/chronic_pain/chronic_pain.htm
National Pain Foundation: www.nationalpainfoundation.org

References

Abeles AM, Pillinger MH, Solitar BM, et al: Narrative review: the pathophysiology of fibromyalgia. Ann Intern Med 146:726–734, 2007

American Academy of Pain Medicine, American Pain Society: The use of opiates for the treatment of chronic pain: a consensus statement. Glenview, IL, American Pain Society, 2008. Available at: http://www.ampainsoc.org/advocacy/opioids.htm. Accessed July 15, 2010.

American Psychiatric Association: Diagnostic and Statistical Manual of Mental Disorders, 2nd Edition. Washington, DC, American Psychiatric Association, 1968

American Psychiatric Association: Diagnostic and Statistical Manual of Mental Disorders, 3rd Edition. Washington, DC, American Psychiatric Association, 1980

American Psychiatric Association: Diagnostic and Statistical Manual of Mental Disorders, 3rd Edition, Revised. Washington, DC, American Psychiatric Association, 1987

American Psychiatric Association: Diagnostic and Statistical Manual of Mental Disorders, 4th Edition. Washington, DC, American Psychiatric Association, 1994

American Psychiatric Association: Diagnostic and Statistical Manual of Mental Disorders, 4th Edition, Text Revision. Washington, DC, American Psychiatric Association, 2000

Angst F, Brioschi R, Main CJ, et al: Interdisciplinary rehabilitation in fibromyalgia and chronic back pain: a prospective outcome study. J Pain 7:807–815, 2006

Aragona M, Bancheri L, Perinelli D, et al: Randomized double-blind comparison of serotonergic (citalopram) versus noradrenergic (reboxetine) reuptake inhibitors in outpatients with somatoform, DSM-IV-TR pain disorder. Eur J Pain 9:33–38, 2005

Argoff CE, Backonja MM, Belgrade MJ, et al: Consensus guidelines: treatment planning and options. Diabetic peripheral neuropathic pain. Mayo Clin Proc 81:S12–S25, 2006

Arnold LM, Hudson JI, Hess EV, et al: Family study of fibromyalgia. Arthritis Rheum 50:944–952, 2004

Baastrup C, Finnerup NB: Pharmacological management of neuropathic pain following spinal cord injury. CNS Drugs 22:455–475, 2008

Bair MJ, Wu J, Damush TM, Sutherland JM, et al: Association of depression and anxiety alone and in combination with chronic musculoskeletal pain in primary care patients. Psychosom Med 70:890–897, 2008

Ballantyne JC, LaForge KS: Opioid dependence and addiction during opioid treatment of chronic pain. Pain 129:235–255, 2007

Bartusch SL, Sanders BJ, D'Alessio JG, et al: Clonazepam for the treatment of lancinating phantom limb pain. Clin J Pain 12:59–62, 1996

Beiske AG, Loge JH, Ronningen A, et al: Pain in Parkinson's disease: prevalence and characteristics. Pain 141:173–177, 2009

Berger A, Dukes EM, Edelsberg J, et al: Use of tricyclic antidepressants in older patients with painful neuropathies. Eur J Clin Pharmacol 62:757–764, 2006

Berrocoso E, Mico JA: Role of serotonin 5-HT1A receptors in the antidepressant-like effect and the antinociceptive effect of venlafaxine in mice. Int J Neuropsychopharmacol 14:1–11, 2008

Beyreuther BK, Freitag J, Heers C, et al: Lacosamide: a review of preclinical properties. CNS Drug Rev 13:21–42, 2007

Blozik E, Stuck AE, Niemann S, et al: Geriatric Pain Measure short form: development and initial evaluation. J Am Geriatr Soc 55: 2045–2050, 2007

Braden JB, Sullivan MD: Suicidal thoughts and behavior among adults with self-reported pain conditions in the national comorbidity survey replication. J Pain 9:1106–1115, 2008

Brattberg G, Parker MG, Thorslund M: A longitudinal study of pain: reported pain from middle age to old age. Clin J Pain 13:144–149, 1997

Brefel-Courbon C, Grolleau S, Thalamas C, et al: Comparison of chronic analgesic drugs prevalence in Parkinson's disease, other chronic diseases and the general population. Pain 141:14–18, 2009

Breslau N, Davis GC: Migraine, physical health and psychiatric disorder: a prospective epidemiologic study in young adults. J Psychiatr Res 27:211–221, 1993

Buffett-Jerrott SE, Stewart SH: Cognitive and sedative effects of benzodiazepine use. Curr Pharm Des 8:45–58, 2002

Burns JW, Kubilus A, Bruehl S, et al: Do changes in cognitive factors influence outcome following multidisciplinary treatment for chronic pain? A cross-lagged panel analysis. J Consult Clin Psychol 71:81–91, 2003

Calandre EP, Hidalgo J, Rico-Villademoros F: Use of ziprasidone in patients with fibromyalgia: a case series. Rheumatol Int 27:473–476, 2007

Cao H, Zhang YQ: Spinal glial activation contributes to pathological pain states. Neurosci Biobehav Rev 32:972–983, 2008

Caplehorn JR, Drummer OH: Fatal methadone toxicity: signs and circumstances, and the role of benzodiazepines. Aust N Z J Public Health 26:358–362, 2002

Carozzi V, Marmiroli P, Cavaletti G: Focus on the role of glutamate in the pathology of the peripheral nervous system. CNS Neurol Disord Drug Targets 7:348–360, 2008

Carville SF, Arendt-Nielsen S, Bliddal H, et al: EULAR evidence-based recommendations for the management of fibromyalgia syndrome. Ann Rheum Dis 67:536–541, 2008

Castel LD, Freburger JK, Holmes GM, et al: Spine and pain clinics serving North Carolina patients with back and neck pain: what do they do, and are they multidisciplinary? Spine 34:615–622, 2009

Charette SL, Ferrell BA: Rheumatic diseases in the elderly: assessing chronic pain. Rheum Dis Clin North Am 33:109–122, 2007

Cheung G, Choi P: The use of the Pain Assessment Checklist for Seniors with Limited Ability to Communicate (PACSLAC) by caregivers in dementia care. N Z Med J 121:21–29, 2008

Chou R, Fanciullo GJ, Fine PG, et al: Opioids for chronic noncancer pain: prediction and identification of aberrant drug-related behaviors: a review of the evidence for an American Pain Society and American Academy of Pain Medicine clinical practice guideline. J Pain 10:131–146, 2009

Ciccone DS, Just N, Bandilla EB, et al: Psychological correlates of opioid use in patients with chronic nonmalignant pain: a preliminary test of the downhill spiral hypothesis. J Pain Symptom Manage 20:180–192, 2000

Cicero TJ, Dart RC, Inciardi JA, et al: The development of a comprehensive risk-management program for prescription opioid analgesics: Researched Abuse, Diversion and Addiction-Related Surveillance (RADARS). Pain Med 8:157–170, 2007

Clark MR, Treisman GJ: Perspectives on pain and depression. Adv Psychosom Med 25:1–27, 2004

Clark MR, Stoller KB, Brooner RK: Assessment and management of chronic pain in individuals seeking treatment for opioid dependence disorder. Can J Psychiatry 53:496–508, 2008

Clough-Gorr KM, Blozik E, Gillmann G, et al: The self-administered 24-item geriatric pain measure (GPM-24-SA): psychometric properties in three European populations of community-dwelling older adults. Pain Med 9:695–709, 2008

Codd EE, Martinez RP, Molino L, et al: Tramadol and several anticonvulsants synergize in attenuating nerve injury-induced allodynia. Pain 134:254–262, 2008

Corran TM, Gibson SJ, Farrell MJ, et al: Comparison of chronic pain experience between young and elderly patients, in Proceedings of the 7th World Congress on Pain, Progress in Pain Research and Management, Vol 2. Seattle, WA, IASP Press, 1994, pp 895–906

Critchley DJ, Ratcliffe J, Noonan S, et al: Effectiveness and cost-effectiveness of three types of physiotherapy used to reduce chronic low back pain disability: a pragmatic randomized trial with economic evaluation. Spine 32:1474–1481, 2007

Crofford LJ: Pain management in fibromyalgia. Curr Opin Rheumatol 20:246–250, 2008

Croft PR, Papageorgiou AC, Ferry S, et al: Psychological distress and low back pain: evidence from a prospective study in the general population. Spine 20:2731–2737, 1996

Cruccu G, Gronseth G, Alksne J, et al: AAN-EFNS guidelines on trigeminal neuralgia management. Eur J Neurol 15:1013–1028, 2008

Culberson JW, Ziska M: Prescription drug misuse/abuse in the elderly. Geriatrics 63:22–31, 2008

Dammen T, Ekeberg O, Arnesen H, et al: Health-related quality of life in non-cardiac chest pain patients with and without panic disorder. Int J Psychiatry Med 38:271–286, 2008

Dellemijn PL, Fields HL: Do benzodiazepines have a role in chronic pain management? Pain 57:137–152, 1994

Dersh J, Polatin PB, Gatchel RJ: Chronic pain and psychopathology: research findings and theoretical considerations. Psychosom Med 64:773–786, 2002

Dersh J, Mayer T, Theodore BR, et al: Do psychiatric disorders first appear preinjury or postinjury in chronic disabling occupational spinal disorders? Spine 32:1045–1051, 2007

Deyo RA, Mirza SK, Turner JA, et al: Overtreating chronic back pain: time to back off? J Am Board Fam Med 22:62–68, 2009

Dick IE, Brochu RM, Purohit Y, et al: Sodium channel blockade may contribute to the analgesic efficacy of antidepressants. J Pain 8:315–324, 2007

Dobscha SK, Corson K, Perrin NA, et al: Collaborative care for chronic pain in primary care: a cluster randomized trial. JAMA 301:1242–1252, 2009

Dodick DW: Clinical practice: chronic daily headache. N Engl J Med 354:158–165, 2006

Dogra S, Beydoun S, Mazzola J, et al: Oxcarbazepine in painful diabetic neuropathy: a randomized, placebo-controlled study. Eur J Pain 9:543–554, 2005

Drage LA, Rogers RS III: Burning mouth syndrome. Dermatol Clin 21:135–145, 2003

Dumas EO, Pollack GM: Opioid tolerance development: a pharmacokinetic/pharmacodynamic perspective. AAPS J 10:537–551, 2008

Dworkin RH, O'Connor AB, Backonja M, et al: Pharmacologic management of neuropathic pain: evidence-based recommendations. Pain 132:237–251, 2007

Dworkin SF, Von Korff M, LeResche L: Multiple pain and psychiatric disturbance: an epidemiologic investigation. Arch Gen Psychiatry 47:239–244, 1990

Edwards RR, Smith MT, Kudel I, et al: Pain-related catastrophizing as a risk factor for suicidal ideation in chronic pain. Pain 126:272–279, 2006

Emanuel EJ, Fairclough DL, Daniels ER, et al: Euthanasia and physician-assisted suicide: attitudes and experiences of oncology patients, oncologists, and the public. Lancet 347:1805–1810, 1996

Esteve R, Ramirez-Maestre C, Lopez-Marinez AE: Adjustment to chronic pain: the role of pain acceptance, coping strategies, and pain-related cognitions. Ann Behav Med 33:179–188, 2007

Evers S, Afra J, Frese A, et al: EFNS guideline on the drug treatment of migraine-report of an EFNS task force. Eur J Neurol 13:560–572, 2006

Finnerup NB: A review of central neuropathic pain states. Curr Opin Anaesthesiol 21:586–589, 2008

Finnerup NB, Otto M, McQuay HJ, et al: Algorithm for neuropathic pain treatment: an evidence based proposal. Pain 118:289–305, 2005

Fishbain DA, Cutler RB, Lewis J, et al: Do the second-generation "atypical neuroleptics" have analgesic properties? A structured evidence-based review. Pain Med 5:359–365, 2004

Fishbain DA, Cole B, Lewis J, et al: What percentage of chronic nonmalignant pain patients exposed to chronic opioid analgesic therapy develop abuse/addiction and/or aberrant drug-related behaviors? A structured evidence-based review. Pain Med 9:444–459, 2008a

Fishbain DA, Lewis JE, Cutler R, et al: Does smoking status affect multidisciplinary pain facility treatment outcome? Pain Med 9:1081–1090, 2008b

Flor H, Fydrich T, Turk DC: Efficacy of multidisciplinary pain treatment centers: a meta-analytic review. Pain 49:221–230, 1992

Folkman S, Lazarus RS, Gruen RJ, et al: Appraisal, coping, health status, and psychological symptoms. J Per Soc Psychol 50:571–579, 1986

Fordyce WE, Fowler RS Jr, Lehmann JF, et al: Operant conditioning in the treatment of chronic pain. Arch Phys Med Rehabil 54:399–408, 1973

Foster G, Taylor SJ, Eldridge SE, et al: Self-management education programmes by lay leaders for people with chronic conditions. Cochrane Database of Systematic Reviews, Issue 4. Art. No.: CD005108. DOI: 10.1002/14651858.CD005108.pub2, 2007

Frese A, Husstedt IW, Ringelstein EB, et al: Pharmacologic treatment of central post-stroke pain. Clin J Pain 22:252–260, 2006

Gagliese L, Melzack R: Chronic pain in elderly people. Pain 70:3–14, 1997

Gallagher RM, Mueller LL, Freitag FG: Divalproex sodium in the treatment of migraine and cluster headaches. J Am Osteopath Assoc 102:92–94, 2002

Gear RW, Miaskowski C, Heller PH, et al: Benzodiazepine mediated antagonism of opioid analgesia. Pain 71:25–29, 1997

Giannopoulos S, Kosmidou M, Sarmas I, et al: Patient compliance with SSRIs and gabapentin in painful diabetic neuropathy. Clin J Pain 23:267–269, 2007

Gibson SJ: IASP global year against pain in older persons: highlighting the current status and future perspectives in geriatric pain. Expert Rev Neurother 7:627–635, 2007

Gibson SJ, Farrell MJ, Katz B, et al: Multidisciplinary management of chronic nonmalignant pain in older adults, in Pain in the Elderly. Edited by Ferrell BR, Ferrell BA. Seattle, WA, IASP Press, 1996, pp 91–99

Gidal BE: New and emerging treatment options for neuropathic pain. Am J Manag Care 12(suppl):S269–S278, 2006

Gilron I, Bailey J, Weaver DF, et al: Patients' attitudes and prior treatments in neuropathic pain: a pilot study. Pain Res Manage 7: 199–203, 2002

Goadsby PJ, Charbit AR, Andreou AP, et al: Neurobiology of migraine. Neuroscience 161:327–341, 2009

Grabe HJ, Meyer C, Hapke U, et al: Somatoform pain disorder in the general population. Psychother Psychosom 72:88–94, 2003

Greenberg J, Burns JW: Pain anxiety among chronic pain patients: specific phobia or manifestations of anxiety sensitivity? Behav Res Ther 41:223–240, 2003

Gronseth G, Cruccu G, Alksne J, et al: Practice parameter: the diagnostic evaluation and treatment of trigeminal neuralgia (an evidence-based review): report of the Quality Standards Subcommittee of the American Academy of Neurology and the European Federation of Neurological Societies. Neurology 71:1183–1190, 2008

Hains BC, Waxman SG: Sodium channel expression and the molecular pathophysiology of pain after SCI. Prog Brain Res 161:195–203, 2007

Han DW, Kweon TD, Lee JS, et al: Antiallodynic effect of pregabalin in rat models of sympathetically maintained and sympathetic independent neuropathic pain. Yonsei Med J 48:41–47, 2007

Hari AR, Wydenkeller S, Dokladal P, et al: Enhanced recovery of human spinothalamic function is associated with central neuropathic pain after SCI. Exp Neurol 216:428–430, 2009

Harpaz R, Ortega-Sanchez IR, Seward JF; Advisory Committee on Immunization Practices Centers for Disease Control and Prevention: Prevention of herpes zoster: recommendations of the Advisory Committee on Immunization Practices (ACIP). MMWR Recomm Rep 57:1–30, 2008

Hasenbring M, Marienfeld G, Kuhlendahl D, et al: Risk factors of chronicity in lumbar disc patients: a prospective investigation of biologic, psychologic, and social predictors of therapy outcome. Spine 19:2759–2765, 1994

Hauser W, Bernardy K, Uceyler N, et al: Treatment of fibromyalgia syndromes with antidepressants: a meta-analysis. JAMA 301: 198–209, 2009

Hein S, Bonsignore M, Barkow K, et al: Lifetime depressive and somatic symptoms as preclinical markers of late-onset depression. Eur Arch Psychiatry Clin Neurosci 253:16–21, 2003

Herr KA, Mobily PR: Comparison of selected pain assessment tools for use with the elderly. Appl Nurs Res 6:39–46, 1993

Hidalgo J, Rico-Villademoros F, Calandre EP: An open-label study of quetiapine in the treatment of fibromyalgia. Prog Neuropsychopharmacol Biol Psychiatry 31:71–77, 2007

Hill A, Niven CA, Knussen C: The role of coping in adjustment to phantom limb pain. Pain 62:79–86, 1995

Holroyd KA, Drew JB: Behavioral approaches to the treatment of migraine. Semin Neurol 26:199–207, 2006

Huge V, Schloderer U, Steinberger M, et al: Impact of a functional restoration program on pain and health-related quality of life in patients with chronic low back pain. Pain Med 7:501–508, 2006

Hulsebosch CE, Hains BC, Crown ED, et al: Mechanisms of chronic central neuropathic pain after spinal cord injury. Brain Res Rev 60:202–213, 2009

Ilgen MA, Zivin K, McCammon RJ, et al: Pain and suicidal thoughts, plans and attempts in the United States. Gen Hosp Psychiatry 30:521–527, 2008

Institute for Clinical Systems Improvement: Assessment and management of acute pain. Bloomington, MN, Institute for Clinical Systems Improvement, 2008. Available at: http://internationalguidelinescenter.businesscatalyst.com/_webapp_1826687/Assessment_and_management_of_acute_ pain. Accessed October 4, 2010.

Jackson JL, Kroenke K: Prevalence, impact, and prognosis of multisomatoform disorder in primary care: a 5-year follow-up study. Psychosom Med 70:430–434, 2008

Jain KK: Current challenges and future prospects in management of neuropathic pain. Expert Rev Neurother 8:1743–1756, 2008

Jenewein J, Moergeli H, Wittmann L, et al: Development of chronic pain following severe accidental injury: results of a 3-year follow-up study. J Psychosom Res 66:119–126, 2009

Jensen MP, Turner JA, Romano JM: Correlates of improvement in multidisciplinary treatment of chronic pain. J Consult Clin Psychol 62:172–179, 1994

Jensen TS, Finnerup NB: Management of neuropathic pain. Curr Opin Support Palliat Care 1:126–131, 2007

Johnson RW: Herpes zoster and postherpetic neuralgia: optimal treatment. Drugs Aging 10:80–94, 1997

Johnson RW, Wasner G, Saddier P, et al: Herpes zoster and postherpetic neuralgia: optimizing management in the elderly patient. Drugs Aging 25:991–1006, 2008

Jones CK, Eastwood BJ, Need AB, et al: Analgesic effects of serotonergic, noradrenergic or dual reuptake inhibitors in the carrageenan test in rats: evidence for synergism between serotonergic and noradrenergic reuptake inhibition. Neuropharmacology 51:1172–1180, 2006

Kainz B, Gulich M, Engel EM, et al: Comparison of three outpatient therapy forms for treatment of chronic low back pain—findings of a multicentre, cluster randomized study. Rehabilitation 45: 65–77, 2006

Karoly P, Ruehlman LS: Psychological "resilience" and its correlates in chronic pain: findings from a national community sample. Pain 123:90–97, 2006

Katz PP, Yelin EH: Prevalence and correlates of depressive symptoms among persons with rheumatoid arthritis. J Rheumatol 20:790–796, 1993

Keefe FJ, Caldwell DS, Williams DA, et al: Pain coping skills training in the management of osteoarthritic knee pain, II: follow-up results. Behav Ther 21:435–447, 1990

Kim HJ, Paek SH, Kim JY, et al: Chronic subthalamic deep brain stimulation improves pain in Parkinson disease. J Neurol 255: 1889–1894, 2008

Kirsh KL, Whitcomb LA, Donaghy K, et al: Abuse and addiction issues in medically ill patients with pain: attempts at clarification of terms and empirical study. Clin J Pain 18(suppl):S52–S60, 2002

Knabl J, Witschi R, Hosl K, et al: Reversal of pathological pain through specific spinal $GABA_A$ receptor subtypes. Nature 451: 330–334, 2008

Kothare SV, Kaleyias J: Zonisamide: review of pharmacology, clinical efficacy, tolerability, and safety. Expert Opin Drug Metab Toxicol 4:493–506, 2008

Kroenke K, Arrington ME, Mangelsdorff AD: The prevalence of symptoms in medical outpatients and the adequacy of therapy. Arch Intern Med 150:1685–1689, 1990

Lake AE III, Saper JR, Hamel RL: Comprehensive inpatient treatment of refractory chronic daily headache. Headache 49:555–562, 2009

Larson SL, Clark MR, Eaton WW: Depressive disorder as a long-term antecedent risk factor for incident back pain: a 13-year follow-up study from the Baltimore Epidemiological Catchment Area sample. Psychol Med 34:211–219, 2004

Lazarus RA, Folkman S: Stress, Appraisal, and Coping. New York, Springer, 1984

Leeuw M, Goossens ME, Linton SJ, et al: The fear-avoidance model of musculoskeletal pain: current state of scientific evidence. J Behav Med 30:77–94, 2007

Leknes S, Tracey I: A common neurobiology for pain and pleasure. Nat Rev Neurosci 9:314–320, 2008

Liebschutz J, Saitz R, Brower V, et al: PTSD in urban primary care: high prevalence and low physician recognition. J Gen Intern Med 22:719–726, 2007

Lin EH, Katon W, Von Korff M, et al: Effect of improving depression care on pain and functional outcomes among older adults with arthritis: a randomized controlled trial. JAMA 290:2428–2429, 2003

Lipton RB, Bigal ME, Diamond M, et al: Migraine prevalence, disease burden, and the need for preventive therapy. Neurology 68:343–349, 2007

Lopez-Lopez A, Montorio I, Izal M, et al: The role of psychological variables in explaining depression in older people with chronic pain. Aging Ment Health 12:735–745, 2008

Love S, Coakham HB: Trigeminal neuralgia: pathology and pathogenesis. Brain 124:2347–2360, 2001

Lynn J, Teno JM, Phillips RS, et al: Perceptions by family members of the dying experience of older and seriously ill patients. SUPPORT Investigators. Study to Understand Prognoses and Preferences for Outcomes and Risks of Treatments. Ann Intern Med 1226:97–106, 1997

Magni G, Rigatti-Luchini S, Fracca F, et al: Suicidality in chronic abdominal pain: an analysis of the Hispanic Health and Nutrition Examination Survey (HHANES). Pain 76:137–144, 1998

Manetto C, McPherson SE: The behavioral-cognitive model of pain. Clin Geriatr Med 12:461–471, 1996

Mantyselka P, Ahonen R, Viinamaki H, et al: Drug use by patients visiting primary care physicians due to nonacute musculoskeletal pain. Eur J Pharm Sci 17:201–206, 2002

Marnitz U, Weh L, Müller G, et al: Multimodal integrated assessment and treatment of patients with back pain: pain related results and ability to work. Schmerz 22:415–423, 2008

McCarthy LH, Bigal ME, Katz M, et al: Chronic pain and obesity in elderly people: results from the Einstein aging study. J Am Geriatr Soc 57:115–119, 2009

McCleane G: Antidepressants as analgesics. CNS Drugs 22:139–156, 2008

McCracken LM: Learning to live with the pain: acceptance of pain predicts adjustment in persons with chronic pain. Pain 74:21–27, 1998

McCracken LM, Hoskins J, Eccleston C: Concerns about medication and medication use in chronic pain. J Pain 7:726–734, 2006

McCracken LM, MacKichan F, Eccleston C: Contextual cognitive-behavioral therapy for severely disabled chronic pain sufferers: effectiveness and clinically significant change. Eur J Pain 11:314–322, 2007

McWilliams LA, Cox BJ, Enns MW: Mood and anxiety disorders associated with chronic pain: an examination in a nationally representative sample. Pain 106:127–133, 2003

Mease PJ, Clauw DJ, Gendreau RM, et al: The efficacy and safety of milnacipran for treatment of fibromyalgia: a randomized, double-blind, placebo-controlled trial. J Rheumatol 36:398–409, 2009

Merskey H, Lindblom U, Mumford JM, et al: Pain terms: a current list with definitions and notes on usage. Pain 27(suppl):S215–S221, 1986

Mico JA, Ardid D, Berrocoso E, et al: Antidepressants and pain. Trends Pharmacol Sci 27:348–354, 2006

Middaugh SJ, Levin RB, Kee WG, et al: Chronic pain: its treatment in geriatric and younger patients. Arch Phys Med Rehabil 69:1021–1026, 1988

Miller JP, Magill ST, Acar F, et al: Predictors of long-term success after microvascular decompression for trigeminal neuralgia. J Neurosurg 110:620–626, 2009

Mitra S: Opioid-induced hyperalgesia: pathophysiology and clinical implications. J Opioid Manag 4:123–130, 2008

Moja L, Cusi C, Sterzi R, et al: Selective serotonin re-uptake inhibitors (SSRIs) for preventing migraine and tension-type headaches. Cochrane Database of Systematic Reviews 2005, Issue 3. Art. No.: CD002919. DOI: 10.1002/14651858.CD002919.pub2

Molton IR, Graham C, Stoelb BL, et al: Current psychological approaches to the management of chronic pain. Curr Opin Anaesthesiol 20:485–489, 2007

Morrison RS, Flanagan S, Fischberg D, et al: A novel interdisciplinary analgesic program reduces pain and improves function in older adults after orthopedic surgery. J Am Geriatr Soc 57:1–10, 2009

Moulin DE, Clark AJ, Gilron I, et al: Pharmacological management of chronic neuropathic pain: consensus statement and guidelines from the Canadian Pain Society. Pain Res Manage 12:13–21, 2007

Muehlbacher M, Nickel MK, Kettler C, et al: Topiramate in treatment of patients with chronic low back pain: a randomized, double-blind, placebo-controlled study. Clin J Pain 22:526–531, 2006

Mulleners WM, Chronicle EP: Anticonvulsants in migraine prophylaxis: a Cochrane review. Cephalalgia 28:585–597, 2008

Munro G, Erichsen HK, Mirza NR: Pharmacological comparison of anticonvulsant drugs in animal models of persistent pain and anxiety. Neuropharmacology 53:609–618, 2007

Nasreddine W, Beydoun A: Oxcarbazepine in neuropathic pain. Expert Opin Investig Drugs 16:1615–1625, 2007

Nicholson BD: Evaluation and treatment of central pain syndromes. Neurology 62:S30–S36, 2004

Noble M, Tregear SJ, Treadwell JR, et al: Long-term opioid therapy for chronic noncancer pain: a systematic review and meta-analysis of efficacy and safety. J Pain Symptom Manage 35:214–228, 2008

Obermann M, Katsarava Z: Update on trigeminal neuralgia. Expert Rev Neurother 9:323–329, 2009

Ohayon MM, Schatzberg AF: Using chronic pain to predict depressive morbidity in the general population. Arch Gen Psychiatry 60:39–47, 2003

Oosterman JM, de Vries K, Dijkerman HC, et al: Exploring the relationship between cognition and self-reported pain in residents of homes for the elderly. Int Psychogeriatr 21:157–163, 2009

Pace MC, Mazzariello L, Passavanti MB, et al: Neurobiology of pain. J Cell Physiol 209:8–12, 2006

Passik SD, Kirsh KL: The interface between pain and drug abuse and the evolution of strategies to optimize pain management while minimizing drug abuse. Exp Clin Psychopharmacol 16:400–404, 2008

Passik SD, Kirsh KL, Whitcomb L, et al: Monitoring outcomes during long-term opioid therapy for noncancer pain: results with the Pain Assessment and Documentation Tool. J Opioid Manag 1:257–266, 2005

Passik SD, Kirsh KL, Donaghy KB, et al: Pain and aberrant drug-related behaviors in medically ill patients with and without histories of substance abuse. Clin J Pain 22:173–181, 2006

Penas CF, Schoenen J: Chronic tension-type headache: what is new? Curr Opin Neurol 22:254–261, 2009

Peng P, Stinson JN, Choiniere M, et al: Role of health care professionals in multidisciplinary pain treatment facilities in Canada. Pain Res Manag 13:484–488, 2008a

Peng P, Tumber P, Stafford M, et al: Experience of methadone therapy in 100 consecutive chronic pain patients in a multidisciplinary pain center. Pain Med 9:786–794, 2008b

Perahia DG, Pritchett YL, Desaiah D, et al: Efficacy of duloxetine in painful symptoms: an analgesic or antidepressant effect? Int Clin Psychopharmacol 21:311–317, 2006

Picavet HS, Vlaeyen JW, Schouten JS: Pain catastrophizing and kinesiophobia: predictors of chronic low back pain. Am J Epidemiol 156:1028–1034, 2002

Pincus T, Burton AK, Vogel S, et al: A systematic review of psychological factors as predictors of chronicity/disability in prospective cohorts of low back pain. Spine 27:E109–E120, 2002

Pinto A, Sollecito TP, DeRossi SS: Burning mouth syndrome: a retrospective analysis of clinical characteristics and treatment outcomes. N Y State Dent J 69:18–24, 2003

Potvin S, Grignon S, Marchand S: Human evidence of a supra-spinal modulating role of dopamine on pain perception. Synapse 63: 390–402, 2009

Prasad S, Galetta S: Trigeminal neuralgia: historical notes and current concepts. Neurologist 15:87–94, 2009

Rahman A, Reed E, Underwood M, et al: Factors affecting self-efficacy and pain intensity in patients with chronic musculoskeletal pain seen in a specialist rheumatology pain clinic. Rheumatology 47:1803–1808, 2008

Reid MC, Papaleontiou M, Ong A, et al: Self-management strategies to reduce pain and improve function among older adults in community settings: a review of the evidence. Pain Med 9:409–424, 2008

Riley J, Eisenberg E, Müller-Schwefe G, et al: Oxycodone: a review of its use in the management of pain. Curr Med Res Opin 24:175–192, 2008

Rojas-Corrales MO, Casas J, Moreno-Brea MR, et al: Antinociceptive effects of tricyclic antidepressants and their noradrenergic metabolites. Eur Neuropsychopharmacol 13:355–363, 2003

Rosenzweig-Lipson S, Beyer CE, Hughes ZA, et al: Differentiating antidepressants of the future: efficacy and safety. Pharmacol Ther 113:134–153, 2007

Rosso AL, Gallagher RM, Luborsky M, et al: Depression and self-rated health are proximal predictors of episodes of sustained change in pain in independently living, community dwelling elders. Pain Med 9:1035–1049, 2008

Rowbotham MC, Goli V, Kunz NR, et al: Venlafaxine extended release in the treatment of painful diabetic neuropathy: a double-blind, placebo-controlled study. Pain 110:697–706, 2004

Saarto T, Wiffen PJ: Antidepressants for neuropathic pain. Cochrane Database of Systematic Reviews 2007, Issue 4. Art. No.: CD005454. DOI: 10.1002/14651858.CD005454.pub2

Sanders SH, Harden RN, Vicente PJ: Evidence-based clinical practice guidelines for interdisciplinary rehabilitation of chronic nonmalignant pain syndrome patients. Pain Pract 5:303–315, 2005

Sandoval JA, Furlan AD, Mailis-Gagnon A: Oral methadone for chronic noncancer pain: a systematic literature review of reasons for administration, prescription patterns, effectiveness, and side effects. Clin J Pain 21:503–512, 2005

Schieir O, Thombs BD, Hudson M, et al: Symptoms of depression predict the trajectory of pain among patients with early inflammatory arthritis: a path analysis approach to assessing change. J Rheumatol 36:231–239, 2009

Schley MT, Wilms P, Toepfner S, et al: Painful and nonpainful phantom and stump sensations in acute traumatic amputees. J Trauma 65:858–864, 2008

Schmidt NB, Santiago HT, Trakowski JH, et al: Pain in patients with pain disorder: relation to symptoms, cognitive characteristics and treatment outcome. Pain Res Manag 7:134–141, 2002

Scudds RJ, McD Robertson J: Empirical evidence of the association between the presence of musculoskeletal pain and physical disability in community-dwelling senior citizens. Pain 75:229–235, 1998

Seidel S, Aigner M, Ossege M, et al: Antipsychotics for acute and chronic pain in adults. Cochrane Database of Systematic Reviews 2008, Issue 4. Art. No.: CD004844. DOI: 10.1002/14651858.CD004844.pub2

Sherman JJ, Turk DC: Nonpharmacologic approaches to the management of myofascial temporomandibular disorders. Curr Pain Headache Rep 5:421–431, 2001

Sherman JJ, Turk DC, Okifuji A: Prevalence and impact of posttraumatic stress disorder-like symptoms on patients with fibromyalgia syndrome. Clin J Pain 16:127–134, 2000

Silberstein SD: Treatment recommendations for migraine. Nat Clin Pract Neurol 4:482–489, 2008

Silberstein SD, Hulihan J, Karim MR, et al: Efficacy and tolerability of topiramate 200 mg/d in the prevention of migraine with/without aura in adults: a randomized, placebo-controlled, double-blind, 12-week pilot study. Clin Ther 28:1002–1011, 2006

Silberstein SD, Loder E, Diamond S, et al: Probable migraine in the United States: results of the American Migraine Prevalence and Prevention (AMPP) study. Cephalalgia 27:220–234, 2007

Simon GE, VonKorff M, Piccinelli M, et al: An international study of the relation between somatic symptoms and depression. N Engl J Med 341:1329–1335, 1999

Skevington SM: Investigating the relationship between pain and discomfort and quality of life, using the WHOQOL. Pain 76:395–406, 1998

Smedstad LM, Vaglum P, Kvien TK, et al: The relationship between self-reported pain and sociodemographic variables, anxiety, and depressive symptoms in rheumatoid arthritis. J Rheumatol 22:514–520, 1995

Solaro C, Messmer UM, Uccelli A, et al: Low-dose gabapentin combined with either lamotrigine or carbamazepine can be useful therapies for trigeminal neuralgia in multiple sclerosis. Eur Neurol 44:45–48, 2000

Stacey BR, Barrett JA, Whalen E, et al: Pregabalin for postherpetic neuralgia: placebo-controlled trial of fixed and flexible dosing regimens on allodynia and time to onset of pain relief. J Pain 9:1006–1017, 2008

Stanos S, Houle TT: Multidisciplinary and interdisciplinary management of chronic pain. Phys Med Rehabil Clin N Am 17:435–450, 2006

Stefan H, Feuerstein TJ: Novel anticonvulsant drugs. Pharmacol Ther 113:165–183, 2007

Stein WM, Ferrell BA: Pain in the nursing home. Clin Geriatr Med 12:601–613, 1996

Stenager EN, Stenager E, Jensen K: Attempted suicide, depression and physical diseases: a one-year follow-up study. Psychother Psychosom 61:65–73, 1994

Stephenson DT, Arneric SP: Neuroimaging of pain: advances and future prospects. J Pain 9:567–579, 2008

Streltzer J, Eliashof BA, Kline AE, et al: Chronic pain disorder following physical injury. Psychosomatics 41:227–234, 2000

Sullivan M, Katon W: Somatization: the path between distress and somatic symptoms. Am Pain Soc J 2:141–149, 1993

Sullivan M, Rodgers WM, Kirsch I: Catastrophizing, depression and expectancies for pain and emotional distress. Pain 91:147–154, 2001

Tack J, Broekaert D, Fischler B, et al: A controlled crossover study of the selective serotonin reuptake inhibitor citalopram in irritable bowel syndrome. Gut 55:1095–1103, 2006

Tanabe M, Takasu K, Takeuchi Y, et al: Pain relief by gabapentin and pregabalin via supraspinal mechanisms after peripheral nerve injury. J Neurosci Res 86:3258–3264, 2008

Tassinari D, Sartori S, Tamburini E, et al: Adverse effects of transdermal opiates treating moderate-severe cancer pain in comparison to long-acting morphine: a meta-analysis and systematic review of the literature. J Palliat Med 11:492–501, 2008

Tassone DM, Boyce E, Guyer J, et al: Pregabalin: a novel gamma-aminobutyric acid analogue in the treatment of neuropathic pain, partial-onset seizures, and anxiety disorders. Clin Ther 29:26–48, 2007

Tavakoli M, Malik RA: Management of painful diabetic neuropathy. Expert Opin Pharmacother 9:2969–2978, 2008

Taylor CP, Angelotti T, Fauman E: Pharmacology and mechanism of action of pregabalin: the calcium channel alpha2-delta subunit as a target for antiepileptic drug discovery. Epilepsy Res 73:137–150, 2007

Todorov AA, Kolchev CB, Todorov AB: Tiagabine and gabapentin for the management of chronic pain. Clin J Pain 21:358–361, 2005

Tofferi JK, Jackson JL, O'Malley PG: Treatment of fibromyalgia with cyclobenzaprine: a meta-analysis. Arthritis Rheum 51:9–13, 2004

Tomlinson DR, Gardiner NJ: Diabetic neuropathies: components of etiology. J Peripher Nerv Syst 13:112–121, 2008

Truini A, Galeotti F, Haanpaa M, et al: Pathophysiology of pain in postherpetic neuralgia: a clinical and neurophysiological study. Pain 140:405–410, 2008

Turk DC, Swanson KS, Tunks ER: Psychological approaches in the treatment of chronic pain patients: when pills, scalpels, and needles are not enough. Can J Psychiatry 53:213–223, 2008

Turner JA, Holtzman S, Mancl L: Mediators, moderators, and predictors of therapeutic change in cognitive-behavioral therapy for chronic pain. Pain 127:197–198, 2007

Tzellos TG, Papazisis G, Amaniti E, et al: Efficacy of pregabalin and gabapentin for neuropathic pain in spinal-cord injury: an evidence-based evaluation of the literature. Eur J Clin Pharmacol 64:851–858, 2008

Ullrich PM: Pain following spinal cord injury. Phys Med Rehabil Clin N Am 18:217–233, 2007

Valet M, Gundel H, Sprenger T, et al: Patients with pain disorder show gray-matter loss in pain-processing structures: a voxel-based morphometric study. Psychosom Med 71:49–56, 2009

Vanotti A, Osio M, Jailland E, et al: Overview on pathophysiology and newer approaches to treatment of peripheral neuropathies. CNS Drugs 21(suppl):3–12, 2007

Van Passel L, Arif H, Hirsch LJ: Topiramate for the treatment of epilepsy and other nervous system disorders. Expert Rev Neurother 6:19–31, 2006

Van Tulder MW, Ostelo R, Vlaeyen JW, et al: Behavioral treatment for chronic low back pain: a systematic review within the framework of the Cochrane Back Review Group. Spine 26:270–281, 2001

Van Wilgen CP, Dijkstra PU, Versteegen GJ, et al: Chronic pain and severe disuse syndrome: long-term outcome of an inpatient multidisciplinary cognitive behavioural programme. J Rehabil Med 41:122–128, 2009

Verbunt JA, Seelen HA, Vlaeyen JW, et al: Disuse and deconditioning in chronic low back pain: concepts and hypotheses on contributing mechanisms. Eur J Pain 7:9–21, 2003

Verdu B, Decosterd I, Buclin T, et al: Antidepressants for the treatment of chronic pain. Drugs 68:2611–2632, 2008

Veves A, Backonja M, Malik RA: Painful diabetic neuropathy: epidemiology, natural history, early diagnosis, and treatment options. Pain Med 9:660–674, 2008

Vinik AI, Tuchman M, Safirstein B, et al: Lamotrigine for treatment of pain associated with diabetic neuropathy: results of two randomized, double-blind, placebo-controlled studies. Pain 128: 169–179, 2007

Volpi A, Gatti A, Pica F, et al: Clinical and psychosocial correlates of post-herpetic neuralgia. J Med Virol 80:1646–1652, 2008

Vorobeychik Y, Chen L, Bush MC, et al: Improved opioid analgesic effect following opioid dose reduction. Pain Med 9:724–727, 2008

Vowles KE, McCracken LM, Eccleston C: Processes of change in treatment for chronic pain: the contributions of pain, acceptance, and catastrophizing. Eur J Pain 11:779–787, 2007

Vowles KE, McCracken LM, Eccleston C: Patient functioning and catastrophizing in chronic pain: the mediating effects of acceptance. Health Psychol 27(suppl):S136–S143, 2008a

Vowles KE, McCracken LM, McLeod C, et al: The Chronic Pain Acceptance Questionnaire: confirmatory factor analysis and identification of patient subgroups. Pain 140:284–291, 2008b

Vuckovic SM, Tomic MA, Stepanovic-Petrovic RM, et al: The effects of alpha2-adrenoceptor agents on anti-hyperalgesic effects of carbamazepine and oxcarbazepine in a rat model of inflammatory pain. Pain 125:10–19, 2006

Wang SJ, Fuh JL, Lu SR, et al: Quality of life differs among headache diagnoses: analysis of SF-36 survey in 901 headache patients. Pain 89:285–292, 2001

Wernicke JF, Pritchett YL, D'Souza DN, et al: A randomized controlled trial of duloxetine in diabetic peripheral neuropathic pain. Neurology 67:1411–1420, 2006

Wiffen PJ, Rees J: Lamotrigine for acute and chronic pain. Cochrane Database of Systematic Reviews 2007, Issue 2. Art. No.: CD006044. DOI: 10.1002/14651858.CD006044.pub2

Williamson GM, Schulz R: Pain, activity restriction and symptoms of depression among community-residing elderly adults. J Gerontol 47:367–372, 1992

Wood PB: Role of central dopamine in pain and analgesia. Expert Rev Neurother 8:781–797, 2008

Wood PB, Schweinhardt P, Jaeger E, et al: Fibromyalgia patients show an abnormal dopamine response to pain. Eur J Neurosci 25: 3576–3582, 2007

Wu CL, Agarwal S, Tella PK, et al: Morphine versus mexiletine for treatment of postamputation pain: a randomized, placebo-controlled, crossover trial. Anesthesiology 109:289–296, 2008

Yucel A, Ozyalcin S, Koknel TG, et al: The effect of venlafaxine on ongoing and experimentally induced pain in neuropathic pain patients: a double blind, placebo controlled study. Eur J Pain 9:407–416, 2005

Ziegler D, Pritchett YL, Wang F, et al: Impact of disease characteristics on the efficacy of duloxetine in diabetic peripheral neuropathic pain. Diabetes Care 30:664–669, 2007

Zin CS, Nissen LM, Smith MT, et al: An update on the pharmacological management of post-herpetic neuralgia and painful diabetic neuropathy. CNS Drugs 22:417–442, 2008

Zochodne DW: Diabetic polyneuropathy: an update. Curr Opin Neurol 21:527–533, 2008

24

Parkinson's Disease and Movement Disorders

Daniel Weintraub, M.D.
Andrew D. Siderowf, M.D., M.S.C.E.
Alexander I. Tröster, Ph.D., A.B.P.P.(CN)
Karen E. Anderson, M.D.

Although Parkinson's disease (PD) is traditionally considered a movement disorder, the high prevalence of psychiatric complications suggests that it is more accurately conceptualized as a neuropsychiatric disease. Affective disorders, cognitive impairment, and psychosis have long been recognized as a part of PD presentation. Other common but less well studied psychiatric disorders evidenced in PD patients include apathy, impulse dyscontrol, disorders of sleep and wakefulness, personality changes, and pathological laughing and crying.

Psychiatric aspects of PD are associated with excess disability, worse quality of life, poorer outcomes, and greater caregiver distress. Yet in spite of the burden and frequent occurrence of these complications, there is incomplete understanding of the epidemiology, phenomenology, risk factors, neuropathophysiology, and optimal treatment strategies for these disorders. Psychiatric aspects are typically multimorbid, and there is great intraindividual and interindividual variability in presentation. Not surprisingly, evidence indicates that psychiatric disorders in PD are underrecognized and undertreated.

The hallmark neuropathophysiological changes that occur in PD plus the association between exposure to dopaminergic medications and certain psychiatric disorders suggest a neurobiological basis for most psychiatric symptoms, but psychological factors are likely involved in the development of affective disorders. Although antidepressants, anxiolytics, antipsychotics, and cognitive-enhancing agents are commonly prescribed for patients with PD, controlled studies demonstrating efficacy and tolerability are lacking. Future research on neuropsychiatric complications in PD should be oriented toward determining modifiable correlates or risk factors and establishing efficacious and effective treatment strategies.

Parkinson's Disease

Motor Symptoms

The features of Parkinson's disease are listed in Table 24–1. The cardinal motor features of PD are resting tremor, cogwheel rigidity, and bradykinesia (slowness or paucity of movement). The typical parkinsonian tremor is a rest tremor that is most prominent when the patient is sitting and relaxed; however, tremor can also be present with postural maneuvers and action. The typical frequency is 3.5–5 Hz. *Rigidity* is defined as resistance to passive movement that occurs in both flexors and extensors throughout the entire range of motion. In PD, rigidity has a cogwheel quality, due to the impression that when an extremity is moved passively, resistance results in stops and starts in a quick repetitive sequence. Bradykinesia, the third cardinal manifestation of PD, is the decreased ability to move rapidly or to alternate rapidly between two different movements. Motor freezing, which is the inability to initiate movements or to continue a movement once it has started, is a particularly problematic type of bradykinesia.

In addition to these cardinal manifestations, masked facies, dysarthria, and gait disturbance are important motor features of PD. Loss of facial expression can create the appearance of apathy and depression, whether or not such affective symptoms are present. The speech of an individual with PD is a "hypokinetic dysarthria," typically monotonal, hypophonic, and muffled. Syllables may be repeated (palilalia), and words and phrases tend to rush together. The characteristic gait of PD is marked by shuffling, stooped posture, and reduced arm swing. Arm and hand tremor may also be accentuated while walking. As the gait disorder progresses, turning may become

TABLE 24–1. Features of Parkinson's disease (PD)

Cardinal manifestations
Tremor
Rigidity
Bradykinesia
Other common motor features
Masked facies
Dysarthria
Stooped posture
Motor features of advancing PD
Postural instability/falls
Motor complications
Dyskinesias
"Wearing off" and "on-off"
Gait freezing
Nonmotor features of PD
Autonomic instability
Loss of sense of smell
Sleep disturbance
Insomnia
Daytime drowsiness
REM behavior disorder
Dementia and cognitive impairment
Mood disturbances
Anxiety
Psychosis
Apathy
Impulse dyscontrol

Note. REM=rapid eye movement.

more difficult. Rather than turning in one smooth movement, a person needs to take multiple steps. This type of turning is referred to as "en bloc turning." Patients may also have difficulty initiating gait (start hesitation) or stopping once started (festination). Postural instability is a late manifestation of PD but is highly disabling. Falling forward (propulsion) and backward (retropulsion) may occur in response to external forces. Spontaneous loss of balance indicates severe balance disturbance.

Motor Complications

Motor complications, including dyskinesias and motor fluctuations, mark the transition from early to moderate or advanced PD and are a significant therapeutic problem. In one early study, dyskinesias had developed in 68% of treated patients after 5 years, and clinically significant motor fluctuations appeared in 50% of the patients over the same time period.

Levodopa-induced dyskinesias are involuntary movements that are usually either choreoathetotic or dystonic in nature; these include facial grimacing, head turning, and ballistic movements of the limbs and trunk. They tend to occur more prominently on the side of the body more affected by parkinsonian symptoms. Peak-dose dyskinesias occur during the time of maximal motor response to levodopa and are primarily choreoathetotic in character. Low-dose dyskinesia, on the other hand, is more likely to be dystonic than is peak-dose dyskinesia. Low-dose dyskinesia occurs either before or after the maximal motor response but most typically occurs when a dose is wearing off. Although generally considered to be the result of chronic therapy with levodopa, the pathophysiological mechanisms underlying drug-induced dyskinesia remain unknown. Changes in receptor sensitivity due to chronic therapy may play a role.

Motor fluctuations are more disabling complications than dyskinesias for most patients. In early PD, patients experience a sustained response to each dose of levodopa. Over time, however, this long-duration response declines, resulting in the so-called "wearing off" phenomenon. Patients with advanced disease may develop sudden changes in magnitude of motor response to a dose of levodopa, referred to as the "on-off" phenomenon. As a result of these wearing off and on-off fluctuations, patients with advanced PD may spend most of the waking day with an unsatisfactory motor response (Fahn 1992).

Differential Diagnosis

Other Disorders Causing Parkinsonian Signs

A range of disorders can cause a syndrome that has clinical features in common with PD. Disorders with parkinsonian features can be classified as degenerative and nondegenerative (Table 24–2). The most difficult differentiation is between idiopathic PD and other degenerative forms of parkinsonism, particularly early in the disease course. In particular, multiple-systems atrophy and progressive supranuclear palsy may be difficult to differentiate from PD. Clinically, multiple-systems atrophy is characterized by early and severe autonomic disturbance, and progressive supranuclear palsy by early falls and oculomotor impairment. However, these features may not be obvious at the time of initial diagnosis.

TABLE 24–2. Differential diagnosis of Parkinson's disease

Neurodegenerative diseases with parkinsonian features
Parkinson's disease
Progressive supranuclear palsy
Multiple-systems atrophy
Shy-Drager syndrome
Striatonigral degeneration
Olivo-pontocerebellar atrophy
Alzheimer's disease
Diffuse Lewy body disease
Corticobasal degeneration
Other causes of parkinsonism or parkinsonian signs
Drug-induced parkinsonism
Neuroleptics, valproate, calcium channel blockers
Toxin-induced parkinsonism
MPTP—selective complex I poison
Pesticides
Heavy metals
Manganese (does not cause typical parkinsonism)
Vascular parkinsonism
Hydrocephalus
Posttraumatic parkinsonism

Note. MPTP=1-methyl-4-phenyl-1,2,3,6-tetrahydropyridine.

Diagnostic Value of Clinical Features

Hoehn and Yahr (1967) found that the most common initial symptom in their patients with "primary parkinsonism" was tremor, occurring in 70.5% of cases. The next most common initial symptom was gait disturbance, followed by slowness, stiffness, muscle pain, and loss of dexterity. Hughes et al. (1992) studied the relative diagnostic value of different parkinsonian signs in reference to pathologically confirmed diagnosis. The most sensitive clinical features were the presence of rest tremor, definite asymmetry of clinical signs, and a markedly positive response to levodopa. Using the conventional diagnostic criteria of presence of two of the three cardinal features of disease (tremor, rigidity, and bradykinesia), very high sensitivity (99%) could be achieved. However, the specificity of this definition for pathologically confirmed PD was quite low.

Research Diagnostic Criteria

Ward and Gibb (1990) proposed the following criteria for PD, largely to minimize the false-positive rate: 1) progressive disorder; 2) presence of at least two of the three cardinal signs of PD; 3) presence of at least two of the following: markedly positive response to levodopa, asymmetric signs, asymmetry at onset, and initial symptom of tremor; 4) absence of clinical characteristics of alternative diagnoses; and 5) absence of etiology known to cause similar features. Larsen et al. (1994) proposed a series of clinical diagnostic criteria at different levels of confidence: definite clinical idiopathic PD, probable clinical idiopathic PD, and possible clinical idiopathic PD. Both the U.K. Brain Bank consortium (Hughes et al. 1993) and Koller (1992) have published inclusion and exclusion criteria for the diagnosis of PD. The consistent themes in all of these schemata are that 1) high sensitivity can be achieved relatively easily; 2) good specificity can also be achieved, but not to the same extent as sensitivity; and 3) trade-offs between sensitivity and specificity are inevitable.

Epidemiology

Frequency

A large number of epidemiological studies measuring the prevalence and incidence of PD have been performed. One study found that the prevalence of "parkinsonian signs" in a community of older people living in Boston, Massachusetts, was 14.9% for people ages 65–74 years, 29.5% for people ages 75–84, and 52.4% for individuals ages 85 and older. By contrast, most studies examining the prevalence of idiopathic PD rather than parkinsonian signs find a lower prevalence. Population-based, door-to-door studies are generally considered the most rigorous measure of prevalence. In such studies, done around the world, the prevalence of PD has ranged from 44 per 100,000 people ages 50 and older in Chinese cities to over 300 per 100,000 persons of all ages in Bombay, India. The prevalence of PD in European populations has been estimated at about 250 per 100,000.

The incidence of PD is harder to establish because case ascertainment methods, such as reviews of hospital records, tend to underestimate the true number of cases. Mayeux et al. (1995) developed a registry of patients with PD, drawing on a diverse group of sources, including hospital and administrative billing records, private practitioner office records, and rosters from senior centers in the geographic area of upper Manhattan, New York. Using this registry, Mayeux and colleagues found an overall incidence of PD of 13 new cases per 100,000 person-years. Other published estimates of the incidence of PD range from 5 to 20 new cases per 100,000 person-years.

Demographic Risk Factors

Increasing age is consistently the strongest risk factor for PD in epidemiological studies. The prevalence of PD in individuals under age 40 is <5 per 100,000; the prevalence in individuals over age 70 is ~700 per 100,000 persons.

After age adjustment, most studies show a modestly increased risk for men compared to women of ~1.2–1.5 to 1. Race also appears to be a risk factor for PD, although this is controversial. The prevalence of PD is reported to be highest in Europe and North America and lowest in Asia and Africa. Several studies have found a slight excess of cases among whites compared to African Americans. However, one community-based study of a biracial county in Mississippi, using a less stringent definition of PD, found similar prevalence rates for blacks and whites.

Etiology: Genetic and Environmental Factors

The etiology of PD remains largely unknown. Investigations of genetic and environmental risk factors have yielded some clues, which suggest that PD may have more than one unifying cause.

Genetic Factors

The revolution in genetics made a substantial impact on knowledge about PD. Since the identification of the first heritable form of parkinsonism in 1997, an expanding list of genes associated with PD, as either heritable traits or genetic risk factors, has been identified. A study involving multiple generations of individuals in Iceland showed that individuals with PD were ~2.5–3 times more likely to be related to another patient with PD than were unaffected individuals. Although surveys of patients with PD show that only about 10% of cases have a family history, understanding the role that various genetic factors play in familial PD may have broader implications for all patients with PD.

At least two genes associated with autosomal dominant PD have been identified. The α-synuclein gene (*SNCA*) was the first gene to be unequivocally linked to PD (Polymeropoulos et al. 1997). Familial PD may be caused by mutations to this gene or by increased copies of a normal *SNCA* gene. Subsequent studies have shown that mutations in *SNCA* are a rare cause of PD. The discovery of the role of *SNCA* has led to important neuropathological studies regarding the role of *SNCA* in sporadic PD and the development of transgenic animal models. The other important autosomal dominant gene associated with PD is the leucine-rich repeat kinase 2 gene (*LRRK2*). This gene is recognized as the most common gene causing autosomal dominant PD, and it may be found in up to 25% of familial cases of PD in some populations, particularly Ashkenazi Jews and North African Arabs.

Several autosomal recessive genetic mutations have been linked to PD. The most common is *parkin*, which causes autosomal recessive juvenile-onset parkinsonism. *Parkin*-related parkinsonism closely resembles sporadic PD, with the exceptions that the age at onset is substantially younger than normal and Lewy bodies have not been found in the majority of cases of *parkin*-related parkinsonism that have come to autopsy. Other genes associated with autosomal recessive parkinsonism include the phosphatase and tensin homolog (PTEN)–induced kinase 1 gene (*PINK1*) and the *DJ-1* gene (also known as *PARK7*).

Risk-factor genes represent a third category of genetic factors related to PD. For example, heterozygous carriers of *parkin* mutations may be at higher risk for typical late-onset PD. Carriers of mutations in the glucocerebrosidase gene (*GBA*) have up to a fivefold higher risk of PD than noncarriers. Genome-wide association studies have identified several other risk-factor genes for PD, including the Rep1 polymorphism in the promoter region for *SNCA* and polymorphisms in the microtubule-associated protein tau gene.

Environmental Factors

The recognition that exposure to the neurotoxin 1-methyl-4-phenyl-1,2,3,6-tetrahydropyridine (MPTP) can cause a syndrome clinically and pathologically similar to idiopathic PD (Langston et al. 1983) continues to foster interest in other environmental risk factors for PD. A number of such risk factors, including heavy metals, well water, pesticides, and rural versus urban residence, have been evaluated. In most cases, the increased risk from these exposures is modest (Tanner and Goldman 1996). The evidence may be strongest in the case of pesticide exposure and most controversial for exposure to heavy metals such as manganese.

Being a nonsmoker has shown the most consistent relationship to PD. In an exhaustive review of the literature, Morens et al. (1995) found that 34 of 35 published studies found an inverse relationship between smoking and PD. The risk-odds ratio for smoking in these studies tended to cluster around 0.5 (i.e., smokers had about half the risk of nonsmokers). In addition, numerous studies have found the risk reduction to be greater for current smokers than for former smokers, suggesting a biological gradient (dose-response) effect. Possible explanations for the observed association include a neuroprotective effect of nicotine or another constituent of cigarette smoke, and a decreased appetite for cigarettes among individuals at risk for PD because of a third, unknown factor.

Caffeine consumption has been associated with a lower risk of PD. In one study, this effect was stronger in men than women. These studies provide a rationale for a possible role of caffeine, as well as the adenosine neurotransmitter system (the site of action of caffeine), in the pathogenesis of PD.

TABLE 24–3. Treatments for motor aspects of Parkinson's disease

Levodopa
Dopamine agonists
Pramipexole
Ropinirole
MAO-B inhibitors
Rasagiline
Selegiline
Catechol O-methyltransferase inhibitors
Entacapone
Tolcapone
Other
Anticholinergics
Amantadine
Deep brain stimulation

Note. MAO-B=monoamine oxidase type B.

Treatment of Motor Aspects

A treatment algorithm for PD is discussed in detail below.

Choice of Initial Therapy

Replacement of dopamine is the cornerstone of symptomatic treatment for PD. This goal can be accomplished in a number of ways (Table 24–3), including providing dopamine in the form of its immediate chemical precursor, levodopa; administering synthetic dopamine agonists (DAs); and giving agents that prevent the catabolism of levodopa or dopamine, such as monoamine oxidase type B (MAO-B) inhibitors and inhibitors of catechol O-methyltransferase (COMT). Dopaminergic treatment is useful throughout the disease course in PD. Surgical treatments, particularly deep brain stimulation (DBS), are generally reserved for patients with advanced PD and disabling motor complications. In addition, nonpharmacological approaches, such as aerobic exercise, are important adjuncts to medications.

Levodopa has been the mainstay of PD treatment since the initial demonstrations of its effectiveness by Cotzias et al. (1969). Levodopa is almost always given with a peripheral dopa decarboxylase inhibitor (e.g., carbidopa, benserazide). Available DAs include pramipexole and ropinirole, which are both effective antiparkinsonian agents. These agents have longer half-lives than levodopa but are somewhat less potent. MAO-B inhibitors, including selegiline and rasagiline, have modest antiparkinsonian effects but have favorable side-effect profiles, and some data suggest that earlier initiation of this class of medication may lead to better outcomes at 12–18 months after treatment initiation. The American Academy of Neurology has issued practice guidelines stating that MAO-B inhibitors, DAs, and levodopa are all appropriate treatments for early PD (Miyasaki et al. 2002) The debate over which medication to use as initial early therapy in patients with more substantial disability focuses on the choice between levodopa (carbidopa/levodopa preparations in the United States) or a DA. Two studies have shown that patients treated with DAs have a lower risk of developing motor complications such as dyskinesias; however, motor performance in patients initially treated with levodopa is somewhat better. In addition, there is a lower risk of side effects, particularly somnolence, in patients treated with levodopa.

Clinical judgment is required to determine which patients are more appropriate for initial therapy with a DA and which should be treated with levodopa. Younger patients and those with milder symptoms should probably be treated with a DA. However, older patients or those with more severe symptoms at presentation should probably be treated with levodopa as initial therapy. Furthermore, the increased frequency of side effects may limit the use of DAs in susceptible individuals.

Treatment of Advanced Parkinson's Disease

Over time, most patients with PD require higher dosages of medication or treatment with combinations of medications to maintain adequate motor function and to avoid disabling dyskinesias. Several options are available to treat motor complications. MAO-B inhibitors, DAs, and COMT inhibitors have all been shown to reduce motor fluctuations in patients treated with levodopa. Many patients also require small, frequent dosages of levodopa to maintain an adequate drug effect without severe dyskinesias. Medical treatment of patients with advanced PD and complex motor complications is challenging and requires frequent rebalancing of dopaminergic medications.

Surgical Therapy for Advanced Parkinson's Disease

Surgical treatment with DBS has been a major step forward in the management of advancing PD with motor complications. DBS has largely replaced lesioning procedures, such as pallidotomy, because of lower morbidity and adjustability of stimulator settings. Stimulators are implanted in either the subthalamic nucleus (STN) or the globus pallidus pars interna (GPi). DBS leads to substantial relief from motor fluctuations and dyskinesia over a sustained period of time (Krack et al. 2003). Stimulation of the STN, but not the GPi, is also associated with reduction in need for dopaminergic medications. Recent controlled investigations have confirmed the results of early case series showing substantial benefit of DBS on motor symptoms of PD and health-related quality of life. Whether the GPi or

STN is a better anatomical target remains an important unanswered question.

Other surgical approaches to PD have not been successful. Two randomized trials of fetal cell transplantation have been performed, using a placebo-controlled sham-surgery approach. In both studies, no consistent benefit of fetal cell implantation was observed, and complications, including severe involuntary movements, were observed in a substantial proportion of treated patients.

Cognitive Impairment and Dementia in Parkinson's Disease

Intellect and senses were said by Parkinson to be preserved in the disease later to bear his name. PD long remained considered a pure movement disorder, and its neurobehavioral manifestations were not widely appreciated until the late twentieth century. Even after neuropsychological studies had moved away from describing effects of postencephalitic and vascular parkinsonism in the 1940s–1960s and the consequences of surgical and pharmacological treatment of PD in the 1950s–1970s, cognitive impairment was thought not to emerge until late in the disease course. Research in the 1980s and 1990s focused on characterization of Parkinson's disease with dementia (PDD) and its differentiation from other dementias. Milder (nondementia) cognitive impairments in PD were appreciated to occur in a small proportion of patients, but only since the early 2000s has there been recognition that up to one-third of patients may already have subtle cognitive changes at the time of diagnosis of PD (Foltynie et al. 2004; Muslimovic et al. 2005). This appreciation of early cognitive changes in a sizable minority of patients, coupled with the expansion of the concept of mild cognitive impairment (MCI) beyond its amnestic prototype to include nonmemory impairments, brought with it recent enthusiasm to import the concept of MCI to better understand, diagnose, and treat PD patients with cognition intermediate between normal and dementia states (Caviness et al. 2007; Janvin et al. 2006). The application of MCI to PD faces challenges (Tröster 2008), and empirical data to answer the question of whether PD-MCI (or specific subtypes) represents a transition state from normal to dementia are lacking. Similarly, little attention has been devoted to the prodrome of dementia with Lewy bodies (DLB), and it is unclear whether the prodromes of PDD and DLB are differentiable. Nonetheless, the process of establishing a diagnosis of MCI may provide a clinically useful heuristic in PD. Before detailing research and diagnosis of MCI in PD, we outline the qualitative features of cognitive impairment in PD without dementia, bearing in mind that studies of these impairments have usually distinguished only between groups of patients with and without dementia.

Characteristics of Nondementia Cognitive Impairment

In this section, we provide a brief summary of the neuropsychological characterization of cognitive impairment in PD. Readers interested in greater detail about relevant studies are referred to Tröster et al. (2008). Studies of PD most reliably reveal compromises in attention/working memory, executive function, processing speed, recall, and visuospatial processes. Patients with PD perform normally on simple attention tests such as span tasks, but they perform poorly on tasks demanding efficient manipulation of information within working memory (a limited-capacity, multicomponent system allowing temporary, online manipulation and storage of information to guide and control action) and set shifting (e.g., digit ordering, Stroop task). Executive functions, including planning, conceptualization, and cognitive flexibility of thought, are often compromised early in patients with PD, as revealed by studies using tower and card sorting tasks. Studies using gambling tasks to evaluate decision making, judgment, and impulsivity have yielded inconsistent findings, perhaps because impairments may be observable only when patients are on dopaminergic medications.

Motor-speech abnormalities (e.g., dysarthria) are not accompanied by aphasia, but subtle alterations in performance on language tasks may occur secondary to diminished attention, working memory, or inefficient strategy use. Visual confrontation naming is preserved in PD, but it becomes more compromised in patients with obvious cognitive impairment. Performance on verbal fluency requiring oral generation of words from certain categories within time limits is typically intact in patients without dementia. Two types of verbal fluency tasks, however, seem especially sensitive to PD: alternating word fluency tasks that require retrieval of consecutive words from alternate categories and verb fluency tasks that require naming of actions. Visuospatial deficits are quite common in PD and occur independently of motor deficits. Thus, facial and line matching tasks reveal impairments in PD.

Impairments in episodic memory may be evident in the earliest stages of PD and at diagnosis (Foltynie et al. 2004; Muslimovic et al. 2005). Learning of new information is slowed in PD. Recognition recall, unlike free recall, is less impaired, but not necessarily intact. The relative preservation of recognition may be related to retrieval deficits. Alternatively, because patients can also have encoding difficulties, encoding may be adequate to support recognition but too shallow to support good recall. Remote memory is typically preserved.

Screening for Cognitive Impairment

The advantages of screening examinations include brevity, simplicity of administration and scoring, patient acceptability, and limited expense. Such screening can be helpful in deciding whether a patient might require full neuropsychological evaluation. Possible disadvantages include the limited information obtained, the use of cutoff scores that may not be adequately corrected for demographics and base rates, and the limited sensitivity and specificity for use across a broad range of disorders. In an American Academy of Neurology practice parameter (Miyasaki et al. 2006), two instruments have been recommended for screening for dementia in PD: the Mini-Mental State Examination (MMSE; Folstein et al. 1975) and the revised Cambridge Cognitive Examination (CAMCOG-R; Roth et al. 1999). As discussed in the following paragraphs, research since publication of that practice parameter, however, suggests that better alternatives are probably available.

The MMSE deemphasizes working memory and executive functions and consequently might lack sensitivity to cognitive changes associated with subcortical-frontal dysfunction. This suspicion was confirmed by a study (Janvin et al. 2003) comparing PD patients with and without MCI (defined by a neuropsychological test battery). The mean MMSE score of the mildly impaired group was only 1.5 points lower than that of the intact group and was in the normal range (mean 28.0, SD 2.1). Similarly, several studies have shown MMSE scores to be higher and less sensitive to MCI than the Montreal Cognitive Assessment (MoCA) scores (Mamikonyan et al. 2009). Nonetheless, the MMSE probably has adequate sensitivity and specificity in detecting impairment among patients with unequivocal dementia and PD. Using DSM-IV dementia criteria (American Psychiatric Association 1994) as the "gold standard," a study of 126 patients with PD found an MMSE cutoff of 23(dementia)/24(no dementia) to have 98% sensitivity and 77% specificity. Annual rate of change in the MMSE is ~1 point for persons with PD without dementia, but ~2–2.5 points for those with dementia.

On the CAMCOG, a cutoff score of 80 points and below to identify dementia in PD had 95% sensitivity and 94% specificity (Hobson and Meara 1999). Cognitively intact patients with PD (MMSE>25) demonstrate an average annual rate of change of ~4 points on the revised version of the instrument (CAMCOG-R). Another commonly used cognitive screening instrument, the Dementia Rating Scale (DRS; Mattis 1973), has been shown to differentiate Lewy body dementias from Alzheimer's disease (AD) and to have 93% sensitivity and 91% specificity in detecting dementia in patients with PD (Llebaria et al. 2008).

Given concerns about assessing patients with PD using cognitive screening examinations designed primarily for use in AD, several groups have developed screening tests emphasizing "frontal" functions or PD cognitive deficits. The Mini-Mental Parkinson (MMP; Mahieux et al. 1995), Frontal/Subcortical Assessment Battery (FSAB; Rothlind and Brandt 1993), Frontal Assessment Battery (FAB; Dubois et al. 2000), Scales for Outcomes of Parkinson's Disease—Cognition (SCOPA-COG; Marinus et al. 2003), Parkinson Neuropsychometric Dementia Assessment (PANDA; Kalbe et al. 2008), and Parkinson's Disease-Cognitive Rating Scale (PD-CRS; Pagonabarraga et al. 2008) show promise as relatively brief, valid screening instruments in PD, but they remain to be validated in independent samples of patients with PD, PD-MCI, and PDD.

Mild Cognitive Impairment

Diagnosis

A flowchart suggesting an algorithm for diagnosing and subtyping MCI is presented in Figure 24–1. Suspicion of MCI is raised when the patient or informants complain of cognitive decline. History taking and a mental status examination (and possibly neuropsychological evaluation if mental status examination and screening test results are ambiguous) are used to determine 1) whether the patient's cognition is normal or abnormal for age and 2) whether the cognitive changes have a significant functional impact. If functioning is relatively normal (which precludes a diagnosis of dementia per DSM criteria or the more recent criteria for PDD) but cognition is abnormal, a provisional diagnosis of MCI can be made. MCI is then subtyped on the basis of 1) whether impairments involve memory and 2) whether impairments are evident in one or more domains of cognition. Although neuropsychological tests are not required to diagnose or subtype MCI because it is a clinical diagnosis, in practice this is commonly done. Particularly because oft-used screening instruments, such as the MMSE, are insensitive to mild cognitive deficits in patients with PD, neuropsychological evaluation or an expanded screening instrument will likely be needed to confirm and subtype MCI in PD.

Mild Cognitive Impairment Subtypes and Risk of Dementia

Janvin et al. (2006) addressed how MCI subtype might be related to subsequent dementia, but unfortunately they used a very limited cognitive assessment (possibly affecting accuracy of MCI identification). In their community study of 72 PD subjects without dementia, 38 were retrospectively diagnosed with MCI (6 with amnestic MCI; 17 with nonamnestic MCI, single domain; and 15 with multiple-domain MCI, unspecified). Fifty-nine patients (82%) completed 4-year follow-up; whereas only 20% of the PD subjects without dementia per DSM-III-R criteria (American Psychiatric Association 1987) completed follow-up, 62% of those with PD-MCI did. Single-domain nonamnestic MCI and multiple-domain MCI were associated with later development of dementia, but amnestic

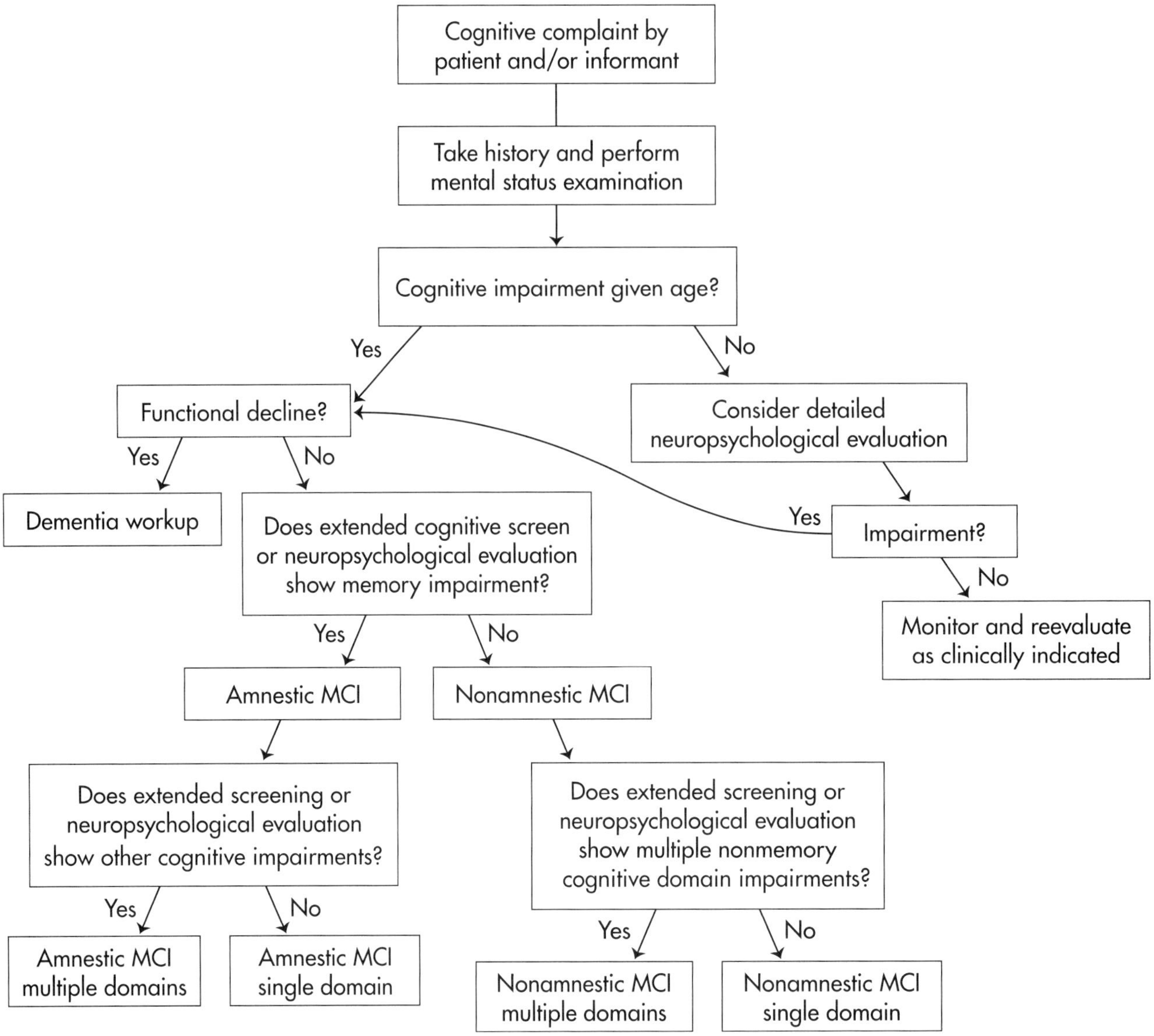

FIGURE 24–1. Diagnostic decision tree for cognitive impairment in Parkinson's disease.

MCI=mild cognitive impairment.

MCI was not. These findings are consistent with the observation that 19% of 196 early, drug-naive PD patients had MCI, and among those, two-thirds had nonamnestic MCI (Aarsland et al. 2009).

The suggestion from the PD-MCI study that non-memory-related deficits may be harbingers of dementia (Janvin et al. 2006) is supported by studies that preceded the MCI approach and instead used an empirical approach to identifying cognitive tests and functions that best predicted subsequent dementia (Jacobs et al. 1995; Janvin et al. 2005; Mahieux 1998; Piccirilli et al. 1989; Reid et al. 1996; Woods and Tröster 2003). The typical design of these studies involves the prospective study of patients who receive neuropsychological evaluations at regular intervals. A consistent finding emerging from such studies is that tests placing a premium on executive functions (and to a lesser extent on memory) are the best predictors of PDD. Thus, tasks and tests associated with subsequent development of PDD include Lurian tasks, nonverbal reasoning, choice reaction time, design memory, digit span backwards, perseverative errors on a card sorting task, immediate word list recall, word list recognition discriminability, category (semantic) and/or letter (phonemic or lexical) verbal fluency, identification of similarities and differences between words and designs, and the interference portion of the Stroop task.

TABLE 24–4. Neuropsychological, disease, and demographic risk factors for dementia in Parkinson's disease (PD)

Neuropsychological and neuropsychiatric factors	Disease factors	Demographic factors
Susceptibility to hallucinations with levodopa or dopamine agonist treatment	Later age at PD onset	Family history of dementia (Alzheimer's disease or PDD)
Poor executive function	Longer disease duration	Advanced age
Poor attention and/or working memory	Postural instability and gait disturbance	Lower educational attainment
Poor episodic memory	Greater disease severity	Lower socioeconomic status
Visuoperceptual deficit		
Depression		
REM sleep behavior disorder		

Note. PDD=Parkinson's disease with dementia; REM=rapid eye movement.

Treatment

Extensive open-label and limited controlled research suggests that treatment of PDD with cholinesterase inhibitors and glutamatergic agents has beneficial effect (Emre 2007), but given the relatively recent concept of MCI in PD, studies have not investigated the use of these agents in PD with MCI. Both uncontrolled and controlled research studies suggest that cognitive rehabilitation treatments may improve executive dysfunction in PD (Sammer et al. 2006; Sinforiani et al. 2004).

Parkinson's Disease With Dementia

Debate continues about whether PDD and DLB are the same or different disorders. The recently proposed convention of referring to PDD and DLB as Lewy body dementias (and to PD, PDD, and DLB as Lewy body disorders) (Lippa et al. 2007) recognizes that the two dementias share pathobiological features but that from a clinical standpoint, the distinction between PDD and DLB remains viable and desirable. This chapter focuses on PDD (DLB is discussed more thoroughly in Chapter 21, "Psychosis").

Prevalence and Incidence

A review of point prevalence rates (Aarsland et al. 2005) found that among the methodologically soundest studies, ~32% of PD patients have dementia, 3%–4% of dementia cases are attributable to PDD, and PDD prevalence is ~0.5% among persons ages 65 and older. The investigators reported a cumulative PDD prevalence rate of 28% after 5 years of follow-up in patients who were followed from initial PD diagnosis; a community-based study found that ~10% had developed dementia within a mean 3.5-year follow-up period after diagnosis; and another long-term community-based study reported a cumulative prevalence rate for PDD of 78% (Aarsland et al. 2003). A study following patients with PD until death (and in whom autopsy was performed) found that 83% of the patients developed dementia (Galvin et al. 2006). Incidence of PDD varies by age, ranging from 3% among patients younger than age 60 to 15% among PD patients older than age 80. Annual incidence figures indicate that ~10% of PD patients per year will develop dementia. A variety of neuropsychological, disease-related, and demographic factors have been identified as increasing the risk for dementia in PD (Table 24–4).

Pathobiology and Neuroimaging Correlates of Cognitive Dysfunction and Dementia

PD involves the loss of pigmented cells from the substantia nigra, and it is estimated that 70%–80% of this system's neurons have been lost when PD motor symptoms emerge, meaning the disease has a considerable prodrome. The neuropathology of this prodrome, as well as the pathological correlates of the clinical progression of PD, occurs in stages described and critically reevaluated by Braak and colleagues (Braak and Del Tredici 2008; Braak et al. 2003). This six-stage model is based on the distribution and severity of α-synuclein-reactive Lewy neuronal inclusions (Lewy bodies and neurites), thought to be related in part to protein misfolding. The model describes pathology progressing from medulla and pontine tegmentum in Stages I and II; to midbrain (including the substantia nigra), prosencephalon, and mesocortex in Stages III and IV; and to neocortex in Stages V and VI. Individuals with clinical PD at autopsy usually have pathology in Stages IV–VI, and cognitive changes, even when assessed with the relatively insensitive MMSE, can be seen as early as Stage III and progress with the more severe pathology of Stages IV–VI.

Dopamine depletion in the striatum is more profound in the putamen than in the caudate. Cell loss and pathology in PD are also evident in the locus coeruleus (noradrenergic), the dorsal raphe nuclei (serotonergic), the nucleus basalis of Meynert (cholinergic), and the dorsal vagal nucleus. Indeed, these nondopaminergic nuclei are already affected by Stage II in the model by Braak and colleagues, lending neuroanatomical plausibility to the notion of early (prodromal) cognitive and behavioral changes in PD. Dysfunction of these nondopaminergic neurotransmitter systems has been linked to cognitive (especially executive) and affective changes in PD. As neocortical pathology increases, the range and severity of cognitive deficits also increase, and the severity of dementia has been associated with cortical Lewy body burden (Hurtig et al. 2000). Furthermore, prefrontal and parietal metabolic abnormalities (consistent with the known executive and visuospatial deficits in PD) increase as patients with PD progress from intact cognition through single- and multiple-domain MCI (Huang et al. 2008).

Diagnosis

DSM criteria for dementia have been criticized regarding their use with patients with PDD and DLB. Concerns include the fact that although memory impairment is required for the diagnosis, memory impairment may be absent or mild in the earliest stages of PDD and DLB. The diagnostic requirement that cognitive impairment underlies the social and occupational functional declines is difficult to ascertain given that functional limitations may be associated with motor impairments and, presumably, with the psychotic features often observed in DLB, but this requirement has been retained in the PDD criteria.

One helpful pointer in determining the etiology of the functional impairment is the observation that limitations in physical activities of daily living (ADLs) are more strongly associated with motor symptoms, whereas impairments in instrumental ADLs (i.e., those allowing a person to remain independent in the community) and capacity to consent to medical treatment are strongly associated with executive dysfunction. Separate diagnostic criteria have been proposed for PDD (Table 24–5) and DLB (Table 24–6). Though arbitrary, the distinction in the temporal sequence of onset of dementia and motor symptoms in PDD and DLB has been maintained. Specifically, in PDD the cognitive impairment lags onset of motor signs by more than 1 year; by contrast, in DLB the dementia precedes the motor signs or occurs within 1 year of their onset. Of importance is that alternative causes of dementia (especially depression and vascular disease) be excluded when dementia appears early in the course of PD.

Neurobehavioral Features

In general, the cognitive impairments in PDD represent an exacerbation of those features described for PD. However, as cognitive impairment progresses in PD, recognition becomes more affected and impairments in remote memory may emerge. In addition, impairments in naming and verbal fluency become obvious, even if less pronounced than in AD. The neurobehavioral features of PDD and DLB are similar (Tröster 2008), although DLB on occasion has been shown to involve greater compromise of attention (especially visual) and executive function than PDD. The neurobehavioral profile of Lewy body dementias, however, is readily distinguished from that of AD, because Lewy body dementias more often involve a subcortical impairment profile and AD typically shows a cortical impairment profile (Table 24–7). Whereas Lewy body dementias manifest more severe attention, executive, and visuospatial impairments than AD, AD shows greater compromise of memory, particularly on recognition testing. PDD is more likely than AD to be accompanied by psychosis, depression, and bradyphrenia.

Treatment

Given the role of cholinergic abnormalities in PDD cognitive deficits, cholinesterase inhibitors might be expected to have a positive effect on these deficits. Relatively few studies have been undertaken, and rivastigmine is currently the only approved drug for dementia in PD, on the basis of the results of a large placebo-controlled study (Emre et al. 2004). That drug has been shown to lead to modest improvements in attention and executive function and to stabilization of ADLs (Emre et al. 2007b). Although use of this drug has been associated with nausea, vomiting, and exacerbation of tremor, the tremor exacerbation may be transient. Fewer and smaller trials have supported the use of donepezil, and modest cognitive and behavioral improvements are sometimes accompanied by gastrointestinal side effects that are unacceptable to patients. Galantamine and memantine have not been subjected to adequate trials in PDD. Before initiation of cholinesterase inhibitors, however, a determination needs to be made regarding the likely cause of the cognitive impairment (Figure 24–2). Medical and psychiatric causes or contributors to cognitive impairment should be documented and treated, and iatrogenic causes, including drug effects, minimized or eliminated. Ancillary services, such as occupational and speech therapy and visits from a social worker, should be made available to the patient and care providers.

Neuropsychiatry of Parkinson's Disease

Depression

Epidemiology

Prevalence estimates for depression in PD (dPD) are typically between 20% and 40% but range from 5% to 75% due to dif-

TABLE 24–5. Clinical diagnostic criteria for Parkinson's disease with dementia (PDD)

Core features (both required for probable or possible PDD)

1. Diagnosis of Parkinson's disease per U.K. Parkinson's Disease Brain Bank (Queen Square Brain Bank) criteria
2. Dementia of insidious onset and slow progression in the presence of PD, defined by:
   a. Impairment of more than one domain of cognition
   b. Impairment representing a decline from premorbid functioning
   c. Impairment in day-to-day functioning not ascribable to motor or autonomic dysfunction

Associated features (typical cognitive profile as outlined below in at least two of the four domains and at least one of the behavioral symptoms required for diagnosis of probable PDD; atypical cognitive profile in one or more domains allows for diagnosis of possible PDD, in which behavioral disturbance may or may not be present)

1. Cognition
   a. Impaired attention, which may fluctuate within or across days
   b. Impaired executive functions (e.g., planning, conceptualization, initiation, rule finding, set maintenance or shifting, bradyphrenia)
   c. Preserved language, but word-finding and complex sentence comprehension deficits may be present
   d. Impaired memory, usually with benefit from cuing and better recognition than recall
2. Behavior
   a. Apathy
   b. Changes in mood and personality, including features of depression and anxiety
   c. Delusions—commonly of the paranoid type
   d. Hallucinations—usually visual, complex, and well formed
   e. Excessive daytime sleepiness/somnolence

Features making the diagnosis of PDD uncertain (none of these features can be present when diagnosing probable PDD; one or both of these features can be present when diagnosing possible PDD)

1. Another abnormality capable of impairing cognition but judged not to be the cause of the dementia (e.g., vascular disease on neuroimaging)
2. Unknown time interval between onset of motor and cognitive symptoms

Features suggesting another condition as causing the mental impairment (if present, PDD cannot be diagnosed)

1. Cognitive and behavioral abnormality occurring solely in the context of other conditions, such as confusional state due to systemic disease or intoxication, or major depressive disorder
2. Features consistent with probable vascular dementia per NINDS-AIREN criteria

Note. NINDS-AIREN=National Institute of Neurological Disorders and Stroke and Association Internationale pour la Recherché et l'Enseignement en Neurosciences; PD=Parkinson's disease.
Source. Emre et al. 2007a; Tröster 2008.

ferences in study populations, definitions of depression, and criteria for symptom attribution. Recent studies using community samples and formal diagnostic criteria have reported that major depression may occur in 5%–10% of patients, with an additional 10%–30% experiencing nonmajor forms of depression (e.g., minor or subsyndromal depression). Although dPD is common, little research has been done into the prevalence of bipolar disorder in PD.

The presence of dPD is associated with excess disability, worse quality of life, increased caregiver distress, and more rapid progression of motor impairment and disability (Starkstein et al. 1992a). It may also be a risk factor for or a correlate of cognitive impairment or dementia (Marder et al. 1995). Additional discussion of dPD can be found in Chapter 19, "Mood Disorders."

TABLE 24–6. Revised clinical diagnostic criteria for dementia with Lewy bodies (DLB)

Central feature: Progressive cognitive decline that interferes with social and occupational function

Core features (any 2=probable DLB; any 1=possible DLB)

1. Fluctuating cognition
2. Recurrent visual hallucinations
3. Spontaneous motor parkinsonism

Suggestive features (1 or more + a core feature=probable DLB; any 1 alone=possible DLB)

1. REM sleep behavior disorder
2. Severe neuroleptic sensitivity
3. Decreased tracer uptake in striatum on SPECT dopamine transporter imaging or on MIBG myocardial scintigraphy

Supportive features (common but lacking diagnostic specificity)

1. Repeated falls and syncope
2. Transient, unexplained loss of consciousness
3. Systematized delusions
4. Hallucinations in other modalities
5. Relative preservation of medial temporal lobe on CT or MRI scan
6. Decreased tracer uptake on SPECT or PET imaging in occipital regions
7. Prominent slow waves on EEG with temporal lobe transient sharp waves

Note. CT=computed tomography; EEG=electroencephalography; MIBG=metaiodobenzylguanidine; MRI=magnetic resonance imaging; PET=positron emission tomography; REM=rapid eye movement; SPECT=single-photon emission computed tomography.
Source. McKeith et al. 2005; Tröster 2008.

Correlates and Risk Factors

Some studies have found that dPD is associated with female sex, a personal history of depression, early-onset PD (i.e., before age 55), and "atypical" parkinsonism (e.g., prominent akinesia and rigidity, extensive vascular disease). Regarding psychiatric symptoms, correlates of dPD include worse cognition, psychosis, anxiety, apathy, fatigue, and insomnia. Most patients with dPD also meet criteria for an anxiety disorder, and PD patients with anxiety disorder often meet criteria for depression (Menza et al. 1993). Although apathy is a distinct psychiatric syndrome, extensive overlap exists between depression and apathy in PD (Starkstein et al. 1992b).

Cognitive impairment and dPD adversely impact each other. Executive impairment, which in particular has been associated with dPD, may be due to the additive effects of PD and depression (Tröster et al. 1995).

Presentation

Evidence suggests that dPD has a slightly different symptom profile than depression without PD, including higher rates of anxiety, pessimism, suicide ideation without suicide behavior, and less guilt and self-reproach. Core nonsomatic symptoms of depression (e.g., suicidal thoughts, feelings of guilt, depressed mood, anhedonia) discriminate highly between depressed and nondepressed patients, whereas somatic symptoms correlate variably with a diagnosis of depression (Leentjens et al. 2003a).

Assessing dPD is challenging, partly as a result of symptom overlap with core PD symptoms (e.g., insomnia, psychomotor slowing, difficulty concentrating, fatigue). In addition, PD patients may withdraw from social activities if they are uncomfortable being in public when experiencing tremors or dyskinesias. Even the appearance of a nondepressed PD patient can be similar to that of someone with severe depression (e.g., bradykinetic movements and flat facies).

Controversy exists over the specific types of dPD. Research findings suggest that nonmajor depression (e.g., minor or subsyndromal depression) is more common than major depression in PD (Reijnders et al. 2008). Also, depressive symptoms can be specifically related to motor symptoms, as in patients who experience temporary dysphoria and anxiety during "off" periods (i.e., when PD medications wear off and lose their effect; Menza et al. 1990). An overview of the phenomenology of dPD is presented in Table 24–8.

Partly due to the issues outlined above, dPD is underrecognized and undertreated, even in specialty care settings (Shulman et al. 2002). For instance, Weintraub et al. (2003) found that one-third of patients evaluated at a movement disorders center met criteria for a depressive disorder, and two-thirds of them were not currently receiving antidepressant treatment.

Etiology and Pathophysiology

It was previously purported that the etiology of dPD either was "reactive" and secondary to the stress of having a chronic disabling disease or was a result of neuropathophysiological changes that occur in PD. At the time of initial PD diagnosis, some patients do develop a depressive disorder, and others experience emotional changes that do not meet criteria for a psychiatric diagnosis as part of an adjustment process. It has also been suggested that the association between depression

TABLE 24–7. A comparison of neurobehavioral features in Parkinson's disease with dementia and in Alzheimer's disease

Feature	Parkinson's disease with dementia	Alzheimer's disease
Attention/working memory	Impaired early	Mildly impaired
Information processing speed	Impaired	Relatively preserved
Executive dysfunction	Disproportionate to overall level of cognitive impairment	Proportionate to overall level of cognitive impairment
Naming	Mildly impaired	Moderately to severely impaired
Verbal fluency	Mildly to moderately impaired (letter more than semantic)	Moderately to severely impaired (semantic more than letter)
Calculation	Preserved	Impaired
Recall	Impaired	Severely impaired
Recognition	Relatively preserved	Severely impaired
Priming (implicit memory)	Relatively preserved	Impaired
Procedural memory	Impaired	Relatively preserved
Remote memory	Intact or mildly impaired with no temporal gradient	Impaired with temporal gradient
Visuospatial-perceptual-constructional processes	Impaired	Moderately impaired
Depression	Common	Less common
Hallucinations	Common (especially well-formed visual)	Less common
Delusions	Less common	Common (especially paranoid)
Apathy	Common	Less common
Motor speech	Relatively intact	Impaired early

and early-onset PD reported in some studies is due to the fact that younger patients experience more significant career, family, and financial disruptions.

However, dPD cannot be explained solely as a psychological process and likely results from a complex interaction of psychological and neurobiological factors. Some research suggests that PD patients are more depressed than patients with other chronic disabling diseases (Brandt-Christensen et al. 2007a, 2007b). In addition, recent research on the association between severity of depression and PD severity has been equivocal. Interesting findings suggesting a biological basis for dPD come from studies reporting that PD patients have a higher lifetime prevalence of depressive disorders than non-PD controls and that non-PD patients with depression are at higher risk of subsequently developing PD than nondepressed controls (Schuurman et al. 2002). These findings implicate depression as a potential risk factor or prodromal symptom of PD.

Biologically, the high frequency of dPD has been explained by dysfunction in 1) subcortical nuclei and the frontal lobes; 2) striatal-thalamic-frontal cortex circuits and the basotemporal limbic circuit; and 3) brain stem monoamine and indolamine systems (i.e., dopamine, serotonin, norepinephrine, acetylcholine). Possibly as significant as the changes in subcortical structures are impairments in the pathways connecting these regions and the frontal cortex. Functional brain imaging studies have reported simultaneous pan-frontal cortex and caudate hypometabolism in dPD, changes that are presumed to reflect neurodegeneration of the cortical-striatal-thalamic-cortical circuits (Mayberg et al. 1990).

Regarding neurotransmitters, disproportionate degeneration of dopamine neurons in the ventral tegmental area has been reported in patients with a history of dPD (Brown and Gershon 1993). In addition, imaging studies in dPD have found both a decrease in signal intensity from neural path-

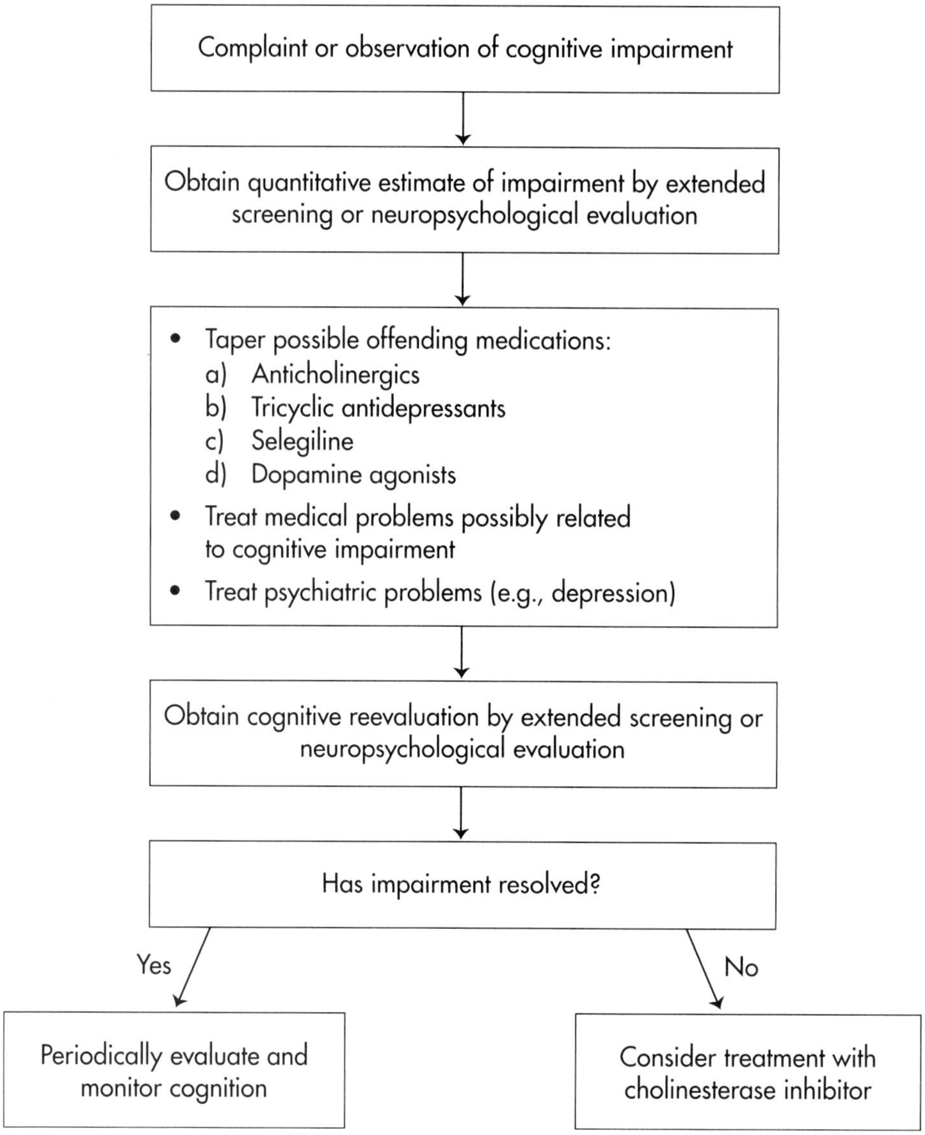

FIGURE 24–2. Clinical management of cognitive impairment in Parkinson's disease.

ways originating in monoaminergic brain stem nuclei and a negative correlation between depression scores and dorsal midbrain serotonin transporter (5-HTT) densities (Berg et al. 1999; Hesse et al. 2009; Murai et al. 2001).

Treatment

Approximately 20%–25% of patients with PD in specialty care are taking an antidepressant at any given time, most commonly a selective serotonin reuptake inhibitor (SSRI; Weintraub et al. 2003). Results of numerous open-label trials using SSRIs and other newer antidepressants in PD suggest a positive effect and good tolerability (Weintraub et al. 2005). Although concern has been raised via case reporting and physician surveys that SSRIs might worsen parkinsonism, mounting clinical experience and the results of open-label studies suggest that most PD patients are able to tolerate SSRI treatment without worsening of their PD. Concern that the combination of selegiline and SSRIs might lead to serotonin syndrome has been somewhat allayed by clinical experience (Richard et al. 1997).

Only several placebo-controlled studies of antidepressant use in dPD have been published. In three studies, tricyclic antidepressants (nortriptyline or desipramine) were found to be superior to placebo (Andersen et al. 1980; Devos et al. 2008; Menza et al. 2009); however, tricyclic antidepressants can be difficult for PD patients to tolerate due to aggravation of PD-associated orthostatic hypotension, constipation, and cognitive problems. Two placebo-controlled SSRI studies were underpowered and reported negative findings (Leentjens et al. 2003b; Wermuth et al. 1998), whereas another small study reported positive findings (Devos et al. 2008).

TABLE 24–8. Clinical features of depression in Parkinson's disease (PD)

Symptom	Comments
Depressed mood or sadness	Specific to PD depression, but variably present
Anhedonia	Diminished pleasure may be more specific to depression than diminished interest, which also occurs in apathy
Fatigue	Daytime fatigue common in PD without depression and as side effect of treatment with dopaminergic agents
Psychomotor changes	Mental slowing common in PD without depression
Decreased concentration	Changes in attention common in PD without depression
Insomnia	Sleep changes almost universally present in PD, although early morning wakening may be more specific to PD depression
Diminished appetite	May be more specific to PD depression compared with other neurovegetative symptoms
Feelings of worthlessness and guilt	Specific to PD depression, but may not be as prevalent as in non-PD depression
Suicidality	Suicide intent or attempts may not be as prevalent, although helplessness and hopelessness are common
Anxiety	Overwhelming majority of depressed PD patients also have clinically significant anxiety

We found that close to half of patients with PD currently taking an antidepressant still met DSM-IV criteria for a depressive disorder (Weintraub et al. 2003). In spite of insufficient data supporting the efficacy of SSRIs in dPD, over 70% of patients with PD in our sample were treated solely with an SSRI. In addition, only 11% of patients taking an antidepressant and still meeting criteria for depression were taking an antidepressant dosage within the highest recommended range, and only 33% had received more than one antidepressant trial. Clearly, dPD is undertreated, even in PD specialty care centers.

Regarding PD medications, levodopa is not thought to have a consistent mood effect, although there have been case reports of levodopa-induced hypomania. Preliminary studies suggest that DAs have antidepressant properties in both non-PD and PD populations. Selegiline, a selective MAO-B inhibitor at lower dosages, has also been reported in a preliminary study to have antidepressant properties in PD.

Electroconvulsive therapy can be effective for severe dPD and also improves parkinsonism, although the motor benefits wear off once treatment is discontinued (Moellentine et al. 1998; see also Chapter 10, "Electroconvulsive Therapy and Related Treatments"). It is unclear whether psychotherapy has a place in the treatment of dPD, either as an alternative first-line treatment or as an adjunct for patients with partial medication response. Anecdotally, many PD patients prefer psychotherapy, do not respond to pharmacotherapy, or are reluctant to take another medication, so cognitive-behavioral therapy and problem-solving therapy are appropriate treatment options for dPD; the latter is particularly useful when cognitive impairment is clinically significant. Given that depressive symptoms in PD are often not severe and can be transient, watchful waiting as a treatment strategy may be appropriate, provided that the patient has regular follow-ups. Regardless of the mode of treatment, we have found that disease education, practical advice, and involving patients' caregivers or significant others in the assessment and treatment process of dPD are helpful.

Clinical Recommendations

PD patients should be screened regularly for depression. Given time constraints, a brief screening instrument that can be self-administered is recommended. For example, the Geriatric Depression Rating Scale—Short Form (GDS-SF) is a 15-item yes/no questionnaire that at a cutoff of 5 has 88% sensitivity and 85% specificity for a DSM-IV diagnosis of depression in PD (Weintraub et al. 2006). Based on the results of open-label trials, psychopharmacological treatment may begin with an SSRI at a dosage recommended for geriatric patients. Due to questions about the efficacy of antidepressants in PD, it is important that dosages within the highest recommended range be used if depressive symptoms persist and treatment is well tolerated.

Other possible first-line or adjunctive antidepressants include nortriptyline, venlafaxine, mirtazapine, or bupropion. In spite of promising preliminary studies, it is premature to recommend using a DA as an antidepressant. A significant percentage of patients with PD may not tolerate, respond to, or want antidepressant treatment, so it is important to have access to and utilize appropriate nonpharmacological treatments for depression in this population.

Anxiety

Up to 40% of patients with PD experience anxiety symptoms or disorders, including generalized anxiety disorder, panic attacks, obsessive-compulsive disorder, and social phobia (Richard et al. 1996). Although patients often avoid public situations so their parkinsonian symptoms (e.g., tremor and dyskinesias) will not be noticed, such behavior does not meet DSM-IV criteria for social phobia. Anecdotal experience indicates that anxiety symptoms are often more upsetting and disabling than depressive symptoms in PD, perhaps due to their intensity, accompanying somatic complaints, and propensity to worsen parkinsonism.

Increasing anxiety and discrete anxiety attacks have been associated with motor complications, particularly the onset of off periods (i.e., periods of decreased mobility). When off periods occur, patients often describe a sensation of feeling "trapped" as they become increasingly immobilized. Anxiety symptoms resolve with improvement in motor symptoms.

Studies have reported an increased prevalence of anxiety disorders up to 20 years before PD onset (Shiba et al. 2000). This research underscores the biological underpinnings of anxiety in PD.

No controlled treatment studies have been done of anxiety in patients with PD to inform clinical decision making (Walsh and Bennett 2001). For patients who experience anxiety as part of an off state, PD medication adjustments can be made in an attempt to decrease the duration and severity of these episodes. Anecdotally, newer antidepressants are commonly used for anxiety disorders, whether or not comorbid depression is present. However, anxiety in PD responds variably to antidepressants, and many patients require treatment with benzodiazepines (most commonly low-dose lorazepam, alprazolam, and clonazepam). Given that these patients frequently have physical and cognitive impairments, benzodiazepines must be used cautiously.

Psychosis

Epidemiology

Psychosis occurs in <10% of *untreated* PD patients, but hallucinations or illusions occur in 15%–40% of *treated* PD patients (Fénelon et al. 2000), and ~5% of patients experience delusions in addition to hallucinations (Wint et al. 2004). Persistent psychotic symptoms are associated with greater functional impairment, caregiver burden, and nursing home placement.

Correlates and Risk Factors

Correlates of psychosis in patients with PD include exposure to PD medications, older age, greater cognitive impairment, increasing severity and duration of PD, comorbid depression or anxiety, increasing daytime fatigue, comorbid sleep disorder, visual impairment, polypharmacy, and delirium.

Presentation

PD patients with psychotic syndromes can be roughly categorized into two phenomenological groups. One group experiences visual illusions or hallucinations only, although auditory hallucinations and more rarely olfactory and tactile hallucinations can also occur. The hallucinations are typically formed animal or human figures and are stereotyped for each patient. These patients typically retain insight into the hallucinations, do not find them troubling, and may not require treatment (i.e., "benign hallucinosis"). The other group experiences complex psychotic symptoms, typically hallucinations and persecutory delusions in the context of dementia, sometimes complicated by delirium. These patients typically do not have insight into their psychosis, may display behavioral changes (including sundowning), and typically require treatment. Rarely, psychosis in PD may manifest as part of a manic episode, and psychosis early in the course of PD suggests a diagnosis of DLB.

Vivid perceptual changes and illogical thinking can also occur in patients with PD as part of vivid dreaming or rapid eye movement (REM) behavior disorder, and the overwhelming majority of psychotic patients with PD also report sleep disturbances (Arnulf et al. 2000). Clinically, it is difficult to distinguish nocturnal psychotic symptoms from sleep-related cognitive and perceptual changes.

Etiology and Pathophysiology

Exposure to dopaminergic therapy has been implicated as the major cause of psychosis in patients with PD (Wolters 2001). Claims have been made that certain agents are less likely than others to induce psychosis, but evidence is anecdotal. Despite the clear association between medication exposure and psychosis in patients with PD, some recent studies reporting that the dosage and duration of antiparkinsonian treatment are not correlated with psychosis indicate that PD psychosis likely results from a complex interaction of medication exposure, PD pathology, aberrant REM-related phenomena, and comorbid vulnerabilities, particularly cognitive impairment and visual disturbances (Fénelon et al. 2008).

Dopaminergic medication exposure may lead to excessive stimulation or hypersensitivity of mesocorticolimbic dopamine D_2 and D_3 receptors and induce psychosis (Wolters 1999). However, the association between psychosis, cognitive impairment, and mood disorders suggests more widespread brain involvement, involving other neurotransmitter systems or neural pathways. For instance, cholinergic deficits and a serotonergic-dopaminergic imbalance have also been implicated in the development of PD psychosis.

Treatment

The treatment of PD patients with psychosis is challenging, because optimizing the management of motor symptoms with dopaminergic medication typically worsens psychosis, whereas treating psychosis with an antipsychotic can worsen parkinsonism. A thorough medical evaluation for delirium should be performed, and any nonessential non-PD medications that might contribute to mental impairment should be discontinued. Next, the risk-benefit ratio of each antiparkinsonian medication should be reviewed. On the basis of clinical experience, medications are usually discontinued (if tolerated from a motor standpoint) in the following order: anticholinergics, selegiline, amantadine, DAs, and COMT inhibitors. Finally, if necessary, levodopa dosage is reduced (Olanow et al. 2001).

In conjunction with the steps outlined above, antipsychotic treatment is initiated for patients with PD and persistent and problematic psychosis. Typical antipsychotics are not recommended for use in this population, because they have been reported to significantly worsen parkinsonism. Clozapine has been shown to be efficacious for PD psychosis in placebo-controlled studies at much lower dosages (mean dosages of 25–36 mg/day) than typically used in psychiatric populations (Parkinson Study Group 1999), but it is usually reserved for treatment-refractory patients. Clinically, quetiapine has become the most commonly used antipsychotic, a preference based on clinical experience, the results of several positive open-label studies, and the adverse impact on parkinsonism reported with other atypical antipsychotics. However, the only two placebo-controlled studies of quetiapine for PD psychosis were negative (Ondo et al. 2005; Rabey et al. 2007), so its efficacy for PD psychosis has not been demonstrated. A review of controlled antipsychotic studies is presented in Table 24–9.

Clinical Recommendations

Assessing psychosis in patients with PD is important, because it is associated with significant caregiver distress and worse outcomes. Screening can be done quickly in the context of a routine clinic visit by inquiring about perceptual changes, particularly the range of visual disturbances that can occur, and administering the brief Parkinson's Psychosis Rating Scale (Friedberg et al. 1998). Treatment with an atypical antipsychotic should occur only if the symptoms are problematic, after acute medical conditions have been ruled out, and after the antiparkinsonian medications have been reviewed. Based on open-label studies and clinical experience, current first-line antipsychotic treatment is quetiapine (starting dosage 12.5–25 mg/day; mean maintenance dosage ~75 mg/day; dosage range 25–300 mg/day), with clozapine reserved for patients who do not respond to or tolerate quetiapine. Monitoring for worsening parkinsonism is important as the antipsychotic dosage is increased. Cholinesterase inhibitors may have antipsychotic effects in patients with PD, and their cognitive-enhancing properties are likely to be of benefit to the large percentage of psychotic patients with comorbid cognitive impairment.

Apathy

Apathy, succinctly defined as a decrease in goal-directed behavior, thinking, and mood, is reported to occur in ~40% of patients with PD (Starkstein et al. 1992b). Although apathy overlaps with depression, delirium, and dementia, apathy also occurs independently of these syndromes. Similar to depression, apathy is associated with impaired function.

Because apathy usually is accompanied by diminished self-awareness, changes typically are noticed and brought to the attention of clinicians by caregivers. A common assumption is that the patient is depressed; however, a lack of endorsement of sad mood and the typical cognitive changes seen in depression (e.g., guilt, helplessness, hopelessness) suggest a diagnosis of apathy instead. It is also important to distinguish between apathy and PD-induced slowness.

Goal-directed behavior is associated with dopaminergic and noradrenergic function and with activation of the frontal cortex and basal ganglia. Studies of apathy in patients with PD have reported associations with executive deficits, verbal memory impairment, and bradyphrenia (Starkstein et al. 2009).

No treatment studies have been reported for apathy in patients with PD. Comorbid psychiatric conditions (e.g., depression) should be treated initially. Anecdotally, psychostimulants (e.g., methylphenidate) and stimulant-related compounds (e.g., modafinil) are used in clinical practice, but their effectiveness for this condition is not known. On the basis of the proposed neuropathophysiology of apathy, antidepressants and other medications that increase dopamine or norepinephrine activity (e.g., DAs, tricyclic antidepressants, dual reuptake inhibitor antidepressants, bupropion, atomoxetine) may be beneficial. In addition to providing pharmacological treatment, the clinician should educate patients and families on the distinction between apathy and depression and should encourage steps that overcome patient inertia, which may lead to improved functioning and quality of life.

TABLE 24–9. Placebo-controlled studies of antipsychotics in Parkinson's disease

Reference	Number of subjects/ completers	Length of study	Active treatment	Setting	Relevant outcome measures and results	Adverse events and comments for study medication
Wolters et al. 1990	6/3	40 days	Clozapine (mean 171 mg/day)	Inpatient	3/6 patients responded by clinical evaluation	Worsening parkinsonism in 3/6 patients and delirium in 4/6 patients treated with clozapine
French Clozapine Parkinson Study Group 1999	60/46	4 weeks	Clozapine (mean 36 mg/day)	Outpatient	Positive treatment effect change in PANSS positive score ($P<0.001$)	Somnolence and worsening parkinsonism more commonly reported as adverse events with clozapine No change in UPDRS motor or MMSE scores with clozapine
Parkinson Study Group 1999	60/54	4 weeks	Clozapine (mean 25 mg/day)	Outpatient	Positive treatment effect for change in BPRS ($P=0.002$) and SAPS ($P=0.01$) scores	Improved tremor with clozapine Leukopenia in one clozapine patient
Breier et al. 2002	87/60	4 weeks	Olanzapine (mean modal 4 mg/day)	Outpatient	No treatment effect for change in BPRS ($P=0.96$) or NPI ($P=0.78$) scores	Higher study discontinuation rate with olanzapine Increased parkinsonism with olanzapine
Breier et al. 2002	78/59	4 weeks	Olanzapine (mean modal 4 mg/day)	Outpatient	No treatment effect for change in BPRS ($P=0.61$) or NPI ($P=0.50$) scores	Increased parkinsonism with olanzapine
Ondo et al. 2002	30/27	9 weeks	Olanzapine (mean 5 mg/day)	Outpatient	No treatment effect for change in UPDRS item 2 ($P=0.16$) or structured interview for hallucinations in PD (no *P* value provided)	Increased parkinsonism with olanzapine
Pollak et al. 2004	60/46	4 weeks	Clozapine (mean 36 mg/day)	Outpatient	Positive treatment effect for change in PANSS positive score ($P<0.001$)	Somnolence, worsening of parkinsonism, and sialorrhea more commonly reported as adverse events with clozapine Neutropenia ($n=2$) and seizures ($n=1$) with clozapine No change in UPDRS motor or MMSE scores with clozapine

TABLE 24–9. Placebo-controlled studies of antipsychotics in Parkinson's disease *(continued)*

Reference	Number of subjects/ completers	Length of study	Active treatment	Setting	Relevant outcome measures and results	Adverse events and comments for study medication
Ondo et al. 2005	31/26	12 weeks	Quetiapine (mean 170 mg/day)	Outpatient	No treatment effect for change in BPRS (no *P* value provided) or Baylor PD Hallucination Questionnaire scores ($P=0.19$)	No change in UPDRS motor scores with quetiapine

Note. BPRS=Brief Psychiatric Rating Scale; MMSE=Mini-Mental State Examination; NPI=Neuropsychiatric Inventory; PANSS=Positive and Negative Syndrome Scale for Schizophrenia; PD=Parkinson's disease; SAPS=Scale for the Assessment of Positive Symptoms; UPDRS=Unified Parkinson's Disease Rating Scale.

Source. Reprinted from Weintraub D, Katz IR: "Pharmacologic Interventions for Psychosis and Agitation in Neurodegenerative Diseases: Evidence About Efficacy and Safety." *Psychiatric Clinics of North America* 28:941–983, 2005. Used with permission.

Impulse-Control Disorders and Related Behaviors

Impulse-control disorders (ICDs), including problem or pathological gambling, compulsive buying, compulsive sexual behavior, and binge or compulsive eating, have been reported to occur in patients with PD (Voon and Fox 2007). These psychiatric disorders, which have both impulsive and compulsive features, are commonly conceptualized as "behavioral" addictions.

Preliminary cross-sectional prevalence estimates for ICDs in PD patients from formal assessment studies have ranged from 1.7% to 6.1% for problem or pathological gambling, from 2.0% to 4.0% for compulsive sexual behavior, and from 0.4% to 3.0% for compulsive buying (Voon and Fox 2007; Weintraub 2008).

Case reporting and cross-sectional studies have suggested an association between DA treatment and ICDs in PD. ICDs in PD have also been reported less commonly in the context of levodopa treatment and after DBS. ICD behaviors before PD onset, personal or familial histories of alcoholism, impulsive or novelty-seeking characteristics, young age, male sex, and early onset of PD have also been associated with ICD development in PD.

ICDs in PD may lead to significant impairments in psychosocial functioning, interpersonal relationships, physical health, and quality of life. Patients may not report such behaviors to a treating physician, perhaps for any of several reasons: embarrassment, lack of suspicion of an association with PD treatment, or ambivalence regarding ceasing the behavior. Evidence indicates that ICDs are underrecognized in clinical practice.

To date, clinical management of ICDs in patients with PD has been suboptimal. Although the aforementioned behaviors can be personally and financially ruinous, clinicians are often slow to recognize the condition and intervene. A trial discontinuation or dosage lowering of the presumed offending medication is the primary initial treatment option, because no evidence suggests that the addition of any class of psychiatric medication helps in the management of this condition. In a recent follow-up of a small group of PD patients with ICD receiving routine clinical care, most patient had either significantly decreased or discontinued their DA treatment over time, and the overwhelming majority of them no longer met diagnostic criteria for an ICD (Mamikonyan et al. 2008).

Disorders of Sleep and Wakefulness

Up to 90% of patients with PD report insomnia, hypersomnia, sleep fragmentation, sleep terrors, nightmares, nocturnal movements, or REM behavior disorder (RBD) (Arnulf et al. 2000). RBD, another disorder that may be a prodrome of PD, is characterized by loss of normal skeletal muscle atonia during REM sleep, prominent motor activity, and dreams (see Chapter 18, "Sleep Disorders," for further discussion).

Other sleep cycle–related disorders in PD are restless legs syndrome and periodic leg movements in sleep, which are overlapping but distinct disorders. In addition, patients with more advanced PD may have an increased frequency of obstructive or central apnea.

RBD and other sleep disturbances have been attributed to both progressive degeneration of the cholinergic pedunculopontine nucleus (Jellinger 1988) and reduced striatal dopaminergic activity (Eisensehr et al. 2000). Associated clinical factors that disrupt sleep are immobility due to nocturnal bradykinesia and rigidity, tremors and dyskinesias, cramps, micturition, pain, and excessive sweating. Sleep disturbances also are correlated with psychosis, depression, and cognitive impairment.

Excessive daytime sleepiness (EDS) or fatigue occurs in 15%–50% of patients with PD (Tandberg et al. 1999), and the two are thought to be overlapping but distinct disorders (Havlikova et al. 2008). EDS has been attributed variably to impairments in the striatal-thalamic-frontal-cortical system, exposure to dopaminergic medications (especially DAs), and nocturnal sleep disturbances. In addition, advanced disease, depression, cognitive impairment, and psychosis are clinical correlates of EDS. Daytime "sleep attacks" (i.e., sudden-onset REM sleep) have been reported rarely in this population, particularly in conjunction with DA treatment, although it remains controversial whether this is a distinct clinical entity beyond excessive sleepiness.

Treatment depends on the specific disorder and its etiology. Sleep disturbances that are due to nocturnal worsening of parkinsonism may respond to adjustments in the PD medication regimen. Restless legs syndrome and periodic leg movements in sleep are commonly treated with dopaminergic medications, and RBD is typically treated with clonazepam. Preliminary studies suggest that EDS can be treated successfully with modafinil, and psychostimulants are also used in clinical practice. The role of other hypnotic or psychiatric medications in the treatment of sleep disturbances in patients with PD has not been evaluated.

Complications of Deep Brain Stimulation Surgery

The impact of DBS, primarily bilateral subthalamic DBS, on nonmotor symptoms appears to be varied and complex (Appleby et al. 2007; Voon et al. 2006). In the immediate wake of electrode implantation, with its route through prefrontal cortex and subcortical white matter, patients have experienced transient abnormalities such as confusional states. Longer-term findings have included executive dysfunction suggestive of a frontal lobe syndrome. Psychiatric findings have also included both overall improvement and occasionally a worsening, either transient or long term, of disorders including depression, anxiety, psychosis, mania, and emotional lability. Among cognitive findings, a meta-analysis (Parsons et al. 2006) of 28 cohort studies identified small declines in cognitive function, with statistical significance for decline in executive functions and in verbal learning and memory—and a more sizable effect on a specific executive measure (semantic and phonemic verbal fluency). Postsurgical psychiatric monitoring is warranted, a need heightened by reports of postsurgical suicidal ideation and completed or attempted suicides (Voon et al. 2008).

Nonmotor Fluctuations

Most patients with PD receiving long-term treatment with levodopa develop motor fluctuations, which include off periods of worsening parkinsonism and on periods of dyskinesias. The majority of patients with motor fluctuations also experience nonmotor fluctuations, including anxiety, slowness of thinking, fatigue, and dysphoria, and these fluctuations can be more disabling than motor fluctuations for a substantial percentage of PD patients (Witjas et al. 2002). In addition, patients may rarely experience hypomanic symptoms during on periods. Nonmotor fluctuations do not appear to be a simple reaction to changes in motor status, because no consistent correlation exists between severity of motor and nonmotor symptoms, and improvements in mood following levodopa infusion in PD patients with motor fluctuations can precede improvements in motor status. It remains to be seen if treatments shown to reduce severity or time of motor fluctuations, such as COMT inhibitors, DAs, and DBS, also lead to improvements in severity or duration of nonmotor fluctuations.

Huntington's Disease

Huntington's disease (HD) is an inherited, progressive neurodegenerative disorder most commonly associated with dramatic abnormal movements, chorea, and dystonia. Aside from the movement disorder, cognitive impairment and psychiatric symptoms occur in virtually all people with HD. Behavioral symptoms are often more troubling to patients and families than the actual movement disorder, and these symptoms can greatly increase the burden placed on families and other care providers.

Clinical Features

Prevalence of HD is estimated at ~5 per 100,000; it is less common among those of non-European ancestry (Folstein et al. 1987). Typically, diagnosis is in the third or fourth decade of life, but onset may occur from childhood through the eighth decade of life (Gilstad and Reich 2003). With the availability of direct genetic testing on individual patients, the diagnosis of HD is now made more frequently in those who have onset of chorea in their 60s or even 70s without a known family history of HD.

Neurological abnormalities include abnormal involuntary movements (chorea and dystonia) and disorders of voluntary movement (gait disorders, impairment of saccades and smooth pursuit, dysarthria, and swallowing impairment). These symptoms progress over the course of 10–15 years, leading in most cases to severe disability. Chorea, the rapid and involuntary writhing movement that is the hallmark of the disease, typically worsens in the middle stages of the illness and then decreases as the patient becomes more debilitated. Dystonia worsens as the disease progresses, as do bradykinesia and rigidity. Those patients with onset later in life generally have a slowly progressive course of illness. These older patients are sometimes misdiagnosed as having a parkinsonian syndrome.

Genetics and Neuropathophysiology

Genetics and Disease Mechanism

The genetic abnormality underlying HD is caused by an abnormal expansion of trinucleotide repeats coding for glutamine at the *N*-terminus of the *huntingtin* protein. The increase occurs in sequences of cytosine, adenine, and guanine (CAG) in exon 1 of the HD gene, which is located on chromosome 4. The gene is expressed throughout the body. The normal function of *huntingtin* is unknown. Excitotoxicity, mitochondrial dysfunction, and dysregulation of gene expression have all been suggested as pathological mechanisms. The HD gene is transmitted as an autosomal dominant trait; each child of an affected individual has a 50% chance of inheriting the gene. Normal individuals have between 9 and 29 CAG repeats. Those who develop clinically apparent symptoms of HD have a higher repeat number, usually 39 or over. The CAG repeat number is inversely correlated with age at symptom onset. Genetic counseling at a certified testing program is recommended by the Huntington's Disease Society of America for those seeking presymptomatic at-risk testing for the HD gene. Adverse outcomes, such as severe depression and suicide attempts, have occurred following genetic testing.

Neuropathological Process

The distinctive neuropathological change seen in HD is the decline in the number of medium spiny striatal neurons. The first neuropathological change in HD is in the associative areas of the striatum (Middleton and Strick 2000). Caudate changes predominate, but cell death also occurs in the globus pallidus. As the disease advances, widespread atrophy occurs (Hedreen et al. 1991).

Brain Imaging Findings

Basal ganglia atrophy correlates positively with CAG repeat length in magnetic resonance imaging (MRI) structural and volumetric studies (Rosas et al. 2001). Generalized atrophy and focal frontal lobe changes occur. Diminished caudate volume has also been reported in presymptomatic at-risk individuals. Cortical thinning and volume reductions in other regions are present even in early stages of HD.

Functional studies show caudate and putamenal hypometabolism, along with some frontal metabolic reductions that correlate with decline in function (Bartenstein et al. 1997). Positron emission tomography (PET) studies of dopamine function have found both striatal and cortical receptor abnormalities (Pavese et al. 2003).

Cognitive Impairment

Visuospatial performance deficits may be some of the earliest cognitive changes seen in HD (Josiassen et al. 1983). Memory deficits in HD include slowed rates of learning and impaired recall. Free recall improves with cuing. Retention is relatively normal in HD, as distinct from AD. Executive dysfunction is also reported consistently in studies of patients with HD (Josiassen et al. 1983). Procedural memory is impaired, as is evident in tests of skill and motor learning. Performance deficits on neuropsychological testing are also seen in carriers of the HD CAG expansion before a clinical diagnosis can be made (Langbehn et al. 2007).

Psychiatric Symptoms

Psychiatric symptoms may occur at any point in the course of HD, perhaps predating the onset of motor abnormalities in some cases (Duff et al. 2007). Overall prevalence of psychiatric symptoms in HD has been reported as anywhere from 30% to over 70% (van Duijn et al. 2007). A study of outpatients using careful evaluation with standard measures and information from caregivers found that 98% of patients with HD had at least one psychiatric symptom, demonstrating that as more evaluations are conducted, most patients are likely to have some behavioral disturbances (Paulsen et al. 2001).

Unlike the somewhat predictable progression of motor and cognitive symptoms, no generalized time course for psychiatric disease has been demonstrated in patients with HD. Apathy is the one possible exception; it may worsen as the illness progresses. CAG repeat length has not been shown to correlate positively with presence of psychiatric symptoms. Severe psychiatric symptoms are one of the main considerations in the decision to institutionalize a patient (Wheelock et al. 2003). Because patients are often amenable to treatment with standard psychopharmacological agents, providing relief from these symptoms can impact greatly on quality of life for both patients and caregivers.

Irritability and Aggression

Irritability is probably the most common behavioral symptom in patients with HD. It is reported in 40%–80% of patients, depending on assessment measures used (van Duijn et al. 2007). Aggression, when it occurs in HD, usually accompanies irritability. In a study of 960 patients with HD, over 60% of the patients or their caregivers reported aggressive patient behavior when questioned at their first visit to an HD clinic (Marder et al. 2000). Chatterjee et al. (2005) found that patient and caregiver irritability ratings did not concur; patients rated themselves as having a lower level of irritability than did caregivers. This discrepancy was seen in relatively cognitively intact patients, suggesting impairment of patient insight with respect to this symptom. A retrospective study found that over one-third of HD patients in nursing homes were aggressive. Irritability and hostility measures have been shown to be significantly elevated in individuals who are presymptomatic but known to carry the HD expansion, compared with those who are at risk but do not have the expansion, suggesting that irritability can appear quite early in the course of the illness.

Burns et al. (1990) reported that 59% of HD patients were aggressive when assessed with a standardized scale. In a clinician-based survey, frequent and severe physical aggression occurred in only 10% of HD patients. Discrepancies in estimates of aggression in patients with HD may be due to selection bias, with institutionalized patients showing higher rates of aggression because this behavior leads to institutionalization.

Behavioral techniques, such as adherence to a schedule to minimize unexpected events, may be helpful in decreasing irritability and aggression (Moskowitz et al. 2001). Education of caregivers in how to identify and avoid situations that trigger irritability and how to minimize its effects if it does occur is extremely important. Careful evaluation to rule out medical illness, delirium, medication toxicity, or physical discomfort should be conducted, especially in patients who have not been disruptive previously or in those who may have impaired communication. Irritability and aggression both respond to pharmacotherapy in many cases, sometimes in combination with behavioral interventions. It is important to start in the lower end of the dosing range for medications when treating any patient with HD. Exceptions may occur if patients are particularly aggressive; individual patients may require high dosages of medication to control these behavioral problems.

Personality Alterations

Nonspecific personality changes are probably one of the most frequent, and least studied, of all behavioral abnormalities in patients with HD. Reports indicate that personality alterations occur in 10%–40% of patients with HD (Saugstad and Odegard 1986). These changes include impulsivity, emotional lability, and lack of empathy for others. Personality changes may occur before clinical diagnosis (Lishman 1998).

Apathy

Apathy is an extremely common and treatment-resistant symptom in patients with HD. Over 50% of HD patients in several studies were found to have apathy (Paulsen et al. 2001), and it has been shown to increase with duration of illness. Apathy is often difficult to differentiate from depression, especially as the disease progresses and communication diminishes due to dysarthria or impaired cognition. Pharmacological interventions are not particularly helpful for apathy. Structuring daily activities may be useful, as for irritability and aggression. Education of family members to promote reasonable expectations for patient interactions is often the most practical and useful approach.

Affective Disorders

Changes in mood are quite common in patients with HD, with studies finding 30%–70% of patients reporting depressed mood (van Duijn et al. 2007). Depression is generally reported to occur either with or following onset of motor abnormalities, arguing against purely reactive mood changes (Paulsen et al. 2001).

Suicide rates in HD are increased fourfold compared with the general population. Completed suicide rates ranging from 3% to 7% have been reported, with over 25% of patients attempting suicide at some point in the illness; suicide risk is particularly increased among patients in their 50s or 60s. Risk factors for suicidal behavior in HD patients are similar to those in the general population and include depression, living alone, childlessness, and being unmarried. HD patients who express suicidal ideation should be evaluated immediately. Suicidal ideation may occur in conjunction with genetic testing in at-risk persons (Almqvist et al. 1999).

The prevalence of mania and hypomania is also increased in HD. From the limited data available, mania appears to occur in ~5% of patients; if hypomania is included, 10% of patients have these symptoms (Folstein 1989).

Treatment of mood disorders in patients with HD is particularly important, given the high rate of suicide seen in the disorder. Many patients will improve greatly with standard dosages of antidepressants. If irritability or psychosis accompanies the depression, addition of a small dosage of an atypical neuroleptic can be helpful.

Anxiety Disorders

Anxiety disorders have received relatively little study in HD. Older studies report anxiety as a frequent prodromal symptom. Obsessive and compulsive symptoms have been found to occur with high frequency in patients with HD. Of patients with HD, 20%–50% have been reported to have obsessive or compulsive symptoms, depending on the measure used for assessment (Anderson et al. 2001). Beglinger et al. (2007) found that the probability of obsessive-compulsive symptoms is more than three times greater by the time a patient shows clearly manifest disease than in at-risk people with no apparent motor symptoms. The possible relationship of obsessive and compulsive symptoms to frontal-striatal changes in HD is supported by PET studies in primary obsessive-compulsive disorder.

Anxiety disorders usually respond to the standard treatments. As in the general population, when antidepressants are used, especially SSRIs, higher dosages may be needed to achieve maximal control of anxiety symptoms. No studies have been reported of behavioral therapy, such as systematic desensitization or cognitive-behavioral therapy, for anxiety disorders in HD.

Psychotic Symptoms

Psychotic symptoms are seen in 3%–11% of patients with HD (van Duijn et al. 2007). Psychosis is generally thought to be more prevalent in patients with younger onset of disease (Paulsen et al. 2001). Delusions of persecution are probably the most common psychotic symptoms.

Psychosis and paranoia in patients with HD respond to pharmacotherapy. Although starting with an atypical neuroleptic is usually preferable, due to the more favorable side-effect profile, standard high-potency agents such as haloperidol may be the first choice in patients who would benefit from suppression of chorea in addition to treatment of psychosis.

Treatment

At this time, no treatment has been proven to prevent symptom onset or slow disease progression in humans with the HD gene expansion. Agents such as omega fatty acids and minocycline have been studied following promising work in animal models, but they have not shown definitive benefits in human clinical trials (Huntington Study Group TREND-HD Investigators 2008). Numerous treatment trials are in progress or about to begin, and hopefully this work will lead to therapies that delay symptom onset or modify the course of manifest HD.

In 2008, tetrabenazine became the first therapy approved by the U.S. Food and Drug Administration (FDA) for symptomatic treatment of HD. Tetrabenazine selectively depletes central monoamines by reversibly binding to the type 2 vesicular monoamine transporter. It has been used in Europe for many years to treat chorea and other movement disorders, and it was shown to be effective in reducing chorea severity in a randomized clinical trial in the United States that served as the basis for FDA approval (Huntington Study Group 2006). In some patients, tetrabenazine is not without significant side effects, including sedation, akathisia, depressed mood, and anxiety. The drug carries a black box warning that because of its mechanism of action, it may exacerbate underlying psychiatric conditions; its use has been linked to suicidal behavior and completed suicide (Huntington Study Group 2006). It is important to stress to patients and families that tetrabenazine has not been shown to modify disease course but is rather a symptomatic treatment for reduction of chorea. Tetrabenazine is beneficial in a select group of patients who are functionally or socially impaired by involuntary movements. Because side effects can be delayed at onset, expertise in dosing escalation and monitoring at maintenance dosage is required.

Treatment of psychiatric symptoms is extremely important and can greatly improve quality of life in patients with HD and reduce the burden on their caregivers. Prior reviews have summarized the limited research on treatment of behavioral symptoms in HD (Anderson and Marder 2002). Anderson and Marder (2002) outlined suggestions for a stepwise approach to evaluation and treatment of various problematic behaviors. Treatment recommendations may also be found in publications from the Huntington's Disease Society of America (Rosenblatt et al. 1999). Many behavioral interventions are extremely useful, especially in later life.

Other measures to improve quality of life and maintain function in patients with HD include physical therapy, speech and swallowing assessment and therapy, dietary interventions to maintain weight, and modification of diet to prevent choking. As in all neurodegenerative illness, maintenance of physical function and independence at the highest possible level may greatly impact overall quality of life and mental outlook.

Key Points

- PD is the second most common neurodegenerative disease in Western countries, after Alzheimer's disease, and its prevalence continues to increase.
- Dementia is a common long-term complication in PD.
- A range of cognitive impairments that do not meet criteria for dementia are common in PD, even early in the disease course.
- A range of neuropsychiatric disorders are relatively common in PD and include depression, anxiety, psychosis, apathy, disorders of sleep and wakefulness, and impulse-control disorders.
- Routine screening for neuropsychiatric disturbances in PD is important because they have an adverse impact on quality of life, function, disease course, and caregiver burden.
- Psychiatric complications, including impulse-control disorders or psychosis, can occur with dopaminergic treatment or following deep brain stimulation surgery. Affective symptoms, including depression and apathy, may fluctuate along with motor symptoms.
- Antidepressants, anxiolytics, antipsychotics, and cholinesterase inhibitors can be helpful when used appropriately in patients with PD, but evidence for their efficacy is limited.
- Cognitive impairment and a range of psychiatric disturbances occur in HD and are associated with caregiver burden and institutionalization.
- Irritability, personality alterations, apathy, affective disturbances, anxiety disorders, and psychosis are particularly common in HD.
- Visuospatial, recognition memory, and executive deficits are common cognitive impairments in HD.
- Research into the treatment of behavioral and cognitive disturbances in HD is very limited, so standard psychiatric treatments are used. For psychosis, this can be either a typical or an atypical antipsychotic.

Recommended Readings and Web Sites

Aarsland D, Andersen K, Larsen JP, et al: Prevalence and characteristics of dementia in Parkinson disease: an 8-year prospective study. Arch Neurol 60:387–392, 2003

Almqvist EW, Block M, Brinkman R, et al: A worldwide assessment of the frequency of suicide, suicide attempts or psychiatric hospitalization after predictive testing for Huntington disease. Am J Hum Genet 64:1293–1304, 1999

Anderson KE, Marder KS: An overview of psychiatric symptoms in Huntington's disease. Curr Psychiatry Rep 3:379–388, 2001

Anderson KE, Louis ED, Stern Y, et al: Cognitive correlates of obsessive and compulsive symptoms in Huntington's disease. Am J Psychiatry 158:799–801, 2001

Emre M, Aarsland D, Albanese A, et al: Rivastigmine for dementia associated with Parkinson's disease. N Engl J Med 351:2509–2518, 2004

Emre M, Aarsland D, Brown R, et al: Clinical diagnostic criteria for dementia associated with Parkinson's disease. Mov Disord 22: 1689–1707, 2007

Huntington Study Group: Tetrabenazine as antichorea therapy in Huntington disease: a randomized controlled trial. Neurology 66:366–372, 2006

Leentjens AF: Depression in Parkinson's disease: conceptual issues and clinical challenges. J Geriatr Psychiatry Neurol 17:120–126, 2004

Miyasaki JM, Shannon K, Voon V, et al: Practice parameter: evaluation and treatment of depression, psychosis, and dementia in Parkinson disease (an evidence-based review). Report of the Quality Standards Subcommittee of the American Academy of Neurology. Neurology 66:996–1002, 2006

Olanow CW, Stern MB, Sethi K: The scientific and clinical basis for the treatment of Parkinson disease. Neurology 72:S1–S136, 2009

Paulsen JS, Ready RE, Hamilton JM, et al: Neuropsychiatric aspects of Huntington's disease. J Neurol Neurosurg Psychiatry 71:310–314, 2001

Ravina B, Marder K, Fernandez HH, et al: Diagnostic criteria for psychosis in Parkinson's disease: report of an NINDS, NIMH work group. Mov Disord 22:1061–1068, 2007

Richard IH: Anxiety disorders in Parkinson's disease. Adv Neurol 96:42–55, 2005

van Duijn E, Kingma EM, van der Mast RC: Psychopathology in verified Huntington's disease gene carriers. J Neuropsychiatry Clin Neurosci 19:441–448, 2007

Voon V, Fox SH: Medication-related impulse control and repetitive behaviors in Parkinson disease. Arch Neurol 64:1089–1096, 2007

Huntington's Disease Society of America: www.hdsa.org

Michael J. Fox Foundation for Parkinson's Research: www.michaeljfox.org

National Parkinson Foundation: www.parkinson.org

Parkinson's Disease Foundation: www.pdf.org

References

Aarsland D, Andersen K, Larsen JP, et al: Prevalence and characteristics of dementia in Parkinson disease: an 8-year prospective study. Arch Neurol 60:387–392, 2003

Aarsland D, Zaccai J, Brayne C: A systematic review of prevalence studies of dementia in Parkinson's disease. Mov Disord 20:1255–1263, 2005

Aarsland D, Bronnick K, Larsen JP, et al: Cognitive impairment in incident, untreated Parkinson disease: The Norwegian ParkWest Study. Neurology 72:1121–1126, 2009

Almqvist EW, Block M, Brinkman R, et al: A worldwide assessment of the frequency of suicide, suicide attempts or psychiatric hospitalization after predictive testing for Huntington disease. Am J Hum Genet 64:1293–1304, 1999

American Psychiatric Association: Diagnostic and Statistical Manual of Mental Disorders, 3rd Edition, Revised. Washington, DC, American Psychiatric Association, 1987

American Psychiatric Association: Diagnostic and Statistical Manual of Mental Disorders, 4th Edition. Washington, DC, American Psychiatric Association, 1994

Andersen J, Aabro E, Gulmann N, et al: Anti-depressive treatment in Parkinson's disease: a controlled trial of the effect of nortriptyline in patients with Parkinson's disease treated with l-dopa. Acta Neurol Scand 62:210–219, 1980

Anderson KE, Marder KS: Huntington's disease, in Current Therapy in Neurologic Disease, 6th Edition. Edited by Johnson RT, Griffin JW, McArthur JC. Philadelphia, PA, Mosby, 2002, pp 282–287

Anderson KE, Louis ED, Stern Y, et al: Cognitive correlates of obsessive and compulsive symptoms in Huntington's disease. Am J Psychiatry 158:799–801, 2001

Appleby BS, Duggan PS, Regenberg A, et al: Psychiatric and neuropsychiatric adverse events associated with deep brain stimulation: a meta-analysis of ten years' experience. Mov Disord 22: 1722–1728, 2007

Arnulf I, Bonnet AM, Damier P, et al: Hallucinations, REM sleep, and Parkinson's disease: a medical hypothesis. Neurology 55:281–288, 2000

Bartenstein P, Weindl A, Spiegel S, et al: Central motor processing in Huntington's disease: a PET study. Brain 120:1553–1567, 1997

Beglinger LJ, Langbehn DR, Duff K, et al: Probability of obsessive and compulsive symptoms in Huntington's disease. Biol Psychiatry 61:415–418, 2007

Berg D, Supprian T, Hofmann E, et al: Depression in Parkinson's disease: brainstem midline alteration on transcranial sonography and magnetic imaging. J Neurol 246:1186–1193, 1999

Braak H, Del Tredici K: Invited article: nervous system pathology in sporadic Parkinson disease. Neurology 70:1916–1925, 2008

Braak H, Del Tredici K, Rüb U, et al: Staging of brain pathology related to sporadic Parkinson's disease. Neurobiol Aging 24:197–210, 2003

Brandt-Christensen M, Kvist K, Nilsson FM, et al: Treatment with antiparkinson and antidepressant drugs: A register-based, pharmaco-epidemiological study. Mov Disord 22:2037–2042, 2007a

Brandt-Christensen M, Lopez AG, Nilsson FM, et al: Parkinson's disease and antidepressant drug treatment: a case-register study. Parkinsonism Relat Disord 13:406–410, 2007b

Breier A, Sutton VK, Feldman PD, et al: Olanzapine in the treatment of dopamimetic-induced psychosis in patients with Parkinson's disease. Biol Psychiatry 52:438–445, 2002

Brown AS, Gershon S: Dopamine and depression. J Neural Transm Gen Sect 91:75–109, 1993

Burns A, Folstein S, Brandt J, et al: Clinical assessment of irritability, aggression, and apathy in Huntington disease and Alzheimer disease. J Nerv Ment Dis 178:20–26, 1990

Caviness JN, Driver-Dunckley E, Connor DJ, et al: Defining mild cognitive impairment in Parkinson's disease. Mov Disord 22: 1272–1277, 2007

Chatterjee A, Anderson KE, Moskowitz CB, et al: A comparison of self-report and caregiver assessment of depression, apathy, and irritability in Huntington's disease. J Neuropsychiatry Clin Neurosci 17:378–383, 2005

Cotzias GC, Papavasiliou PS, Gellene R: Modification of Parkinsonism—chronic treatment with L-dopa. N Engl J Med 280: 337–345, 1969

Devos D, Dujardin K, Poirot I, et al: Comparison of desipramine and citalopram treatments for depression in Parkinson's disease: a double-blind, randomized, placebo-controlled study. Mov Disord 23:850–857, 2008

Dubois B, Slachevsky A, Litvan I, et al: The FAB: a Frontal Assessment Battery at bedside. Neurology 55:1621–1626, 2000

Duff K, Paulsen JS, Beglinger LF, et al: Psychiatric symptoms in Huntington's disease before diagnosis: the predict-HD study. Biol Psychiatry 62:1341–1346, 2007

Eisensehr I, Linke R, Noachtar S, et al: Reduced striatal dopamine transporters in idiopathic rapid eye movement sleep behavior disorder: comparison with Parkinson's disease and controls. Brain 123:1155–1160, 2000

Emre M: Treatment of dementia associated with Parkinson's disease. Parkinsonism Relat Disord 13(suppl):S457–S461, 2007

Emre M, Aarsland D, Albanese A, et al: Rivastigmine for dementia associated with Parkinson's disease. N Engl J Med 351:2509–2518, 2004

Emre M, Aarsland D, Brown R, et al: Clinical diagnostic criteria for dementia associated with Parkinson's disease. Mov Disord 22: 1689–1707, 2007a

Emre M, Cummings JL, Lane RM: Rivastigmine in dementia associated with Parkinson's disease and Alzheimer's disease: similarities and differences. J Alzheimers Dis 11:509–519, 2007b

Fahn S: Adverse effects of levodopa, in The Scientific Basis for the Treatment of Parkinson's Disease. Edited by Olanow CW, Lieberman AN. Carnforth, UK, Parthenon, 1992, pp 89–112

Fénelon G: Psychosis in Parkinson's disease: phenomenology, frequency, risk factors, and current understanding of pathophysiologic mechanisms. CNS Spectr13 (suppl 4):18–25, 2008

Fénelon G, Mahieux F, Huon R, et al: Hallucinations in Parkinson's disease: prevalence, phenomenology, and risk factors. Brain 123: 733–745, 2000

Folstein MF, Folstein SE, McHugh PR: "Mini-mental state": a practical method for grading the cognitive state of patients for the clinician. J Psychiatr Res 12:189–198, 1975

Folstein SE: Huntington Disease: A Disorder of Families. Baltimore, MD, Johns Hopkins University Press, 1989

Folstein SE, Chase GA, Wahl WE, et al: Huntington's disease in Maryland: clinical aspects of racial variation. Am J Hum Genet 41: 168–179, 1987

Foltynie T, Brayne CEG, Robbins TW, et al: The cognitive ability of an incident cohort of Parkinson's patients in the UK: the CamPaIGN study. Brain 127:550–560, 2004

French Clozapine Parkinson Study Group: Clozapine in drug-induced psychosis in Parkinson's disease. Lancet 353:2041–2042, 1999

Friedberg G, Zoldan J, Weizman A, et al: Parkinson Psychosis Rating Scale: a practical instrument for grading psychosis in Parkinson's disease. Clin Neuropharmacol 21:280–284, 1998

Galvin JE, Pollack J, Morris J: Clinical phenotype of Parkinson disease dementia. Neurology 67:1605–1611, 2006

Gilstad J, Reich SG: Chorea in an octogenarian. Neurologist 9:165–166, 2003

Havlikova E, van Dijk JP, Rosenberger J, et al: Fatigue in Parkinson's disease in not related to excessive sleepiness or quality of sleep. J Neurol Sci 270:107–113, 2008

Hedreen JC, Peyser CE, Folstein SE, et al: Neuronal loss in layers V and VI of cerebral cortex in Huntington's disease. Neurosci Lett 133:257–261, 1991

Hesse S, Meyer PM, Strecker K, et al: Monoamine transporter availability in Parkinson's disease patients with or without depression. Eur J Nucl Med Mol Imaging 36:428–435, 2009

Hobson P, Meara J: The detection of dementia and cognitive impairment in a community population of elderly people with Parkinson's disease by use of the CAMCOG neuropsychological test. Age Ageing 28:39–43, 1999

Hoehn MH, Yahr MD: Parkinsonism: onset, progression, and mortality. Neurology 17:427–442, 1967

Huang C, Mattis P, Perrine K, et al: Metabolic abnormalities associated with mild cognitive impairment in Parkinson disease. Neurology 70:1470–1477, 2008

Hughes AJ, Ben-Shlomo Y, Daniel SE, et al: What features improve the accuracy of clinical diagnosis in Parkinson's disease: a clinicopathologic study. Neurology 42:1142–1146, 1992

Hughes AJ, Daniel SE, Lees AJ: The clinical features of Parkinson's disease in 100 histologically proven cases. Adv Neurol 60:595–599, 1993

Huntington Study Group: Tetrabenazine as antichorea therapy in Huntington disease: a randomized controlled trial. Neurology 66:366–372, 2006

Huntington Study Group TREND-HD Investigators: Randomized controlled trial of ethyl-eicosapentaenoic acid in Huntington disease: the TREND-HD study. Arch Neurol 65:1582–1589, 2008

Hurtig HI, Trojanowski JQ, Galvin J, et al: Alpha-synuclein cortical Lewy bodies correlate with dementia in Parkinson's disease. Neurology 54:1916–1921, 2000

Jacobs DM, Marder K, Cote LJ, et al: Neuropsychological characteristics of preclinical dementia in Parkinson's disease. Neurology 45:1691–1696, 1995

Janvin C, Aarsland D, Larsen JP, et al: Neuropsychological profile of patients with Parkinson's disease without dementia. Dement Geriatr Cogn Disord 15:126–131, 2003

Janvin CC, Aarsland D, Larsen JP: Cognitive predictors of dementia in Parkinson's disease: a community-based, 4-year longitudinal study. J Geriatr Psychiatry Neurol 18:149–154, 2005

Janvin CC, Larsen JP, Aarsland D, et al: Subtypes of mild cognitive impairment in Parkinson's disease: progression to dementia. Mov Disord 21:1343–1349, 2006

Jellinger K: The pedunculopontine nucleus in Parkinson's disease. J Neurol Neurosurg Psychiatry 51:540–543, 1988

Josiassen RC, Curry LM, Mancall EL: Development of neuropsychological deficits in Huntington's disease. Arch Neurol 40:791–796, 1983

Kalbe E, Calabrese P, Kohn N, et al: Screening for cognitive deficits in Parkinson's disease with the Parkinson neuropsychometric dementia assessment (PANDA) instrument. Parkinsonism Relat Disord 14:93–101, 2008

Koller WC: How accurately can Parkinson's disease be diagnosed? Neurology 42:6–16, 1992

Krack P, Batir A, Van Blercom N, et al: Five-year follow-up of bilateral stimulation of the subthalamic nucleus in advanced Parkinson's disease. N Engl J Med 13:1925–1934, 2003

Langbehn DR, Paulsen JS; Huntington Study Group: Predictors of diagnosis in Huntington disease. Neurology 68:1710–1717, 2007

Langston JW, Ballard PA, Tetrud JW, et al: Chronic parkinsonism in humans due to a product of meperidine analog synthesis. Science 219:979–980, 1983

Larsen JP, Dupont E, Tandberg E: Clinical diagnosis of Parkinson's disease: proposal of diagnostic subgroups classified at different levels of confidence. Acta Neurol Scand Suppl 89:242–251, 1994

Leentjens AF, Marinus J, Van Hilten JJ, et al: The contribution of somatic symptoms to the diagnosis of depression in Parkinson's disease: a discriminant analytic approach. J Neuropsychiatry Clin Neurosci 15:74–77, 2003a

Leentjens AF, Vreeling FW, Luijckx GJ, et al: SSRIs in the treatment of depression in Parkinson's disease. Int J Geriatr Psychiatry 18: 552–554, 2003b

Lippa CF, Duda JE, Grossman M, et al: DLB and PDD boundary issues: diagnosis, treatment, molecular pathology, and biomarkers. Neurology 68:812–819, 2007

Lishman WA: Senile dementias, presenile dementias, and pseudodementias, in Organic Psychiatry: The Psychological Consequences of Cerebral Disorder, 3rd Edition. Oxford, UK, Blackwell Science, 1998, pp 428–506

Llebaria G, Pagonabarraga J, Kulisevsky J, et al: Cut-off score of the Mattis Dementia Rating Scale for screening dementia in Parkinson's disease. Mov Disord 23:1546–1550, 2008

Mahieux F, Michelet D, Manifacier MJ, et al: Mini-Mental Parkinson: first validation study of a new bedside test constructed for Parkinson's disease. Behav Neurol 8:15–22, 1995

Mahieux F, Fénelon G, Flahault A, et al: Neuropsychological prediction of dementia in Parkinson's disease. J Neurol Neurosurg Psychiatry 64:178–183, 1998

Mamikonyan E, Siderowf AD, Duda JE, et al: Long-term follow-up of impulse control disorders in Parkinson's disease. Mov Disord 23:75–80, 2008

Mamikonyan E, Moberg PJ, Siderowf AD, et al: Mild cognitive impairment is common in Parkinson's disease patients with normal Mini-Mental State Examination (MMSE) scores. Parkinsonism Relat Disord 15:226–231, 2009

Marder K, Tang M-X, Cote L, et al: The frequency and associated risk factors for dementia in patients with Parkinson's disease. Arch Neurol 52:695–701, 1995

Marder K, Zhao H, Myers RH, et al: Rate of functional decline in Huntington's disease. Huntington Study Group. Neurology 54: 452–458, 2000

Marinus J, Visser M, Verwey NA, et al: Assessment of cognition in Parkinson's disease. Neurology 61:1222–1228, 2003

Mattis S: Dementia Rating Scale Professional Manual. Odessa, FL, Psychological Assessment Resources, 1973

Mayberg HS, Starkstein SE, Sadzot B, et al: Selective hypometabolism in the inferior frontal lobe in depressed patients with Parkinson's disease. Ann Neurol 28:57–64, 1990

Mayeux R, Marder K, Cote LJ, et al: The frequency of idiopathic Parkinson's disease by age, ethnic group, and sex in northern Manhattan, 1988–1993. Am J Epidemiol 142:820–827, 1995

McKeith IG, Dickson DS, Lowe J, et al: Diagnosis and management of dementia with Lewy bodies: third report of the DLB consortium. Neurology 65:1863–1872, 2005

Menza MA, Sage J, Marshall E, et al: Mood changes and "on-off" phenomena in Parkinson's disease. Mov Disord 5:148–151, 1990

Menza MA, Robertson-Hoffman DE, Bonapace AS: Parkinson's disease and anxiety: comorbidity with depression. Biol Psychiatry 34:465–470, 1993

Menza MA, Dobkin RD, Marin H, et al: A controlled trial of antidepressants in patients with Parkinson's disease and depression. Neurology 72:886–892, 2009

Middleton FA, Strick PL: Basal ganglia and cerebellar loops: motor and cognitive circuits. Brain Res Rev 31:236–250, 2000

Miyasaki JM, Martin W, Suchowersky O, et al: Practice parameter: initiation of treatment for Parkinson's disease: an evidence-based review: report of the Quality Standards Subcommittee of the American Academy of Neurology. Neurology 58:11–17, 2002

Miyasaki JM, Shannon K, Voon V, et al: Practice parameter: evaluation and treatment of depression, psychosis, and dementia in Parkinson disease (an evidence-based review). Report of the Quality Standards Subcommittee of the American Academy of Neurology. Neurology 66:996–1002, 2006

Moellentine C, Rummans T, Ahlskog JE, et al: Effectiveness of ECT in patients with parkinsonism. J Neuropsychiatry Clin Neurosci 10:187–193, 1998

Morens DM, Grandinetti A, Reed D, et al: Cigarette smoking and protection from Parkinson's disease: false association or etiologic clue. Neurology 45:1041–1051, 1995

Moskowitz CB, Marder K: Palliative care for people with late-stage Huntington's disease. Neurol Clin 19:849–865, 2001
Murai T, Muller U, Werheid K, et al: In vivo evidence for differential association of striatal dopamine and midbrain serotonin systems with neuropsychiatric symptoms in Parkinson's disease. J Neuropsychiatry Clin Neurosci13:222–228, 2001
Muslimovic D, Post B, Speelman JD, et al: Cognitive profile of patients with newly diagnosed Parkinson disease. Neurology 65: 1239–1245, 2005
Olanow CW, Watts RL, Koller WC: An algorithm (decision tree) for the management of Parkinson's disease (2001): treatment guidelines. Neurology 56(suppl):S1–S88, 2001
Ondo WG, Levy JK, Vuong KD, et al: Olanzapine treatment for dopaminergic-induced hallucinations. Mov Disord 17:1031–1035, 2002
Ondo WG, Tintner R, Voung KD, et al: Double-blind, placebo-controlled, unforced titration parallel trial of quetiapine for dopaminergic-induced hallucinations in Parkinson's disease. Mov Disord 20:958–963, 2005
Pagonabarraga J, Kulisevsky J, Llebaria G, et al: Parkinson's disease-cognitive rating scale: a new cognitive scale specific for Parkinson's disease. Mov Disord 23:998–1005, 2008
Parkinson Study Group: Low-dose clozapine for the treatment of drug-induced psychosis in Parkinson's disease. N Engl J Med 340:757–763, 1999
Parsons TD, Rogers SA, Braaten AJ, et al: Cognitive sequelae of subthalamic nucleus deep brain stimulation in Parkinson's disease: a meta-analysis. Lancet Neurol 5:578–588, 2006
Paulsen JS, Ready RE, Hamilton JM, et al: Neuropsychiatric aspects of Huntington's disease. J Neurol Neurosurg Psychiatry 71:310–314, 2001
Pavese N, Andrews TC, Brooks DJ, et al: Progressive striatal and cortical dopamine receptor dysfunction in Huntington's disease: a PET study. Brain 126:1127–1135, 2003
Piccirilli M, D'Alessandro P, Finali G, et al: Frontal lobe dysfunction in Parkinson's disease: prognostic value for dementia? Eur Neurol 29:71–76, 1989
Pollak P, Tison F, Rascol O, et al: Clozapine in drug induced psychosis in Parkinson's disease: a randomised, placebo controlled study with open follow up. J Neurol Neurosurg Psychiatry 75:689–695, 2004
Polymeropoulos MH, Lavedan C, Leroy E, et al: Mutation in the alpha-synuclein gene identified in families with Parkinson's disease. Science 276:2045–2047, 1997
Rabey JM, Prokhorov T, Miniovitz A, et al: Effect of quetiapine in psychotic Parkinson's disease patients: a double-blind labeled study of 3 months' duration. Mov Disord 22:313–318, 2007
Reid WG, Hely MA, Morris JG, et al: A longitudinal study of Parkinson's disease: clinical and neuropsychological correlates of dementia. J Clin Neurosci 3:327–333, 1996
Reijnders JS, Ehrt U, Weber WE, et al: A systematic review of prevalence studies of depression in Parkinson's disease. Mov Disord 23:183–189, 2008
Richard IH, Schiffer RB, Kurlan R: Anxiety and Parkinson's disease. J Neuropsychiatry Clin Neurosci 8:383–392, 1996
Richard IH, Kurlan R, Tanner C, et al: Serotonin syndrome and the combined use of deprenyl and an antidepressant in Parkinson's disease. Neurology 48:1070–1077, 1997
Rosas HD, Goodman J, Chen YI, et al: Striatal volume loss in HD as measured by MRI and the influence of CAG repeat. Neurology 57:1025–1028, 2001
Rosenblatt A, Ranen NG, Nance MA, et al: A Physician's Guide to the Management of Huntington's Disease, 2nd Edition. New York, Huntington's Disease Society of America, 1999
Roth M, Huppert F, Mountjoy C, et al: The Cambridge Examination for Mental Disorders of the Elderly—Revised. Cambridge, UK, Cambridge University Press, 1999
Rothlind JC, Brandt J: A brief assessment of frontal and subcortical functions in dementia. J Neuropsychiatry Clin Neurosci 5:73–77, 1993
Sammer G, Reuter I, Hullmann K, et al: Training of executive functions in Parkinson's disease. J Neurol Sci 248:115–119, 2006
Saugstad L, Odegard O: Huntington's chorea in Norway. Psychol Med 16:39–48, 1986
Schuurman AG, van den Akker M, Ensinck KT, et al: Increased risk of Parkinson's disease after depression. Neurology 58:1501–1504, 2002
Shiba M, Bower JH, Maraganore DM, et al: Anxiety disorders and depressive disorders preceding Parkinson's disease: a case-control study. Mov Disord 15:669–677, 2000
Shulman LM, Taback RL, Rabinstein AA, et al: Non-recognition of depression and other non-motor symptoms in Parkinson's disease. Parkinsonism Relat Disord 8:193–197, 2002
Sinforiani E, Banchieri L, Zucchella C, et al: Cognitive rehabilitation in Parkinson's disease. Arch Gerontol Geriatr Suppl 9:387–391, 2004
Starkstein SE, Mayberg HS, Leiguarda R, et al: A prospective longitudinal study of depression, cognitive decline, and physical impairments in patients with Parkinson's disease. J Neurol Neurosurg Psychiatry 55:377–382, 1992a
Starkstein SE, Mayberg HS, Preziosi TJ, et al: Reliability, validity, and clinical correlates of apathy in Parkinson's disease. J Neuropsychiatry Clin Neurosci 4:134–139, 1992b
Starkstein SE, Merello M, Jorge R, et al: The syndromic validity and nosological position of apathy in Parkinson's disease. Mov Disord 24:1211–1216, 2009
Tandberg E, Larsen JP, Karlsen K: Excessive daytime sleepiness and sleep benefit in Parkinson's disease: a community-based study. Mov Disord 14:922–927, 1999
Tanner CM, Goldman SM: Epidemiology of Parkinson's disease. Neurol Clin 14:317–333, 1996
Tröster AI: Neuropsychological characteristics of dementia with Lewy bodies and Parkinson's disease with dementia: differentiation, early detection, and implications for "mild cognitive impairment" and biomarkers. Neuropsychol Rev 18:103–119, 2008
Tröster AI, Fields JA: Parkinson's disease, progressive supranuclear palsy, corticobasal degeneration, and related disorders of the frontostriatal system, in Textbook of Clinical Neuropsychology. Edited by Morgan JE, Ricker JH. New York, Psychology Press, 2008, pp 536–577

Tröster AI, Stalp LD, Paolo AM, et al: Neuropsychological impairment in Parkinson's disease with and without depression. Arch Neurol 52:1164–1169, 1995

van Duijn E, Kingma EM, van der Mast RC: Psychopathology in verified Huntington's disease gene carriers. J Neuropsychiatry Clin Neurosci 19:441–448, 2007

Voon V, Fox SH: Medication-related impulse control and repetitive behaviors in Parkinson disease. Arch Neurol 64:1089–1096, 2007

Voon V, Kubu C, Krack P, et al: Deep brain stimulation: neuropsychological and neuropsychiatric issues. Mov Disord 21(suppl): S305–S326, 2006

Voon V, Krack P, Lang AE, et al: A multicentre study on suicide outcomes following subthalamic stimulation for Parkinson's disease. Brain 131:2720–2728, 2008

Walsh K, Bennett G: Parkinson's disease and anxiety. Postgrad Med J 77:89–93, 2001

Ward CD, Gibb WR: Research diagnostic criteria for Parkinson's disease. Adv Neurol 53:245–249, 1990

Weintraub D: Dopamine and impulse control disorders in Parkinson's disease. Ann Neurol 64(suppl):S93–S100, 2008

Weintraub D, Moberg PJ, Duda JE, et al: Recognition and treatment of depression in Parkinson's disease. J Geriatr Psychiatry Neurol 16:178–183, 2003

Weintraub D, Morales KH, Moberg PJ, et al: Antidepressant studies in Parkinson's disease: a review and meta-analysis. Mov Disord 20:1161–1169, 2005

Weintraub D, Oehlberg KA, Katz IR, et al: Test characteristics of the 15-item geriatric depression scale and Hamilton depression rating scale in Parkinson's disease. Am J Geriatr Psychiatry 14:169–175, 2006

Wermuth L, Sørensen PS, Timm S, et al: Depression in idiopathic Parkinson's disease treated with citalopram: a placebo-controlled trial. Nord J Psychiatry 52:163–169, 1998

Wheelock VL, Tempkin T, Marder K, et al: Predictors of nursing home placement in Huntington disease. Neurology 60:998–1001, 2003

Wint DP, Okun MS, Fernandez HH: Psychosis in Parkinson's disease. J Geriatr Psychiatry Neurol 17:127–136, 2004

Witjas T, Kaphan E, Azulay JP, et al: Nonmotor fluctuations in Parkinson's disease: frequent and disabling. Neurology 59:408–413, 2002

Wolters EC: Dopaminomimetic psychosis in Parkinson's disease patients: diagnosis and treatment. Neurology 52(suppl):S10–S13, 1999

Wolters EC: Intrinsic and extrinsic psychosis in Parkinson's disease. J Neurol 248(suppl):22–27, 2001

Wolters EC, Hurwitz TA, Mak E, et al: Clozapine in the treatment of parkinsonian patients with dopaminomimetic psychosis. Neurology 40:832–834, 1990

Woods SP, Tröster AI: Prodromal frontal/executive dysfunction predicts incident dementia in Parkinson's disease. J Int Neuropsychol Soc 9:17–24, 2003

25

Cerebrovascular Disease

Robert G. Robinson, M.D.
Ricardo E. Jorge, M.D.

The group of cerebrovascular diseases that includes both 1) sudden-onset ischemia of the brain due to thrombosis or emboli and 2) hemorrhagic bleeds within the brain parenchyma or subdural or epidural regions usually due to aneurysms or trauma constitutes some of the most common life-threatening problems among the elderly population in the United States. Stroke, defined as a sudden loss of blood supply to the brain leading to permanent tissue damage caused by thrombotic, embolic, or hemorrhagic events, ranks as the third leading cause of death (behind only heart disease and cancer) in patients over age 50 (Lloyd-Jones et al. 2010). Stroke is the leading cause of long-term disability in the world and accounts for half of all the acute hospitalizations for neurological disorder. According to the American Heart Association (2010), there are 795,000 strokes annually in the United States and 6.4 million stroke survivors. Among individuals over age 75 years, 10% are stroke survivors (Thom et al. 2006). Although the annual incidence of stroke declined from about 1945 to 1975, due to improved control of hypertension, several investigators have reported increased incidence of stroke in the 1980s and 1990s. Pessah-Rasmussen et al. (2003), for example, reported in 1998 that the age-standardized incidence of stroke in Malmö, Sweden, was 647 per 100,000 for men and 400 per 100,000 for women. The annual incidence had increased by 3.1% in men and 2.9% in women between 1989 and 1998.

The psychiatric complications of stroke lesions, although recognized for more than 100 years (Kraepelin 1921), have never received the attention that has been devoted to poststroke motor deficits, language problems, or intellectual disturbances. These behavioral and emotional disorders, however, have been shown to significantly impair the physical (Parikh et al. 1990) and cognitive recovery and to increase the long-term mortality (House et al. 2001) of stroke patients. Everson et al. (1998) examined the association between depression symptoms and stroke mortality in a prospective 29-year study of behavioral, social, and psychological factors related to health and mortality in a community sample. They confirmed a significant relationship between depressive symptoms and stroke mortality.

In this chapter, we discuss the most frequent emotional-behavioral sequelae of stroke lesions. Some of these psychiatric complications of stroke, such as depression, have been the focus of intense research, whereas other complications, such as anxiety or emotional lability, have not been characterized as well.

Poststroke Depression

Diagnosis

The method for diagnosis of depression among patients with stroke is to conduct a structured or semistructured mental status examination using instruments such as the Structured Clinical Interview for DSM-IV (SCID; Spitzer et al. 1995) or the Composite International Diagnostic Interview (CIDI; Robins et al. 1988). The type of symptoms elicited by either of these structured interviews and the severity and duration of symptoms are applied to DSM-IV (American Psychiatric Association 1994) diagnostic criteria for *mood disorder due to a general medical condition with major depressive-like episode.* This diagnosis requires the presence of either depressed mood or loss of interest and a total of five of the nine criteria used for diagnosis of major depression with distress or impairment in social, occupational, or other functioning and not related to bereavement. Although DSM-IV includes a second subtype—*mood disorder due to a general medical condition with depressive features*—this does not require any specific diagnostic criteria, and we have therefore chosen not to use this very nonspecific diagnostic category.

To diagnose patients with less severe depressive disorders, we have used the research criteria from DSM-IV for *minor depression.* This subsyndromal form of major depression requires at least two but fewer than five symptoms of major depression, as well as the other duration and functional impairment diagnostic criteria. Symptoms must have lasted for at least 2 weeks, and at least one of the symptoms is either depressed mood or loss of interest or pleasure. Spalletta et al. (2005) compared the frequency of specific depressive symptoms among 50 patients with major depression, 62 with minor depression, and 88 nondepressed patients. Symptoms were elicited using the Structured Clinical Interview for DSM-IV Axis I Disorders—Patient Edition (SCID-P). Results showed that the three groups differed significantly in the frequency of every symptom. After correction for multiple comparisons, however, symptoms of self-blame and guilt failed to differentiate the three groups, although all other symptoms did. Furthermore, patients with minor depression had significantly higher frequency of depressed mood, loss of energy, insomnia, and psychomotor disturbance compared with nondepressed patients with stroke. Thus, we believe the most useful categories for poststroke depression (PSD) are 1) mood disorder due to stroke with major depressive-like episode and 2) mood disorder due to stroke with minor depression.

Prevalence

The prevalence of PSD (both major and minor depression) has been assessed in a large number of patients throughout the world who have been examined in various clinical settings. Based on the world's literature, the current number of patients who were examined for depression following stroke exceeds 6,000. Several factors, however, have complicated the assessment of prevalence rates:

- The first is the setting in which patients were examined. Community studies have generally reported somewhat lower prevalence rates than studies done in rehabilitation hospitals, outpatient settings, or acute hospital settings.
- Second, patients with comprehension deficits due to fluent or global aphasias have been excluded from some or all studies of PSD. Furthermore, patients with hemorrhagic rather than ischemic stroke, decreased level of consciousness, fatigue, atypical strokes, or other systemic illness have often been excluded. Although some investigators have tried to estimate the frequency of depression in some of these patients, such as those with comprehension deficits due to fluent global aphasia (Damecour and Caplan 1991), no reliable method has been devised to examine patients who are unable to reliably respond to verbal interview. Examiners' judgments about whether a patient is depressed, depending on observations of the patient's behavior—such as having difficulty falling asleep, waking up early in the morning, not eating, losing weight, frequent tearfulness, social withdrawal, or acts of self-harm—are often unreliable and have not been validated as a method of diagnosing depression.
- The third factor that has led to variability in reported prevalence rates for PSD is the use of cutoff scores on depression rating scales to determine the existence of depression.

The gold standard for diagnosis of depression is conducting a structured interview and applying the findings to established diagnostic criteria.

The prevalence rates from depression studies reported in the literature, grouped according to the setting in which the patient was examined, are shown in Table 25–1. The lowest prevalence rates were depressive disorder found in patients studied in community settings, where 14% of the patients were found to have major depression and 9% to have minor depression. In acute hospitals or rehabilitation hospitals, the mean prevalence rates were 22% for major depression and 20% for minor depression. In outpatient settings, in which patients were studied for 3 months to 3 or more years following stroke, the prevalence rates for both major and minor depression were 24%.

Based on prevalence estimates by the American Heart Association, there are 6.4 million U.S. stroke survivors (Lloyd-Jones et al. 2010), suggesting that there may be 2.6 million patients presently with PSD in the United States—almost half of these cases being major depression. Also, more than 3 million of these patients likely have been depressed at some time since their initial stroke. Although the financial impact of this number of patients impaired by stroke and depression has not been studied, the enormity of the problem is obvious from these findings.

Duration of Depression

Morris et al. (1990) found that among a group of 99 patients in a stroke rehabilitation hospital in Australia, those with major depression had a mean duration of 40 weeks, whereas those with minor depression (termed *adjustment disorder* by Morris et al.) had a mean duration of only 12 weeks. Aström et al. (1993) found that among 80 patients with acute stroke, 27 (34%) developed major depression in the hospital or by 3-month follow-up. Of these patients with major depression, 15 (60%) had recovered by 1-year follow-up, but only 1 more patient had recovered by 3-year follow-up. This finding indicates that a significant minority of patients may develop severe and prolonged depressive episodes following stroke.

Two factors have been identified that influence the natural course of PSD: 1) treatment of depression with antidepressants and 2) lesion location. Treatment with antidepressants is

TABLE 25–1. Prevalence studies of poststroke depression

Investigators	Patient population	*N*	Criteria	Major depression (%)	Minor depression (%)	Total (%)
Community studies						
Wade et al. 1987	Community	379	Cutoff score			22
House et al. 1991	Community	89	PSE, DSM-III	11	12	23
Burvill et al. 1995	Community	294	PSE, DSM-III	15	8	23
Kotila et al. 1998	Community	321	Cutoff score			44
Hayee et al. 2001	Community	161	Cutoff score, BDI, 3 months			41
		156	Cutoff score, BDI, 12 months			42
Stewart et al. 2001	Community	287	Cutoff score, GDS			19
Desmond et al. 2003	Community	421	Cutoff score, SIGH-D			11
Pooled data means for community studies		2,108		14.1	9.1	25.9
Acute hospital studies						
Robinson et al. merged data (1983–1990)	Acute hospital	278	PSE, DSM-IV	27	20	47
Ebrahim et al. 1987	Acute hospital	149	Cutoff score			23
Aström et al. 1993	Acute hospital	80	DSM-III	25	NR	25[a]
Herrmann et al. 1993	Acute hospital	21	RDC	24	14	38
Andersen et al. 1994b	Acute hospital or outpatient	285	Cutoff score, Ham-D	10	11	21
Shima et al. 1994	Hospital 1–2 months			9		9
Gonzalez-Torrecillas et al. 1995	Hospital	130	SADS, RDC	26	11	37
Gainotti et al. 1999	Acute or rehabilitation hospital	153	PSDRS	31	NR	31
Kauhanen et al. 1999	Stroke unit 3 months	106	DSM-III-R	9	44	53

TABLE 25–1. Prevalence studies of poststroke depression *(continued)*

Investigators	Patient population	*N*	Criteria	Major depression (%)	Minor depression (%)	Total (%)
Acute hospital studies (*continued*)						
Palomäki et al. 1999	Hospital	100	DSM-III-R	6		6
Singh et al. 2000	Acute hospital 3 months	81	Cutoff score, ZDS, MADRS	26	27	53
House et al. 2001	Acute hospital	448	ICD-10	22	NR	22+
Aben et al. 2002	Acute hospital	190	SCID, DSM-IV	23	16	39
Berg et al. 2003	Acute hospital 2 weeks	89	Cutoff score, BDI			27
Pooled data means for acute hospital studies		2,178		22.1	17.3	31.6
Rehabilitation hospital studies						
Folstein et al. 1977	Rehabilitation hospital	20	PSE and items			45
Finklestein et al. 1982	Rehabilitation hospital	25	Cutoff score			48
Sinyor et al. 1986	Rehabilitation hospital	64	Cutoff score			47
Eastwood et al. 1989	Rehabilitation hospital	87	SADS, RDC	10	40	50
Finset et al. 1989	Rehabilitation hospital	42	Cutoff score			36
Morris et al. 1990	Rehabilitation hospital	99	CIDI, DSM-III	14	21	35
Schubert et al. 1992	Rehabilitation hospital	18	DSM-III-R	28	44	72
Schwartz et al. 1993	Rehabilitation hospital	91	DSM-III	40	NR	40[a]
Cassidy et al. 2004	Rehabilitation hospital	50	DSM-IV	20	NR	20+
Pooled data for rehabilitation hospital studies		591		19.3	30.4	40.8+
Pooled data for acute and rehabilitation hospital studies		2,769		21.6	20.0	33.6

TABLE 25–1. Prevalence studies of poststroke depression *(continued)*

Investigators	Patient population	*N*	Criteria	Major depression (%)	Minor depression (%)	Total (%)
Outpatient studies						
Feibel and Springer 1982	Outpatient 6 months	91	Nursing evaluation			26
Robinson and Price 1982	Outpatient 6 months–10 years	103	Cutoff score			29
Robinson et al. 1983–1990	Merged data 3 months	77	DSM-IV	17	27	44
	6 months	79	DSM-IV	20	27	47
	12 months	70	DSM-IV	10	24	34
	24 months	66	DSM-IV	24	15	39
Collin et al. 1987	Outpatient	111	Cutoff score			42
Aström et al. 1993	Outpatient 3 months	77	DSM-III	31	NR	31[a]
	1 year	73	DSM-III	16	NR	16[a]
	2 years	57	DSM-III	19	NR	19[a]
	3 years	49	DSM-III	29	NR	29[a]
Castillo et al. 1995	Outpatient 3 months	77	PSE, DSM-III	20	13	33
	6 months	80	PSE, DSM-III	21	21	42
	1 year	70	PSE, DSM-III	11	16	27
	2 years	67	PSE, DSM-III	18	17	35
Herrmann et al. 1998	Outpatient	150	MADRS, ZDS			27
Pohjasvaara et al. 1998	Outpatient	277	PSE, DSM-III-R	26	14	40
Gainotti et al. 1999	Outpatient <2 months	58	DSM-III-R	27	NR	27+
	2–4 months	52	DSM-III-R	27	NR	27
	>4 months	43	DSM-III-R	40	NR	40+
Kauhanen et al. 1999	Outpatient 1 year	92	DSM-III-R	16	26	42

TABLE 25–1. Prevalence studies of poststroke depression *(continued)*

Investigators	Patient population	*N*	Criteria	Major depression (%)	Minor depression (%)	Total (%)
Outpatient studies (*continued*)						
Palomäki et al. 1999	Outpatient 12 months	44	DSM-III-R	11	NR	11
	18 months	44	DSM-III-R	16	NR	16
Kim and Choi-Kwon 2000	Outpatient 2–4 months	148	DSM-IV, BDI, poststroke emotional incontinence	18	NR	18
Singh et al. 2000	Outpatient 1 year	136	Cutoff score, MADRS, ZDS			22
Pooled data for outpatient studies		2,191		24.0	23.9	31.5+
Pooled data for all studies		7,068		21.7	19.5	30.6

Note. BDI=Beck Depression Inventory; CIDI=Composite International Diagnostic Interview; DSM-III=Diagnostic and Statistical Manual of Mental Disorders, 3rd Edition; DSM-III-R=Diagnostic and Statistical Manual of Mental Disorders, 3rd Edition, Revised; DSM-IV=Diagnostic and Statistical Manual of Mental Disorders, 4th Edition; GDS= Geriatric Depression Scale; Ham-D=Hamilton Rating Scale for Depression; ICD-10= International Statistical Classification of Diseases and Related Health Problems, 10th Revision; MADRS= Montgomery-Åsberg Depression Rating Scale; NR=not reported; PSDRS=Poststroke Depression Rating Scale; PSE=Present State Examination; RDC=Research Diagnostic Criteria; SADS=Schedule for Affective Disorders and Schizophrenia; SCAN=Schedules for Clinical Assessment in Neuropsychiatry; SCID= Structured Clinical Interview for DSM-IV; SIGH-D=Structured Interview Guide for the Hamilton Depression Rating Scale; ZDS=Zung Self-Rating Depression Scale.

[a]Because minor depression was not included, these values may be low.

Source. Robinson RG: *The Clinical Neuropsychiatry of Stroke: Cognitive, Behavioral and Emotional Disorders Following Vascular Brain Injury,* Second Edition. New York, Cambridge University Press, 2006. Copyright © 2006 R. Robinson. Reprinted with permission of Cambridge University Press.

discussed later in this chapter in "Association With Physical Impairment" and "Association With Cognitive Impairment." Regarding lesion location, Starkstein et al. (1988a) compared two groups of depressed patients. One group had spontaneously recovered from depression by 6 months after stroke (n=6), whereas the other group remained depressed through the 6-month follow-up (n=10). There were no known significant between-group differences in background variables such as age, sex, and education, and both groups had similar levels of social functioning and degrees of cognitive impairment. There were, however, two significant between-group differences. One was lesion location: the recovered group had a higher frequency of subcortical and cerebellar or brain stem lesions, whereas the nonrecovered group had a higher frequency of cortical lesions (P<0.01). Impairments in activities of daily living (ADLs) were also significantly different between the two groups. The nonrecovered group had significantly more impairments in ADLs in the hospital than did the recovered group.

Thus, PSD is not a transient but is usually a prolonged depression with a natural course of 9–10 months for most cases of major depression, although depression lasting more than 3 years does occur in some patients with major or minor depression. Lesion location and severity of associated impairments may influence the longitudinal course of PSD.

Relationship to Lesion Variables

The relationship between depressive disorder and lesion location has been perhaps the most controversial area of research in the field of PSD. Although establishing an association between specific clinical symptoms and lesion location is one of the fundamental goals in neurology, this has rarely been the case in psychiatric disorders. Numerous studies, however, have found a significant association between lesion location and the development of PSD, particularly during the first few months following stroke (Aström et al. 1993; Morris et al. 1996). Furthermore, based on both structural and functional imaging studies of patients with mood disorders not associated with stroke, a hypothesis has emerged that the cortical-basal ganglia-thalamic circuits are the likely mediators of mood disorders among patients with or without brain injury. Inputs from the dorsal lateral cortex, the orbital frontal cortex, the anterior cingulate, the temporal cortex, and the amygdala and hippocampus are known to have input to the striatum with connections through the pallidum to the thalamus and back to the frontal cortical regions. Similarly, treatment studies utilizing rapid transcranial magnetic stimulation or electroconvulsive therapy (ECT) have both found that stimulation of the left hemisphere produces a significantly better response than unilateral stimulation of the right hemisphere (Fregni et al. 2006). These findings have generally supported the original observation in patients with stroke that mood disorders involve injury or dysfunction to frontal regions of the left hemisphere.

The first report of a significant correlation between lesion location and PSD was an investigation by Robinson and Szetela (1981) examining 29 patients with left hemisphere brain injury secondary to stroke (n=18) or traumatic brain injury (n=11). Based on localization of lesion by computed tomography, a significant inverse correlation was found between the severity of depression and the distance of the anterior border of the lesion from the frontal pole in the left hemisphere (r=−0.76). A number of other studies have subsequently found similar correlations. A meta-analysis by Narushima et al. (2003) found eight independent studies of severity of depression and proximity of lesion to the left or right frontal pole that were conducted within 6 months following stroke. Of the 163 patients with left hemisphere stroke, the combined correlation coefficient was −0.53 using fixed and −0.59 using random model assumptions (P<0.001). For the 106 patients with right hemisphere lesions, the combined correlation between severity of depression and distance of the lesion from the right frontal pole was nonsignificant (r=−0.20 fixed model; r=−0.23 random model).

Lesion location has also been found to be related to the prevalence of depression following stroke. In a study of 45 patients who were on average 2–3 weeks poststroke with single lesions restricted to either subcortical or cortical structures in either the right or left hemisphere, Starkstein et al. (1987b) found that 44% of patients with left cortical lesions were depressed, whereas 39% with left subcortical lesions, 11% with right cortical lesions, and 14% with right subcortical lesions were depressed. In a subsequent study, Starkstein et al. (1988b) examined the relationship between lesions of specific subcortical nuclei and depression. Basal ganglia (caudate and or putamen) lesions produced major depression in 7 of 8 patients with lesions in the left hemisphere, compared with only 1 of 7 patients having a similar lesion location in the right hemisphere and none of the 10 patients with thalamic lesions (P<0.001). On the basis of these findings and those of other investigators, Robinson (2006) conducted a meta-analysis of studies done within 2 months following stroke comparing the frequency of major depression among patients with left anterior versus left posterior lesions and left anterior versus right anterior lesions. Among 128 patients in the left anterior versus left posterior comparison, the odds ratio for depression was 2.29 (95% confidence interval [CI], 1.6–3.4, P<0.001) using the fixed model assumptions and the odds ratio was 2.29 (95% CI, 1.5–3.4, P<0.001) using the random model assumptions. Similarly, the comparison of left and right anterior lesions had an odds ratio of 2.18 for the fixed model (95% CI, 1.4–3.3, P<0.001) and 2.16 for the random model (95% CI 1.3–3.6, P<0.004).

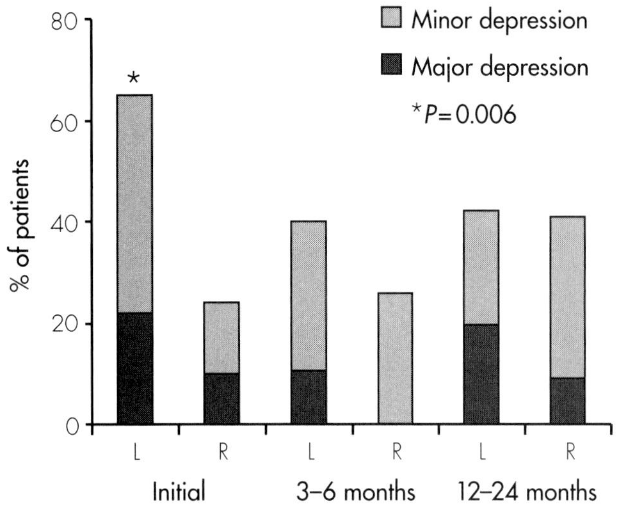

FIGURE 25–1. Frequency of major and minor depression defined by DSM-IV criteria associated with single lesions of the left (L) or right (R) hemisphere during the acute stroke period and at follow-up.

The lateralized effect of left hemisphere lesions on both major and minor depression was found only during the acute stroke period. At 3–6 months and 12–24 months follow-up, there were no hemispheric lesion effects on the frequency of depression.

Source. Robinson RG: *The Clinical Neuropsychiatry of Stroke: Cognitive, Behavioral and Emotional Disorders Following Vascular Brain Injury,* Second Edition. New York, Cambridge University Press, 2006. Copyright © 2006 R. Robinson. Reprinted with permission of Cambridge University Press.

Robinson's (2006) meta-analysis suggested that the failure of some investigators to replicate the association of left anterior lesion location with an increased frequency of depression may, in most cases, be related to time since stroke. The lateralized effect of left anterior lesions on both major and minor depression is a phenomenon of the acute poststroke period (Figure 25–1), when patients are less than 2 months poststroke. A review of stroke by Bhogal et al. (2004) concluded that the association between left hemisphere lesion location and PSD depended on both when patients were examined following stroke (i.e., within the first 2 months or during the chronic poststroke period) and whether patients were examined as inpatients or community patients (i.e., the severity of stroke impairment is significantly greater among inpatients than among patients living in the community).

Association With Physical Impairment

Numerous investigators have reported a significant association between depression and functional physical impairment (i.e., ADLs). Of 18 studies involving 3,281 patients, 15 (83%) found a statistically significant relationship between the severity or existence of PSD and severity of impairment in ADLs. Whether this association is construed as the severe functional impairment producing depression or alternatively as the severe depression producing greater severity of functional impairment has not been determined. Studies, in fact, support both interpretations. Sinyor et al. (1986) was the first to report that depression influenced recovery in ADLs. Nondepressed stroke patients were found to show either a slight improvement or no change in functional status from the acute poststroke period to 1-month follow-up, whereas depressed patients showed a significant decline in ADLs during the first month. In another study, Parikh et al. (1990) compared a consecutive series of 25 patients with major or minor depression during the acute stroke period with 38 nondepressed stroke patients and examined their amount of recovery at 2-year follow-up. Although both groups had similar impairments in ADLs during the time they were in the hospital, the depressed patients had significantly less improvement at the 2-year follow-up than did the nondepressed patients. This finding was independent of the type and amount of in-hospital rehabilitation therapy, size or location of the lesion, patients' demographic characteristics, nature of the stroke, occurrence of another stroke during the follow-up period, and patients' medical history. Similar results were reported by Pohjasvaara et al. (2001), who found that among 256 patients, those with depression at 3 months had a Rankin Scale score of >2 (i.e., significant residual motor impairment) at 15 months compared with nondepressed patients (odds ratio [OR] 2.5, 95% CI, 1.6–3.8, $P<0.01$). A review by Hackett and Anderson (2005) reported that 9 of 11 studies that assessed physical disability found that greater physical impairment was significantly associated with a greater frequency of depression compared with no depression following stroke.

The effect of treatment on recovery in ADLs was examined by Narushima and Robinson (2003), who compared 34 patients who received antidepressant treatment with either nortriptyline (100 mg/day) or fluoxetine (40 mg/day) for 12 weeks beginning 19±25 (±SD) days after stroke, and 28 patients who received the same antidepressants but began at 140±28 days poststroke. There were no significant differences between the groups in age, education, lesion volume, lesion location, or amount of rehabilitation services. During the period from 6 to 24 months following stroke, the two groups were matched for time since stroke. There was a significant group×time interaction using either intention to treat or efficacy analysis (Figure 25–2). The early-treatment group continued to show gradual recovery in ADLs over 2 years, whereas the late-treatment group showed gradual deterioration between 12-month and 24-month follow-ups. Logistic regression analysis examining the effects of diagnosis (i.e., depressed or nondepressed), medication (i.e., fluoxetine or nortriptyline), presence of severe motor impairment (i.e., National Institutes of Health Stroke Scale rating of greater or less than 15), presence or absence of prior psychiatric history, use of antidepressants beyond the 12-week study period, and use of early versus late antidepressant treatment, showed that only early versus late antidepressant use was an independent predictor of ADL scores at 2-year follow-up.

Thus, antidepressant treatment of depression appears to significantly influence recovery in ADLs; however, early treatment within the first month poststroke appears to be significantly more effective than delayed treatment. It should also be noted that this effect was independent of the existence of depression. Thus, both depressed and nondepressed patients given antidepressants within the first month after stroke improved in their ADLs more than did patients given antidepressants after the first month following stroke.

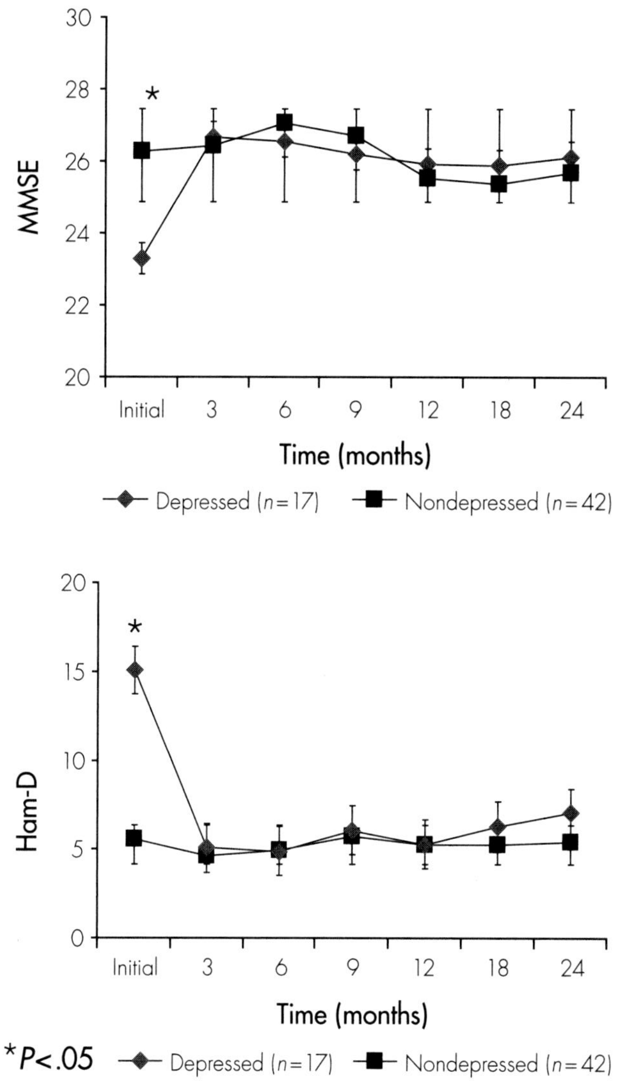

FIGURE 25–2. Scores over 2 years on the Mini-Mental State Examination (MMSE) and Hamilton Rating Scale for Depression (Ham-D) for patients whose poststroke depression remitted after treatment and for nondepressed stroke patients.

*Repeated-measures analysis of variance showed significant group-by-time interactions for scores on both the MMSE ($F_{6,52}$=2.46, P=0.04) and Ham-D ($F_{6,52}$=13.99, P<0.01).

Source. Reprinted from Narushima K, Chan KL, Kosier JT, et al.: "Does Cognitive Recovery After Treatment of Poststroke Depression Last? A 2-Year Follow-Up of Cognitive Function Associated With Poststroke Depression." *American Journal of Psychiatry* 160:1157–1162, 2003. Copyright © 2003 American Psychiatric Association. Used with permission.

Association With Cognitive Impairment

Numerous investigators have reported that elderly patients with functional major depression (i.e., depression without brain injury) have cognitive deficits that improve with treatment of depression (i.e., dementia of depression). Among patients with PSD, this issue was examined by Robinson et al. (1986), who found that patients with major depression following a left hemisphere stroke had significantly more impairment on the Mini-Mental State Examination (MMSE) than did a comparable group of nondepressed patients. Both the size of the patient's lesion and the severity of depression correlated independently with severity of cognitive impairment. In a follow-up study, Starkstein et al. (1988c) reported that stroke patients with major depression, who were matched for both lesion location and lesion volume with nondepressed patients who had comparable levels of education, had significantly lower (i.e., more impaired) MMSE scores.

Morris et al. (1990), Downhill and Robinson (1994), and Spalletta et al. (2002) also reported a similar phenomenon. In Spalletta et al.'s (2002) study, among 153 patients with first ever stroke lesions of the left (n=87) or right (n=66) hemisphere who were <1 year poststroke, patients with left hemisphere lesions and major depression (n=30) showed significantly more impairment on the MMSE than did nondepressed patients with left hemisphere lesions (n=27) (Figure 25–3).

Treatment studies of PSD have consistently failed to show an improvement in cognitive function even when poststroke mood disorders responded to antidepressant therapy. Kimura et al. (2000), however, examined this issue in a study of patients with major (n=33) or minor (n=14) PSD, comparing patients taking nortriptyline or placebo using double-blind methodology. When patients were divided into those who responded to treatment (i.e., >50% decline in Hamilton Rating Scale for Depression [Ham-D] score) and those who did not respond, there was a significantly greater improvement in MMSEs among patients who responded to treatment (n=24) than among patients who did not respond to treatment (n=23). A repeated-measures analysis of variance (ANOVA) demonstrated a signif-

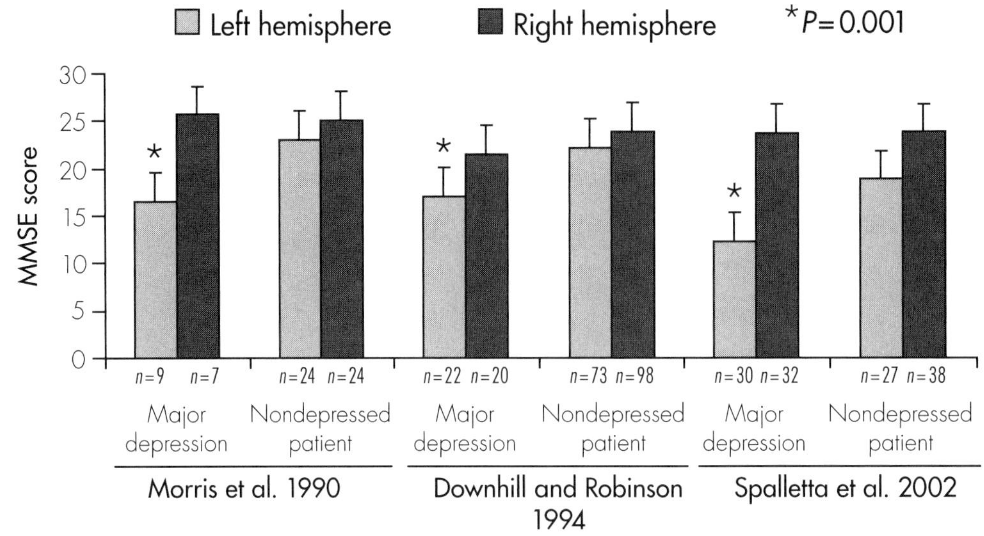

FIGURE 25–3. Mini-Mental State Examination (MMSE) scores following acute stroke in three studies among patients with major or no mood disturbance grouped according to the hemisphere of ischemia.

In all three studies, there was a significant difference between patients with major depression following left hemisphere stroke and nondepressed patients with similar lesions (P=0.001). Major depression following right hemisphere lesions did not lead to the same phenomenon.

Source. Robinson RG: *The Clinical Neuropsychiatry of Stroke: Cognitive, Behavioral and Emotional Disorders Following Vascular Brain Injury,* Second Edition. New York, Cambridge University Press, 2006. Copyright © 2006 R. Robinson. Reprinted with permission of Cambridge University Press.

icant group×time interaction, with responders having significantly less impaired MMSE scores than nonresponders at nortriptyline dosages of 75 mg (P=0.036) and 100 mg (P=0.024). When the effect of major versus minor depression was examined, patients with major depression who responded to treatment (n=15) showed significantly greater improvement in MMSE scores than did patients with major depression who did not respond (n=18, P=0.009). Among patients with minor depression (9 responders and 5 nonresponders), a repeated-measures ANOVA of MMSE scores showed no significant group ×time interaction.

The fact that earlier treatment studies did not show a significant effect of treatment of depression on cognitive function was the result of effect size. When nortriptyline-treated patients, some of whom responded to treatment and some of whom did not, were compared with those taking placebo, some of whom responded and some of whom did not, the effect size was only 0.16 (Kimura et al. 2000). When patients were divided into those who responded and those who did not respond, the effect size increased to 0.96, thus allowing a significant difference to be demonstrated with a much smaller group size.

Association With Mortality

Increased mortality is perhaps the ultimate validation of the importance of depression in the prognosis following stroke. The first study to examine mortality associated with PSD was reported by Morris et al. (1993). At 10-year follow-up, mortality status was obtained for 91 of 103 patients who were initially examined following acute stroke. The 48 (53%) patients who had died were compared with those who had survived. Patients with acute PSD were three to four times more likely to have died during 10 years of follow-up than were patients who were not depressed after the acute stroke (OR=3.4, 95% CI=1.4–8.4, P=0.007). Furthermore, the frequency of death among patients with a diagnosis of major versus minor depression at the time of the acute stroke was identical (i.e., 70%). The survival curves for the depressed and nondepressed patients over 10-year follow-up are shown in Figure 25–4. A differential rate of mortality was evident as early as the first year following stroke and continued to diverge for ~7 years before the survival curves were parallel from years 7 to 10. Because many factors may be associated with mortality following stroke, a multiple logistic regression was carried out examining factors of age, marital status, gender, social class, social ties, social functioning, MMSE score, ADLs, alcohol use, medical comorbidity, type of stroke, hemispheric and cortical-subcortical lesion location, volume of lesion, severity of impairment, and severity of depression on the likelihood of survival over 10 years. After controlling for these variables, depression severity was independently associated with mortality

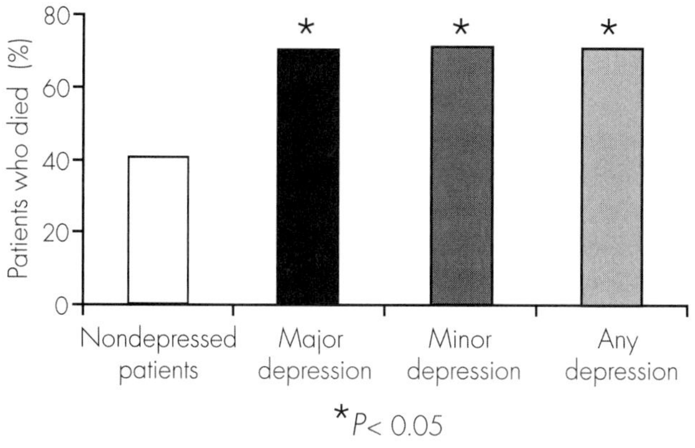

FIGURE 25–4. Percentage of patients with stroke who died within 10 years following stroke.

Patients are grouped according to their depression diagnosis at the time of the initial poststroke evaluation. Both major and minor depression were associated with significantly more deaths compared with no depression, even though by 2-year follow-up, patients with in-hospital major depression and nondepressed patients were not significantly different in their Hamilton depression scores.

Source. Robinson RG: *The Clinical Neuropsychiatry of Stroke: Cognitive, Behavioral and Emotional Disorders Following Vascular Brain Injury,* Second Edition. New York, Cambridge University Press, 2006. Copyright © 2006 R. Robinson. Reprinted with permission of Cambridge University Press.

(adjusted OR=3.7, 95% CI=1.1–12.2, P=0.03). Furthermore, depression and fewer social ties had added effects on mortality. Patients who were both depressed and had fewer social ties had the highest mortality (12 of 13 patients, 92%). Patients who were not depressed and had a higher-than-average number of social ties had the lowest mortality (15 of 39 patients, 38%). The other independent factors associated with mortality were history of alcohol abuse and lesion volume.

House et al. (2001) examined 448 hospitalized patients 1 month following acute stroke with follow-up at 12 and 24 months. Mood symptoms were assessed using the semistructured Present State Examination (PSE) and the 28-item General Health Questionnaire (GHQ-28). At 12-month follow-up, 45 of the 446 patients who could be identified had died. Causes of death included recurrent stroke (37.8%), cardiovascular disease (22.2%), and other causes (40%). The odds ratio for mortality was 3.1 between the lowest and the highest scoring quartiles based on GHQ-28 scores, with a mortality rate of 5% in the lowest quartile (i.e., least depressed) and 14% in the highest quartile. Furthermore, those scoring 1 or more on the depression subscale of the GHQ-28 (i.e., the 3 items examining depressive symptoms) had an odds ratio of mortality 2.4 times greater than patients who scored zero on the depression subscale. Multiple logistic regression showed that a GHQ-28 severe depression subscale score above 0, greater age, lower MMSE scores, and lower poststroke scores on the Barthel Index were all independently associated with risk of dying within 12 months following stroke. At 24 months, 65% of the remaining 446 who could be identified had died. A similar multiple logistic regression analysis found that a GHQ-28 severe depression subscale score of ≥1 remained statistically significantly related to mortality, as did older age and MMSE scores of <24.

The largest poststroke mortality risk study was a retrospective study conducted by Williams et al. (2004), who reviewed the records of 151,119 veterans hospitalized for ischemic stroke who survived more than 30 days. Within 3 years following stroke, 2,405 had a diagnosis of depression and 2,257 had other psychiatric diagnoses (primarily substance abuse or anxiety disorder). Of the depressed patients, 59% were alive at 6 years, whereas 58.7% of the patients with substance abuse and anxiety disorders and 63% of the patients with no depression or substance abuse diagnosis were alive (hazard ratio 1.13, 95% CI, 1.06–1.21, P<0.01 for depression). Other factors associated with mortality were younger age, white race, and heart disease such as myocardial infarction, congestive heart failure, and atrial fibrillation. The obvious shortcoming of this retrospective review is the low rate of depression (5%), which suggests that depression was missed in many patients.

Thus, PSD appears to be a significant risk factor for increased death as early as 1 year and as late as 7 years following stroke. The mechanism that produces these increased death rates has not been determined, although significant evidence among patients with heart disease suggests that depression leading to decreased heart rate variability, which then leads to fatal cardiac arrhythmia, seems to play a significant role in the increased death rate among patients with depression and heart disease such as myocardial infarction (Carney et al. 1995).

Treatment

Eight placebo-controlled, randomized, double-blind treatment studies have been done on the efficacy of single antidepressant treatment of PSD (Table 25–2). In the earliest such study, conducted by Lipsey et al. (1984), 14 patients were treated with nortriptyline and 20 patients were given placebo. The 11 patients treated with nortriptyline who completed the 6-week study with dosages increasing from 25 to 100 mg showed significantly greater improvement in Ham-D scores than did the 15 placebo-treated patients who completed the study (P<0.01). Successfully treated patients had serum nortriptyline levels of 50–150 ng/mL. Three patients experienced side effects (delirium confusion, drowsiness, agitation) that were severe enough to require the discontinuation of the

TABLE 25–2. Double-blind, placebo-controlled treatment studies of poststroke depression

Study	*N*	Medication (*n*, max dose)	Duration	Evaluation method	Results	Response rate	Completion rate
Lipsey et al. 1984	34	NTP (14, 100 mg)	6 weeks	Ham-D, ZDS	Intent to treat and efficacy: NTP>placebo	Completers: 100% NTP 33% placebo	11 of 14 NTP 15 of 20 placebo
Reding et al. 1986	27	TRZ (7, 200 mg) Placebo (9)	32+6 days	ZDS	Efficacy: TRZ >placebo on Barthel ADL for patients with abnormal DST	NR	
Andersen 1994a	66	CIT (33, 20 mg, 10 mg >65 years) Placebo (33)	6 weeks	Ham-D, MES	Intent to treat: CIT>placebo	Completers: 61% CIT 29% placebo	26 of 33 CIT 31 of 33 placebo
Grade et al. 1998	21	MPH (10, 30 mg) Placebo (11)	3 weeks	Ham-D	Intent to treat: MPH>placebo	NR	9 of 10 MPH 10 of 11 placebo
Wiart et al. 2000	31	FLX (16, 20 mg) Placebo (15)	6 weeks	MADRS	Intent to treat: FLX>placebo	62% FLX 33% placebo	14 of 16 FLX 15 of 15 placebo
Robinson et al. 2000	56	FLX (23, 40 mg) NTP (16, 100 mg) Placebo (17)	12 weeks	Ham-D	Intent to treat: NTP>placebo=FLX=placebo	14% FLX 77% NTP 31% placebo	14 of 23 FLX 13 of 16 NTP 13 of 17 placebo
Fruehwald et al. 2003	54	FLX (28, 20 mg) Placebo (26)	12 weeks	BDI, Ham-D	Ham-D>15 FLX=placebo Ham-D scores	69% FLX Ham-D≤13 75% placebo Ham-D ≤13	26 of 28 FLX 24 of 26 placebo
Rampello et al. 2005	31	RBX (16, 4 mg) Placebo (15)	16 weeks	BDI, Ham-D	RBX>placebo for patients with "retarded" depression	NR	NR

Note. Barthel ADL=Barthel's Index of Activities of Daily Living; BDI=Beck Depression Inventory; CIT=citalopram; DST=dexamethasone suppression test; FLX=fluoxetine; Ham-D=Hamilton Rating Scale for Depression; MADRS=Montgomery-Åsberg Depression Rating Scale; MES=Melancholia Scale; MPH=methylphenidate; NR=not reported; NTP=nortriptyline; RBX=reboxetine; TRZ=trazodone; ZDS=Zung Self-Rating Depression Scale.

Source. Robinson RG: *The Clinical Neuropsychiatry of Stroke: Cognitive, Behavioral and Emotional Disorders Following Vascular Brain Injury,* Second Edition. New York, Cambridge University Press, 2006. Copyright © 2006 R. Robinson. Reprinted with permission of Cambridge University Press.

study medication. In the first study to use a selective serotonin reuptake inhibitor (SSRI), Andersen et al. (1994a) compared citalopram with placebo. Patients receiving active treatment ($n=33$) showed a significantly greater reduction in Ham-D scores at both 3 weeks and 6 weeks compared with the patients given placebo ($n=33$).

Nortriptyline was also compared with fluoxetine and placebo in a double-blind, randomized three-arm trial (Robinson et al. 2000). Patients with either major or minor depression were enrolled in the study and randomly assigned to fluoxetine ($n=23$), nortriptyline ($n=16$), or placebo ($n=17$). Patients in the fluoxetine group were treated with 10 mg for the first 3 weeks, and the dosage was then increased to 20 mg for weeks 4–6, to 30 mg for weeks 6–9, and to 40 mg for weeks 9–12. The patients in the nortriptyline group were given 25 mg for the first week, 50 mg for weeks 2 and 3, then 75 mg for weeks 3–6, and finally 100 mg for weeks 6–12. Intention-to-treat analysis demonstrated a significant time × treatment interaction at 12 weeks of treatment, with nortriptyline-treated patients showing a significantly greater decline in Ham-D scores than patients taking either placebo or fluoxetine. Intention-to-treat response rates were 10 of 16 (62%) for nortriptyline, 2 of 23 (9%) for fluoxetine, and 4 of 17 (24%) for placebo. There were no significant differences found between the fluoxetine and placebo groups.

In a double-blind, placebo-controlled study, Rampello et al. (2005) compared reboxetine and placebo in PSD patients with psychomotor retardation. Over the 16-week trial, the 16 patients given reboxetine (4 mg/day) had a significantly greater decline in mean scores (±SD) on Ham-D (24.1±1.5 to 9.3±2.1) and Beck Depression Inventory (BDI; 20.6±2.2 to 8.1±3.4) compared with patients taking placebo (Ham-D 24.0±1.3 to 22.7±2.4; BDI 19.9±1.5 to 18.4±3.3). The number of completers and the relative rates of response and remission were not given.

On the basis of available data, nortriptyline remains the most extensively investigated treatment for PSD and is recommended for patients with no contraindications, such as heart block, cardiac arrhythmia, narrow-angle glaucoma, sedation, or orthostatic hypotension. Dosages of nortriptyline should be increased slowly, and blood levels should be monitored with a goal of achieving serum concentrations between 50 and 150 ng/mL. For patients with contraindications to the use of nortriptyline, alternative choices are citalopram (20 mg for patients under age 66 and 10 mg for patients ages 66 and older) or reboxetine (2 mg bid).

Although it has not been used in a randomized controlled trial, ECT has also been reported to be effective in treating PSD (Murray et al. 1986). ECT caused few side effects and no neurological deterioration. Psychostimulants have also been reported to be effective for the treatment of PSD in open-label trials. Finally, psychological treatment using cognitive-behavioral therapy in 123 stroke patients has been found by Lincoln and Flannaghan (2003) to be no more effective than attention (i.e., placebo) treatment ($n=39$, CBT completers; $n=43$, placebo completers).

Poststroke Anxiety

Although anxiety is one of the most frequent complaints in the general population, it has rarely been the focus of empirical research among stroke patients.

Phenomenology and Frequency

In a study on the prevalence of anxiety disorders in stroke patients, Castillo et al. (1995) examined 309 patients admitted to the hospital with acute stroke using DSM-III-R (American Psychiatric Association 1987) criteria for generalized anxiety disorder. Results indicated that 78 patients (26.9%) met criteria for generalized anxiety disorder, whereas the prevalence of anxiety in the chronic stage was 23%. In a 3-year longitudinal study, Åström (1996) found a prevalence of anxiety in the acute poststroke period of 28%, and there was no significant decrease through the 3 years of follow-up. However, the presence of anxiety was strongly associated with the presence of depression; 58 of 78 stroke patients meeting criteria for generalized anxiety disorder in the study by Castillo et al. (1995) were also depressed. Thus, although generalized anxiety disorder is a common finding among stroke patients, it frequently coexists with depression. A study by Shimoda and Robinson (1998) demonstrated a significant interaction of depression and anxiety in stroke. In this study, compared with nondepressed patients, patients with both anxiety and depression had greater impairment in ADLs at long-term follow-up (Figure 25–5) and worse recovery in social functioning.

Clinical Correlates and Mechanism

In the study of 309 patients with acute stroke, Castillo et al. (1995) examined the clinical and lesion correlates of anxiety and depression. The anxious and nonanxious groups were not significantly different in demographic backgrounds or neurological findings. The nondepressed anxious patients, however, had a significantly higher frequency of alcoholism than did the nonanxious patients (26% generalized anxiety disorder vs. 8% nonanxious, $P<0.05$). When patients with both generalized anxiety disorder and depression were compared to patients with depression only (Starkstein et al. 1990a), patients with anxiety and depression had a significantly higher frequency of cortical lesions (mainly left frontal), whereas the patients with depression had a significantly higher frequency of subcortical lesions (mainly left basal ganglia) (Figure 25–6).

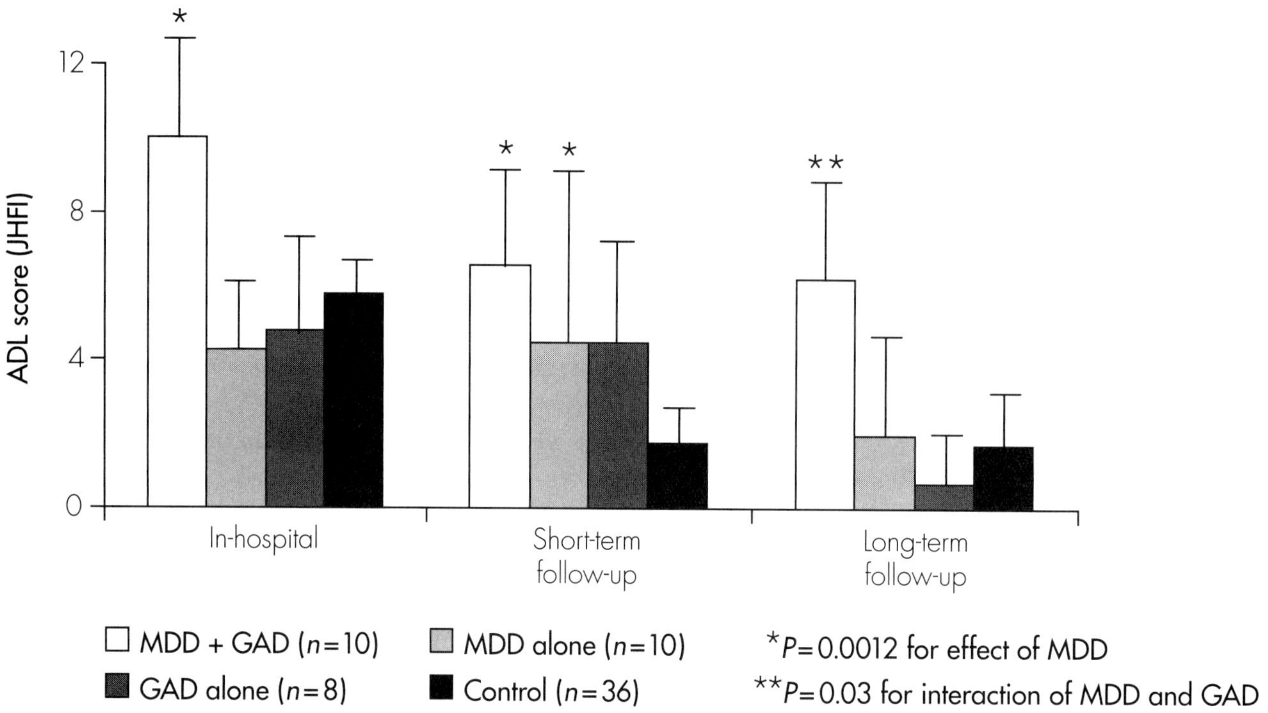

FIGURE 25–5. Activities of daily living (ADL) scores (mean±SEM) in patients with major depressive disorder (MDD) and/or generalized anxiety disorder (GAD) in-hospital.

Patients with MDD had significantly more impaired ADL scores at short-term follow-up (3–6 months). At long-term follow-up (1–2 years), there was an effect of MDD (P=0.02) and a significant interaction of MDD and GAD (P=0.03). Thus, the long-term recovery in ADLs was significantly worse in patients with MDD and GAD in-hospital than patients without this combination of disorders. JHFI=Johns Hopkins Functioning Inventory.

Source. Robinson RG: *The Clinical Neuropsychiatry of Stroke: Cognitive, Behavioral and Emotional Disorders Following Vascular Brain Injury,* Second Edition. New York, Cambridge University Press, 2006. Copyright © 2006 R. Robinson. Reprinted with permission of Cambridge University Press.

Among the anxious patients without depression, 67% had right hemisphere lesions compared with 43% of the anxious depressed patients (P=0.04). Finally, among patients with right hemisphere lesions, the anxious patients had lesions that were significantly more posterior than those of the nonanxious patients (P=0.038). Aström (1996) found that at the acute stage after stroke, anxiety plus depression was associated with left hemisphere lesions, whereas anxiety alone was associated with right hemisphere lesions.

Although the mechanism of anxiety is still unknown, several studies have reported a significant decrease in cortical metabolic activity with increased anxiety, as well as a lack of correlation between the severity of anxiety and subcortical metabolic rate. These results are in agreement with our finding of significantly more severe anxiety after cortical lesions than after subcortical lesions and suggest a critical role for cortical-subcortical interaction in the modulation of anxious states (Starkstein et al. 1990a). No controlled trials of treatment of poststroke anxiety disorders have been reported. Kimura et al. (2003), however, found that nortriptyline produced a greater decline in Hamilton Anxiety Scale (Ham-A) scores among 13 patients with depression plus generalized anxiety disorder than among 14 similar patients given placebo (Figure 25–7). The administration of benzodiazepines to reduce anxiety symptoms among the elderly and frail population should be discouraged because of the increased risk of falls and impaired cognitive functioning associated with their use. The efficacy of other anxiolytic medications such as buspirone has not been demonstrated among stroke patients.

Poststroke Apathy

Apathy, or the absence or lack of feeling, emotion, interest, or concern, has been reported frequently among stroke patients. Starkstein et al. (1993a) examined a consecutive series of 80 patients with single stroke lesions and no significant impairment in comprehension using the Apathy Scale. Both the validity and

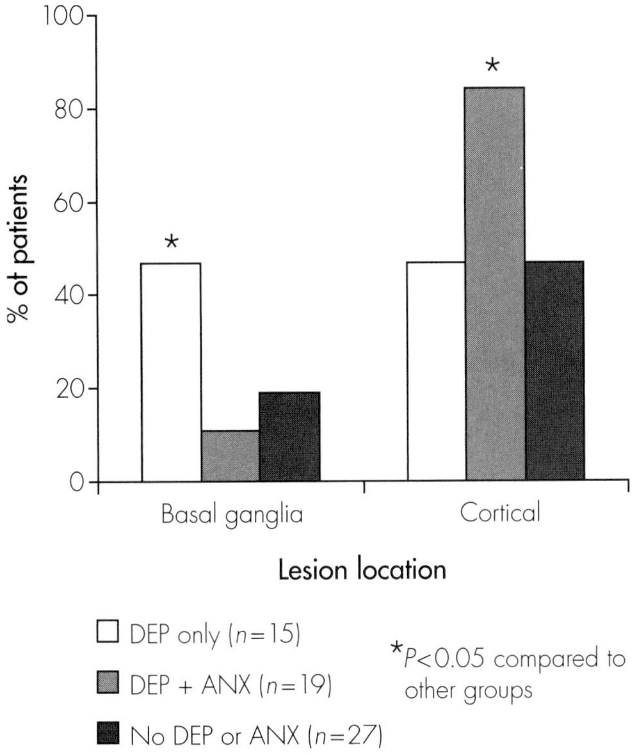

FIGURE 25–6. Comparison of basal ganglia and cortical lesions among patients with major depression only (DEP only), major depression plus generalized anxiety disorder (DEP+ANX), and no mood or anxiety disorder (No DEP or ANX).

Major depression alone was associated with basal ganglia lesions while major depression plus generalized anxiety disorder was associated with cortical lesions.

Source. Robinson RG: *The Clinical Neuropsychiatry of Stroke: Cognitive, Behavioral and Emotional Disorders Following Vascular Brain Injury,* Second Edition. New York, Cambridge University Press, 2006. Copyright © 2006 R. Robinson. Reprinted with permission of Cambridge University Press.

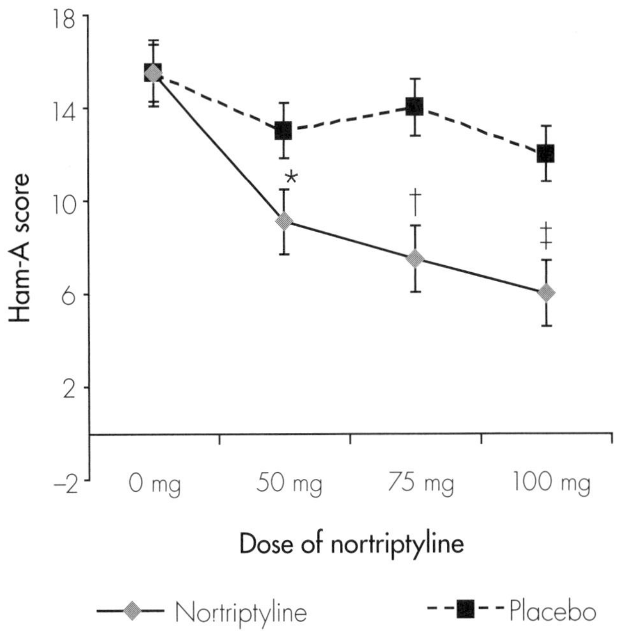

FIGURE 25–7. Mean Hamilton Anxiety Scale (Ham-A) scores among patients with generalized anxiety disorder (GAD) and comorbid depression following stroke at increasing doses of nortriptyline.

The nortriptyline group ($n=13$) showed significantly greater improvement in anxiety symptoms than the placebo group ($n=14$) ($P=0.002$). Error bars represent standard errors of the mean.

$^*P<0.05$, $^†P<0.01$, $^‡P<0.02$.

Source. Reprinted with permission from Kimura M, Tateno A, Robinson RG: "Treatment of Poststroke Generalized Anxiety Disorder Comorbid With Poststroke Depression: Merged Analysis of Nortriptyline Trials." *American Journal of Geriatric Psychiatry* 11: 320–327, 2003.

reliability of this scale were demonstrated in the assessment of apathy in patients with cerebrovascular lesions (Starkstein et al. 1993a). A score of 14 on this scale separated apathetic from nonapathetic patients with high sensitivity and specificity.

Prevalence and Clinical Correlates

In a study of poststroke apathy, Starkstein et al. (1993a) found that 9 of 80 patients (11%) showed apathy as their only psychiatric disorder, whereas another 11% had both apathy and depression. The only demographic correlate of apathy was age: apathetic patients (with or without depression) were significantly older than were nonapathetic patients. Also, apathetic patients showed significantly more severe deficits in ADLs, and there was a significant interaction between depression and apathy (i.e., Johns Hopkins Functioning Inventory [JHFI] scores were 4.8±4.0 for patients with no disorder, 6.21±3.9 for depressed patients, 7.6±5.8 for apathetic patients, and 13.7±5.5 for depressed and apathetic patients; effect of apathy $P<0.001$, effect of depression $P<0.002$, and interaction $P=0.05$).

Clinical-Pathological Correlates and Mechanism of Poststroke Apathy

Compared with patients with no apathy, patients with apathy (without depression) showed a significantly higher frequency of lesions involving the posterior limb of the internal capsule (Starkstein et al. 1993a) (Figure 25–8). Lesions in the internal globus pallidus and the posterior limb of the internal capsule have been reported to produce important behavioral changes, such as motor neglect, psychic akinesia, and akinetic mutism.

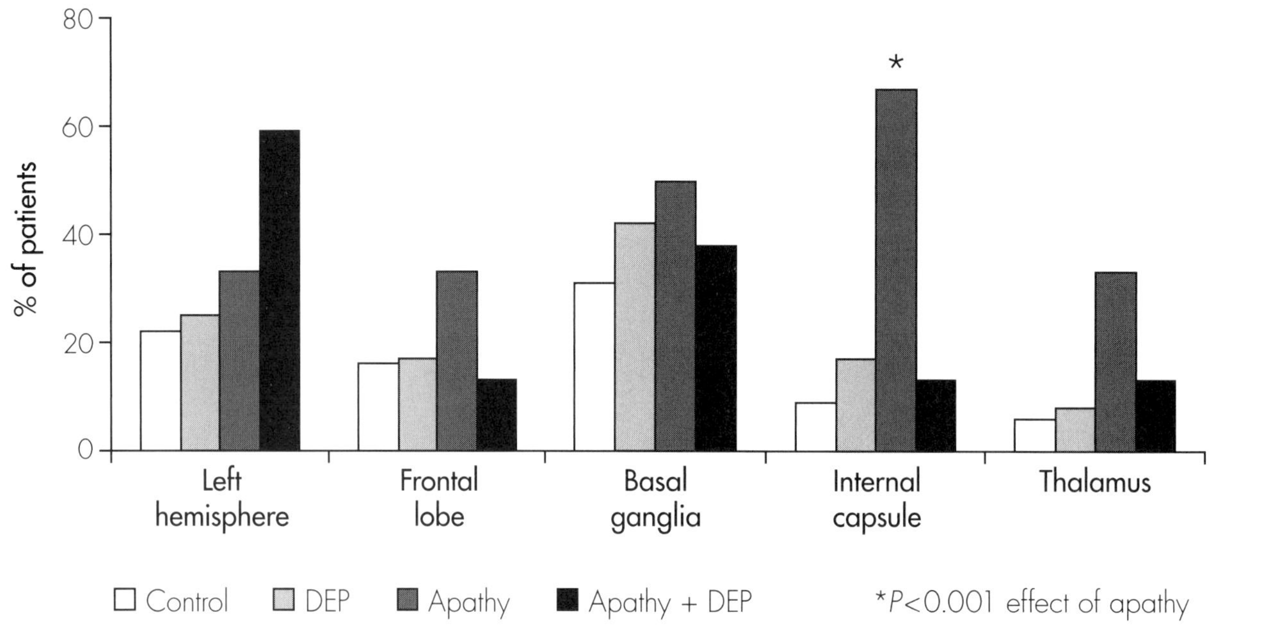

FIGURE 25–8. Frequency of specific lesion locations in patients with apathy and/or depression (DEP).

The only lesion location that was significantly more frequent in patients with apathy compared to the other groups was the posterior arm of the internal capsule. This may reflect the interruption of pallidomesencephalic fibers from the inner pallidum to the pedunculopontine nucleus, which in cats and rodents plays an important role in goal-oriented locomotion.

Source. Robinson RG: *The Clinical Neuropsychiatry of Stroke: Cognitive, Behavioral and Emotional Disorders Following Vascular Brain Injury,* Second Edition. New York, Cambridge University Press, 2006. Copyright © 2006 R. Robinson. Reprinted with permission of Cambridge University Press.

The ansa lenticularis is one of the main internal pallidal outputs, and it ends in the pedunculopontine nucleus after going through the posterior limb of the internal capsule. In rodents, this pathway has a prominent role in goal-oriented behavior, and dysfunction of this system may explain the presence of apathy in stroke patients.

Treatment

Although no prospective trials of treatment of apathy in patients with stroke have been reported, Robinson et al. (2009) examined 137 stroke patients with major depression, of whom 70 (51.1%) also met published diagnostic criteria for apathy. Patients were randomly assigned to 600 mg/day or 900 mg/day of nefiracetam or to placebo and received at least 4 weeks of treatment. A repeated-measures ANOVA of Apathy Scale scores demonstrated a significant time×treatment interaction ($F_{6,128}=2.3$, $P=0.05$). Patients who received 900 mg of nefiracetam had a 7.5±8.5 (±SD) point change in Apathy Scale score, whereas patients who received 600 mg of nefiracetam had a score change of 3.5±6.6 and those receiving placebo had a score change of 2.0±7.0 (Figure 25–9). Although this was a secondary analysis of a study intended to assess the utility of nefiracetam for the treatment of depression, it represents the first double-blind, randomized controlled treatment trial of apathy.

Nefiracetam is an experimental drug that has not been approved by the U.S. Food and Drug Administration for any indication in the United States but represents a possible new treatment for poststroke apathy. Nefiracetam is a novel pyrrolidone-type nootropic that enhances aminergic, glutaminergic, and cholinergic neurotransmission by stimulating nicotinic acetylcholine receptors, activating protein kinase C, and reducing magnesium block of the *N*-methyl-D-aspartate (NMDA) receptor. The majority of treatment studies in apathy are small or anecdotal reports of the utility of stimulants and dopamine agonists. These drugs have been shown to improve arousal and speed of information processing, reduce distractibility, and improve some aspects of motivation and executive function. There is some evidence that amantadine and donepezil may improve motivation among patients with apathetic symptoms and dementia.

Poststroke Psychosis

The phenomenon of hallucinations and delusions in stroke patients has been called agitated delirium, acute atypical psychosis, peduncular hallucinosis, release hallucinations, or acute organic psychosis. The term *secondary hallucinations* refers to sensory perceptions in the absence of appropriate stimuli, with

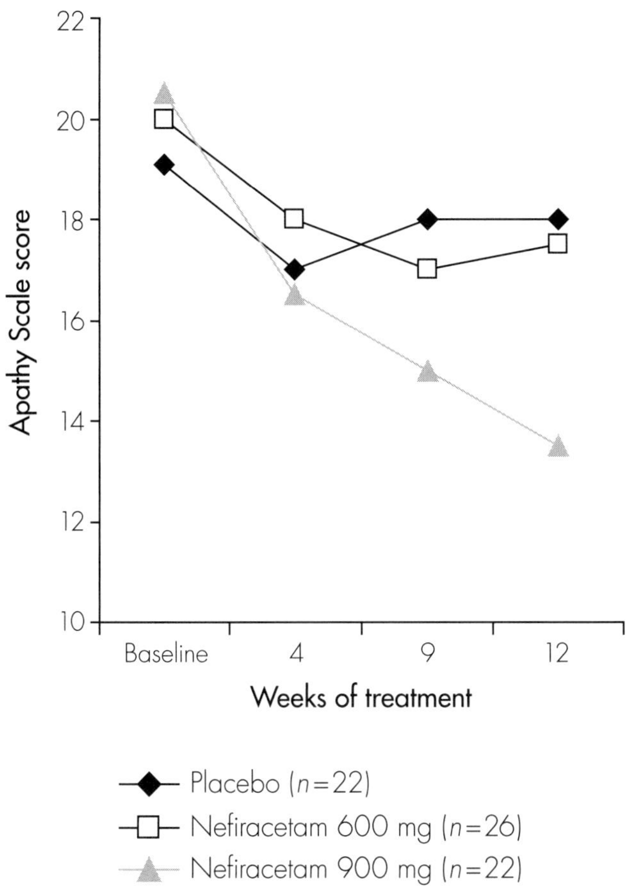

FIGURE 25–9. Patients who received 900 mg/day of nefiracetam had a significant reduction on apathy scores over 12 weeks than patients treated with placebo or 600 mg/day of nefiracetam.

Source. Reprinted from Robinson RG, Jorge RE, Clarence-Smith K, et al: "Double-Blind Treatment of Apathy in Patients With Poststroke Depression Using Nefiracetam." *The Journal of Neuropsychiatry and Clinical Neurosciences* 21:144–151, 2009. Used with permission. Copyright © 2009 American Psychiatric Publishing.

the important qualifications that 1) the patient believes the (nonexistent) sensory perception is real and 2) this disorder started after a brain lesion. The term *secondary hallucinosis* refers to a perception without a stimulus, when the patient does *not* believe the (nonexistent) sensory perception is real and the disorder occurs after a brain lesion. In this section, the term *secondary psychosis* refers to patients who develop either secondary hallucinations or delusions after stroke lesions.

Prevalence and Clinical-Pathological Correlates

In a study of secondary psychosis after stroke lesions, Rabins et al. (1991) found a very low prevalence of this phenomenon among stroke patients (only 5 in more than 300 consecutive admissions). All 5 patients had right hemisphere lesions, primarily involving frontoparietal regions. When compared with 5 age-matched patients with cerebrovascular lesions in similar locations but no psychosis (Rabins et al. 1991), patients with secondary psychosis had significantly greater subcortical atrophy, as manifested by significantly larger areas of both the frontal horn of the lateral ventricle and the body of the lateral ventricle (measured on the side contralateral to the brain lesion; Figure 25–10). Several other investigators have reported a high frequency of seizures among patients with secondary psychosis (e.g., Levine and Finklestein 1982). These seizures usually started after the brain lesion but before the onset of psychosis. Rabins et al. (1991) also found seizures in 3 of 5 patients with poststroke psychosis, compared with none of 5 poststroke nonpsychotic control subjects.

Mechanism

Three factors appear to be important in the mechanism of secondary psychosis, hallucination type: a right hemisphere lesion involving the temporoparietal cortex, seizures, and subcortical brain atrophy. The mechanism of secondary hallucinosis is even less clear than secondary hallucinations. Although in the literature most patients with secondary hallucinosis had peduncular lesions, patients with lesions in other brain areas, such as the diencephalon, also showed the phenomenon. These lesions have frequently been found to involve primary sensory pathways, mainly visual and auditory. Thus, secondary hallucinosis may be a "release phenomenon" secondary to damage to reticular activating brain stem pathways, and the presence of primary sensory deficits in these patients may be a necessary predisposing factor.

Treatment

Although no controlled medication trials in patients with poststroke psychosis have been reported, it is generally accepted that atypical antipsychotics such as olanzapine, quetiapine, or aripiprazole are reasonable choices because they are less likely to produce extrapyramidal symptoms than typical neuroleptics. However, some evidence suggests that the newer antipsychotics may increase the risk of stroke and death among elderly patients with neurological disease (Schneider et al. 2006). Overall, clinicians should adopt a judicious approach, pondering the safest therapeutic alternatives and using antipsychotics in small dosages and for limited intervals.

Anosognosia

The term *anosognosia* was coined to describe the lack of awareness of hemiplegia, but it was later used to refer to the unawareness of other poststroke deficits, such as cortical blindness, hemianopia, and amnesia.

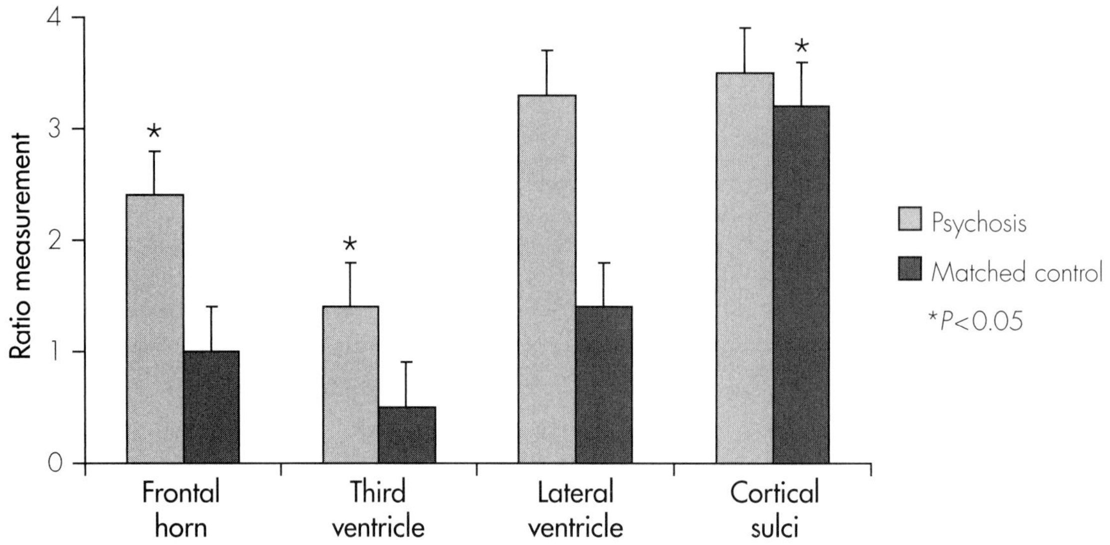

FIGURE 25–10. Measurements of cortical sulci and ventricular-brain ratios in patients who developed delusions and hallucinations following stroke and lesion and age-matched controls who were nonpsychotic.

Although the psychotic patients had higher mean±SEM ratios on all measures, the significant differences were found in the frontal horn ratio (distance between the frontal horns of the lateral ventricles divided by the width of the brain at that level) and the third ventricle ratio (area of the third ventricle divided by the transpineal width). These findings indicate that the psychotic patients had greater subcortical atrophy than nonpsychotic patients. This atrophy probably preceded the stroke, suggesting that these patients may have had a premorbid vulnerability that was brought out by the right hemisphere stroke.

Source. Robinson RG: *The Clinical Neuropsychiatry of Stroke: Cognitive, Behavioral and Emotional Disorders Following Vascular Brain Injury,* Second Edition. New York, Cambridge University Press, 2006. Copyright © 2006 R. Robinson. Reprinted with permission of Cambridge University Press.

Prevalence and Clinical Correlates

Starkstein et al. (1992) examined the prevalence of anosognosia in a consecutive series of 80 patients with single acute stroke lesions. They developed an anosognosia questionnaire, which they used to determine the existence of anosognosia. To rate the severity of this phenomenon, they also developed the Denial of Illness Scale, which allows the classification of patients into those with mild, moderate, or severe anosognosia. Patients with aphasia were included only if they had intact verbal comprehension as measured by their ability to complete Part 1 of the Token Test. The assessment of anosognosia, however, examined only motor, sensory, and visual field disturbances and did not evaluate anosognosia for aphasia.

The first important finding from this study was that about one-third of this consecutive series of patients had anosognosia (19% mild, 11% moderate, and 13% severe; Starkstein et al. 1992). The investigators also examined potential correlates of anosognosia and found this phenomenon to be significantly associated with the presence of a neglect syndrome (i.e., failure to respond to or orient to stimuli contralateral to the lesion), as well as deficits in recognizing facial emotions and the emotional content of speech (prosody). There also was a significant association between anosognosia and right hemisphere lesions involving the temporal and parietal lobes, thalamus, and basal ganglia (Figure 25–11).

Two important negative findings should be noted. First, the frequency of depression was similar among patients with and without anosognosia. Thus, the existence of anosognosia does not preclude stroke patients from experiencing or reporting depressive feelings. Second, patients with anosognosia did not show more severe sensory deficits than did patients without anosognosia; that is, anosognosia is not related to the presence of sensory deficits (Starkstein et al. 1992).

Mechanism

Starkstein et al. (1992) found that brain atrophy, probably preexisting the brain lesion, may have been an important predisposing factor for anosognosia, because patients with anosognosia had significantly more frontal subcortical and diencephalic atrophy (but not cortical atrophy) than did patients with no anosognosia (Figure 25–12). Moreover, patients with anosognosia had significantly more deficits in frontal lobe–related cognitive tasks than did patients with no anosognosia but with lesions in similar brain areas (Figure 25–13).

These findings suggest that lesions in specific cortical and subcortical areas of the right hemisphere, although necessary,

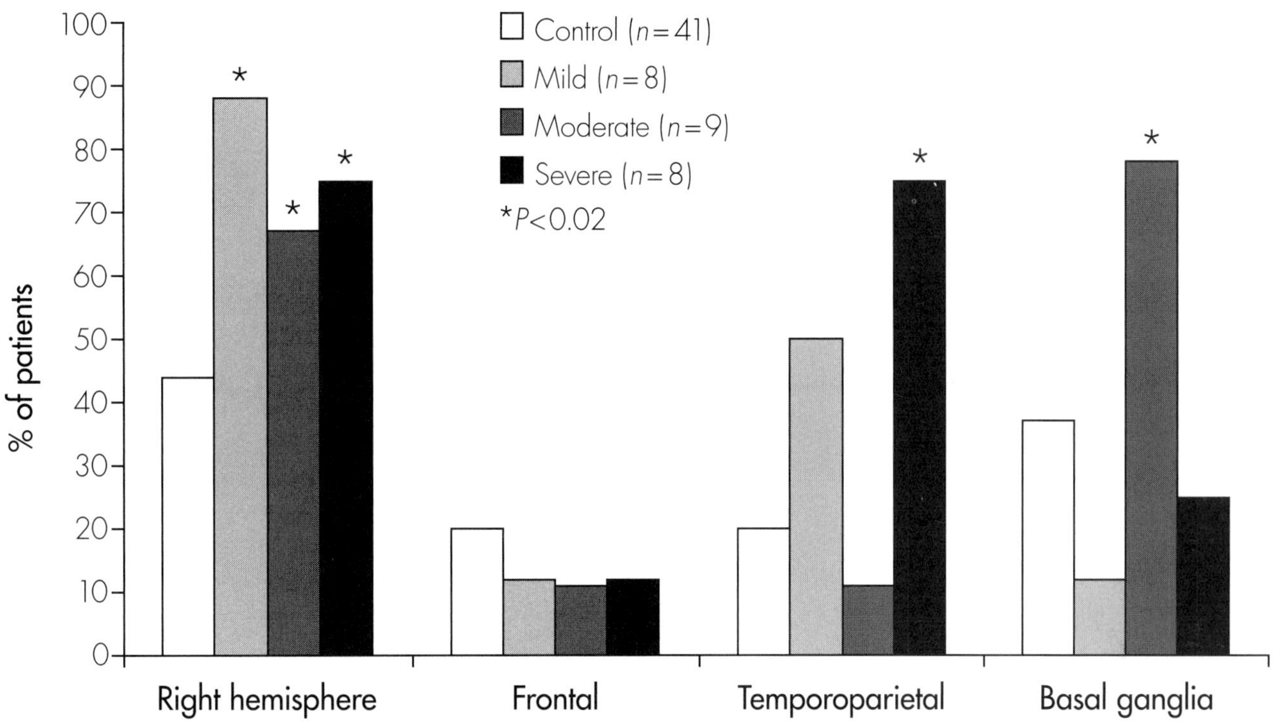

FIGURE 25–11. Frequency of lesion locations in patients with and without anosognosia.

The strongest association was between anosognosia and right hemisphere lesions. Patients with severe anosognosia were more likely to have temporoparietal lesions than any other group while moderate severe anosognosia was associated with basal ganglia lesions. Note that frontal lesions were not associated with the existence of anosognosia in this population.

Source. Robinson RG: *The Clinical Neuropsychiatry of Stroke: Cognitive, Behavioral and Emotional Disorders Following Vascular Brain Injury,* Second Edition. New York, Cambridge University Press, 2006. Copyright © 2006 R. Robinson. Reprinted with permission of Cambridge University Press.

may not be sufficient to produce anosognosia. Concomitant frontal lobe dysfunction (as expressed by frontal subcortical atrophy and deficits in frontal lobe–related cognitive tasks) may be necessary to produce the syndrome.

Heilman and Valenstein (1993) proposed that anosognosia may result from a dysfunction of a system that monitors the intention to move as well as the actual performance of movements. This mismatch between the intention to move and the (lack of) movement may convey the impression that the movement was actually performed and that the limb is normal. The systems monitoring single sensory and motor modalities may be located in the right parietal lobe, whereas the frontal lobe may constitute a supramodal monitoring structure.

Catastrophic Reaction

Catastrophic reaction is a term coined by Goldstein (1948) to describe the inability of the organism to cope when faced with physical or cognitive deficits. It is expressed as anxiety, tears, aggressive behavior, swearing, displacement, refusal, renouncement, and sometimes compensatory boasting.

Prevalence and Clinical Correlates

The catastrophic reaction has been reported to be a frequent finding among patients with aphasia and has been given the status of a separate neuropsychiatric syndrome. However, there are no empirical studies regarding the construct validity of the catastrophic reaction, and it is possible that the catastrophic reaction may represent a symptom of a major depressive syndrome or anxiety disorder in stroke patients. To empirically examine this issue, Starkstein et al. (1993b) evaluated a consecutive series of 62 patients using the Catastrophic Reaction Scale (CRS), which the investigators developed to assess the existence and severity of the catastrophic reaction. The CRS was demonstrated to be a reliable instrument in the measurement of catastrophic reaction symptoms.

Starkstein et al. (1993b) identified the catastrophic reaction in 12 of 62 consecutive patients (19%) with acute stroke lesions. Three major findings emerged from this study. First, patients with catastrophic reaction were found to have a significantly higher frequency of familial and personal history of psychiatric disorders (mostly depression) than were patients without the catastrophic reaction. Second, catastrophic reac-

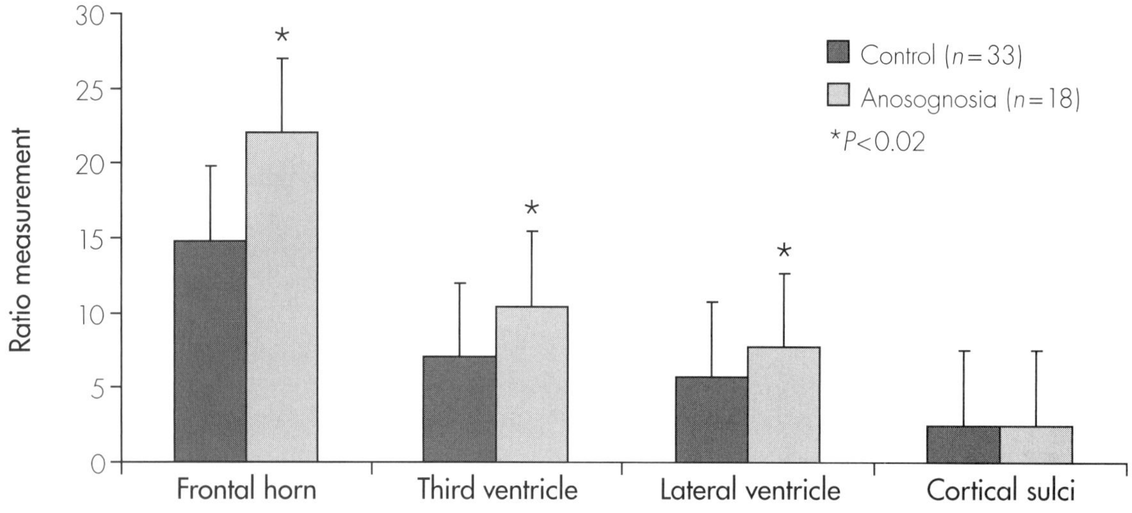

FIGURE 25–12. Ventricle–brain size ratios for patients with anosognosia compared with those for patients without anosognosia.

Ventricle–brain size ratios for patients with anosognosia were significantly larger than those for patients without anosognosia. The cortical measures were not different between groups, indicating that patients with unawareness of their physical impairment following a stroke have more subcortical brain atrophy (which probably preceded the stroke). Compromised subcortical function in the right hemisphere may mediate this phenomenon of anosognosia.

Source. Robinson RG: *The Clinical Neuropsychiatry of Stroke: Cognitive, Behavioral and Emotional Disorders Following Vascular Brain Injury,* Second Edition. New York, Cambridge University Press, 2006. Copyright © 2006 R. Robinson. Reprinted with permission of Cambridge University Press.

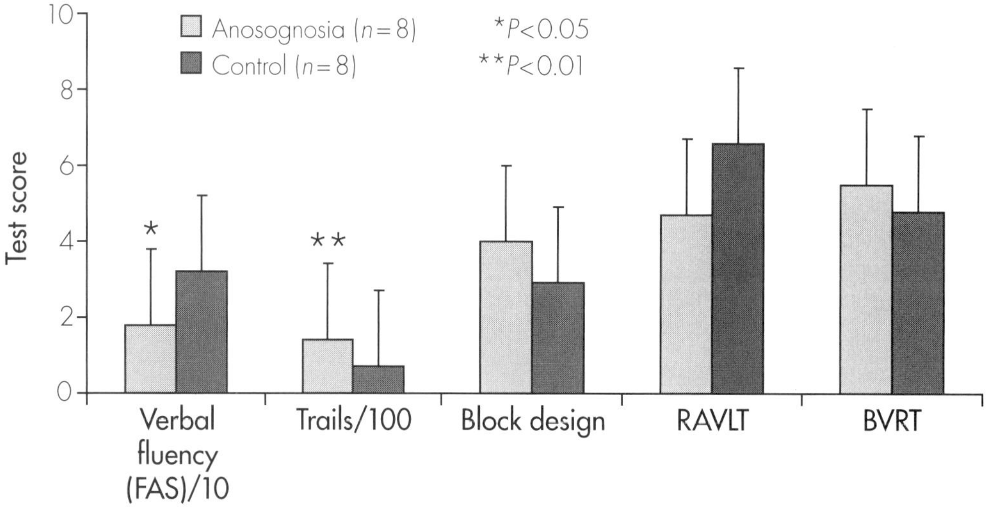

FIGURE 25–13. Performance of patients with and without anosognosia who were matched for lesion location on several neuropsychological examinations.

Patients with anosognosia were significantly more impaired than controls on verbal fluency (FAS) and Trails A and B but not on any of the other construction, attention, learning, or memory tasks. These findings suggest that anosognosia is associated with frontal lobe dysfunction. BVRT=Benton Visual Retention Test; RAVLT=Rey Auditory Verbal Learning Test.

Source. Robinson RG: *The Clinical Neuropsychiatry of Stroke: Cognitive, Behavioral and Emotional Disorders Following Vascular Brain Injury,* Second Edition. New York, Cambridge University Press, 2006. Copyright © 2006 R. Robinson. Reprinted with permission of Cambridge University Press.

tion was not significantly more frequent among patients with aphasia than among patients without aphasia, which does not support the suggestion that catastrophic reaction is more frequent among "frustrated" patients with aphasia. Third, of the 12 patients with catastrophic reaction, 9 (75%) also had major depression, 2 (17%) had minor depression, and only 1 (8%) was not depressed. On the other hand, among patients without catastrophic reaction (i.e., 50 patients), 7 (14%) had major depression, 6 (12%) had minor depression, and 37 (74%) were not depressed. Thus catastrophic reaction was significantly associated with major depression (χ^2=20.9, *df*=2, *P*=0.0001). Moreover, patients with a catastrophic reaction had significantly higher scores on the Ham-A and Ham-D than did patients with no catastrophic reaction.

Mechanism

Patients with a catastrophic reaction had a significantly higher frequency of lesions involving the basal ganglia (Starkstein et al. 1993b) (Figure 25–14). When 10 depressed patients with a catastrophic reaction were compared with 10 depressed patients without a catastrophic reaction, the catastrophic reaction group showed significantly more anterior lesions, which were located mostly in subcortical regions (8 of 9 depressed patients with catastrophic reaction had subcortical lesions; 3 of 9 depressed patients without catastrophic reaction had subcortical lesions) (χ^2=5.84, *df*=1, *P*=0.01).

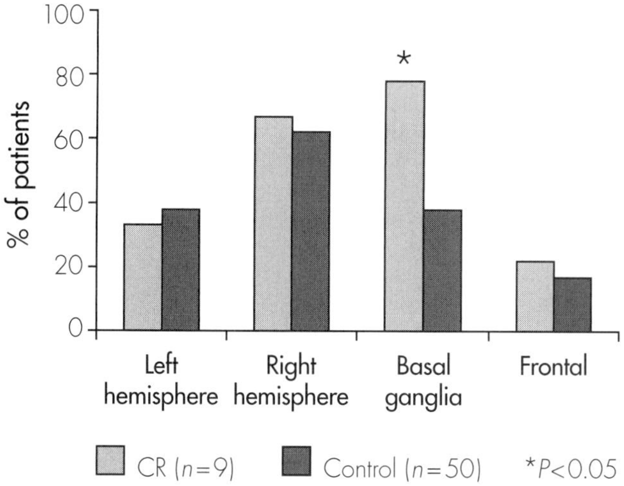

FIGURE 25–14. Lesion locations found on computed tomography scans in 59 patients with or without catastrophic reactions (CR).

Source. Robinson RG: *The Clinical Neuropsychiatry of Stroke: Cognitive, Behavioral and Emotional Disorders Following Vascular Brain Injury,* Second Edition. New York, Cambridge University Press, 2006. Copyright © 2006 R. Robinson. Reprinted with permission of Cambridge University Press.

These findings suggest that the catastrophic reaction is not merely a behavioral response of patients confronted with their limitations, because patients with and without a catastrophic reaction showed a similar frequency of aphasia and physical impairments. On the contrary, the catastrophic reaction seems to characterize a specific type of poststroke major depression (i.e., major depressions associated with anterior subcortical lesions). Anterior brain lesions (both cortical and subcortical) have been consistently associated with PSD. Subcortical damage, however, has usually been hypothesized to underlie the "release" of emotional display by removing inhibitory input to the limbic areas of the cortex.

Pathological Emotions

Pathological emotional expression is a common complication of stroke lesions. It is a more severe form of emotional lability and is characterized by episodes of laughing and/or crying that are not appropriate to the context. They may appear spontaneously or may be elicited by nonemotional events and do not correspond to underlying emotional feelings. Other terms that have been applied to these disorders are *emotional incontinence* and *pseudobulbar affect.*

Prevalence and Clinical Correlates

Robinson et al. (1993) examined the clinical correlates and treatment of pathological laughter and crying in 28 patients with either acute or chronic stroke. They developed a Pathological Laughter and Crying Scale (PLACS) to assess the existence and severity of emotional lability. The investigators demonstrated in 18 treatment patients and 54 acute stroke patients the reliability and validity of this instrument in the assessment of emotional lability (Robinson et al. 1993). They also found that PLACS scores did not correlate with Ham-D scores, MMSE scores, ADL scores, or Social Ties scores, indicating that the PLACS was assessing a factor other than the ones being measured by these other instruments.

A double-blind drug trial of nortriptyline was conducted in 31 patients with emotional lability (Robinson et al. 1993). After randomization, patients were given active drug or placebo in a single bedtime dose. Patients were first given 25 mg of nortriptyline for 1 week, then 50 mg for 2 weeks, 70 mg for 1 week, and 100 mg for the last 2 weeks of the study. One patient dropped out during the study, and two patients withdrew before initiation of the study; therefore, 28 completed the 6-week protocol. Patients receiving nortriptyline showed significant improvements in PLACS scores compared with the placebo-treated patients; these differences became statistically significant at weeks 4 and 6. Although a significant improvement in depression scores also was observed, improvements in PLACS scores were significant for both depressed and nondepressed patients with pathological laughing and crying, indicating that treatment response was not related simply to an improvement in depression. Four additional double-blind trials have further demonstrated the utility of antidepressant medication in the treatment of pseudobulbar affect (Andersen et al. 1993; Brown et al. 1998; Burns et al. 1999; Robinson et al. 1993) (Figure 25–15). In addition, more recent studies suggest that treatment with a combination of dextromethorphan and quinidine is also effective for treating this condition among patients with other neurological disorders (Brooks et al. 2004; Panitch et al. 2006). A combination product of dextromethorphan and quinidine (Nuedexta) is the first treatment approved by the U.S. Food and Drug Administration with an indication for pseudobulbar affect (correspondence with Avanir Pharmaceuticals, November 2010).

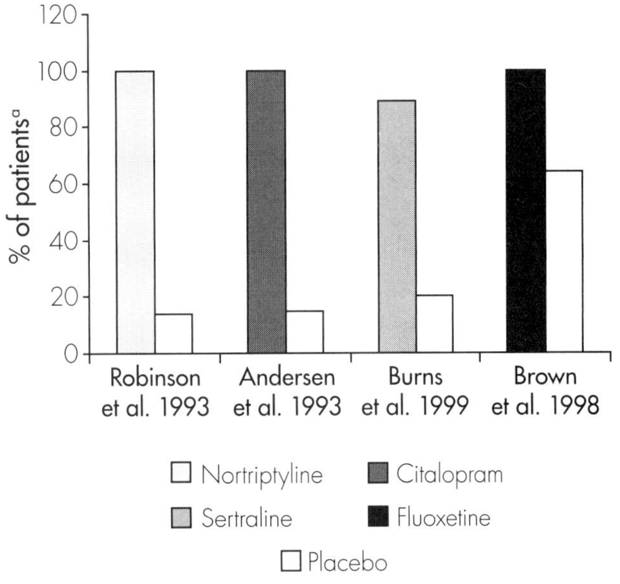

FIGURE 25–15. Comparison of double-blind treatment studies using nortriptyline, citalopram, sertraline, or fluoxetine in patients with pathological crying.

The mean pooled data response rates were 96% for active medication and 27.5% for placebo. These findings suggest that all of the medications are effective in the treatment of poststroke pathological crying.

[a]With >50% reduction in severity score or crying episodes.

Source. Robinson RG: *The Clinical Neuropsychiatry of Stroke: Cognitive, Behavioral and Emotional Disorders Following Vascular Brain Injury,* Second Edition. New York, Cambridge University Press, 2006. Copyright © 2006 R. Robinson. Reprinted with permission of Cambridge University Press.

Mechanism

Pseudobulbar affect has classically been explained as being secondary to the bilateral interruption of neocortical upper motor neuron innervation of bulbar motor nuclei. The finding that emotional lability can be successfully treated with tricyclic drugs suggests that biogenic amine systems may also play a role in the pathogenesis of this disorder. Anderson et al. (1993) reported that stroke patients with relatively large bilateral pontine lesions had more severe pathological crying than did patients with cortical or subcortical hemisphere lesions; the researchers speculated that pathological crying may result from partial destruction of the serotonergic raphe nuclei or their ascending projections to the hemispheres.

Mania

Prevalence and Clinical Correlates

Mania is a relatively rare consequence of acute stroke lesions. Using DSM-IV-TR criteria for mood disorder, manic type (American Psychiatric Association 2000), we found only three cases of secondary mania among a consecutive series of 309 acute stroke patients in an unpublished study (Robinson 2006). On the other hand, secondary mania is more frequent among patients with traumatic brain injury. In a study of 66 patients with acute traumatic brain injury, we found six cases (9%) of secondary mania (Jorge et al. 1993). Patients with traumatic brain injury frequently sustain damage to orbitofrontal and basotemporal cortical areas, which may be related to the mechanism of mania. These brain areas are rarely damaged in stroke patients, and this difference in the frequency of frontal and temporal cortical injury between those with traumatic brain injury and those with ischemic brain injury may explain the different prevalence of mania in these two populations. Cummings and Mendez (1984) found right thalamic stroke lesions in two cases of secondary mania.

In a series of 17 patients with post–brain injury mania, Robinson et al. (1988) reported a high frequency of lesions involving the basal and polar areas of the right temporal lobe and subcortical areas of the right hemisphere, such as the head of the caudate nucleus and right thalamus. Similar lesion location was also reported in patients with bipolar affective disorder. In a study using positron emission tomography (PET) with 18F-fluorodeoxyglucose, Starkstein et al. (1990b) examined metabolic abnormalities in three patients with mania following right basal ganglia strokes. The patients had focal hypometabolic deficits in the right basotemporal cortex. This finding suggested that lesions leading to secondary mania may do so through their distant effects on the right basotemporal cortex. This phenomenon of lesions producing distant effects

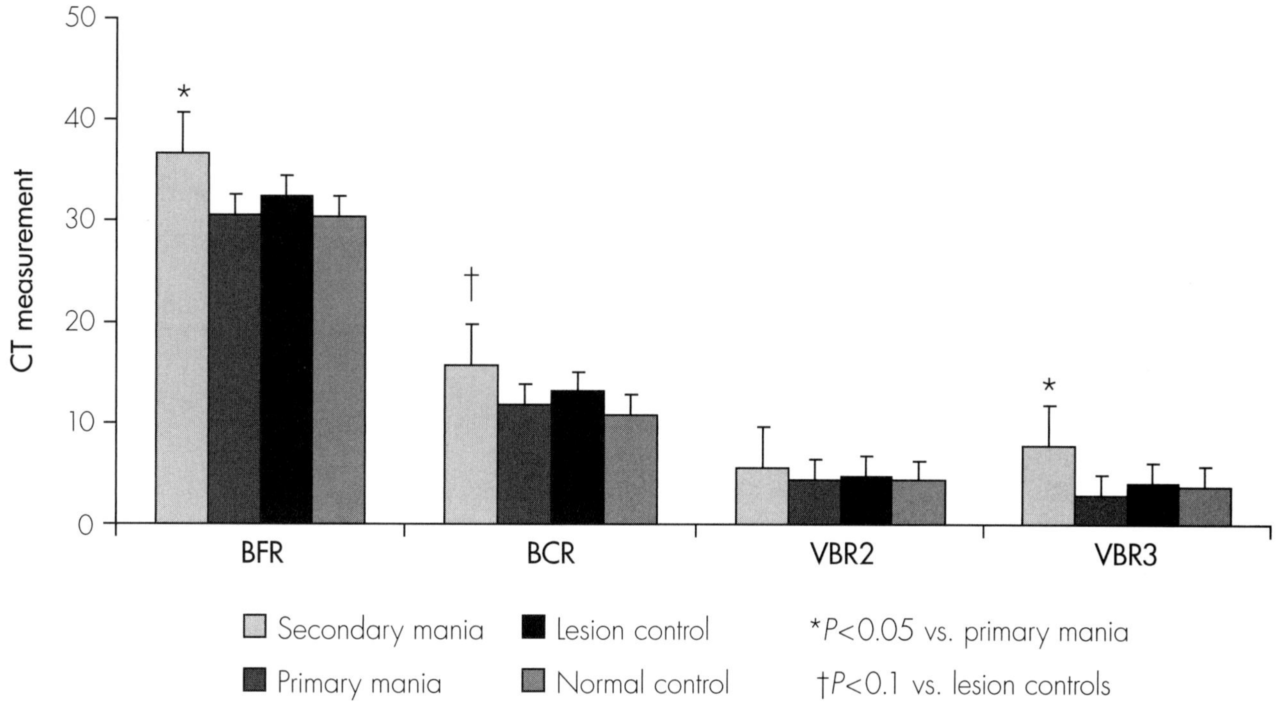

FIGURE 25–16. Measurements taken from computed tomography (CT) scans (mean±SEM) of patients with mania after brain injury (secondary mania); of patients with mania without brain injury (primary mania); of patients matched with secondary manic patients for age, lesion size, and location (lesion control); and of nonlesion (normal) control subjects, age-matched to secondary manic patients.

The bifrontal ratio (BFR) and third ventricle–brain size ratio (VBR3) were significantly greater in the secondary mania patients compared to each of the other groups. BCR=bicaudate ratio; VBR2=lateral ventricle–brain size ratio. This suggests that patients who developed mania following brain injury had subcortical atrophy, which was probably present before the injury and made them more vulnerable to becoming manic following injury.

Source. Robinson RG: *The Clinical Neuropsychiatry of Stroke: Cognitive, Behavioral and Emotional Disorders Following Vascular Brain Injury,* Second Edition. New York, Cambridge University Press, 2006. Copyright © 2006 R. Robinson. Reprinted with permission of Cambridge University Press.

is a well-recognized consequence of some brain lesions and has been termed *diaschisis.*

Because not every patient with a right orbitofrontal or basotemporal lesion develops a manic syndrome, investigators have also looked for potential predisposing factors for secondary mania (Robinson et al. 1988; Starkstein et al. 1987a). In these studies, patients with secondary mania had a significantly higher frequency of familial history of psychiatric disorders, as well as significantly more subcortical brain atrophy (as determined by increased ventricular-brain ratios), than did patients with similar brain lesions but no mania (Figure 25–16). Interestingly, those patients without a genetic predisposition had significantly more subcortical atrophy than did secondary mania patients with a genetic burden, suggesting that subcortical atrophy and genetic predisposition may be independent risk factors for mania following brain injury.

Mechanism

Two clinical-pathological correlations appear to be important in mania secondary to stroke. First, most lesions associated with secondary mania involve, directly or indirectly, limbic or limbic-related areas of the brain. Second, virtually all of these lesions are localized to the right hemisphere.

The basotemporal cortex appears to be a crucial area in the production of mania (Figure 25–17). This paralimbic area receives projections from secondary sensory and multimodal association regions (e.g., the frontal, temporal, and parietal association areas), limbic regions, and paralimbic areas (e.g., the insula and the parahippocampal gyrus). The basotemporal cortex is strongly connected to the orbitofrontal cortex through the uncinate fasciculus, and both may exert a tonic inhibitory control over limbic and dorsal cortical regions. Thus, lesions or dysfunction of these areas may result in mo-

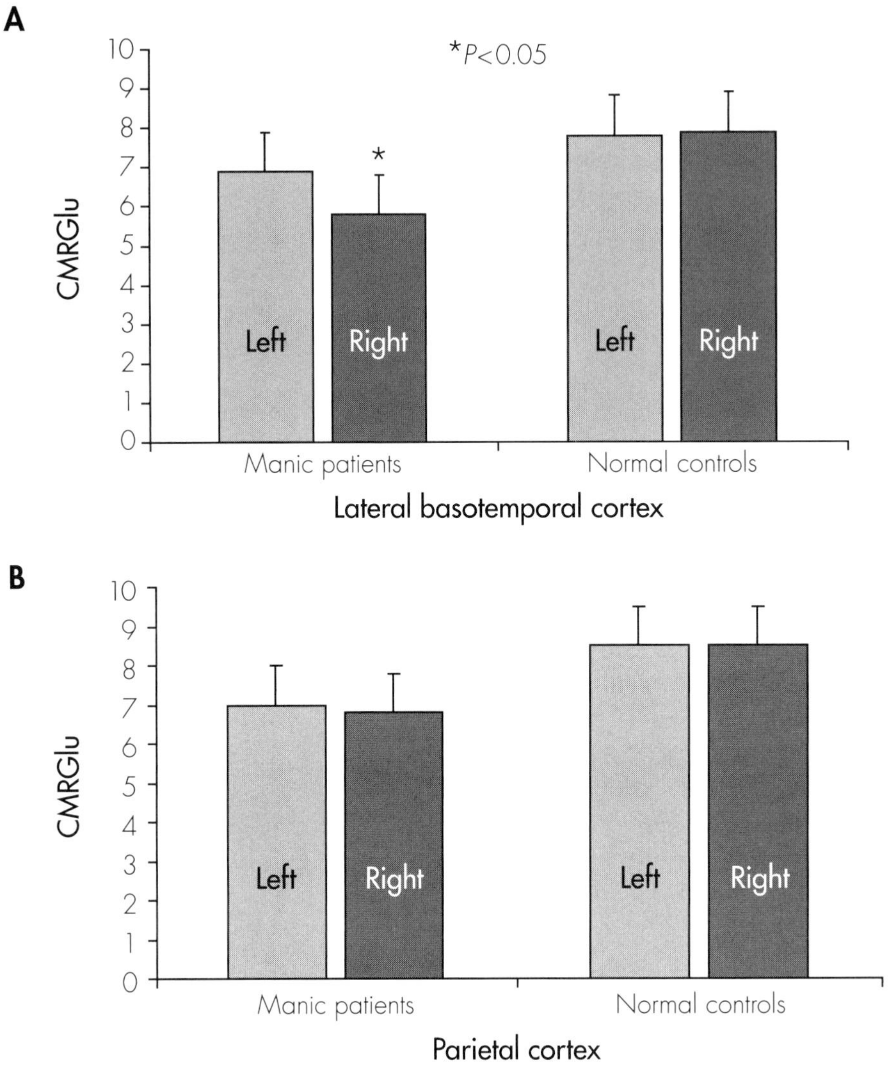

FIGURE 25–17. Regional rates of glucose metabolic rates among three patients with mania following subcortical brain lesions and seven age-comparable normal controls.

Data are means and standard deviations. **Panel A:** Patients with mania had significantly lower metabolic activity in the right basotemporal cortex compared to controls ($P<0.05$). There was no significant difference in the left temporal cortex of patients and controls. **Panel B:** Patients with mania were not significantly different from the controls in terms of metabolic activity in the parietal cortex. CMRGlu=Cerebral glucose metabolic rate in milligrams of glucose per 100 g tissue per minute.

Source. Robinson RG: *The Clinical Neuropsychiatry of Stroke: Cognitive, Behavioral and Emotional Disorders Following Vascular Brain Injury,* Second Edition. New York, Cambridge University Press, 2006.

tor disinhibition (i.e., hyperactivity and pressured speech), intellectual disinhibition (i.e., flight of ideas and grandiose delusions), and instinctive disinhibition (i.e., hyperphagia and hypersexuality).

The second finding that needs to be incorporated into any explanation of poststroke mania is that the manias almost always occur following right hemisphere lesions. In laboratory studies of the neurochemical and behavioral effects of brain lesions in rats, Pearlson and Robinson (1981) found that small suction lesions in the right (but not left) frontal cortex of rats produced a significant increase in locomotor activity. Similar abnormal behavior was also found after electrolytic lesions of the right (but not left) nucleus accumbens (which is considered part of the ventral striatum) (Kubos et al. 1987). Moreover, right frontocortical suction lesions also produced a significant increment in dopaminergic turnover in the nucleus accumbens that was not seen with left hemisphere lesions (Belcheva et al. 1990). Therefore, it is possible that in the presence of predisposing factors such as a genetic burden or subcortical atrophy, significant increments in biogenic amine turnover in the nucleus accumbens produced by specific right hemisphere lesions may be part of the mechanism that results in a manic syndrome.

Treatment

No controlled trials of the efficacy of different mood stabilizers to treat poststroke mania have been reported. Sodium valproate, carbamazepine, and to a lesser extent lithium should be considered as the initial treatment options. However, we emphasize the need for close monitoring of side effects that might occur among stroke patients with mania, particularly extrapyramidal side effects, cognitive impairment, and hematological toxicity.

Conclusion

We have discussed several emotional and behavioral disorders that occur following cerebrovascular lesions. Depression occurs in about 40% of stroke patients, with approximately equal distributions of major depression and minor depression. Patients with PSD often have a greater degree of cognitive impairment (i.e., dementia of depression) and significantly less recovery in ADLs than do patients who never develop depression. Poststroke depression is significantly associated with left frontal and left basal ganglia lesions and may be successfully treated with antidepressants. Anxiety, which is present in about 27% of stroke patients, is associated with depression in the vast majority of cases. Among the few patients with poststroke anxiety and no depression, there was a high frequency of alcoholism and lesions of the right hemisphere. Apathy is present in about 20% of stroke patients. It is associated with older age, more severe deficits in ADLs, and a significantly higher frequency of lesions involving the posterior limb of the internal capsule.

Hallucinations and hallucinosis are rare complications of stroke lesions. Poststroke hallucinations are associated with right hemisphere temporoparietal lesions, subcortical brain atrophy, and seizures. Poststroke hallucinosis is associated with damage to reticular activating and primary sensory pathways. Anosognosia is present in about 30% of patients with acute stroke lesions. It is associated with right hemisphere temporoparietal, basal ganglia, and thalamic lesions; neglect; and subcortical brain atrophy.

Catastrophic reactions occur in about 20% of stroke patients; they are not related to the severity of impairment or the presence of aphasia but may represent a defining symptom for one clinical type of poststroke major depression. Catastrophic reactions are associated with anterior subcortical lesions and may result from a "release" of emotional display in depressed patients. Pathological emotional expression is another common complication of stroke lesions that sometimes coexists with depression and may be successfully treated with antidepressants. Finally, mania is a rare complication of stroke lesions. It is strongly associated with right hemisphere damage involving the orbitofrontal cortex, basal temporal cortex, thalamus, or basal ganglia. Risk factors for mania include a family history of psychiatric disorders and subcortical atrophy.

Key Points

- Many neuropsychiatric disorders are associated with stroke and range from depression and mania to apathy, pathological emotion, psychoses, anxiety disorders, and catastrophic reactions.
- Major depression occurs in about 20% of patients following acute stroke, and another 20% of patients develop minor (subsyndromal) depression.
- Depression following stroke is associated with impaired physical and cognitive recovery, as well as increased mortality.
- Treatment with antidepressant medication improves mood in many patients with poststroke depression but also improves recovery and decreases mortality.
- Anxiety occurs in more than half of patients with poststroke depression. Apathy, catastrophic reactions, and pathological emotions are comorbid with depression in about half of the cases.

Recommended Readings

Andersen G, Vestergaard K, Lauritzen L: Effective treatment of poststroke depression with the selective serotonin reuptake inhibitor citalopram. Stroke 25:1099–1104, 1994

Bhogal SK, Teasell R, Foley N, et al: Lesion location and poststroke depression: systematic review of the methodological limitations in the literature. Stroke 35:794–802, 2004

Robinson RG: The Clinical Neuropsychiatry of Stroke. New York, Cambridge University Press, 2006

Robinson RG, Jorge RE, Moser DJ, et al: Escitalopram and problem-solving therapy for prevention of poststroke depression: a randomized controlled trial. JAMA 299:2391–2400, 2008

Spalletta G, Guida G, De Angelis D, et al: Predictors of cognitive level and depression severity are different in patients with left and right hemispheric stroke within the first year of illness. J Neurol 249:1541–1551, 2002

Starkstein SE, Fedoroff JP, Price TR, et al: Apathy following cerebrovascular lesions. Stroke 24:1625–1630, 1993

Whyte EM, Mulsant BH: Post stroke depression: epidemiology, pathophysiology, and biological treatment. Biol Psychiatry 52: 253–264, 2002

References

Aben I, Verhey F, Lousberg R, et al: Validity of the Beck depression inventory, Hospital anxiety and depression scale, SCL-90, and Hamilton depression rating scale as screening instruments for depression in stroke patients. Psychosomatics 43:386–393, 2002

American Heart Association: Heart Disease and Stroke Statistics—2010 Update. Dallas, Texas, American Heart Association, 2010

American Psychiatric Association: Diagnostic and Statistical Manual of Mental Disorders, 3rd Edition. Washington, DC, American Psychiatric Association, 1980

American Psychiatric Association: Diagnostic and Statistical Manual of Mental Disorders, 3rd Edition, Revised. Washington, DC, American Psychiatric Association, 1987

American Psychiatric Association: Diagnostic and Statistical Manual of Mental Disorders, 4th Edition. Washington, DC, American Psychiatric Association, 1994

American Psychiatric Association: Diagnostic and Statistical Manual of Mental Disorders, 4th Edition, Text Revision. Washington, DC, American Psychiatric Association, 2000

Andersen G, Vestergaard K, Riis J: Citalopram for poststroke pathological crying. Lancet 342:837–839, 1993

Andersen G, Vestergaard K, Lauritzen L: Effective treatment of poststroke depression with the selective serotonin reuptake inhibitor citalopram. Stroke 25:1099–1104, 1994a

Andersen G, Vestergaard K, Riis JO, et al: Incidence of poststroke depression during the first year in a large unselected stroke population determined using a valid standardized rating scale. Acta Psychiatr Scand 90:190–195, 1994b

Aström M: Generalized anxiety disorder in stroke patients: a 3-year longitudinal study. Stroke 27:270–275, 1996

Aström M, Adolfsson R, Asplund K: Major depression in stroke patients: a 3-year longitudinal study. Stroke 24:976–982, 1993

Belcheva I, Starkstein SE, Honig M, et al: Hemispheric asymmetry in behavioral response to Dl and D2 receptor agonists in the nucleus accumbens. Brain Res 533:286–291, 1990

Berg A, Psych L, Palomäki H, et al: Poststroke depression: an 18-month follow-up. Stroke 34:138–143, 2003

Bhogal SK, Teasell R, Foley N, et al: Lesion location and poststroke depression: systematic review of the methodological limitations in the literature. Stroke 35:794–802, 2004

Brooks BR, Thisted RA, Appel SH, et al: Treatment of pseudobulbar affect in ALS with dextromethorphan/quinidine: a randomized trial. Neurology 63:1364–1370, 2004

Brown KW, Sloan RL, Pentland B: Fluoxetine as a treatment for poststroke emotionalism. Acta Psychiatr Scand 98:455–458, 1998

Burns A, Russell E, Stratton-Powell H, et al: Sertraline in stroke-associated lability of mood. Int J Geriatr Psychiatry 14:681–685, 1999

Burvill PW, Johnson GA, Jamrozik KD, et al: Prevalence of depression after stroke: the Perth Community Stroke Study. Br J Psychiatry 166:320–327, 1995

Carney RM, Saunders RD, Freedland KE, et al: Association of depression with reduced heart rate variability in coronary artery disease. Am J Cardiol 76:562–564, 1995

Cassidy E, O'Connor R, O'Keane V: Prevalence of poststroke depression in an Irish sample and its relationship with disability and outcome following inpatient rehabilitation. Disabil Rehabil 26: 71–77, 2004

Castillo CS, Schultz SK, Robinson RG: Clinical correlates of early onset and late-onset poststroke generalized anxiety. Am J Psychiatry 152:1174–1179, 1995

Collin SJ, Tinson D, Lincoln NB: Depression after stroke. Clin Rehabil 1:27–32, 1987

Cummings JL, Mendez MF: Secondary mania with focal cerebrovascular lesions. Am J Psychiatry 141:1084–1087, 1984

Damecour CL, Caplan D: The relationship of depression to symptomatology and lesion site in aphasic patients. Cortex 27:385–401, 1991

Desmond DW, Remien RH, Moroney JT, et al: Ischemic stroke and depression. J Int Neuropsychol Soc 9:429–439, 2003

Downhill JE Jr, Robinson RG: Longitudinal assessment of depression and cognitive impairment following stroke. J Nerv Ment Dis 182: 425–431, 1994

Eastwood MR, Rifat SL, Nobbs H, et al: Mood disorder following cerebrovascular accident. Br J Psychiatry 154:195–200, 1989

Ebrahim S, Barer D, Nouri F: Affective illness after stroke. Br J Psychiatry 151:52–56, 1987

Everson SA, Roberts RE, Goldberg DE, et al: Depressive symptoms and increased risk of stroke mortality over a 29-year period. Arch Intern Med 158:1133–1138, 1998

Feibel JH, Springer CJ: Depression and failure to resume social activities after stroke. Arch Phys Med Rehabil 63:276–278, 1982

Finklestein S, Benowitz LI, Baldessarini RJ, et al: Mood, vegetative disturbance, and dexamethasone suppression test after stroke. Ann Neurol 12:463–468, 1982

Finset A, Goffeng L, Landro NI, et al: Depressed mood and intrahemispheric location of lesion in right hemisphere stroke patients. Scand J Rehabil Med 21:1–6, 1989

Folstein MF, Maiberger R, McHugh PR: Mood disorder as a specific complication of stroke. J Neurol Neurosurg Psychiatry 40:1018–1020, 1977

Fregni F, Boggio PS, Valle AC, et al: A sham-controlled trial of a 5-day course of repetitive transcranial magnetic stimulation of the unaffected hemisphere in stroke patients. Stroke 37:2115–2122, 2006

Fruehwald S, Gatterbauer E, Rehak P, et al: Early fluoxetine treatment of poststroke depression: a three-month double-blind placebo-controlled study with an open-label long-term follow up. J Neurol 250:347–351, 2003

Gainotti G, Azzoni A, Marra C: Frequency, phenomenology and anatomical-clinical correlates of major poststroke depression. Br J Psychiatry 175:163–167, 1999

Goldstein K: Language and Language Disturbances. New York, Grune & Stratton, 1948

Gonzalez-Torrecillas JL, Mendlewicz J, Lobo A: Effects of early treatment of poststroke depression on neuropsychological rehabilitation. Int Psychogeriatr 7:547–560, 1995

Grade C, Redford B, Chrostowski J, et al: Methylphenidate in early poststroke recovery: a double-blind, placebo-controlled study. Arch Phys Med Rehabil 79:1047–1050, 1998

Hackett ML, Anderson CS: Predictors of depression after stroke: a systematic review of observational studies. Stroke 36:2296–2301, 2005

Hayee MA, Akhtar N, Haque A, et al: Depression after stroke-analysis of 297 stroke patients. Bangladesh Med Res Counc Bull 27:96–102, 2001

Heilman KM, Valenstein E: Clinical Neuropsychology, 3rd Edition. Oxford, UK, Oxford University Press, 1993

Herrmann M, Bartles C, Wallesch CW: Depression in acute and chronic aphasia: symptoms, pathoanatomical-clinical correlations and functional implications. J Neurol Neurosurg Psychiatry 56:672–678, 1993

Herrmann N, Black SE, Lawrence J, et al: The Sunnybrook Stroke Study: a prospective study of depressive symptoms and functional outcome. Stroke 29:618–624, 1998

House A, Dennis M, Mogridge L, et al: Mood disorders in the year after first stroke. Br J Psychiatry 158:83–92, 1991

House A, Knapp P, Bamford J, et al: Mortality at 12 and 24 months after stroke may be associated with depressive symptoms at 1 month. Stroke 32:696–701, 2001

Jorge RE, Robinson RG, Starkstein SE, et al: Secondary mania following traumatic brain injury. Am J Psychiatry 150:916–921, 1993

Kauhanen M, Korpelainen JT, Hiltunen P, et al: Poststroke depression correlates with cognitive impairment and neurological deficits. Stroke 30:1875–1880, 1999

Kim JS, Choi-Kwon S: Poststroke depression and emotional incontinence: correlation with lesion location. Neurology 54:1805–1810, 2000

Kimura M, Robinson RG, Kosier T: Treatment of cognitive impairment after poststroke depression: a double-blind treatment trial. Stroke 31:1482–1486, 2000

Kimura M, Tateno A, Robinson RG: Treatment of poststroke generalized anxiety disorder comorbid with poststroke depression: merged analysis of nortriptyline trials. Am J Geriatr Psychiatry 11:320–327, 2003

Kotila M, Numminen H, Waltimo O, et al: Depression after stroke: results of the FINNSTROKE study. Stroke 29:368–372, 1998

Kraepelin E: Manic Depressive Insanity and Paranoia. Edinburgh, UK, E & S Livingstone, 1921

Kubos KL, Moran TH, Robinson RG: Differential and asymmetrical behavioral effects of electrolytic or 6-hydroxydopamine lesions in the nucleus accumbens. Brain Res 401:147–151, 1987

Levine DN, Finklestein S: Delayed psychosis after right temporoparietal stroke or trauma: relation to epilepsy. Neurology 32: 267–273, 1982

Lincoln NB, Flannaghan T: Cognitive behavioral psychotherapy for depression following stroke: a randomized controlled trial. Stroke 34:111–115, 2003

Lipsey JR, Robinson RG, Pearlson GD, et al: Nortriptyline treatment of poststroke depression: a double-blind study. Lancet 1:297–300, 1984

Lloyd-Jones D, Adams RJ, Brown TM, et al: Heart disease and stroke statistics—2010 update: a report from the American Heart Association. Circulation 121:e46–e215, 2010

Morris PL, Robinson RG, Raphael B: Prevalence and course of depressive disorders in hospitalized stroke patients. Int J Psychiatry Med 20:349–364, 1990

Morris PL, Robinson RG, Andrzejewski P, et al: Association of depression with 10-year poststroke mortality. Am J Psychiatry 150: 124–129, 1993

Morris PL, Robinson RG, Raphael B, et al: Lesion location and poststroke depression. J Neuropsychiatry Clin Neurosci 8:399–403, 1996

Murray GB, Shea, V, Conn DK: Electroconvulsive therapy for poststroke depression. J Clin Psychiatry 47:258–260, 1986

Narushima K, Robinson RG: The effect of early versus late antidepressant treatment on physical impairment associated with poststroke depression: is there a time-related therapeutic window? J Nerv Ment Dis 191:645–652, 2003

Narushima K, Kosier JT, Robinson RG: A reappraisal of poststroke depression, intra- and inter-hemispheric lesion location using meta-analysis. J Neuropsychiatry Clin Neurosci 15:422–430, 2003

Palomäki H, Kaste M, Berg A, et al: Prevention of poststroke depression: 1 year randomised placebo controlled double blind trial of mianserin with 6 month follow up after therapy. J Neurol Neurosurg Psychiatry 66:490–494, 1999

Panitch HS, Thisted RA, Smith RA, et al: Randomized, controlled trial of dextromethorphan/quinidine for pseudobulbar affect in multiple sclerosis. Ann Neurol 59:780–787, 2006

Parikh RM, Robinson RG, Lipsey JR, et al: The impact of poststroke depression on recovery in activities of daily living over two year follow-up. Arch Neurol 47:785–789, 1990

Pearlson GD, Robinson RG: Suction lesions of the frontal cerebral cortex in the rat induce asymmetrical behavioral and catecholaminergic responses. Brain Res 218:233–242, 1981

Pessah-Rasmussen H, Engstrom G, Jerntorp I, et al: Increasing stroke incidence and decreasing case fatality, 1989–1998: a study from the Stroke Register in Malmö, Sweden. Stroke 34:913–918, 2003

Pohjasvaara T, Leppavuori A, Siira I, et al: Frequency and clinical determinants of poststroke depression. Stroke 29:2311–2317, 1998

Pohjasvaara T, Vataja R, Leppavuori A, et al: Depression is an independent predictor of poor long-term functional outcome poststroke. Eur J Neurol 8:315–319, 2001

Rabins PV, Starkstein SE, Robinson RG: Risk factors for developing atypical (schizophreniform) psychosis following stroke. J Neuropsychiatry Clin Neurosci 3:6–9, 1991

Rampello L, Alvano A, Chiechio S, et al: An evaluation of efficacy and safety of reboxetine in elderly patients affected by "retarded" poststroke depression: a random, placebo-controlled study. Arch Gerontol Geriatr 40:275–285, 2005

Reding MJ, Orto LA, Winter SW, et al: Antidepressant therapy after stroke: a double-blind trial. Arch Neurol 43:763–765, 1986

Robins LN, Wing J, Wittchen HU, et al: The Composite International Diagnostic Interview: an epidemiologic instrument suitable for use in conjunction with different diagnostic systems and in different cultures. Arch Gen Psychiatry 45:1069–1077, 1988

Robinson RG: The Clinical Neuropsychiatry of Stroke: Cognitive, Behavioral and Emotional Disorders Following Vascular Brain Injury, 2nd Edition. New York, Cambridge University Press, 2006

Robinson RG, Price TR: Post-stroke depressive disorders: a follow-up study of 103 outpatients. Stroke 13:635–641, 1982

Robinson RG, Szetela B: Mood change following left hemispheric brain injury. Ann Neurol 9:447–453, 1981

Robinson RG, Bolla-Wilson K, Kaplan E, et al: Depression influences intellectual impairment in stroke patients. Br J Psychiatry 148: 541–547, 1986

Robinson RG, Boston JD, Starkstein SE, et al: Comparison of mania and depression after brain injury: causal factors. Am J Psychiatry 145:172–178, 1988

Robinson RG, Parikh RM, Lipsey JR, et al: Pathological laughing and crying following stroke: validation of measurement scale and double-blind treatment study. Am J Psychiatry 150:286–293, 1993

Robinson RG, Schultz SK, Castillo C, et al: Nortriptyline versus fluoxetine in the treatment of depression and in short term recovery after stroke: a placebo controlled, double-blind study. Am J Psychiatry 157:351–359, 2000

Robinson RG, Jorge RE, Clarence-Smith K, et al: Double-blind treatment of apathy in patients with poststroke depression using nefiracetam. J Neuropsychiatry Clin Neurosci 21:144–151, 2009

Schneider LS, Dagerman K, Insel PS: Efficacy and adverse effects of atypical antipsychotics for dementia: meta-analysis of randomized, placebo-controlled trials. Am J Geriatr Psychiatry 14:191–210, 2006

Schubert DSP, Taylor C, Lee S, et al: Physical consequences of depression in the stroke patient. Gen Hosp Psychiatry 14:69–76, 1992

Schwartz JA, Speed NM, Brunberg JA, et al: Depression in stroke rehabilitation. Biol Psychiatry 33:694–699, 1993

Shima S, Kitagawa Y, Kitamura T, et al: Poststroke depression. Gen Hosp Psychiatry 16:286–289, 1994

Shimoda K, Robinson RG: Effects of anxiety disorder on impairment and recovery from stroke. J Neuropsychiatry Clin Neurosci 10: 34–40, 1998

Singh A, Black SE, Herrmann N, et al: Functional and neuroanatomic correlations in poststroke depression: the Sunnybrook Stroke Study. Stroke 31:637–644, 2000

Sinyor D, Cooper E, Sartorius N: Relationship to functional impairment coping strategies and rehabilitation outcome. Stroke 17: 1102–1107, 1986

Spalletta G, Guida G, De Angelis D, et al: Predictors of cognitive level and depression severity are different in patients with left and right hemispheric stroke within the first year of illness. J Neurol 249:1541–1551, 2002

Spalletta G, Ripa A, Caltagirone C: Symptom profile of DSM-IV major and minor depressive disorders in first-ever stroke patients. Am J Geriatr Psychiatry 13:108–115, 2005

Spitzer RL, Williams JBW, Gibbon M: Structured Clinical Interview for DSM-IV (SCID). New York, Biometrics Research, New York State Psychiatric Institute, 1995

Starkstein SE, Pearlson GD, Boston J, et al: Mania after brain injury: a controlled study of causative factors. Arch Neurol 44:1069–1073, 1987a

Starkstein SE, Robinson RG, Price TR: Comparison of cortical and subcortical lesions in the production of poststroke mood disorders. Brain 110:1045–1059, 1987b

Starkstein SE, Robinson RG, Berthier ML, et al: Differential mood changes following basal ganglia versus thalamic lesions. Arch Neurol 45:725–730, 1988a

Starkstein SE, Robinson RG, Price TR: Comparison of patients with and without poststroke major depression matched for size and location of lesion. Arch Gen Psychiatry 45:247–252, 1988b

Starkstein SE, Robinson RG, Price TR: Comparison of spontaneously recovered versus non-recovered patients with post-stroke depression. Stroke 19:1491–1496, 1988c

Starkstein SE, Cohen BS, Fedoroff P, et al: Relationship between anxiety disorders and depressive disorders in patients with cerebrovascular injury. Arch Gen Psychiatry 47:785–789, 1990a

Starkstein SE, Mayberg HS, Berthier ML, et al: Mania after brain injury: neuroradiological and metabolic findings. Ann Neurol 27:652–659, 1990b

Starkstein SE, Fedoroff JP, Price TR, et al: Anosognosia in patients with cerebrovascular lesions: a study of causative factors. Stroke 23:1446–1453, 1992

Starkstein SE, Fedoroff JP, Price TR, et al: Apathy following cerebrovascular lesions. Stroke 24:1625–1630, 1993a

Starkstein SE, Fedoroff JP, Price TR, et al: Catastrophic reaction after cerebrovascular lesions: frequency, correlates, and validation of a scale. J Neurol Neurosurg Psychiatry 5:189–194, 1993b

Stewart R, Prince M, Richards M, et al: Stroke, vascular risk factors and depression: cross-sectional study in a UK Caribbean-born population. Br J Psychiatry 178:23–28, 2001

Thom T, Haase N, Rosamond W, et al: Heart disease and stroke statistics—2006 update: a report from the American Heart Association Statistics Committee and Stroke Statistics Subcommittee. Circulation 113:e85–e151, 2006

Wade DT, Legh-Smith J, Hewer RA: Depressed mood after stroke, a community study of its frequency. Br J Psychiatry 151:200–205, 1987

Wiart L, Petit H, Joseph PA, et al : Fluoxetine in early poststroke depression: a double-blind placebo-controlled study. Stroke 31: 1829–1832, 2000

Williams LS, Ghose SS, Swindle RW: Depression and other mental health diagnoses increase mortality risk after ischemic stroke. Am J Psychiatry 161:1090–1095, 2004

26

Traumatic Brain Injury

Richard B. Ferrell, M.D.
Thomas W. McAllister, M.D.

Traumatic brain injury (TBI) is a significant health problem among older adults, both as a matter of personal and family suffering and as a public health issue. The topic deserves special attention because of its human cost, but also because a significant number of such injuries might be prevented by personal and public safety measures and by attention to treatable health problems that are also risk factors. The Centers for Disease Control and Prevention has called TBI a "silent epidemic" (National Center for Injury Prevention and Control 2003) and this term is widely used. Falls are the leading cause of TBI for older-aged persons, and injuries from falls may be less obvious than from causes such as motor vehicle accidents (MVAs), so TBI in older adults might be underdiagnosed (Langlois et al. 2003). Although TBI in older adults shares many causes and consequences with TBI in younger persons, there are differences. Outcome in TBI is generally worse for older persons than for younger persons. For example, Bouras et al. (2007) collected data from 1,926 head trauma cases. Patients older than age 65 had worse outcomes than younger persons, and victims ages 65–74 fared better than persons older than 75.

Neuropsychiatrists and geriatric psychiatrists are most likely to encounter older patients with a history of TBI after they have recovered from the acute injury and possibly after a period of rehabilitation. Clinicians may be asked to consult, evaluate, treat, and offer prognosis regarding various complaints and conditions. Among these are 1) cognitive changes, such as poor memory or concentration; 2) personality changes; 3) irritability or apathy; 4) behavioral changes, especially disinhibited or aggressive behavior; and 5) psychiatric complaints. Depression, psychosis, anxiety disorders, obsessive-compulsive symptoms, and manic syndromes sometimes occur for the first time after TBI.

The National Institutes of Health Consensus Development Panel on Rehabilitation of Persons With Traumatic Brain Injury (1999) estimated that the incidence of TBI in the general population is 100 per 100,000. Prevalence is estimated at 2.5–6.5 million individuals. Other estimates include about 1.4 million injuries per year, with 50,000 deaths and 235,000 hospitalizations. The highest age of risk is 15–24 years, but the second highest risk group includes persons ages 64 and older. The incidence rate climbs more steeply after age 70. One estimate for persons ages 65–75 is 200 TBIs per 100,000 persons. This is twice the rate for the overall population but less than that of young adults.

Mild TBI, which can be a very significant problem for older adults, is probably underdiagnosed. Mild TBI, as defined by criteria such as a Glasgow Coma Scale score between 13 and 15 (Teasdale and Jennett 1974), loss of consciousness of ≤30 minutes, and duration of posttraumatic amnesia of <24 hours, can still result in substantial functional and cognitive disability and personality change. Although full recovery is the outcome of most mild TBI, all brain injuries can result in lifelong impairment of a person's physical, cognitive, and psychosocial function. These epidemiological figures are a rough guide to the magnitude of the problem, but they give only a glimpse at the cost in terms of the suffering of those injured and their families.

In the United States and much of the world, MVAs are the leading cause of brain trauma in young adults, but for persons ages 65 and older, falls are the predominant cause. Young men experience brain injury about twice as often as young women, but after age 65, the numbers are more equal. Certain age-related anatomical changes dispose older persons to greater risk of extra-axial hemorrhage, especially subdural hematoma.

Risk Factors

Many factors influence the risk of TBI among older adults (Table 26–1). Older individuals often have medical or neuro-

TABLE 26–1. Risk factors for falls

Reduced visual acuity, dark adaptation, and perception
Reduced hearing
Vestibular dysfunction
Musculoskeletal disorders
Foot disorders (calluses, bunions, deformities, loss of normal dorsiflexion)
Postural hypotension
Preexisting neurological disease
Proprioceptive dysfunction, cervical degenerative disorders, and peripheral neuropathy
Stroke
Alzheimer's disease and other dementias
Postural hypotension
Parkinson's disease
Weakness and frailty

psychiatric conditions that predispose them to falls or MVAs. Orthopedic illnesses, such as degenerative joint disease, and neurological disorders, such as impairment from stroke or Parkinson's disease, are common examples of illnesses that increase the risk of falling. Other risk factors include vision impairment, hearing impairment, vestibular disease, proprioceptive dysfunction, foot disorders, and postural hypotension.

Iatrogenic factors can increase risk of falls. Of principal importance are the risks associated with sedating or blood pressure–lowering drugs such as benzodiazepines, phenothiazines, older heterocyclic antidepressant drugs, and antihypertensive drugs. This iatrogenic risk factor can be especially common in nursing home patients, because drugs with sedating properties are often used to manage agitation (Ferrell 2000). Prudent pharmacotherapy, using a careful analysis of likely risks and benefits, the lowest effective dosages of medicine, and minimal polypharmacy, is a good approach when dealing with this difficult clinical dilemma.

Types and Mechanisms

To understand the common neuropsychiatric sequelae of TBI, it is helpful to consider the common underlying mechanisms of injury and the profile of damage that often results from these mechanisms. Two broad categories of forces result in brain injury: 1) contact or impact and 2) inertial acceleration or deceleration. Contact injuries result when the brain comes into contact with an object, which might be the skull or an external object. Contact mechanisms often result in damage to the scalp, the skull, and the brain surface (e.g., contusions, lacerations, hematomas) (Gennarelli and Graham 2005). The configuration of the external surface of the brain, the brain's position in the skull, and the uneven topography of the inner surface of certain skull regions are factors that result in heightened vulnerability to impact forces for certain brain regions (anterior and middle cranial fossae) (Bigler 2007; see Figure 26–1). Frequent sites of such injury are the anterior temporal poles, the lateral and inferior temporal cortices, the frontal poles, and the orbital frontal cortices.

Inertial injury results from rapid acceleration or deceleration of the brain that produces shear, tensile, and compression forces. These forces have maximum impact on axons and blood vessels, resulting in axonal injury, tissue tears, and intracerebral hematoma. These mechanisms also produce more widespread or diffuse injury to white matter, including diffuse axonal injury, also referred to as diffuse traumatic injury. Although damage can be diffuse, areas of greater vulnerability include the corpus callosum, the rostral brain stem, and the subfrontal white matter (Gennarelli and Graham 2005).

In older individuals, these forces frequently cause damage to cerebral blood vessels, with hemorrhage resulting. The classification of intracranial hemorrhages is based on the location of the bleeding. Traumatic hemorrhage between the skull and the dura mater, or epidural hemorrhage, is usually a result of severe trauma causing skull fracture and arterial rupture. Subdural hemorrhage or hematoma typically results from falls, MVAs, and assaults but can also occur after injuries without impact, such as whiplash injuries, or after very mild head bumps. Subdural hematoma, which results from rupture of the bridging veins in the subdural space between the brain and the dural venous sinuses (Figure 26–2), is common in older people. Age-related brain atrophy causes these bridging veins to be stretched and therefore more vulnerable to tearing (Chung and Caplan 2007) (Figure 26–3).

Intracerebral hematomas—that is, hematomas not in contact with the surface of the brain—are most frequently found in the frontal and temporal regions. Their exact pathogenesis is not clearly understood, but they might result from blood vessel rupture at the time of injury. In addition, tissue-tear hemorrhages can occur. These are often small, ranging in size from miniscule petechiae to 1-cm lesions. They are characteristically located in the parasagittal portion of the brain, are associated with diffuse axonal injury, and are caused by acceleration-induced brain damage (Gennarelli and Graham 2005).

In addition to the impact and inertial forces, mechanical distortion of neurons results in massive release of neurotransmitters, with subsequent triggering of complex excitotoxic in-

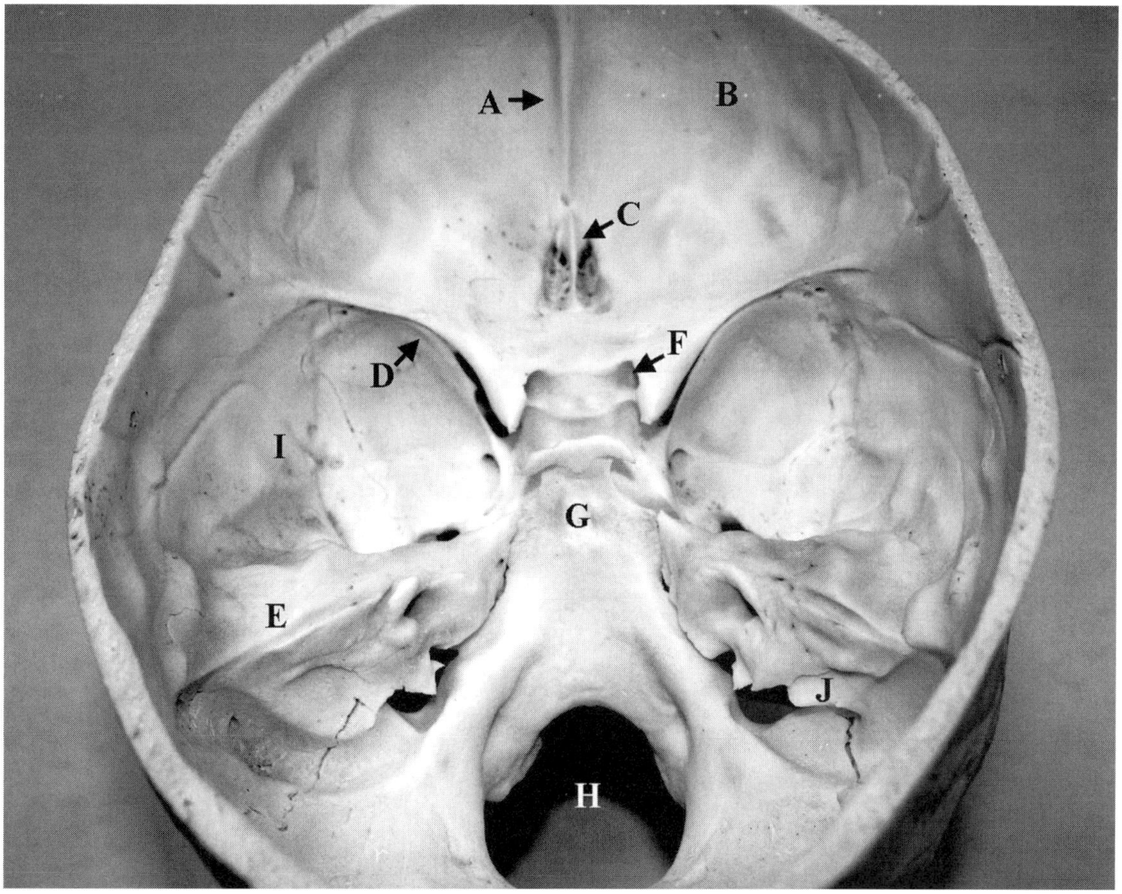

FIGURE 26–1. Skull base.

The skull cap has been removed, exposing the inner surface of the ventral base of the skull, with the various anatomical structures with the three cranial fossae clearly defined. The uneven surface of each fossa is clearly observable. The general location of the hippocampus (medial wall of the middle cranial fossa) and where the base of the frontal lobe is located (anterior cranial fossa) are depicted. A=frontal crest; B=anterior cranial fossa; C=crista galli with cribriform plate beneath; D=sphenoid bone; E=petrous temporal bone; F=clinoid bone and area of the sella turcica; G=clivus; H=foramen magnum; I=middle cranial fossa; J=posterior cranial fossa.

Source. Bigler ED: "Anterior and Middle Cranial Fossa in Traumatic Brain Injury: Relevant Neuroanatomy and Neuropathology in the Study of Neuropsychological Outcome." *Neuropsychology* 21:520, 2007.

jury cascades (Raghupathi et al. 2000). Although this probably occurs throughout the brain, the excitotoxic cascades and other forms of secondary injury, such as hypoxia and ischemia, have a disproportionate effect on certain brain regions, such as the hippocampus, even in the context of an otherwise fairly mild injury (Umile et al. 2002).

Although not particularly relevant to older persons, the use of explosive devices, particularly "improvised explosive devices" (a primary method of attack in the conflicts in Iraq and Afghanistan and in hostilities elsewhere) has called attention to the effects of "blast injury." Explosions generate a rapidly moving wave of overheated, overpressurized air, followed by a low-pressure trough. These waves are particularly damaging to air- and fluid-filled organs and cavities and can be associated with significant brain injury (Cernak et al. 2001; Mayorga 1997; Warden 2006). These blast-created pressurized waves probably cause injury by distorting vascular or neural tissue or both. Other injury mechanisms that often occur in blast injuries include impact effects from the head coming into contact with an object, rapid acceleration or deceleration of the brain causing inertial injury, and penetrating injuries from shrapnel or debris.

Thus, the typical profile of injury involves a combination of primary injury, which occurs at the time of application of force, and secondary injury, which evolves over time after the primary injury, with a combination of focal and diffuse injury. In a fall, damage usually results from a combination of impact force from the skull and brain hitting a hard surface and iner-

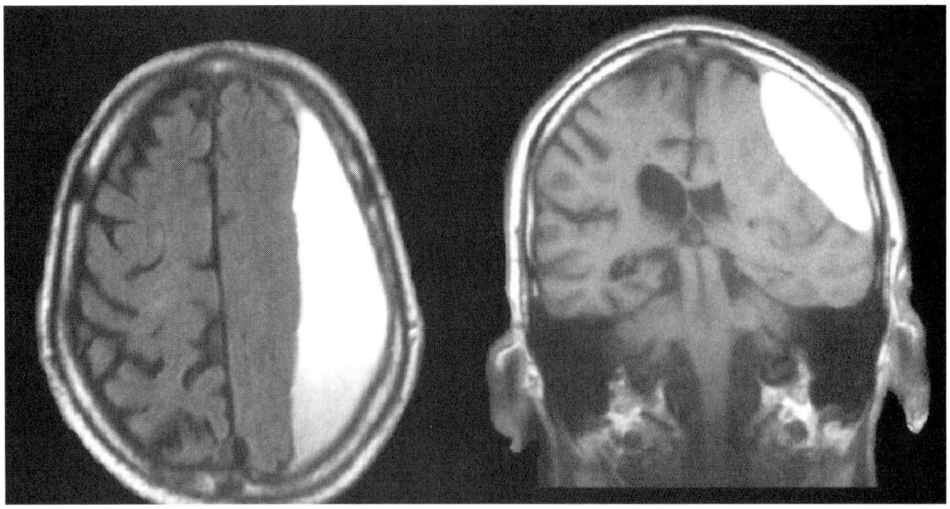

FIGURE 26–2. Subdural hematoma—unilateral acute.

Source. Reprinted with permission from Preston DC, Shapiro BE: *Neuroimaging in Neurology: An Interactive CD.* Philadelphia, PA, WB Saunders/Elsevier Health Sciences, 2007. Copyright © 2007 Elsevier. www.elsevierhealth.com.

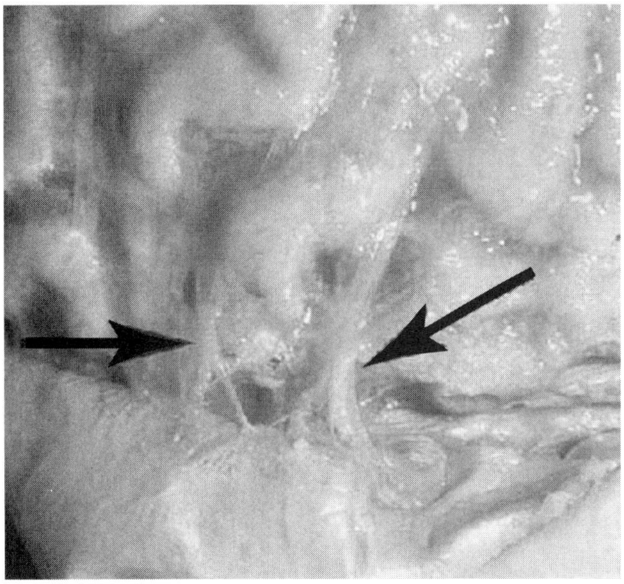

FIGURE 26–3. Bridging veins with dura mater reflected.

Source. Reprinted with permission from Newton BW: "Anatomy of the Spinal Cord and Brain," in *Neuroscience in Medicine.* Edited by Conn PM. Totowa, NJ, Humana Press, 2008, p. 47. Copyright © 2008 Springer Science+Business Media.

tial force from rapid deceleration, with subsequent stress and strain on white matter and cerebral vasculature. Although the damage may be diffuse or multifocal, certain brain regions are highly vulnerable to injury. These vulnerable regions include the frontal cortex and subfrontal white matter, the deeper midline structures including the basal ganglia, the rostral brain stem, and the temporal lobes including the hippocampi. Injuries to these areas probably account for both the high rate of challenging behavior and the increased rates of psychiatric illness that are associated with TBI.

In addition to the profile of regional brain injury described above, certain neurotransmitter systems, particularly the catecholaminergic and cholinergic systems, are altered in TBI. Both of these systems play critical roles in a variety of domains important in behavioral homeostasis, including arousal, cognition, reward behavior, and mood regulation (Charney 1998; McAllister 2000; Smeets and Gonzalez 2000). For example, there is significant evidence for dysfunction of catecholaminergic systems associated with TBI (McAllister et al. 2004; McIntosh 1994; McIntosh et al. 1998). TBI results in activation of the sympathoadrenomedullary axis, with subsequent alterations in hemodynamic parameters and cardiopulmonary function. Plasma norepinephrine levels are elevated after TBI, and this elevation correlates with injury severity indicators (Jennett and Teasdale 1981). Circulating levels of dopamine, norepinephrine, and epinephrine may be markers of injury severity and likelihood of recovery (McIntosh 1994; McIntosh et al. 1998). Animal models of TBI have also shown a relationship between injury severity, increasing circulating levels of epinephrine and norepinephrine, and secondary complications such as cardiac arrhythmias (Prasad et al. 1993). Transient hypoxia, common in more severe injuries, can result in dramatic releases of hippocampal norepinephrine (Globus et al. 1989). Animal studies suggest that alterations in dopamine, norepinephrine, and epinephrine levels can be prolonged after TBI and can be associated with alterations in catecholaminergic receptors in damaged cortical areas that can impair catecholaminergic function after trauma (McIntosh 1994; Prasad et al. 1993). Administration of certain catecholaminergic agents may enhance recovery from brain injury (Feeney and Hovda 1983; Feeney and Sutton 1987; Feeney et al. 1981), even after one-time doses (Boyeson and Feeney 1984; Feeney et al. 1981; Romhanyi et al. 1990; Tandian et al. 1990). Conversely, catecholaminergic *antagonists* can slow rate of recovery from certain types of brain injury (Sutton and Feeney 1992).

Likewise, several lines of evidence suggest acute and chronic disturbances in the central cholinergic system. Cerebral cholinergic neurons and their ascending projections are vulnerable to trauma (Arciniegas 2003). Acutely, cholinergic neurons release large amounts of acetylcholine, which probably plays a role in triggering the excitotoxic cascades. In fact, cholinergic antagonists can be neuroprotective in models of TBI (see Arciniegas 2003 for review). After the acute injury, long-term reductions in cerebral acetylcholine levels have been shown (Dixon et al. 1995).

This described profile of structural and neurochemical injury plays a direct role in the common neurobehavioral sequelae associated with TBI outlined in the next section below ("Neuropsychiatric Sequelae of TBI"), including problems in cognition and in emotional and behavioral regulation and increased rates of psychiatric disorders.

Neuropsychiatric Sequelae

Changes in Cognition

Challenges with cognition are the most common complaints voiced after TBI (Lovell and Franzen 1994; Whyte et al. 1996) and are the major barrier to normal life regarding independent living, social adaptation, family life, and work (Ben-Yishay and Diller 1993; Cicerone et al. 2000). Several cognitive domains are predictably impaired in patients with TBI, including frontal executive functions such as problem solving, set shifting, impulse control, and self-monitoring (Freedman et al. 1987; Lehtonen et al. 2005; Mattson and Levin 1990). Other common cognitive symptoms include impaired attention (Binder 1986, 1997; Binder et al. 1997; Cripe 1987; Gentilini et al. 1989; Gronwall 1989, 1991; Hart et al. 2006; Leininger et al. 1990; Levin and Grossman 1978; Levin et al. 1987a, 1987b, 1988; Mathias and Wheaton 2007), short-term memory and learning (Cripe 1987; Levin et al. 1987b, 1988; McMillan and Glucksman 1987; Ruff et al. 1989; Stuss et al. 1985; Vakil 2005), speed of information processing (Cripe 1987; Gronwall 1989; Leininger et al. 1990; Levin et al. 1987b; Mathias and Wheaton 2007; McMillan and Glucksman 1987; O'Jile et al. 2006; Rassovsky et al. 2006; Stuss et al. 1985), and speech and language functions (Ewing-Cobbs and Barnes 2002; Jackson and Moffat 1987; Levin et al. 1987b; Ross and Rush 1981; Weintraub et al. 1981). These are not completely independent domains. A mixture of deficits across these mental functions is typical.

Postconcussion syndrome is a term that refers to common symptoms that occur after TBI, usually after mild TBI. Although cognitive symptoms such as decreases in memory, attention, and concentration are particularly prominent, somatic symptoms such as headache, fatigue, insomnia, dizziness, tinnitus, and sensitivity to noise or light frequently co-occur, and emotional complaints such as depression, irritability, and anxiety are also common. These symptoms typically show significant improvement after approximately 3 months but may last longer (Grafman and Salazar 2000). It is not at all clear that this is truly a syndrome as opposed to a list of symptoms common after brain injury with variable recovery trajectories. Furthermore, the use of the term does not imply a single cause or suggest that there might be a single treatment; neither has been shown to be true, nor has it been our clinical experience. For these reasons, it seems more prudent to think in terms of persistent postconcussive symptoms and consider causes and treatments separately.

Changes in Personality

Persons with TBI and their families and caregivers frequently describe alterations in emotional and behavioral regulation as "changes in personality." Many of the distressing changes in personality after TBI are the result of impaired executive function and can be referred to as "dysexecutive syndromes." A full discussion of the neuroanatomical substrates of these behaviors is beyond the scope of this chapter, but the link between the injury profile in a typical TBI and some of these behaviors is fundamentally understood and warrants some thought and discussion (see McDonald et al. 2002 for review).

Five major frontal-subcortical circuits have been identified, of which three have significant roles in nonmotor forms of behavior (Cummings 1993; Mega and Cummings 2001). Each of these three circuits can affect motivated behavior, though in somewhat different ways. Damage to the dorsolateral prefrontal cortex and its circuitry impairs executive functions such as working memory, decision making, problem solving, and mental flexibility. Damage to the orbitofrontal cortex and related nodal points impairs intuitive reflexive social behaviors and the capacity to self-monitor and self-correct within a social context. Damage to anterior cingulate and related circuitry impairs motivated and reward-related behaviors. Damage to medial temporal regions further impairs other aspects of memory and the smooth integration of emotional memory with current experience and real-time assessment of salience of stimuli. The frontal-subcortical circuits responsible for these critical domains of higher intellectual function and empathic, motivated, nuanced human behavior are highly vulnerable to injury in the typical TBI.

As a result of the damage frequently sustained to components of these frontal-subcortical circuits, an array of common symptoms can be seen in TBI survivors (McAllister 2007). These include impulsivity, irritability, affective instability, awareness deficits, and apathy.

Impulsivity

Impulse-control problems may be evident in verbal utterances, physical actions, snap decisions, and poor judgment derived from failure to consider the implications of an action. Impulsivity is closely related to the concept of being stimulus bound, in which the individual responds to the most salient cue in the environment or attaches exaggerated importance to a particular cue.

Irritability

Family members may describe patients with TBI as more irritable or more easily angered than before injury. Although a particular stimulus for anger might be perceived as a legitimate aggravation, the response is commonly exaggerated. Responses can range from oral outbursts to dangerous assaultive behavior. The person's capacity to modulate such behavior is what has changed.

Affective Instability

Injured persons and their families and caregivers frequently describe exaggerated displays of emotional expression, out of proportion to the precipitating stimulus and to the preinjury range of responses to similar stimuli. Cues that previously elicited momentary sadness now precipitate weeping or crying. Events that in the past might have provoked a frown or an irritated reply now result in loud angry outbursts associated with marked sympathetic arousal. The main features of this affective instability are a paroxysmal onset, brief duration, and exaggerated intense response that is excessive for the precipitating stimulus. This phenomenon is common to many central nervous system disorders and has been variably called pathological affect, affective lability, pseudobulbar affect, affective incontinence, and more recently, involuntary emotional expression disorder.

Awareness Deficits

The burden of the changes in personality and behavior that accompany TBI is often increased by lack of awareness of the impairment. The injured person might not appreciate that his or her behavior is different since the injury, whereas family members are greatly distressed and describe fundamental ways in which the injured individual has changed. Some individuals with TBI, however, may have a sense that they are different or "not who I used to be." They may struggle to describe exactly how their behavior or personality has changed. Persons with TBI are less likely to be aware of changes in behavior and executive function than of changes in physical domains such as motor function. The extent of awareness of impairment correlates with functional and vocational outcome in many (Ezrachi et al. 1991; Sherer et al. 1998a, 1998b; Trudel et al. 1996) but not all (Cavallo et al. 1992) studies. Current literature suggests that lack of awareness of illness is not simply a function of global cognitive deficits but is likely to be related to frontal executive dysfunction (Cuesta and Peralta 1994; Cuesta et al. 1995; David et al. 1995; Lysaker and Bell 1994; McEvoy et al. 1989; Mohamed et al. 1999; Young et al. 1993). In individuals with TBI, this unawareness is frequently a prominent family and caregiver concern (Ford 1976; McAllister 1992; Miller and Stern 1965; Oddy et al. 1985; Ota 1969; Prigatano 1991). Even when the individual with TBI admits to some difficulties, he or she is often unable to comprehend the implications of these deficits in social situations.

Apathy

The underlying deficit associated with apathy is in the realm of motivated behavior (Marin 1991). Although apathy is not as overtly disturbing as some of the other changes described in this section, it can be a concern and is a common reason that individuals with TBI do not progress in rehabilitation programs. Apathy is often misinterpreted as laziness or depression and may be linked paradoxically to aggression when, for example, attempts to engage the individual in activities for which he or she has little interest can precipitate assaultive behavior (McAllister 2000).

Apathy is quite common after TBI. Kant et al. (1998) found that apathy mixed with depression occurred in 60% of their sample. Andersson et al. (1999) found that almost half of individuals with TBI in their study had significant apathy. Deficits in motivated behavior can occur in association with injury to the circuitry of "reward" (Chau et al. 2004; McAllister 2000). Key nodal points in this circuitry include the amygdala, hippocampus, caudate, entorhinal and cingulate cortices, ventral tegmental area, and medial forebrain bundle. Catecholaminergic systems, most notably the mesolimbic dopaminergic system, appear to play critical roles in the modulation of this reward system (Chau et al. 2004; McAllister 2000).

Relationship to Psychiatric Disorders

A significant body of evidence suggests that in addition to causing changes in cognition, behavior, and personality, TBI results in an increased relative risk of developing various psychiatric disorders, including mood and anxiety disorders, substance abuse disorders, and psychotic syndromes (Deb et al. 1998; Hibbard et al. 1998; Koponen et al. 2002; van Reekum et al. 2000). For example, Koponen et al. (2002) studied 60 individuals 30 years after TBI and found that 48% developed a new Axis I psychiatric disorder after their injury. The most common diagnoses were depression, substance abuse, and anxiety disorders. Rates of lifetime and current depression (26% and 10%, respectively), panic disorder (8% and 6%), and psychotic disorders (8% and 8%) were significantly higher than base rates found in the Epidemiologic Catchment Area (ECA) study (Silver et al. 2001). Hibbard et al. (1998) studied 100 adults on average 8 years after TBI. A significant number of the individuals had Axis I disorders before injury. After TBI, the most frequent diagnoses were major depression and anxiety disorders such as posttraumatic stress disorder (PTSD), obsessive-compulsive disorder, and panic disorder. Almost half (44%) of the individuals had two or more disorders. More recently, these investigators reported a longitudinal study of 188 individuals enrolled within 4 years of injury and assessed at yearly intervals on at least two occasions (Hibbard et al. 2004). Once again, they found elevated rates when compared with population base rates as reported in the ECA study of psychiatric disorders, such as depression and substance abuse, before injury. After TBI, individuals had increased rates of depression, PTSD, and other anxiety disorders. This was particularly true of those with preinjury psychiatric disorders. Furthermore, the rates were greatest at the initial assessment point after injury and stabilized or decreased over time. In a careful review of the literature about the relationship of TBI to psychiatric disorders, van Reekum et al. (2000) concluded that TBI was associated with an increase in the relative risk for several psychiatric disorders. Others have also reported increased indicators of psychiatric illness after TBI and increased medical costs associated with those indicators (Fann et al. 2004; Wei et al. 2005). Fujii and Ahmed (2002) analyzed case studies of psychosis after TBI. Delusions and hallucinations were common, but negative symptoms were generally not present, so the clinical profile was different in this respect from that typically seen in schizophrenia.

Like those with other potentially disabling conditions, individuals with TBI experience symptoms and feelings such as discouragement, frustration, fatigue, and anxiety. Not all of these symptoms will rise to the level of a disorder, but symptoms that are sustained for several weeks and that interfere with social or occupational function or quality of life are legitimately considered disorders. The consistent observation that individuals who sustain a TBI have higher base rates of psychopathology before injury also suggests that there is a reciprocal interaction: psychopathology predisposes to TBI, and TBI in turn increases vulnerability to psychiatric disorders. Because many of these studies were done in younger populations, it is not clear if this interaction between injury and psychopathology holds true for older individuals. Nevertheless, an elevated index of suspicion for the development of psychiatric illness, in the context of changing or worsening behavioral challenges after a TBI, is justified.

Relationship to Alzheimer's Disease

Many individuals with moderate or severe TBI with significant impairment in memory and executive function meet the diagnostic criteria for dementia as a direct result of injury. A critical issue is whether TBI increases the risk of a progressive dementing disorder such as Alzheimer's disease (AD) later in life. The relationship between TBI and AD is complicated and not completely understood.

There is reason to be concerned about a potential link between AD and TBI. Van Den Heuvel et al. (2007) wrote an excellent review of this topic. This issue was probably first raised by the clinical observation that boxers with repetitive brain injury developed a progressive dementia referred to as dementia pugilistica (Martland 1928). Pathological examination of individuals with this syndrome initially showed predominant neurofibrillary tangles and then subsequently showed amyloid plaques similar to those found in AD and other neurodegenerative disorders (Roberts et al. 1990). Subsequent investigations found that TBI-associated disruption of axonal transport results in the rapid accumulation of amyloid precursor protein (APP) in both animals (Van Den Heuvel et al. 1999, 2007) and humans (Blumbergs et al. 1995; Graham et al. 1995). Furthermore, the APP colocalizes with enzymes that process APP to β-amyloid (Aβ), as well as with Aβ itself, in both animals and humans (Smith et al. 1999, 2003). Evidence of abnormal APP as well as Aβ plaques has been found after a single TBI both acutely (Ikonomovic et al. 2004) and years after the injury (Rudelli et al. 1982). Current evidence suggests that APP, Aβ, and other proteins associated with AD and other neurodegenerative disorders accumulate quite rapidly after TBI (Chen et al. 2009; Uryu et al. 2004, 2007) and that in some, but not all, individuals, these abnormal deposits can be chronic. Some, but not all, studies have shown increased amyloid plaques and neurofibrillary tangles in autopsy studies of individuals with TBI, suggesting that although acute changes in the amyloid cascades may be quite common, not all individuals will have chronic abnormalities (Braak and Braak 1997; Chen et al. 2009).

Related to the variability in findings of AD-like pathology in human cohorts, investigators have explored whether genetic factors play a role in individual susceptibility differences. For example, some evidence suggests that for people with a genetic vulnerability to AD, TBI may increase the risk of developing AD at an earlier age (Friedman et al. 1999; Gedye et al.

1989; Mayeux et al. 1993, 1995; Nicoll et al. 1995). Mayeux et al. (1995) compared 138 persons ages 65 and older who were diagnosed with AD and 193 healthy persons of comparable age without dementia. Based on this comparison, the investigators analyzed the relative weight for each of the risk factors for AD found in the histories of these individuals. They found that the odds ratio for AD associated with TBI was 3.7. When TBI occurred after age 70, the risk for AD was even greater, with a 19.1 odds ratio (Mayeux et al. 1993).

In a later study, Mayeux et al. (1995) retrospectively studied 113 older adults with AD, comparing them with a control group of 123 healthy older individuals without dementia. They found that a history of TBI alone did not increase the risk of AD but that the presence of the apolipoprotein E (*APOE*) ε4 allele alone increased the risk twofold. Most important, a combination of the ε4 allele and a history of TBI increased the risk of AD by a factor of 10.

Related to these observations, persons with the *APOE* ε4 allele might have a worse outcome after TBI than those without the ε4 allele, regardless of the presence or absence of dementia (Friedman et al. 1999; Teasdale et al. 1997). For example, Teasdale et al. (1997) prospectively studied individuals with TBI and found that persons with the ε4 allele had a significantly worse outcome 6 months after brain injury than did individuals without the ε4 allele but with similar demographic and brain injury variables (Teasdale et al. 1997). In this study, worse outcome meant being in a vegetative state, being severely disabled based on the Glasgow Outcome Score, or death.

Another study found that those with the ε4 allele had worse short-term outcome, meaning a low Glasgow Coma Scale score and loss of consciousness lasting more than 7 days after TBI, and worse outcome 6–8 months after the TBI (Friedman et al. 1999). Although TBI might increase the risk of AD for people who have the ε4 allele, TBI by itself does not appear to be an independent risk factor for developing AD (Mayeux et al. 1993, 1995; Mehta et al. 1999). In other words, TBI alone is neither a necessary nor a sufficient cause of AD.

Not all studies agree that TBI increases the risk of developing AD in people with the *APOE* ε4 allele. A prospective population-based study of 6,645 individuals, who were ages 55 and older and free of dementia at baseline, found that mild brain trauma was not a major risk factor for the development of AD. Moreover, brain trauma did not appear to increase the risk of developing AD in people carrying the ε4 allele (Mehta et al. 1999). In the same study, however, the investigators found a trend toward a higher risk of dementia with an increasing number of brain injuries and with a history of loss of consciousness lasting more than 15 minutes following head injury. Another possibility is that diminished cognitive reserve associated with TBI might facilitate earlier manifestation of dementia symptoms in individuals already at risk for AD (Starkstein and Jorge 2005). Thus, despite some compelling scientific reasons to consider the relationship of TBI to AD and other neurodegenerative disorders, as well as some strong evidence suggesting clinical associations, the relationship between TBI and dementia needs further study.

Neuropsychiatric Assessment

Careful evaluation of neurobehavioral problems is an important part of the rehabilitation of older persons with TBI. The pattern of sequelae should make sense from the injury. A good neuropsychiatric evaluation is based on the principle of understanding the profile of brain injury and then evaluating the current signs and symptoms in the context of what is known about the injury to assess goodness of fit. If signs and symptoms are not accounted for by the profile of injury, then an explanation other than TBI should be sought. The clinical picture should make sense in the context of the brain damage. Several points are worth highlighting.

Use Multiple Sources of Information

Obtaining the most accurate information possible is essential. The cognitive deficits that frequently accompany a TBI can affect the injured person's ability to give an accurate history. Short-term memory deficits, problems with sequencing events in time, and difficulties with self-awareness can make clear and accurate history giving difficult. The clinician must then seek other sources of information, such as family members, friends, employers, medical records, and school or work records, that can clarify the history and current clinical presentation. This may be particularly challenging for elderly patients, who may be living alone and may have been struggling with memory problems even before their TBI.

Assess Preinjury Baseline

Assessment of the effects of an injury starts with a thorough understanding of what the individual was like before the injury. Without such information, there is a risk of mistaken attribution of lifelong traits, characteristics, and behaviors to the brain injury. Such baseline information is best obtained shortly after the injury. The more time that has passed from the injury, the greater is the tendency to incorrectly attribute more and more symptoms and complaints to the injury.

Assess Postinjury Changes

Once the baseline picture is complete, the clinician can more accurately assess the changes that have occurred since the injury. It is important to carefully review the functional domains that are frequently affected by injury, including cognition, personality, mood regulation, speech and language, mobility, and higher-order functional areas such as vocational performance and performance of one's role within the family or other social context.

Attempt to Determine Etiology

We emphasize that temporal association does not guarantee causality. Neurobehavioral change can be associated with brain injury in several ways. Change may be a direct effect of the insult to neural tissue, with subsequent disruption of the functions subserved by the damaged tissue. Assessment of this possibility requires accurate, sometimes fine-grained knowledge of the profile of regional brain injury—that is, the "neural component"—and its relationship to the functional change in question. Alternatively, the reported change could reflect the development of a new illness or disorder that causes behavioral change. For example, an individual could be affected by a "biological component," such as endocrine complications of a brain injury related to pituitary damage, or could have chronic pain from orthopedic injuries. Behavioral change also could be caused by the emotional meaning of the accident or injury—that is, a "psychological component"—such as a loss of self-esteem resulting from a disfiguring injury, loss of mobility or other physical disability, or unemployment. Finally, changes in the patient's environment, such as the patient's living situation, a change in caregivers, or a change in routine or the flow and continuity of daily life, can affect the behavior and adaptation of a person with brain injury or other neuropsychiatric illness; these changes constitute the "social component."

Development of a Formulation and Interpretation of Events

Brain injury can involve all the above-mentioned etiological components (e.g., biological, psychological, social). For example, the individual would not have endocrine abnormalities without the injury-related pituitary damage. Depression might not have developed without the injury. The degree of linkage to neural tissue damage, however, varies among these components. An individual showing new aggressive outbursts associated with a change in residential care providers might be better helped by further training of the residential provider rather than by the aggressive use of medications. However, if this patient has clear evidence of orbitofrontal damage, his or her threshold for tolerating frustration might be lowered so that both treatment with medication and improved environmental support are needed.

Assessment and formulation of the relative contribution of each of these components to the development of the behavior change frame a neurobiopsychosocial paradigm. This approach is different from traditional psychiatric assessment with respect to the critical importance placed on understanding the profile of regional brain injury, as well as the array of complex behavioral circuitry that this profile would reasonably disrupt. The work of the neuropsychiatric assessment can be summarized as the process of matching the profile of brain injury with the changes that have occurred in cognition, behavior, and overall function, and gauging the "goodness of fit" between predicted and actual outcomes. The clinician then assigns relative weights to the various contributions of neural, biological, psychological, and social components. This formulation provides a rational basis for treatment and intervention.

Even experienced clinicians can make mistakes in this process because of the complexity of clinical presentations and the difficulty in obtaining complete data. The final critical component in this process is therefore regular reevaluation of the efficacy of treatment. Each formulation should have an underlying hypothesis. Each intervention should flow logically from the hypothesis and should then be empirically tested by clinical response (e.g., "I believe the increase in aggression is part of a depressive disorder; therefore, I will prescribe an antidepressant"). Poor or incomplete response to the intervention should lead to a reevaluation and to formulation of a new hypothesis to be tested. It is acceptable to be wrong, but it is not acceptable to engage in sloppy thinking.

Principles in Treatment

Prevention and General Treatment Concepts

Because no cure exists for TBI once it has occurred, prevention is of great importance. As is the case in prevention of most illnesses, education is of paramount importance. This includes informing the public about the reality of TBI risk in older people, including risk of falls. A point not often mentioned in the literature, and perhaps an idealistic one, is that a routine of physical conditioning and fitness on the part of older individuals would likely significantly decrease risk of TBI from accidental falling. Once injury has occurred, treatment consists of physical and cognitive rehabilitation, social and psychotherapeutic support, and careful use of pharmacotherapy to treat specific neuropsychiatric symptoms or syndromes. All treatment should be directed to the needs of older persons. With regard to psychopharmacotherapy, this means using geriatric prescribing principles, such as starting with low dosages, making small changes, having as clear an indication as possible for each medicine, and persisting with a particular regimen long enough to give it a good chance to work. Pessimism with regard to recovery of older individuals from TBI is not justified, especially in the case of mild or moderate injury. The general trend of reported data is toward a worse outcome for older than for younger individuals with TBI, but individuals are not statistics. Each person, regardless of age, should receive concerted rehabilitative treatment aimed at maximum functional recovery.

Use of Medications

Atypical Clinical Presentations

Clinical presentations of common psychiatric disorders may not meet standard diagnostic criteria as outlined in DSM-IV-TR (American Psychiatric Association 2000) because cognitive and sensorimotor deficits associated with TBIs can distort the picture. Having "relaxed-fit" criteria when approaching diagnoses in individuals with TBI is therefore reasonable.

Trait Versus State Presentations

Two broad factors contribute to the neurobehavioral sequelae of TBI: 1) the injury-induced changes in personality and 2) the associated increased rate of psychiatric disorders. A problem occurs when the patient with a psychiatric disorder presents with a heightening or worsening of personality change. For example, an individual with TBI can have a baseline of increased irritability or lowered frustration tolerance. If depression or mania or another psychiatric disorder then occurs, these traits can be exaggerated. If the clinician does not carefully tease out the postinjury baseline and clearly ascertain if a change has occurred in the frequency and intensity of the challenging behaviors, the behavior can easily be misattributed to a dysexecutive syndrome only, instead of to a dysexecutive syndrome that is being made significantly worse by the presence of a treatable psychiatric disorder, such as depression. An important therapeutic opportunity is then lost.

Importance of Diagnostic Hypothesis

When possible, the clinician should treat syndromes or disorders rather than symptoms and should try to establish a diagnosis before beginning treatment. Designing a treatment plan should follow, not precede, an earnest attempt to formulate a differential diagnosis and propose a most-likely diagnostic hypothesis. Many clinicians, however, are inclined to prescribe antipsychotics or selective serotonin reuptake inhibitors (SSRIs) without formulating a hypothesis about what they are treating. This symptomatic approach is similar to treating a fever associated with a bacterial infection with acetaminophen but not antibiotics. In the neuropsychiatric arena, a symptomatic approach should be used only after having carefully ruled in or out 1) the presence of an Axis I disorder, such as depression, mania, or psychosis; 2) neuromedical conditions that might account for the behavior, such as complex partial seizures, pain, iatrogenic complications, or medication side effects; and 3) factors in the environment that might cause the change in behavioral symptoms.

Role of Behavioral Metaphors

When data are difficult to obtain or when the neurological deficits through which challenging behaviors are being expressed are particularly severe, a clinician may be at a loss to account for the etiology of a given behavior or cluster of behaviors, or to be clear about a treatment strategy. A fallback position is to conceptualize the behaviors as if they were a particular syndrome or as if they represented what Tariot and colleagues have termed a "behavioral metaphor" (Tariot 1999; Tariot et al. 2002). For example, a person expressing increased negativism, loss of interest in activities, or self-destructive or self-injurious behavior might be viewed as having a depressive syndrome and thus could reasonably be prescribed an antidepressant regimen. An individual with increased irritability, increased arousal and activation, and a significant reduction in sleep might be regarded as having an irritable mania-like syndrome and thus could reasonably be started on an anticycling regimen of mood stabilizers. The critical point is that these are testable hypotheses and should be treated as such. Target behaviors and baseline frequencies should be identified before treatment, and an adequate but time-limited trial of treatment should be prescribed. If the anticipated goal is not achieved in a reasonable time, the treatment should be discontinued and an alternative hypothesis should be considered. Individuals with cognitive impairment, including individuals with TBI, often have heightened sensitivity to medications, as well as to their environments.

Predictability of Response

Both injured and noninjured individuals base decisions and actions on their predictions of how others will respond to a given action. Persons with TBI often have great difficulty with this type of prediction and may be confused, anxious, or agitated as a result.

Summary

For the clinician performing a neuropsychiatric assessment, ignoring the patient's environment and factors that may be provoking challenging behaviors will greatly reduce the efficacy of any prescribed medication, even if it is the proper medication. Conversely, without properly prescribed medication, even heroic efforts at applied behavioral analysis and environmental manipulation may be in vain. The therapeutic question then should not be framed as "Do we prescribe a drug or write a behavioral plan?" but rather as "Which medicine prescribed in the context of what changes in environment and strategies for shaping behavior has the best potential for success?"

Conclusion

Older adults are at significant risk for TBI. Although TBI can be devastating at any age, older individuals are at heightened risk for death and for disability of all types. Possible neuropsychiatric complications include cognitive disability, affective illness or instability, impaired judgment, psychosis, disinhibited or maladaptive behavior, and anxiety disorders. Falls are the leading cause of TBI in older persons. Because of age-related changes in the brain and its vasculature, older adults are especially vulnerable to extra-axial hemorrhage, such as subdural hematoma. Risk factors for falls include preexisting orthopedic or neurological disorders, weakness, problems with balance or vision, other general medical conditions, and iatrogenic factors. Convalescence and rehabilitation after TBI may be slower for older persons than for younger persons. Despite greater risk for worse outcomes, older adults with neuropsychiatric complaints deserve careful and compassionate neuropsychiatric evaluation and treatment.

Key Points

- Falls are the leading cause of traumatic brain injury (TBI) in older adults, so efforts aimed at fall prevention are the most important protective measures.
- TBI can result in cognitive impairment and personality changes, including impulsivity, irritability, affective instability, lack of awareness of deficits, and apathy.
- TBI heightens risk for psychiatric disorders, including affective disorders, anxiety disorders, substance abuse disorders, and psychotic syndromes.
- Recovery for older adults may be slower or less complete than for younger people, but older people still deserve concerted efforts to enhance their rehabilitation and to diagnose and treat associated neuropsychiatric symptoms.

Recommended Web Sites

Brain Injury Association of America: www.biausa.org/index.html. Includes information about finding a Brain Injury Association by state, as well as information about careers, living with brain injury, and how to get involved.

Brain Injury Resource Center: www.headinjury.com. This site is maintained by the Brain Injury Resource Center and is an excellent source for best practices in the field of traumatic brain injury. The site advocates that "proactive involvement, knowledge, self-awareness, and self-advocacy are key to quality of life following brain injury."

Centers for Disease Control and Prevention, Traumatic Brain Injury page: www.cdc.gov/traumaticbraininjury. Provides information on all types of head injury, with particularly good sections regarding fall risk and prevention in older people.

References

American Psychiatric Association: Diagnostic and Statistical Manual of Mental Disorders, 4th Edition, Text Revision. Washington, DC, American Psychiatric Association, 2000

Andersson S, Krogstad JM, Finset A: Apathy and depressed mood in acquired brain damage: relationship to lesion localization and psychophysiological reactivity. Psychol Med 29:447–456, 1999

Arciniegas DB: The cholinergic hypothesis of cognitive impairment caused by traumatic brain injury. Curr Psychiatry Rep 5:391–399, 2003

Ben-Yishay Y, Diller L: Cognitive remediation in traumatic brain injury: update and issues. Arch Phys Med Rehabil 74:204–213, 1993

Bigler ED: Anterior and middle cranial fossa in traumatic brain injury: relevant neuroanatomy and neuropathology in the study of neuropsychological outcome. Neuropsychology 21:515–531, 2007

Binder LM: Persisting symptoms after mild head injury: a review of the post-concussive syndrome. J Clin Exp Neuropsychol 8:323–346, 1986

Binder LM: A review of mild head trauma, part II: clinical implications (review). J Clin Exp Neuropsychol 19:432–457, 1997

Binder LM, Rohling ML, Larrabee J: A review of mild head trauma, part I: meta-analytic review of neuropsychological studies. J Clin Exp Neuropsychol 19:421–431, 1997

Blumbergs PC, Scott G, Manavis J, et al: Topography of axonal injury as defined by amyloid precursor protein and the sector scoring method in mild and severe closed head injury. J Neurotrauma 12: 565–572, 1995

Bouras T, Stranjalis G, Korfias S, et al: Head injury mortality in a geriatric population: differentiating an "edge" age group with better potential for benefit than older poor-prognosis patients. J Neurotrauma 24:1355–1361, 2007
Boyeson MG, Feeney DM: The role of norepinephrine in recovery from brain injury. Abstr Soc Neurosci 10:68, 1984
Braak H, Braak E: Frequency of stages of Alzheimer-related lesions in different age categories. Neurobiol Aging 18:351–357, 1997
Cavallo MM, Kay T, Ezrachi O: Problems and changes after traumatic brain injury: differing perceptions within and between families. Brain Inj 6:327–335, 1992
Cernak I, Wang Z, Jiang J, et al: Ultrastructural and functional characteristics of blast injury-induced neurotrauma. J Trauma 50: 695–706, 2001
Charney DS: Monoamine dysfunction and the pathophysiology and treatment of depression. J Clin Psychiatry 59(suppl):11–14, 1998
Chau DT, Roth RM, Green AI: The neural circuitry of reward and its relevance to psychiatric disorders. Curr Psychiatry Rep 6:391–399, 2004
Chen X, Johnson V, Uryu K, et al: A lack of amyloid beta plaques despite persistent accumulation of amyloid beta in axons of long-term survivors of traumatic brain injury. Brain Pathol 19:214–223, 2009
Chung CS, Caplan LR: Stroke and other neurovascular disorders, in Textbook of Clinical Neurology, 3rd Edition. Edited by Goetz C. Philadelphia, PA, WB Saunders, 2007
Cicerone K, Dahlberg C, Kalmar K, et al: Evidence-based cognitive rehabilitation: recommendations for clinical practice. Arch Phys Med Rehabil 81:1596–1615, 2000
Cripe LI: The neuropsychological assessment and management of closed head injury: general guidelines. Cognitive Rehabilitation 5:18–22, 1987
Cuesta MJ, Peralta V: Lack of insight in schizophrenia. Schizophr Bull 20:359–366, 1994
Cuesta MJ, Peralta V, Caro F, et al: Is poor insight in psychotic disorders associated with poor performance on the Wisconsin Card Sorting Test? Am J Psychiatry 152:1380–1382, 1995 (erratum in Am J Psychiatry 153:270, 1996)
Cummings JL: Frontal-subcortical circuits and human behavior. Arch Neurol 50:873–880, 1993
David A, Van Os J, Jones P, et al: Insight and psychotic illness: cross-sectional and longitudinal associations. Br J Psychiatry 167:621–628, 1995
Deb S, Lyons I, Koutzoukis C: Neuropsychiatric sequelae one year after a minor head injury. J Neurol Neurosurg Psychiatry 65:899–902, 1998
Dixon CE, Liu SJ, Jenkins LW, et al: Time course of increased vulnerability of cholinergic neurotransmission following traumatic brain injury in the rat. Behav Brain Res 70:125–131, 1995
Ewing-Cobbs L, Barnes M: Linguistic outcomes following traumatic brain injury in children. Semin Pediatr Neurol 9:209–217, 2002
Ezrachi O, Ben-Yishay Y, Kay T, et al: Predicting employment in traumatic brain injury following neuropsychological rehabilitation. J Head Trauma Rehabil 6:71–84, 1991
Fann JR, Burington B, Leonetti A, et al: Psychiatric illness following traumatic brain injury in an adult health maintenance organization population. Arch Gen Psychiatry 61:53–61, 2004 (comment in Evid Based Ment Health 7:88, 2004)
Feeney DM, Hovda DA: Amphetamine and apomorphine restore tactile placing after motor cortex injury in the cat. Psychopharmacology 79:67–71, 1983
Feeney DM, Sutton RL: Pharmacotherapy for recovery of function after brain injury. Crit Rev Neurobiol 3:135–197, 1987
Feeney DM, Boyeson MG, Linn RT, et al: Responses to cortical injury, 1: methodology and local effects of contusions in the rat. Brain Res 211:67–77, 1981
Ferrell R: Pharmacotherapy of disruptive behaviors associated with brain disease. Semin Clin Neuropsychiatry 5:283–289, 2000
Ford B: Head injuries: what happens to survivors. Med J Aust 1:603–605, 1976
Freedman PE, Bleiberg J, Freedland K, et al: Anticipatory behaviour deficits in closed head injury. J Neurol Neurosurg Psychiatry 50:398–401, 1987
Friedman SD, Brooks WM, Jung RE, et al: Quantitative proton MRS predicts outcome after traumatic brain injury. Neurology 52: 1384–1391, 1999
Fujii D, Ahmed I: Characteristics of psychotic disorder due to traumatic brain injury: an analysis of case studies in the literature. J Neuropsychiatry Clin Neurosci 14:130–140, 2002
Gedye A, Beattie B, Tuokko H, et al: Severe head injury hastens age of onset of Alzheimer's disease. J Am Geriatr Soc 37:970–973, 1989
Gennarelli T, Graham D: Neuropathology, in Textbook of Traumatic Brain Injury. Edited by Silver J, McAllister T, Yudofsky S. Washington, DC, American Psychiatric Publishing, 2005, pp 27–50
Gentilini M, Nichelli P, Schoenhuber R: Assessment of attention in mild head injury, in Mild Head Injury. Edited by Levin H, Eisenberg H, Benton A. New York, Oxford University Press, 1989, pp 163–175
Globus M, Busto R, Dietrich W, et al: Direct evidence for acute and massive norepinephrine release in the hippocampus during transient ischemia. J Cereb Blood Flow Metab 9:892–896, 1989
Grafman J, Salazar A: Traumatic brain inury, in Synopsis of Neuropsychiatry. Edited by Fogel B, Schiffer R, Rao S. Philadelphia, PA, Lippincott Williams & Wilkins, 2000, pp 491–501
Graham DI, Gentleman SM, Lynch A, et al: Distribution of beta-amyloid protein in the brain following severe head injury. Neuropathol Appl Neurobiol 21:27–34, 1995
Gronwall D: Cumulative and persisting effects of concussion on attention and cognition, in Mild Head Injury. Edited by Levin H, Eisenberg H, Benton A. New York, Oxford University Press, 1989, pp 153–162
Gronwall D: Minor head injury. Neuropsychology 5:253–265, 1991
Hart T, Whyte J, Millis S, et al: Dimensions of disordered attention in traumatic brain injury: further validation of the Moss Attention Rating Scale. Arch Phys Med Rehabil 87:647–655, 2006
Hibbard MR, Uysal S, Kepler K, et al: Axis 1 psychopathology in individuals with traumatic brain injury. J Head Trauma Rehabil 13:24–39, 1998

Hibbard MR, Ashman TA, Spielman LA, et al: Relationship between depression and psychosocial functioning after traumatic brain injury. Arch Phys Med Rehabil 85(4 suppl 2):S43–S53, 2004

Ikonomovic MD, Uryu K, Abrahamson EE, et al: Alzheimer's pathology in human temporal cortex surgically excised after severe brain injury. Exp Neurol 190:192–203, 2004

Jackson HF, Moffat NJ: Impaired emotional recognition following severe head injury. Cortex 23:293–300, 1987

Jennett B, Teasdale G: Management of head injuries. Contemp Neurol 20:114–140, 1981

Kant R, Duffy JD, Pivovarnik A: Prevalence of apathy following head injury. Brain Inj 12:87–92, 1998

Koponen S, Taiminen T, Portin R, et al: Axis 1 and 2 psychiatric disorders after traumatic brain injury: a 30-year follow-up study. Am J Psychiatry 159:1315–1321, 2002

Langlois J, Kegler S, Butler J, et al: Traumatic brain injury–related hospital discharges: results from a 14-state surveillance system, 1997. MMWR Surveill Summ 52:1–20, 2003

Lehtonen S, Stringer AY, Millis S, et al: Neuropsychological outcome and community re-integration following traumatic brain injury: the impact of frontal and non-frontal lesions. Brain Inj 19:239–256, 2005

Leininger BE, Gramling SE, Farrell AD, et al: Neuropsychological deficits in symptomatic minor head injury patients after concussion and mild concussion. J Neurol Neurosurg Psychiatry 53: 293–296, 1990 (comment in J Neurol Neurosurg Psychiatry 54: 846–847)

Levin HS, Grossman RG: Behavioral sequelae of closed head injury. Arch Neurol 35:720–727, 1978

Levin HS, Amparo EG, Eisenberg HM, et al: Magnetic resonance imaging and computerized tomography in relation to the neurobehavioral sequelae of mild and moderate head injuries. J Neurosurg 66:706–713, 1987a

Levin HS, Mattis S, Ruff RM, et al: Neurobehavioral outcome following minor head injury: a three-center study. J Neurosurg 66:234–243, 1987b

Levin HS, Goldstein FC, High WM, et al: Disproportionately severe memory deficit in relation to normal intellectual functioning after closed head injury. J Neurol Neurosurg Psychiatry 51:1294–1301, 1988

Lovell M, Franzen M: Neuropsychological assessment, in Neuropsychiatry of Traumatic Brain Injury. Edited by Silver JM, Yudofsky SC, Hales RE. Washington, DC, American Psychiatric Press, 1994, pp 133–160

Lysaker P, Bell M: Insight and cognitive impairment in schizophrenia: performance on repeated administrations of the Wisconsin Card Sorting Test. J Nerv Ment Dis 182:656–660, 1994

Marin RS: Apathy: a neuropsychiatric syndrome. J Neuropsychiatry Clin Neurosci 3:243–254, 1991

Martland H: Punch drunk. JAMA 91:1103–1107, 1928

Mathias JL, Wheaton P: Changes in attention and information-processing speed following severe traumatic brain injury: a meta-analytic review. Neuropsychology 21:212–223, 2007

Mattson AJ, Levin HS: Frontal lobe dysfunction following closed head injury: a review of the literature. J Nerv Ment Dis 178:282–291, 1990

Mayeux R, Ottman R, Tang MX, et al: Genetic susceptibility and head injury as risk factors for Alzheimer's disease among community-dwelling elderly persons and their first-degree relatives. Ann Neurol 33:494–501, 1993

Mayeux R, Ottman R, Maestre G, et al: Synergistic effects of traumatic head injury and apolipoprotein-epsilon 4 in patients with Alzheimer's disease. Neurology 45:555–557, 1995

Mayorga MA: The pathology of primary blast overpressure injury. Toxicology 121:17–28, 1997

McAllister TW: Neuropsychiatric sequelae of head injuries. Psychiatr Clin North Am 15:395–413, 1992

McAllister TW: Apathy. Semin Clin Neuropsychiatry 5:275–282, 2000

McAllister TW: Neuropsychiatric aspects of TBI, in Brain Injury Medicine: Principles and Practice. Edited by Zasler N, Katz D, Zafonte R. New York, Demos Medical Publishing, 2007, pp 835–864

McAllister TW, Flashman LA, Sparling MB, et al: Working memory deficits after traumatic brain injury: catecholaminergic mechanisms and prospects for treatment—a review. Brain Inj 18:331–350, 2004

McDonald BC, Flashman LA, Saykin AJ: Executive dysfunction following traumatic brain injury: neural substrates and treatment strategies. NeuroRehabilitation 17:333–344, 2002

McEvoy JP, Apperson LJ, Applebaum PS, et al: Insight into schizophrenia: its relationship to acute psychopathology. J Nerv Ment Dis 177:43–47, 1989

McIntosh TK: Neurochemical sequelae of traumatic brain injury: therapeutic implications. Cerebrovasc Brain Metab Rev 6:109–162, 1994

McIntosh TK, Juhler M, Wieloch T: Novel pharmacologic strategies in the treatment of experimental traumatic brain injury: 1998. J Neurotrauma 15:731–769, 1998

McMillan TM, Glucksman EE: The neuropsychology of moderate head injury. J Neurol Neurosurg Psychiatry 50:393–397, 1987

Mega MS, Cummings JL: Frontal subcortical circuits, in The Frontal Lobes and Neuropsychiatric Illness. Edited by Salloway S, Malloy PF, Duffy JD. Washington, DC, American Psychiatric Publishing, 2001, pp 15–32

Mehta K, Ott A, Kalmijn S, et al: Head trauma and risk of dementia and Alzheimer's disease: the Rotterdam Study. Neurology 53: 1959–1962, 1999

Miller H, Stern G: The long-term prognosis of severe head injury. Lancet 1:225–229, 1965

Mohamed S, Fleming S, Penn DL, et al: Insight in schizophrenia: its relationship to measures of executive functions. J Nerv Ment Dis 187:525–531, 1999

National Center for Injury Prevention and Control: Report to Congress on Mild Traumatic Brain Injury in the United States: Steps to Prevent a Serious Public Health Problem. Atlanta, GA, Centers for Disease Control and Prevention, 2003. Available at: http://www.cdc.gov/ncipc/pub-res/mtbi/report.htm. Accessed February 7, 2011.

National Institutes of Health Consensus Development Panel on Rehabilitation of Persons With Traumatic Brain Injury: Consensus conference: rehabilitation of persons with traumatic brain injury. JAMA 282:974–983, 1999

Nicoll J, Roberts G, Graham D: Apolipoprotein E epsilon 4 allele is associated with deposition of amyloid beta-protein following severe head injury. Nat Med 1:135–137, 1995

Oddy M, Coughlan T, Tyerman A, et al: Social adjustment after closed head injury: a further follow-up seven years after injury. J Neurol Neurosurg Psychiatry 48:564–568, 1985

O'Jile JR, Ryan LM, Betz B, et al: Information processing following mild head injury. Arch Clin Neuropsychol 21:293–296, 2006

Ota Y: Psychiatric studies on civilian head injuries, in The Late Effects of Head Injury. Edited by Walker AE, Caveness WF, Critchley M. Springfield, IL, Charles C Thomas, 1969, pp 110–119

Prasad MR, Tzigaret C, Smith DH, et al: Decreased alpha-adrenergic receptors after experimental brain injury. J Neurotrauma 9:269–279, 1993

Prigatano GP: Disturbances of self-awareness of deficit after traumatic brain injury, in Awareness of Deficit After Brain Injury. Edited by Prigatano GL, Schacter DL. New York, Oxford University Press, 1991, pp 111–126

Raghupathi R, Graham DI, McIntosh TK: Apoptosis after traumatic brain injury. J Neurotrauma 17:927–938, 2000

Rassovsky Y, Satz P, Alfano MS, et al: Functional outcome in TBI, II: verbal memory and information processing speed mediators. J Clin Exp Neuropsychol 28:581–591, 2006

Roberts GW, Allsop D, Bruton C: The occult aftermath of boxing. J Neurol Neurosurg Psychiatry 53:373–378, 1990

Romhanyi R, Tandian D, Hovda DA, et al: Catecholaminergic stimulation enhances recovery of function following concussive brain injury. J Neurotrauma 9:164, 1990

Ross ED, Rush AJ: Diagnosis and neuroanatomical correlates of depression in brain-damaged patients: implications for a neurology of depression. Arch Gen Psychiatry 38:1344–1354, 1981

Rudelli R, Strom JO, Welch PT, et al: Post-traumatic premature Alzheimer's disease. Arch Neurol 39:570–575, 1982

Ruff RM, Levin HS, Mather S, et al: Recovery of memory after mild head injury: a three center study, in Mild Head Injury. Edited by Levin HS, Eisenberg HM, Benton AL. New York, Oxford University Press, 1989, pp 176–188

Sherer M, Bergloff P, Levin E, et al: Impaired awareness and employment outcome after traumatic brain injury. J Head Trauma Rehabil 13:52–61, 1998a

Sherer M, Boake C, Levin E, et al: Characteristics of impaired awareness after traumatic brain injury. J Int Neuropsychol Soc 4:380–387, 1998b

Silver JM, Kramer R, Greenwald S, et al: The association between head injuries and psychiatric disorders: findings from the New Haven NIMH Epidemiologic Catchment Area Study. Brain Inj 15:935–945, 2001

Smeets WJ, Gonzalez A: Catecholamine systems in the brain of vertebrates: new perspectives through a comparative approach. Brain Res Brain Res Rev 33:308–379, 2000

Smith DH, Chen XH, Nonaka M, et al: Accumulation of amyloid beta and tau and the formation of neurofilament inclusions following diffuse brain injury in the pig. J Neuropathol Exp Neurol 58:982–992, 1999

Smith DH, Chen XH, Iwata A, et al: Amyloid beta accumulation in axons after traumatic brain injury in humans. J Neurosurg 98: 1072–1077, 2003

Starkstein SE, Jorge R: Dementia after traumatic brain injury. Int Psychogeriatr 17(suppl):S93–S107, 2005

Stuss DT, Ely P, Hugenholtz H, et al: Subtle neuropsychological deficits in patients with good recovery after closed head injury. Neurosurgery 17:41–47, 1985

Sutton RL, Feeney DM: Alpha-noradrenergic agonists and antagonists affect recovery and maintenance of beam-walking ability after sensorimotor cortex ablation in the rat. Restor Neurol Neurosci 4:1–11, 1992

Tandian D, Romhanyi R, Hovda DA, et al: Amphetamine enhances both behavior and metabolic recovery following fluid percussion brain injury. J Neurotrauma 9:174, 1990

Tariot PN: The older patient: the ongoing challenge of efficacy and tolerability. J Clin Psychiatry 60(suppl):29–33, 1999

Tariot PN, Loy R, Ryan JM, et al: Mood stabilizers in Alzheimer's disease: symptomatic and neuroprotective rationales. Adv Drug Deliv Rev 54:1567–1577, 2002

Teasdale G, Jennett B: Assessment of coma and impaired consciousness: a practical scale. Lancet 2:81–84, 1974

Teasdale G, Nicoll J, Murray G, et al: Association of apolipoprotein E polymorphism with outcome after head injury. Lancet 350: 1069–1071, 1997

Trudel TM, Tryon WW, Purdum CM: Closed head injury, awareness of disability and long term outcome. Presented at the New Hampshire Brain Injury Association Annual Meeting, Manchester, NH, May 1996

Umile EM, Sandel ME, Alavi A, et al: Dynamic imaging in mild traumatic brain injury: support for the theory of medial temporal vulnerability. Arch Phys Med Rehabil 83:1506–1513, 2002

Uryu K, Chen XH, Graham DJ: Short-term accumulation of beta-amyloid in axonal pathology following traumatic brain injury in humans. Neurobiol Aging 25(suppl):P2–P250, 2004

Uryu K, Chen X, Martinez D, et al: Multiple proteins implicated in neurodegenerative diseases accumulate in axons after brain trauma in humans. Exp Neurol 208:185–192, 2007

Vakil E: The effect of moderate to severe traumatic brain injury (TBI) on different aspects of memory: a selective review. J Clin Exp Neuropsychol 27:977–1021, 2005

Van Den Heuvel C, Blumbergs PC, Finnie JW, et al: Upregulation of amyloid precursor protein messenger RNA in response to traumatic brain injury: an ovine head impact model. Exp Neurol 159:441–450, 1999

Van Den Heuvel C, Thornton E, Vink R: Traumatic brain injury and Alzheimer's disease: a review. Prog Brain Res 161:303–316, 2007

van Reekum R, Cohen T, Wong J: Can traumatic brain injury cause psychiatric disorders? J Neuropsychiatry Clin Neurosci 12:316–327, 2000

Warden D: Military TBI during the Iraq and Afghanistan wars. J Head Trauma Rehabil 21:398–402, 2006

Wei W, Sambamoorthi U, Crystal S, et al: Mental illness, traumatic brain injury, and Medicaid expenditures. Arch Phys Med Rehabil 86:905–911, 2005

Weintraub S, Mesulam MM, Kramer L: Disturbances in prosody: a right-hemisphere contribution to language. Arch Neurol 38: 742–744, 1981

Whyte J, Polansky M, Cavallucci C, et al: Inattentive behavior after traumatic brain injury. J Int Neuropsychol Soc 2:274–281, 1996

Young DA, Davila R, Scher H: Unawareness of illness and neuropsychological performance in chronic schizophrenia. Schizophr Res 10:117–124, 1993

27

Epilepsy

Mario F. Mendez, M.D., Ph.D.

Epilepsy is associated with neuropsychiatric conditions that may be especially severe in elderly people. Seizure disorders can have psychosocial consequences, neuropsychological effects, seizure-related (ictally related) behavioral changes, and between-seizure or interictal psychopathology (Table 27–1). The most well-established interictal psychopathology is depression, but one-fourth or more of patients with epilepsy experience a range of psychopathology, including anxiety disorders and interictal dysphoric disorder, personality changes, and several forms of psychosis. In this chapter, I explore the behavioral aspects of epilepsy that might affect elderly patients and conclude with a discussion of management issues.

Demography and Definitions

Seizures result from abnormal neuronal discharges in the brain. They are sudden, involuntary behavioral events due to excessive or hypersynchronous electrical discharges often from hyperexcitable neurons. Seizures can be primary, secondary to a brain lesion, or symptomatic from acute situational conditions such as sleep deprivation or drug withdrawal. The term *epilepsy* refers specifically to recurrent unprovoked seizures and includes primary and secondary epileptic seizures but excludes symptomatic ones. Seizures can be *generalized* (characterized by an initial widespread bihemispheric involvement) or *partial* (characterized by an initial focal onset in part of one hemisphere) (Table 27–2).

Epilepsy is particularly common among elderly persons. Among persons ages 75 years and older living in the community, the prevalence of epilepsy is about 15/1,000, compared to 5–8/1,000 for the population overall (Annegers 1997; Hauser et al. 1991). Among over a million U.S. veterans ages 65 and older, over 20,000 (18%) had a diagnosis of epilepsy (Peruccca et al. 2006; Pugh et al. 2004). The incidence of new-onset epilepsy corresponds to a U-shaped curve, with its highest incidence in the first year of life, dropping to a minimum in individuals in their 30s through 50s, and rising to peak again among those ages 60 and older (Cloyd et al. 2006). Among persons ages 75 and older, the incidence of epilepsy is about 101/100,000 patient-years, compared to 30–50/100,000 for the population overall (Annegers 1997; Hussain et al. 2006). This incidence is even higher among elderly patients residing in nursing homes compared to those living in the community. Some studies show that about 9% of nursing home residents have epilepsy or seizures (Garrard et al. 2000).

Although two-thirds of epilepsy in young adults is idiopathic, most elderly patients with epilepsy have a known cause (Hauser 1992). Of those over age 65 years, 30%–40% have a cerebrovascular etiology for their seizures; 10%–15% have brain tumors; and up to 23% have neurodegenerative disease, trauma, or other secondary lesions (Hauser 1997; Sanders and Murray 1991). Persons with mild Alzheimer's disease (AD) had a cumulative incidence of unprovoked seizure risk of 8%, with a particularly high risk among those with early-onset AD (Amatniek et al. 2006). No known cause was found for the remaining one-third of elderly patients with recent-onset seizures; however, many of these patients have cerebrovascular risk factors and subcortical small vessel disease on neuroimaging (Ramsay et al. 2004).

Clinical Aspects

In adults, the three most common types of seizures are 1) generalized tonic-clonic seizures (GTCSs), with convulsions (also known as grand mal seizures); 2) complex partial seizures (CPSs), with an alteration of consciousness; and 3) simple partial seizures (SPSs), with isolated motor, somatosensory, autonomic, or psychic symptoms. SPSs that evolve to CPSs are considered auras, and CPSs that evolve to GTCSs are secondarily generalized. Although about one-third of all epileptic patients have CPSs, about one-half of elderly patients with epilepsy have CPSs, reflecting the increased specific focal

TABLE 27–1. Behavioral disorders in epilepsy

Psychosocial
Low self-esteem, dependency, and helplessness
Fear of loss of control
Stigmatization
Loss of independence
Associated marital, job, transportation, and related problems
Neuropsychological
From seizures
From underlying lesions/disease
From antiepileptic drugs
Ictally related
Prodromal symptoms (e.g., dysphoria, apprehension)
Ictal automatisms and psychic symptoms
Nonconvulsive status (e.g., simple partial seizures, complex partial seizures, absence seizures, and periodic lateralizing epileptiform discharges)
Postictal confusion and other postictal behaviors
Ictal-postictal intermixed behaviors (e.g., twilight states)
Psychotic episodes related to the ictus
Interictal
Depression and suicidality
Anxiety disorders and dysphoria
"Heightened significance" and other personality changes
Interictal schizophreniform psychosis
Hyposexuality
Other (e.g., dissociative states)

TABLE 27–2. International classification of epileptic seizures

I. Partial (focal, local) seizures
   A. Simple partial seizures
      Motor, somatosensory, autonomic, or psychic symptoms
   B. Complex partial seizures
      1. Begin with symptoms of simple partial seizure but progress to impairment of consciousness
      2. Begin with impairment of consciousness
   C. Partial seizures with secondary generalization
      1. Begin with simple partial seizure
      2. Begin with complex partial seizure (including those with symptoms of simple partial seizures at onset)

II. Generalized seizures (convulsive or nonconvulsive)
   A. Absence (typical and atypical)
   B. Myoclonus
   C. Clonic
   D. Tonic
   E. Tonic-clonic
   F. Atonic/akinetic

III. Unclassified

Source. Adapted from Commission on Classification and Terminology of the International League Against Epilepsy 1981.

causes of their epilepsy (Hauser 1992). In addition, variants of childhood absence (petit mal) seizures, which result in brief lapses of consciousness, occur occasionally in elderly patients.

Seizures in elderly patients differ from seizures in young patients. The CPSs in elderly patients usually lack the classic features of CPSs of temporal lobe origin (*temporal lobe epilepsy* [TLE]) seen in younger adults. Because their seizure focus is often extratemporal or frontal from strokes or other lesions, seizures in the elderly may manifest as blackout spells, altered mental status, memory lapses, episodes of confusion, or syncope (Ramsay et al. 2004). Auras and automatisms are less common or specific in elderly patients than in young adults. The occurrence of secondary generalized convulsions is only 25.9% in elderly patients, compared with 65% in young adults (Cloyd et al. 2006). When there are GTCSs, the postictal confusional state may last for hours, days, or even weeks in the elderly patients, compared with 5–15 minutes in young adults.

The evaluation of new-onset seizures in elderly patients includes the identification of cerebrovascular, neoplastic, and other acquired neuropathology; the exclusion of acute symptomatic seizures; and the characterization of any epileptiform discharges. On electroencephalograms (EEGs), seizure disorders may have interictal spikes and other markers of abnormal electrical activity. EEGs are more likely to define the type of epileptiform changes if the patient attains drowsiness or sleep during the tracing. Patients with new-onset seizures also need neuroimaging of the brain, preferably magnetic resonance imaging with its superior resolution for most parenchymal lesions. Routine X-ray and laboratory studies help exclude the presence of symptomatic seizures. In addition, a lumbar puncture is indicated in the presence of a persistent alteration of consciousness, especially if it is accompanied by fever and meningeal signs.

Epileptic seizures must be differentiated from symptomatic seizures, syncope, and psychogenic nonepileptic seizures.

Symptomatic seizures are common in older people and may result from electrolyte imbalance, hypoglycemia or hyperglycemia, or a range of metabolic disturbances. An important consideration is a symptomatic seizure due to syncope (convulsive syncope) from lack of circulation to the brain. Patients with brief lapses of consciousness but without typical ictal features or postictal confusion usually have syncope from a cardiovascular, toxic-metabolic, or cerebrovascular cause; however, these lapses could be atypical seizures, particularly of frontal lobe origin. Psychogenic nonepileptic seizures are the most frequent conversion reactions among seizure patients. Although nonepileptic seizures are most common in young women with psychological stressors and poor coping skills, they have occurred in elderly patients (Behrouz et al. 2006). Nonepileptic seizures are characterized by a sudden collapse or by motor activity that does not fit a typical CPS or GTCS, ictal durations of ≥2 minutes, occurrence in the presence of a witness, possible induction with injections or suggestion, poor responsiveness to antiepileptic drugs (AEDs), and lack of a seizure-induced rise in serum prolactin levels (Reuber 2008).

Neuropsychiatric Aspects

The neuropsychiatric aspects of epilepsy include four categories: psychosocial, neuropsychological, ictally related behavioral alterations, and interictal psychopathology (see Table 27–1). Psychosocial aspects are those directly due to the stress of having a seizure disorder, and neuropsychological aspects refer to persistent disturbances in cognitive abilities. Temporary behavior changes also occur before, during, or after a seizure as a direct result of ictal or seizure discharges. A final group of behaviors manifests as sustained psychopathology during the interictal or seizure-free period. Although these categories overlap and some behaviors are eventually reclassified as underlying mechanisms are identified, these categories are useful for discussing the neuropsychiatric aspects of epilepsy.

Psychosocial Impact of Seizures

The presence of a seizure disorder in later life has important psychosocial implications (see Table 27–1). Quality of life is worse for patients with epilepsy than for the general population or those with other chronic conditions (Berto 2002). Epilepsy is associated with low self-esteem, a sense of decreased control and self-efficacy, and the perception of being stigmatized (Berto 2002; Collings 1994). Patients with epilepsy are subject to low self-esteem, particularly arising from the greater dependency that the disorder engenders. Self-esteem problems can be greater in elderly individuals, who already may be heavily reliant on family and others. The possibility of having a seizure at any time results in feelings of loss of control. Elderly subjects tend to be cautious and conservative, and the potential for public loss of control can be particularly distressing. In addition to an overall increased sense of vulnerability is a very real fear of falling and sustaining incapacitating hip fractures or other trauma. Also, stigmatization from the disorder continues, and people often misunderstand and fear those with epilepsy. This can lead to housing problems; some nursing homes do not accept elderly patients with seizures.

The independence of elderly patients may already be impaired or tenuous, and epilepsy further narrows their ability to function independently. Seizures may critically compromise the function of elderly individuals who are still able to keep a job, provide their own transportation, maintain their economic status, and perform other independent activities. Although seizures by themselves rarely result in institutionalization, in an already impaired elder, seizures may be the final condition that terminates independent living. In addition, given the higher frequency of secondary epilepsy in elderly individuals, these patients are often already disabled from underlying neurological disorders such as stroke or dementia.

Neuropsychological Impact of Seizures

Neuropsychological functions are vulnerable to the effects of seizures. Prolonged seizures can result in metabolic and direct electrical injury to the brain. By age 70, significant loss of neuronal tissue has occurred, as well as a decline in cognitive efficiency, particularly on time-dependent tasks and in memory retrieval. With this decreased neuronal reserve, elderly patients have a greater neuropsychological decline from neuronal damage as a result of ongoing seizure activity than do younger patients. Most studies indicate that patients with a long history of poorly controlled seizures have a mild intellectual decline, particularly in memory (Vingerhoets 2006). Moreover, in older patients with secondary epilepsy, seizures are often associated with disorders that impair cognition, such as strokes, vascular dementia, or AD, and further seizures exacerbate their cognitive impairments (Mendez and Cummings 2003).

Although most seizures can be controlled with AEDs, these medications have potential neuropsychological side effects (Ortinski and Meador 2004). Elderly patients have a slowed elimination of these drugs, require lower dosages, are often taking multiple interacting medications, and are therefore more likely to experience AED toxicity (Leppik 2006). In patients with already significant susceptibility to confusional states and the memory decline of the aged brain, the addition of AEDs greatly increases the possibility of cognitive worsening (Aldenkamp et al. 2003; Mendez and Lim 2003). Even at therapeutic levels, some drugs can cause specific problems. For example, barbiturates may need to be discontinued because of drug-induced depression, suicidal ideation, sedation, psychomotor slowing, and paradoxical hyperactivity. In general, the older AEDs are worse than the newer AEDs; however, drugs such as topiramate have significant effects on attention and verbal function (Aldenkamp et al. 2003; Ortinski and Meador 2004). The added susceptibility to AED-induced toxicity in elderly patients indicates the need for close monitoring, especially of AED serum levels, the effects of polypharmacy, renal and liver function test values, and AED-induced hyponatremia.

Ictally Related Behavioral Alterations

Ictally related behavioral alterations (see Table 27–1) occur before, during, and after seizures. First, a prodrome of dysphoria, insomnia, anxiety, or build up of tension may precede seizures or be relieved by them. Second, ictal discharges can produce both reactive automatisms involving semipurposeful activity and psychic manifestations producing affective, cognitive, language, memory, and perceptual changes. Examples of automatisms include ictal laughter from left hemisphere discharges and ictal crying from right hemisphere discharges (Dark et al. 1996). Examples of psychic manifestations include affective changes, such as ictal fear and depression, and cognitive changes, such as derealization and depersonalization. Even a recurrent uninvited thought can be a seizure manifestation (Mendez 2009). Moreover, prolonged alterations of responsiveness may result from nonconvulsive status epilepticus or from recurrent electrical discharges with electroencephalographic complexes known as *periodic lateralizing epileptiform discharges.* Third, the postictal period includes a confusional state lasting minutes to hours or, occasionally, days. The postictal period can be particularly prolonged in elderly patients, who may take longer to recover from the disruption of seizures (Ramsay et al. 2004). Although semidirected ictally related aggression is extremely rare, nondirected destructive behavior frequently occurs during the postictal confusional state as a response to attempts at restraint. Finally, occasional protracted periods with intermixed ictal and postictal changes can produce twilight states; compulsive wandering, or poriomania; an agitated state; and depressive delirium (Mendez 2009).

During the postictal period, patients may have neuropsychiatric symptoms such as depression, anxiety, hypomania, and psychosis (Kanner et al. 2004). Most dramatically, brief psychotic episodes may follow a flurry of seizures or may occasionally alternate with seizures (Kanemoto et al. 1996; Sachdev 1998). These episodes involve days to weeks of agitated, hallucinatory, paranoid, and impulsive behaviors, often with sudden mood swings and suicide attempts. Most patients develop their psychotic episodes 12–48 hours after a flurry of seizures and may occasionally continue to display psychotic symptoms for an extended period of time. Another group develops psychotic episodes after seizures are controlled, and this "alternating psychosis" promptly resolves once the seizures recur. *Forced or paradoxical normalization* refers to this subgroup with an antagonism between psychotic episodes and the seizures or EEG discharges (Landolt 1958).

Interictal Psychopathology

Patients with epilepsy are susceptible to psychopathology during the seizure-free periods (see Table 27–1). These behavioral disorders usually occur in patients with long-standing, incompletely controlled seizures, particularly CPSs of TLE origin. Community epidemiological studies have shown a high prevalence of interictal psychiatric problems among patients with epilepsy (Mendez 2009). The percentage of patients with epilepsy in psychiatric hospitals has ranged from 5% to 10%, significantly higher than the prevalence of epilepsy in the general population (Mendez et al. 1986). Of patients attending epilepsy clinics, about 30% have had a prior psychiatric hospitalization, and about 18% were on at least one psychotropic drug (Mendez 2009). Studies report more psychopathology among patients with epilepsy than among control subjects with other neurological disorders (Mendez et al. 1986, 1993a). Finally, although CPSs from TLE are less prevalent in elderly patients than in young adults, elderly patients, particularly those with long-standing seizures, remain susceptible to interictal depression and suicidality, anxiety disorders and dysphoria, personality changes, psychosis, hyposexuality, and other psychopathology.

Depression and Suicidality

Less well known than interictal psychosis is the problem of depression in epilepsy. Depression is undoubtedly a frequent neuropsychiatric disturbance in older patients with seizures. Depression occurs in up to 75% of patients with epilepsy, and there are elevations in depressive traits in patients with epilepsy compared with those in control groups (Barry et al. 2008; Mendez 2009). Depression is also the main reason for the psychiatric hospitalization of patients with epilepsy (Mendez et al. 1986). Furthermore, there may be a twofold or greater frequency of interictal depression among outpatients with seizures, particularly those with CPSs, than among disabled individuals with other handicaps (Mendez et al. 1986).

Patients with epilepsy who have depression most commonly have a chronic interictal depression or dysthymia that is distinct from ictal depression (Mendez 2009; Robertson et al. 1994). This interictal depression frequently has endogenous features, paranoia, and other symptoms suggesting a continuum with schizoaffective disorder (Mendez et al. 1986). According to most investigators, seizures relieve depression in patients with epilepsy (similar to the effects of electroconvulsive therapy [ECT]), whereas better seizure control or decreased secondarily generalized seizures make it worse (Mendez et al. 1993a). A few investigators have also reported depression with increased seizure activity or no relationship between depression and seizure frequency (Mendez 2009). Depression is specifically associated with CPSs from left-sided temporal foci, suggesting a neurobiologically based organic mood disorder rather than a nonspecific psychosocial reaction to a chronic disability (Mendez et al. 1986). Conversely, most studies have not confirmed the proposed association of right hemisphere foci with the much rarer cases of mania found in epilepsy.

Elderly individuals with epilepsy are at greater risk for suicide than those without epilepsy. The lifetime prevalence rate of suicide for people with epilepsy is about 12%, compared with 1.1%–1.2% in the general population (Jones et al. 2003). About one-third of all patients with epilepsy have attempted suicide at some point in time. A comparison of suicide attempts among patients with epilepsy and impaired control subjects with other handicaps and without epilepsy revealed suicide attempts by 30% of the subjects with epilepsy but only 7% of the control subjects (Mendez et al. 1986); this increased risk of suicide continued even long after temporal lobectomy and successful control of seizures. Patients with epilepsy are likely to attempt suicide not only because of psychosocial stress, but also because of increased interictal psychopathology such as depression, psychosis, and borderline personality characteristics. They are most likely to complete suicide when they have psychosis with paranoid hallucinations, agitated compunction to kill themselves, and occasional ictal command hallucinations to commit suicide (Mendez and Doss 1992).

Anxiety Disorders and Dysphoria

Anxiety disorders are common among patients with epilepsy. Mensah et al. (2007) reported anxiety rates of 20.5% in one community sample of 515 people with epilepsy. Anxiety disorders often coexist with the interictal depression or dysthymia observed among many patients with epilepsy (Kanner 2009). Anxiety disorders are also associated with AED side effects, chronic ill health, and psychosocial stressors such as unemployment, but surprisingly are not associated with seizure variables, except perhaps with a right-sided TLE focus (Satishchandra et al. 2003). The presence of a TLE focus also has a greater association with obsessionality and obsessive-compulsive behavior than does idiopathic generalized epilepsy (Monaco et al. 2005).

In addition to having an association with defined anxiety disorders, such as generalized anxiety and obsessive-compulsive behavior, epilepsy has an association with less well-defined dysphoria and irritability (Blumer et al. 2004). The dysphoric episodes are composed of variable periods of heightened irritability with anxiety and sometimes of outbursts of "episodic dyscontrol" (intermittent explosive disorder with ictal-like features). Like epileptic patients with anxiety disorders, epileptic patients with dysphoria may also have comorbid depression. Most directed aggression by patients with epilepsy correlates with outbursts of reactive episodic dyscontrol, as well as subnormal intelligence, lower socioeconomic status, prior head injuries, and possible orbital frontal damage (Mendez et al. 1993b).

Personality Characteristics

Patients with epilepsy have a high prevalence of personality disorders (Perini et al. 1996; Swanson et al. 1995). Patients with epilepsy who have personality disorders show dependent and avoidant personality traits. Those with epilepsy are stigmatized, feared, and subject to difficulties obtaining a job, driving an automobile, and maintaining a marriage. Those psychosocial difficulties, along with underlying neurobiological factors, may predispose patients with epilepsy to personality disorders.

Although no specific epileptic personality exists, a group of traits termed the *Gastaut-Geschwind syndrome* occurs in a subset of patients with CPSs. Because in most studies the Minnesota Multiphasic Personality Inventory (MMPI) proved insensitive to the personality traits attributed to epilepsy, the Bear-Fedio Inventory was developed to assess these traits (Bear and Fedio 1977). According to Bear and Fedio, patients with CPSs of TLE origin have a personality characterized by a sense of "heightened significance," as indicated by sobriety and humorlessness, tenaciousness or "viscosity" in interpersonal encounters, a deepened affect, a pronounced sense of personal destiny, and an intense interest in religious, moral, and philosophical issues. Such patients are circumstantial, give overly detailed background information, and write copiously about their thoughts and feelings. In addition, Bear and Fedio reported that patients with left-sided temporal foci tend to maximize their problems, whereas those with right-sided foci minimize them. Conclusive proof that patients with CPSs are prone to the Gastaut-Geschwind syndrome has remained elusive. Other applications of the Bear-Fedio Inventory found the same "personality" characteristics in patients without epilepsy who had psychiatric disorders or comparable physical disabilities (Mendez 2009).

Interictal Psychosis

The best-known psychiatric disorder in epilepsy is the chronic schizophreniform psychosis (Sachdev 1998). The influential study by Slater and Beard (1963) reported on 69 patients with both epilepsy and an interictal schizophrenic disorder and concluded that these two disorders occurred together more frequently than expected by chance. Although some investigators have interpreted this association as reflecting selective sampling, most subsequent studies indicate that 7%–12% of patients with epilepsy develop a psychotic disorder, usually a chronic interictal schizophrenic illness (Trimble 1991). For example, in a controlled investigation of 1,611 outpatients with epilepsy, interictal schizophrenic disorders were 9–10 times more common among patients with epilepsy than among control subjects with other neurological disorders (Mendez et al. 1993c). Moreover, on the MMPI, patients with epilepsy had more elevated schizophrenia and paranoia scale scores than did patients with other neurological disabilities (Dikmen et al. 1983).

The schizophrenic disorder may be especially associated with CPSs. One study found psychosis in 12% of 1,675 patients with CPSs of TLE origin, especially those with left-sided foci, compared with less than 1% of 6,671 patients with generalized epilepsy (Gibbs 1951), and a psychotic illness occurred in 9 (10%) of 87 children with TLE followed for up to 30 years (Lindsay et al. 1979). In conclusion, patients with epilepsy have a several-fold greater risk for a chronic schizophrenic illness than does the general population, and the risk is particularly high for CPS patients, regardless of age. Finally, some investigators suggest that low folate levels and high plasma homocysteine levels may be related to interictal psychosis among patients with epilepsy (Monji et al. 2005).

Unlike ictally related psychotic episodes, this chronic interictal schizophrenic disorder has no direct relationship to individual seizures (Mendez et al. 1993c). Although the exact relationship of seizure activity and schizophrenia is debated (Sachdev 1998), these patients often had an 11- to 15-year history of poorly controlled seizures (Slater and Beard 1963). Furthermore, the schizophrenic symptoms commonly increase with increased CPSs or with AED withdrawal (Mendez et al. 1993c; Figure 27–1). CPSs of left TLE origin may particularly predispose patients to this psychotic disorder (Mendez et al. 1993c); however, removal of the seizure focus does not prevent the development of psychosis (Manchanda et al. 1996).

The schizophrenic disorder resembles an episodic schizoaffective psychosis with prominent paranoia, positive symptoms, relatively preserved affect, and normal premorbid personality (Slater and Beard 1963). Compared with patients who have process schizophrenia, patients with schizophrenic disorder may have more hallucinations and religiosity and less social withdrawal, systematized delusions, Schneiderian first-rank symptoms, and family history of schizophrenia. However, these features are not clearly atypical or unique, and most schizophrenic syndromes in epilepsy can correspond to typical schizophrenic disorder categories (Mendez et al. 1993c). Some studies even indicate that the perceived differences in symptomatology between interictal psychosis and schizophrenia are just quantitatively less in the interictal psychosis (Matsuura et al. 2004).

Hyposexuality and Other Behavioral Disorders

Incompletely treated patients with epilepsy experience hyposexuality (Mendez 2009), a problem that can affect elderly patients. Both men and women experience disturbances of sexual arousal and a lowered sexual drive (Morrell and Guldner 1996; Murialdo et al. 1995). Patients with epilepsy appear to lack libido and may experience impotence or frigidity. This hyposexuality improves after seizures are controlled. Other patients with epilepsy experience physiological signs of decreased sexual arousal and possible subclinical hypogonadotropic hypogonadism (Murialdo et al. 1995).

A great many other interictal behavioral disturbances have occurred among individuals with epilepsy, but their association with epilepsy is not clear. For example, case reports have described dissociative states in epilepsy (e.g., multiple personality disorder, possession and fugue states, and psychogenic amnesia) (Ahern et al. 1993), and epileptic patients may have aggressive tendencies and paraphilias. These behaviors, however, are not established as part of the neuropsychiatry of epilepsy.

Etiology and Pathology

Current theories of the psychopathology of epilepsy emphasize a physiological disturbance in the temporal limbic system rather than psychodynamic processes. As previously described, depression, anxiety disorders and dysphoria, personality disorders, psychosis, and hyposexuality are two to three times more common in patients with CPSs (most of whom have a temporal focus) than in patients with GTCSs. The most common pathological findings in patients with epilepsy are mediobasal temporal lobe lesions involving limbic structures, but the limbic system may also be involved through its frontal and diencephalic connections. Stimulation and ablation studies in animals and humans link limbic structures to emotional behavior. Psychotic-like behavior in animal subjects has followed repeated application of epileptic agents to kindle limbic structures (Smith and Darlington 1996); patients with schizophrenia have had limbic discharges on depth electrode monitoring (Heath 1982); and disinhibition of the mesolimbic dopamine system has resulted from kindling in the limbic system (Stevens and Livermore 1978).

Several specific mechanisms are potentially responsible for psychiatric disturbances in epilepsy. First, the underlying brain lesions could be the source of both seizures and behavioral changes. Psychosis may be more common with left temporal lobe pathology such as hamartomas or gangliogliomas, and depression is associated with strokes and other hypoactive lesions in the left hemisphere. Second, ictal discharges could kindle behavioral changes by facilitating limbic-sensory associations and other neuronal connections. The schizophrenic psychosis is associated with increased frequencies of CPSs, and personality disorders may occur in patients with auras (Mendez et al. 1993c). Third, decreased function, such as the focal interictal hypometabolism observed on positron emission tomography (PET), may lead to interictal behavioral changes. Depression often follows seizure control sufficient to inhibit secondary generalization to GTCSs (i.e., the surrounding hypometabolism may result in depression by preventing the spread of temporal

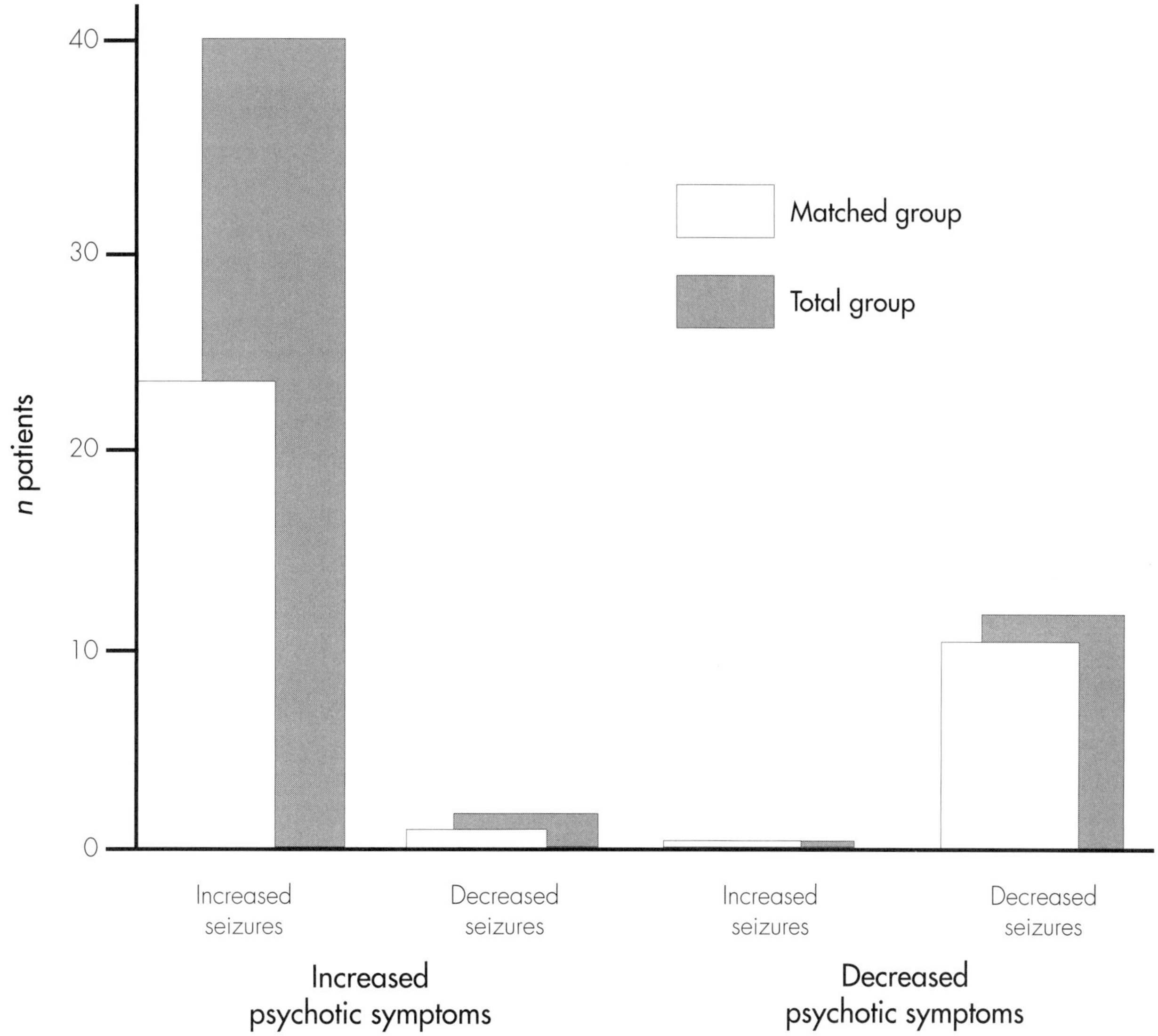

FIGURE 27–1. Correspondence of psychotic symptoms to seizure frequency.

Increased psychotic symptoms: Total schizophrenic epilepsy group (n=149): increased seizures in 42 and decreased seizures in 2 (χ^2=40.56, df=1, P<0.001). Matched schizophrenic epilepsy group (n=62): increased seizures in 24 and decreased seizures in 1 (χ^2=24.25, df=1, P<0.001. *Decreased psychotic symptoms:* Total group: increased seizures in 9 and decreased seizures in 0 (χ^2=7.33, df=1, P<0.007). Matched group: increased seizures in 8 and decreased seizures in 0 (χ^2=6.55, df=1, P<0.001).

Source: Reprinted with permission from Mendez MF, Grau R, Doss RC, et al.: "Schizophrenia in Epilepsy: Seizure and Psychosis Variables." *Neurology* 43:1073–1077, 1993.

limbic epileptic foci). Fourth, seizures may result in neuroendocrine or neurotransmitter changes, including increased dopaminergic or inhibitory transmitters, decreased prolactin, increased testosterone, and increased endogenous opioids. These changes probably explain, at least in part, the hyposexuality of some patients with epilepsy. Finally, physiological factors may be potentiated by psychodynamic factors. For example, a proposed role for auras in personality disorders or psychosis may relate to their impact on reality testing (Mendez et al. 1993c).

Treatment

The treatment of epilepsy requires knowledge of the use of AEDs (Table 27–3). These medications are commonly prescribed for elderly patients. In the United States, approximately 1.5% of community-dwelling elderly and 9%–10% of nursing home residents are taking AEDs (Garrard et al. 2003; Pugh et al. 2004). About 7%–8% are taking AEDs at the time of nursing home admission, and another 2%–3% begin taking AEDs soon after admission (Garrard et al. 2003). This means that as many as 150,000 elderly nursing home residents may be taking AEDs. In one study, the most commonly reported AEDs taken by elderly patients in the United States were phenytoin (61%), phenobarbital (18%), and carbamazepine (10%) (Pugh et al. 2004). In other countries, the AEDs most commonly taken by elderly patients differ; for example, in Germany carbamazepine is most frequently prescribed, followed by valproic acid (Huying et al. 2006).

Clinicians prescribing AEDs for elderly patients require knowledge of age-related physiological changes that result in lower AED metabolism and the need for lower dosages and closer monitoring (Mendez and Lim 2003). Aging is associated with decreased albumin and serum protein, altered drug absorption and distribution, changes in hepatic metabolism, and decreased renal elimination. The most significant concern is the decrease in drug protein binding. As serum albumin levels fall, the likelihood increases that drug binding will decrease, and the measurement of total concentration is misleading. Some of the traditional AEDs (phenytoin, valproic acid) are highly protein bound; hence, in elderly patients the therapeutic dosage of medications such as phenytoin is often lower than that for young adults. Aging is associated with decreased hepatic mass and blood flow, with decreased hepatic drug metabolism, particularly oxidative metabolism (cytochrome P450). Aging is also associated with a decreased renal glomerular filtration rate. AEDs such as gabapentin and levetiracetam are primarily excreted unmetabolized through the kidneys. Other potential pharmacokinetic factors include poor drug absorption from decreased gastric motility and gastric atrophy and an increased fat-lean mass ratio, resulting in wider distribution of fat-soluble drugs.

When choosing among AEDs, clinicians also need to be aware of potential side effects. Cognitive and behavioral impairments are the most frequent side effects from AEDs. Elderly patients are particularly vulnerable to cognitive side effects (Table 27–4). The most common cognitive effect is a mild slowing of mental speed. The older AEDs have greater cognitive effects than the newer AEDs. Of the newer AEDs, topiramate can result in significant cognitive impairments, and oxcarbazepine has a high risk of hyponatremia. Lamotrigine is a particularly good drug for elderly patients because of its low cognitive side effects and tolerability (Brodie et al. 1999; Rowan et al. 2005). Levetiracetam is another newer AED that is well tolerated by elderly patients (Cramer et al. 2003). Of the AEDs taken by psychiatric patients, lamotrigine and oxcarbazepine have the fewest side effects, and topiramate, valproic acid, and carbamazepine have the most (Gualtieri and Johnson 2006).

Most epileptic seizures respond to AEDs. Phenytoin, carbamazepine, and valproate are older AEDs for partial seizures and GTCSs (see Table 27–3), the main seizures of adulthood. In the treatment of patients with epilepsy who are psychiatrically disturbed, a first consideration is the use of psychoactive AEDs (Pollack and Scott 1997) (Table 27–5). These medications may relieve some behavioral symptoms either through direct psychotropic properties or through their effects on seizure control. The psychotropic properties of AEDs are particularly important in the management of depression. If possible, the clinician should discontinue phenobarbital and other barbiturates, which may promote depression in elderly patients, and use lamotrigine, carbamazepine, or valproate, all of which stabilize mood and provide prophylaxis against recurrent depressive episodes. Lamotrigine, carbamazepine, valproate, and gabapentin have significant antimanic properties, probably through mood stabilization effects. These medications may also ameliorate some dyscontrolled, aggressive behavior in patients with brain injury. Clonazepam, in addition to its anxiolytic properties, can serve as a supplement to other antimanic therapies. Gabapentin also decreases anxiety and improves general well-being in some patients with epilepsy. Both carbamazepine and ethosuximide may have value for patients with borderline personality disorder.

Encephalopathic changes occur at toxic levels of all AEDs. Even at therapeutic levels, barbiturates may need to be discontinued because of drug-induced depression, suicidal ideation, sedation, psychomotor slowing, and paradoxical hyperactivity in very young and very old patients. Gabapentin may induce aggressive behavior or hypomania, and vigabatrin may precipitate depression and psychosis. In addition, clinicians need to be aware of the potential emergence of psychopathology when patients stop taking AEDs (Ketter et al. 1994). Anxiety and depression are the most common emergent symptoms, but psychosis and other behaviors may also occur.

Another therapeutic consideration is the seizure threshold–lowering effect of psychotropic medications (Table 27–6). This is usually not a problem but can occasionally reach clinical significance. Psychotropic drugs are most likely to produce convulsions when introduced rapidly or given in high doses; clozapine and bupropion, particularly in combination, may be especially problematic. For example, clozapine has induced seizures in 1%–4.4% of patients when the dose was rapidly increased (Mendez 2009). When initiating psychotropic therapy, it is best to start low and go slow while monitoring AED levels and EEGs.

The potential exists for interaction of AEDs and psychotropic medications. Attention to drug interactions is particularly important in treating elderly patients, who are often taking multiple medications. In addition to increasing the metabolism of other AEDs, the addition of an AED most commonly increases the metabolism of psychotropic drugs, with a consequent decrease in their therapeutic effectiveness. The

TABLE 27–3. Antiepileptic drugs (AEDs)

AEDs (trade name)	Indications	Half-life (hours)	Therapeutic level (mg/L)	Usual adult dose (mg/day)	Dosing regimens
Primary drugs					
Carbamazepine (Tegretol, Epitol)	CPS, SPS, GTCS	11–32	4–12	600–1,200	tid
Ethosuximide (Zarontin)	Absence	30–60	40–100	1,000–2,000	tid–qid
Phenytoin (Dilantin)	CPS, SPS, GTCS	10–34	10–20	300–500	bid–qd
Valproic acid (Depakene), divalproex sodium (Depakote)	CPS, SPS, GTCS, absence, atonic, myoclonic	5–20	40–50	1,000–3,000	tid–qid bid (Depakote only)
Secondary drugs					
Clonazepam (Klonopin)	Absence, atonic, myoclonic	20–40	0.005–0.07	2–6	tid–qid
Gabapentin (Neurontin)	CPS, SPS, 2°GTCS	4–7	2–20	900–3,600	tid
Lamotrigine (Lamictal)	CPS, SPS, 2°GTCS	15–24	2–20	75–600	bid
Phenobarbital (various)	CPS, SPS, GTCS	46–140	15–40	90–120	bid–qd
Primidone (Mysoline)	CPS, SPS, GTCS	5–18	5–12	750–1,000	tid–qid
Tiagabine (Gabitril)	CPS, SPS, 2°GTCS	6–8	NE	32–56	bid
Topiramate (Topamax)	CPS, SPS, 2°GTCS	12–30	NE	200–400	bid
Vigabatrin (Sabril)	CPS, SPS, 2°GTCS	4–8	NE	1,000–6,000	bid–qd

Note. CPS=complex partial seizure; GTCS=generalized tonic-clonic seizure; 2°GTCS=secondary generalized tonic-clonic seizure; NE=not established; SPS=simple partial seizure.

TABLE 27–4. Cognitive effects of antiepileptic drugs

Anticonvulsant medication	Impaired cognition at therapeutic doses	Cognitive areas potentially impaired
Benzodiazepines	++++	Mental speed, attention, memory
Carbamazepine	+ to ++	Mental speed, attention, memory
Gabapentin	0	
Lamotrigine	0	
Levetiracetam	0	
Oxcarbazepine	0	
Phenobarbital	+++++	Mental speed, attention, memory
Phenytoin	+++	Mental speed, attention, memory
Primidone	++++	Mental speed, attention, memory
Tiagabine	0	
Topiramate	+++	Mental speed, attention, memory, word naming
Valproic acid	++	Mental speed, attention, memory
Vigabatrin	+	Mental speed
Zonisamide	0	

Note. Strength of effect represented on scale of 0 (no effect) to +++++ (marked effect).
Source. Aldenkamp 2001; Mendez and Lim 2003.

TABLE 27–5. Psychiatric effects of antiepileptic drugs

Antiepileptic drugs	Psychiatric effects
Carbamazepine	Mood stabilizer, antimanic, mild antidepressant
Clonazepam	May cause hyperactivity and additional deficits
Ethosuximide	May cause psychosis
Gabapentin	Mood stabilizer; treatment for bipolar, panic, and general anxiety disorders
Lamotrigine	Mood stabilizer; treatment for bipolar disorder and depression; may cause psychosis
Phenobarbital/primidone	May cause depression, hyperactivity, conduct disorder, and additional deficits
Phenytoin	May cause depression
Tiagabine	May cause depression and psychosis
Topiramate	May cause depression and psychosis
Valproic acid	Antimanic; possibly a mild antidepressant
Vigabatrin	May cause depression and psychosis

TABLE 27–6. Seizure threshold effect of psychotropic medications

Potential	Antipsychotic	Antidepressant	Other psychotropic
		Proconvulsant	
High	Chlorpromazine Clozapine	Amitriptyline Amoxapine Bupropion Imipramine Maprotiline Nortriptyline	—
Moderate	Most piperazines Thiothixene	Clomipramine Protriptyline	Lithium
Low	Aripiprazole Fluphenazine Haloperidol Loxapine Molindone Pimozide Quetiapine Risperidone Thioridazine	Desipramine Doxepin Fluoxetine Sertraline Trazodone Trimipramine Other selective serotonin reuptake inhibitors	Ethchlorvynol Glutethimide Hydroxyzine Meprobamate Methaqualone
		Anticonvulsant	
High	—	Barbiturates	—
Low	Dextroamphetamine Methylphenidate	Monoamine oxidase inhibitors	Oral benzodiazepine

exception is the addition of valproic acid, which can increase psychotropic levels, rarely to a toxic range. Withdrawal of AEDs can precipitate rebound elevations in psychotropic levels. Alternatively, antipsychotics can reduce the threshold for seizures. The initiation of a psychotropic can result in competitive inhibition of AED metabolism with elevations of AED levels to toxicity.

Conclusion

The neuropsychiatric aspects of epilepsy in elderly patients include a broad range of behavioral changes. The incidence of seizure disorders is higher in persons over age 65 than at any age since infancy; consequently, clinicians need to understand the particular psychosocial impact of seizures on older people. In later life, neuropsychological effects from seizures increase, both from the causative brain lesions and from AEDs. Older patients can experience an increased severity of ictally related behavioral disturbances, such as prolonged periods of postictal confusion. Moreover, patients with epilepsy have an increased frequency of interictal psychiatric disturbances, such as depression and suicidality, anxiety disorders and dysphoria, personality changes, psychosis, and hyposexuality. Management of these behavioral disorders requires attention to the behavioral effects of AEDs, the seizure threshold–lowering effects of psychotropic medications, and the interactions between them.

Key Points

- Elderly patients with epilepsy may have neuropsychiatric symptoms.
- Ictally-related behavioral disturbances may be severe.
- Interictally-related behavioral disturbances include depression, psychosis, and personality changes.
- Management includes awareness and monitoring of behavioral aspects of AEDs.
- Management requires attention to the convulsant risks of psychotropic medications.

Recommended Reading

Mendez MF: Neuropsychiatric aspects of epilepsy, in Kaplan and Sadock's Comprehensive Textbook of Psychiatry, 9th Edition. Edited by Sadock BJ, Sadock VA, Ruiz P. New York, Williams & Wilkins, 2009, pp 377–390

References

Ahern GL, Herring AM, Tackenberg J, et al: The association of multiple personality and temporolimbic epilepsy: intracarotid amobarbital test observations. Arch Neurol 50:1020–1025, 1993

Aldenkamp AP: Effects of antiepileptic drugs on cognition. Epilepsia 42 (suppl 1):46–49, discussion 50–51, 2001

Aldenkamp AP, De Krom M, Reijs R: Newer antiepileptic drugs and cognitive issues. Epilepsia 44 (suppl 4):21–29, 2003

Amatniek JC, Hauser WA, DelCastillo-Castaneda C, et al: Incidence and predictors of seizures in patients with Alzheimer's disease. Epilepsia 47:867–872, 2006

Annegers JF: Epidemiology of epilepsy, in The Treatment of Epilepsy: Principles and Practice, 2nd Edition. Edited by Wyllie E. Baltimore, MD, Williams & Wilkins, 1997, pp 157–164

Barry JJ, Ettinger AB, Friel P, et al: Consensus statement: the evaluation and treatment of people with epilepsy and affective disorders. Epilepsy Behav 13 (suppl 1):S1–S29, 2008

Bear D, Fedio P: Quantitative analysis of interictal behavior in temporal lobe epilepsy. Arch Neurol 34:454, 1977

Behrouz R, Heriaud L, Benbadis SR: Late-onset psychogenic nonepileptic seizures. Epilepsy Behav 8:649–650, 2006

Berto P: Quality of life in patients with epilepsy and impact of treatments. Pharmacoeconomics 20:1039–1059, 2002

Blumer D, Montouris G, Davies K: The interictal dysphoric disorder: recognition, pathogenesis, and treatment of the major psychiatric disorder of epilepsy. Epilepsy Behav 5:826–840, 2004

Brodie MJ, Overstall PW, Giorgi L: Multicentre, double-blind, randomised comparison between lamotrigine and carbamazepine in elderly patients with newly diagnosed epilepsy. The UK Lamotrigine Elderly Study Group. Epilepsy Res 37:81–87, 1999

Cloyd J, Hauser W, Towne A, et al: Epidemiological and medical aspects of epilepsy in the elderly. Epilepsy Res 68 (suppl 1):S39–S48, 2006

Collings JA: International differences in psychosocial well-being: a comparative study of adults with epilepsy in three countries. Seizure 3:183–190, 1994

Commission on Classification and Terminology of the International League Against Epilepsy: Proposal for revised clinical and electroencephalographic classification of epileptic seizures. Epilepsia 22:489–501, 1981

Cramer JA, Leppik IE, De Rue K, et al: Tolerability of levetiracetam in elderly patients with CNS disorders. Epilepsy Res 56:135–145, 2003

Dark Fl, McGrath JJ, Ron MA: Pathological laughing and crying. Aust N Z J Psychiatry 30:472–479, 1996

Dikmen S, Hermann BP, Wilensky AJ, et al: Validity of the Minnesota Multiphasic Personality Inventory (MMPI) to psychopathology in patients with epilepsy. J Nerv Ment Dis 171:114–122, 1983

Garrard J, Cloyd J, Gross C, et al: Factors associated with antiepileptic drug use among elderly nursing home residents. J Gerontol A Biol Sci Med Sci 55:M384–M392, 2000

Garrard J, Harms S, Hardie N, et al: Antiepileptic drug use in nursing home admissions. Ann Neurol 54:75–85, 2003

Gibbs FA: Ictal and non-ictal psychiatric disorders in temporal lobe epilepsy. J Nerv Ment Dis 113:522–528, 1951

Gualtieri CT, Johnson LG: Comparative neurocognitive effects of 5 psychotropic anticonvulsants and lithium. MedGenMed 8:46, 2006

Hauser WA: Seizure disorders: the changes with age. Epilepsia 33 (suppl 4):S6–S14, 1992

Hauser WA: Epidemiology of seizures in the elderly, in Seizures and Epilepsy in the Elderly. Edited by Rowan AJ, Ramsay RE. Boston, MA, Butterworth-Heinemann, 1997, pp 7–18

Hauser WA, Annegers JP, Kurland LT: Prevalence of epilepsy in Rochester, Minnesota: 1940–1980. Epilepsia 32:429–445, 1991

Heath RG: Psychosis and epilepsy: similarities and differences in the anatomic-physiologic substrate. Advances in Biological Psychiatry 8:106–116, 1982

Hussain SA, Haut SR, Lipton RB, et al: Incidence of epilepsy in a racially diverse, community-dwelling, elderly cohort: results from the Einstein aging study. Epilepsy Res 71:195–205, 2006

Huying F, Klimpe S, Werhahn KJ. Antiepileptic drug use in nursing home residents: a cross-sectional, regional study. Seizure 15:194–197, 2006

Jones JE, Hermann BP, Barry JJ, et al: Rates and risk factors for suicide, suicidal ideation, and suicide attempts in chronic epilepsy. Epilepsy Behav 4 (suppl 3):S31–S38, 2003

Kanemoto K, Kawasaki J, Kawai I: Postictal psychosis: a comparison with acute interictal and chronic psychoses. Epilepsia 37:551–556, 1996

Kanner AM: Psychiatric issues in epilepsy: the complex relation of mood, anxiety disorders, and epilepsy. Epilepsy Behav 15: 83–87, 2009

Kanner AM, Soto A, Gross-Kanner H: Prevalence and clinical characteristics of postictal psychiatric symptoms in partial epilepsy. Neurology 62:708–713, 2004

Ketter TA, Malow BA, Flamini R, et al: Anticonvulsant withdrawal-emergent psychopathology. Neurology 44:55–61, 1994

Landolt H: Serial electroencephalographic investigations during psychotic episodes in epileptic patients and during schizophrenic attacks, in Lectures on Epilepsy. Edited by de Haas L. New York, Elsevier Science, 1958, pp 91–133

Leppik IE: Antiepileptic drug trials in the elderly. Epilepsy Res 68:45–48, 2006

Lindsay J, Ounsted C, Richards P: Long-term outcome in children with temporal lobe seizures, III: psychiatric aspects in childhood and adult life. Dev Med Child Neurol 21:630–636, 1979

Manchanda R, Schaefer B, McLachlan RS, et al: Psychiatric disorders in candidates for surgery for epilepsy. J Neurol Neurosurg Psychiatry 61:82–89, 1996

Matsuura M, Adachi N, Oana Y, et al: A polydiagnostic and dimensional comparison of epileptic psychosis and schizophrenia spectrum disorders. Schizophr Res 69:189–201, 2004

Mendez MF: Neuropsychiatric aspects of epilepsy, in Kaplan and Sadock's Comprehensive Textbook of Psychiatry, 9th Edition. Edited by Sadock BJ, Sadock VA, Ruiz P. New York, Williams & Wilkins, 2009, pp 377–390

Mendez MF, Cummings JL: Dementia: A Clinical Approach, 3rd Edition. Philadelphia, PA, Butterworth-Heinemann, 2003

Mendez MF, Doss RC: Ictal and psychiatric aspects of suicide among epileptics. Int J Psychiatry Med 22:231–237, 1992

Mendez MF, Lim TH: Seizures in elderly patients with dementia: epidemiology and management. Drugs Aging 20:791–803, 2003

Mendez MF, Cummings JL, Benson DF: Depression in epilepsy: significance and phenomenology. Arch Neurol 43:766–770, 1986

Mendez MF, Doss RC, Taylor JL, et al: Interictal depression in epilepsy: relationship to seizure variables. J Nerv Ment Dis 181:444–447, 1993a

Mendez MF, Doss RC, Taylor JL: Interictal violence in epilepsy: relationship to behavior and seizure variables. J Nerv Ment Dis 181:566–569, 1993b

Mendez MF, Grau R, Doss RC, et al: Schizophrenia in epilepsy: seizure and psychosis variables. Neurology 43:1073–1077, 1993c

Mensah SA, Beavis JM, Thapar AK, et al: A community study of the presence of anxiety disorder in people with epilepsy. Epilepsy Behav 11:118–124, 2007

Monaco F, Cavannna A, Magli E, et al: Obsessionality, obsessive-compulsive disorder and temporal lobe epilepsy. Epilepsy Behav 7:491–496, 2005

Monji A, Yanagimoto K, Maekawa T, et al: Plasma folate and homocysteine levels may be related to interictal "schizophrenia-like" psychosis in patients with epilepsy. J Clin Psychopharmacol 25:3–5, 2005

Morrell MJ, Guldner GT: Self-reported sexual function and sexual arousability in women with epilepsy. Epilepsia 37:1204–1210, 1996

Murialdo G, Galimberti CA, Funzi S, et al: Sex hormones and pituitary function in male epileptic patients with altered or normal sexuality. Epilepsia 36:360–365, 1995

Ortinski P, Meador KJ: Cognitive side effects of antiepileptic drugs. Epilepsy Behav 5 (suppl 1):S60–S65, 2004

Perini GL, Tosin C, Carraro C, et al: Interictal personality disorders in temporal lobe epilepsy and juvenile myoclonic epilepsy. J Neurol Neurosurg Psychiatry 61:601–605, 1996

Peruccca E, Berlowitz D, Birnbaum A, et al: Pharmacological and clinical aspects of antiepileptic drug use in the elderly. Epilepsy Res 68 (suppl 1):S49–S63, 2006

Pollack MIL, Scott FL: Gabapentin and lamotrigine: novel treatments for mood and anxiety disorders. CNS Spectr 2:56–61, 1997

Pugh MJ, Cramer J, Knoefel J, et al: Potentially inappropriate antiepileptic drugs for elderly patients with epilepsy. J Am Geriatr Soc 52:417–422, 2004

Ramsay RE, Rowan AJ, Pryor FM: Special considerations in treating the elderly patient with epilepsy. Neurology 62 (suppl 2):S24–S29, 2004

Reuber M: Psychogenic nonepileptic seizures: answers and questions. Epilepsy Behav 12:622–635, 2008

Robertson MM, Channon S, Baker J: Depressive symptomatology in a general hospital sample of outpatients with temporal lobe epilepsy: a controlled study. Epilepsia 35:771–777, 1994

Rowan AJ, Ramsay RE, Collins JF, et al: New onset geriatric epilepsy: a randomized study of gabapentin, lamotrigine, and carbamazepine. Neurology 64:1868–1873, 2005

Sachdev P: Schizophrenia-like psychosis and epilepsy: the status of the association. Am J Psychiatry 155:325–336, 1998

Sanders KM, Murray GB: Geriatric epilepsy: a review. J Geriatr Psychiatry Neurol 4:98–105, 1991

Satishchandra P, Krishnamoorthy ES, van Elst LT, et al: Mesial temporal structures and comorbid anxiety in refractory partial epilepsy. J Neuropsychiatry Clin Neurosci 15:450–452, 2003

Slater E, Beard A: The schizophrenia-like psychosis of epilepsy: psychiatric aspects. Br J Psychiatry 109:95–150, 1963

Smith PF, Darlington CL: The development of psychosis in epilepsy: a re-examination of the kindling hypothesis. Behav Brain Res 75:59–66, 1996

Stevens JR, Livermore A: Kindling of the mesolimbic dopamine system: animal model of psychosis. Neurology 28:36–46, 1978

Swanson SJ, Rao SM, Grafman J, et al: The relationship between seizure subtype and interictal personality: results from the Vietnam Head Injury Study. Brain 118:91–103, 1995

Trimble MR: The Psychosis of Epilepsy. New York, Raven Press, 1991

Vingerhoets G: Cognitive effects of seizures. Seizure 15:221–226, 2006

28

Neoplastic, Demyelinating, Infectious, and Inflammatory Brain Disorders

Douglas W. Scharre, M.D.

A variety of acquired disorders of the brain are common in the geriatric population. Although motor and sensory symptoms and signs may be obvious features of these disorders, the neuropsychiatric complications often inflict the greatest disabilities and in some cases may be the sole manifestations of the brain dysfunction. In this chapter, I discuss the neuropsychiatric manifestations of the major neoplastic, demyelinating, infectious, and inflammatory disorders of the brain.

Neoplastic Disorders

Demographics

Primary and metastatic neoplasms of the central nervous system (CNS) are common in the geriatric population. The overall incidence of CNS tumors is 14.6/100,000 per year in adults and increases with age (Arora et al. 2009). Eighty-five percent of all primary neoplasms occur intracranially; the rest are intraspinal. In clinical series, 45% of intracranial tumors are gliomas, 15%–18% are meningiomas, 7%–13% are pituitary adenomas, and 6% are metastases (Kleinschmidt-DeMasters et al. 2003; Tyler and Byrne 1992). However, many tumors go unrecognized during life, and in autopsy series meningiomas account for up to 40% and metastatic tumors up to 18% of all intracranial neoplasms (Kurtzke and Kurland 1983). The most common cancers to metastasize to the brain are lung cancer (40%–50% of total metastases), breast cancer (15%–25%), and melanoma (5%–20%). Less common metastases occur from kidney, colon, testis, and lymphatic system cancers (Alvord and Shaw 1991). Eighty percent of all brain metastases occur in the cerebral hemispheres and 20% infratentorially (Eichler and Loeffler 2007).

Physiology

CNS neoplasms impact brain function in multiple ways. Direct invasion and compression produce focal neurological deficits or neuropsychiatric symptoms. Vasogenic brain edema is produced in many neoplasms secondary to capillary leakage across a defective blood-brain barrier. This edema in conjunction with the mass effect of the tumor not only leads to compression effects but also often leads to increased intracranial pressure. The typical signs and symptoms of increased intracranial pressure are headache, nausea, vomiting, papilledema, sixth cranial nerve palsies, and mental status changes. The neuropsychiatric profile of patients with increased intracranial pressure consists of diminished arousal, impaired attention, impaired cognition, irritability, emotional lability, and psychomotor retardation (Wen et al. 2006). In the late stages, severe increased intracranial pressure results in bradycardia, hypertension, and herniation syndromes.

Neurological and neuropsychiatric manifestations vary greatly depending on the location of the tumor. Tumors located near the ventricular system often cause obstructive hydrocephalus, resulting in headache, slow processing speed, forgetfulness, cognitive decline, incontinence, and gait disturbances. Tumors obstructing the arterial or venous circulation may result in ischemic infarctions, hemorrhages, and increased intracranial pressure. Cortically located tumors, particularly in temporal and frontal locations, have a higher risk of producing focal or generalized seizures. Primary brain tumors result in focal seizures with secondary generalization in 20%–45% of patients (Rajneesh and Binder 2009).

Histopathology

Intracranial neoplasms consist of rapidly growing tumor cells, tumor-related blood vessel growth, and necrotic tissue. Astrocytomas are classified as low grade, intermediate grade, or high grade (glioblastoma multiforme) according to the degree of nuclear atypism, mitosis, endothelial proliferation, and necrosis exhibited (Kleihues et al. 1993). Elderly individuals tend to have higher-grade astrocytomas. Oligodendrogliomas frequently contain calcifications and may bleed. Meningiomas are derived from cells of the arachnoid, pia mater, and dura mater and do not invade the brain parenchyma. Pituitary adenomas arise from one of several cell types in the anterior lobe of the pituitary. Most of the pituitary adenomas in the geriatric age range are nonfunctional chromophobe types (Alvord and Shaw 1991). Metastatic tumors have the histopathology of the primary tumor.

Laboratory Evaluations

Lumbar puncture is generally avoided because of the risk of precipitating a herniation syndrome when there is a mass lesion in the brain. When cerebrospinal fluid (CSF) is collected, it typically reveals a mild pleocytosis, elevated protein, and normal glucose in patients with brain neoplasms (Cummings and Benson 1992). CSF cytology is helpful in cases of meningeal carcinomatosis, but large CSF volumes and repeated taps are often required before positive cytology is found. Increased protein, decreased glucose, increased lactate, a high opening pressure, and positive cytology for malignancy are the typical findings in carcinomatous meningitis (Zeller et al. 2002) (Table 28–1).

Electroencephalography in patients with a brain tumor is usually abnormal, revealing either focal or generalized slowing, sharp waves and spikes, or frank epileptiform activity. Conventional angiography or magnetic resonance angiography can demonstrate tumor vascularity (stain), tumor mass effect, and tumor-related vessels (Tsuchiya et al. 2004). The amount of tumor vascularity, particularly in gliomas, is often correlated with tumor growth rate. Angiography of meningiomas often shows a meningeal blood supply and a distinct vascular blush (Tyler and Byrne 1992).

Magnetic resonance imaging (MRI) and computed tomography (CT) may reveal evidence of mass processes, edema, midline shifts, hydrocephalus, and hemorrhage. Contrast enhancement greatly improves tumor detection. MRI is more sensitive than CT in the detection of small tumors, but CT can demonstrate calcifications and bony erosions better. Unfortunately, neither CT nor MRI can accurately define intraparenchymal tumor boundaries. For most intracranial tumors, MRI shows increased signal on T_2-weighted and gadolinium-enhanced T_1-weighted images. Measuring the apparent diffusion coefficient on diffusion-weighted MRI images can assist with predicting the preoperative grading of astrocytomas (E.J. Lee et al. 2008). Diffusion tensor imaging provides fiber tracking information on how critical brain regions are connected or are disrupted by a tumor (Tummala et al. 2003). MRI spectroscopy can provide information about the makeup of the tumor and can help distinguish tumor from infection or identify the most malignant portion of a large tumor, guiding the surgeon to a preferred site for biopsy (Hollingworth et al. 2006). Meningiomas exhibit an extra-axial location, dural base, and marked enhancement with contrast agents. Cerebral metastases often appear as multiple ring-enhancing nodular masses on MRI images (Eichler and Loeffler 2007). MRIs of a glioblastoma multiforme and a meningioma are shown in Figures 28–1 and 28–2, respectively.

Single-photon emission computed tomography (SPECT) and positron emission tomography (PET) can provide information on tumor blood flow, grade, recurrence, and response to treatment (Tyler and Byrne 1992). PET is also useful to find metabolically active areas to biopsy (Wong et al. 2002) and can be useful in following tumors over time for changes in tumor behaviors (Hustinx et al. 2005). Functional MRI (fMRI) can map critical speech and motor brain regions that may be adjacent to the tumor. This may be particularly useful for planning surgical resection or biopsy (Hall et al. 2009).

Treatment and Prognosis

Treatment decisions are based primarily on prognostic factors, including the patient's age and health, to maximize survival and neurological function while avoiding unnecessary or risky therapies. The location and type of CNS neoplasms also determine the approach to treatment. Surgical removal, debulking, chemotherapy, and radiation therapy are often used in some combination. In patients with less favorable prognoses, such as those with multiple metastases, active extracranial disease, and/or poor functional status, whole brain radiotherapy is the treatment of choice (Eichler and Loeffler 2007). For patients with limited brain involvement and a more favorable prognosis, stereotactic surgery or radiosurgery is often used. The combination of surgery or stereotactic radiosurgery and whole brain radiation is common in those with single brain metastases. Chemotherapy agents depend on the breakdown of the blood-brain barrier at the tumor site for selective drug delivery. Molecularly targeted therapies are favored (Soffietti et al. 2008). The complications of radiation therapy include hypothalamic-pituitary dysfunction with resultant hypothyroidism, hypogonadism, or panhypopituitarism (Constine et al. 1993). Approaches that avoid cognitive

TABLE 28–1. Cerebrospinal fluid profiles of various conditions

Condition	White cells (cells/mm^3)	Protein (mg/dL)	Glucose (mg/dL)	Miscellaneous
Carcinomatous meningitis	Normal	↑	↓	↑ lactate, ↑ OP, cytology
Paraneoplastic syndrome/limbic encephalitis	30–40 lymphocytosis	50–100	Normal	IgG ↑, OCB (occasional)
Multiple sclerosis	0–20 lymphocytosis	Normal to 100	Normal	OCB, IgG ↑
Acute disseminated encephalomyelitis	10–4,000 PMN, lymphocytes	Normal to 344	Normal	↑ pressure, OCB (occasional)
Creutzfeldt-Jakob disease	0–15 lymphocytosis	Normal, 50–120	Normal	IgG ↑ (occasional), 14–3–3 brain protein, tau, neuron-specific enolase
Herpes simplex encephalitis	50–1,000 lymphocytosis	50–400	Normal	Culture, PCR
West Nile encephalitis	0–1,800 lymphocytosis	45–80	Normal	IgM ELISA
Aseptic meningoencephalitis	5–1,000 lymphocytosis	45–80	20–40, normal	Culture, IgM ELISA
HIV-1 dementia complex	0–8 lymphocytosis	<80	↓ (occasional)	IgG ↑, culture, HIV RNA, HIV viral load
Progressive multifocal leukoencephalopathy	0–8 lymphocytosis	<80	Normal	PCR for JC virus DNA
Acute bacterial meningitis	100–60,000 PMN	100–1,000	5–40	Culture, antigen detection
Brain abscess	0–500 PMN, lymphocytes	40–100	↓ (occasional)	
Fungal meningitis	5–800 lymphocytosis	45–500	10–40, normal	Culture, cryptococcal antigen, cryptococcal PCR
Neurosyphilis	5–1,000 lymphocytosis	50–100	<40, normal	VDRL, IgG ↑
Neuroborreliosis (Lyme disease)	0–150 lymphocytosis	40–100	Normal	IgG ↑, PCR, intrathecal antibodies
Isolated angiitis of the CNS	0–800 lymphocytosis	40–600	↓ (occasional)	IgG ↑ (occasional)
Lymphomatoid granulomatosis	0–225 atypical lymphocytes	40–780	Normal	OCB (occasional)
Behçet's syndrome	0–500 lymphocytosis	Normal to 160	Normal	IgG ↑ (occasional), BBB

TABLE 28–1. Cerebrospinal fluid profiles of various conditions *(continued)*

Condition	White cells (cells/mm^3)	Protein (mg/dL)	Glucose (mg/dL)	Miscellaneous
Systemic lupus erythematosus	0–50 lymphocytosis	Normal to 100	Normal	OCB, IgG ↑, BBB, antineuronal antibodies
Sjögren's syndrome	Mild lymphocytosis	Normal to 100	Normal	OCB, IgG ↑

Note. BBB=blood-brain barrier breakdown; CNS=central nervous system; HIV-1= human immunodeficiency virus type 1; IgG=immunoglobulin G; IgM ELISA=immunoglobulin M antibody capture enzyme-linked immunosorbent assay; OCB=oligoclonal bands; OP=opening pressure; PCR=polymerase chain reaction; PMN=polymorphonuclear cells; VDRL=Venereal Disease Research Laboratory.

Source. Akman-Demir et al. 1999; Alexander 1993; Ances et al. 2005; Bale 1991; Bossolasco et al. 2005; Darnell and Posner 2003; Davis et al. 2008; Fishman 1992; Geerts et al. 1991; Goodall et al. 2006; Green et al. 2001; Hoffman and Weber 2009; Hsich et al. 1996; Joffe 2007; Kleinschmidt-DeMasters et al. 2003; Pandori et al. 2006; Paraskevas et al. 2007; Paschoal et al. 2004; Patsalides et al. 2005; Rupprecht and Pfister 2009; Sampathkumar 2003; Schmidt et al. 2006; Spudich et al. 2005; West et al. 1995; Younger et al. 1988; Zeller et al. 2002.

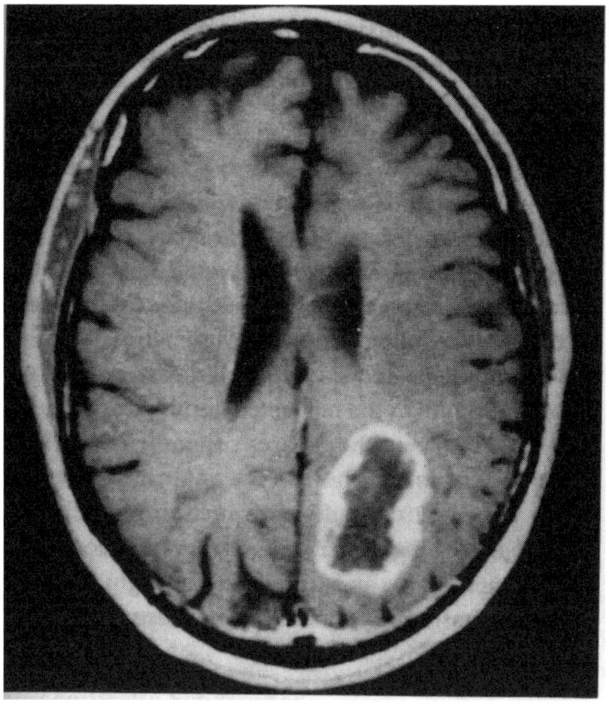

FIGURE 28–1. Gadolinium-enhanced, T_1-weighted magnetic resonance image (MRI) of a 56-year-old man with a left parieto-occipital glioblastoma multiforme.

MRI reveals a ring-enhancing mass with a necrotic center.

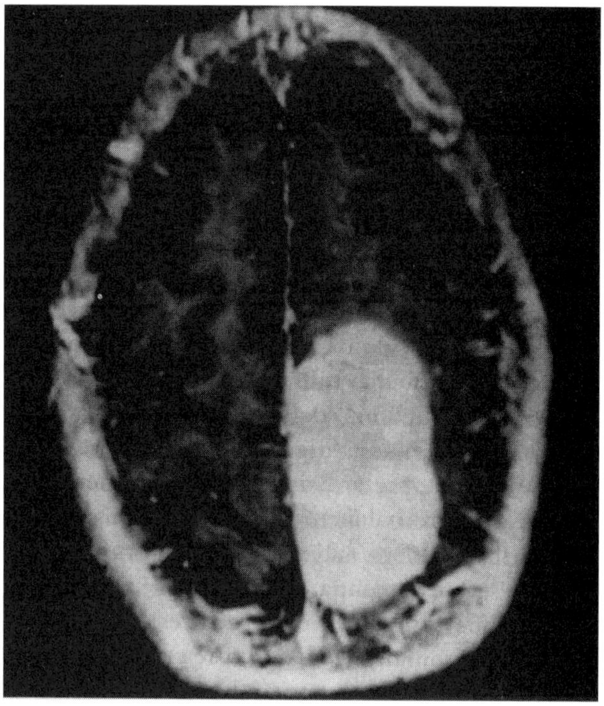

FIGURE 28–2. T_1-weighted magnetic resonance image (MRI) of a 56-year-old woman with a left-sided posterior falx meningioma.

A large dural-based, extra-axial mass is homogeneously enhanced with gadolinium.

impairment are now being stressed because such impairment relates significantly to quality of life. Radiation and chemotherapy leukoencephalopathy complications are discussed in the section "Demyelinating Disorders" later in this chapter.

Corticosteroids are useful in reducing cerebral edema secondary to CNS neoplasms and thereby also aid in the reduction of any associated increased intracranial pressure. Anticonvulsants are given to prevent seizures. A more complete tumor resection and shorter preoperative duration of epilepsy increase a patient's chances of being seizure free (Rajneesh and Binder 2009). Treatment of neuropsychiatric symptoms should avoid aggravating cognitive deficits. Psychosis is best treated with very low dosages of an atypical antipsychotic that is increased slowly until an adequate response is achieved. Depression is treated with antidepressants, usually a selective serotonin reuptake inhibitor (SSRI). Mania is treated with divalproex sodium, carbamazepine, or an atypical antipsychotic; lithium is usually avoided because of its potential for exacerbating seizures (Price et al. 2008). Apathy and psychomotor retardation may be helped with methylphenidate or pemoline.

Astrocytomas and oligodendrogliomas are treated with surgery, radiation therapy, and/or chemotherapy, depending on their degree of malignancy. In approximately 90% of cases, meningiomas can be completely removed surgically but have a high rate of recurrence. Pituitary microadenomas are removed through a transphenoidal approach or are treated with chemotherapy. Macroadenomas with extensive extraglandular extension often require craniotomies for removal and postsurgical hormonal replacement. Brain metastases treatment options include surgery, surgery plus radiation, chemotherapy, and stereotactic radiosurgery (Modha et al. 2005). The 5-year survival rates are as follows: 27.6% for malignant brain tumors overall, 63% for oligodendroglioma, 56% for meduloblastoma, 87% for pilocytic astrocytoma, and 31% for anaplastic astrocytoma; the median survival for glioblastoma multiforme is about 1 year, with only 8.8% of patients surviving 2 years (Davis et al. 1999).

Neuropsychiatric Manifestations

Frontal Lobe Tumors

Frontal lobe tumors produce few focal neurological findings and usually manifest with personality changes or as a dementing condition. The neuropsychiatric symptoms of apathy, disinhibition, impulsivity, childishness, sexually inappropriate behaviors, and impaired insight are the hallmarks of frontal involvement (Hoffer et al. 2007). Euphoria or depression, irritability, lack of concern, poor judgment, disorientation, and poor attention are additional frequent early findings. Psychosis with paranoia, delusions, and hallucinations can also be observed. Patients with right frontal tumors may display more euphoria, mania, and impulsivity, whereas those with left frontal tumors may display more depression and abulia (Belyi 1987). The dementia is characterized by impaired word list generation and aphasia with dominant hemisphere tumors, decreased design fluency with nondominant hemisphere tumors, constructional deficits, motor programming deficits, perseveration, forgetfulness, poor abstraction, and psychomotor retardation. Tumors located in mesial frontal regions may produce somnolence and akinetic mutism. Large subfrontal meningiomas, gliomas spreading to both frontal lobes, and frontal-predominant metastatic tumors frequently result in severe dementia. Fifty percent of patients with frontal lobe tumors develop seizures, usually focal motor (Jacksonian) type, and a few develop hydrocephalus due to obstruction of the interventricular foramen. Tumors located in the posterofrontal region produce hemiparesis, olfactory groove meningiomas produce anosmia, sphenoid ridge meningiomas produce unilateral exophthalmos and cranial nerve palsies, prefrontal tumors often produce a grasp reflex, and tumors involving the frontal eye fields produce a conjugate deviation of the eyes toward the side of the tumor.

Temporal Lobe Tumors

Temporal lobe tumors cause the highest frequency of psychiatric symptoms. These tumors may cause personality changes, irritability, euphoria, depression, anxiousness, psychosis, hallucinations (auditory, formed visual, and simple olfactory or gustatory), or cognitive impairment early in their course. Dominant hemisphere tumors can produce aphasia and verbal memory deficits (amnesia), whereas nondominant hemisphere tumors produce nonverbal memory deficits. Hydrocephalus may result from obstruction of the third ventricle or compression of the midbrain with obstruction of the cerebral aqueduct. Partial complex seizures are frequent and manifest with staring, blinking, complex motor activity, déjà vu phenomena, visual distortions, hallucinations, and other psychomotor disturbances.

Parietal Lobe Tumors

Tumors located in the anterior parietal area may produce somatosensory disturbances, including deficits in two-point discrimination; identification of finger writing (agraphesthesia); identification of objects by their shape, size, texture, or weight (astereognosis); simultaneous identification of bilateral stimulation (inattention); and localization of tactile stimuli (atopognosia). Parietal lobe tumors may cause a contralateral lower-quadrant field cut due to disruption of the superior optic radiations. Apraxia, difficulties in drawing, and focal sensory seizures may also occur with parietal lobe lesions.

Tumors involving the nondominant parietal lobe are most likely to cause a neglect syndrome of the contralateral body and extrapersonal space (inattention). In the full-blown condition, patients will not see, dress, shave, or groom the neglected side of the body and do not respond to stimuli in the neglected hemispace. They may deny a contralateral hemiparesis (anosognosia). Dominant parietal lobe tumors in the angular gyrus region cause Gerstmann's syndrome, characterized by difficulties with writing (dysgraphia), finger identification, calculations (acalculia), and distinguishing right from left. Often, aphasia and constructional disturbances are also present.

Occipital Lobe Tumors

Occipital lobe tumors commonly produce contralateral homonymous visual field deficits, simple visual seizures with generalization, and visual hallucinations consisting of unformed images such as flashes, streaks, or simple geometric patterns. Bilateral medial occipitotemporal tumors may cause a disturbance in visual recognition of objects (visual agnosia), identification of familiar faces (prosopagnosia), or recognition of familiar environments (environmental agnosia). Occasionally, right-sided lesions alone may produce some of these syndromes.

Deep Midline Tumors

Deep midline tumors often cause bihemispheric dysfunction due to invasion or brain compression by surrounding edema. Tumors within or near the third ventricle can obstruct the interventricular foramen or the cerebral aqueduct and cause hydrocephalus. Tumors within the ventricle (e.g., colloid cysts of the third ventricle) can cause intermittent obstruction, resulting in severe headaches and vomiting that are position dependent.

Corpus callosum tumors, especially within the inferior and posterior parts of the corpus callosum, may manifest with psychiatric symptoms that include psychosis, dementia, and somnolence.

Pituitary and hypothalamic area tumors often cause bitemporal hemianopsia, optic atrophy, endocrine disturbances, diabetes insipidus, somnolence, personality changes, and cognitive decline. Excessive somnolence, rage attacks, and hyperphagia are occasionally seen with direct hypothalamic involvement.

Pineal tumors compress the superior colliculus, producing aqueduct occlusion, hydrocephalus, and Parinaud's syndrome with paralysis of upward gaze and ptosis.

Thalamic tumors may produce amnestic memory loss, confabulation, confusional states, emotional lability, depression, somnolence, hemiparesis, and hemihypesthesia with hemianesthesia (Dejerine-Roussy syndrome). Basal ganglia tumors result in impaired attention, memory loss, personality changes, depression, and movement disorders including chorea, dystonia, and rigidity.

Posterior Fossa Tumors

Tumors in the posterior fossa can obstruct the fourth ventricle or the outflow into the basal cisterns, resulting in hydrocephalus. Prominent signs and symptoms include headache, vomiting, mental status changes, cranial nerve palsies, nystagmus, ataxia, dysmetria, hypotonia, and intention tremor. Brain stem tumors produce cranial nerve deficits, long tract signs, cerebellar symptoms, and hydrocephalus. Personality changes, lethargy, disorientation, memory impairment, and mutism may also occur (Cummings and Benson 1992).

Paraneoplastic Syndromes

The remote effects of carcinoma on the nervous system are nearly all due to an immune-mediated process. Paraneoplastic syndromes involving the brain are rare, affecting only about 1 in every 10,000 patients with cancer (Darnell and Posner 2003). The symptoms usually develop rapidly over days to a few weeks; they may occur before the discovery of the neoplasm or arise in the setting of asymptomatic cancer. The tumor often is found months or years later. The most likely pathogenesis of these syndromes is onconeuronal autoantibodies directed against antigens shared by both the cancer and the nervous system (Darnell and Posner 2003). Several syndromes affecting the brain have been described.

Subacute cerebellar degeneration syndrome is characterized by ataxia, dysarthria, nystagmus, and diplopia and is caused by antibodies directed against Purkinje cell cytoplasm (anti-Yo, usually associated with ovarian cancer, or anti-Tr, usually associated with Hodgkin's disease) or against Purkinje cell neuronal nuclei (anti-Hu, also known as type 1 antineuronal nuclear antibodies [ANNA-1], usually associated with small cell lung cancer) (Bernal et al. 2003; Darnell and Posner 2003).

Uncontrolled eye movements characterize opsoclonus paraneoplastic syndrome, usually with cerebellar ataxia due to antibodies against neuronal nuclei of probably brain stem regions (anti-Ri, also known as type 2 antineuronal nuclear antibodies [ANNA-2], usually associated with gynecological or breast cancers). Memory disturbances have also been described with anti-Ri syndromes (Fadare and Hart 2004). Retinal degeneration paraneoplastic syndrome (cancer-associated retinopathy) typically produces scotomas, blindness, and visual hallucinations due to anti–recoverin antibodies of retina photoreceptors (Posner 1997).

Of all the paraneoplastic syndromes, limbic encephalitis is the one most associated with neuropsychiatric symptoms. Anti-Ma and anti-Ta antibodies have both been implicated in causing encephalopathy symptoms. Anti-Ta antibodies are found in young men with limbic encephalitis and testicular germ cell tumors (Hoffmann et al. 2008). Limbic encephalitis is also seen commonly with small cell lung carcinoma and Hodgkin's disease. Other associations include carcinoma of the breast, uterus, ovary, prostate, and kidney; multiple myeloma; lymphosarcoma; reticulum cell sarcoma; neuroblastoma; and acute leukemia. The age at onset for anti-Ma associated limbic and brain stem encephalitis is typically 50–80 years (Hoffmann et al. 2008). Antibodies against neuronal surface antigens, voltage-gated potassium channels, and *N*-methyl-D-aspartate (NMDA) receptors are also common in limbic encephalitis (Graus et al. 2008). Limbic encephalitis is characterized by an amnestic memory disturbance, cognitive decline, depression, anxiety, personality changes, paranoia, hallucinations, psychosis, and diminished alertness. When anti-Hu antibodies are involved, a severe sensory neuropathy is present. Occasionally, complex partial seizures, cerebellar deficits, brain stem signs, myelopathy, and autonomic failure are observed (Dalmau et al. 1992).

In patients with limbic encephalopathy, neuronal loss and perivascular inflammatory infiltrates are found at autopsy, particularly in the medial temporal areas (Newman et al. 1990). Sometimes, the cerebellum, brain stem, spinal cord, dorsal root ganglia, and autonomic ganglia are involved. Neuroimaging is typically unrevealing. However, MRI may demonstrate increased signal on T_2-weighted images in the frontal and temporal lobes (Ances et al. 2005). CSF examination usually shows mild transient lymphocytic pleocytosis and persistent elevated protein, increased immunoglobulin G (IgG), and oligoclonal banding (Ances et al. 2005) in this and in most paraneoplastic neurological syndromes (see Table 28–1). Dramatic responses have been observed clinically with immunotherapy or tumor resection (thereby removing the source of antigen) in patients with limbic encephalitis and in those with cancer-associated autoimmune retinopathies (Ances et al. 2005; Darnell and Posner 2003; Ferreyra et al. 2009). However, those individuals with intracellular antigens do not respond well to immunotherapy (Graus et al. 2008). Additionally, patients with paraneoplastic syndromes causing neuronal loss and death will be unlikely to recover significant function.

Demyelinating Disorders

Although demyelinating conditions are more common in young individuals, there are many examples of these disorders with late survival or presentation in the elderly population. A comprehensive list of both common and rare white matter disorders is presented in Table 28–2. Primary demyelination involves the loss of the myelin sheath, leaving the axon intact but denuded. Dysmyelinating conditions involve impairment in the formation or development of the myelin sheath. These two types of myelin disease give similar clinical and neuropsychiatric features.

TABLE 28–2. Causes of demyelinating disorders in elderly patients

Autoimmune
Multiple sclerosis
Behçet's syndrome
Systemic lupus erythematosus
Sjögren's syndrome
Acute disseminated encephalomyelitis
Vogt-Koyanagi-Harada syndrome
Postinfectious encephalomyelitis
Vascular
Binswanger's disease (subcortical arteriosclerotic encephalopathy)
Toxic-metabolic
Marchiafava-Bignami disease
Central pontine myelinolysis
Vitamin B_{12} deficiency
Folate deficiency
Thiamine (vitamin B_1) deficiency
Vitamin B_6 deficiency
Vitamin E deficiency
Anoxic/hypoxic leukoencephalopathy
Radiation leukoencephalopathy
Chemotherapy-related leukoencephalopathy
Hereditary-metabolic
Metachromatic leukodystrophy
Adrenoleukodystrophy
Cerebrotendinous xanthomatosis
Membranous lipodystrophy
Hereditary adult-onset leukodystrophy
Globoid cell leukodystrophy, late onset
Infectious
HIV-1-associated cognitive/motor complex
Progressive multifocal leukoencephalopathy
Lyme disease
Neoplastic
Lymphoma of the central nervous system
Paraneoplastic syndromes

Multiple Sclerosis

Multiple sclerosis (MS) is the most common demyelinating disorder of the CNS. Although it typically manifests in young adults, 0.6% of the patients do not have their first symptom until age 60 or later (Hooge and Redekop 1992). The prevalence at age 70 is about 50/100,000 (Kurtzke and Kurland 1983). MS is rare in the tropics, but its frequency increases in more northern latitudes. Women are affected more than men by a 2:1 ratio.

Clinical Features

The clinical course of MS has several forms, all of which show lesion dissemination in time and space: relapsing-remitting, secondary progressive, primary progressive, and progressive relapsing. The relapsing-remitting type is characterized by symptoms that may evolve over a few days and then partially or totally resolve over weeks. The secondary progressive form is characterized by a steady progression of neurological damage after an initial relapsing-remitting course. When there have never been relapses or remissions on the steadily progressive course, a patient's MS is termed primary progressive. A progressive relapsing course shows steady neurological worsening interspersed with acute exacerbations that remit. The most common pattern, particularly in those with onset over age 40, is secondary progressive.

Brain stem and spinal cord regions are frequently affected and may cause internuclear ophthalmoplegia, diplopia, trigeminal neuralgia, vertigo, myelopathy, acute transverse myelitis, bladder dysfunction, constipation, autonomic dysfunction, sensory disturbances, gait imbalance, and pain syndromes. Brain demyelination often results in visual impairment (optic neuritis), spastic weakness, gait disturbance, ataxia, movement disorders, sensory dysfunction, paroxysmal disorders, and neuropsychiatric syndromes. Most patients with symptom onset after age 50 have a slowly progressive myelopathy with spastic paraparesis, gait imbalance, and bladder impairment (Hooge and Redekop 1992; Noseworthy et al. 1983).

Neuropsychiatric Aspects

Cognitive and psychiatric symptoms may be the presenting complaint in MS, or they may coexist with other neurological deficits. Like other motor and sensory disturbances, they may also exacerbate and remit or may be continuously present after onset. Treatment with steroids and other medications can complicate and contribute to the neuropsychiatric disturbances. Table 28–3 lists the principal neuropsychiatric manifestations of MS and their approximate frequencies.

Fatigue, a sense of tiredness or lack of energy that is greater than expected for the effort required for a task or the degree of disability evidenced by the patient, occurs in up to 75% of pa-

TABLE 28–3. Frequency of neuropsychiatric manifestations in multiple sclerosis

Neuropsychiatric manifestation	Frequency
Fatigue	75%
Sexual dysfunction	50% (women); 75% (men)
Hypersexuality	4%
Sleep disturbance	58%
Emotional lability	10%
Depression	50%
Euphoria	25%
Mania	13%
Personality changes	40%
Psychosis	1%–3%
Cognitive dysfunction	30%–70%

tients with MS, often preventing normal activities (Bakshi 2003). Fatigue must be differentiated from symptoms of depression, weakness, lack of rest, or excessive exercise. In MS patients, fatigue is exacerbated by heat and improves with cooler temperatures (Krupp et al. 1988).

About 75% of men and 50% of women with MS report sexual dysfunction that increases over time (Stenager et al. 1992). In men, two-thirds have erectile dysfunction and one-third report decreased libido. In women, painful genital dysesthesias, inability to achieve orgasm, and decreased libido are common. Nearly 90% of men have neurogenic causes for their erectile dysfunction (Beits et al. 1994). Hypersexuality is uncommon but has been reported in 4% of patients with MS (Mahler 1992; Yang et al. 2004).

Sleep disturbances are common in MS patients, with 42% having early insomnia, 58% having late insomnia, and 32% having excessive daytime sleepiness (Stanton et al. 2006). The sleep disturbance may be associated with depression, fatigue, spasticity, bladder difficulties, or periodic leg movements.

It is important to distinguish between how the patient subjectively feels (mood) and the outward expression of his or her emotion (affect). About 10% of patients with MS have difficulties regulating their emotional expression, resulting in rapid mood swings or inappropriate emotional responses (Lantz 2005). Many patients have depressed moods in spite of a euphoric affect.

Compared with patients with other chronic neurological diseases, MS patients have significantly more depression (Patten et al. 2003). About half of all patients with MS experience at least one major depression during their illness. No association has been found between their depression and a family history of depression, duration of illness, age, gender, or socioeconomic status (Minden et al. 1987). Depression is associated with recent exacerbations of MS symptoms requiring steroid therapy, but not with severity of disability or cognitive impairment in most studies (Schiffer and Caine 1991).

Euphoria, a cheerful affect inappropriate to the situation, occurs in about 25% of patients with MS (Rabins 1990). It is not associated with steroid use and does not have other features of hypomania. In fact, many euphoric patients have a depressed mood. Euphoria appears to be produced by bilateral subfrontal demyelination (Minden and Schiffer 1990), and MS patients with euphoria have more neurological and cognitive deficits than those who do not (Rabins 1990).

Mania occurs in up to 13% of MS patients (Joffe et al. 1987), and MS patients have twice the risk of developing bipolar disorder as the general population. Human leukocyte antigen analysis and family history studies suggest a genetic predisposition for bipolar disorder in patients with MS who manifest manic behavior (Schiffer et al. 1988). Drugs, including steroids, baclofen, dantrolene, and tizanidine, can also induce mania.

Up to 40% of MS patients have been observed to have personality changes, including apathy, lack of concern over their disabilities, lack of initiation, impaired insight, irritability, and poor judgment (Mahler 1992). These changes may be related to frontal lobe dysfunction (Mendez 1995).

Psychosis in MS, including auditory or visual hallucinations, delusions, or paranoia, is seen in about 1%–3% of patients, and it occurs at a later age than in patients with idiopathic schizophrenia (Feinstein et al. 1992; Ron and Logsdail 1989). It can occur without steroid use and without a family history of schizophrenia. Psychosis in MS is associated with increased temporal and temporoparietal lobe abnormalities that are evident on MRI (Feinstein et al. 1992; Reiss et al. 2006; Ron and Logsdail 1989).

Cognitive dysfunction occurs in up to 70% of patients with MS (Rao 1996; Wallin et al. 2006), with most investigators emphasizing memory, attention, and information processing speed impairments. About 20%–30% of patients with MS meet criteria for a dementia syndrome, with deficits primarily involving poor retrieval memory, slowed information processing, visuospatial abnormalities, and frontal-executive dysfunction; this pattern is suggestive of a subcortical dementia syndrome because specific aphasic conditions are absent (Mackenzie and Green 2009; Rao 1986). Corpus callosal atrophy seen on MRI and increased plaque volume correlate with the severity of cognitive impairment, but not as much as do central atrophy measures (Benedict et al. 2004). The cognitive deficits increase with duration of the disease and in those with progressive MS subtypes (Amato et al. 2001; Piras et al. 2003). The cognitive changes correlate weakly with physical disability in some studies (Amato et al. 2001) but not in others (Wishart and Sharpe 1997).

Both verbal and nonverbal memory is impaired, with spatial memory being more severely affected in most studies (Grafman et al. 1990). The memory deficit is a retrieval abnormality with contextual encoding deficits and not a true amnesia (Rao 1986; Thornton et al. 2002). Remote memory is usually spared. Verbal IQ is generally better preserved than performance IQ, and motor speech impairments are common (Mackenzie and Green 2009; Rao 1986). However, verbal fluency (the number of words beginning with a certain letter produced in 1 minute or the number of animals named per minute) is decreased and is one of the most sensitive and earliest measures of cognitive impairment seen in patients with MS (Henry and Beatty 2006). Although specific aphasic syndromes are rarely described, patients with chronic progressive MS do develop global expressive and receptive language disturbances (Mackenzie and Green 2009). Executive functions, including planning, abstraction, concept formation, set shifting, sustained attention, and organizational skills, are affected in patients with MS and suggest frontal lobe dysfunction (Arnett et al. 1997; Mendozzi et al. 1993). Frontal white matter lesions on MRI have been correlated with apathy, diminished spontaneity of speech, executive dysfunction, and slowed information processing speed (Comi et al. 1995; Huber et al. 1992).

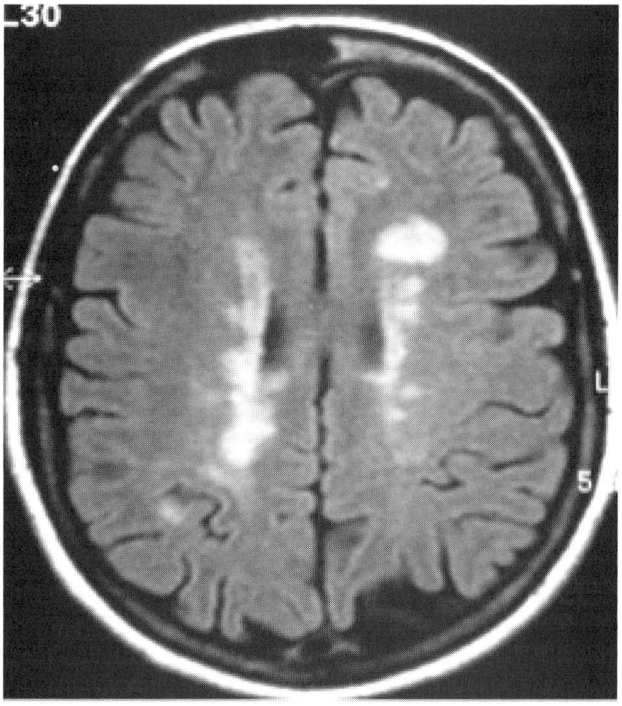

FIGURE 28–3. Magnetic resonance image (MRI) of a patient with chronic progressive multiple sclerosis.

MRI shows multiple areas of increased signal on the proton density–weighted image in the right and left periventricular regions.

Pathophysiology and Diagnosis

MS is believed to be caused by an immune-mediated response triggered by exposure to an unknown environmental agent in the genetically predisposed individual. This results in multifocal discrete inflammatory demyelinated areas scattered throughout the white matter that can be seen as plaques on MRI (Frohman et al. 2003). The plaques are typically seen in the periventricular white matter, corpus callosum, gray-white junction regions, cortex, and spinal cord (Bakshi et al. 2004). MRI shows these plaques in the white matter as areas of high signal on T_2-weighted images (Figure 28–3), and gadolinium contrast can distinguish active from inactive plaques (Bastianello et al. 1990). Diagnosis is aided by finding increased IgG production and oligoclonal bands in the CSF (see Table 28–1) and by prolonged latencies on evoked potential testing (Gronseth and Ashman 2000).

Treatment

Therapies for MS are aimed at modifying the immune processes thought to be responsible for the pathogenesis of MS. Prednisone and methylprednisolone appear to speed the recovery of an acute exacerbation. Reduction of the frequency of clinical relapses in patients with relapsing-remitting MS has been shown with immunotherapies, including intravenous immunoglobulin (Achiron et al. 1996; Goodin et al. 2002), glatiramer acetate (K.P. Johnson et al. 1995), and interferon beta-1b (Interferon beta-1b in the treatment of multiple sclerosis 1995; Lublin et al. 1996). Interferon beta-1a agents have also been shown to delay the accumulation of physical disability in patients with relapsing-remitting MS (Clanet et al. 2004; Jacobs et al. 1996; Panitch et al. 2002). These agents have had some effect on diminishing the number and size of lesions observed on MRI. Neutralizing antibodies can develop to interferon beta treatments, but less so for interferon beta-1a agents, and high titers are associated with a reduction in the therapeutic effect of these agents (Goodin et al. 2007). Mitoxantrone has demonstrated reduction of neurological disability and/or the frequency of clinical relapses in patients with secondary progressive, progressive relapsing, or worsening relapsing-remitting MS (Goodin et al. 2003; Millefiorini et al. 1997), but more studies are needed. The first selective adhesion molecule inhibitor for MS, natalizumab, a monoclonal antibody designed to prevent immune cells from escaping into the tissue of the brain, has been demonstrated to reduce measures of disease activity and improve measures of disease severity in patients with relapsing-remitting MS (Miller et al. 2003; O'Conner et al. 2004); however, due to development of progressive multifocal leukoencephalopathy (PML) in about 1/1,000 cases (Yousry et al. 2006), natalizumab should be reserved for selected patients with relapsing-remitting disease who have failed other therapies or who have a particularly aggressive initial disease course (Goodin et al. 2008). New evidence has suggested that B-lymphocytes may be involved in MS pathogenesis. A single course of rituximab, a monoclonal antibody that depletes specific B-lymphocytes, reduced inflammatory brain lesions and clinical relapses for 48 weeks in patients with relapsing-remitting MS (Hauser et al. 2008).

Unfortunately, many of the immunotherapies can produce neuropsychiatric and other adverse effects. If used longer term, adrenocorticosteroids may cause serious infections, electrolyte disturbances, peptic ulcers, osteoporosis, myopathy, cataracts, and Cushing's habitus. Behavior disturbances include nervousness, insomnia, depression, mania, and psychosis. Immunosuppressive agents may also cause serious infections, increases risk of neoplasia, and multiple organ toxicities. The most common side effects of the immune-modifying agents (interferon betas and glatiramer) are injection site reactions. Postinjection flushing, palpitations, throat constriction, urticaria, and dyspnea can also occur. Dizziness, hypertonia, and tremor are seen with glatiramer, and seizures have been reported with the interferons. Neuropsychiatric side effects include fatigue, anxiety, depression, psychotic depression, and suicide. Depression is a common reason for discontinuation of the interferon betas and glatiramer (Copaxone prescribing insert; Neilley et al. 1996). Although only 1% of patients spontaneously report depression after taking interferon beta-1b, in one study, 40% of patients were experiencing new or increased symptoms of depression within 6 months of initiating therapy, and treatment of the depression significantly reduced discontinuation of the interferon beta-1b (Mohr et al. 1997).

Management of specific symptoms may contribute to improved patient functioning. Spasticity is treated with a combination of physical therapy, tizanidine (Nance et al. 1997), baclofen, benzodiazepines, botulinum toxin, or dantrolene. Paroxysmal disorders respond to anticonvulsants. Anticholinergics, self-catheterization, and prophylactic antibiotics reduce bladder disorders and urinary tract infections.

Treatments for the neuropsychiatric manifestations are also available. Cognitive impairment may be helped with cholinesterase inhibitors (Krupp et al. 2004; Parry et al. 2003) or the use of memory aids, lists, routinization of daily activities, and other cognitive retraining strategies. Pathological laughing or crying can be treated with antidepressants, including low-dose amitriptyline, SSRIs, or a combination of dextromethorphan with quinidine (Lantz 2005). Depression is treated with SSRIs with low side effects and usually very high response rates, except in those patients with executive dysfunction (Julian and Mohr 2006). Bipolar disorder and manic symptoms are treated with lithium, mood stabilizers, and/or atypical antipsychotics. Low dosages of atypical antipsychotics are also the treatment of choice for psychotic symptoms (Jefferies 2006). Anticholinergic agents may impair cognition but aid bladder symptoms; the choice of treatment in any single individual will depend on the relative anticholinergic effect desired. Fatigue may be ameliorated by amantadine (Murray 1985), pemoline (Weinshenker et al. 1992), or modafinil (Rammohan et al. 2002; Stankoff et al. 2005), or with steroids if associated with an acute exacerbation. Sleep disturbances can be improved by sleeping aids and control of pain, nocturia, depression, and periodic leg movements of sleep. Erectile dysfunction is aided by sildenafil citrate (Fowler et al. 2005). Pharmacotherapy reassessment is essential to eliminate agents no longer needed. Support groups and psychotherapy are useful for information exchange, social interaction, stress reduction, and emotional support.

Acute Disseminated Encephalomyelitis

Acute disseminated encephalomyelitis and its many variations, including acute necrotizing hemorrhagic, postinfectious, postvaccinal, multiphasic, and recurrent encephalomyelitis, represent an immune-mediated condition resulting in CNS demyelination (Tenembaum et al. 2007). The condition can occur at any age. It is typically, but not exclusively, a monophasic illness manifesting with fever, headache, and altered consciousness and is typically preceded days or weeks earlier by either viral illness or vaccination (Geerts et al. 1991). The hemorrhagic form is usually, but not always, rapidly fatal. If the individual survives the acute condition, gradual recovery over days to weeks ensues. Hemiparesis, sensory deficits, seizures, dysarthria, or dysphasia may be present initially (Geerts et al. 1991). The neuropsychiatric residua vary depending on the degree of injury and extent of recovery. A subcortical dementia syndrome similar to that seen in MS is typical. Inflammation, demyelination, and variable hemorrhage occur in the white matter. Neuroimaging studies show multifocal abnormalities and large lesions that often involve the cortex with very little periventricular or callosal involvement (Kesselring et al. 1990). CSF cultures are negative (see Table 28–1). A brain biopsy may be required to rule out infection or tumor. Treatment is supportive and may require reduction of increased intracranial pressure. Immunosuppression has been used with some success (Seales and Greer 1991), and in those patients not responding, a combination of immunosuppressants with intravenous immunoglobulin (Straussberg et al. 2001) or plasmapheresis may help (Lin et al. 2004).

Binswanger's Disease

Binswanger's disease, also called subcortical arteriosclerotic encephalopathy, is a vascular dementia resulting from hypoxic ischemia involving the small penetrating vessels supplying the deep white matter of the cerebral hemispheres. It occurs in elderly individuals, most with a history of chronic hypertension. A gradually progressive course of dementia with frontal features and personality change is typical. Neuropsychiatric findings include memory deficits, executive impairment, decreased attention, poor judgment, lack of spontaneity, reduced drive, apathy, perseveration, pseudobulbar palsy, emotional incontinence, and at times euphoria, elation, and aggressiveness (Babikian and Ropper 1987; McPherson and Cummings 1996). Weakness, ataxia, rigidity, small-stepped gait, frequent falls, frontal release signs, dysarthria, and urinary incontinence are typical neurological abnormalities. White matter demyelination is seen pathologically, and MRI reveals hyperintensities on T_2-weighted images in the periventricular and deep white matter regions. Binswanger's disease and lacunar state commonly co-occur (Jellinger 2007).

Marchiafava-Bignami Disease

Marchiafava-Bignami disease is characterized by demyelination of the corpus callosum and adjacent white matter. It is rare and occurs mostly in middle-aged and older men with chronic alcoholism. Many of these individuals exhibit a chronic dementia syndrome that progresses over months to years (Kohler et al. 2000). Remissions are possible. Severe cases present in stupor or coma, and the patient dies rapidly.

The neuropsychiatric features vary widely across cases. The CNS manifestations include dementia, aphasia, slow information processing, frontal release signs (grasp and suck), dysarthria, paratonia, hemiparesis, apraxic gait, incontinence, seizures, and signs of corpus callosum interhemispheric disconnection, such as left-sided limb apraxia, left-hand anomia, and agraphia (Kohler et al. 2000). Personality changes, apathy, violence, and sexual deviations have also been reported.

The characteristic pathology of Marchiafava-Bignami disease is demyelination of the corpus callosum with relative sparing of the splenium and absence of inflammatory changes. Less often involved are the anterior or posterior commissures, centrum semiovale, superior cerebellar peduncles, or white matter of the pons. MRI scans show demyelination essentially limited to the callosum, with the severity of involvement correlating to the severity of the clinical course (Heinrich et al. 2004). Alcohol abstinence and proper nutrition are recommended. In a few cases, acute steroid treatment showed initial clinical improvement (Gerlach et al. 2003).

Vitamin B_{12} Deficiency

Vitamin B_{12} deficiency may be secondary to pernicious anemia, malabsorption syndromes, acquired immunodeficiency, stomach or small bowel resections, stomach acid–reducing agents, or in rare cases dietary B_{12} deficiency (Swain 1995). Both folate and vitamin B_{12} deficiency can produce a megaloblastic anemia and demyelination in the spinal cord and brain, causing peripheral neuropathy, myelopathy, gait disturbance, incontinence, visual impairment, dementia, and neuropsychiatric syndromes. Vitamin B_{12} deficiency is common in elderly people, and B_{12} levels should be checked routinely in the evaluation of anyone with dementia (Knopman et al. 2001). The incidence of low vitamin B_{12} levels among dementia patients has been found to range between 29% and 47%, but some studies have not found a correlation between dementia and low serum B_{12} levels because some cognitively normal people may have low levels (Goebels and Soyka 2000).

Confusion, memory impairment, slow reaction time, and perseveration are common cognitive findings with vitamin B_{12} deficiency (Cummings and Benson 1992; van Goor et al. 1995). The dementia may occasionally precede other systemic manifestations of the vitamin deficiency (Karnaze and Carmel 1990). Neuropsychiatric manifestations include apathy, depression, personality changes, agitation, aggression, paranoia, delusions, and hallucinations (Clementz and Schade 1990; Lindenbaum et al. 1988). Numbness, tingling, lower-extremity weakness, and gait disturbance may progress to flaccid paralysis and incontinence.

The dorsal and lateral columns of the spinal cord and the white matter in the brain show areas of spongiform degenerative demyelination. Electroencephalography reveals generalized slowing in patients with vitamin B_{12} deficiency and dementia. A low serum B_{12} level is usually diagnostic. When the vitamin B_{12} level is within about 100 pg/mL of the lower laboratory limit of normal, it may not accurately reflect B_{12} levels in the individual. In those cases, serum methylmalonic acid and homocysteine levels (increased as a metabolic consequence of vitamin B_{12} deficiency) should be assessed; if both are elevated, the patient likely has a vitamin B_{12} deficiency (van Goor et al. 1995). If such a deficiency is suspected, a Schilling test could be performed to evaluate for malabsorption or the lack of intrinsic factor, a protein required for sufficient absorption of vitamin B_{12} across the intestinal mucosa. Administration of vitamin B_{12} may reverse or stop the progression of the neurological symptoms and dementia (Cunha et al. 1995). The recommended dosage is 1,000 μg of cobalamin administered intramuscularly daily for 1 week, weekly for 1 month, and then monthly (Martin 1988).

Postanoxic/Posthypoxic States

Elderly individuals are particularly prone to anoxia/hypoxia from cardiopulmonary failure or sleep apnea. Chronic hypoxia results in a slowly progressive dementia syndrome, whereas acute anoxia can lead to profound neuronal injury and death. Postanoxic myoclonus status epilepticus is a poor prognostic factor in these settings (Hui et al. 2005). Rarely, patients may develop extensive white matter demyelination a few weeks after apparent recovery from an acute anoxic insult. The delayed symptoms include slowed responses, somnolence, irritability, depression, inattentiveness, disorientation, forgetfulness, pseudobulbar palsy, mutism, incontinence, gait disturbances, and spasticity (H.B. Lee and Lyketsos 2001). Death often occurs, but moderate recovery has been observed. Postanoxic demyelination is seen diffusely over both cerebral hemispheres on MRI.

Radiation- and Chemotherapy-Related Leukoencephalopathy

Neoplastic conditions are very common in the geriatric population, and both radiation therapy and chemotherapy are often used either alone or in combination to treat the tumors. These therapies can be used either to reduce the tumor burden or as a prophylactic to reduce the likelihood of potential brain or spinal cord metastases. However, both may also lead to a delayed demyelination of the CNS occurring from 3 months to 5 years after the treatment. The neurological complications of cranial irradiation include memory loss, cognitive decline, abulia, gait disturbance, ataxia, long tract signs, and tremors. Patients may become severely disabled with dementia and paresis (B.E. Johnson et al. 1985). Prophylactic cranial irradiation also has been associated with cases of dementia (D'Ambrosio et al. 2007).

Chemotherapeutic agents cause a delayed demyelination thought to be secondary to oligodendrocyte neurotoxicity. The cognitive findings are similar to the delayed effects of radiation treatment (Silberfarb 1983). Methotrexate is the most notable example of such an agent, especially when given intrathecally (Ojeda 1982). Cyclosporine (de Groen et al. 1987), cytosine arabinoside (Y.Y. Lee et al. 1986), and 5-fluorouracil combined with levamisole (Hook et al. 1992) have all been reported to cause demyelination. The combination of radiation therapy and chemotherapy, particularly when using methotrexate, cisplatin, lomustine, or amphotericin B, appears to enhance the neurotoxicity (So et al. 1987; Walker and Rosenblum 1992).

Demyelination with necrosis is the pathological finding seen with the delayed effects of radiation on the CNS. Demyelination with or without necrosis has also been reported with the use of chemotherapeutic agents (Hook et al. 1992; Ojeda 1982). Diffuse symmetrical low attenuation of the white matter, cerebral atrophy, ventricular dilatation, and occasionally mass effect are seen with CT scanning of the head (So et al. 1987). MRI reveals increased signal on the T_2-weighted images in the periventricular white matter in a diffuse, symmetrical, and confluent pattern. Scattered focal lesions that enhance with gadolinium are also common (Hook et al. 1992; So et al. 1987).

Metachromatic Leukodystrophy

Metachromatic leukodystrophy is a dysmyelinating disorder with infantile, juvenile, and adult forms. The adult form may manifest from ages 16 to 40 and will usually last 5–20 years, but occasionally as long as 40 years. The enzyme that is deficient in this autosomal recessive inheritable disorder is arylsulfatase A; this deficiency leads to sulfatide accumulation in brain and peripheral nerves (Hageman et al. 1995). Personality changes and cognitive decline mark the insidious onset of the adult form (Estrov et al. 2000; Fukutani et al. 1999). Disinhibition, poor judgment, dishevelment, inappropriate affect, emotional lability, looseness of associations, diminished attention span, memory deficits, abstraction and calculation difficulties, spatial disorientation, and constructional problems are seen (Baumann et al. 2002; Merriam et al. 1990). The disorder may progress to psychosis (in more than 50% of cases), occasional mania, and dementia (Hyde et al. 1992; Kumperscak et al. 2005). Spasticity, ataxia, and seizures are often present. Resting and postural tremors, choreoathetosis, and dystonia have occasionally been described (Baumann et al. 2002; Merriam et al. 1990). Peripheral neuropathy, in the adult form, may not be clinically evident though present electrophysiologically. Sulfatide deposits are present around both central and peripheral nerves and in viscera. Demyelination sparing the arcuate fibers (U-fibers) is present in the cerebral hemispheres and evident on neuroimaging (Baumann et al. 2002). Motor and sensory nerve conduction velocities are mildly slowed, and increased CSF protein is occasionally found. Diagnosis is made by measuring the enzyme deficiency in leukocytes or measuring the amount of sulfatide in urine (Baumann et al. 2002). Genetic counseling is indicated.

Adrenoleukodystrophy

Adrenoleukodystrophy (ALD) is an X-linked (X-q28) dysmyelinating disorder featuring a deficiency of a peroxisomal enzyme, which results in the excessive storage of very long chain fatty acids (VLCFAs) (Moser 1997). There are neonatal, juvenile, adolescent, and adult cerebral forms, as well as an X-linked adrenomyeloneuropathy (AMN) form. The adult cerebral form, representing about 3% of all cases, may manifest from ages 18 to 57 (Weller et al. 1992).

The initial finding in the adult cerebral form of ALD is usually dementia. Most of the neurological and psychiatric symptoms begin when individuals reach age 30. Other neurological findings include upper motor neuron signs, paresis, ataxia, gait apraxia, dysarthria, homonymous hemianopsia, impaired visual acuity leading to cortical blindness, ocular movement disorders, and hearing loss. Seizures are a late finding. Psychiatric features are seen in nearly 40% of patients, often occur early in the course, and include hypomania and mania, disinhibition, emotional lability, depression, hyperactivity, physical and sexual aggression, and psychosis (Kitchin et al. 1987; Rosebush et al. 1999). Adrenal insufficiency and a bronze discoloration of the skin typically become evident after the neurological symptoms begin. The AMN form begins with a progressive spastic paraparesis and a mild peripheral neuropathy, with 20% eventually developing dementia. Emotional lability and depression have also been observed (Naidu and Moser 1990). In ALD, there is demyelination of cerebral white matter, sparing the arcuate fibers. Increased signal on T_2-weighted images is present in the periventricular white matter on MRI scanning, typically starting occipitally and progressing anteriorly (Rosebush et al. 1999). CSF protein is increased. Diagnosis is made by assaying VLCFAs in plasma or skin fibroblasts. A low cortisol level or a reduced adrenal response to stimulation indicates adrenal insufficiency.

Treatment using a low-VLCFA diet with erucic and oleic acid is not encouraging, and immunosuppressants have also been tried (Rosebush et al. 1999). Adrenal steroids are used for the adrenal dysfunction, and atypical antipsychotics and/or mood stabilizers are most effective for the psychotic and manic symptoms (Rosebush et al. 1999).

Cerebrotendinous Xanthomatosis

Cerebrotendinous xanthomatosis is an autosomal recessive disorder that results in impaired hepatic synthesis of bile salts, leading to markedly increased levels of cholestanol. Onset occurs between infancy and the seventh decade. The clinical features include cataracts, tuberous and tendon xanthomas, dementia, ataxia, pyramidal tract signs, spasticity, dysarthria, seizures, depression, and a demyelinating neuropathy. Early atherosclerosis with coronary artery disease is also common. The tendon xanthomas often begin between ages 20 and 40. Cognitive decline can appear in childhood or be delayed until well past middle age. A frontotemporal dementia phenotype has also been described (Guyant-Maréchal et al. 2005). Spasticity and ataxia progress; in the terminal stage, incontinence and pseudobulbar palsy are present. Pathology shows extensor tendon xanthomas and brain deposition of high-density lipoprotein. CSF examination demonstrates a mildly elevated protein. CT and MRI scanning reveal atrophy, focal tuberous xanthomas, and demyelination in the cerebellum and cerebrum (Hokezu et al. 1992). Diagnosis is confirmed by finding elevated levels of cholestanol in plasma or bile. Early treatment with chenodeoxycholic acid to reduce the formation of cholestanol may reverse and prevent the clinical findings.

Infectious Disorders

Infectious conditions producing neuropsychiatric signs and symptoms are common in the elderly population. Certain systemic signs, such as fever, may not be present in older people, whereas other nonspecific symptoms, such as confusion, headache, malaise, generalized weakness, and diminished appetite, may be more prominent. Progression to an acute confusional state or delirium with hallucinations, delusions, paranoia, impaired attention, disorientation, cognitive deficits, sleep disturbance, and tremors may occur rapidly. Consideration of infectious etiologies at an early stage enables prompt diagnosis and treatment. Determining the specific pathogen may require neuroimaging with MRI or CT, followed by lumbar puncture and potentially brain biopsy. Common CNS infections of the geriatric age group are listed in Table 28–4.

Prion Infections

Prions are proteinaceous infectious particles consisting of protein without nucleic acid. They can cause transmissible diseases, can be inherited on chromosome 20 in 10%–15% of cases, or may occur sporadically (DeArmond and Prusiner 2003). The normal prion protein is converted post-translationally from an α-helix to an abnormal β-sheet conformation that is insoluble to detergents and tends to aggregate. The abnormal configuration can induce normal prion proteins to change their conformation to the abnormal form, causing accumulation of prions to sufficient levels to cause a progressive neurodegenerative disease state (Prusiner and Hsiao 1994).

Creutzfeldt-Jakob Disease

Creutzfeldt-Jakob disease (CJD) has a worldwide incidence of approximately one per million. About 90% of CJD cases arise sporadically; 5%–15% are familial, with an autosomal dominant inheritance; and only rare transmitted cases have occurred (Lang et al. 1995; Mendell et al. 2000; Rappaport 1987; Will et al. 1996). The usual age at onset is between 50 and 70 years. The clinical course is typically very rapid, and death usually occurs within several months to 1 year. Occasionally, individuals have survived for several years.

Initially, the patient has complaints of generalized fatigue, anxiety, sleep disturbance, appetite change, depression, impaired concentration, and forgetfulness. After a few weeks, a progressive dementia ensues with aphasia, amnesia, apraxia, and agnosia (Geschwind et al. 2008). Myoclonus, chorea, tremor, ataxia, cerebellar signs, pyramidal signs, spasticity, rigidity, and seizures typically occur after the dementia has started (Brown et al. 1986; Cummings and Benson 1992). Widespread cortical and subcortical multifocal processes contribute to the cognitive deficits, aphasia, and motor abnormalities. Akinetic mutism is a frequent clinical feature in the end stage and is suggestive of mesial frontal lobe involvement.

Pathology shows a spongiform state in the cortical and subcortical gray matter, with loss of neurons and gliosis. Frontal, temporal, and occipital lobes may be more affected than parietal lobes. Some CJD patients have amyloid plaques in the cerebellum and cerebrum similar to those found in kuru. Diffusion-weighted MRI shows multifocal cortical and subcortical hyperintensities in the gray matter (Mendez et al. 2003). PET and SPECT show multiple diffuse areas of hypometabo-

TABLE 28–4. Causes of central nervous system infections in elderly patients

Prions
Creutzfeldt-Jakob disease
Variant Creutzfeldt-Jakob disease
Gerstmann-Sträussler-Scheinker syndrome
Fatal familial insomnia
Kuru
Viruses
Acute
Herpes simplex encephalitis
Other meningoencephalitides
Chronic
HIV-1
Progressive multifocal leukoencephalopathy
Bacteria
Acute bacterial meningitis
Tuberculosis meningitis
Brain abscess
Subdural empyema
Whipple's disease
Fungus
Chronic meningitis
Spirochetes
Neurosyphilis
Lyme disease
Parasites
Toxoplasma
Cysticercosis
Amoeba

lism or hypoperfusion in both cortical and subcortical regions (Goldman et al. 1993; Watanabe et al. 1996). CSF showing a positive immunoassay for the 14–3–3 brain protein is supportive of CJD; however, neuronal injury from other conditions may cause spurious results, and many patients with autopsy-proven CJD are negative for this protein (Geschwind et al. 2003; Hsich et al. 1996; Knopman et al. 2001). Elevated CSF levels of neuron-specific enolase and tau or p-tau protein can be suggestive but not diagnostic of CJD (Goodall et al. 2006; Green et al. 2001) (see Table 28–1). The electroencephalogram (EEG) shows background slowing and a very characteristic periodic polyspike discharge (Chiofalo et al. 1980). No evidence supports the genetic analysis of the prion gene as being of value in the diagnosis of suspected CJD (Knopman et al. 2001). Diagnosis can be made by the clinical features, neuroimaging, EEG, and CSF and is confirmed by brain biopsy if the features are atypical. The diagnostic criteria based on the clinical phenotype are very accurate in predicting new cases (Poser et al. 1999). Treatment is not available except for supportive care.

Variant Creutzfeldt-Jakob Disease

First presenting in the United Kingdom in 1994, the still rare condition called variant Creutzfeldt-Jakob disease (vCJD) is caused by dietary exposure to meat that contains brain or spinal cord tissue infected with the prion responsible for bovine spongiform encephalopathy (Croes and van Duijn 2003). In contrast to CJD, vCJD begins with behavioral symptoms, including dysphoria, insomnia, apathy, and withdrawal, that suggest early frontal lobe involvement. A few months later, dementia, gait imbalance, dysarthria, and sensory symptoms occur (Spencer et al. 2002). Bilateral hyperintensities on MRI in the pulvinar regions of the thalami are characteristic (Collie et al. 2001). Neuropathology shows florid plaques with vacuoles (Ironside 2000). The key is prevention of transmission from eating contaminated meat products or receiving blood transfusions from infected persons (Llewelyn et al. 2004).

Gerstmann-Sträussler-Scheinker Syndrome

Gerstmann-Sträussler-Scheinker (GSS) syndrome is a rare autosomal dominant disorder caused by a range of mutations of the prion protein gene on chromosome 20 and with onset between ages 40 and 60 (Collins et al. 2001). Eight known point mutations in the prion protein gene can result in the GSS syndrome (Panegyres et al. 2001; Prusiner 1996). GSS syndrome is characterized by a mild dementia, with pyramidal, extrapyramidal, and cerebellar signs (Farlow et al. 1989). Gaze palsies, deafness, and blindness may occur.

Fatal Familial Insomnia

Fatal familial insomnia (FFI) is also caused by a range of mutations of the prion protein gene on chromosome 20 (Collins et al. 2001). FFI does not appear to be transmissible and has a course and presentation similar to CJD but with the addition of progressive insomnia and dysautonomia. Onset usually occurs at about age 50, followed by a 12- to 13-month course to death. Patients often develop dysarthria, ataxia, myoclonus, pyramidal tract signs, insomnia, and autonomic disturbances, including hyperhidrosis, hyperthermia, tachycardia, and hypertension. Although in FFI the neuropathology of neuronal loss and gliosis seems mostly restricted to the anterior and dorsal medial thalamic nuclei, these nuclei have tremendous connections with specific frontal lobe regions, and neuropsychological evaluation of these patients reveals significant executive dysfunction, including difficulties with working memory, attention, sequencing, and planning abilities (Gallassi et al. 1992). PET imaging shows prominent hypometabolism in bilateral thalami (Bar et al. 2002; Harder et al. 2004).

Kuru

Kuru is a transmissible prion disease seen in certain New Guinea tribes that practice ritualistic cannibalism. Progressive dementia, cerebellar ataxia, and tremors are typical. Brain pathology reveals spongiform change, neuronal loss, and amyloid (kuru) plaques in approximately 75% of cases (Collins et al. 2001).

Viral Infections

Viral infections can be classified as either acute, with a rapid onset of symptoms, or chronic, with a course over months to years (see Table 28–4). The clinical features of the infection relate to the selective vulnerability of certain cell types to the particular virus.

Herpes Simplex Encephalitis

Herpes simplex encephalitis (HSE) is an acute infection that often affects the temporal and frontal lobes, and although it is treatable, mortality is high (Kapur et al. 1994; Schmutzhard 2001). Half of all cases occur in persons ages 50 and older (Whitley 1991). Initial clinical features include headache, fever, stiff neck, and photophobia. HSE progresses over a few days to produce lethargy, mental status changes, memory impairment, aphasia, focal neurological deficits, seizures, and eventually coma (Whitley 1991). Frontal lobe injury may cause grasp reflexes, frontal release signs, motor impersistence, disinhibition, impulsivity, psychomotor hyperactivity, hyperoral behavior, apathy, echolalia, mutism, anomia, inattention, and utilization behaviors (Brazzelli et al. 1994). Temporal lobe damage often causes amnesia, hallucinations, and, if bilateral, the Klüver-Bucy syndrome, which is characterized by hyperoral behavior, dietary changes, hypersexuality, placidity, visual agnosia, and hypermetamorphosis (excessive tactile exploration of the environment) (Cummings and Benson 1992). Dementia occurs in about 13% of acute encephalitis cases (Hokkanen and Launes 1997).

Hemorrhagic necrosis and petechial hemorrhages are seen at autopsy in the brains of people with HSE. The medial temporal, insular, cingulate, and orbitotemporal regions are the areas most commonly involved. Common regions in the frontal lobes include the mesial prefrontal and basal forebrain regions (Kapur et al. 1994). Periodic lateralized epileptiform discharges are the usual focal EEG abnormality, seen in 80% of patients (Bale 1991). MRI scans often show focal areas of increased T_2 signal in the temporal/insular or frontal regions (Figure 28–4). The lumbar puncture usually suggests a viral infection, and application of polymerase chain reaction (PCR) can confirm a specific diagnosis of herpes simplex virus infection in the brain (Pandori et al. 2006) (see Table 28–1). Brain biopsy has been replaced by PCR because of the 3% risk of serious morbidity.

Therapy with acyclovir (10–15 mg/kg every 6–8 hours for 10–14 days) is started empirically and immediately, because toxic effects are minimal and mortality is reduced from 70% to 19% (Whitley 1991). Recovery may be complete or partial. Considerable cognitive improvement occurs in most patients during follow-up, and the cognitive recovery can be substantial in those treated with acyclovir (Hokkanen and Launes 1997).

Other Meningoencephalitides

The arboviruses are major causes of meningoencephalitis in the elderly population (Davis et al. 2008). All are mosquito or tick borne, and all have seasonal and geographical preferences. West Nile encephalitis is now the most common type in the United States, ahead of St. Louis encephalitis. West Nile virus causes a meningoencephalitis in 1 out of every 150 cases. Adults over age 50 are most susceptible. Western and Eastern equine encephalitis viruses are common particularly in young children and the elderly. Rubella, mumps, measles, coxsackieviruses, polio, and adenoviruses typically occur in younger age groups (Bale 1991).

The acute prodromes of viral meningoencephalitides are all similar to that described for HSE. The specific neurological deficits depend on the extent and distribution of the infection. Lethargy, mental status changes, focal neurological deficits, seizures, and coma may occur. The typical clinical features of West Nile encephalitis include encephalopathy, acute flaccid paralysis, myelitis involving the anterior gray matter, optic neuritis, tremors, myoclonus, ataxia, postural instability, and seizures (Guharoy et al. 2004). Thalami and basal ganglia are most frequently involved in West Nile infections, but frontal lobe impairment also occurs, with personality changes and agitation. Permanent postencephalitic intellectual deficits have been observed with several arbovirus infections, including Western equine, Eastern equine, Japanese, and St. Louis encephalitis viruses (Cummings and Benson 1992).

CSF shows lymphocytic-predominant pleocytosis, mild to moderately elevated protein, and normal glucose. Serum or CSF immunoglobulin M (IgM) antibody capture enzyme-linked immunosorbent assay (ELISA) is diagnostic for all of the common arboviruses (Sampathkumar 2003; Tunkel et al. 2008; see Table 28–1). Current therapy is supportive. Treatment with intravenous immunoglobulin has been suggested for West Nile infection (Roos 2004), but primary prevention can be achieved with insect repellants containing *N,N*-Diethyl-*m*-toluamide (DEET).

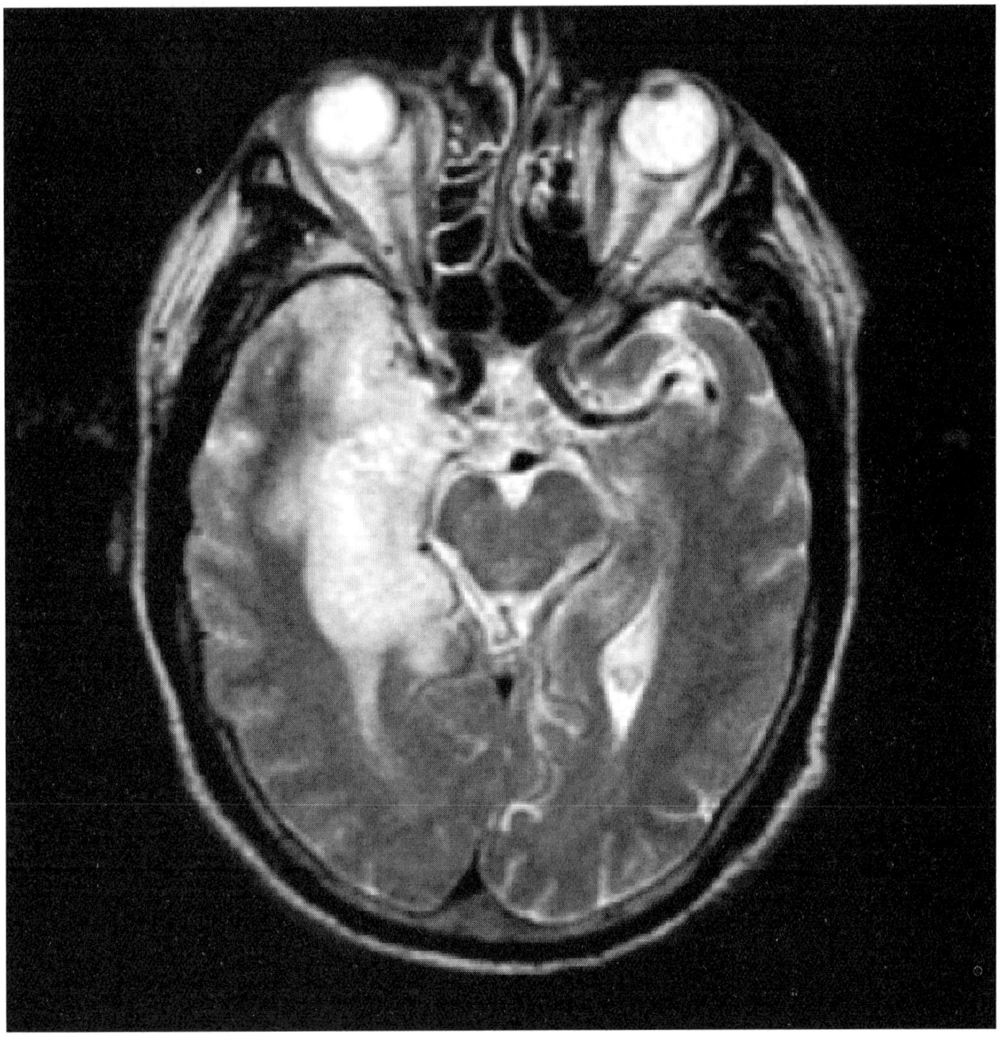

FIGURE 28–4. Magnetic resonance image (MRI) of a man with an acute onset of headaches, fevers, impaired attention, and memory loss.

He became more lethargic over 2 days and developed frontal release signs. MRI revealed left mesial temporal, frontal, and insular region signal abnormalities. Cerebrospinal fluid polymerase chain reaction confirmed herpes simplex virus infection.

Human Immunodeficiency Virus Type 1

Human immunodeficiency virus type 1 (HIV-1) is a retrovirus that preferentially infects T helper cells (Pantaleo et al. 1993). As the number of T helper cells declines, acquired immunodeficiency syndrome (AIDS) occurs, making the individual susceptible to numerous opportunistic infections (Centers for Disease Control 1992). Although this disease is most prevalent among men ages 25–44, an increasing number of cases have been identified in the geriatric population. The median period of time between the initial infection and the development of AIDS is 10 years. Elderly individuals, however, have a more rapid course.

The most common signs and symptoms of HIV-1 infection include fever, lethargy, rash, headache, lymphadenopathy, pharyngitis, myalgias, arthralgias, diarrhea, vomiting, and night sweats (Kahn and Walker 1998). Neurological and neuropsychiatric symptoms occur early, and opportunistic infections account for many additional clinical syndromes (Table 28–5).

At the time of seroconversion, some individuals develop a primary HIV-1 meningitis consisting of fever, headache, meningismus, and CSF pleocytosis (Cooper et al. 1985). Diagnosis of HIV-1 infection is made by detecting serum antibodies to HIV-1 proteins using ELISA techniques (Kahn and Walker 1998). Individuals may then become asymptomatic or have mild (Bornstein et al. 1992) abnormalities on neuropsycho-

TABLE 28–5. Neurological disorders in human immunodeficiency virus type 1 (HIV-1) infection

Primary HIV-1 infection

Aseptic meningitis

HIV-1-associated minor cognitive/motor disorder

HIV-1-associated dementia complex

HIV-1-associated myelopathy

HIV-1-associated acute inflammatory demyelinating polyradiculoneuropathy (HIV-1–associated Guillain-Barré syndrome)

Chronic inflammatory demyelinating polyneuropathy

HIV-1-associated predominately sensory polyneuropathy

Mononeuritis multiplex

HIV-1-associated myopathy

Vasculitis (stroke)

Opportunistic infections

Viral

- Cytomegalovirus (meningoencephalitis, retinitis, myelitis)
- Papovavirus (progressive multifocal leukoencephalopathy)
- Herpes simplex virus (myelitis, encephalitis)
- Varicella zoster virus (myelitis, encephalitis)

Opportunistic infections *(continued)*

Nonviral

- *Toxoplasma gondii* (meningoencephalitis)
- Mycobacteria (meningitis)
- *Cryptococcus neoformans* (meningitis, brain abscess)
- *Aspergillus fumigatus* (meningitis, brain abscess)
- *Histoplasma capsulatum* (meningitis, brain abscess)
- *Candida albicans* (meningitis, brain abscess)
- *Coccidioides immitis* (meningitis, brain abscess)
- *Nocardia asteroides* (brain abscess)
- Mucormycosis (brain abscess)
- *Listeria monocytogenes* (meningitis)
- *Escherichia coli* (meningitis)
- Syphilis (meningovascular)
- Amebic infections (brain abscess)

Opportunistic neoplasms

Primary central nervous system lymphoma

Metastatic systemic lymphoma

Metastatic Kaposi's sarcoma

Other conditions

Stroke (endocarditis, tumor hemorrhage)

Drug intoxication or withdrawal

logical testing. However, once systemic findings appear (lymphadenopathy syndrome or AIDS-related complex), 50% of these individuals have neurological signs or symptoms, and 50% have abnormalities on neuropsychological testing (Janssen et al. 1988). Mental and motoric slowness (Kieburtz and Schiffer 1989), referred to as the HIV-1-associated minor cognitive/motor disorder, is the most common abnormality (American Academy of Neurology AIDS Task Force 1991). Impaired memory, poor reasoning skills, and slow information processing speed are common (Rao 1996). By the time AIDS has been diagnosed, neurological complications are seen in 60% of individuals (Kieburtz and Schiffer 1989).

The HIV-1-associated dementia (HIVD) has been described by many names, including subacute encephalopathy, HIV encephalopathy, or AIDS dementia complex. HIVD affects 15%–20% of all AIDS patients (Ghafouri et al. 2006; Power and Johnson 1995), and it is the initial manifestation in nearly one-fifth of patients ages 74 and older (Janssen et al. 1992). It is characterized by progression over weeks to months of a subcortical dementia syndrome with mental slowness, impaired concentration, forgetfulness, cognitive abnormalities, apathy, social withdrawal, slowed motor skills, ataxia, and weakness, potentially resulting in severe global cognitive dysfunction, paraplegia, mutism, and incontinence (American Academy of Neurology AIDS Task Force 1991; Price et al. 1988). Behavioral symptoms such as agitation, delusions, and hallucinations may occur (Cummings and Benson 1992). Neuropsychological testing reveals deficits particularly in nonverbal tasks and frontal lobe tasks, including Trails B and verbal fluency (Hestad et al. 1993; Power and Johnson 1995). CT and MRI scans show generalized cerebral atrophy and periventricular white matter abnormalities (Bakshi 2004). CSF is abnormal but nonspecific, and CSF HIV RNA does not correlate with the severity of dementia or abnormal neurological performance (Spudich et al. 2005) (see Table 28–1). The pathology of the HIVD consists of reactive gliosis and microglial nodules, especially in the subcortical white and gray matter. Loss of cortical neurons occurs in the orbitofrontal, temporal, and parietal cortical regions but does not correlate well with the severity of dementia (Masliah et al. 1992). More recent studies suggest that HIV-associated cognitive impairment correlates with activated and not necessarily infected brain microglia and macrophages, which in turn appear to cause indirect neuronal injury and death (Ghafouri et al. 2006).

An effective therapy for HIV/AIDS, known as highly active antiretroviral therapy (HAART), became available in 1995. HAART consists of a combination of at least three drugs blocking different aspects of viral replication, including reverse transcriptase inhibitors and protease inhibitors. HAART can restore immune function and suppress viral replication, consequently ameliorating HIV-related symptoms in the CNS and preventing opportunistic conditions. With the use of HAART by patients with HIV, dementia incidence decreased from 30% to 10% (Chang and Tyring 2004; Lawrence and Major 2002). Some of these treatments have neuropsychiatric side effects: fatigue, malaise, myopathy, and confusion with zidovudine; dosage-related, occasionally painful peripheral neuropathy with stavudine, didanosine, and zalcitabine; and paresthesias with ritonavir ("Drugs for HIV Infection" 1997).

Opportunistic infections and neoplasms involving the CNS in patients with HIV-1 are listed in Table 28–5. PML is discussed in the following subsection, and cryptococcal meningitis is discussed later in "Fungal Infections." Cytomegalovirus encephalitis in its severe forms causes diffuse, bilateral cerebral dysfunction with impaired alertness. Neuroimaging can occasionally show subependymal enhancement (Offiah and Turnbull 2006). Cerebral toxoplasmosis and primary CNS lymphoma can be diagnosed based on clinical presentation, neuroimaging, and a treatment trial or occasionally a brain biopsy (Contini 2008; Noy 2006). Cerebral toxoplasmosis evolves in only a few days, with focal neurological findings and enhancing lesions with mass effect and edema evident on MRI (Offiah and Turnbull 2006) (Figure 28–5). It can also mimic an HIVD course (Arendt et al. 1991). Primary CNS lymphoma also causes focal neurological deficits but progresses more slowly, and diffusion-weighted MRI is helpful in its identification (Reiche et al. 2007). Treatment with HAART lowers the frequency and mortality of opportunistic infections, including CNS lymphoma (Skiest and Crosby 2003). Specific treatments are also available for many of the opportunistic infections and neoplasms.

Intracerebral hemorrhages, embolic infarctions from nonbacterial thrombotic endocarditis, strokes due to vasculitis, and medication effects also contribute to the neurological deficits seen with HIV-1 infection.

Progressive Multifocal Leukoencephalopathy

PML caused by the human papovavirus JC virus typically occurs in patients with deficits in cell-mediated immunity (Berger and Major 1999). Onset is usually between ages 30 and 70 and typically progresses over several weeks or months to death in less than 1 year (Bale 1991).

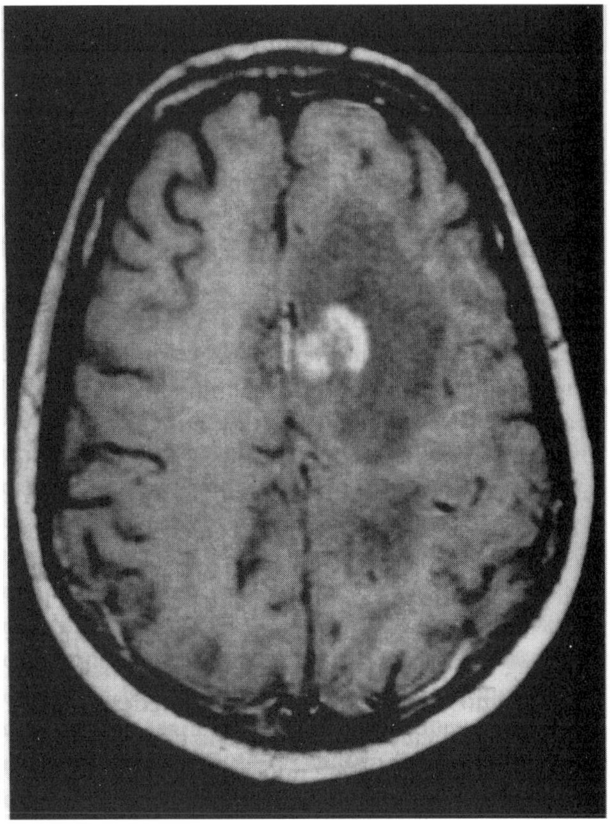

FIGURE 28–5. Gadolinium-enhanced T_1-weighted magnetic resonance image (MRI) of an individual with acquired immunodeficiency syndrome (AIDS) and a cerebral abscess resulting from toxoplasmosis.

MRI reveals a mass lesion in the left medial frontal region with surrounding edema.

Typical cognitive deficits include impaired concentration, visuospatial deficits, memory impairment, aphasia, calculation deficits, and slowed information processing speed (Zunt et al. 1997). PML often causes hemiparesis, ataxia, or hemianopsia, but dementia may be its only manifestation. Depression and agitation have been reported (Stagno et al. 1990). Fever or other systemic signs are not present.

Pathologically, the JC virus infects oligodendrocytes, resulting in demyelination, particularly in the frontal and parieto-occipital regions (Whiteman et al. 1993). MRI shows multifocal demyelination in the subcortical white matter without mass effect or contrast enhancement (Sakai et al. 2009). CSF may confirm PML by PCR detection of the JC virus DNA (Bossolasco et al. 2005) (see Table 28–1). Diagnosis is also made by brain biopsy. Treatment is mostly supportive, but HAART treatment can restore the immune system functioning and improves survival of PML patients (Clifford et al. 1999). However, some patients treated with HAART develop an inflammatory reaction in the area of their PML, and use of steroids may be helpful (Tan et al. 2009).

Bacterial Infections

Acute Bacterial Meningitis

The incidence of bacterial meningitis is 5/100,000 per year (van de Beek et al. 2006). Mortality can be as high as 35% in individuals over age 65 (Behrman et al. 1989). Common organisms causing acute bacterial meningitis in the elderly population are *Streptococcus pneumoniae* and *Neisseria meningitides,* which account for up to 80% of all cases, and *Listeria monocytogenes, Haemophilus influenzae* type B, and other gram-negative bacilli, which account for smaller percentages (Hoffman and Weber 2009). Predisposing conditions such as diabetes, cancer, recent craniotomy, sinus surgery, skull fractures, or immunosuppressive therapy are present in about 35% of cases, and concurrent infections occur in approximately 40% of cases (Behrman et al. 1989).

The initial symptoms of bacterial meningitis are fever, headache, stiff neck, photophobia, nausea, and occasionally vomiting. Agitation, lethargy, and often, especially in elderly patients, acute confusional states follow. Mental status changes are more common than meningismus or headache (Behrman et al. 1989). Focal neurological deficits, including hemiparesis, visual field defects, aphasia, and cranial nerve palsies, as well as seizures are usually due to cerebrovascular complications or acute obstructive hydrocephalus (Bentley et al. 2007; Muller et al. 1995; Zoons et al. 2008). Long-term sequelae include dementia, aphasia, personality changes, hydrocephalus, seizures, and persistent focal neurological deficits (Hoogman et al. 2007; Schmidt et al. 2006).

CT or MRI may show evidence of hydrocephalus, edema, or infarct. CSF is diagnostic, revealing increased intracranial pressure, polymorphonuclear pleocytosis, elevated protein, hypoglycorrhachia, positive cultures, and bacterial antigen detection, with a 5% chance of brain herniation (Joffe 2007) (see Table 28–1). Purulent meningitis and brain edema are seen at autopsy. Early antibiotic use improves outcomes. Adjunctive steroid use can reduce the bacterial toxin–induced inflammation in the host and improve outcomes (Greenwood 2007). Vaccination protects against *Streptococcus pneumoniae* and possible meningitis. It is cost-effective and recommended for every person over age 65 (Advisory Committee on Immunization Practices 2009).

Brain Abscess and Epidural Abscess

Abscesses consist of collections of purulent material that may be present in brain parenchyma, subdural space, or epidural space. The incidence of brain abscess is about six per million per year (Mamelak et al. 1995). Fifteen percent of all brain abscesses and 25% of all spinal epidural abscesses occur in patients over age 60 (Wispelwey and Scheld 1992). Typical organisms causing brain abscesses include aerobic and anaerobic *Streptococcus, Staphylococcus, Bacteroides, Fusobacterium,* and *Clostridium* species (Carpenter et al. 2007). In immunocompromised individuals, various fungal species, cysticercosis, and toxoplasmosis are prevalent (Wispelwey and Scheld 1992). *Staphylococcus aureus,* anaerobic bacteria, and gram-negative organism infections are frequent causes of brain abscesses after extension of a frontal sinusitis or following neurosurgery (Carpenter et al. 2007). Causes of abscesses include infections from direct extension from sinuses, ear, or the oral cavity; sepsis; and penetrating head trauma (Bernardini 2004).

Headache, fever, mental status changes, and focal neurological signs are common initial symptoms of brain abscesses (Carpenter et al. 2007). Seizures and increased intracranial pressure may occur. Neuropsychiatric manifestations may suggest a frontal lobe location. Long-term sequelae include late seizures and persistent focal neurological deficits. Fluid-attenuated inversion recovery (FLAIR) MRI and diffusion-weighted MRI are very helpful in differentiating empyemas and brain abscesses from lesions of other etiologies (Kastrup et al. 2005), and electroencephalography usually shows focal delta activity. Lumbar puncture may precipitate a herniation syndrome and is contraindicated for patients with brain abscesses (see Table 28–1). Treatments for brain abscesses include broad-coverage antibiotics and surgical drainage (Carpenter et al. 2007).

Fungal Infections

Half of all chronic fungal meningitis infections occur in individuals with depressed immune systems or chronic debilitation (Cummings and Benson 1992); therefore, these infections are frequent among the geriatric population. Cryptococcal meningitis is the most common fungal infection (Jones and Nathwani 1995). Other causative organisms include *Coccidioides, Histoplasma, Candida, Blastomyces,* and *Aspergillus.*

Fungal meningitis often begins insidiously and progresses slowly over weeks to months. Although headache, fever, and stiff neck are common, they may not always be present. Mental status changes occur frequently; these include lethargy, apathy, disorientation, poor concentration, memory deficits, and aphasia. Focal neurological deficits, cranial nerve dysfunction, gait imbalance, dementia, and hydrocephalus also may occur (Cummings and Benson 1992). CSF examination reveals lymphocytic pleocytosis, increased protein, and hypoglycorrhachia (see Table 28–1). Cryptococcal antigen and PCR for cryptococcosis in the CSF are specific for cryptococcal meningitis (Fishman 1992; Paschoal et al. 2004). Cultures or titers are necessary for diagnosis of other fungal infections. Fluconazole and other newer azole antifungal agents are safe and effective as first-line therapies without the severe toxicity seen with amphotericin B (Saag et al. 2000).

Spirochete Infections

Neurosyphilis

Syphilis, caused by the spirochete *Treponema pallidum*, is spread by intimate contact. Although CNS invasion may occur, most patients are asymptomatic (Scheck and Hook 1994). The annual incidence of syphilis of all types was 15/100,000 in the United States in 2008 (Centers for Disease Control and Prevention 2009). Primary syphilis manifests as a chancre that heals in several weeks and is followed by a diffuse skin rash indicative of the bacteremia of secondary syphilis. Meningeal neurosyphilis may be seen at this early stage. Tertiary syphilis occurs 1–50 years after the primary infection; typical types include cardiovascular (aortitis), meningovascular, paretic, and tabetic. The tabetic form does not involve the brain, and the meningovascular form manifests by causing strokes. Because of the long incubation times, neurosyphilis frequently begins between ages 30 and 60 (Cummings and Benson 1992). Increasingly, HIV-1 patients are getting syphilis (Fox et al. 2000). Over the last 25 years, the typical forms of neurosyphilis are becoming rare, and more cases with atypical clinical features featuring neuropsychiatric symptoms are being identified (Mitsonis et al. 2008).

General paresis results from syphilitic invasion into the brain parenchyma. Before penicillin treatment, general paresis accounted for up to 20% of all admissions to mental hospitals (Hook and Marra 1992), but now it is extremely uncommon. Many of the clinical features of general paresis suggest frontal lobe involvement; these features include inattention, dementia, anomia, tremulous speech, impaired judgment, irritability, pseudobulbar palsy, paralysis, tremor, ataxia, incontinence, optic atrophy, and Argyll Robertson pupils. Mania is seen in 20%–40% of patients; depression in 6%; and grandiose delusions, paranoia, and hallucinations in 3%–6% (Cummings and Benson 1992; Mitsonis et al. 2008).

The pathology of syphilis is varied and includes meningitis, stroke, vasculitis, inflammatory infiltrates, neuronal loss, gliosis, and rarely gumma formation (Morshed et al. 2008). MRI shows bilateral frontal and/or temporal lobe atrophy and subcortical abnormalities (Offiah and Turnbull 2006; Zifko et al. 1996). Because neurosyphilis is becoming rare, screening should be done only if 1) the patient has some specific risk factor or evidence of prior syphilitic infection or 2) the patient resides in one of the few areas in the United States (southern states and some regions of the Midwest; St. Louis and Wasserheit 1998) with a high number of syphilis cases (Knopman et al. 2001). Testing should be done using the fluorescent treponemal antibody absorption (FTA-ABS) test because other screening tests may be nonreactive in tertiary syphilis (Simon 1985). False positives can occur with systemic lupus erythematosus and some infectious conditions (Hook and Marra 1992). If the FTA-ABS test is positive, a lumbar puncture is indicated. CSF in neurosyphilis shows lymphocytic pleocytosis, elevated protein, a positive Venereal Disease Research Laboratory (VDRL) test, occasional hypoglycorrhachia, increased IgG, and increased tau (Paraskevas et al. 2007) (see Table 28–1). Penicillin is the treatment of choice for all forms of syphilis, with the intravenous route and longer duration of treatment required for patients with neurosyphilis and syphilis associated with HIV-1 (Hook and Marra 1992). Desensitization is recommended for patients with penicillin allergies (Centers for Disease Control and Prevention et al. 2006). Treatment of neuropsychiatric symptoms typically includes the use of atypical antipsychotics, mood stabilizers, and antidepressants (Sanchez and Zisselman 2007).

Lyme Disease

Lyme disease is caused by the tick-borne spirochete *Borrelia burgdorferi*. After the tick bite, an acute localized erythema chronicum migrans (ECM) rash and a viral-like syndrome occur. Dissemination occurs within a few weeks to months, with symptoms including a multifocal ECM rash, acute arthritis, cardiac conduction block, myocarditis, myositis, hepatitis, meningitis, or radiculoneuritis. Some individuals develop a chronic course, leading to chronic arthritis, radiculoneuritis, seventh nerve palsies, encephalomyelitis, or encephalopathy.

Early neurological manifestations occur in 10%–15% of patients and may include bilateral seventh nerve palsies, oculomotor disturbances, other cranial neuropathies, radiculopathies, mononeuritis multiplex, myopathy, or acute lymphocytic meningitis with headache, photophobia, and meningismus (Halperin 2008). Chronic neurological features typically include memory loss, anomia, cognitive deficits, and mild dementia. Deficits in executive function, attention, organization, initiation, abstract concept formation, and verbal fluency are also typical and suggest frontal lobe dysfunction (Fallon and Nields 1994; Waniek et al. 1995). Behavioral disturbances include depression, emotional lability, sleep disturbances, anorexia nervosa, fatigue, irritability, psychosis with paranoia and hallucinations, and violent outbursts (Fallon and Nields 1994). Rarely, patients develop focal CNS deficits including paresis, ataxia, seizures, or a severe dementia with CSF evidence of an encephalitis (Halperin 2008).

In patients with Lyme disease, neuropathological findings include vasculitis, focal demyelination, and, in the late stages, neuronal loss, gliosis, and signs of brain parenchyma infection. MRI may reveal multifocal regions of increased signal in the white matter that are consistent with demyelination (Halperin 2008). Diagnosis is made with a positive serology in the setting of appropriate clinical findings. Demonstration of intrathecal antibody production and CSF PCR for the spirochete may help with diagnosis (Rupprecht and Pfister 2009) (see Table 28–1). Intravenous antibiotics—usually ceftriaxone or cefotaxime for 2–4 weeks—can prevent or halt the neurological complications of Lyme disease and may lead to significant improvement (Halperin 2008).

Inflammatory Disorders

Inflammatory disorders that affect the brain include the vasculitides, the collagen vascular diseases, and certain other conditions. Most of these diseases can manifest at any age, but some are particularly prevalent in elderly individuals. Causes of inflammatory disorders involving the CNS in the geriatric age group are listed in Table 28–6. Of the collagen vascular disorders, scleroderma, rheumatoid arthritis, and Cogan's syndrome only rarely affect the CNS. Some of these conditions have been addressed earlier in this chapter.

Vasculitides

Giant Cell (Temporal) Arteritis

Giant cell (temporal) arteritis is a systemic vasculitis that nearly always occurs in patients over age 50 and affects women twice as often as men (Calvo-Romero 2003). The incidence is as high as 7/100,000 per year (Boesen and Sorensen 1987), and it rises dramatically with increasing age to over 25/100,000 per year in persons over age 80. Constitutional symptoms are prominent and include fever, weight loss, anorexia, and malaise. The classic features of polymyalgia rheumatica syndrome, including pain and stiffness in the muscles of the neck, shoulders, and pelvis, are seen in 50% of those with giant cell arteritis (Salvarani et al. 2008). Headache, jaw claudication, scalp tenderness, and tenderness and nodularity of the superior temporal artery are common (Bhatti and Tabandeh 2001). The headache is characterized by a stabbing or throbbing pain, which is centered over the temple and radiates over the scalp and face. Scalp necrosis, muscular wasting, and angina occur infrequently.

Except for visual disturbance, CNS involvement is infrequent. Blurred vision, amaurosis fugax, and diplopia are reported, and blindness occurs, usually without warning, in 8%–23% of cases (Caselli and Hunder 1997). Multiple infarcts, more common in the posterior circulation territories, have been reported, but dementia syndromes unexplained by strokes are also seen (Nesher et al. 2004). Less frequently, facial neuralgia, vertigo, and neuropathy occur. Depression is the most common psychiatric manifestation, and psychosis is observed in rare cases (H. Johnson et al. 1997).

Pathology shows a patchy giant cell arteritis frequently involving the branches of the external carotid, ophthalmic, and vertebral arteries. The large- and medium-sized arteries throughout the body are also involved but are rarely symptomatic. Involvement of the intracranial arteries is uncommon. Multinucleated giant cells with destruction of the internal elastic lamina are seen. Anemia is common, and an elevated Westergren sedimentation rate (>50 mm/hour and often >100 mm/hour) is almost always found. A superior temporal artery biopsy should be done in all suspected cases (Hall and Balcer 2004). MRI has been used to help with diagnosis, with high specificity (Khoury et al. 2008). Negative biopsies should not dissuade treatment for patients with the typical clinical features. Treatment should be initiated without waiting for biopsy confirmation; prednisone, typically in dosages of 60–80 mg/day, has been shown to be effective for those without visual and neurological symptoms, and intravenous methylprednisolone is useful for those with such symptoms (Hall and Balcer 2004). Slow taper over months is suggested due to high recurrence rates.

Polyarteritis Nodosa

Polyarteritis nodosa (PAN) is an acute systemic necrotizing vasculitis. Immune complex deposition in PAN causes a relapsing and remitting vasculitis that eventually leads to infarction or hemorrhage in multiple organs (Pettigrew et al. 2007). The incidence of PAN is about 0.2/100,000 per year, with males affected twice as often as females. Age at onset ranges from 6 to 80 years, with a mean of about 45 years. Common systemic findings include fever, weight loss, headache, anorexia, asthma, dyspnea, proteinuria, hypertension, arthralgias, skin rash, congestive heart failure, and gastrointestinal pain.

Neurological manifestations occur in up to 80% of cases, mostly resulting from peripheral nervous system involvement, giving rise to mononeuritis multiplex, polyneuropathy, cranial neuropathy, or myopathy. CNS involvement is seen in about 40% of cases and typically occurs later in the course, with dementia, encephalopathy, psychosis, seizures, or strokes (Moore and Calabrese 1994). Specific neuropsychiatric symptoms occur in about 20% of cases and include disorientation, attentional deficits, memory impairment, cognitive deterioration, visual hallucinations, mania, paranoia, and hypoarousal progressing to coma. Hemiparesis, homonymous hemianopsia, and ataxia occur secondary to the strokes.

Pathology shows a necrotizing vasculitis of the small- and medium-sized muscular arteries (Pettigrew et al. 2007). Elevated sedimentation rate, anemia, leukocytosis, and thrombocytosis are common. Angiography reveals aneurysms and arteriopathy. MRI and CT may reveal evidence of infarction (Provenzale and Allen 1996). CSF shows increased pressure, elevated protein, lymphocytic pleocytosis, and occasionally

TABLE 28–6. Causes of inflammatory disorders involving the central nervous system in elderly patients

Vasculitides
Giant cell (temporal) arteritis
Polyarteritis nodosa
Churg-Strauss angiitis
Isolated angiitis of the central nervous system
Wegener's granulomatosis
Lymphomatoid granulomatosis
Takayasu's arteritis
Behçet's syndrome
Collagen vascular diseases
Systemic lupus erythematosus
Antiphospholipid antibody syndrome
Sneddon's syndrome
Sjögren's syndrome
Scleroderma
Rheumatoid arthritis
Cogan's syndrome
Mixed connective tissue disease
Other
Paraneoplastic disorders
Acute disseminated encephalomyelitis
Neuromyelitis optica
Neoplastic-related disorders
Infectious-related disorders
Drug- and toxin-induced disorders
Sarcoid

subarachnoid bleeding. Diagnosis is made clinically and confirmed by tissue biopsy (muscle, skin, sural nerve, or kidney) and angiography. Corticosteroids and immunosuppressive agents are the treatments of choice and often lead to remissions or recovery (Bonsib 2001).

Isolated Angiitis of the Central Nervous System

Isolated angiitis of the CNS, also known as granulomatous angiitis, occurs at any age and is confined to the CNS. Lymphoma, sarcoidosis, and herpes zoster conditions are occasionally associated with this vasculitis. Fever and weight loss are noted in 25% of cases. Usually, an initial subacute presentation with severe headache and encephalopathy is followed gradually by focal deficits, including strokes, and progressing to a vascular dementia syndrome affecting medium and small vessels (Vollmer et al. 1993).

Other common manifestations include seizures, aphasia, hemiparesis, supranuclear cranial nerve palsies, cerebellar signs, myelopathy, and neuropsychiatric symptoms (Block and Reith 2003). Increased intracranial pressure may occur, leading to papilledema and potentially coma and brain stem herniation. Dementia and behavioral changes, including mood disturbance and psychosis, are commonly seen (Hocaoglu and Tan 2005).

A segmental vasculitis with fibrinoid necrosis and giant cells is found in the medium and small arteries, capillaries, and veins of the CNS. The sedimentation rate is increased in 60% of these patients but only to a mean of about 35 mm/hour. CT or MRI may be normal or reveal focal, occasionally enhancing, lesions, hemorrhage, or edema, all of which are found most commonly in the temporal and frontal cortical regions (Vollmer et al. 1993) (Figure 28–6). Angiography may show vasculopathy but usually does not. CSF findings are nonspecific (see Table 28–1). Diagnosis is made clinically and confirmed by brain biopsy. Treatment with prednisone and cyclophosphamide is often ineffective, and there is an 87% mortality rate, with deaths occurring a mean of 6 months after onset of symptoms (Alreshaid and Powers 2003; Younger et al. 1988).

Wegener's Granulomatosis

Wegener's granulomatosis is a systemic necrotizing granulomatosis vasculitis always affecting the respiratory tract and often the kidneys. Typical systemic clinical manifestations include fever, weight loss, sinusitis, otitis media, saddle-nose deformity, cough, hemoptysis, pleuritis, glomerulonephritis, visual symptoms, ulcerative or papular skin lesions, arthralgias, myalgias, and pericarditis (Duna et al. 1995).

Neurological involvement occurs in about one-third of cases and consists mostly of cranial and peripheral neuropathies, including mononeuritis multiplex. The brain can be affected by infarction, hemorrhage, diffuse periventricular white matter lesions, meningeal inflammation, or granulomatous mass lesions causing seizures, focal deficits, and encephalopathy (Nishino et al. 1993). Contiguous extension of granulomatous inflammation from the paranasal sinuses to the brain and often the frontal lobes is typical (Nishino et al. 1993).

Vasculitis, necrosis, and granulomas are seen pathologically on biopsy. Diagnosis is made by cytoplasmic antineutrophil cytoplasmic antibodies (c-ANCA) with a sensitivity and specificity of about 90% (Duna et al. 1995). Angiography is not very helpful, neuroimaging is useful but nonspecific, and CSF can rule out infection. Corticosteroids and cytotoxic agents are needed for successful treatment.

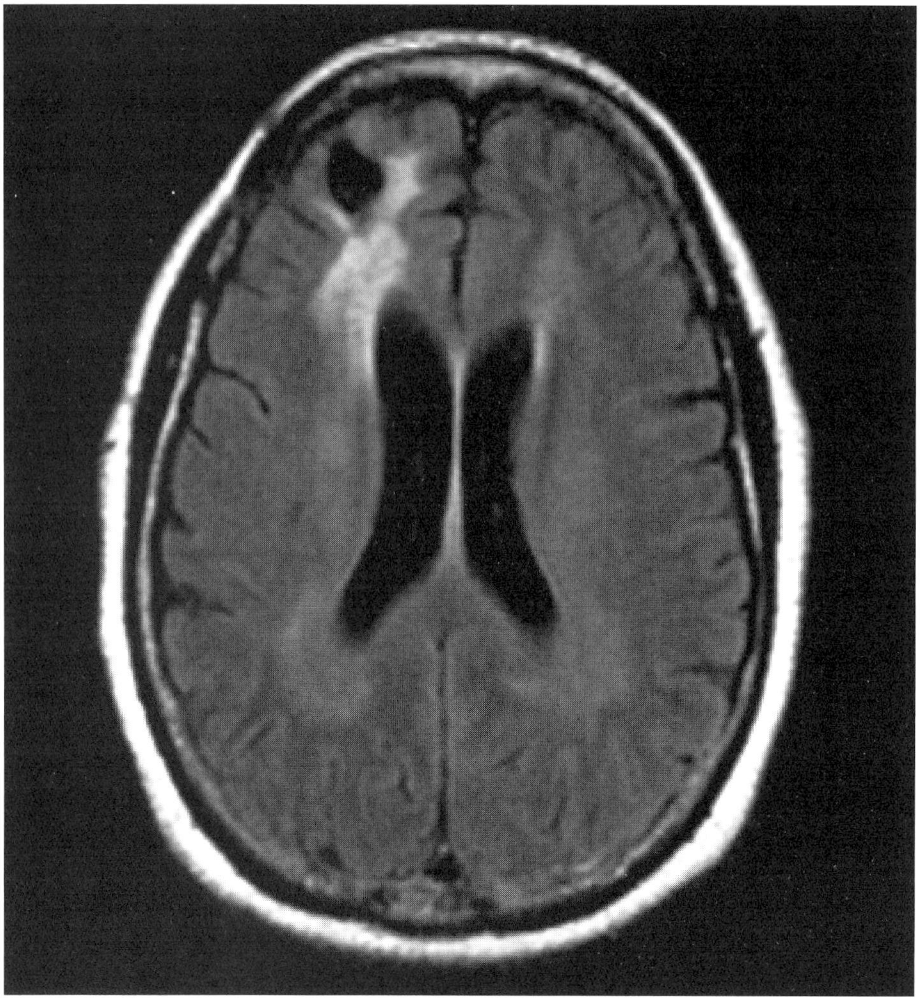

FIGURE 28–6. MRI of a 60-year-old woman after a brain biopsy of the left frontal lobe revealed a vasculitis consistent with isolated angiitis of the central nervous system.

She presented with intermittent headaches and an acute confusional state. Her sedimentation rate was only 32 mm/hour, and her cerebrospinal fluid showed <5 lymphocytes and a protein of 65 mg/dL.

Lymphomatoid Granulomatosis

Lymphomatoid granulomatosis is a rare condition that typically affects the lungs, skin, and nervous system. It is a B-cell lymphoproliferative disorder that appears to be related to Epstein-Barr infection (Muzino et al. 2003), at least when it occurs systemically. However, the rare primary cerebral cases seem not to be associated with Epstein-Barr infection (Lucantoni et al. 2009). Common manifestations include fever, weight loss, cough, chest pain, skin ulcers and papules, and peripheral neuropathies.

CNS dysfunction occurs in 20%–40% of cases and includes a broad spectrum of deficits, such as monocular blindness, internuclear ophthalmoplegia, dysphagia, dysarthria, spasticity, paraparesis, hemiparesis, ataxia, aphasia, encephalopathy, and dementia. Behavioral symptoms reported in these patients include personality change, irritability, disinhibition, impulsivity, distractibility, and mood disturbance (Bushunow et al. 1996).

CSF shows pleocytosis with atypical B cells (Patsalides et al. 2005) (see Table 28–1). Angiography may show a vasculitic pattern, and neuroimaging may show mass lesions, enhancement, or white matter changes (Patsalides et al. 2005). Treatment with prednisone and cyclophosphamide is usually necessary to maintain prolonged remissions. Adjunctive radiotherapy or chemotherapy can also be effective. Rituximab has been successful in some cases (Ishiura et al. 2008).

Behçet's Syndrome

Behçet's syndrome is an inflammatory disorder of uncertain etiology characterized by recurrent oral and genital ulcers, uveitis, thrombophlebitis, and arthritis (Kurokawa and Suzuki 2003). Fever and gastrointestinal complaints are also common. Prevalence is uncertain, with reports ranging from 4 to 100 per 100,000.

The CNS is affected in approximately 40% of Behçet's syndrome cases; the most common manifestation is a relapsing focal meningoencephalitis affecting the brain stem and causing headache, cranial neuropathies, dysarthria, long tract signs, and bulbar and pseudobulbar palsies (Siva et al. 2004). Seizures and increased intracranial pressure have also been reported. A dementia syndrome with memory deficits, aphasia, and cognitive impairment can occur. Personality changes, disinhibition, emotional disturbances, apathy, and akinetic mutism are frequently described behaviors (Hirohata et al. 1998; Yamamori et al. 1994).

A chronic small-vessel vasculitis is seen pathologically, often involving the brain stem, spinal cord, globus pallidus, hypothalamus, cerebral white matter, retina, and skin (Yamamori et al. 1994). Meningeal inflammation is also common. MRI sometimes reveals venous thrombosis and frequently shows deep subcortical and brain stem abnormalities with edema along long tracts in the brain stem and thalamus that may help to differentiate it from other vasculitides (Koçer et al. 1999). Angiography is usually normal, and CSF examination shows a nonspecific lymphocytic pleocytosis with elevated protein (Akman-Demir et al. 1999) (see Table 28–1). Diagnosis is based on clinical features. Treatment for CNS disease includes high-dose steroids and immunosuppressive agents and possibly interferon alfa or thalidomide (Kotter et al. 2004; Kurokawa and Suzuki 2003).

Collagen Vascular Diseases

Systemic Lupus Erythematosus

An immunological disorder affecting multiple organ systems, systemic lupus erythematosus (SLE) is characterized by the presence of many autoantibodies that participate in immunologically mediated tissue injury. The incidence of SLE is about 3/100,000 per year (McCarty et al. 1995), and the prevalence is about 100/100,000 (Ward 2004). Women are nine times more affected than men, and African Americans are three times more affected than whites (McCarty et al. 1995; Ward 2004). Although SLE is a disease primarily of young to middle-aged adults, it can also occur in very old people. Systemic manifestations may include fever, anorexia, rash, lymphadenopathy, arthralgias, pericarditis, valvular disease, pleuritis, Raynaud's phenomenon, alopecia, renal insufficiency, nephrotic syndrome, and hypertension (Gill et al. 2003). Diagnosis of SLE is based on clinical features, a positive antinuclear antibody test, and other specific antibody tests (Tan et al. 1982).

Neuropsychiatric and focal CNS manifestations, often occurring early in the disease course, are seen in 40%–80% of SLE cases and represent the highest incidence for any of the collagen vascular disorders (Brey et al. 2002). CNS dysfunction may occur from primary involvement of the brain or secondarily from complications of the disease, including infection often associated with immunosuppression, seizures, strokes, embolism from endocarditis, steroid treatment toxicity, uremia, and severe hypertension. Nearly 80% of cases develop memory deficits, impaired attention/acute confusional states, and other cognitive deficits (Brey et al. 2002). Up to 60% of patients have symptoms of psychosis with hallucinations and delusions, depression, mania, phobias, and/or anxiety (Fukui et al. 2000; S. Lee et al. 2004). Neuropsychological testing shows deficits in information processing, cognitive flexibility, working memory, visuospatial learning, memory, attention, and verbal fluency (Benedict et al. 2008). Focal CNS involvement and non-neuropsychiatric symptoms are seen in up to 35% of cases and result in supranuclear cranial nerve deficits, chorea, ataxia, parkinsonism, transverse myelitis, and focal paresis (Greenberg 2009; Joseph et al. 2007).

Occasionally associated with SLE is the antiphospholipid (APL) antibody syndrome, characterized by the presence of APL antibodies (particularly lupus anticoagulant and anticardiolipin antibodies), venous or arterial thrombotic strokes or ischemia, recurrent spontaneous abortions, and thrombocytopenia (Miyakis et al. 2006; Sanna et al. 2003a). Myelopathy, deep vein thrombosis, Guillain-Barré syndrome, migraine, chorea, and seizures have also been associated with this syndrome (Cervera et al. 2002). APL antibodies are present in up to 50% of patients with SLE. Sneddon's syndrome—recurrent strokes often causing dementia in patients with livedo reticularis—is also associated with APL antibodies.

The main pathological feature of SLE is a small-vessel vasculopathy that results in microinfarcts and microhemorrhages, which usually cannot be identified with angiography. An autoimmune process with antineuronal antibodies may be an important cause of neuropsychiatric lupus and CNS involvement. Serum antiribosomal P-protein antibodies have a high specificity but a low sensitivity for neuropsychiatric lupus patients with psychosis and depression (Karassa et al. 2006), and they do not correlate well with cognitive symptoms (Reichlin 2003). Although MRI is useful in localizing strokes, findings are often normal even in patients with neuropsychiatric symptoms and CNS involvement (neuropsychiatric lupus). However, magnetization transfer imaging appears to show correlation with cognitive dysfunction, and diffusion-weighted MRI may be able to differentiate ischemic changes from inflammatory lesions (Peterson et al. 2003; Valdes-Ferrer et al. 2008). Fluorodeoxyglucose (FDG) PET is a sensitive tool for detecting manifest or subclinical CNS involvement in SLE. PET consistently shows multiple hypoperfusion abnormalities, most commonly in the parieto-occipital regions of patients with neuropsychiatric SLE, and these findings correlate well with the clinical course of disease (Weiner et al. 2000). Nearly all individuals with neuropsychiatric lupus have abnormal CSF findings, including IgG index, oligoclonal bands, and/or CSF antineuronal antibodies, which may improve with response to therapy (West et al. 1995) (see Table 28–1). CSF antineuronal antibodies have a high specificity and average sensitivity and correlate with CNS symptoms (Zhang et al. 2007).

Treatments for neuropsychiatric symptoms include nonsteroidal anti-inflammatory agents, steroids, and immunosuppressive agents (Bertsias et al. 2008). Rituximab, a chimeric antibody directed against CD20 on B-lymphocytes, has benefited neurological symptoms in patients with SLE (Thatayatikom and White 2006). Plasmapheresis is used in refractory cases, and intrathecal methotrexate with dexamethasone has been successful in patients with severe CNS disease (Sanna et al. 2003b). Oral anticoagulants are advisable to prevent the recurrent thrombotic events seen with APL antibodies and may be more successful than immunotherapies for focal thrombotic disease (Bertsias et al. 2008; Sanna et al. 2003b). Low-dose aspirin should be used for primary prevention of thrombosis in those with APL antibodies (Bertsias et al. 2008). Atypical antipsychotics are used for psychosis, antidepressants for mood symptoms, and anticonvulsants for seizures.

Sjögren's Syndrome

Sjögren's syndrome, seen mostly in women, is a systemic autoimmune disorder characterized by symptoms of dry eyes and dry mouth and may involve the lungs, liver, kidneys, heart, blood vessels, skin, muscles, joints, peripheral nerves, spinal cord, and brain. CNS manifestations, reported in up to 50% of patients in some centers, include cognitive dysfunction (based on neuropsychological testing), mood disorders, anxiety disorders, dementia, and seizures (Harboe et al. 2009). Migraine, focal neurological deficits, intracerebral hemorrhage, subarachnoid hemorrhage, myelitis, aseptic meningitis, and neuropathy are also observed (Alexander 1993; Harboe et al. 2009).

The dementia syndrome has subcortical features, with deficits noted in attention, concentration, memory, and executive abilities (Alexander 1993; Belin et al. 1999). The psychiatric symptoms include mood disturbances, depression, and obsessive-compulsive traits (Alexander 1993; Belin et al. 1999; Harboe et al. 2009).

Lymphocytic infiltration of the exocrine glands causes dry eyes and dry mouth. In Sjögren's syndrome, small-caliber cerebral blood vessels are affected by a vasculopathy much more often than are larger vessels; angiography shows a vasculitis in only 20% of cases because it is not as sensitive to disease of the small cerebral vessels (Alexander 1993). Laboratory evaluations are frequently positive for antinuclear antibodies and occasionally for anti-SSA (Ro) (seen with more serious CNS disease) and anti-SSB (La) antibodies. Autoantibodies to cerebral muscarinic acetylcholine receptors may play a role in cognitive impairment (Reina et al. 2004). CSF is often abnormal but nonspecific (see Table 28–1). Biopsy of a minor salivary gland is diagnostic. MRI shows nonspecific subcortical and periventricular white matter lesions in 80% of cases. SPECT is a more sensitive tool and shows cortical hypoperfusion in regions where MRI is normal in those patients with neuropsychiatric dysfunction (Chang et al. 2002). Corticosteroids and rarely other immunosuppressive agents are used for treatment.

Conclusion

Acquired brain conditions occur frequently in the geriatric population. Some conditions have onset in late life, whereas other conditions have chronic courses and persist into advanced age. Diagnosis and treatment of these disorders in elderly patients are complicated by the frequent co-occurrence of other chronic medical conditions, multiple medication regimens, and the normal physiological changes that accompany aging.

Neoplastic, demyelinating, infectious, and inflammatory conditions are commonly seen in neuropsychiatry practice. Many of these disorders are treatable, and some are reversible. A thorough history, including all neuropsychiatric symptoms, physical examination, and detailed evaluation of mental status, is essential for accurate diagnosis. Basic laboratory assessments, CSF evaluation, and neuroimaging are indicated in many cases to aid diagnosis, detect reversible causes, and assist in management. These brain disorders are a great source of disability in individuals, and physicians must make an accurate and early diagnosis of them to facilitate appropriate treatment and care and to improve the quality of life for the patient and caretakers.

Key Points

- In geriatric patients, diagnosis and treatment of specific maladies are complicated by the frequent co-occurrence of other chronic conditions and aging physiology.
- Do not overlook the value of cerebrospinal fluid analysis when appropriate.

- Specific neuropsychiatric symptoms provide important clues to diagnosis and localization of disease.
- Be mindful of treatment-induced behavioral and cognitive disturbances.
- Neuropsychiatric complaints often produce the greatest disabilities, and their treatment greatly improves quality of life for patient and caregiver.

References

Achiron A, Barak Y, Goren M, et al: Intravenous immune globulin in multiple sclerosis: clinical and neuroradiological results and implications for possible mechanisms of action. Clin Exp Immunol 104 (suppl 1):67–70, 1996

Advisory Committee on Immunization Practices: Recommended adult immunization schedule: United States, 2009. Ann Intern Med 150:40–44, 2009

Akman-Demir G, Serdaroglu P, Tasçi B: Clinical patterns of neurological involvement in Behçet's disease: evaluation of 200 patients. The Neuro-Behçet Study Group. Brain 122:2171–2182, 1999

Alexander EL: Neurologic disease in Sjogren's syndrome: mononuclear inflammatory vasculopathy affecting central/peripheral nervous system and muscles, a clinical review and update of immunopathogenesis. Rheum Dis Clinic North Am 19:869–908, 1993

Alreshaid AA, Powers WJ: Prognosis of patients with suspected primary CNS angiitis and negative brain biopsy. Neurology 61:831–833, 2003

Alvord EC Jr, Shaw C-M: Neoplasms affecting the nervous system of the elderly, in The Pathology of the Aging Human Nervous System. Edited by Duckett S. Philadelphia, PA, Lea & Febiger, 1991, pp 210–286

Amato MP, Ponziani G, Siracusa G, et al: Cognitive dysfunction in early onset multiple sclerosis: a reappraisal after 10 years. Arch Neurol 58:1602–1606, 2001

American Academy of Neurology AIDS Task Force: Nomenclature and research case definitions for neurologic manifestations of human immunodeficiency virus-type 1 (HIV-1) infection. Neurology 41:778–785, 1991

Ances BM, Vitaliani R, Taylor RA, et al: Treatment-responsive limbic encephalitis identified by neuropil antibodies: MRI and PET correlates. Brain 128:1764–1777, 2005

Arendt G, Hefter H, Figge C, et al: Two cases of cerebral toxoplasmosis in AIDS patients mimicking HIV-related dementia. J Neurol 238:439–442, 1991

Arnett PA, Rao SM, Grafman J, et al: Executive functions in multiple sclerosis: an analysis of temporal ordering, semantic encoding, and planning abilities. Neuropsychology 11:535–544, 1997

Arora RS, Alston RD, Eden TO, et al: Age-incidence patterns of primary CNS tumors in children, adolescents, and adults in England. Neuro Oncology 11:403–413, 2009

Babikian V, Ropper AH: Binswanger's disease: a review. Stroke 18:2–12, 1987

Bakshi R: Fatigue associated with multiple sclerosis: diagnosis, impact and management. Mult Scler 9:219–227, 2003

Bakshi R: Neuroimaging of HIV and AIDS related illnesses: a review. Front Biosci 9:632–646, 2004

Bakshi R, Hutton GJ, Miller JR, et al: The use of magnetic resonance imaging in the diagnosis and long-term management of multiple sclerosis. Neurology 63 (suppl 5):S3–S11, 2004

Bale JF Jr: Encephalitis and other virus-induced neurologic disorders, in Clinical Neurology, Vol 2. Edited by Baker AB, Joynt RJ. New York, Harper & Row, 1991, pp 1–86

Bar KJ, Hager F, Nenadic I, et al: Serial positron emission tomographic findings in an atypical presentation of fatal familial insomnia. Arch Neurol 59:1815–1818, 2002

Bastianello S, Pozzilli C, Bernardi S, et al: Serial study of gadolinium-DPTA MRI enhancement in multiple sclerosis. Neurology 40: 591–595, 1990

Baumann N, Turpin JC, Lefevre M, et al: Motor and psycho-cognitive clinical types in adult metachromatic leukodystrophy: genotype/phenotype relationships? J Physiol (Paris) 96:301–306, 2002

Behrman RE, Myers BR, Mendelson MH, et al: Central nervous system infections in the elderly. Arch Intern Med 149:1596–1599, 1989

Beits CD, Jones SJ, Fowler CG, et al: Erectile dysfunction in multiple sclerosis: associated neurological and neurophysiological deficits, and treatment of the condition. Brain 117:1303–1310, 1994

Belin C, Moroni C, Caillat-Vigneron N, et al: Central nervous system involvement in Sjögren's syndrome: evidence from neuropsychological testing and HMPAO-SPECT. Ann Med Interne (Paris) 50:598–604, 1999

Belyi BI: Mental impairment in unilateral frontal tumors: role of the laterality of the lesion. Int J Neurosci 32:799–810, 1987

Benedict RH, Carone DA, Bakshi R: Correlating brain atrophy with cognitive dysfunction, mood disturbances, and personality disorder in multiple sclerosis. J Neuroimaging 14(suppl):36S–45S, 2004

Benedict RH, Shucard JL, Zivadinov R, et al: Neuropsychological impairment in systemic lupus erythematosus: a comparison with multiple sclerosis. Neuropsychol Rev 18:149–166, 2008

Bentley P, Qadri F, Wild EJ, et al: Vasculitic presentation of staphylococcal meningitis. Arch Neurol 64:1788–1789, 2007

Berger JR, Major EO: Progressive multifocal leukoencephalopathy. Semin Neurol 19:193–200, 1999

Bernal F, Shams'ili S, Rojas I, et al: Anti-Tr antibodies as markers of paraneoplastic cerebellar degeneration and Hodgkin's disease. Neurology 60:230–234, 2003

Bernardini GL: Diagnosis and management of brain abscess and subdural empyema. Curr Neurol Neurosci Rep 4:448–456, 2004

Bertsias G, Ioannidis JP, Boletis J, et al; Task Force of the EULAR Standing Committee for International Clinical Studies Including Therapeutics: EULAR recommendations for the management of systemic lupus erythematosus. Ann Rheum Dis 67:195–205, 2008

Bhatti MT, Tabandeh H: Giant cell arteritis: diagnosis and management. Curr Opin Ophthalmol 12:393–399, 2001

Block F, Reith W: Isolated vasculitis of the central nervous system. Der Radiologe 40:1090–1097, 2003

Boesen P, Sorensen SF: Giant cell arteritis, temporal arteritis, and polymyalgia rheumatica in a Danish county: a prospective investigation, 1982–1985. Arthritis Rheum 30:294–299, 1987

Bonsib SM: Polyarteritis nodosa. Semin Diagn Pathol 18:14–23, 2001

Bornstein RA, Nasrallah HA, Para MF, et al: Neuropsychological performance in asymptomatic HIV infection. J Neuropsychiatry Clin Neurosci 4:386–394, 1992

Bossolasco S, Calori G, Moretti F: Prognostic significance of JC virus DNA levels in cerebrospinal fluid of patients with HIV-associated progressive multifocal leukoencephalopathy. Clin Infect Dis 40:738–744, 2005

Brazzelli M, Colombo N, Della Sala S, et al: Spared and impaired cognitive abilities after bilateral frontal damage. Cortex 30:27–51, 1994

Brey RL, Holliday SL, Saklad AR, et al: Neuropsychiatric syndromes in lupus: prevalence using standardized definitions. Neurology 58:1214–1220, 2002

Brown P, Cathala F, Castaigne P, et al: Creutzfeldt-Jakob disease: clinical analysis of a consecutive series of 230 neuropathologically verified cases. Ann Neurol 20:597–602, 1986

Bushunow PW, Casas V, Duggan DB: Lymphomatoid granulomatosis causing central diabetes insipidus: case report and review of the literature. Cancer Invest 14:112–119, 1996

Calvo-Romero JM: Giant cell arteritis. Postgrad Med J 79:511–515, 2003

Carpenter J, Stapleton S, Holliman R: Retrospective analysis of 49 cases of brain abscess and review of the literature. Eur J Clin Microbiol Infect Dis 26:1–11, 2007

Caselli RJ, Hunder GG: Giant cell (temporal) arteritis. Neurol Clin 15:893–902, 1997

Centers for Disease Control: 1993 revised classification system for HIV infection and expanded surveillance case definition for AIDS among adolescents and adults. MMWR Recomm Rep 41 (RR-17):1–19, 1992

Centers for Disease Control and Prevention, Workowski KA, Berman SM: Sexually transmitted diseases treatment guidelines, 2006. MMWR Recomm Rep 55 (RR-11):1–94, 2006

Centers for Disease Control and Prevention: 2008 Sexually Transmitted Diseases Surveillance, Table 1: Cases of sexually transmitted diseases reported by state health departments and rates per 100,000 population: United States, 1941–2008. Atlanta, GA, Centers for Disease Control and Prevention, November 16, 2009. Available at: http://www.cdc.gov/std/stats08/tables/1.htm. Accessed November 7, 2010.

Cervera R, Piette JC, Font J, et al: Antiphospholipid syndrome: clinical and immunologic manifestations and patterns of disease expression in a cohort of 1,000 patients. Arthritis Rheum 46:1019–1027, 2002

Chang CP, Shiau YC, Wang JJ, et al: Abnormal regional cerebral blood flow on 99mTc ECD brain SPECT in patients with primary Sjögren's syndrome and normal findings on brain magnetic resonance imaging. Ann Rheum Dis 61:774–778, 2002

Chang YC, Tyring SK: Therapy of HIV infection. Dermatol Ther 17:449–464, 2004

Chiofalo N, Fuentes A, Galvez S: Serial EEG findings in 27 cases of Creutzfeldt-Jakob disease. Arch Neurol 37:143–145, 1980

Clanet M, Kappos L, Hartung HP, et al: Interferon beta-1a in relapsing remitting multiple sclerosis: four-year extension of the European IFNbeta-1a Dose Comparison Study. Mult Scler 10:139–144, 2004

Clementz GL, Schade SG: The spectrum of vitamin B12 deficiency. Am Fam Physician 41:150–162, 1990

Clifford DB, Yiannoutsos C, Glicksman M, et al: HAART improves prognosis in HIV-associated progressive multifocal leukoencephalopathy. Neurology 52:623–625, 1999

Collie DA, Sellar RJ, Zeidler M, et al: MRI of Creutzfeldt-Jakob disease: imaging features and recommended MRI protocol. Clin Radiol 56:726–739, 2001

Collins S, McLean CA, Masters CL: Gerstmann-Sträussler-Scheinker syndrome, fatal familial insomnia, and kuru: a review of these less common human transmissible spongiform encephalopathies. J Clin Neurosci 8:387–397, 2001

Comi G, Filippi M, Martinelli V, et al: Brain MRI correlates of cognitive impairment in primary and secondary progressive multiple sclerosis. J Neurol Sci 132:222–227, 1995

Constine LS, Woolf PD, Cann D, et al: Hypothalamic-pituitary dysfunction after radiation for brain tumors. N Engl J Med 328:87–94, 1993

Contini C: Clinical and diagnostic management of toxoplasmosis in the immunocompromised patient. Parassitologia 50:45–50, 2008

Cooper DA, Gold J, MacLean P, et al: Acute AIDS retrovirus infection. Lancet 1:537–540, 1985

Croes EA, van Duijn CM: Variant Creutzfeldt-Jakob disease. Eur J Epidemiol 18:473–477, 2003

Cummings JL, Benson DF: Dementia: A Clinical Approach, 2nd Edition. Stoneham, MA, Butterworth, 1992

Cunha UG, Rocha FL, Peixoto JM, et al: Vitamin B12 deficiency and dementia. Int Psychogeriatr 7:85–88, 1995

Dalmau J, Graus F, Rosenblum MK, et al: Anti-Hu-associated paraneoplastic encephalomyelitis/sensory neuronopathy: a clinical study of 71 patients. Medicine 71:59–72, 1992

D'Ambrosio DJ, Cohen RB, Glass J, et al: Unexpected dementia following prophylactic cranial irradiation for small cell lung cancer: case report. J Neurooncol 85:77–79, 2007

Darnell RB, Posner JB: Paraneoplastic syndromes involving the nervous system. N Engl J Med 349:1543–1554, 2003

Davis FG, McCarthy BJ, Freels S, et al: The conditional probability of survival of patients with primary malignant brain tumors. Cancer 75:485–491, 1999

Davis LE, Beckham JD, Tyler KL: North American encephalitic arboviruses. Neurol Clin 26:727–757, 2008

DeArmond SJ, Prusiner SB: Perspectives on prion biology, prion disease pathogenesis, and pharmacologic approaches to treatment. Clin Lab Med 23:1–41, 2003

de Groen PC, Aksamit AJ, Rakela J, et al: Central nervous system toxicity after liver transplantation: the role of cyclosporine and cholesterol. N Engl J Med 317:861–866, 1987

Drugs for HIV infection. Med Lett Drugs Ther 39:111–116, 1997

Duna GF, Galperin C, Hoffman GS: Wegener's granulomatosis. Rheum Dis Clin North Am 21:949–986, 1995

Eichler A, Loeffler J: Multidisciplinary management of brain metastases. Oncologist 12:884–898, 2007

Estrov Y, Scaglia F, Bodamer OA: Psychiatric symptoms of inherited metabolic disease. J Inherit Metab Dis 23:2–6, 2000

Fadare O, Hart HJ: Anti-Ri antibodies associated with short-term memory deficits and a mature cystic teratoma of the ovary. Int Semin Surg Oncol 1:11, 2004

Fallon BA, Nields JA: Lyme disease: a neuropsychiatric illness. Am J Psychiatry 151:1571–1583, 1994

Farlow MR, Yee RD, Dlouhy SR, et al: Gerstmann-Sträussler-Scheinker disease, I: extending the clinical spectrum. Neurology 39: 1446–1452, 1989

Feinstein A, du Boulay G, Ron MA: Psychotic illness in multiple sclerosis: a clinical and magnetic resonance imaging study. Br J Psychiatry 161:680–685, 1992

Ferreyra HA, Jayasundera T, Khan NW, et al: Management of autoimmune retinopathies with immunosuppression. Arch Ophthalmol 127:390–397, 2009

Fishman RA: Cerebrospinal Fluid in Diseases of the Nervous System, 2nd Edition. Philadelphia, PA, WB Saunders, 1992

Fowler C, Miller J, Sharief M, et al: A double blind, randomized study of sildenafil citrate for erectile dysfunction in men with multiple sclerosis. J Neurol Neurosurg Psychiatry 76:700–705, 2005

Fox PA, Hawkins DA, Dawson S: Dementia following an acute presentation of meningovascular neurosyphilis in an HIV-1 positive patient. AIDS 14:2062–2063, 2000

Frohman EM, Goodin DS, Calabresi PA et al: The utility of MRI in suspected MS: report of the Therapeutics and Technology Assessment Subcommittee of the American Academy of Neurology. Neurology 61:602–611, 2003

Fukui T, Kawamura M, Hasegawa Y, et al: Multiple cognitive impairments associated with systemic lupus erythematosus and antiphospholipid antibody syndrome: a form of progressive vascular dementia? Eur Neurol 43:115–116, 2000

Fukutani Y, Noriki Y, Sasaki K, et al: Adult-type metachromatic leukodystrophy with a compound heterozygote mutation showing character change and dementia. Psychiatry Clin Neurosci 53: 425–428, 1999

Gallassi R, Morreale A, Montagna P, et al: Fatal familial insomnia: neuropsychological study of a disease with thalamic degeneration. Cortex 28:175–187, 1992

Geerts Y, Dehaene I, Lammens M: Acute hemorrhagic leucoencephalitis. Acta Neurol Belg 91:201–211, 1991

Gerlach A, Oehm E, Wattchow J, et al: Use of high-dose cortisone in a patient with Marchiafava-Bignami disease. J Neurol 250:758–760, 2003

Geschwind MD, Martindale J, Miller D, et al: Challenging the clinical utility of the 14–3–3 protein for the diagnosis of sporadic Creutzfeldt-Jakob disease. Arch Neurol 60:813–816, 2003

Geschwind MD, Shu H, Hasman A, et al: Clinical update: rapidly progressive dementia. Ann Neurol 64:97–108, 2008

Ghafouri M, Amini S, Khalili K, et al: HIV-1 associated dementia: symptoms and causes. Retrovirology 3:28–38, 2006

Gill JM, Quisel AM, Rocca PV, et al: Diagnosis of systemic lupus erythematosus. Am Fam Physician 68:2179–2186, 2003

Goebels N, Soyka M: Dementia associated with vitamin B12 deficiency. J Neuropsychiatry Clin Neurosci 12:389–394, 2000

Goldman S, Liard A, Flament-Durand J, et al: Positron emission tomography and histopathology in Creutzfeldt-Jakob disease. Neurology 43:1828–1830, 1993

Goodall CA, Head MW, Everington D, et al: Raised CSF phospho-tau concentrations in variant Creutzfeldt-Jakob disease: diagnostic and pathological implications. J Neurol Neurosurg Psychiatry 77:89–91, 2006

Goodin DS, Frohman EM, Garmany GP, et al: Disease modifying therapies in multiple sclerosis: Subcommittee of the American Academy of Neurology and the MS Council for Clinical Practice Guidelines. Neurology 58:169–178, 2002

Goodin DS, Arnason BG, Coyle PK, et al: The use of mitoxantrone (Novantrone) for the treatment of multiple sclerosis: report of the Therapeutics and Technology Assessment Subcommittee of the American Academy of Neurology. Neurology 61:1332–1338, 2003

Goodin DS, Frohman EM, Hurwitz B, et al: Neutralizing antibodies to interferon beta: assessment of their clinical and radiographic impact: an evidence report: report of the Therapeutics and Technology Assessment Subcommittee of the American Academy of Neurology. Neurology 68:977–984, 2007

Goodin DS, Cohen BA, O'Conner P, et al: The use of natalizumab (Tysabri) for the treatment of multiple sclerosis (an evidence-based review): report of the Therapeutics and Technology Assessment Subcommittee of the American Academy of Neurology. Neurology 71:766–773, 2008

Grafman J, Rao SM, Litvan I: Disorders of memory, in Neurobehavioral Aspects of Multiple Sclerosis. Edited by Rao SM. New York, Oxford University Press, 1990, pp 102–117

Graus F, Salz A, Lai M, et al: Neuronal surface antigen antibodies in limbic encephalitis. Neurology 71:930–936, 2008

Green AJ, Thompson EJ, Stewart GE, et al: Use of 14–3–3 and other brain-specific proteins in CSF in the diagnosis of variant Creutzfeldt-Jakob disease. J Neurol Neurosurg Psychiatry 70: 744–748, 2001

Greenberg BM: The neurologic manifestations of systemic lupus erythematosus. Neurologist 15:115–121, 2009

Greenwood BM: Corticosteroids for acute bacterial meningitis. N Engl J Med 357:2507–2509, 2007

Gronseth GS, Ashman EJ: Practice parameter: the usefulness of evoked potentials in identifying silent lesions in patients with suspected multiple sclerosis (an evidence-based review): report of the Quality Standards Subcommittee of the American Academy of Neurology. Neurology 54:1720–1725, 2000

Guharoy R, Gilroy SA, Noviasky JA, et al: West Nile virus infection. Am J Health Syst Pharm 61:1235–1241, 2004

Guyant-Maréchal L, Verrips A, Girard C, et al: Unusual cerebrotendinous xanthomatosis with fronto-temporal dementia phenotype. Am J Med Genet A 139A:114–117, 2005

Hageman AT, Gabreels FJ, de Jong JG, et al: Clinical symptoms of adult metachromatic leukodystrophy and arylsulphatase pseudodeficiency. Arch Neurol 52:408–413, 1995

Hall JK, Balcer LJ: Giant cell arteritis. Curr Treat Options Neurol 6:45–53, 2004

Hall WA, Kim P, Truwit CL: Functional magnetic resonance imaging-guided brain tumor resection. Top Magn Reson Imaging 19:205–212, 2009

Halperin JJ: Nervous system Lyme disease. Infect Dis Clin North Am 22:261–274, 2008

Harboe E, Tjensvoll AB, Maroni S, et al: Neuropsychiatric syndromes in patients with systemic lupus erythematosus and primary Sjögren syndrome: a comparative population-based study. Ann Rheum Dis 68:1541–1546, 2009

Harder A, Gregor A, Wirth T, et al: Early age of onset in fatal familial insomnia: two novel cases and review of the literature. J Neurol 251:715–724, 2004

Hauser SL, Waubant E, Arnold DL, et al; HERMES Trial Group: B-cell depletion with rituximab in relapsing-remitting multiple sclerosis. N Engl J Med 358:676–688, 2008

Heinrich A, Runge U, Khaw AV: Clinicoradiologic subtypes of Marchiafava-Bignami disease. J Neurol 251:1050–1059, 2004

Henry JD, Beatty WW: Verbal fluency deficits in multiple sclerosis. Neuropsychologia 44:1166–1174, 2006

Hestad K, McArthur JH, Dal Pan GJ, et al: Regional brain atrophy in HIV-1 infection: association with specific neuropsychological test performance. Acta Neurol Scand 88:112–118, 1993

Hirohata S, Suda H, Hashimoto T: Low-dose weekly methotrexate for progressive neuropsychiatric manifestations in Behçet's disease. J Neurological Sci 159:181–185, 1998

Hocaoglu C, Tan M: Isolated angiitis of the central nervous system: a case presented with atypical psychiatric symptoms. Prog Neuropsychopharmacol Biol Psychiatry 29:627–631, 2005

Hoffer ZS, Allen SL, Mathews M: Treatment of psychiatric symptoms associated with a frontal lobe tumor through surgical resection. Am J Psychiatry 164:877–882, 2007

Hoffman O, Weber JR: Review: pathophysiology and treatment of bacterial meningitis. Ther Adv Neurol Disord 2:401–412, 2009

Hoffmann LA, Jarius S, Pellkofer HL, et al: Anti-Ma and anti-Ta associated paraneoplastic neurological syndromes: 22 newly diagnosed patients and review of previous cases. J Neurol Neurosurg Psychiatry 79:767–773, 2008

Hokezu Y, Kuriyama M, Kubota R, et al: Cerebrotendinous xanthomatosis: cranial CT and MRI studies in eight patients. Neuroradiology 34:308–312, 1992

Hokkanen L, Launes J: Cognitive recovery instead of decline after acute encephalitis: a prospective follow up study. J Neurol Neurosurg Psychiatry 63:222–227, 1997

Hollingworth W, Medina LS, Lenkinski RE, et al: A systemic literature review of magnetic resonance spectroscopy for the characterization of brain tumors. AJNR Am J Neuroradiol 27:1404–1411, 2006

Hooge JP, Redekop WK: Multiple sclerosis with very late onset. Neurology 42:1907–1910, 1992

Hoogman M, van de Beek D, Weisfelt M, et al: Cognitive outcome in adults after bacterial meningitis. J Neurol Neurosurg Psychiatry 78:1092–1096, 2007

Hook CC, Kimmel DW, Kvols LK, et al: Multifocal inflammatory leukoencephalopathy with 5-fluorouracil and levamisole. Ann Neurol 31:262–267, 1992

Hook EW III, Marra CM: Acquired syphilis in adults. N Engl J Med 326:1060–1069, 1992

Hsich G, Kenney K, Gibbs CJ, et al: The 14–3–3 brain protein in cerebrospinal fluid as a marker for transmissible spongiform encephalopathies. N Engl J Med 335:924–930, 1996

Huber SJ, Bornstein RA, Rammohan KW, et al: Magnetic resonance imaging correlates of executive function impairments in multiple sclerosis. Neuropsychiatry Neuropsychol Behav Neurol 5:33–36, 1992

Hui ACF, Cheng C, Lam A, et al: Prognosis following postanoxic myoclonus status epilepticus. Eur Neurol 54:10–13, 2005

Hustinx R, Pourdehnad M, Kaschten B, et al: PET imaging for differentiating recurrent brain tumor from radiation necrosis. Radiol Clin North Am 43:35–47, 2005

Hyde TM, Ziegler JC, Weinberger DR: Psychiatric disturbances in metachromatic leukodystrophy: insights into the neurobiology of psychosis. Arch Neurol 49:401–406, 1992

Interferon beta-1b in the treatment of multiple sclerosis: final outcome of the randomized controlled trial. IFNB Multiple Sclerosis Study Group and University of British Columbia MS/MRI Analysis Group. Neurology 45:1277–1285, 1995

Ironside JW: Pathology of variant Creutzfeldt-Jakob disease. Arch Virol Suppl 16:143–151, 2000

Ishiura H, Morikawa M, Hamada M, et al: Lymphomatoid granulomatosis involving central nervous system successfully treated with rituximab alone. Arch Neurol 65:662–665, 2008

Jacobs LD, Cookfair DL, Rudick RA, et al: Intramuscular interferon beta-1a for disease progression in relapsing multiple sclerosis. Ann Neurol 39:285–294, 1996

Janssen RS, Saykin AJ, Kaplan JE, et al: Neurological complication of human immunodeficiency virus infection in patients with lymphadenopathy syndrome. Ann Neurol 23:49–55, 1988

Janssen RS, Nwanyanwu OC, Selik RM, et al: Epidemiology of human immunodeficiency virus encephalopathy in the United States. Neurology 42:1472–1476, 1992

Jefferies K: The neuropsychiatry of multiple sclerosis. Adv Psychiatr Treat 12:214–220, 2006

Jellinger KA: The enigma of vascular cognitive disorder and vascular dementia. Acta Neuropathol 113:349–388, 2007

Joffe AR: Lumbar puncture and brain herniation in acute bacterial meningitis: a review. J Intensive Care Med 22:194–207, 2007

Joffe RT, Lippert GP, Gray TA, et al: Mood disorder and multiple sclerosis. Arch Neurol 44:376–378, 1987

Johnson BE, Becker B, Goff WB II, et al: Neurologic, neuropsychologic and computed cranial tomography scan abnormalities in 2- to 10-year survivors of small-cell lung cancer. J Clin Oncol 3: 1659–1667, 1985

Johnson H, Bouman W, Pinner G: Psychiatric aspects of temporal arteritis: a case report and review of the literature. J Geriatr Psychiatry Neurol 10:142–145, 1997

Johnson KP, Brooks BR, Cohen JA, et al: Copolymer 1 reduces relapse rate and improves disability in relapsing-remitting multiple sclerosis: results of a phase III multicenter, double-blind, placebo-controlled trial. Neurology 45:1268–1276, 1995

Jones GA, Nathwani D: Cryptococcal meningitis. Br J Hosp Med 54:439–445, 1995

Joseph FG, Lammie GA, Scolding NJ: CNS lupus: a study of 41 patients. Neurology 69:644–654, 2007

Julian LJ, Mohr DC: Cognitive predictors of response to treatment for depression in multiple sclerosis. J Neuropsychiatry Clin Neurosci 18:356–363, 2006

Kahn JO, Walker BD: Acute human immunodeficiency virus type 1 infection. N Engl J Med 339:33–39, 1998

Kapur N, Barker S, Burrows EH, et al: Herpes simplex encephalitis: long term magnetic resonance imaging and neuropsychological profile. J Neurol Neurosurg Psychiatry 57:1334–1342, 1994

Karassa FB, Afeltra A, Ambrozic A, et al: Accuracy of anti-ribosomal P protein antibody testing for the diagnosis of neuropsychiatric systemic lupus erythematosus: an international meta-analysis. Arthritis Rheum 54:312–324, 2006

Karnaze DS, Carmel R: Neurologic and evoked potential abnormalities in subtle cobalamin deficiency states, including deficiency without anemia and with normal absorption of free cobalamin. Arch Neurol 47:1008–1012, 1990

Kastrup O, Wanke I, Maschke M: Neuroimaging of infections. NeuroRx 2:324–332, 2005

Kesselring J, Miller DH, Robb SA, et al: Acute disseminated encephalomyelitis: MRI findings and the distinction from multiple sclerosis. Brain 113:291–302, 1990

Khoury JA, Hoxworth JM, Mazlumzadeh M, et al: The clinical utility of high resolution magnetic resonance imaging in the diagnosis of giant cell arteritis: a critically appraised topic. Neurologist 14:330–335, 2008

Kieburtz K, Schiffer RB: Neurologic manifestations of human immunodeficiency virus infections. Neurol Clin 7:447–468, 1989

Kitchin W, Cohen-Cole SA, Mickel SF: Adrenoleukodystrophy: frequency of presentation as a psychiatric disorder. Biol Psychiatry 22:1375–1387, 1987

Kleihues P, Burger PC, Scheithauer BW: The new WHO classification of brain tumours. Brain Pathology 3:255–268, 1993

Kleinschmidt-DeMasters BK, Lillehei KO, Breeze RE: Neoplasms involving the central nervous system in the older old. Hum Pathol 34:1137–1147, 2003

Knopman DS, DeKosky ST, Cummings JL, et al: Practice parameter: diagnosis of dementia (an evidence-based review): report of the Quality Standards Subcommittee of the American Academy of Neurology. Neurology 56:1143–1153, 2001

Koçer N, Islak C, Siva A, et al: CNS involvement in neuro-Behçet syndrome: an MR study. Am J Neuroradiol 20:1015–1024, 1999

Kohler CG, Ances BM, Coleman AR, et al: Marchiafava-Bignami disease: literature review and case report. Neuropsychiatry Neuropsychol Behav Neurol 13:67–76, 2000

Kotter I, Gunaydin I, Zierhut M, et al: The use of interferon alpha in Behçet's disease: review of the literature. Semin Arthritis Rheum 33:320–325, 2004

Krupp LB, Alvarez LA, LaRocca NG, et al: Fatigue in multiple sclerosis. Arch Neurol 45:435–437, 1988

Krupp LB, Christodoulou C, Melville P, et al: Donepezil improved memory in multiple sclerosis in a randomized clinical trial. Neurology 63:1579–1585, 2004

Kumperscak HG, Paschke E, Gradisnik P, et al: Adult metachromatic leukodystrophy: disorganized schizophrenia-like symptoms and postpartum depression in two sisters. J Psychiatry Neurosci 30:33–36, 2005

Kurokawa MS, Susuki N: Behçet's disease. Clin Exp Med 3:10–20, 2003

Kurtzke JF, Kurland LT: The epidemiology of neurologic disease, in Clinical Neurology, Vol IV. Edited by Baker AB, Joynt RJ. New York, Harper & Row, 1983, pp 1–143

Lang CJ, Schuler P, Engelhardt A, et al: Probable Creutzfeldt-Jakob disease after a cadaveric dural graft. Eur J Epidemiol 11:79–81, 1995

Lantz MS: Pathologic laughing and crying in multiple sclerosis. Clin Geriatr 13:14–17, 2005

Lawrence DM, Major EO: HIV-1 and the brain: connections between HIV-1-associated dementia, neuropathology and neuroimmunology. Microbes Infect 4:301–308, 2002

Lee EJ, Lee SK, Agid R, et al: Preoperative grading of presumptive low-grade astrocytomas on MR imaging: diagnostic value of minimum apparent diffusion coefficient. AJNR Am J Neuroradiol 29:1872–1877, 2008

Lee HB, Lyketsos CG: Delayed post-hypoxic leukoencephalopathy. Psychosomatics 42:530–533, 2001

Lee S, Jeon H, Yoo W: Reversible dementia in systemic lupus erythematosus without antiphospholipid antibodies or cerebral infarction. Rheumatol Int 24:305–308, 2004

Lee YY, Nauert C, Glass JP: Treatment-related white matter changes in cancer patients. Cancer 57:1473–1482, 1986

Lin CH, Jeng JS, Yip PK: Plasmapheresis in acute disseminated encephalomyelitis. J Clin Apher 19:154–159, 2004

Lindenbaum J, Healton EB, Savage DG, et al: Neuropsychiatric disorders caused by cobalamin deficiency in the absence of anemia or macrocytosis. N Engl J Med 318:1720–1728, 1988

Llewelyn CA, Hewitt PE, Knight RSG, et al: Possible transmission of variant Creutzfeldt-Jakob disease by blood transfusion. Lancet 363:417–421, 2004

Lublin FD, Whitaker JN, Eidelman BH, et al: Management of patients receiving interferon beta-1b for multiple sclerosis: report of a consensus conference. Neurology 46:12–18, 1996

Lucantoni C, De Bonis P, Doglietto F, et al: Primary cerebral lymphomatoid granulomatosis: report of four cases and literature review. J Neurooncol 94:235–242, 2009

Mackenzie C, Green J: Cognitive-linguistic deficit and speech intelligibility in chronic progressive multiple sclerosis. Int J Lang Commun Disord 44:401–420, 2009

Mahler ME: Behavioral manifestations associated with multiple sclerosis. Psychiatr Clin North Am 15:427–438, 1992

Mamelak AN, Mampalam TJ, Obana WG, et al: Improved management of multiple brain abscesses: a combined surgical and medical approach. Neurosurgery 36:76–85, 1995

Martin DC: B12 and folate deficiency dementia. Clin Geriatr Med 4:841–852, 1988

Masliah E, Achim CL, Ge N, et al: Spectrum of human immunodeficiency virus-associated neocortical damage. Ann Neurol 32:321–329, 1992

McCarty DJ, Manzi S, Medsger TA Jr, et al: Incidence of systemic lupus erythematosus: race and gender differences. Arthritis Rheum 38:1260–1270, 1995

McPherson SE, Cummings JL: Neuropsychological aspects of vascular dementia. Brain Cogn 31:269–282, 1996

Mendell JR, Beversdorf DQ, Scharre DW: Inherited neurological disorders: relevant considerations and new aspects, in Clinical Neurology, Vol 4. Edited by Joynt RJ, Griggs RC. Philadelphia, PA, Lippincott-Raven, 2000, pp 1–48

Mendez MF: The neuropsychiatry of multiple sclerosis. Int J Psychiatry Med 25:123–130, 1995

Mendez OE, Shang J, Jungreis CA, et al: Diffusion-weighted MRI in Creutzfeldt-Jakob disease: a better diagnostic marker than CSF protein 14–3–3? J Neuroimaging 13:147–151, 2003

Mendozzi L, Pugnetti L, Saccani M, et al: Frontal lobe dysfunction in multiple sclerosis as assessed by means of Lurian tasks: effect of age at onset. J Neurol Sci 115(suppl):S42–S50, 1993

Merriam AE, Hegarty AM, Miller A: The mental disabilities of metachromatic leukodystrophy: implications concerning the differentiation of cortical, subcortical gray, and white matter dementias. Neuropsychiatry Neuropsychol Behav Neurol 3:217–225, 1990

Millefiorini E, Gasperini C, Pozzilli C, et al: Randomized placebo-controlled trial of mitoxantrone in relapsing-remitting multiple sclerosis: 24-month clinical and MRI outcome. J Neurol 244: 153–159, 1997

Miller DH, Khan OA, Sheremata WA, et al: A controlled trial of natalizumab for relapsing multiple sclerosis. N Engl J Med 348:15–23, 2003

Minden SL, Schiffer RB: Affective disorders in multiple sclerosis: review and recommendations for clinical research. Arch Neurol 47:98–104, 1990

Minden SL, Orav J, Reich P: Depression in multiple sclerosis. Gen Hosp Psychiatry 9:426–434, 1987

Mitsonis Ch, Kararizou E, Dimopoulos N, et al: Incidence and clinical presentation of neurosyphilis: a retrospective study of 81 cases. Int J Neurosci 118:1251–1257, 2008

Miyakis S, Lockshin MD, Atsumi T, et al: International consensus statement on an update of the classification criteria for definite antiphospholipid syndrome (APS). J Thromb Haemost 4:295–306, 2006

Modha A, Shepard SR, Gutin PH: Surgery of brain metastases: is there still a place for it? J Neurooncol 75:21–29, 2005

Mohr DC, Goodkin DE, Likosky W, et al: Treatment of depression improves adherence to interferon beta-1b therapy for multiple sclerosis. Arch Neurol 54:531–533, 1997

Moore PM, Calabrese LH: Neurologic manifestations of systemic vasculitides. Semin Neurol 14:300–306, 1994

Morshed MG, Lee MK, Maguire J, et al: Neurosyphilitic gumma in a homosexual man with HIV infection confirmed by polymerase chain reaction. Int J STD AIDS 19:568–569, 2008

Moser HW: Adrenoleukodystrophy: phenotype, genetics, pathogenesis and therapy. Brain 120:1485–1508, 1997

Muller M, Merkelbach S, Huss GP, et al: Clinical relevance and frequency of transient stenoses of the middle and anterior cerebral arteries in bacterial meningitis. Stroke 26:1399–1403, 1995

Murray TJ: Amantadine therapy for fatigue in multiple sclerosis. Can J Neurol Sci 12:251–254, 1985

Muzino T, Takanashi Y, Onodera H, et al: A case of lymphomatoid granulomatosis/angiocentric immunoproliferative lesion with a long clinical course and diffuse brain involvement. J Neurol Sci 213:67–76, 2003

Naidu S, Moser HW: Peroxisomal disorders. Neurol Clin 8:507–519, 1990

Nance PW, Sheremata WA, Lynch SG, et al: Relationship of the antispasticity effect of tizanidine to plasma concentration in patients with multiple sclerosis. Arch Neurol 54:731–736, 1997

Neilley LK, Goodin DS, Goodkin DE, et al: Side effect profile of interferon beta 1-b (Betaseron). Neurology 46:552–554, 1996

Nesher G, Berkun Y, Mates M, et al: Low-dose aspirin and prevention of cranial ischemic complications in giant cell arteritis. Arthritis Rheum 50:1332–1337, 2004

Newman NJ, Bell IR, McKee AC: Paraneoplastic limbic encephalitis: neuropsychiatric presentation. Biol Psychiatry 27:529–542, 1990

Nishino H, Rubino FA, DeRemee RA, et al: Neurological involvement in Wegener's granulomatosis: an analysis of 324 consecutive patients at the Mayo Clinic. Ann Neurol 33:4–9, 1993

Noseworthy J, Paty D, Wonnacott T, et al: Multiple sclerosis after age 50. Neurology 33:1537–1544, 1983

Noy A: Update in HIV lymphoma. Curr Opin Oncol 18:449–455, 2006

O'Conner PW, Goodman A, Willmer-Hulme AJ, et al: Randomized multicenter trial of natalizumab in acute MS relapses: clinical and MRI effects. Neurology 62:2038–2043, 2004

Offiah CE, Turnbull IW: The imaging appearances of intracranial CNS infections in adult HIV and AIDS patients. Clin Radiol 61:393–401, 2006

Ojeda VJ: Necrotizing leucoencephalopathy associated with intrathecal/intraventricular methotrexate therapy. Med J Aust 2:289–293, 1982

Pandori MW, Lei J, Wong EH, et al: Real-time PCR for detection of herpes simplex virus without nucleic acid extraction. BMC Infect Dis 6:104, 2006

Panegyres PK, Toufexis K, Kakulas BA, et al: A new PRNP mutation (G131V) associated with Gerstmann-Sträussler-Scheinker disease. Arch Neurol 58:1899–1902, 2001

Panitch H, Goodin DS, Francis G, et al: Randomized, comparative study of interferon beta-1a treatment regimens in MS: the EVIDENCE trial. Neurology 59:1496–1506, 2002

Pantaleo G, Graziosi C, Fauci AS: The immunopathogenesis of human immunodeficiency virus infection. N Engl J Med 328:327–335, 1993

Paraskevas GP, Kapaki E, Kararizou E, et al: Cerebrospinal fluid tau protein is increased in neurosyphilis: a discrimination from syphilis without nervous system involvement? Sex Transm Dis 34:220–223, 2007

Parry AMM, Scott RB, Palace J, et al: Potentially adaptive functional changes in cognitive processing for patients with multiple sclerosis and their acute modulation by rivastigmine. Brain 126: 2750–2760, 2003

Paschoal RC, Hirata MH, Hirata RC, et al: Neurocryptococcosis: diagnosis by PCR method. Rev Inst Med Trop Sao Paulo 46:203–207, 2004

Patsalides AD, Atac G, Hedge U, et al: Lymphomatoid granulomatosis: abnormalities of the brain at MR imaging. Radiology 237: 265–273, 2005

Patten SB, Beck CA, Williams JVA, et al: Major depression in multiple sclerosis: a population-based perspective. Neurology 61: 1524–1527, 2003

Peterson PL, Howe FA, Clark CA, et al: Quantitative magnetic resonance imaging in neuropsychiatric systemic lupus erythematosus. Lupus 12:897–902, 2003

Pettigrew HD, Teuber SS, Gershwin ME: Polyarteritis nodosa. Compr Ther 33:144–149, 2007

Piras MR, Magnano I, Canu ED, et al: Longitudinal study of cognitive dysfunction in multiple sclerosis: neuropsychological, neuroradiological, and neurophysiological findings. J Neurol Neurosurg Psychiatry 74:878–885, 2003

Poser S, Mollenhauer B, Kraubeta A, et al: How to improve the clinical diagnosis of Creutzfeldt-Jakob disease. Brain 122:2345–2351, 1999

Posner JB: Paraneoplastic syndromes affecting the central nervous system. Annu Rev Med 48:157–166, 1997

Power C, Johnson RT: HIV-1 associated dementia: clinical features and pathogenesis. Can J Neurol Sci 22:92–100, 1995

Price RW, Sidtis JJ, Navia BA, et al: The AIDS dementia complex, in AIDS and the Nervous System. Edited by Rosenblum ML, Levy RM, Bredesen DE. New York, Raven, 1988, pp 203–219

Price TR, Goetz KL, Lovell MR: Neuropsychiatric aspects of brain tumors, in The American Psychiatric Publishing Textbook of Neuropsychiatry and Behavioral Neurosciences, 5th Edition. Edited by Yudofsky SC, Hales, RE. Washington, DC, American Psychiatric Publishing, 2008, pp 735–764

Provenzale JM, Allen NB: Neuroradiologic findings in polyarteritis nodosa. Am J Neuroradiol 17:1119–1126, 1996

Prusiner SB: Human prion diseases and neurodegeneration. Curr Top Microbiol Immunol 207:1–17, 1996

Prusiner SB, Hsiao KK: Human prion diseases. Ann Neurol 35:385–395, 1994

Rabins PV: Euphoria in multiple sclerosis, in Neurobehavioral Aspects of Multiple Sclerosis. Edited by Rao SM. New York, Oxford University Press, 1990, pp 180–185

Rajneesh K, Binder D: Tumor-associated epilepsy. Neurosurg Focus 27:E4–E4, 2009

Rammohan KW, Rosenberg JH, Lynn DJ, et al: Efficacy and safety of modafinil (Provigil) for the treatment of fatigue in multiple sclerosis: a two centre phase 2 study. J Neurol Neurosurg Psychiatry 72:179–183, 2002

Rao SM: Neuropsychology of multiple sclerosis: a critical review. J Clin Exp Neuropsychol 8:503–542, 1986

Rao SM: White matter disease and dementia. Brain Cogn 31:250–268, 1996

Rappaport EB: Iatrogenic Creutzfeldt-Jakob disease. Neurology 37:1520–1522, 1987

Reiche W, Hagen T, Schuchardt V, et al: Diffusion-weighted MR imaging improves diagnosis of CNS lymphomas: a report of four cases with common and uncommon imaging features. Clin Neurol Neurosurg 109:92–101, 2007

Reichlin M: Ribosomal P antibodies and CNS lupus. Lupus 12:916–918, 2003

Reina S, Sterin-Borda L, Orman B, et al: Autoantibodies against cerebral muscarinic cholinoceptors in Sjögren syndrome: functional and pathological implications. J Neuroimmunol 150:107–115, 2004

Reiss JP, Sam D, Sareen J: Psychosis in multiple sclerosis associated with left temporal lobe lesions on serial MRI scans. J Clin Neurosci 13:282–284, 2006

Ron MA, Logsdail SJ: Psychiatric morbidity in multiple sclerosis: a clinical and MRI study. Psychol Med 19:887–895, 1989

Roos KL: West Nile encephalitis and myelitis. Curr Opin Neurol 17:343–346, 2004

Rosebush PI, Garside S, Levinson AJ, et al: The neuropsychiatry of adult-onset adrenoleukodystrophy. J Neuropsychiatry Clin Neurosci 11:315–327, 1999

Rupprecht TA, Pfister HW: What are the indications for lumbar puncture in patients with Lyme disease? Curr Probl Dermatol 37:200–206, 2009

Saag MS, Graybill RJ, Larsen RA, et al: Practice guidelines for the management of cryptococcal disease. Infectious Diseases Society of America. Clin Infect Dis 30:710–718, 2000

St. Louis ME, Wasserheit JN: Elimination of syphilis in the United States. Science 281:353–354, 1998

Sakai M, Inoue Y, Aoki S, et al: Follow-up magnetic resonance imaging findings in patients with progressive multifocal leukoencephalopathy: evaluation of long-term survivors under highly active antiretroviral therapy. Jpn J Radiol 27:69–77, 2009

Salvarani C, Cantini F, Hunder GG: Polymyalgia rheumatica and giant-cell arteritis. Lancet 372:234–245, 2008

Sampathkumar P: West Nile virus: epidemiology, clinical presentation, diagnosis, and prevention. Mayo Clin Proc 78:1137–1144, 2003

Sanchez FM, Zisselman MH: Treatment of psychiatric symptoms associated with neurosyphilis. Psychosomatics 48:440–445, 2007

Sanna G, Bertolaccini ML, Cuadrado MJ, et al: Neuropsychiatric manifestations in systemic lupus erythematosus: prevalence and association with antiphospholipid antibodies. J Rheumatol 30:985–992, 2003a

Sanna G, Bertolaccini ML, Mathieu A: Central nervous system lupus: a clinical approach to therapy. Lupus 12:935–942, 2003b

Scheck DN, Hook EW III: Neurosyphilis. Infect Dis Clin North Am 8:769–795, 1994

Schiffer RB, Caine ED: The interaction between depressive affective disorder and neuropsychological test performance in multiple sclerosis patients. J Neuropsychiatry Clin Neurosci 3:28–32, 1991

Schiffer RB, Weitkamp LR, Wineman NM, et al: Multiple sclerosis and affective disorder: family history, sex, and HLA-DR antigens. Arch Neurol 45:1345–1348, 1988

Schmidt H, Heimann B, Djukic M, et al: Neuropsychological sequelae of bacterial and viral meningitis. Brain 129:333–345, 2006

Schmutzhard E: Viral infections of the CNS with special emphasis on herpes simplex infections. J Neurol 248:469–477, 2001

Seales D, Greer M: Acute hemorrhagic leukoencephalitis: a successful recovery. Arch Neurol 48:1086–1088, 1991

Silberfarb PM: Chemotherapy and cognitive deficits in cancer patients. Ann Rev Med 34:35–46, 1983

Simon RP: Neurosyphilis. Arch Neurol 42:606–613, 1985

Siva A, Altintas A, Saip S: Behçet's syndrome and the nervous system. Curr Opin Neurol 17:347–357, 2004

Skiest DJ, Crosby C: Survival is prolonged by highly active antiretroviral therapy in AIDS patients with primary central nervous system lymphoma. AIDS 17:1787–1793, 2003

So NK, O'Neill BP, Frytak S, et al: Delayed leukoencephalopathy in survivors with small cell lung cancer. Neurology 37:1198–1201, 1987

Soffietti R, Rudá R, Trevisan E: Brain metastases: current management and new developments. Curr Opin Oncol 20:676–684, 2008

Spencer MD, Knight RSG, Will RG: First hundred cases of variant Creutzfeldt-Jakob disease retrospective case note review of early psychiatric and neurological features. Br J Med 324:1479–1482, 2002

Spudich SS, Nilsson AC, Lollo ND, et al: Cerebrospinal fluid HIV infection and pleocytosis: relation to systemic infection and antiretroviral treatment. BMC Infect Dis 5:98–116, 2005

Stagno SJ, Naugle RI, Roca C, et al: Progressive multifocal leukoencephalopathy appearing as language disturbance. Neuropsychiatry Neuropsychol Behav Neurol 3:283–289, 1990

Stankoff B, Waubant E, Confavreux C, et al; French Modafinil Study Group: Modafinil for fatigue in MS: a randomized placebo-controlled double-blind study. Neurology 64:1139–1143, 2005

Stanton BR, Barnes F, Silber E: Sleep and fatigue in multiple sclerosis. Mult Scler 12:481–486, 2006

Stenager E, Stenager EN, Jensen K: Sexual aspects of multiple sclerosis. Semin Neurol 12:120–124, 1992

Straussberg R, Schonfeld T, Weitz R, et al: Improvement of atypical acute disseminated encephalomyelitis with steroids and intravenous immunoglobulins. Pediatr Neurol 24:139–143, 2001

Swain R: An update of vitamin B12 metabolism and deficiency states. J Fam Prac 41:595–600, 1995

Tan EM, Cohen AS, Fries JF, et al: The 1982 revised criteria for the classification of systemic lupus erythematosus. Arthritis Rheum 25:1271–1277, 1982

Tan K, Roda R, Ostrow L, et al: PML-IRIS in patients with HIV infection: clinical manifestations and treatment with steroids. Neurology 72:1458–1464, 2009

Tenembaum S, Chitnis T, Ness J, et al: Acute disseminated encephalomyelitis. Neurology 68 (suppl 2):S23–S36, 2007

Thatayatikom A, White AJ: Rituximab: a promising therapy in systemic lupus erythematosus. Autoimmun Rev 5:18–24, 2006

Thornton AE, Raz N, Tucke KA: Memory in multiple sclerosis: contextual encoding deficits. J Int Neuropsychol Soc 8:395–409, 2002

Tsuchiya K, Aoki C, Katase S, et al: MR digital subtraction angiography with three-dimensional data acquisition in the diagnosis of brain tumors: preliminary experience. Magn Reson Imaging 22:149–153, 2004

Tummala RP, Chu RM, Liu H, et al: Application of diffusion tensor imaging to magnetic-resonance-guided brain tumor resection. Pediatr Neurosurg 39:39–43, 2003

Tunkel AR, Glaser CA, Bloch KC, et al: The management of encephalitis: clinical practice guidelines by the Infectious Diseases Society of America. Clin Infect Dis 47:303–327, 2008

Tyler JL, Byrne TN: Neoplastic disorders, in Clinical Brain Imaging: Principles and Applications. Edited by Mazziotta JC, Gilman S. Philadelphia, PA, FA Davis, 1992, pp 166–216

Valdez-Ferrer SI, Vega F, Cantu-Brito C, et al: Cerebral changes in SLE with or without antiphospholipid syndrome: a case-control MRI study. J Neuroimaging 18:62–65, 2008

van de Beek D, de Gans J, Tunkel AR, et al: Community-acquired bacterial meningitis in adults. N Engl J Med 354:44–53, 2006

van Goor L, Woiski MD, Lagaay AM, et al: Review: cobalamin deficiency and mental impairment in elderly people. Age Aging 24:536–542, 1995

Vollmer TL, Guarnaccia J, Harrington W, et al: Idiopathic granulomatous angiitis of the central nervous system. Arch Neurol 50: 925–930, 1993

Walker RW, Rosenblum MK: Amphotericin B-associated leukoencephalopathy. Neurology 42:2005–2010, 1992

Wallin MT, Wilken JA, Kane R: Cognitive dysfunction in multiple sclerosis: assessment, imaging, and risk factors. J Rehabil Res Dev 43:63–72, 2006

Waniek C, Prohovnik I, Kaufman MA, et al: Rapidly progressive frontal-type dementia associated with Lyme disease. J Neuropsychiatry Clin Neurosci 7:345–347, 1995

Ward MM: Prevalence of physician-diagnosed systemic Lupus erythematosus in the United States: results from the Third National Health and Nutrition Examination Survey. J Womens Health 13:713–718, 2004

Watanabe N, Seto H, Shimizu M, et al: Brain SPECT of Creutzfeldt-Jakob disease. Clin Nucl Med 21:236–241, 1996

Weiner S, Otte A, Schumacher M, et al: Diagnosis and monitoring of central nervous system involvement in systemic lupus erythematosus: value of F-18 fluorodeoxyglucose PET. Ann Rheum Dis 59:377–385, 2000

Weinshenker BG, Penman M, Bass B, et al: A double-blind, randomized, crossover trial of pemoline in fatigue associated with multiple sclerosis. Neurology 42:1468–1471, 1992

Weller M, Liedtke W, Petersen D, et al: Very-late-onset adrenoleukodystrophy: possible precipitation of demyelination by cerebral contusion. Neurology 42:367–370, 1992

Wen PY, Schiff D, Kesari S, et al: Medical management of patients with brain tumors. J Neurooncol 80:313–332, 2006

West SG, Emlen W, Wener MH, et al: Neuropsychiatric lupus erythematosus: a 10-year prospective study on the value of diagnostic tests. Am J Med 99:153–163, 1995

Whiteman MLH, Post MJD, Berger JR, et al: Progressive multifocal leukoencephalopathy in 47 HIV-seropositive patients: neuroimaging with clinical and pathologic correlation. Radiology 187: 233–240, 1993

Whitley RJ: Herpes simplex virus infections of the central nervous system: encephalitis and neonatal herpes. Drugs 42:406–427, 1991

Will RG, Ironside JW, Zeidler M, et al: A new variant of Creutzfeldt-Jakob disease in the UK. Lancet 347:921–925, 1996

Wishart H, Sharpe D: Neuropsychological aspects of multiple sclerosis: a quantitative review. J Clin Exp Neuropsychol 19:810–824, 1997

Wispelwey B, Scheld WM: Brain abscess. Semin Neurol 12:273–278, 1992

Wong T, van der Westhuizen G, Coleman R: Positron emission tomography imaging of brain tumors. Neuroimaging Clin N Am 12:615–626, 2002

Yamamori C, Ishino H, Inagaki T, et al: Neuro-Behçet disease with demyelination and gliosis of the frontal white matter. Clin Neuropathol 13:208–215, 1994

Yang CC, Severson B, Bowen JD: Hypersexual sensations and behavior in a multiple sclerosis exacerbation: a case report. Int J Impot Res 16:382–384, 2004

Younger DS, Hays AP, Brust JCM, et al: Granulomatous angiitis of the brain: an inflammatory reaction of diverse etiology. Arch Neurol 45:514–518, 1988

Yousry TA, Major EO, Ryschkewitsch C, et al: Evaluation of patients treated with natalizumab for progressive multifocal leukoencephalopathy. N Engl J Med 354:924–933, 2006

Zeller J, Zunker P, Witt K, et al: Unusual presentation of carcinomatous meningitis: case report and review of typical CSF findings. Neurol Res 24:652–654, 2002

Zhang X, Shu H, Zhang F, et al: Cell-ELISA detection of antineuronal antibodies in central nervous system involvement in systemic lupus erythematosus. Ann Rheum Dis 66:530–532, 2007

Zifko U, Wimberger D, Lindner K, et al: MRI in patients with general paresis. Neuroradiology 38:120–123, 1996

Zoons E, Weisfelt M, de Gans J, et al: Seizures in adults with bacterial meningitis. Neurology 70:2109–2115, 2008

Zunt JR, Tu RK, Anderson DM, et al: Progressive multifocal leukoencephalopathy presenting as human immunodeficiency virus type 1 (HIV)-associated dementia. Neurology 49:263–265, 1997

29

Neuropsychiatric Disorders Associated With General Medical Therapies

M. Justin Coffey, M.D.
Stacey Gramann, D.O., M.P.H.

This chapter is designed to guide clinicians through two common scenarios. In the first scenario, the clinician is evaluating a patient with an identified disturbance in mood (or cognition or motor behavior) and wonders whether that disturbance could be a result of a treatment the patient is currently receiving for heart disease, arthritis, cancer, or some other general medical condition. In the second scenario, the clinician is (considering) prescribing some therapy for a patient's heart disease, arthritis, cancer, or some other general medical condition and would like to know what potential neuropsychiatric effects that therapy may have on the patient. In both scenarios, the clinician will want to know how to manage any such behavioral side effects of general medical treatment.

Because most readers of this volume are neuropsychiatrists (and not cardiologists, rheumatologists, or oncologists), we organize the chapter around neuropsychiatric syndromes. We then organize the sections describing each syndrome around the common general medical therapies associated with it. The focus is on medications, but we also discuss nonpharmacological treatments that are increasingly recognized as having potential neuropsychiatric effects. We tabulate the level of evidence linking certain therapies with common neuropsychiatric syndromes. At the end of the chapter, we include an extensive appendix of pharmacological treatments and neuropsychiatric syndromes (Appendix 29–1) that provides a healthy redundancy of the information discussed in the text, but this information is organized so that the cardiologist, rheumatologist, or oncologist can easily find the information sought. Our final goal is to achieve both efficiency and comprehensiveness by referring the reader at relevant points throughout the chapter to other important topics covered elsewhere in this volume.

Epidemiology and Classification

Of the individuals receiving Medicare, 20% have at least five chronic health conditions (American Geriatrics Society 2010). Not only these conditions themselves but also their treatments can be associated with neuropsychiatric syndromes. Treatment-associated disturbances in mood, cognition, and behavior are sources of mortality and morbidity for patients and distress for family members and caregivers. They are also an important and challenging focus of clinical attention for all types of geriatricians because the very nature of chronic general medical conditions is that they often require long-term treatment. As a result, polypharmacy may be unavoidable, placing patients at risk for adverse drug effects (Steinman and Hanlon 2010). Most elderly persons have one or more unnecessary or "high-risk" drugs prescribed (Tamblyn et al. 1994). More than one-third of ambulatory patients taking five scheduled medications per day experience an adverse drug effect (Hanlon et al. 1997). Some of these effects lead to emergency department and hospital care, and many are preventable (Thomsen et al. 2007). These data do not include the untoward effects of the over-the-counter and other nonprescription drugs that elderly patients self-administer, nor do they account for the potential adverse effects of nonpharmacological therapies (e.g., surgery, radiation).

The precise incidence and prevalence of treatment-induced neuropsychiatric disorders are not clearly established (Hybels and Blazer 2003). There are minimal epidemiological descriptions of substance-induced disorders or disorders due to a general medical condition (or their treatment). More clearly established is that the incidence and prevalence of neuropsychiatric symptoms and "minor" syndromes increase with age (Hybels and Blazer 2003). Whenever an atypical or minor syndrome is diagnosed, clinicians will recognize the importance of reviewing the patient's list of current therapies for any potential contributions to the patient's behavioral disturbance.

Neurobiology and the Effects of Aging

Other sections of this text offer detailed discussions of the neurobiology of aging as it relates to prescribing treatments in the elderly. The principles and practice of psychopharmacology in the geriatric population are discussed in Chapter 9, "Geriatric Neuropsychopharmacology." Chapter 10, "Electroconvulsive Therapy and Related Treatments," and Chapter 11, "Brain Stimulation Therapies," provide discussion of the principles and practice of these respective therapies. Substance abuse, including misuse of prescription medications, is discussed in Chapter 17, "Addiction." Chapter 22, "Contemporary Personality Psychology," and Chapter 8, "Psychosocial Therapies," contain discussions of the patient's experience of illness and how to manage responses to illness that may be unhealthy.

Etiology and Pathophysiology

To determine a causal link between a prescribed therapy and an unintended effect, the clinician should use a formal scientific approach (Nebeker et al. 2004). If such an approach is not feasible, then the clinician should attempt to follow a challenge-dechallenge-rechallenge protocol (Spitzer 1986), in which a therapy is initiated, discontinued, and then reinitiated while the patient is assessed for adverse effects. In the case of drug therapy, a temporal relation between the emergence of neuropsychiatric symptoms and the initiation of a medication or a change in its pharmacokinetics suggests a causal link. Once the medication is discontinued, symptoms should be reduced within five times the drug's half-life (the time to reach steady-state serum concentration) or longer in older persons. Otherwise, the behavioral disturbance should be treated as a primary neuropsychiatric syndrome. In practice, these temporal relations may be difficult to confirm, particularly given the pharmacodynamic changes associated with normal aging (see Chapter 9, "Geriatric Neuropsychopharmacology") and the physiological complexity of persons with multiple general medical conditions and multiple active treatments. Moreover, the rules of pharmacology do not apply to nonpharmacological treatments, but in such circumstances the history elicited from the patient should still explore any temporal connections between symptoms and treatment (e.g., surgery, radiation therapy).

Clinical Syndromes

Disturbances in Mood

The literature describing mood disturbances associated with general medical therapies is poorly developed (Patten and Barbui 2004). Published reports generally lack descriptions of psychopathology more specific than "depressive symptoms" or "self-reported depression and anxiety." Terms such as *hypomania,* unless elucidated, may be equally nonspecific, particularly in the neuropsychiatric population in which frontal lobe disinhibition syndromes must be distinguished from idiopathic manic episodes. In addition, the published literature consists mainly of case reports and other observational data rather than controlled or epidemiological studies. Data specific to elderly populations are even more limited (Kotlyar et al. 2005). From such data, it is nearly impossible to determine causal relations that link certain therapies to specific symptoms (Table 29–1). In this section, we discuss only those general medical therapies for which a clinically meaningful amount of data exists or those that are so commonly prescribed that even rare behavioral side effects are of clinical concern.

The lack of controlled data makes it difficult to estimate prevalence of therapy-induced mood disturbances (Kotlyar et al. 2005; Patten and Love 1994). No evidence shows that age is an independent risk factor for treatment-associated mood syndromes (Ganzini et al. 1993). However, elderly persons are the largest consumers of prescribed medications, leading to a presumably increased incidence of medication-associated mood effects in the elderly (Wood et al. 1988). It is not clear whether a personal or family history of primary mood disorder is a true risk factor (Beers and Passman 1990; Patten et al. 1995) or instead represents a "response modifier" of the association between a general medical therapy and specific mood symptoms.

The phenomenology of treatment-associated mood syndromes varies (Levenson 1979; Patten and Lamarre 1992). In general, medication-induced mood syndromes represent apathy syndromes rather than primary depressive illness (Patten and Barbui 2004). Fatigue, lassitude, and reduced emotional expression are common features (Zelnik 1987). Melancholic signs (e.g., unremitting apprehension or gloom, psychomotor disturbance, vegetative signs, cognitive impairment) typically are absent (Taylor and Fink 2006). Perceptual disturbances and delusions, if present, likely indicate the presence of delirium with mood changes rather than a psychotic mood disorder.

Finally, it is important to recognize that both the treatment of general medical conditions and the experience of having the illness itself can affect a patient's emotional experience. Chapter 19, "Mood Disorders," describes the nonpathological low mood state termed *demoralization* and how to distinguish it from pathological mood disturbances arising from a general

TABLE 29–1. Strength of evidence associating prescribed therapies with depressive symptoms or syndromes

Therapy	Level of evidence	Notes
Corticosteroids	Level I	
Antihypertensives	Level II	Level II data are conflicting.
H_2-blockers	Level II	Level II evidence supports no association.
Interferons	Level II	Data in the elderly are lacking.
Dopaminergic drugs	Level III	
Hormone therapies	Level III	
Benzodiazepines	Level III	Level III data are conflicting.
Chemotherapy	Level III	
Deep brain stimulation	Level II	
Implantable cardiac devices	Level III	
Radiation therapy	Level III	

Note. Level I=at least one properly designed randomized controlled trial; Level II=nonrandomized controlled trials, well-designed cohort or case-control studies, or multiple time series; Level III=opinions of respected authorities, based on clinical experience, descriptive studies, or reports of expert committees.

medical condition or its treatment. Chapter 22, "Contemporary Personality Psychology," discusses the psychological responses to illness (or to normal aging) that a patient may have.

Corticosteroids

Results from randomized controlled trials leave no doubt that exogenous corticosteroid therapy can cause adverse neuropsychiatric effects (Conn and Poynard 1994). The estimated incidence is about 5% (Patten and Neutel 2000), with higher rates in women and persons with malignancy or systemic lupus erythematosus (Lewis and Smith 1983; Stiefel et al. 1989). The term *steroid psychosis* is a misnomer because the most prominent adverse effects are mood disturbances (Sirois 2003). Prospective and pharmacoepidemiological studies indicate that steroids may induce both depressive and maniclike disinhibition syndromes (Patten and Neutel 2000). Depressive syndromes occur in 40% of persons who develop neuropsychiatric side effects; may occur in the first week of steroid therapy or on discontinuation; and typically involve irritability, dysphoria, anxiety, and apathy (Fardet et al. 2007). Maniclike syndromes occur in approximately 30% of patients and may be more common than depressive syndromes (Warrington and Bostwick 2006). Prominent features include euphoria and disinhibition. Although some data suggest that maniclike symptoms are more likely to occur earlier in the course of steroid therapy, whereas depressive symptoms are more likely with longer-term treatment, the mood effects of steroids are notoriously unpredictable (Patten and Neutel 2000). When the patient's presentation involves delusions or obsessions, they are typically part of a mood syndrome; the presence of abnormal perceptions indicates the presence of delirium (Ling et al. 1981). Typically, steroid-induced mood syndromes last 2–6 weeks (Vincent 1995). In most cases, symptoms resolve with drug discontinuation (Brown 2003).

Data specific to elderly populations are limited, but age itself does not appear to be a risk factor (Cerullo 2008; Wood et al. 1988). The most predictive factor is steroid dose. Only 2% of patients receiving less than a dose equivalent of 40 mg/day of prednisone develop neuropsychiatric symptoms, compared with 5% who receive 41–80 mg/day and nearly 20% who receive greater than 80 mg/day (Vincent 1995). The pathophysiology of these effects is not fully understood, but neuroendocrine and neurotransmitter theories have been offered (Schacke et al. 2002).

Early recognition and management of these adverse effects are crucial. In one series of 79 patients, 93% had a full recovery, but 4% had chronic symptoms or recurrence, and 3% committed suicide (Lewis and Smith 1983). Interventions found to be safe and effective include antidepressant, anticonvulsant, and antipsychotic drugs, as well as electroconvulsive therapy (ECT) (Brown 2003). In persons at high risk, prophylactic treatment with lithium has been helpful (Sabet-Sharghi and Hutzler 1990).

In persons requiring long-term steroid therapy, a strategy of alternate-day dosing may be beneficial (Sharfstein et al. 1982).

Antihypertensive Medications

The literature associating antihypertensive medications with depression is extensive yet unconvincing. Thorough reviews of this literature do not support a causal link between major depression and β-blockers (Ko et al. 2002; Kohn 2001; Ried et al. 1998; Steffensmeier et al. 2006), α-agonists (Ko et al. 2002; Patten 1990; Paykel et al. 1982), thiazide diuretics (Patten and Love 1997), hydralazine (Beers and Passman 1990), calcium channel blockers (Beers and Passman 1990), angiotensin converting enzyme (ACE) inhibitors (Kotlyar et al. 2005), or 3-hydroxy-3-methylglutaryl coenzyme A (HMG-CoA) reductase inhibitors (i.e., statins) (Feng et al. 2008). The oft-cited exceptions are α-methyldopa (a potent α_2-agonist rarely used in elderly persons) and reserpine (a catecholamine-depleting drug rarely used in clinical practice). Still, numerous case reports describe the onset of depressive symptoms following the administration of these agents, especially propranolol (Patten and Barbui 2004). The precise incidence is not known, but a retrospective cohort study suggested that propranolol is associated with a two- to fourfold increase in risk of developing a depressive syndrome (Thiessen et al. 1990). The predominant symptoms are fatigue and lassitude (Petrie et al. 1982), not melancholic signs. Symptoms typically resolve within 1 week of discontinuing the medication (Zelnik 1987). Risk factors are not clearly identified. Biogenic amine depletion is the proposed pathophysiological mechanism through which these symptoms may emerge (Beers and Passman 1990).

The potential risk of developing fatigue or lassitude from these medications must be weighed against their potential benefits. β-Blockers are widely prescribed and have multiple indications, for both cardiovascular disease and psychiatric disorders. They have established benefits on mortality when given to elderly persons in the post–myocardial infarction period, a high-risk period for the onset of depression (Aronow 1997). Prospective data confirm no increased risk of depression for up to 1 year after patients are prescribed a β-blocker in the postinfarction period (van Melle et al. 2006).

Histamine H_2 Antagonists

Cimetidine is infamous as an inhibitor of many cytochrome P450 isoenzymes, and geriatricians are cautious of its potential to cause adverse drug-drug interactions. Several case reports have suggested an association between cimetidine (Hails 1982) or ranitidine (Stocky 1991) and depressive symptoms, an association more commonly reported in younger adults than in persons older than age 65 (Feng et al. 2008). Controlled data, however, offer no evidence that either cimetidine (Hails 1982; Patten and Love 1997) or ranitidine (Patten and Barbui 2004) causes depressive syndromes. Data specific to older persons are sparse (Wood et al. 1988).

Interferons

Interferon therapy can be used to treat multiple sclerosis (interferon beta), hepatitis C (interferon alfa), and certain malignancies. A fair amount of data links interferon therapy with disturbances in emotional experience (Patten 2006). No causal association has been statistically determined, and data specific to the elderly are limited. Depressive syndromes are most common and are more likely with interferon alfa than with interferon beta (Patten 2006). The syndromes are not well characterized, but fatigue and lethargy are prominent features (Van Gool et al. 2003). "Sickness behavior" and patient requests to stop treatment also have been described. Rarely, disinhibition, euphoria, and pathological laughing and crying have been reported (Patten 2006). Symptoms may occur at any time during the course of interferon treatment, and incidence estimates vary too widely (0%–70%) to be statistically meaningful (Trask et al. 2000). The pathophysiology is not understood. An individual history of depression may be a risk factor (Goeb et al. 2006), and it is worth noting that the early clinical trials of interferon beta in multiple sclerosis included one suicide and other suicide attempts (Feinstein 2004). Thus, ongoing monitoring for the surfacing of depressive symptoms is imperative. Typically, emergent depressive symptoms can be managed without fully discontinuing interferon therapy, and antidepressant medication, if necessary, can be used safely and effectively (Feinstein 2004). Data do not consistently show that prophylactic use of antidepressant medications is beneficial (Crone et al. 2004).

Levodopa and Dopaminergic Drugs

In persons with Parkinson's disease (PD), treatment with levodopa and dopaminergic drugs (e.g., bromocriptine, entacapone) is associated with increased anxiety (10%–15%), euphoria (10%), and maniclike disinhibition (1%) (Cummings 1991). No clear evidence indicates that levodopa causes depression (Patten and Love 1997). Symptom improvement typically occurs with medication dose reduction. However, these symptoms must be distinguished from the variety of similar behavioral syndromes that stem from PD itself. Early case reports suggesting this relation were likely confounded by the comorbidity of mood syndromes in PD. The pathophysiology of these symptoms is not fully understood but probably relates to the stimulatory effects dopaminergic drugs have on D_2 dopamine receptors (Lewitt 2008). Elderly persons and those with dementia may be most vulnerable to these types of adverse effects. In persons whose motor symptoms demand ongoing drug treatment, lithium and ECT may be safe and effective treatment options.

Other neuropsychiatric effects of treatment for PD, including impulse-control disorders, are discussed in more detail in Chapter 24, "Parkinson's Disease and Movement Disorders."

Hormone Therapy

Gonadotropin-releasing hormone (GnRH) agonists (e.g., leuprolide and goserelin, both used to treat prostate cancer) and progestin-releasing implanted contraceptives (e.g., Norplant) have both been linked to depressive symptoms (Patten and Barbui 2004). The literature is limited to case reports, and the incidence is unknown. The phenomenology is consistent with apathy and atypical depressive syndromes, the symptoms of which resolve after the drug is discontinued. The pathophysiology is not understood but has been proposed to involve disturbed tryptophan metabolism because of drug-induced vitamin B deficiency that affects serotonin synthesis (Patten and Love 1993).

Oral contraceptives containing relatively high doses of estrogen, typically prescribed to younger women, have been associated with depressive symptoms through a mechanism involving alterations in tryptophan metabolism (Bucci 1972; Rao 1974). Modern low-estrogen preparations have a more favorable neuropsychiatric side-effect profile (Patten and Lamarre 1992). No evidence indicates that selective estrogen receptor–modifying drugs cause adverse mood effects (Kotlyar et al. 2005). These drugs are used to treat breast cancer, osteoporosis, and menopausal symptoms and include tamoxifen and raloxifene. Indeed, hormone replacement therapy may actually alleviate mild symptoms of depressed mood (Zweifel and O'Brien 1997).

Benzodiazepines

No definitive empirical evidence indicates that benzodiazepines induce depressive syndromes (Patten and Love 1993). An early report of high doses (>40 mg/day) of diazepam resulting in a state of apprehension and suicidal ideation (Hall and Joffe 1972) was followed by other case reports that also suggested a link between high doses of benzodiazepines and depressive symptoms (Smith and Salzman 1991). Other studies disagreed and, instead, concluded that the effects of benzodiazepines unmask the psychomotor signs of melancholic depressive illness (Tiller and Schweitzer 1992).

A separate collection of case reports described a "paradoxical reaction" in persons taking benzodiazepines. The prominent clinical features of this "reaction" are talkativeness, restlessness, and "emotional release," but in rare cases patients may show hostility and rage (Hall and Zisook 1981). Careful reviews of this literature find the reaction to be very rare (<1% incidence) and idiosyncratic (Dietch and Jennings 1988), and it should not preclude the use of these agents acutely (as in catatonia). Aggressive or combative behavior is described exclusively in persons with underlying bipolar disorder or antisocial behavior (Mancuso et al. 2004). The cases involving elderly persons are few, and none describe dangerous behavior (Mancuso et al. 2004).

Chemotherapy

Several case reports associated various chemotherapeutic agents with depressive symptoms (Fawzy et al. 2002). This list of drugs includes vincristine, vinblastine, procarbazine, L-asparaginase, and amphotericin B. The most common feature described is lethargy, and this symptom more likely represents delirium (rather than a mood disorder) given the deliriogenic properties of these toxic drugs.

Deep Brain Stimulation

In persons with advanced PD, deep brain stimulation (DBS) improves motor symptoms and quality of life (see Chapter 24, "Parkinson's Disease and Movement Disorders"). It is also associated with a range of adverse neuropsychiatric side effects, including suicide (Voon et al. 2009). Although reduced verbal fluency and other subtle cognitive effects have been observed, the most prominent and concerning untoward effects involve disturbances in emotional experience (Voon et al. 2006). In the early postoperative period, patients may develop syndromes of apathy, off-period depression, disinhibition (hypomania), affective lability, pathological laughing and crying, hedonistic homeostatic dysregulation (i.e., levodopa abuse), obsessionality, phobia of device failure, and generalized anxiety (Voon et al. 2006). Mood syndromes arising much later than the first few months after DBS surgery are less likely to be related to either the surgery itself or the synergy between direct electrical stimulation and dopaminergic stimulation. Pathological mood disturbances may be more likely with bilateral subthalamic nuclei (STN) stimulation than with pallidal stimulation (Follett et al. 2010). This potential difference in surgical target has led to the hypothesis that increased STN activity ("off" stimulation) may lead to reduced emotional expression, whereas decreased STN activity ("on" stimulation) may lead to excessive or dysregulated emotional expression (Voon et al. 2006). The full pathophysiology, however, is likely more complex and remains unknown. Risk factors for developing neuropsychiatric side effects from DBS are not clear and are likely multifactorial. Treatment options involving drug therapy are being explored because turning the deep brain stimulators off is expected to lead to worsened motor symptoms. In our experience, standard pharmacological treatments closely coordinated within the multidisciplinary team are successful.

Implantable Cardiac Devices

Patients with various forms of heart disease may be vulnerable to behavioral side effects of the implantable cardiac devices

(ICDs) that have supplanted antiarrhythmic drugs as the first-line prevention of sudden cardiac arrest. After the device is implanted, patients may develop two identified anxiety syndromes. The first is characterized by unnecessary avoidant behavior suggestive of agoraphobia and may occur in more than half of the persons receiving ICDs (Lemon et al. 2004). The second is reminiscent of posttraumatic stress that develops in response to ICD discharges, either therapeutic or malfunctional (Pauli et al. 1999). Both ICD-related anxiety syndromes are linked to an increased rate of ventricular tachyarrhythmia (van den Broek et al. 2009), device firing (Kuhl et al. 2006), and sudden cardiac death (Ladwig et al. 2008). The precise incidence of these anxiety syndromes is not known. The pathophysiology is not well understood and may share features with panic and posttraumatic stress disorders. Treatment options are not well studied.

Radiation Therapy

Anticancer radiation therapy is associated with profound fatigue and lassitude that can mimic depressive illness (Greenberg et al. 1992). Fatigue tends to peak after 1 month of radiation. Radiation therapy for brain tumors, benign or malignant, may result in necrosis of cerebral tissue. Radiation necrosis has been linked to several neuropsychiatric side effects that may occur transiently in the postradiation period or several years later. These side effects are poorly understood but may be life-threatening, such as coma or seizures, or less severe, such as depression, personality changes, agitation, and cognitive impairment (al-Mefty et al. 1990). The incidence of these side effects is not known. Treatment may require surgical resection of necrotic tissue.

Delirium and Cognitive Impairment

Nearly every class of medication has been linked to the new onset of cognitive deficits in elderly persons. The literature supporting these associations, however, is poorly developed. Most reports are anecdotal and limited to hospitalized patients with multiple active general medical conditions (Table 29–2); tools used to assess cognition may not be standardized; and with only two exceptions (Inouye and Charpentier 1996; Marcantonio et al. 1994), studies do not measure *incident* cognitive impairment or delirium. The exception is the literature on medications with anticholinergic properties, in which prospective cohort studies and pathophysiological investigations pointed to a stronger link between anticholinergic drugs and cognitive impairment. Still, research findings are controversial (see the section "Anticholinergic Agents" below).

For the most part, new-onset cognitive deficits attributed to a medication arise as part of a delirium syndrome characterized by acute or subacute onset; fluctuating course or severity; and impaired ability to focus, shift, or sustain attention (Cole 2004). Significant inattention can lead to deficits in other cognitive domains as well. Emotional disturbances including fear, anxiety, and apathy are common. Psychomotor behavior can be characterized as hypoactive or hyperactive, although most patients have mixed motor features (Peterson et al. 2006). The presence of perceptual disturbances, such as hallucinations, misperceptions, and photo- and phonophobia, may reflect delirium severity. The clinical features of delirium do not necessarily reflect its etiology (e.g., medication, infection, metabolic derangement), although certain signs and symptoms may suggest recognizable syndromes (e.g., alcohol withdrawal delirium, anticholinergic toxicity). In cases of delirium due to a drug or drug toxicity, discontinuing the offending agent should lead to swift symptom improvement. Among the elderly, however, delirium may take weeks or months to resolve fully (Inouye 2006). This type of protracted delirium blurs the line between delirium and dementia. Indeed, long-term use of medications has been associated with more chronic cognitive impairment that may be subtler than frank delirium. This syndrome is sometimes referred to as *medication-associated dementia,* although the impairment reverses with drug discontinuation and is not associated with irreversible lesions or neurodegeneration.

Among elderly hospital patients, between 11% and 30% of cases of delirium are attributed to medications (Moore and O'Keeffe 1999). Risk factors for medication-associated delirium are difficult to distinguish from those predisposing to delirium from nonpharmacological causes. In elderly persons, the leading risk factor for delirium is dementia (Inouye 2006). Age itself is also a predisposing factor and has been attributed to imbalances in neurotransmitters (i.e., acetylcholine) and age-related alterations in pharmacokinetics and pharmacodynamics (Gray et al. 1999). Studies also consistently identify polypharmacy, illness severity, metabolic and electrolyte derangements, and functional impairment as additional risk factors (Gray et al. 1999). Depending on the patient's level of vulnerability, medications may precipitate delirium via the benign insult of a single dose of a medication or the more severe effects of medication toxicity.

In Chapter 15, "Delirium," the authors discuss this syndrome in detail, including tools for assessment. The dementias are discussed in Chapter 16, "Alzheimer's Disease and the Frontotemporal Dementia Syndromes."

Anticholinergic Agents

The evidence supporting a causal link between anticholinergic medications and cognitive impairment in the elderly is persuasive but not irrefutable. Three well-controlled, cross-sectional population-based studies (one of which included subjects with dementia) found a significant association between anticholinergic drug use and cognitive impairment (as

TABLE 29–2. Strength of evidence associating prescribed therapies with cognitive impairment

Therapy	Level of evidence	Notes
Anticholinergic drugs	Level II	Level II data are conflicting.
Benzodiazepines	Level II	Data are limited to hospitalized persons.
Tricyclic antidepressants	Level II	Level II data are conflicting.
Opioids	Level II	Strongest evidence is for meperidine.
Antihypertensives	Level I	Level I data support no association.
Antiarrhythmics	Level III	
H_2-blockers	Level II	Level II data support no association.
Chemotherapy	Level III	
Anesthesia or surgery	Level II	Controlled studies are difficult to conduct.
Deep brain stimulation	Level I	

Note. Level I=at least one properly designed randomized controlled trial; Level II=nonrandomized controlled trials, well-designed cohort or case-control studies, or multiple time series; Level III=opinions of respected authorities, based on clinical experience, descriptive studies, or reports of expert committees.

measured by the Mini-Mental State Examination) (Cancelli et al. 2008; Cao et al. 2008; Lechevallier-Michel et al. 2005). Three other studies had negative findings (Francis et al. 1990; Marcantonio et al. 1994; Schor et al. 1992). Two longitudinal studies have been conducted, the results of which were mixed (Ancelin et al. 2006; Bottiggi et al. 2006). To our knowledge, no prospective randomized controlled studies have been carried out.

Other lines of evidence supporting a direct relation include findings that there is a correlation between serum anticholinergic activity and delirium (Flacker et al. 1998) (leading to the cholinergic hypothesis of the etiology of delirium), that exposure to anticholinergic medications independently predicts delirium severity (Han et al. 2001), and that the cholinesterase inhibitor physostigmine can reverse the symptoms of delirium associated with anticholinergic medications (Inouye 2006). Some research findings, however, cloud this picture. Reduced or impaired cholinergic transmission is seen in normal aging and is implicated in the presentation of neuropsychiatric symptoms of Alzheimer's disease, dementia is a major predisposing factor to anticholinergic-induced delirium, and serum anticholinergic activity has been found to be elevated in patients with delirium who have not been exposed to anticholinergic medications (Cancelli et al. 2009b; Flacker et al. 1998).

Thus, whether reduced cholinergic activity is a pathogenetic mechanism of delirium or simply an epiphenomenon remains unclear. Altogether, the data suggest that total anticholinergic load, whether from exogenous medications or endogenous pathological mechanisms or some combination, may ultimately determine whether cognitive impairment or delirium manifests in any one individual (Moore and O'Keeffe 1999), a balance that may be mediated by the effects of cortisol (Plaschke et al. 2010).

The complex interplay between potential predisposing and precipitating factors, added to the fact that numerous medications have anticholinergic properties, makes it nearly impossible to identify the precise incidence of cognitive impairment associated with anticholinergic medication. Of the 25 most common medications prescribed to the elderly, 14 have anticholinergic side effects (Cancelli et al. 2009b). Common anticholinergic medications in the elderly include antihistamines, antihypertensive agents, benzodiazepines, tricyclic antidepressants (TCAs), antipsychotics, corticosteroids, H_2-blockers, immunosuppressive agents, and antibiotics (Tune 2001). At toxic levels, these drugs can produce a recognizable syndrome characterized by severe delirium and peripheral anticholinergic effects such as pupillary dilation, tachycardia, piloerection, urinary retention, constipation, flushing (i.e., vasodilation), and anhidrosis. However, in elderly persons with cognitive impairment resulting from anticholinergic medications, accompanying signs of peripheral autonomic anticholinergic activity may or may not be observed (Tune 2001). Although hallucinosis has been independently observed with anticholinergic medications (Cancelli et al. 2009a), the presence of perceptual disturbances likely represents hallucinations as part of delirium or misperception and misinterpretation of actual environmental stimuli that result from cognitive impairment (Cancelli et al. 2009b).

The major risk factors contributing to anticholinergic overload include use of other medications with anticholinergic properties (including over-the-counter medications), impaired baseline cognitive functioning, and impaired hepatic metabolism (Moore and O'Keeffe 1999). Specific populations of elderly persons such as those with PD and Alzheimer's disease may be more susceptible to anticholinergic effects. Treatment of anticholinergic delirium begins with stopping or decreasing the dosage of the suspected anticholinergic agent. If symptoms of delirium are severe or do not resolve, then treatment with physostigmine can be used, watching for potential cholinergic side effects (Moore and O'Keeffe 1999).

Sedative-Hypnotics

Few, if any, studies have investigated the cognitive effects of sedative-hypnotic agents taken for therapeutic reasons by healthy elderly persons in outpatient settings. Nearly all the data linking these drugs to delirium come from studies of hospitalized patients prescribed benzodiazepines, and the results of these studies are mixed (Gray et al. 1999). Studies with positive findings describe such effects as anterograde amnesia, impaired new learning, reduced vigilance, and slowed psychomotor performance (Moore and O'Keeffe 1999). These deficits are not fully explained by the direct sedative effects of these medications (Wolkowitz et al. 1987), and healthy elderly persons may develop tolerance to these side effects. Short-acting benzodiazepines are presumed to be safer, but no head-to-head comparison studies have been done. Short-acting benzodiazepines carry a risk of withdrawal delirium characterized by motor hyperactivity, florid hallucinations, and marked autonomic activity. Long-acting benzodiazepines are more slowly metabolized and excreted in elderly persons, leading to less risk of acute withdrawal but increased risk of toxicity and hypoactive delirium (Moore and O'Keeffe 1999). In some cases, long-term benzodiazepine use may be associated with persistent neurocognitive deficits that may improve on drug withdrawal (Gray et al. 1999). Epidemiological data are insufficient to determine the prevalence or incidence of any of these potential effects.

It is important to note the increasing use of nonbenzodiazepine short-acting hypnotics that are perceived to be cognitively safer than benzodiazepines (Declerk and Bisserbe 1997). Very few studies have examined the cognitive effects of these agents in the elderly (Gray et al. 1999).

Antidepressants

Major challenges exist in assessing the cognitive effects of antidepressant medications in elderly persons. Depressive syndromes are highly comorbid with dementing illnesses, and even in elderly persons without dementia, depressive illness commonly manifests with cognitive deficits (i.e., pseudodementia) or functional impairment (see Chapters 16, "Alzheimer's Disease and the Frontotemporal Dementia Syndromes," and 19, "Mood Disorders"). In either case, treatment of late-life depression improves cognitive and executive functioning (Butters et al. 2000). Studies of antidepressant medications must control for these factors to be clinically meaningful. Controlled studies of lithium in the elderly are lacking.

Data from randomized controlled trials indicate an association between TCAs and cognitive impairment, but similar studies have not confirmed this finding (Gray et al. 1999; Oxman 1996). Amitriptyline has been associated with reduced cognitive reaction time, impaired retrieval from secondary memory, and impaired information processing (Gray et al. 1999). It has been suggested that the cognitive effects of TCAs, particularly the tertiary TCAs, are likely caused by their anticholinergic properties, which may be dose dependent (Gray et al. 1999; Oxman 1996). However, TCAs with lower anticholinergic properties, such as nortriptyline, also have been associated with impaired cognitive performance (Gray et al. 1999). When compared with TCAs, selective serotonin reuptake inhibitor (SSRI) antidepressants may produce less cognitive impairment because of less anticholinergic effect, but results are mixed (Oxman 1996), and TCAs remain a well-tolerated and especially effective therapy for melancholic depression. Both SSRIs and monoamine oxidase inhibitors (MAOIs) appear to be well tolerated in patients with mild cognitive impairment and dementia (Gray et al. 1999; Oxman 1996). It has been suggested that MAOIs may actually improve cognitive functioning through a mechanism separate from their antidepressant effects (Oxman 1996). However, serotonergic activity is not entirely benign. Serotonin toxicity results in a potentially life-threatening delirium syndrome (toxic serotonin syndrome) that has not been well studied in the elderly (Boyer and Shannon 2005). The prevalence of each of these effects is unknown, and risk factors are similar to those for delirium in general.

Analgesics

The evidence linking opioid use to delirium in elderly persons comes from prospective studies of hospitalized patients that were inadequately controlled for confounding factors such as pain and use of other psychotropic medications (Deiner and Silverstein 2009; Mantz et al. 2010). The results are mixed, with three of five trials finding an association between opioid use and delirium (Gray et al. 1999). Meperidine is the only opioid consistently identified as potentially deliriogenic. The mechanism is unclear but may relate to the effects of meperidine's active metabolite or to the anticholinergic effects of meperidine itself (Eisendrath et al. 1987). Signs of somnolence and hypoactive psychomotor behavior dominate the clinical picture. Risk factors are not established, but renal insufficiency may lead to accumulation of active metabolites. Administering the medication through patient-controlled analgesia may reduce the likelihood of adverse cognitive effects when compared with the epidural or intramuscular route (Gray et al. 1999). Morphine, fentanyl, oxycodone, and codeine have not been shown to have a statistically significant association with delirium.

Nonopioid analgesics (e.g., acetaminophen, salicylates) may produce delirium but only at toxic levels. Despite the widespread use of nonsteroidal anti-inflammatory drugs (NSAIDs), neuropsychiatric side effects are not well characterized and are believed to be quite rare. Case series suggest that persons with underlying psychiatric illness may be vulnerable to exacerbations of those illnesses when prescribed indomethacin or sulindac (Browning 1996; Jiang and Chang 1999). The pathophysiology of this reaction is not understood and may involve the structural similarity of the indolic moiety of indomethacin to serotonin. No evidence suggests that age is a risk factor independent of its association with greater general medical comorbidity (Solomon and Gurwitz 1997). Epidemiological studies of the cognitive effects of NSAID use among the elderly have been mixed and inconclusive (Gray et al. 1999).

Cardiovascular Agents

The evidence linking antiarrhythmic medications to delirium in elderly persons is limited to case reports (Keller and Frishman 2003). The oft-cited example is digitalis, which was described in 1784 as precipitating "deliere digitalique," a delirium due to digitalis toxicity. The clinical features of the syndrome are indistinguishable from those of delirium due to other causes, although visual disturbances (e.g., yellow or green halos, blurry vision, scotoma, misperceptions, hallucinations) may be more common (King 1950). Although digitalis is used more judiciously today, it is important to note that elderly persons can develop neuropsychiatric side effects when the drug is at therapeutic serum levels (Pascualy and Veith 1989). Quinine toxicity (cinchonism) is associated with a delirium involving visual disturbances, tinnitus, vertigo, and a lichenoid rash (Keller and Frishman 2003). Tocainide, another class I antiarrhythmic, has been reported to cause confusion, paranoia, impaired concentration, fearfulness, weeping, and "childlike behavior" (Keller and Frishman 2003).

Antihypertensive medications have been sufficiently studied and do not cause cognitive impairment (Gray et al. 1999). Clonidine's central catecholamine effects are theorized to be a cause of cognitive impairment, but minimal data exist to support this conclusion. Frank delirium has been reported with various antihypertensive agents, but data are limited to case reports. Metoprolol and other β-blockers have been associated with lethargy, fatigue, drowsiness, sleep disturbances, anxiety, confusion, visual hallucinations, and nightmares (Keller and Frishman 2003). Distinct cases of patients experiencing hallucinations without changes in arousal and sensorium also have been reported (Sirois 2006). ACE inhibitors, calcium channel blockers, hydralazine, and thiazides all have been reported to cause delirium with visual hallucinations (Keller and Frishman 2003). Statin drugs do not seem to carry a risk of delirium. The prevalence of these adverse effects is unknown but is believed to be rare given the common use of cardiovascular medications in the elderly. Risk factors are not established. The mechanism of these adverse effects is not understood, but medication effects must be distinguished from the consequences of reduced perfusion and other signs of compromised cardiac function.

Histamine Antagonists

Although all histamine H_2 receptor antagonists have been associated with delirium, prospective studies have not confirmed this relation (Cantu and Korek 1991; Moore and O'Keeffe 1999). Cimetidine has been cited in the literature as having the greatest potential for producing central nervous system toxicity, but literature reviews have found no differences among various H_2 receptor antagonist agents (Cantu and Korek 1991). Observational studies have indicated that 1%–2% of all hospital patients and 15%–20% of intensive care patients receiving such medications develop delirium when these drugs reach toxic levels (Moore and O'Keeffe 1999). Reported symptoms include confusion, agitation, lassitude, and hallucinations (Picotte-Prillmayer et al. 1995). Symptoms typically develop within the first 2 weeks of therapy and resolve within 3 days of drug withdrawal (Cantu and Korek 1991). Most of these drug reactions occur in elderly patients, particularly those with underlying renal dysfunction (Moore and O'Keeffe 1999). The specific mechanism by which H_2 receptor antagonists cause these effects is unknown. However, the reversal of H_2 antagonist–induced delirium by physostigmine suggests that anticholinergic effects may play a role (Moore and O'Keeffe 1999).

Diphenhydramine, a histamine H_1 receptor antagonist, also has been associated with impaired attention, short-term verbal memory deficits, and reduced concentration and reaction time in elderly persons (Gray et al. 1999). Second-generation antihistamines (e.g., loratadine) are therefore preferred.

Chemotherapy

Cognitive impairment experienced by some patients receiving chemotherapeutic agents has been referred to as *chemobrain*. Cognitive areas affected include attention, visual and verbal memory, and psychomotor functioning (Nelson et al. 2007). In one prospective observational study, elderly subjects were found to have cognitive impairment in the areas of verbal learning, verbal fluency, and memory within the first days of treatment (Eberhardt et al. 2006). The underlying physiological mechanism remains unknown. It is suspected that chemotherapeutic drugs may be associated with oxidative damage and vascular injury, inflammation, direct injury to neurons, autoimmune processes, anemia, and the expression of the apolipoprotein E4 (*APOE*) gene (Nelson et al. 2007). Despite such findings, evidence indicating a direct association between chemotherapy and cognitive impairment is mixed (Hermelink et al. 2007). The incidence is not known.

General Anesthesia and Surgery

Major and minor surgery carry risks of adverse cognitive effects that increase with age (Fong et al. 2006). Reports of these effects describe two main syndromes—postoperative delirium and postoperative cognitive decline (Fong et al. 2006). *Postoperative delirium* is an acute change in alertness and attention that occurs in the immediate postoperative period and has a fluctuating course that typically resolves in a few days. *Postoperative cognitive decline* is a less-well-validated postoperative syndrome with more subtle deficits in thinking and memory that persist for weeks to months. Although postoperative cognitive decline is reportedly distinct from postoperative delirium, descriptions of postoperative cognitive decline include impairments in concentration, sustained attention, memory, and executive function that are all consistent with a mild, persistent delirium (Ramaiah and Lam 2009). The pathophysiology of both syndromes is multifactorial. Among elderly persons, the incidence of postoperative delirium is 10%–60% following noncardiac surgery and 3%–47% following cardiac surgery, whereas the incidence rates of postoperative cognitive decline are 7%–26% and 24%–80%, respectively (Fong et al. 2006). The wide ranges of reported incidence likely reflect overlapping syndromes and poorly defined phenomenology. Relative to their younger counterparts, elderly persons are at greater risk for developing these syndromes because of difficulty accommodating perioperative volume changes related to decreased cardiac and pulmonary reserves (Singh and Antognini 2010). Among elderly persons, dementia is the leading risk factor (Robinson et al. 2009). Other risk factors include increasing age, depressive illness, and a host of perioperative factors, such as longer duration of anesthesia, pain, and general medical comorbidity, but not factors such as intraoperative hypotension, use of regional (versus general) anesthesia, and intravenous (versus epidural) routes of analgesia administration (Fong et al. 2006). The only perioperative medication consistently associated with an increased risk of postoperative delirium is meperidine.

Deep Brain Stimulation

When used as a treatment for PD, DBS of the STN is associated with deficits in verbal fluency and executive function (Halpern et al. 2009). The source of these side effects is believed to be disruption of frontal-striatal-thalamic circuitry associated with DBS surgery. Older persons with PD and mild cognitive impairment may be most vulnerable to these cognitive changes (Halpern et al. 2009). Conclusions are limited, however, because outcomes in cognition in the "on" and "off" phases of DBS have not been compared (Halpern et al. 2009). In Chapter 11, "Brain Stimulation Therapies," and Chapter 24, "Parkinson's Disease and Movement Disorders," the authors discuss DBS as a treatment for PD in greater detail.

Delusions and Perceptual Disturbances

Overwhelmingly, the presence of delusions or perceptual disturbances attributed to a general medical therapy indicates the presence of delirium or impending delirium. (The effects of illicit drugs are not discussed in this chapter.) Hallucinosis, the presence of hallucinations in the absence of impaired attention or altered arousal, is very rare and generally limited to identifiable neuropsychiatric syndromes that are unrelated to a specific medication or therapy (Coffey et al. 2010). The main exception to this rule is the case of dopamine replacement medications or dopamine receptor agonists in persons with PD (see subsection "Levodopa and Dopaminergic Medications" later in this chapter). Only limited case reports exist of isolated hallucinations associated with other medications; these include anticholinergic medications (particularly in persons with dementia), ACE inhibitors, and β-blockers (Wood et al. 1988). Visual hallucinations are the perceptual aberration typically reported, although it is not clear that the possibility of hallucinations in other sensory modalities was investigated.

Delusions can be difficult to assess in persons with delirium, and studies of medication-associated psychosis do not sufficiently describe such assessment. Altered levels of arousal or impairment in attention and concentration can confound the person's subjective report of his or her symptoms. Furthermore, certain experiences may not be recognized as pathological at all. The delusions of delirium are vague or poorly developed. They may not be truly fixed false beliefs but instead reflect a misunderstanding or misattribution of abnormal perceptual experiences (e.g., hallucinations). Social behaviors suggestive of delusional thought processes also may be misleading. These behaviors include fear, suspiciousness, or defensiveness and may reflect a person's attempts to make sense of abnormal perceptions in the context of acute or chronic (or acute-on-chronic) cognitive impairment.

Levodopa and Dopaminergic Medications

Psychotic symptoms may occur spontaneously in persons with PD (see Chapter 24, "Parkinson's Disease and Movement Disorders") but occur more frequently in patients receiving dopamine receptor agonists (Young et al. 1997). Although it is not clear if these medications have a direct causal link with psychotic symptoms, there is little doubt that they serve as a risk factor for the development of psychotic symptoms (Zahodne and Fernandez 2008). With these medications, rates of psychosis range between 10% and 50% (Factor et al. 1995). Of the psychotic symptoms observed, visual hallucinations and paranoid delusions were the most prominent (Factor et al. 1995). Hallucinosis occurs at a rate of 30% (Factor et al. 1995). Visual hallucinations are described as vivid images of humans, animals, and inanimate objects. In the earliest phases of development, the images appear as benign illusions (Kuzuhara 2001). They occur frequently during nighttime hours and are stereotyped. They are often accompanied by sleep disturbances, with altered, vivid dreaming. The hallucinations may be initially benign but can progress to more distressing symptoms associated with auditory hallucinations (Kuzuhara 2001). The risk is greater in patients with underlying dementia, sleep disturbances, more severe PD, and depressive illness (Zahodne and Fernandez 2008). The mechanism for drug-induced psychotic illness is unknown but is proposed to involve the serotonergic system and dopaminergic activity in the mesolimbic system (Factor et al. 1995). Treatment of psychosis induced by antiparkinsonian medication involves a series of steps aimed at balancing the desirable motor effects with the undesirable nonmotor effects of these drugs. Quetiapine and clozapine may be beneficial in severe cases (Fernandez et al. 2003; Friedman and Factor 2000).

Movement Disorders and Falls

Dopamine Antagonists

Findings from multiple well-controlled trials that included elderly subjects support a causal relation between movement disorders and dopamine-blocking drugs (Caligiuri et al. 2000). Compared with their younger counterparts, elderly persons are at increased risk for drug-induced parkinsonism, tardive dyskinesia, tardive tremor, and catatonia (Detweiler et al. 2007). The mechanism conferring this increased risk is not fully understood (Casey 2004), but it likely involves deranged dopaminergic transmission or loss of dopaminergic cell bodies from the substantia nigra associated with aging (Palmer and DeKosky 1993). The prevalence of drug-induced parkinsonism may be as high as 75% (Casey 1996), whereas that of tardive dyskinesia is 35% (Yassa et al. 1992). The prevalence of akathisia is about equal to that in younger populations, whereas the occurrence of dystonia in elderly persons is low (Caligiuri et al. 2000). Risk factors are not well established (Casey 1996), although persons with Alzheimer's disease appear to be at highest risk (Lee et al. 2005). Both typical and atypical antipsychotics can cause these effects, as well as any of the dopamine-blocking antiemetic drugs (e.g., chlorpromazine, prochlorperazine, metoclopramide).

Drug-induced parkinsonism is characterized by bradykinesia, rigidity, and tremor. The nature of the tremor helps distinguish drug-induced parkinsonism from idiopathic PD. The classic resting ("pill-rolling") tremor of idiopathic PD is replaced in drug-induced parkinsonism by a postural or kinetic tremor of the upper extremities. A perioral lip tremor ("rabbit syndrome") is an equally uncommon finding in drug-induced parkinsonism. Most parkinsonian signs are present within 3 months after initiating treatment with or increasing the dose of a dopamine-blocking drug, although symptoms may be detectable as early as within 96 hours (Mamo et al. 1999). In elderly persons, the symptoms may persist for several weeks, even if the offending medication is discontinued. Furthermore, the presence of antipsychotic drug–induced parkinsonism is a known risk factor for the development of tardive dyskinesia (Mamo et al. 1999). Monitoring should occur regularly during the early course of treatment and then may decrease after 3 months of therapy (Sweet and Pollock 1995).

In general, prescribing antipsychotics in the elderly should begin by following consensus guidelines (Alexopoulos et al. 2004), although we use extra caution given the nature, risk of, and difficulty managing the adverse effects from these agents. Treatment of untoward motor effects is imperative because elderly persons with drug-induced parkinsonism are also at increased risk for dependency, urinary incontinence, and mortality (Wilson and MacLennan 1989). If the offending drug cannot be discontinued, then amantadine may ameliorate untoward motor symptoms. Anticholinergic drugs are also effective but may be less well tolerated in the elderly. Prophylactic treatment is not recommended and does not prevent the emergence of tardive dyskinesia (Mamo et al. 1999).

Antidepressants and Benzodiazepines

Nearly a third of community-dwelling elderly persons have at least one fall per year, with the rate even higher among those living in nursing homes (Cumming 1998). Some of these falls result in fractures, including hip fractures. The evidence supporting a link between medications and falls is substantial but consists mainly of observational epidemiological studies. The risk of falls conferred by medications is highest for antidepressants, for which the increased risk is twofold (Cumming 1998). The mechanism of this effect is not clear but may relate to the sedating properties of some of these agents. However, it is not clear that any particular class of antidepressants (e.g., SSRI vs. TCA) confers a relatively higher risk.

Observational studies also link the risk of falls to the use of benzodiazepines, although few of these studies were designed specifically to investigate this risk (Monane and Avorn 1996). Whether long-acting benzodiazepines confer a higher risk than short-acting ones is not clear. It may be that total daily dose, rather than drug half-life, is the most important factor (Cumming 1998). For all classes of medications associated with an increased risk of falls, management follows core principles of geriatric medicine: optimizing the patient's functional status and mobility, adhering to principles of geriatric pharmacology, and reducing polypharmacy (Monane and Avorn 1996).

β-Adrenergic Agonists

Age is the most important risk factor for drug-induced tremor (Morgan and Sethi 2005), and several other medications are associated with it; these include lithium, SSRIs, TCAs, valproate, amiodarone, cyclosporine, and benzodiazepine or alcohol withdrawal (Diederich and Goetz 1998). β-Agonist drugs, including caffeine, are well-established culprits of medication-induced tremor (Morgan and Sethi 2005). The tremor is an enhanced physiological tremor, such that it is typically postural and kinetic rather than resting (Bhagwath 2001). Examination maneuvers that involve relevant tasks (e.g., drinking a glass of water or writing a sentence) may be more helpful than finger-nose testing. The voice and head (i.e., titubation) are rarely involved and, if present, suggest a diagnosis of nonmedication-related essential tremor. Emotional stress or excitement may exacerbate the tremor, whereas alcohol may alleviate it. In general, drug-induced tremor resolves after the offending drug is discontinued. In severe cases, β-blockers or primidone may be helpful (Detweiler et al. 2007).

Key Points

- With a few exceptions, the evidence establishing direct causal relations between a general medical therapy and a neuropsychiatric syndrome in the elderly is limited to small bodies of uncontrolled data.
- Compared with younger populations, the elderly are at increased risk for adverse drug effects.
- Polypharmacy among elderly persons is consistently identified as a risk factor for adverse drug effects.
- Neuropsychiatric side effects are not limited to drug therapy and also may be observed following surgical, radiation, and brain stimulation therapies.
- Characteristic features of depression associated with general medical therapies include fatigue, lassitude, and other nonmelancholic signs.
- Delusions and abnormal perceptions associated with general medical therapies generally represent signs of delirium.
- The total anticholinergic load, whether from exogenous medications or endogenous pathophysiological mechanisms or some combination, may be the main driver of cognitive impairment observed in persons taking anticholinergic drugs.
- All dopamine-blocking drugs can cause untoward motor effects in the elderly, and antidepressants and sedatives are the medications most closely associated with falls.
- Strategies for managing multiple medications and other nonpharmacological treatments in elderly persons should follow a patient-centered biopsychosocial approach.

References

al-Mefty O, Kersh JE, Routh A, et al: The long-term side effects of radiation therapy for benign brain tumors in adults. J Neurosurg 73:502–512, 1990

Alexopoulos GS, Streim J, Carpenter D, et al: Using antipsychotic agents in older patients. J Clin Psychiatry 65 (suppl 2):5–99; discussion 100–102; quiz 103–104, 2004

American Geriatrics Society: Fact Sheet: The American Geriatrics Society (AGS). New York, American Geriatrics Society, 2010. Available at: http://www.americangeriatrics.org/about_us/who_we_are/faq_fact_sheet. Accessed November 30, 2010.

Ancelin ML, Artero S, Portet F, et al: Non-degenerative mild cognitive impairment in elderly people and use of anticholinergic drugs: longitudinal cohort study. BMJ 332:455–459, 2006

Aronow WS: Postinfarction use of beta-blockers in elderly patients. Drugs Aging 11:424–432, 1997

Beers MH, Passman LJ: Antihypertensive medications and depression. Drugs 40:792–799, 1990

Bhagwath G: Tremors in elderly persons. Hosp Physician 49:31–37, 2001

Bottiggi KA, Salazar JC, Yu L, et al: Long-term cognitive impact of anticholinergic medications in older adults. Am J Geriatr Psychiatry 14:980–984, 2006

Boyer EW, Shannon M: The serotonin syndrome. N Engl J Med 352:1112–1120, 2005

Brown ES: Management of psychiatric side effects associated with corticosteroids. Expert Rev Neurother 3:69–75, 2003

Browning CH: Nonsteroidal anti-inflammatory drugs and severe psychiatric side effects. Int J Psychiatry Med 26:25–34, 1996

Bucci L: Drug-induced depression and tryptophan metabolism. Dis Nerv Syst 33:105–108, 1972

Butters MA, Becker JT, Nebes RD, et al: Changes in cognitive functioning following treatment of late-life depression. Am J Psychiatry 157:1949–1954, 2000

Caligiuri MR, Jeste DV, Lacro JP: Antipsychotic-induced movement disorders in the elderly: epidemiology and treatment recommendations. Drugs Aging 17:363–384, 2000

Callahan CM: Psychiatric syndromes in elderly patients due to medications. Annu Rev Gerontol Geriatr 12:41–75, 1992

Cancelli I, Gigli GL, Piani A, et al: Drugs with anticholinergic properties as a risk factor for cognitive impairment in elderly people: a population-based study. J Clin Psychopharmacol 28:654–659, 2008

Cancelli I, Beltrame M, D'Anna L, et al: Drugs with anticholinergic properties: a potential risk factor for psychosis onset in Alzheimer's disease? Expert Opin Drug Saf 8:549–557, 2009a

Cancelli I, Beltrame M, Gigli GL, et al: Drugs with anticholinergic properties: cognitive and neuropsychiatric side effects in elderly patients. Neurol Sci 30:87–92, 2009b

Cantu TG, Korek JS: Central nervous system reactions to histamine-2 receptor blockers. Ann Intern Med 114:1027–1034, 1991

Cao YJ, Mager DE, Simonsick EM, et al: Physical and cognitive performance and burden of anticholinergics, sedatives, and ACE inhibitors in older women. Clin Pharmacol Ther 83:422–429, 2008

Casey DE: Side effect profiles of new antipsychotic agents. J Clin Psychiatry 57 (suppl 11):40–45; discussion 46–52, 1996

Casey DE: Pathophysiology of antipsychotic drug-induced movement disorders. J Clin Psychiatry 65 (suppl 9):25–28, 2004

Cerullo MA: Expect psychiatric side effects from corticosteroid use in the elderly. Geriatrics 63:15–18, 2008

Coffey MJ, Taylor MA, London ZN: Neurologic disorders presenting with behavioral signs and symptoms, in MedLink Neurology. Gilman S, editor-in-chief. San Diego, CA, MedLink Corporation, March 9, 2010. Available at: http://www.medlink.com/medlinkcontent.asp. Accessed November 30, 2010.

Cole MG: Delirium in elderly patients. Am J Geriatr Psychiatry 12:7–21, 2004

Conn HO, Poynard T: Corticosteroids and peptic ulcer: meta-analysis of adverse events during steroid therapy. J Intern Med 236: 619–632, 1994

Crone CC, Gabriel GM, Wise TN: Managing the neuropsychiatric side effects of interferon-based therapy for hepatitis C. Cleve Clin J Med 71 (suppl 3):S27–S32, 2004

Cumming RG: Epidemiology of medication-related falls and fractures in the elderly. Drugs Aging 12:43–53, 1998

Cummings JL: Clinical Neuropsychiatry. New York, Grune & Stratton, 1985

Cummings JL: Organic psychoses: delusional disorders and secondary mania. Psychiatr Clin North Am 9:293–311, 1986

Cummings JL: Behavioral complications of drug treatment of Parkinson's disease. J Am Geriatr Soc 39:708–716, 1991

Declerk A, Bisserbe J: Short-term safety profile of zolpidem: objective measures of cognitive effects. Eur Psychiatry 12 (suppl 1):15–20, 1997

Deiner S, Silverstein JH: Postoperative delirium and cognitive dysfunction. Br J Anaesth 103 (suppl 1):i41–i46, 2009

Detweiler MB, Kalafat N, Kim KY: Drug-induced movement disorders in older adults: an overview for clinical practitioners. Consult Pharm 22:149–165, 2007

Diederich NJ, Goetz CG: Drug-induced movement disorders. Neurol Clin 16:125–139, 1998

Dietch JT, Jennings RK: Aggressive dyscontrol in patients treated with benzodiazepines. J Clin Psychiatry 49:184–188, 1988

Eberhardt B, Dilger S, Musial F, et al: Short-term monitoring of cognitive functions before and during the first course of treatment. J Cancer Res Clin Oncol 132:234–240, 2006

Eisendrath SJ, Goldman B, Douglas J, et al: Meperidine-induced delirium. Am J Psychiatry 144:1062–1065, 1987

Estroff TW, Gold MS: Medication-induced and toxin-induced psychiatric disorders, in Medical Mimics of Psychiatric Disorders. Edited by Extein I, Gold MS. Washington, DC, American Psychiatric Press, 1986, pp 163–198

Factor SA, Molho ES, Podskalny GD, et al: Parkinson's disease: drug-induced psychiatric states. Adv Neurol 65:115–138, 1995

Fardet L, Kassar A, Cabane J, et al: Corticosteroid-induced adverse events in adults: frequency, screening and prevention. Drug Saf 30:861–881, 2007

Fawzy FI, Servis ME, Greenberg DB: Oncology and psychooncology, in The American Psychiatric Publishing Textbook of Consultation-Liaison Psychiatry: Psychiatry in the Medically Ill, 2nd Edition. Edited by Wise MG, Rundell JR. Washington, DC, American Psychiatric Publishing, 2002, pp 657–678

Feinstein A: The neuropsychiatry of multiple sclerosis. Can J Psychiatry 49:157–163, 2004

Feng L, Tan CH, Merchant RA, et al: Association between depressive symptoms and use of HMG-CoA reductase inhibitors (statins), corticosteroids and histamine H(2) receptor antagonists in community-dwelling older persons: cross-sectional analysis of a population-based cohort. Drugs Aging 25:795–805, 2008

Fernandez HH, Trieschmann ME, Friedman JH: Treatment of psychosis in Parkinson's disease: safety considerations. Drug Saf 26:643–659, 2003

Flacker JM, Cummings V, Mach JR Jr, et al: The association of serum anticholinergic activity with delirium in elderly medical patients. Am J Geriatr Psychiatry 6:31–41, 1998

Follett KA, Weaver FM, Stern M, et al: Pallidal versus subthalamic deep-brain stimulation for Parkinson's disease. N Engl J Med 362:2077–2091, 2010

Fong HK, Sands LP, Leung JM: The role of postoperative analgesia in delirium and cognitive decline in elderly patients: a systematic review. Anesth Analg 102:1255–1266, 2006

Francis J, Martin D, Kapoor WN: A prospective study of delirium in hospitalized elderly. JAMA 263:1097–1101, 1990

Friedman JH, Factor SA: Atypical antipsychotics in the treatment of drug-induced psychosis in Parkinson's disease. Mov Disord 15:201–211, 2000

Ganzini L, Walsh JR, Millar SB: Drug-induced depression in the aged: what can be done? Drugs Aging 3:147–158, 1993

Gardner BK, O'Connor DW: A review of the cognitive effects of electroconvulsive therapy in older adults. J ECT 24:68–80, 2008

Goeb JL, Even C, Nicolas G, et al: Psychiatric side effects of interferon-beta in multiple sclerosis. Eur Psychiatry 21:186–193, 2006

Gray SL, Lai KV, Larson EB: Drug-induced cognition disorders in the elderly: incidence, prevention and management. Drug Saf 21: 101–122, 1999

Greenberg DB, Sawicka J, Eisenthal S, et al: Fatigue syndrome due to localized radiation. J Pain Symptom Manage 7:38–45, 1992

Hails KC: Neuropsychiatric side effects of cimetidine. Pa Med 85:43–47, 1982

Hall RC, Joffe JR: Aberrant response to diazepam: a new syndrome. Am J Psychiatry 129:738–742, 1972

Hall RC, Zisook S: Paradoxical reactions to benzodiazepines. Br J Clin Pharmacol 11 (suppl 1):99S–104S, 1981

Hall RC, Stickney SK, Garner ER: Behavioral toxicity of neuropsychiatric drugs, in Psychiatric Presentations of Mental Illness. Edited by Hall CW. New York, Spectrum Publication, 1980, pp 337–349

Halpern CH, Rick JH, Danish SF, et al: Cognition following bilateral deep brain stimulation surgery of the subthalamic nucleus for Parkinson's disease. Int J Geriatr Psychiatry 24:443–451, 2009

Han L, McCusker J, Cole M, et al: Use of medications with anticholinergic effect predicts clinical severity of delirium symptoms in older medical inpatients. Arch Intern Med 161:1099–1105, 2001

Hanlon JT, Schmader KE, Koronkowski MJ, et al: Adverse drug events in high risk older outpatients. J Am Geriatr Soc 45:945–948, 1997

Hermelink K, Untch M, Lux MP, et al: Cognitive function during neoadjuvant chemotherapy for breast cancer: results of a prospective, multicenter, longitudinal study. Cancer 109:1905–1913, 2007

Hybels CF, Blazer DG: Epidemiology of late-life mental disorders. Clin Geriatr Med 19:663–696, v, 2003

Ingram A, Saling MM, Schweitzer I: Cognitive side effects of brief pulse electroconvulsive therapy: a review. J ECT 24:3–9, 2008

Inouye SK: Delirium in older persons. N Engl J Med 354:1157–1165, 2006

Inouye SK, Charpentier PA: Precipitating factors for delirium in hospitalized elderly persons: predictive model and interrelationship with baseline vulnerability. JAMA 275:852–857, 1996

Jiang HK, Chang DM: Non-steroidal anti-inflammatory drugs with adverse psychiatric reactions: five case reports. Clin Rheumatol 18:339–345, 1999

Keller S, Frishman WH: Neuropsychiatric effects of cardiovascular drug therapy. Cardiol Rev 11:73–93, 2003

King JT: Digitalis delirium. Ann Intern Med 33:1360–1372, 1950

Ko DT, Hebert PR, Coffey CS, et al: Beta-blocker therapy and symptoms of depression, fatigue, and sexual dysfunction. JAMA 288: 351–357, 2002

Kohn R: Beta-blockers an important cause of depression: a medical myth without evidence. Med Health R I 84:92–95, 2001

Kotlyar M, Dysken M, Adson DE: Update on drug-induced depression in the elderly. Am J Geriatr Pharmacother 3:288–300, 2005

Kuhl EA, Dixit NK, Walker RL, et al: Measurement of patient fears about implantable cardioverter defibrillator shock: an initial evaluation of the Florida Shock Anxiety Scale. Pacing Clin Electrophysiol 29:614–618, 2006

Kuzuhara S: Drug-induced psychotic symptoms in Parkinson's disease: problems, management and dilemma. J Neurol 248 (suppl 3):III28–III31, 2001

Ladwig KH, Baumert J, Marten-Mittag B, et al: Posttraumatic stress symptoms and predicted mortality in patients with implantable cardioverter-defibrillators: results from the prospective living with an implanted cardioverter-defibrillator study. Arch Gen Psychiatry 65:1324–1330, 2008

Lechevallier-Michel N, Molimard M, Dartigues JF, et al: Drugs with anticholinergic properties and cognitive performance in the elderly: results from the PAQUID Study. Br J Clin Pharmacol 59: 143–151, 2005

Lee PE, Sykora K, Gill SS, et al: Antipsychotic medications and drug-induced movement disorders other than parkinsonism: a population-based cohort study in older adults. J Am Geriatr Soc 53:1374–1379, 2005

Lemon J, Edelman S, Kirkness A: Avoidance behaviors in patients with implantable cardioverter defibrillators. Heart Lung 33:176–182, 2004

Levenson A: Neuropsychiatric Side Effects of Drugs in the Elderly. New York, Raven, 1979

Lewis DA, Smith RE: Steroid-induced psychiatric syndromes: a report of 14 cases and a review of the literature. J Affect Disord 5:319–332, 1983

Lewitt PA: Levodopa for the treatment of Parkinson's disease. N Engl J Med 359:2468–2476, 2008

Ling MH, Perry PJ, Tsuang MT: Side effects of corticosteroid therapy: psychiatric aspects. Arch Gen Psychiatry 38:471–477, 1981

Mamo DC, Sweet RA, Keshavan MS: Managing antipsychotic-induced parkinsonism. Drug Saf 20:269–275, 1999

Mancuso CE, Tanzi MG, Gabay M: Paradoxical reactions to benzodiazepines: literature review and treatment options. Pharmacotherapy 24:1177–1185, 2004

Mantz J, Hemmings HC Jr, Boddaert J: Case scenario: postoperative delirium in elderly surgical patients. Anesthesiology 112:189–195, 2010

Marcantonio ER, Juarez G, Goldman L, et al: The relationship of postoperative delirium with psychoactive medications. JAMA 272:1518–1522, 1994

Monane M, Avorn J: Medications and falls: causation, correlation, and prevention. Clin Geriatr Med 12:847–858, 1996

Moore AR, O'Keeffe ST: Drug-induced cognitive impairment in the elderly. Drugs Aging 15:15–28, 1999

Morgan JC, Sethi KD: Drug-induced tremors. Lancet Neurol 4:866–876, 2005

Morrison RL, Katz IR: Drug-related cognitive impairment: current progress and recurrent problems, in Annual Review of Gerontology and Geriatrics, Vol 9. Edited by Lawton MP. New York, Springer, 1989, pp 232–279

Nebeker JR, Barach P, Samore MH: Clarifying adverse drug events: a clinician's guide to terminology, documentation, and reporting. Ann Intern Med 140:795–801, 2004

Nelson CJ, Nandy N, Roth AJ: Chemotherapy and cognitive deficits: mechanisms, findings, and potential interventions. Palliat Support Care 5:273–280, 2007

O'Connor DW, Gardner B, Eppingstall B, et al: Cognition in elderly patients receiving unilateral and bilateral electroconvulsive therapy: a prospective, naturalistic comparison. J Affect Disord 124: 235–240, 2010

Oxman TE: Antidepressants and cognitive impairment in the elderly. J Clin Psychiatry 57 (suppl 5):38–44, 1996

Palmer AM, DeKosky ST: Monoamine neurons in aging and Alzheimer's disease. J Neural Transm Gen Sect 91:135–159, 1993

Pascualy M, Veith R: Depression as an adverse drug reaction, in Aging and Clinical Practice: Depression and Coexisting Disease. Edited by Robinson R, Rabins P. New York, Igaku-Shoin, 1989, pp 132–151

Patten SB: Non-psychiatric therapeutic medications in the etiology of organic depression. Psychiatr J Univ Ott 15:150–155, 1990

Patten SB: Psychiatric side effects of interferon treatment. Curr Drug Saf 1:143–150, 2006

Patten SB, Barbui C: Drug-induced depression: a systematic review to inform clinical practice. Psychother Psychosom 73:207–215, 2004

Patten SB, Lamarre CJ: Can drug-induced depressions be identified by their clinical features? Can J Psychiatry 37:213–215, 1992

Patten SB, Love EJ: Can drugs cause depression? A review of the evidence. J Psychiatry Neurosci 18:92–102, 1993

Patten SB, Love EJ: Drug-induced depression: incidence, avoidance and management. Drug Saf 10:203–219, 1994

Patten SB, Love EJ: Drug-induced depression. Psychother Psychosom 66:63–73, 1997

Patten SB, Neutel CI: Corticosteroid-induced adverse psychiatric effects: incidence, diagnosis and management. Drug Saf 22:111–122, 2000

Patten SB, Williams JV, Love EJ: Self-reported depressive symptoms in association with medication exposures among medical inpatients: a cross-sectional study. Can J Psychiatry 40:264–269, 1995

Pauli P, Wiedemann G, Dengler W, et al: Anxiety in patients with an automatic implantable cardioverter defibrillator: what differentiates them from panic patients? Psychosom Med 61:69–76, 1999

Paykel ES, Fleminger R, Watson JP: Psychiatric side effects of antihypertensive drugs other than reserpine. J Clin Psychopharmacol 2:14–39, 1982

Peterson JF, Pun BT, Dittus RS, et al: Delirium and its motoric subtypes: a study of 614 critically ill patients. J Am Geriatr Soc 54: 479–484, 2006

Petrie WM, Maffucci RJ, Woosley RL: Propranolol and depression. Am J Psychiatry 139:92–94, 1982

Picotte-Prillmayer D, DiMaggio JR, Baile WF: H2 blocker delirium. Psychosomatics 36:74–77, 1995

Plaschke K, Kopitz J, Mattern J, et al: Increased cortisol levels and anticholinergic activity in cognitively unimpaired patients. J Neuropsychiatry Clin Neurosci 22:433–441, 2010

Ramaiah R, Lam AM: Postoperative cognitive dysfunction in the elderly. Anesthesiol Clin 27:485–496, 2009

Rao AV: Drug induced depression. J Indian Med Assoc 63:55–57, 1974

Ried LD, McFarland BH, Johnson RE, et al: Beta-blockers and depression: the more the murkier? Ann Pharmacother 32:699–708, 1998

Robinson TN, Raeburn CD, Tran ZV, et al: Postoperative delirium in the elderly: risk factors and outcomes. Ann Surg 249:173–178, 2009

Sabet-Sharghi F, Hutzler JC: Prophylaxis of steroid-induced psychiatric syndromes. Psychosomatics 31:113–114, 1990

Schacke H, Docke WD, Asadullah K: Mechanisms involved in the side effects of glucocorticoids. Pharmacol Ther 96:23–43, 2002

Schor JD, Levkoff SE, Lipsitz LA, et al: Risk factors for delirium in hospitalized elderly. JAMA 267:827–831, 1992

Sharfstein SS, Sack DS, Fauci AS: Relationship between alternate-day corticosteroid therapy and behavioral abnormalities. JAMA 248:2987–2989, 1982

Singh A, Antognini JF: Perioperative pharmacology in elderly patients. Curr Opin Anaesthesiol 23:449–454, 2010

Sirois F: Steroid psychosis: a review. Gen Hosp Psychiatry 25:27–33, 2003

Sirois FJ: Visual hallucinations and metoprolol. Psychosomatics 47:537–538, 2006

Smith BD, Salzman C: Do benzodiazepines cause depression? Hosp Community Psychiatry 42:1101–1102, 1991

Solomon DH, Gurwitz JH: Toxicity of nonsteroidal anti-inflammatory drugs in the elderly: is advanced age a risk factor? Am J Med 102:208–215, 1997

Spitzer WO: Importance of valid measurements of benefit and risk. Med Toxicol 1 (suppl 1):74–78, 1986

Steffensmeier JJ, Ernst ME, Kelly M, et al: Do randomized controlled trials always trump case reports? A second look at propranolol and depression. Pharmacotherapy 26:162–167, 2006

Steinman MA, Hanlon JT: Managing medications in clinically complex elders: "There's got to be a happy medium." JAMA 304: 1592–1601, 2010

Stiefel FC, Breitbart WS, Holland JC: Corticosteroids in cancer: neuropsychiatric complications. Cancer Invest 7:479–491, 1989

Stocky A: Ranitidine and depression. Aust N Z J Psychiatry 25:415–418, 1991

Sultzer DL, Cummings JL: Drug-induced mania: causative agents, clinical characteristics, and management: a retrospective analysis of the literature. Medical Toxicology and Adverse Drug Experience 4:127–143, 1989

Sweet RA, Pollock BG: Neuroleptics in the elderly: guidelines for monitoring. Harv Rev Psychiatry 2:327–335, 1995

Tamblyn RM, McLeod PJ, Abrahamowicz M, et al: Questionable prescribing for elderly patients in Quebec. CMAJ 150:1801–1809, 1994

Taylor MA, Fink M: Melancholia: The Diagnosis, Pathophysiology, and Treatment of Depressive Illness. Cambridge, UK, Cambridge University Press, 2006

Thiessen BQ, Wallace SM, Blackburn JL, et al: Increased prescribing of antidepressants subsequent to beta-blocker therapy. Arch Intern Med 150:2286–2290, 1990

Thomsen LA, Winterstein AG, Sondergaard B, et al: Systematic review of the incidence and characteristics of preventable adverse drug events in ambulatory care. Ann Pharmacother 41:1411–1426, 2007

Tiller JW, Schweitzer I: Benzodiazepines: depressants or antidepressants? Drugs 44:165–169, 1992

Trask PC, Esper P, Riba M, et al: Psychiatric side effects of interferon therapy: prevalence, proposed mechanisms, and future directions. J Clin Oncol 18:2316–2326, 2000

Tune LE: Anticholinergic effects of medication in elderly patients. J Clin Psychiatry 62 (suppl 21):11–14, 2001

van den Broek KC, Nyklicek I, van der Voort PH, et al: Risk of ventricular arrhythmia after implantable defibrillator treatment in anxious type D patients. J Am Coll Cardiol 54:531–537, 2009

Van Gool AR, Kruit WH, Engels FK, et al: Neuropsychiatric side effects of interferon-alfa therapy. Pharm World Sci 25:11–20, 2003

van Melle JP, Verbeek DE, van den Berg MP, et al: Beta-blockers and depression after myocardial infarction: a multicenter prospective study. J Am Coll Cardiol 48:2209–2214, 2006

Vincent FM: The neuropsychiatric complications of corticosteroid therapy. Compr Ther 21:524–528, 1995

Voon V, Kubu C, Krack P, et al: Deep brain stimulation: neuropsychological and neuropsychiatric issues. Mov Disord 21 (suppl 14):S305–S327, 2006

Voon V, Krack P, Lang AE, et al: Parkinson's disease, DBS and suicide: a role for serotonin? Brain June 24, 2009 [Epub ahead of print]

Warrington TP, Bostwick JM: Psychiatric adverse effects of corticosteroids. Mayo Clin Proc 81:1361–1367, 2006

Williams L, Caranasos GJ: Neuropsychiatric effects of drugs in the elderly. J Fla Med Assoc 79:371–375, 1992

Wilson JA, MacLennan WJ: Review: drug-induced parkinsonism in elderly patients. Age Ageing 18:208–210, 1989

Wolkowitz OM, Weingartner H, Thompson K, et al: Diazepam-induced amnesia: a neuropharmacological model of an "organic amnestic syndrome." Am J Psychiatry 144:25–29, 1987

Wood KA, Harris MJ, Morreale A, et al: Drug-induced psychosis and depression in the elderly. Psychiatr Clin North Am 11:167–193, 1988

Yassa R, Nastase C, Dupont D, et al: Tardive dyskinesia in elderly psychiatric patients: a 5-year study. Am J Psychiatry 149:1206–1211, 1992

Young BK, Camicioli R, Ganzini L: Neuropsychiatric adverse effects of antiparkinsonian drugs: characteristics, evaluation and treatment. Drugs Aging 10:367–383, 1997

Zahodne LB, Fernandez HH: Pathophysiology and treatment of psychosis in Parkinson's disease: a review. Drugs Aging 25:665–682, 2008

Zelnik T: Depressive effects of drugs, in Presentations of Depression: Depressive Symptoms in Medical and Other Psychiatric Disorders. Edited by Cameron OG. New York, Wiley, 1987, pp 355–389

Zweifel JE, O'Brien WH: A meta-analysis of the effect of hormone replacement therapy upon depressed mood. Psychoneuroendocrinology 22:189–212, 1997

APPENDIX 29–1. Medical therapies

	Depression	Mania	Anxiety or agitation	Delirium	Psychosis	Visual hallucinations	Dementia-like syndrome
Antihypertensive drugs							
Clonidine	✓	✓	✓	✓			✓
Oxprenolol	✓						
Propranolol	✓	✓		✓	✓	✓	
Reserpine	✓						
Methyldopa	✓			✓	✓		
Guanethidine	✓						
Hydralazine	✓			✓			
Bethanidine	✓						
Captopril		✓	✓				
Nifedipine	✓						
Prazosin	✓						
Cardiac glycosides	✓	✓		✓	✓	✓	✓
Antiarrhythmics							
Procainamide	✓	✓		✓	✓		
Lidocaine	✓			✓	✓		
Quinidine				✓			
Disopyramide				✓	✓		
Antiparkinsonian drugs							
Amantadine	✓		✓	✓	✓	✓	
Bromocriptine	✓	✓	✓	✓	✓	✓	
Levodopa	✓	✓	✓	✓	✓	✓	✓
Pergolide					✓		
Lisuride		✓			✓		
Piribedil		✓					
Trihexyphenidyl				✓		✓	
Procyclidine				✓		✓	
Biperiden				✓		✓	
Analgesics							
NSAIDs	✓			✓	✓		
Salicylates			✓	✓	✓		
Narcotics	✓		✓	✓		✓	
Ibuprofen					✓		
Phenacetin	✓				✓		
Naproxen					✓		
Indomethacin	✓	✓			✓	✓	

APPENDIX 29–1. Medical therapies *(continued)*

	Depression	Mania	Anxiety or agitation	Delirium	Psychosis	Visual hallucinations	Dementia-like syndrome
Anticonvulsants							
Carbamazepine	✓	✓		✓	✓		
Valproate				✓			✓
Phenytoin	✓			✓	✓	✓	✓
Barbiturates	✓		✓	✓			✓
Ethosuximide	✓		✓		✓	✓	
Clonazepam					✓		✓
Phenacemide					✓		
Sedative-hypnotics							
Benzodiazepines	✓	✓	✓	✓	✓		✓
Chloral hydrate	✓			✓			✓
Ethanol	✓			✓			✓
Clomethiazole	✓			✓			✓
Clorazepate	✓			✓			✓
Meprobamate				✓	✓		✓
Anticholinergics/antispasmodics							
Atropine				✓	✓	✓	✓
Benztropine				✓	✓	✓	✓
Propantheline				✓	✓	✓	✓
Scopolamine				✓	✓	✓	✓
Dicyclomine				✓	✓	✓	✓
Hyoscyamine				✓	✓	✓	✓
Lithium		✓		✓			✓
Antidepressants							
TCAs		✓	✓	✓	✓	✓	✓
MAOIs		✓			✓		
Bupropion			✓				
Trazodone		✓			✓		
Fluoxetine		✓	✓	✓			
Sertraline		✓					
Maprotiline						✓	
Neuroleptics							
Butyrophenones	✓			✓			✓
Phenothiazines	✓			✓	✓		✓
Clozapine				✓			
Thiothixene				✓			
Molindone				✓			

APPENDIX 29–1. Medical therapies *(continued)*

	Depression	Mania	Anxiety or agitation	Delirium	Psychosis	Visual hallucinations	Dementia-like syndrome
Antidiarrheals							
Diphenoxylate/ atropine				✓			
Loperamide				✓			
Antimicrobial agents							
Podophyllin					✓		
Penicillins	✓		✓			✓	
Sulfamethoxazole	✓			✓			
Clotrimazole	✓						
Cycloserine	✓		✓	✓	✓		
Dapsone	✓	✓	✓				
Ethionamide	✓						
Tetracycline	✓					✓	
Griseofulvin	✓						
Metronidazole	✓						
Streptomycin	✓						
Nitrofurantoin	✓						
Nalidixic acid	✓						
Antimalarials					✓	✓	
Sulfonamides	✓		✓			✓	
Procaine penicillin	✓		✓	✓	✓		
Thiocarbanilide	✓						
Acyclovir	✓			✓			
Isoniazid	✓	✓	✓		✓	✓	
Mefloquine				✓			
Iproniazid		✓			✓	✓	
Cephalosporins				✓	✓		
Ciprofloxacin				✓			
Amphotericin B				✓			
Antihistamines (H_1 blocking agents)							
Diphenhydramine				✓			
Chlorpheniramine				✓			
H_2 blockers							
Cimetidine	✓	✓		✓	✓	✓	
Ranitidine	✓			✓			
Drugs for urinary incontinence							
Oxybutynin				✓			
Flavoxate				✓			
Hyoscyamine				✓			

APPENDIX 29–1. Medical therapies *(continued)*

	Depression	Mania	Anxiety or agitation	Delirium	Psychosis	Visual hallucinations	Dementia-like syndrome
Withdrawal syndromes							
Barbiturates			✓	✓		✓	
Alcohol	✓		✓	✓	✓	✓	
Benzodiazepines			✓	✓	✓	✓	
Amphetamines	✓	✓	✓	✓	✓		
Chloral hydrate			✓	✓		✓	
Corticosteroids	✓		✓	✓			
Propranolol		✓	✓				
Reserpine		✓	✓				
MAOIs		✓	✓				
TCAs		✓	✓				
Caffeine			✓				
Meprobamate			✓			✓	
Opiates			✓		✓	✓	
Hallucinogens							
Phencyclidine		✓			✓	✓	
Indole hallucinogens	✓	✓			✓	✓	
Cannabinols			✓		✓	✓	
Ketamine						✓	
Nitrous oxide						✓	
Antineoplastic drugs							
Azathioprine	✓						✓
L-Asparaginase	✓			✓	✓		
Plicamycin (mithramycin)	✓						
Vincristine	✓						
6-Azauridine	✓						
Bleomycin	✓						
Trimethoprim	✓						
Interferon	✓		✓	✓			
Endocrine agents							
Corticosteroids	✓	✓		✓	✓	✓	
ACTH		✓					
Oral contraceptives	✓						
Thyroid hormones		✓	✓		✓	✓	

APPENDIX 29–1. Medical therapies *(continued)*

	Depression	Mania	Anxiety or agitation	Delirium	Psychosis	Visual hallucinations	Dementia-like syndrome
Endocrine agents *(continued)*							
Triamcinolone	✓						
Norethisterone	✓						
Danazol	✓						
Clomiphene citrate					✓		
Central nervous system stimulants							
Cocaine		✓	✓				
Sympathomimetics		✓	✓		✓	✓	
Amphetamine	✓	✓	✓		✓		
Fenfluramine	✓		✓				
Diethylpropion	✓		✓		✓		
Phenmetrazine	✓		✓				
Caffeine			✓	✓			
Methylphenidate		✓	✓		✓		
Pseudoephedrine		✓	✓		✓		
Pemoline		✓	✓				
Isoetharine		✓	✓				
Phenylpropanolamine		✓	✓		✓		
Ephedrine		✓	✓		✓		
Phenylephrine		✓	✓		✓		
Epinephrine			✓				
Isoproterenol			✓				
Miscellaneous drugs							
Acetazolamide	✓						
Albuterol					✓		
Anticholinesterase	✓		✓	✓			
Aprindine					✓		
Arsenic			✓		✓	✓	✓
Aspartame		✓					
Baclofen	✓	✓			✓		
Benzene			✓				
Bromide		✓			✓	✓	✓
Calcium		✓					
Carbon disulfide			✓		✓		✓
Carbon monoxide					✓		✓
Choline	✓						
Cocaine		✓	✓		✓		

APPENDIX 29–1. Medical therapies *(continued)*

	Depression	Mania	Anxiety or agitation	Delirium	Psychosis	Visual hallucinations	Dementia-like syndrome
Miscellaneous drugs (*continued*)							
Cyclobenzaprine		✓		✓			
Cyclosporin A		✓					
Cyproheptadine	✓	✓					
Diethyl-*m*-toluamide		✓					
Diltiazem	✓	✓					
Diphenoxylate	✓						
Disulfiram	✓	✓		✓	✓	✓	✓
Flutamide		✓					
Halothane	✓						
Heavy metals			✓		✓	✓	✓
Isosafrole					✓		
L-Glutamine		✓					
Manganese					✓		✓
Mebeverine	✓						
Meclizine	✓						
Mepacrine		✓					
Mercury			✓		✓		✓
Methoserpidine	✓						
Methysergide	✓						
Metoclopramide	✓	✓		✓			
Metrizamide		✓			✓	✓	
Organophosphates			✓				✓
Oxandrolone		✓					
Oxymetholone		✓					
Pentazocine					✓		
Phenindione	✓						
Phosphorous			✓				
Pizotifen	✓						
Procaine	✓			✓			
Procarbazine		✓					
Procyclidine		✓					
Propafenone		✓					

APPENDIX 29–1. Medical therapies *(continued)*

	Depression	Mania	Anxiety or agitation	Delirium	Psychosis	Visual hallucinations	Dementia-like syndrome
Miscellaneous drugs *(continued)*							
Salbutamol	✓						
Tetrabenazine	✓						
Thallium					✓		✓
Theophylline		✓	✓				
Tryptophan		✓					
Veratrum	✓						
Yohimbine		✓	✓				
Zidovudine (AZT)		✓					

Note. ACTH=adrenocorticotropic hormone; H_1=histamine subtype 1 receptor; H_2=histamine subtype 2 receptor; MAOIs=monoamine oxidase inhibitors; NSAIDs=nonsteroidal anti-inflammatory drugs; TCAs=tricyclic antidepressants.

Source. Adapted from Callahan 1992; Cummings 1985, 1986; Estroff and Gold 1986; Hall et al. 1980; Levenson 1979; Morrison and Katz 1989; Pascualy and Veith 1989; Sultzer and Cummings 1989; Williams and Caranasos 1992; Wood et al. 1988.

Index

Page numbers printed in **boldface** type refer to tables or figures.